Review of
Dermatology

Ali Alikhan, MD
Dermatologist
Department of Dermatology
Sutter Medical Foundation
Sacramento, CA, USA

Thomas L.H. Hocker, MD, PCEO
Mohs Surgeon
Dermatopathologist and Dermatologist
Surgical Director
Department of Dermatology
University of Missouri Kansas City
Overland Park, KS, USA

Review of Dermatology

SECOND EDITION

Section Editors

Monisha N. Dandekar, MD
Linda T. Doan, MD, PhD
Nada Elbuluk, MD, MSc
Ronda S. Farah, MD
Phillip C. Hochwalt, MD, FACMS
Julia S. Lehman, MD
Alexander Maley, MD
Roberto A. Novoa, MD
Brea Prindaville, MD
Anand Rajpara, MD
Christopher Sayed, MD
Tiffany C. Scharschmidt, MD
Jennifer J. Schoch, MD
Jonathan I. Silverberg, MD, PhD, MPH
Olayemi Sokumbi, MD

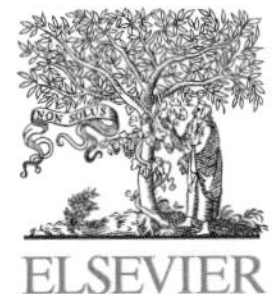
ELSEVIER

Elsevier
1600 John F. Kennedy Blvd.
Ste 1800
Philadelphia, PA 19103-2899

REVIEW OF DERMATOLOGY, SECOND EDITION ISBN: 978-0-323-65386-2

Notice

Practitioners and researchers must always rely on their own experience and knowledge in evaluating and using any information, methods, compounds or experiments described herein. Because of rapid advances in the medical sciences, in particular, independent verification of diagnoses and drug dosages should be made. To the fullest extent of the law, no responsibility is assumed by Elsevier, authors, editors or contributors for any injury and/or damage to persons or property as a matter of products liability, negligence or otherwise, or from any use or operation of any methods, products, instructions, or ideas contained in the material herein.

Previous edition copyrighted 2017.

Senior Content Strategist: Charlotta Kryhl
Senior Content Development Specialist: Rae L. Robertson
Publishing Services Manager: Shereen Jameel
Project Manager: Vishnu T. Jiji
Senior Designer: Renee Duenow

Printed in India

Last digit is the print number: 9 8 7 6 5 4 3 2

Dedications

To my wife, for her unwavering and unconditional love and support

To my grandmother (Amma), who taught me the meaning of sacrifice

To my parents, who have always been the best role models

To my son, whose curiosity and determination continue to amaze me

Ali Alikhan, MD

To Anjali, Avani, and Akari, and Jeevan: daddy loves you unconditionally, and I am inspired constantly by your curiosity, intelligence, relentless drive, and kind hearts. God blessed me with the most amazing kids I could hope for, and blessed you with the unique abilities and talents to achieve anything you set your mind to! Be a force for good.

To my family: your love and support is the light that brightens even the darkest of nights.

To my mentors at Harvard (Dr. Harley Haynes and Hensin Tsao), Mayo (esp. Drs. Pittelkow, Camilleri, and Roenigk), and the entire University of Michigan Dermpath group: thank you for your immense personal support and for shaping my dermatologic world view!

Thomas L. H. Hocker, MD, PCEO

Contributors

Ali Alikhan, MD
Dermatologist
Department of Dermatology
Sutter Medical Foundation
Sacramento, CA, USA

Section Editor for Section 2, Dermatopharmacology
2.1 Antihistamines
2.2 Retinoids
2.3 Corticosteroids
2.4 Immunomodulatory Agents
2.5 Oncologic Agents in Dermatology
2.6 Antimicrobial Agents
2.7 Phototherapy
2.8 Miscellaneous Agents
2.9 Drug Interactions and the Cytochrome P-450 System
2.10 Drug Reactions

Section Editor for Section 3, General Dermatology
3.1 Papulosquamous Dermatoses
3.2 Eczematous Dermatoses
3.3 Interface Dermatitis
3.4 Blistering Diseases
3.5 Connective Tissue Diseases (CTDs) and Sclerosing Dermopathies
3.6 Granulomatous/Histiocytic Disorders
3.7 Monoclonal Gammopathies of Dermatologic Interest
3.8 Xanthomas
3.9 Urticaria and Angioedema
3.10 Neutrophilic Dermatoses
3.11 Eosinophilic Disorders
3.12 Figurate Erythemas
3.13 Follicular and Eccrine/Apocrine Disorders
3.14 Drug Reactions
3.15 Photodermatoses and Other Physical Dermatoses
3.16 Amyloidoses
3.17 Neurodermatology and Psychodermatology
3.18 Palmoplantar Keratodermas
3.19 Nutritional Disorders in Dermatology
3.20 Depositional and Calcification Disorders Not Discussed Elsewhere
3.21 Ulcers
3.22 Vasculitides, Vasculopathies, and Other Vascular Disorders
3.23 Panniculitides and Lipodystrophies
3.24 Dermatoses of Pregnancy
3.25 Hair, Nail, and Mucosal Disorders
3.26 Pigmentary Disorders

Section Editor for Section 5, Infectious Diseases
5.1 Viral Diseases
5.2 HIV/AIDS Dermatology
5.3 Bacterial Infections
5.4 Fungal Diseases
5.5 Parasites and Other Creatures

Monisha N. Dandekar, MD
Dermatopathologist
MAWD Pathology
Lenexa, KS, USA

Section Editor for Section 6, Neoplastic Dermatology
6.1 Keratinocytic Neoplasms
6.2 Cysts
6.3 Melanocytic Neoplasms
6.4 Adnexal Neoplasms and Hamartomas
6.5 Hair Follicle Neoplasms/Hamartomas
6.6 Sebaceous Proliferations
6.7 Neural Neoplasms
6.8 Smooth Muscle Neoplasms
6.9 Hematolymphoid Neoplasms
6.10 Fibrohistiocytic Neoplasms
6.11 Vascular Proliferations
6.12 Neoplasms of Adipocytic Lineage
6.13 Dermoscopy

Linda T. Doan, MD, PhD
Assistant Professor of Dermatology and Pathology
University of California, Irvine
Irvine, CA, USA

Section Editor for Section 1, Basic Science
1.1 Structure and Function of the Skin
1.2 Embryology
1.3 Wound Healing
1.4 Genetics
1.5 Ultraviolet Light
1.6 Immunology
1.6.1 Innate Versus Adaptive Immunity
1.6.2 Immunologic Mediators
1.6.3 Cells of Significance
1.6.4 Major Histocompatibility Complex
1.7 Laboratory Techniques

Nada Elbuluk, MD, MSc
Associate Professor of Dermatology
University of Southern California
Los Angeles, CA, USA

Section Editor for Section 10, Cutaneous Manifestations of Internal Disease and Metastases
10.1 Cardiovascular/Cardiopulmonary
10.2 Endocrine
10.3 Gastroenterology
10.4 Neurology
10.5 Renal
10.6 Paraneoplastic Syndromes

Ronda S. Farah, MD
Assistant Professor of Dermatology
University of Minnesota
Minneapolis, MN, USA

Section Editor for Section 9, Cosmetic Dermatology
9.1 Lasers
9.2 Botulinum Toxin
9.3 Dermal Fillers
9.4 Liposuction and Fat Reduction
9.5 Sclerotherapy
9.6 Cosmeceuticals, Nutraceuticals, and Other Supplements
9.7 Hair Transplantation
9.8 Chemical Peels
9.9 Other Esthetic Procedures and Scales

Phillip C. Hochwalt, MD, FACMS
Mohs and Reconstructive Surgeon
Department of Dermatology
Confluence Health
Wenatchee, WA, USA

Section Editor for Section 6, Neoplastic Dermatology
6.1 Keratinocytic Neoplasms
6.2 Cysts
6.3 Melanocytic Neoplasms
6.4 Adnexal Neoplasms and Hamartomas
6.5 Hair Follicle Neoplasms/Hamartomas
6.6 Sebaceous Proliferations
6.7 Neural Neoplasms
6.8 Smooth Muscle Neoplasms
6.9 Hematolymphoid Neoplasms
6.10 Fibrohistiocytic Neoplasms
6.11 Vascular Proliferations
6.12 Neoplasms of Adipocytic Lineage
6.13 Dermoscopy

Section Editor for Section 8, Dermatologic Surgery
8.1 Surgical Anatomy
8.2 Local Anesthetics and Perioperative Pain Control
8.3 Surgical Instruments and Needles
8.4 Suture Techniques
8.5 Wound Closure Materials
8.6 Antisepsis and Sterilization
8.7 Electrosurgery
8.8 Cryosurgery
8.9 Excisions
8.10 Mohs Surgery
8.11 Flaps
8.12 Grafts
8.13 Surgical Complications and Measures to Avoid Them
8.14 Scar Improvement
8.15 Nail Surgery
8.16 Wound Dressings

Thomas L.H. Hocker, MD, PCEO
Mohs Surgeon
Dermatopathologist and Dermatologist
Surgical Director
Department of Dermatology
University of Missouri Kansas City
Overland Park, KS, USA

Section Editor for Section 5, Infectious Diseases
5.1 Viral Diseases
5.2 HIV/AIDS Dermatology
5.3 Bacterial Infections
5.4 Fungal Diseases
5.5 Parasites and Other Creatures

Section Editor for Section 8, Dermatologic Surgery
8.1 Surgical Anatomy
8.2 Local Anesthetics and Perioperative Pain Control
8.3 Surgical Instruments and Needles
8.4 Suture Techniques
8.5 Wound Closure Materials
8.6 Antisepsis and Sterilization
8.7 Electrosurgery
8.8 Cryosurgery
8.9 Excisions
8.10 Mohs Surgery
8.11 Flaps
8.12 Grafts
8.13 Surgical Complications and Measures to Avoid Them
8.14 Scar Improvement
8.15 Nail Surgery
8.16 Wound Dressings

Julia S. Lehman, MD
Professor of Dermatology, Laboratory Medicine, and Pathology
Laboratory Director, Immunodermatology
Mayo Clinic
Rochester, MN, USA

Section Editor for Section 3, General Dermatology
3.4 Blistering Diseases

Section Editor for Section 7, Dermatopathology
7.1 Essential Concepts in Dermatopathology
7.2 High-Yield Dermatopathology Diagnoses at a Glance
7.3 High-Yield Dermatopathology Differential Diagnoses

Alexander Maley, MD
Dermatologist
Aurora Healthcare
Milwaukee, WI, USA

Section Editor for Section 2, Dermatopharmacology
2.1 Antihistamines
2.2 Retinoids
2.3 Corticosteroids
2.4 Immunomodulatory Agents
2.5 Oncologic Agents in Dermatology
2.6 Antimicrobial Agents
2.7 Phototherapy
2.8 Miscellaneous Agents
2.9 Drug Interactions and the Cytochrome P-450 System
2.10 Drug Reactions

Section Editor for Section 11, Epidemiology, Statistics, Study Design, Public Health Principles, and Billing
11.6 Billing

Roberto A. Novoa, MD
Clinical Associate Professor of Pathology and Dermatology
Stanford University
Stanford, CA, USA

Section Editor for Section 6, Neoplastic Dermatology
6.1 Keratinocytic Neoplasms
6.2 Cysts
6.3 Melanocytic Neoplasms
6.4 Adnexal Neoplasms and Hamartomas
6.5 Hair follicle Neoplasms/Hamartomas
6.6 Sebaceous Proliferations
6.7 Neural Neoplasms
6.8 Smooth Muscle Neoplasms
6.9 Hematolymphoid Neoplasms
6.10 Fibrohistiocytic Neoplasms
6.11 Vascular Proliferations
6.12 Neoplasms of Adipocytic Lineage
6.13 Dermoscopy

Section Editor for Section 7, Dermatopathology
7.1 Essential Concepts in Dermatopathology
7.2 High-Yield Dermatopathology Diagnoses at a Glance
7.3 High-Yield Dermatopathology Differential Diagnoses

Brea Prindaville, MD
Assistant Professor of Dermatology
Pediatric Dermatologist
Brown University
Providence, RI, USA

Section Editor for Section 4, Pediatric Dermatology
4.1 Neonatal Dermatology
4.2 Viral Exanthems and Select Infectious Disorders of Childhood
4.3 Inherited Pigmentary Disorders
4.4 Epidermolysis Bullosa
4.5 Tumor Syndromes
4.6 Vascular Tumors, Malformations, and Related Vascular Disorders
4.7 Disorders of Hair and Nails
4.8 Inherited Metabolic and Nutritional Disorders
4.9 Inherited Connective Tissue Disorders
4.10 Autoinflammatory Disorders (Periodic Fever Syndromes)
4.11 Neurocutaneous Syndromes

4.12 Premature Aging Syndromes and DNA Repair Disorders
4.13 Primary Immunodeficiency Disorders with Cutaneous Manifestations
4.14 Disorders of Cornification
4.15 Miscellaneous Pediatric Dermatologic Disorders

Anand Rajpara, MD
Residency Program Director and Associate Professor
Department of Dermatology
Kansas University Medical Center
Kansas City, KS, USA

Section Editor for Section 3, General Dermatology
3.1 Papulosquamous Dermatoses
3.2 Eczematous Dermatoses
3.3 Interface Dermatitis
3.4 Blistering Diseases
3.5 Connective Tissue Diseases (CTDs) and Sclerosing Dermopathies
3.6 Granulomatous/Histiocytic Disorders
3.7 Monoclonal Gammopathies of Dermatologic Interest
3.8 Xanthomas
3.9 Urticaria and Angioedema
3.10 Neutrophilic Dermatoses
3.11 Eosinophilic Disorders
3.12 Figurate Erythemas
3.13 Follicular and Eccrine/Apocrine Disorders
3.14 Drug Reactions
3.15 Photodermatoses and Other Physical Dermatoses
3.16 Amyloidoses
3.17 Neurodermatology and Psychodermatology
3.18 Palmoplantar Keratodermas
3.19 Nutritional Disorders in Dermatology
3.20 Depositional and Calcification Disorders Not Discussed Elsewhere
3.21 Ulcers
3.22 Vasculitides, Vasculopathies, and Other Vascular Disorders
3.23 Panniculitides and Lipodystrophies
3.24 Dermatoses of Pregnancy
3.25 Hair, Nail, and Mucosal Disorders
3.26 Pigmentary Disorders

Christopher Sayed, MD
Professor of Dermatology
University of North Carolina
Chapel Hill, NC, USA

Section Editor for Section 3, General Dermatology
3.1 Papulosquamous Dermatoses
3.2 Eczematous Dermatoses
3.3 Interface Dermatitis
3.4 Blistering Diseases
3.5 Connective Tissue Diseases (CTDs) and Sclerosing Dermopathies
3.6 Granulomatous/Histiocytic Disorders
3.7 Monoclonal Gammopathies of Dermatologic Interest
3.8 Xanthomas
3.9 Urticaria and Angioedema
3.10 Neutrophilic Dermatoses
3.11 Eosinophilic Disorders
3.12 Figurate Erythemas
3.13 Follicular and Eccrine/Apocrine Disorders
3.14 Drug Reactions
3.15 Photodermatoses and Other Physical Dermatoses
3.16 Amyloidoses
3.17 Neurodermatology and Psychodermatology
3.18 Palmoplantar Keratodermas
3.19 Nutritional Disorders in Dermatology
3.20 Depositional and Calcification Disorders not Discussed Elsewhere
3.21 Ulcers
3.22 Vasculitides, Vasculopathies, and Other Vascular Disorders
3.23 Panniculitides and Lipodystrophies
3.24 Dermatoses of Pregnancy
3.25 Hair, Nail, and Mucosal Disorders
3.26 Pigmentary Disorders

Tiffany C. Scharschmidt, MD
Associate Professor of Dermatology
University of California
San Francisco, CA, USA

Section Editor for Section 1, Basic Science
1.1 Structure and Function of the Skin
1.2 Embryology
1.3 Wound Healing
1.4 Genetics
1.5 Ultraviolet Light
1.6 Immunology
1.6.1 Innate Versus Adaptive Immunity
1.6.2 Immunologic Mediators
1.6.3 Cells of Significance
1.6.4 Major Histocompatibility Complex
1.7 Laboratory Techniques

Jennifer J. Schoch, MD
Associate Professor of Dermatology
University of Florida
Gainesville, FL, USA

Section Editor for Section 4, Pediatric Dermatology
4.1 Neonatal Dermatology
4.2 Viral Exanthems and Select Infectious Disorders of Childhood
4.3 Inherited Pigmentary Disorders
4.4 Epidermolysis Bullosa
4.5 Tumor Syndromes
4.6 Vascular Tumors, Malformations, and Related Vascular Disorders
4.7 Disorders of Hair and Nails
4.8 Inherited Metabolic and Nutritional Disorders
4.9 Inherited Connective Tissue Disorders
4.10 Autoinflammatory Disorders (Periodic Fever Syndromes)
4.11 Neurocutaneous Syndromes
4.12 Premature Aging Syndromes and DNA Repair Disorders
4.13 Primary Immunodeficiency Disorders with Cutaneous Manifestations
4.14 Disorders of Cornification
4.15 Miscellaneous Pediatric Dermatologic Disorders

Jonathan I. Silverberg, MD, PhD, MPH
Professor of Dermatology
George Washington University School of Medicine and Health Sciences
Baltimore, MD, USA
Director, Clinical Research and Contact Dermatitis
Washington, DC, USA

Section Editor for Section 11, Epidemiology, Statistics, Study Design, Public Health Principles, and Billing
11.1 Epidemiological Definitions
11.2 Epidemiologic Principles
11.3 Types of Studies and Their Limitations
11.4 Types of Bias
11.5 Maintenance of Certification for the American Board of Dermatology

Olayemi Sokumbi, MD
Associate Professor of Dermatology and Laboratory Medicine & Pathology
Mayo Clinic
Jacksonville, FL, USA

Section Editor for Section 3, General Dermatology
3.1 Papulosquamous Dermatoses
3.2 Eczematous Dermatoses
3.3 Interface Dermatitis
3.4 Blistering Diseases
3.5 Connective Tissue Diseases (CTDs) and Sclerosing Dermopathies
3.6 Granulomatous/Histiocytic Disorders
3.7 Monoclonal Gammopathies of Dermatologic Interest
3.8 Xanthomas
3.9 Urticaria and Angioedema
3.10 Neutrophilic Dermatoses
3.11 Eosinophilic Disorders
3.12 Figurate Erythemas
3.13 Follicular and Eccrine/Apocrine Disorders
3.14 Drug Reactions
3.15 Photodermatoses and Other Physical Dermatoses
3.16 Amyloidoses
3.17 Neurodermatology and Psychodermatology
3.18 Palmoplantar Keratodermas
3.19 Nutritional Disorders in Dermatology
3.20 Depositional and Calcification Disorders Not Discussed Elsewhere
3.21 Ulcers
3.22 Vasculitides, Vasculopathies, and Other Vascular Disorders
3.23 Panniculitides and Lipodystrophies
3.24 Dermatoses of Pregnancy
3.25 Hair, Nail, and Mucosal Disorders
3.26 Pigmentary Disorders

Acknowledgments

Our thanks to Dr. Christopher Sayed, Dr. Julia Lehman, Dr. Phillip Hochwalt, and Dr. Anwar Qais Saadoon as they each contributed photos to the cover.

We would also like to thank Elsevier as well as our terrific Section Editors for making this book possible.

Preface

Purpose of this book

We envision this book serving as a comprehensive review for dermatology residents and practicing dermatologists. We hope that the book is used not only in the United States, but all over the world.

How the book should be used

The book can be used in many ways:

- As a resource for practicing dermatologists preparing for recertification examinations or simply as a quick reference.
- As a resource for dermatology residents preparing for board examinations, in-service examinations, or simply as a quick reference (it could even be used throughout residency as a place to compile notes and facts learned from reading textbooks and journal articles, much the way First Aid© was used during medical school).

How the book should NOT be used

There is NO substitution for reading textbooks and journal articles during residency. This book should serve as a review or a syllabus of dermatology, but should not take the place of textbooks and original literature. Many great resources to truly learn dermatology exist—our favorites are *Dermatology* (commonly referred to as "Bolognia"), *Andrews' Diseases of the Skin*, *Comprehensive Dermatologic Drug Therapy* (commonly referred to as "Wolverton"), *The Requisites in Dermatology Series* (particularly dermatopathology and dermatologic surgery), *Practical Dermatopathology* (commonly referred to as "Rapini"), and *Hurwitz Clinical Pediatric Dermatology*.

Other information

Please remember that space was limited for this book, as it is for all books—we had to make important choices to leave certain information out of the book.

We are extremely grateful to the authors and editors of the textbooks listed above, as well as those of *McKee's Pathology of the Skin* and *Weedon's Skin Pathology*, as nearly all of the figures came from these resources.

Despite reading and re-reading this text many times, we imagine that some errors may have snuck by. We encourage you to email us at reviewofdermatology@gmail.com with any errors or suggestions so we can correct these for our third edition. Please also email us if you have ideas to improve the book or would like to contribute to future editions.

Contents

1 **BASIC SCIENCE** 1
Linda T. Doan and Tiffany C. Scharschmidt

1.1 **Structure and Function of the Skin** 1
1.2 **Embryology** 13
1.3 **Wound Healing** 13
1.4 **Genetics** 15
1.5 **Ultraviolet Light** 17
1.6 **Immunology** 18
1.7 **Laboratory Techniques** 28

2 **DERMATOPHARMACOLOGY** 39
Alexander Maley and Ali Alikhan

2.1 **Antihistamines** 39
2.2 **Retinoids** 40
2.3 **Corticosteroids** 42
2.4 **Immunomodulatory Agents** 46
2.5 **Oncologic Agents in Dermatology** 54
2.6 **Antimicrobial Agents** 57
2.7 **Phototherapy** 65
2.8 **Miscellaneous Agents** 67
2.9 **Drug Interactions and the Cytochrome P-450 System** 70
2.10 **Drug Reactions** 71

3 **GENERAL DERMATOLOGY** 79
Christopher Sayed, Ali Alikhan, Olayemi Sokumbi, Anand Rajpara, and Julia S. Lehman

3.1 **Papulosquamous Dermatoses** 79
3.2 **Eczematous Dermatoses** 86
3.3 **Interface Dermatitis** 96
3.4 **Blistering Diseases** 107
3.5 **Connective Tissue Disease (CTD) and Sclerosing Dermopathies** 119
3.6 **Granulomatous/Histiocytic Disorders** 149
3.7 **Monoclonal Gammopathies of Dermatologic Interest** 161
3.8 **Xanthomas** 164
3.9 **Urticaria and Angioedema** 166
3.10 **Neutrophilic Dermatoses** 169
3.11 **Eosinophilic Disorders** 172
3.12 **Figurate Erythemas** 173
3.13 **Follicular and Eccrine/Apocrine Disorders** 176
3.14 **Drug Reactions** 184
3.15 **Photodermatoses and Other Physical Dermatoses** 184
3.16 **Amyloidoses** 188
3.17 **Neurodermatology and Psychodermatology** 189
3.18 **Palmoplantar Keratodermas** 192
3.19 **Nutritional Disorders in Dermatology** 192
3.20 **Depositional and Calcification Disorders Not Discussed Elsewhere** 194
3.21 **Ulcers** 194
3.22 **Vasculitides, Vasculopathies, and Other Vascular Disorders** 194
3.23 **Panniculitides and Lipodystrophies** 210
3.24 **Dermatoses of Pregnancy** 212
3.25 **Hair, Nail, and Mucosal Disorders** 212
3.26 **Pigmentary Disorders** 220

4 **PEDIATRIC DERMATOLOGY** 229
Brea Prindaville and Jennifer J. Schoch

4.1 **Neonatal Dermatology** 229
4.2 **Viral Exanthems and Select Infectious Disorders of Childhood** 229

4.3 Inherited Pigmentary Disorders 240
4.4 Epidermolysis Bullosa 244
4.5 Tumor Syndromes 248
4.6 Vascular Tumors, Malformations, and Related Vascular Disorders 250
4.7 Disorders of Hair and Nails 255
4.8 Inherited Metabolic and Nutritional Disorders 258
4.9 Inherited Connective Tissue Disorders 263
4.10 Autoinflammatory Disorders (Periodic Fever Syndromes) 269
4.11 Neurocutaneous Syndromes 271
4.12 Premature Aging Syndromes and DNA Repair Disorders 275
4.13 Primary Immunodeficiency Disorders With Cutaneous Manifestations 278
4.14 Disorders of Cornification 278
4.15 Miscellaneous Pediatric Dermatologic Disorders 281

5 INFECTIOUS DISEASES 293
Ali Alikhan and Thomas L.H. Hocker

5.1 Viral Diseases 293
5.2 HIV/AIDS Dermatology 301
5.3 Bacterial Infections 304
5.4 Fungal Diseases 322
5.5 Parasites and Other Creatures 329

6 NEOPLASTIC DERMATOLOGY 337
Monisha N. Dandekar, Roberto A. Novoa, Phillip C. Hochwalt, and Spyros M. Siscos

Neoplastic Dermatology 337
6.1 Keratinocytic Neoplasms 337
6.2 Cysts 343
6.3 Melanocytic Neoplasms 344
6.4 Adnexal Neoplasms and Hamartomas 351
6.5 Hair Follicle Neoplasms/Hamartomas 359
6.6 Sebaceous Proliferations 363
6.7 Neural Neoplasms 364
6.8 Smooth Muscle Neoplasms 367
6.9 Hematolymphoid Neoplasms 368
6.10 Fibrohistiocytic Neoplasms 373
6.11 Vascular Proliferations 378
6.12 Neoplasms of Adipocytic Lineage 382
6.13 Dermoscopy 382

7 DERMATOPATHOLOGY 391
Julia S. Lehman and Roberto A. Novoa

7.1 Essential Concepts in Dermatopathology 391
7.2 High-Yield Dermatopathology Diagnoses at a Glance 415
7.3 High-Yield Dermatopathology Differential Diagnoses 415

8 DERMATOLOGIC SURGERY 443
Phillip C. Hochwalt and Thomas L.H. Hocker

8.1 Surgical Anatomy 443
8.2 Local Anesthetics and Perioperative Pain Control 450
8.3 Surgical Instruments and Needles 454
8.4 Suture Techniques 455
8.5 Wound Closure Materials 455
8.6 Antisepsis and Sterilization 458
8.7 Electrosurgery 458
8.8 Cryosurgery 461
8.9 Excisions 461
8.10 Mohs Surgery 463
8.11 Flaps 463
8.12 Grafts 472
8.13 Surgical Complications and Measures to Avoid Them 473
8.14 Scar Improvement 476
8.15 Nail Surgery 477
8.16 Wound Dressings 479

9 COSMETIC DERMATOLOGY 481
Ronda S. Farah

9.1 Lasers 481
9.2 Botulinum Toxin 488
9.3 Dermal Fillers 491
9.4 Liposuction and Fat Reduction 494
9.5 Sclerotherapy and Vein Management 494
9.6 Cosmeceuticals, Nutraceuticals, and Other Supplements 497
9.7 Hair Transplantation 498
9.8 Chemical Peels 498
9.9 Other Esthetic Procedures and Scales 500

10 CUTANEOUS MANIFESTATIONS OF INTERNAL DISEASE AND METASTASES 505
Nada Elbuluk

10.1 Cardiovascular/Cardiopulmonary 505
10.2 Endocrine 512
10.3 Gastroenterology 514
10.4 Neurology 519
10.5 Renal 519
10.6 Paraneoplastic Syndromes 520

11 EPIDEMIOLOGY, STATISTICS, STUDY DESIGN, PUBLIC HEALTH PRINCIPLES, AND BILLING 527
Jonathan I. Silverberg and Alexander Maley

11.1 Epidemiologic Definitions 527
11.2 Epidemiologic Principles 527
11.3 Types of Studies and Their Limitations 528
11.4 Types of Bias 530
11.5 Maintenance of Certification for the American Board of Dermatology 530
11.6 Billing 530
Index 535

1 Basic Science

Linda T. Doan and Tiffany C. Scharschmidt

CONTENTS LIST

1.1 STRUCTURE AND FUNCTION OF THE SKIN
1.2 EMBRYOLOGY
1.3 WOUND HEALING
1.4 GENETICS
1.5 ULTRAVIOLET LIGHT
1.6 IMMUNOLOGY
1.7 LABORATORY TECHNIQUES

1.1 STRUCTURE AND FUNCTION OF THE SKIN

- Functions: interfaces with environment, collects sensory data, protects against infection and chemical penetration, temperature regulation, water retention, and excretion of drugs/waste
- Composed of three layers: epidermis, dermis, and subcutis

Epidermis

Cellular biology of the epidermis

- Squamous epithelium composed of keratinocytes connected by desmosomes, adherens junctions, tight junctions, and gap junctions (Table 1.1)
  - Intercellular junctions
    - **Desmosomes**: primary keratinocyte intercellular junction
      - Provide structure and integrity to the epidermis by anchoring/attaching to **keratins**
      - Components (see Table 1.1)
      - Desmocollins, desmogleins, and other cadherins are **calcium-dependent**
    - **Adherens junctions**: also mediate tight intercellular binding (Fig. 1.1)
      - Anchor/attach to **actin** filaments
      - Consist of α-catenin (cytoplasmic), β-catenin (cytoplasmic), plakoglobin (cytoplasmic), and classic cadherins (E and P; transmembrane)
    - **Tight junctions**: composed of claudins and occludin; form tight seal against water loss in granular layer
    - **Gap junctions**: facilitate intercellular communication; composed of **connexons** (tubular channels composed of **six connexins**)
- Cells originate in the cuboidal basal layer and flatten out as they ascend to the surface—four to five layers/strata (deep to superficial): **s. basale, s. spinosum, s. granulosum, s. lucidum** (only on palmoplantar surfaces), and **s. corneum** (Table 1.2)
- An increasing total (intra- and extracellular) calcium gradient is present in the epidermis, with low levels of calcium in the stratum basale and increasingly higher levels of calcium toward the stratum granulosum
  - Multiple calcium-dependent processes in the epidermis are driven by the calcium gradient including keratinocyte maturation, desmosome formation, transglutaminase function, cleavage of profilaggrin, and extrusion and degradation of keratohyalin granules
- **Stratum basale**: mitotically active cuboidal cells from which the upper layers of the epidermis are derived
  - Attached to dermis by hemidesmosomes
  - Cellular proliferation stimulated by various factors, including trauma and UV (↑ **ornithine decarboxylase** expression is associated with (a/w) proliferative states)
    - Ornithine decarboxylase is inhibited by corticosteroids, retinoids, and vitamin D3
  - 10% of cells in the basal layer are stem cells, which give rise to other **stem cells**, and to **transient amplifying cells** that will replicate for a few cycles until they

Table 1.1 Intercellular Junction Proteins

Junction Type	Protein Family	Protein	Disease State
Desmosome *Anchor/attach to* ***keratin filaments***	Cadherin (transmembrane) *Cadherins are calcium-dependent transmembrane proteins.*	Desmoglein 1	Autoimmune: pemphigus foliaceus, PNP, PV (mucocutaneous form), IgA pemphigus (intraepidermal neutrophilic type) Inherited: **striate PPK** Infectious: bullous impetigo and SSSS
		Desmoglein 3	Pemphigus vulgaris (mucosal-predominant and mucocutaneous forms), PNP, IgA pemphigus (intraepidermal neutrophilic type)
		Desmoglein 4	**Monilethrix** (autosomal recessive form), autosomal recessive hypotrichosis
		Desmocollin 1	IgA pemphigus (SPD type)
		Desmocollin 2	Carvajal-like phenotype in one family
		Desmocollin 3	Hypotrichosis
	Plakin (cytoplasmic)	Desmoplakin	**Carvajal syndrome**
	Armadillo (cytoplasmic)	Plakophilin	Ectodermal dysplasia with skin fragility
Desmosome and adherens junction	Armadillo (catenin) (cytoplasmic)	Plakoglobin	**Naxos syndrome**
Adherens junction *Attach to* ***actin*** *filaments*	Cadherin (transmembrane)	E-Cadherin	Somatic mutations in many neoplasms
	Armadillo (cytoplasmic)	β-Catenin	Somatic mutations in many neoplasms, including **pilomatricomas;** also may be seen in **myotonic dystrophy and Rubinstein-Taybi**
Gap junction *Facilitate intercellular communication. Important for calcium regulation*	Connexin (transmembrane)	Connexin 26 (GJB2)	**Vohwinkel** syndrome, **KID** syndrome, **Bart-Pumphrey** syndrome, **PPK with deafness**; also common in non-syndromic deafness!
		Connexin 30 (GJB6)	**Hidrotic ectodermal dysplasia**
		Connexin 30.3 (GJB 4)	**Erythrokeratoderma variabilis**
		Connexin 31 (GJB 3)	**Erythrokeratoderma variabilis**

PNP, paraneoplastic pemphigus; *PV*, pemphigus vulgaris; *PPK*, palmoplantar keratosis; *SSSS*, staph scalded skin syndrome; *SPD*, subcorneal pustular dermatosis; *KID*, keratosis ichthyosis deafness syndrome

differentiate and move upward, eventually desquamating
  - Transit time from basal layer to stratum corneum = **14 days**; transit through the stratum corneum/desquamation = **14 days** (**total** = **28 days** from basal layer to desquamation)
- **Stratum spinosum**: named for the "spiny" appearance of intercellular desmosomal connections on microscopy
  - Contains multiple types of intercellular junctions
  - Terminal keratinocyte differentiation 2° to ↑ **calcium** in suprabasal epidermis
  - **Odland bodies** (lamellar granules) are produced by Golgi bodies in spinous layer
    - Primarily contain **ceramide** (**most important lipid** involved in epidermal barrier function), along with glycoproteins, glycolipids, and phospholipids
    - Are specialized lysosomes that exert most of their action in the stratum corneum, by discharging ceramides and other lipids into the extracellular space of the junction between the stratum granulosum and stratum corneum → **ceramides help form the cornified cell envelope** (see below), and eventually replace the cell membrane
- **Stratum granulosum**: flattened cells with prominent basophilic **keratohyalin granules**, which contain **profilaggrin** (converted to filaggrin at the junction of stratum granulosum and stratum corneum), **loricrin**, keratin intermediate filaments, and involucrin
  - Cells begin to lose nuclei, but keep overall structure
  - **Cornified cell envelope** production primarily takes place in the granular layer (Fig. 1.2)
    - Cross-linked protein and lipid structure encased in extracellular lipids forming a strong polymer that eventually replaces the plasma membrane
      - Process starts with envoplakin, periplakin, and involucrin scaffolding along the inner cell membrane (which is eventually replaced by ceramides from lamellar granules)
      - Further reinforcement by cross-linking **loricrin (a major component of cornified envelope**, first appears in granular layer; mutated in **Vohwinkel** syndrome variant lacking deafness), small proline-rich proteins, keratin, and filaggrin
      - **Cross-linking occurs via transglutaminase 1** → γ-glutamyl lysine isopeptide bonds (**Boards factoids:** TG-1 is mutated in lamellar ichthyosis; TG-3 is antigenic target in dermatitis herpetiformis)
      - Other components include envoplakin (helps connect desmosomes to cornified envelope), periplakin, elafin, and others
      - Outer surface of the cornified envelope is ultimately surrounded by lipids (primarily ceramide) = **cornified lipid envelope**
      - Ultimately provides strong water-impermeable outer barrier
- **Stratum corneum**: outermost layer, which serves as a mechanical barrier between the epidermis and the environment

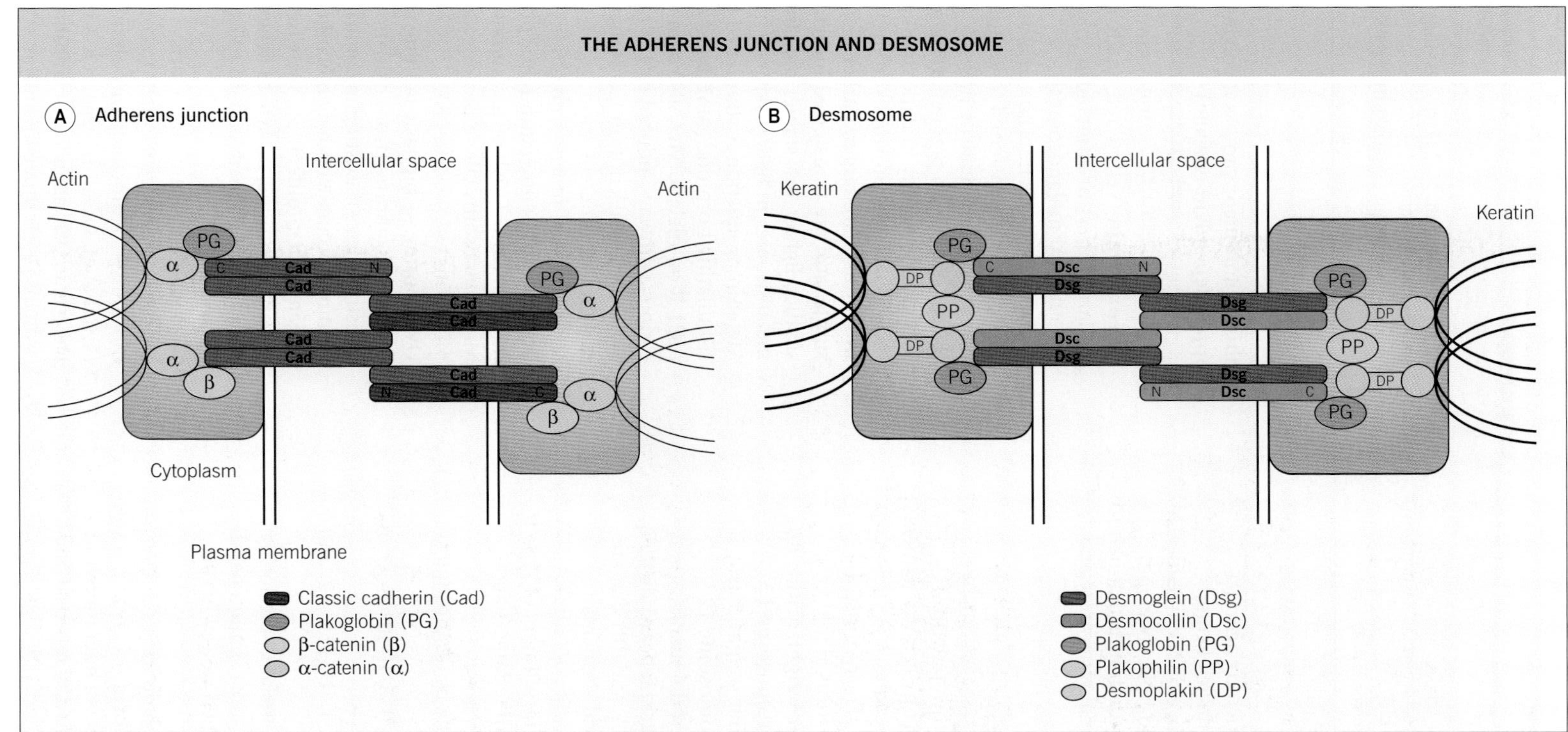

Fig. 1.1 The adherens junction and desmosome. (A) The adherens junction complex contains classic cadherins as transmembrane constituents, and α-catenins, β-catenins, and plakoglobin as cytoplasmic constituents. A classic cadherin is directly coupled through its cytoplasmic tail to β-catenin or plakoglobin, which in turn is linked to β-catenin, which binds to actin. (B) The desmosome complex includes desmogleins and desmocollins as transmembrane constituents, and plakoglobin, plakophilin, and desmoplakin as cytoplasmic constituents. Desmogleins and desmocollins associate with plakoglobin, which in turn binds to desmoplakin and links keratin to the membrane. *C,* Carboxy-terminus. *N,* amino-terminus. (From Amagai M. Pemphigus. In: Bolognia JL, Schaffer JV, Cerroni L, eds. *Dermatology*. 4th ed. Philadelphia: Elsevier; 2018:494–509.)

Table 1.2 Layers of the Epidermis

Epidermal Layer	Stage of Maturation	Products of Significance	Associated Diseases
S. basale	10% of cells in basal layer are stem cells	Keratin 5/14	Epidermolysis bullosa simplex
S. spinosum	Terminal keratinocyte differentiation secondary to ↑ **intracellular calcium**	Keratin 1/10 Odland bodies (lamellar granules) *Contains ceramides*	Epidermolytic ichthyosis Flegel's and Harlequin's ichthyosis are 2° to ↓ lamellar granules. X-Linked ichthyosis 2° to absent steroid sulfatase in lamellar granules
S. granulosum	Cells lose nuclei, flatten, produce keratohyalin granules (KHG) which contributes to the cornified cell envelope which forms beginning in this layer	KHG which contain **profilaggrin, loricrin**, keratin IF, and involucrin	Ichthyosis vulgaris (filaggrin) Atopic dermatitis (filaggrin) Vohwinkel without deafness (loricrin)
S. corneum	Anucleate, protein-rich corneocytes		

- Composed primarily of protein-rich corneocytes ("bricks"; normally contain NO nuclei; keratin filaments attached to cornified envelope) embedded in a lipid matrix ("mortar," cornified lipid envelope)
- Serves as a barrier to water loss (conditions that perturb the skin barrier → ↑ transepidermal water loss) and toxins/infectious agents

Epidermal cells of importance

- <u>Keratinocytes:</u> the primary cells of the epidermis; responsible for producing proteins (e.g., keratin filaments) and lipids important for barrier function
  - Keratins: intermediate filaments that comprise the primary cytoskeleton of the epidermis (Table 1.3)
    - Type I keratins: **low molecular weight**; **acidic**; **K9-28**, K31-40 (hair keratins); **chromosome 17**
    - Type II keratins: **high molecular weight; basic**; **K1-8**, K81-86 (hair keratins); **chromosome 12**
    - Basic structure is an α-helical rod domain (consisting of heptad amino acid repeats) divided into four segments (1A, 1B, 2A, and 2B) that are interrupted by three non-helical segments ("linkers")
    - Functional unit consists of **heterodimers of type I and type II** filaments that form tetramers and ultimately filaments
    - Anchored to plasma membrane by desmosomes
    - 40 to 70 kD
  - Keratinocytes produce IL-1, IL-6, IL-8, IL-10, IL-12, and **TNF-α**, among others
  - Keratinocytes respond to IL-2, IL-4, IL-13, IL-22, and TNF-α, among others
- <u>Melanocytes:</u> **Neural crest-derived,** melanin-producing cells; dendritic morphology; found in the stratum basale in~1:10 ratio with keratinocytes (when viewed in two-dimensional plane)
  - **c-kit** activation is needed for melanocyte development/migration; **piebaldism** occurs as a result of c-kit loss → impaired melanocyte migration and proliferation; **c-kit mutations** are a/w mucosal and acral melanoma
  - Each melanocyte interfaces with ~**36 keratinocytes** when analyzed three-dimensionally **(epidermal melanin unit)**
  - Melanin is produced in melanosomes (lysosome-type organelles) from its precursor, tyrosine, through a multistep enzymatic process involving **tyrosinase (copper-dependent enzyme)**
    - Tyrosine $\xrightarrow{\text{(tyrosinase-dependent step)}}$ DOPA $\xrightarrow{\text{(tyrosinase-dependent step)}}$ DOPAquinone → **pheomelanin** (yellow/red; made by round melanosomes) or **eumelanin** (black/brown; made by elliptical melanosomes)
    - Melanosomes are transported along the dendritic processes and transferred to keratinocytes through phagocytosis of dendrite tips
    - Racial variation in pigmentation: identical melanocyte density in dark- and light-skinned individuals; **melanosomes in darker-skinned individuals are larger, darker (↑ melanin), more stable, and are transferred individually** (vs. smaller, lighter, less stable, and **clustered** melanosomes in lighter-skinned individuals)
    - Melanin production is stimulated by melanocyte-stimulating hormone **(MSH)** and **ACTH** activity on **MC1-R** on melanocytes; also stimulated through various pathways induced by UV radiation
    - SOX10 is a transcription factor that controls melanocyte differentiation
    - **MC1-R loss** of function mutations → ↑ **pheomelanin:eumelanin** ratio (phenotype = **red hair**/fair skin, ↑ **risk of melanoma)**
    - Melanin absorbs UV → protects against UV-induced mutations
    - UV exposure → biphasic tanning response: immediate tanning (from oxidation and redistribution of existing melanin) and delayed tanning (occurs with new melanin synthesis, melanocytic proliferation, increased transfer of melanin from melanocyte to keratinocyte). (See Section 1.5 for discussion on roles of UVA and UVB in tanning).
  - Other high-yield examination facts:
    - Defects in enzymes required to convert tyrosine to melanin → **oculocutaneous albinism**; OCA1 (*Tyrosinase*), OCA2 (*P gene*), OCA3 (*TRP-1*)
    - Defects in packaging of melanosome-specific proteins → **Hermansky-Pudlak** syndrome (HPS1 > HPS3 > other gene mutations)
    - Defects in lysosome and melanosome trafficking to dendrites → **Griscelli** (*MYO5A*, *RAB27A*, and *MLPH* mutations) and **Chédiak-Higashi syndrome** (*LYST* mutations)

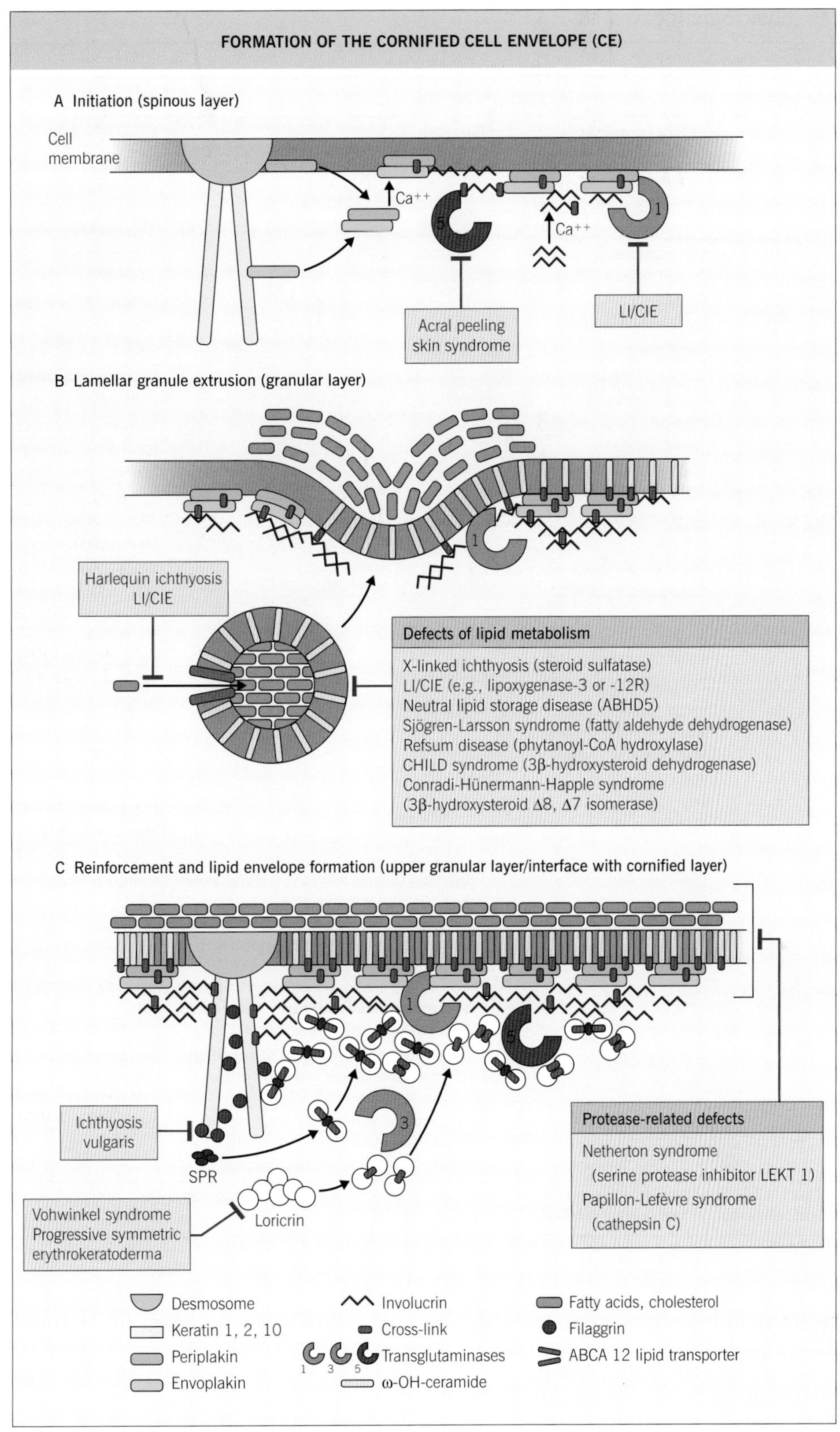

Fig. 1.2 Formation of the cornified cell envelope *(CE)*. Terminal differentiation of keratinocytes is triggered by an increase in the intracellular Ca^{2+} concentration of the suprabasal epidermis. CE assembly is initiated in the upper spinous layer via formation of a cross-linked scaffold composed of envoplakin, periplakin, and involucrin along the inner surface of the cell membrane (A). This is followed by (or perhaps coincident with) extrusion of lamellar granules into the extracellular space (B). Specialized ω-hydroxyceramides are delivered to, and eventually replace, the cell membrane, where they become linked to scaffold proteins. Reinforcement occurs via cross-linking and translocation to the cell periphery of loricrin (accounts for > 80% of the mass of the CE) and small proline-rich proteins *(SPRs)* (C). Complexes of keratin and filaggrin also become cross-linked to the CE. In addition, proteases play important roles in processing of CE proteins and the proteolysis of corneodesmosomes that is required for desquamation. A mature and terminally differentiated cornified cell thus consists of keratin filaments covalently attached to the CE, which is composed of protein and lipid envelope components and is imbedded in the extracellular lipid lamellae. Defects in transglutaminases, lipid metabolism, CE structural proteins, and proteases lead to a variety of diseases characterized by ichthyosis and/or keratoderma (1–3). *CHILD, C*ongenital *h*emidysplasia with *i*chthyosiform erythroderma and *l*imb *d*efects; *CIE,* congenital ichthyosiform erythroderma; *LI,* lamellar ichthyosis. (From Arin MJ, Roop DR, Koch PJ, Koster MI. Biology of keratinocytes. In: Bolognia JL, Schaffer JV, Cerroni L, eds. *Dermatology*. 4th ed. Philadelphia: Elsevier; 2018:876–887. Courtesy, Julie V Schaffer, MD.)

Table 1.3 Protein Components of the Epidermis (Including Nonepidermal Keratins)

Protein	Site of Synthesis	Function	Disease State
Keratin 1	Suprabasal keratinocytes (produced in spinous layer)	Primary keratinocyte cytoskeleton	Epidermolytic ichthyosis (preferred new name for EHK), epidermolytic and nonepidermolytic (Unna-Thost) PPK, ichthyosis hystrix of Curth-Macklin[a]
Keratin 2	Granular layer		Superficial epidermolytic ichthyosis (Siemens)
Keratin 3	Cornea		Meesmann's corneal dystrophy
Keratin 4	Mucosal epithelium		White sponge nevus
Keratin 5	Basal keratinocytes		EBS, Dowling-Degos disease[a]
Keratin 6a	Outer root sheath of hair		Pachyonychia congenita I[a]
Keratin 6b	Nail bed epithelium		Pachyonychia congenita II
Keratin 9	Palmoplantar suprabasal keratinocytes		Vorner (epidermolytic) PPK
Keratin 10	Suprabasal keratinocytes (produced in spinous layer)		Epidermolytic ichthyosis[a]
Keratin 11	Granular layer		
Keratin 12	Cornea		Meesmann's corneal dystrophy
Keratin 13	Mucosal epithelium		White sponge nevus
Keratin 14	Basal keratinocytes		EBS, Naegeli-Franceschetti-Jadassohn syndrome, dermatopathia pigmentosa reticularis
Keratin 16	Outer root sheath of hair		Pachyonychia congenita I[a]
Keratin 17	Nail bed epithelium		Pachyonychia congenita II, steatocystoma multiplex
Keratin 19	Stem cells of basal layer		
Keratin 71, 73, 74	Hair inner root sheath		Wooly hair
Keratin 32, 35, 82, 85	Hair cuticle		
Keratin 17, 33, 34, 36, 37, 75, 81	Hair medulla		Pseudofolliculitis barbae
Keratins 31–38, 81, 83, 85, 86	Hair cortex		Monilethrix (*KRT81, KRT83, KRT86* most commonly; also *DSG4*)
Filaggrin/profilaggrin	Granular layer	Aggregates keratin, flattening granular layer cells. Degraded in the stratum corneum into **urocanic acid** and pyrrolidone carboxylic acid, which **help block/absorb UV radiation**. Urocanic acid is also a component of **natural moisturization factor**—helps keep stratum corneum hydrated/moist	Ichthyosis vulgaris, atopic dermatitis
Loricrin	Granular layer	**Most abundant component of cornified cell envelope**. Cross-linked to involucrin by transglutaminase 1.[b]	Vohwinkel syndrome with ichthyosis (NO deafness) Decreased in psoriasis
Involucrin	Granular layer	Component of cornified cell envelope. Proteins are cross-linked together by transglutaminase 1 → strong border	Increased in psoriasis

[a]*In psoriasis and other hyperproliferative states, keratin 6 and 16 are upregulated and keratin 1 and 10 are downregulated.*
[b]*Transglutaminase 1 mutations → lamellar ichthyosis and NBCIE.*

- Langerhans cells (LCs): major antigen-presenting cells (APCs) of the skin
  - Dendritic histiocytes characterized by **reniform** (kidney-shaped) nuclei, and tennis racket-shaped **Birbeck granules** seen on electron microscopy
  - Interact with keratinocytes via E-cadherin
  - Positive immunostains: **CD207 (langerin**; most sensitive immunohistochemical stain; specific for Birbeck granules), **CD1a**, **S100**, CD34, vimentin, and actin
  - Originate from CD34+ progenitor cells in bone marrow like other monocytes/macrophages
  - Found mainly in stratum spinosum, where it first encounters and processes antigens, and **subsequently migrates to the lymph nodes** to activate T cells
  - **Downregulated in skin after UV exposure** → ↓ immune surveillance
  - See p. 27 for further discussion of immunologic function
- Merkel cells: slow-adapting mechanoreceptors enriched in the fingertips, lips, oral cavity, and hair follicle outer root sheath
  - Found in stratum basale; communicate with neurons
  - **CK20⁺ in paranuclear dot pattern** sensitive/specific for Merkel cells; also (+) for neurofilament, S100, synaptophysin, chromogranin A, vasoactive intestinal peptide, neuron-specific enolase, and calcitonin gene-related peptide

Basement membrane zone (BMZ) (Fig. 1.3, Table 1.4)

- Semipermeable barrier between epidermis and dermis that also serves to adhere basal keratinocytes to the underlying dermis
- Key steps within each location:
  - Basal keratinocyte/hemidesmosome: intracellular keratin filaments (**K5** and **K14**) attach to electron-dense hemidesmosomal plaques (**plectin** and **BPAG1 [BP230]**) on the basal plasma membrane → hemidesmosomal plaque proteins bind to intracellular portions of the anchoring filaments (BPAG2 and $\alpha6\beta4$ integrin)
  - Lamina lucida: extracellular portion of **anchoring filaments (BPAG2, $\alpha6\beta4$ integrin**, and **laminin 332)** extend from the hemidesmosome down to the lamina densa; the thin filaments result in an electron-lucent region; is the weakest portion of BMZ → is zone of separation in **salt-split skin** and also in **suction blisters**
  - Lamina densa: anchoring filaments attach to **type IV collagen** (major component) and other proteins (laminin 332, laminin 331, and nidogen) in the lamina densa → attachment between basal keratinocyte and lamina densa. Several proteoglycans present, including heparin sulfates and chondroitin sulfates. Proteoglycans can bind collagen IV, laminins, and nidogen. **Perlecan** (a type of heparin sulfate proteoglycan) is the most prominent proteoglycan
  - Sublamina densa: loops of **type VII collagen (anchoring fibrils)** arise from the underside of lamina densa, extend down into the dermis, hook around dermal **type I and III collagen fibers**, and then loop back up to reattach to lamina densa (or anchoring plaques in dermis) → firmly anchors the lamina densa (and all aforementioned structures) to the papillary dermis
- BMZ also functions as a permeability barrier: proteoglycans are **negatively charged** and are a major contributor to the permeability barrier

Dermis

- Located below the epidermis, derived from mesoderm, and divided into papillary dermis (superficial) and reticular dermis (deep)

Dermal cells of importance

- Fibroblasts: create extracellular matrix (ECM) and are involved in wound healing
- Mononuclear phagocytes: discussed on p. 25
- Mast cells: discussed on p. 27
- Glomus cells: specialized smooth muscle cells derived from **Sucquet-Hoyer canals**, which surround vessels and assist in thermoregulation by allowing for blood **shunting** from arterioles to venules (bypassing capillaries); found mainly in the **palms/soles**
  - Overproduction → glomus tumor (favors acral sites because of ↑ glomus cell density)

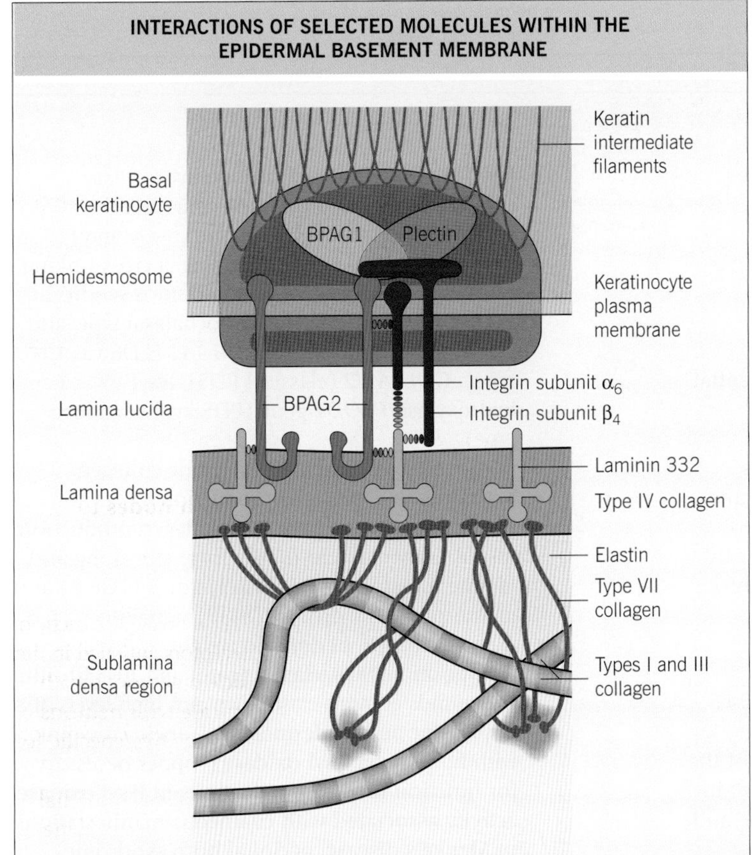

Fig. 1.3 Interactions of selected molecules within the epidermal basement membrane. These interactions promote epidermal adhesion and also play a key role in a number of dermatologic diseases. Important molecular interactions include those between: (1) plakin family members, BPAG1, and plectin, with keratin intermediate filaments; (2) the former with BPAG2 and integrin $\alpha_6\beta_4$ (specifically the large cytoplasmic domain of integrin subunit β_4); (3) the cytoplasmic domains of BPAG2 and integrin subunit β_4; (4) the extracellular domains of BPAG2 and integrin subunit α_6 as well as laminin 332 (formerly laminin 5); (5) integrin $\alpha_6\beta_4$ in hemidesmosomes and laminin 332 in the lamina densa; (6) laminin 332 and type VII collagen; (7) type VII collagen with type IV collagen, fibronectin, and type I collagen in the sublamina densa region. (From Yancey KB. The biology of the basement membrane. In: Bolognia JL, Schaffer JV, Cerroni L, eds. *Dermatology*. 4th ed. Philadelphia: Elsevier; 2018:483–493.)

Table 1.4 Basement Membrane Zone Proteins

Protein	Site	Source	Family	Function	Disease State
BPAg1 (230 kD)	Hemidesmosome/keratinocyte	Keratinocyte	Plakin	Binds keratins and integrins; intracellular/part of attachment plaque	BP, EB simplex
BPAg2 (180 kD)	Hemidesmosome/ keratinocyte → lamina lucida Amino terminus is intracellular and carboxy terminus is extracellular NC16A domain is closer to amino terminus but is extracellular	Keratinocyte	Collagen (XVII)	Transmembrane protein and one of the anchoring filaments; interacts with BPAg1, laminin 5, β4 integrin, and plectin	**N16A terminus:** BP, pemphigoid gestationis, linear IgA bullous disease **Carboxy terminus:** Cicatricial pemphigoid
α6β4 Integrin	Hemidesmosome/ keratinocyte → lamina lucida	Keratinocyte	Integrin	Interacts with keratins, laminin 5, plectin, BPAg1, BPAg2; part of the anchoring filaments	**Ocular** cicatricial pemphigoid (antibodies to **β4**), **EB with pyloric atresia** (85%)
Laminin 332 (laminin 5, epiligrin)	Lamina lucida → Lamina densa	Keratinocyte	Laminin	Connects other anchoring filaments (BPAg2 and α6β4 integrin) to collagen VII; part of the anchoring filaments	**Antiepiligrin pemphigoid** (a/w malignancy), **JEB-Herlitz**
Plectin	Hemidesmosome	Keratinocyte	Plakin	Binds keratins and integrins; intracellular/part of attachment plaque	**EB with muscular dystrophy**, EB with pyloric atresia (15%)
Nidogen (entactin)	Lamina densa	Unclear	Nidogen	Adaptor between laminin 1 and collagen IV in lamina densa; stabilizes proteins of lamina densa	
Collagen IV	Lamina densa	Unclear	Collagen	Anchors laminins in lamina densa → structural support; also a component of **anchoring plaques** in dermis, which attach collagen VII to collagen I and III	Goodpasture disease, Alport syndrome
Collagen VII	Sublamina densa	Fibroblasts	Collagen	Major component of **anchoring fibrils**	**Dystrophic EB, bullous lupus, EB acquisita**
Heparan sulfate proteoglycan	Lamina densa	Fibroblasts	Proteoglycans	Contribute to matrix of and give an overall **negative charge** (**creating a permeability barrier**) to the basement membrane	

BP, bullous pemphigoid; *BPAg*, bullous pemphigoid antigen; *EB*, epidermolysis bullosa

- Dermal DCs: bone marrow–derived APCs that reside within dermis; **highly phagocytic**

Structural components and cell biology of the dermis

- Extracellular matrix
  - Provides structure and support to the dermis; essential for water retention and for signal transduction
  - Synthesized by dermal fibroblasts
  - Composed of collagens, elastin, fibrillins, fibulins, integrins, laminins, glycoproteins, and proteoglycans (Fig. 1.4)
    - Collagens are **triple helices** formed by amino acid chains where every third residue is **glycine (Gly-X-Y),** with a high likelihood of **proline** and **hydroxyproline/hydroxylysine** in the X and Y positions, respectively
      - Accounts for **75%** of dry weight of the skin; #1 component of the dermis
      - **Collagen I is the primary collagen** (85%) of the ECM; type III (10%; important and prevalent in **blood vessels**, fetal skin, GI tract, new scars, and **keloids**) and V are also present
      - **Lysyl hydroxylase** and proline hydroxylase catalyze cross-linking of collagen; **vitamin C-dependent process** (deficiency → scurvy)
      - Defects in collagen and/or collagen cross-linking result in most forms of Ehlers-Danlos syndrome (EDS): ***COL1A1/2*** (EDS arthrochalasia type, and osteogenesis imperfecta); ***COL3A1*** (EDS vascular type); ***COL5A1/2*** (classical EDS); lysyl hydroxylase/***PLOD1*** gene (EDS kyphoscoliosis type)
      - Matrix metalloproteinases degrade collagen
      - Retinoids → ↑ collagen production
      - Corticosteroids and UV → ↓ collagen production
    - Elastic fibers provide resilience from stretching and modulate transforming growth factor-β (TGF-β) and bone morphogenic protein (BMP) signaling
      - Account for **4%** of dry skin weight
      - Composition: **90% elastin** (core) and **10% fibrillin** (surrounds elastin); elastin contains high levels of **desmosine** and **isodesmosine** → these cross-link with fibrillin via **lysyl oxidase (copper necessary for function function; reductions in lysyl oxidase activity associated with cuatneous manifestations of Menke's disease, occipital horn syndrome)**

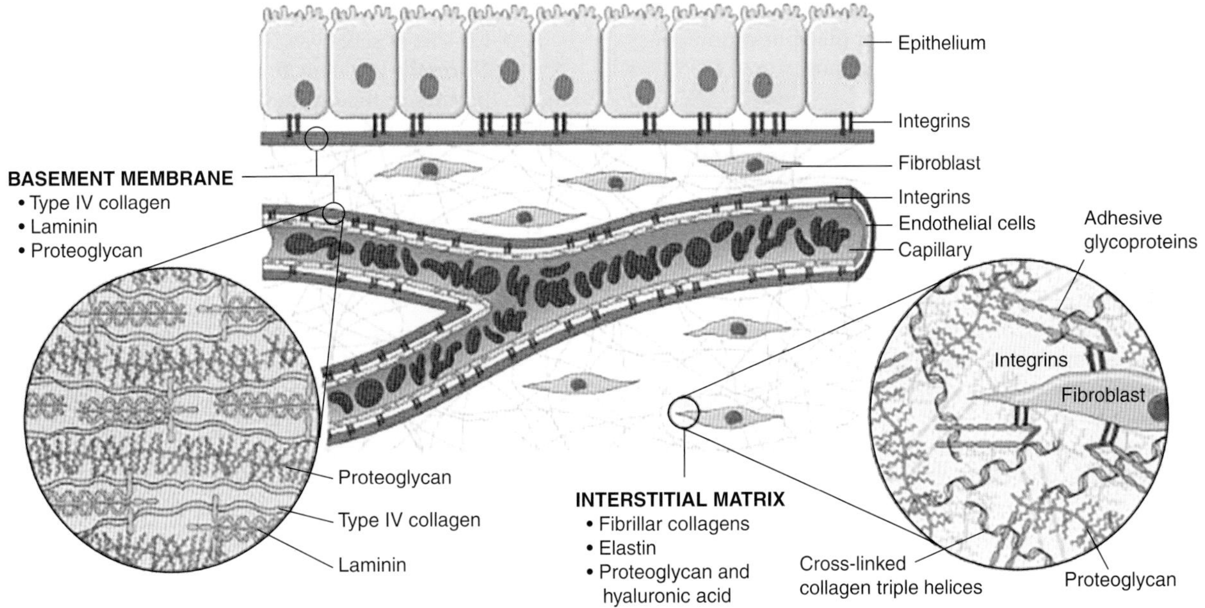

Fig. 1.4 Major extracellular matrix molecules composing the basal lamina and interstitial matrix of healthy skin. (From Kumar V, Abbas A, Aster J. *Robbins & Cotran Pathologic Basis of Disease*. 9th ed. Philadelphia: Elsevier; 2015.)

- ◆ Notable defects/mutations in elastic tissue: ***Fibrillin 1*** (Marfan's syndrome); ***Fibrillin 2*** (congenital contractural arachnodactyly); ***Fibulin 5*** (cutis laxa; gene defect results in decreased desmosine); ***LEMD3*** (Buschke-Ollendorff syndrome; defect results in increased desmosine); ***ABCC6*** (pseudoxanthoma elasticum; mutation results in fragmentation and calcification of elastic fibers)
- ◆ **Elaunin** fibers run horizontal/parallel in reticular dermis and **oxytalan** fibers run vertical/perpendicular to dermo-epidermal junction (DEJ) in papillary dermis; mnemonic: "stand (= vertical) up-high (= high in dermis) with OXYgen (= OXYtalan)"
- ◆ UV radiation → damage of elastic fibers

- ▪ All aforementioned fibers are set in a matrix of proteoglycans and glycosaminoglycans (**GAGs**) that **retain large quantities of water** (up to 1000× their volume!) = ground substance
  - ○ Most important GAGs = **hyaluronic acid**, chondroitin sulfate, dermatan sulfate, and heparan sulfate
  - ○ GAGs are broken down by lysosomal hydrolases

- • Cutaneous vasculature
  - ▪ Cutaneous vasculature important for metabolic support of the skin and maintenance of body temperature
    - ○ Two vascular plexuses: superficial (→ vessels of the reticular dermis) and deep (→ follicles, glands)
    - ○ **VEGF** is the primary mediator of **vasculogenesis**
      - ◆ ↑ VEGF: most cancers, psoriasis, **POEMS syndrome**, and other diseases with increased vasculature
    - ○ Lymphatic vessels collect fluid and proteins from interstitium and direct it into the lymph circulation
    - ○ **Prox1**, **Podoplanin (D2-40)**, **LYVE-1**, and VEGFR-3 are lymphatic vessel markers
- • Cutaneous neurology and neurobiology
  - ▪ Nerves of the skin are responsible for detecting touch/pressure, pain, itch, and other sensations
  - ▪ Cutaneous sensory nerves are divided into free nerve endings and corpuscular nerve endings (round/globular collection of neural and other cells)
    - ○ Free nerve endings
      - ◆ **Itch and pain: A-δ** (larger; myelinated) and **C-polymodal nociceptor** afferent fibers (smaller; unmyelinated)
      - ◆ End in the epidermis/superficial dermis
    - ○ Specialized nerve receptors
      - ◆ Krause end bulbs: **genitalia**, perianal region, and vermillion lips; mnemonic "Kinky **Krause ends** on erotic areas"
      - ◆ Meissner's corpuscle: superficial (dermal papillae) mechanoreceptor of **digits**; fast adapting; suited for pressure/**light touch**
      - ◆ Pacinian corpuscle: deep (deep dermis/fat) mechanoreceptor of palmoplantar skin, nipples, and genital region; fast adapting; suited for **vibration** and deeper pressure
      - ◆ Merkel nerve ending: superficial (basal epidermis) mechanoreceptor most concentrated in fingertips, lips, and external genitalia; slow adapting; suited for pressure/touch. Resident Merkel cells are not distinguishable on routine H&E except in cases of proliferation (Merkel cell carcinomas).
      - ◆ Ruffini corpuscle: deep (fat) mechanoreceptor most concentrated around fingernails; slow adapting; suited for **sustained pressure**

- Innervation of cutaneous appendages:
  - Adrenergic control: **vascular smooth muscle, apocrine glands**, and arrector pili contraction
  - Cholinergic control: eccrine glands
- Adnexal structures
  - Eccrine glands
    - Secretory exocrine gland primarily responsible for **thermoregulation** and waste excretion
    - Found on all cutaneous surfaces except: external auditory canal, lips, glans penis, clitoris, and labia minora
    - Highest concentration = palms and soles
    - Controlled by hypothalamus; innervated by **postganglionic sympathetic fibers**, which synapse with **muscarinic acetylcholine receptors** on the glands
    - Isotonic sweat secreted in secretory gland → NaCl reabsorbed in duct → **hypotonic sweat** is delivered to surface under normal conditions
      - ↑ rate of sweating → more isotonic solution (less time to reabsorb NaCl in duct)
      - Maximal rate of sweating ~ 3 L/hr
      - Merocrine secretion
    - Components (deep to superficial): secretory coil (deep dermis), intradermal/straight duct (eosinophilic cuticle seen on histology), and acrosyringium (intraepidermal portion; spiral duct that opens onto the skin surface)
    - Stains for S100, keratin (CK5/6, CK7), and CEA
  - Apocrine glands
    - Secretory exocrine glands with unclear function in humans; in animals they mediate sexual attraction through pheromone release
      - Activity begins around puberty
    - Located primarily in **anogenital skin, axillae**, external ear canal (ceruminous), vermillion border, **periumbilical region**, eyelid margin (Moll's), and breast (mammary)
    - Empty into follicular infundibulum (above sebaceous duct)
    - Secretory control unclear → glands non-innervated, but do have **β-adrenergic receptors**, which are likely **stimulated by circulating catecholamines**
    - Secretory products released through **decapitation secretion**: cholesterol and cholesterol esters, triglycerides, squalene, and fatty acids
      - **Lipofuscin** = pigmented mixture of lipids and proteins → responsible for yellow-brown color of **chromhidrosis**
    - Initially odorless secretions → later modified by surface bacteria → results in body odor
    - Ectopic or modified apocrine glands: **mammary glands**, ceruminous glands of the external auditory canal, and **Moll's gland of the eyelids**
      - These empty directly to the surface
  - Sebaceous glands
    - Secretory exocrine glands found primarily on the scalp, face, and upper anterior trunk ("seborrheic areas")
      - NOT on the palms/soles
    - Functions include water retention and innate immune defense
    - Consist of sebocytes, which contain lipid vacuoles
    - **Normally a/w hair follicles** and empty into inferior portion of the infundibulum
    - Pubertal androgen production is major signal for sebaceous gland maturation (under adrenergic control)
      - Transient maternal androgen stimulation present in infancy
    - Other endocrine factors stimulating maturation and sebum production: MSH, CRH, and substance P
    - Secretory products released through **holocrine secretion** (entire cell lyses to release contents):
      - **Triglycerides (#1 component**; ≈50%) > wax esters (#2) > squalene (#3)
      - Others: cholesterol esters, cholesterol, antimicrobial peptides, androgens, and cytokines
    - **Ectopic sebaceous glands**: Meibomian glands on eyelid tarsal plate (secretes oily meibum to prevent evaporation of tear film on eyeball), Fordyce spots (vermillion lip/oral mucosa), Montgomery tubercles (areolae/nipples), Tyson glands (labia minora/prepuce), and Zeis glands (services eyelashes, not truly ectopic as Zeis glands are a/w eyelash follicle; located close to Moll's gland)
      - A stye (hordeolum) is a result of an occlusion/inflammation of the Zeis/eyelash unit, and is typically painful. A chalazion is a deeper occlusion of a meibomian gland, and is typically asymptomatic at first.
  - Hair
    - Epithelial-derived appendage important for temperature regulation, protection of other structures (nasal mucosa, eyes, and ears), social and sexual cues, and tactile sensory input
    - Three types of hairs:
      - Lanugo: fine hairs shed late in gestation and during the first month of life; may be seen in adults in context of certain types of hypertrichosis
      - Vellus: fine hairs over face, trunk, and extremities early in life; most numerous hairs on body
      - Terminal: coarse, darker hairs of scalp, eyebrows, and eyelashes; postpubertal androgens induce switch to terminal hairs in other sites
    - Hair density: ~100,000 hairs on scalp; more in blonde and fewer in red-haired individuals
    - Anatomy: Table 1.5, Fig. 1.5
    - Follicular layers: Fig. 1.6
      - Cortex is where most hair keratins are located
      - Cuticle helps keeps hair intact—damage → split ends (trichoptilosis)
      - Cuticle from hair shaft and inner root sheath merge
    - Dermal papilla: mesenchymal structure (from embryonic mesoderm) containing vasculature; contributes to hair cycle regulation
    - Hair cycle: Table 1.6
      - Anagen: phase of growth
        - ➔ Length of anagen phase determines hair length

Table 1.5 Hair Anatomy

Portion of Hair	Description
Hair bulb	Lowermost portion of the hair follicle
Hair matrix	Rapidly proliferating keratinocytes that terminally differentiate to produce the hair shaft
Infundibulum	Region extending from the skin surface down to the point where the sebaceous gland opens into the hair follicle; ORS displays cornification similar to that of the interfollicular epidermis (i.e., contains **keratohyalin granules**). The most superficial portion of the hair follicle—mnemonic: "It's always more 'fun' on top"
Isthmus	Region located between the opening of the sebaceous gland, down to the site of insertion of the arrector pili muscle; ORS displays **trichilemmal keratinization** (keratinizes without a granular layer; IRS shed before this point)
Lower hair follicle	Region located between hair bulb to proximal isthmus; encapsulates DP; has inner and outer root sheaths; **critical line of Auber** is the widest area
Arrector pili muscle	Inserts at the level of the bulge; pulls up hair ("goose bumps")
Bulge	Segment of the ORS located at the level of arrector pili muscle insertion; major seat of epithelial **stem cells of the hair follicle**
Secondary hair germ	Additional seat of epithelial and also of melanocyte stem cells; located between club hair and DP in telogen hair follicle
Connective tissue sheath (CTS)	Special mesenchymal follicular sheath that is tightly attached to the hair follicle basement membrane and is continuous with the follicular DP
Follicular dermal papilla (DP)	Onion-shaped, closely packed, specialized fibroblast population with inductive and morphogenic properties; **provides signals that stimulate hair matrix to proliferate**; hair cycle-dependent fibroblast trafficking occurs between CTS and DP; **volume of DP determines the size of hair bulb and, thus, hair shaft diameter**
Inner root sheath (IRS)	Packages and guides the hair shaft; cornifies normally with **trichohyalin granules**; stains red secondary to citrulline; **not present in telogen hairs**; is present in lower hair follicle but not in the isthmus/infundibulum (IRS is shed at the beginning of the isthmus)
Outer root sheath (ORS)	Merges distally into the epidermis and proximally into the hair bulb; provides slippage plane, nutrition, regulatory molecules, and stem cells
Critical line of Auber	**Widest section of the hair bulb** and where most mitotic activity essential for hair growth occurs
Adamson's fringe	Anatomic point marking the upper boundary of the follicular bulb; point at which IRS and hair shaft begin to keratinize.
Follicle pigmentary unit	Melanin-producing hair follicle melanocytes located up and around the upper one-third of the DP; transfer pheomelanosomes or eumelanosomes to differentiating hair follicle keratinocytes in the precortical matrix; goes largely into apoptosis during each catagen phase, regenerated from melanocyte stem cells in hair germ during anagen

Modified from Wang E, de Berker D, Christiano AM. Biology of hair and nails. In: Bolognia JL, Schaffer JV, Cerroni L, eds. Dermatology. *4th ed. Philadelphia: Elsevier; 2018:1144–1161. Courtesy John P. Sundberg, DVM, PhD.*

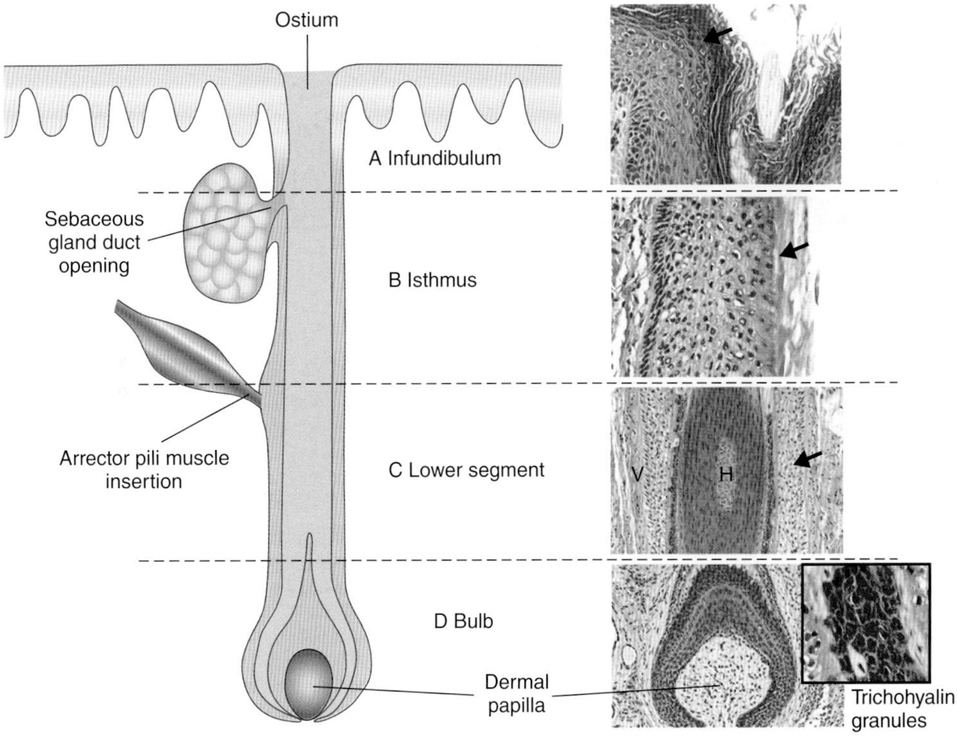

Fig. 1.5 Follicular microanatomy: follicular segments. (A) The infundibulum extends from follicular ostia to the opening of the sebaceous ducts. Note the infundibular epithelium is identical to interfollicular epidermis in that keratinization occurs with a granular layer (*arrow*). (B) The isthmus is located between the opening of the sebaceous duct and the insertion of the arrector pili muscle. The cells of the outer root sheath (ORS) are increasingly pale due to increased glycogen content. Note that the ORS keratinizes without an intervening granular layer at the isthmus (trichilemmal keratinization) (*arrow*). The inner root sheath (IRS) may be seen desquamating at this level (not shown). (C) The lower segment extends from the lower isthmus to the hair bulb. In this segment, the ORS has abundant glycogen observed as pale cytoplasm (*arrow*), and the vitreous layer is prominent *(V)*. Hair shaft *(H)*. (D) Hair bulb. Note the IRS contains trichohyalin granules (*insert*). (Photographs courtesy of Dr. Diego Morales.)

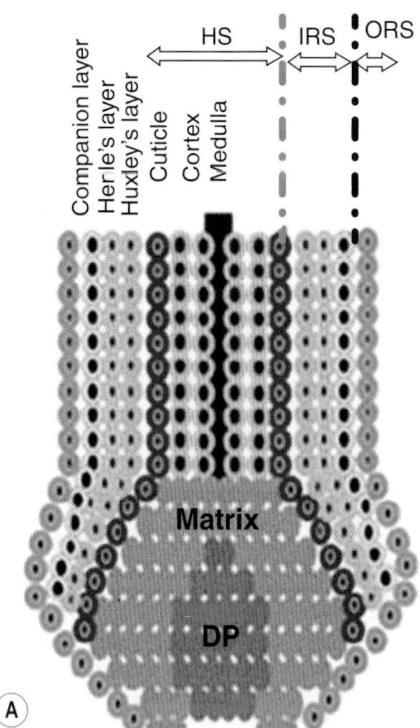

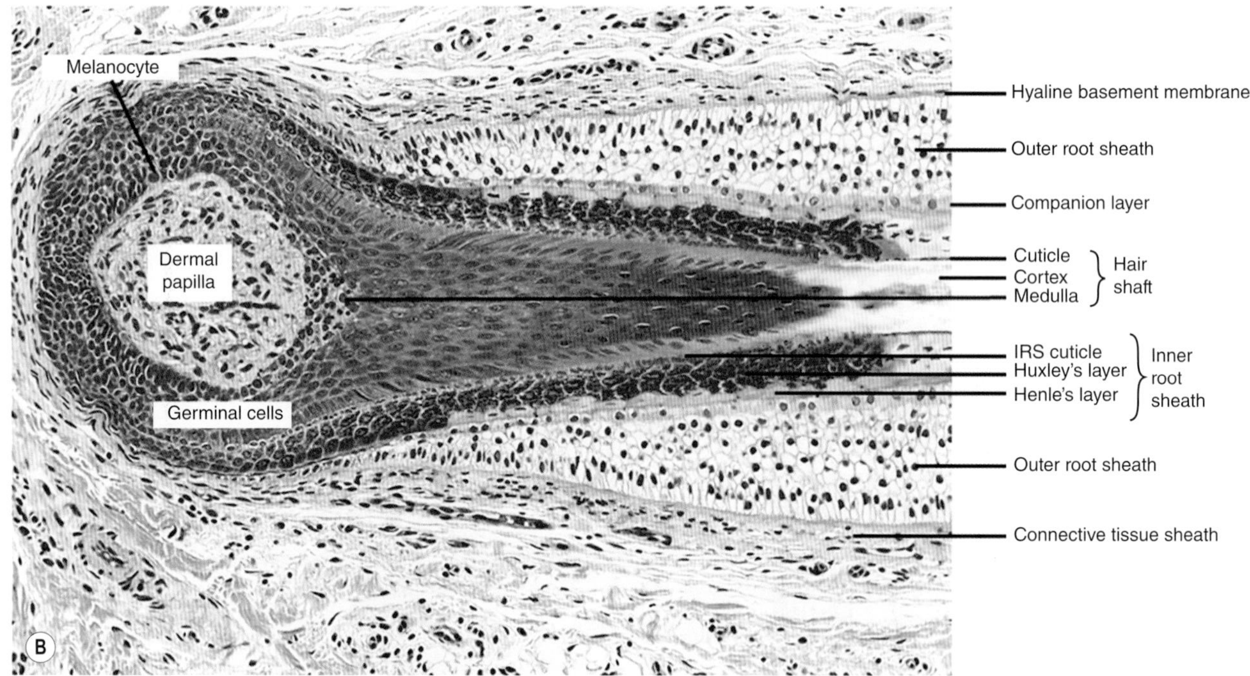

Fig. 1.6 (A) and (B) Follicular microanatomy: layers of the suprabulbar region. From inner to outer layer: hair shaft (*HS*; cuticle, cortex, and medulla), inner root sheath (*IRS*; Henle's layer, Huxley's layer, and cuticle), outer root sheath (*ORS*), and glassy membrane. *DP,* Dermal papilla. (*A,* From Mahjour SB, Ghaffarpasand F, Wang H. Hair follicle regeneration in skin grafts: current concepts and future perspectives. *Tissue Eng Part B Rev.* 2012;18(1):15–23; *B,* Photograph courtesy of Dr. Diego Morales.)

Table 1.6 Hair Growth Cycle

	Anagen	Catagen	Telogen (Club Hairs)
Phase activity	Growth (~**0.4 mm/day** or ~1 cm/month on scalp); follicular melanocytes only active in anagen phase)	Regression (**melanocytes in matrix undergo apoptosis;** inner root sheath lost)	Resting
Duration	2–6 years	2–3 weeks	3 months
Percentage (%) of scalp hairs	85–90	1–2	10–15

- ➔ Bimatoprost works by prolonging the anagen phase, and increasing percentage of hairs in anagen phase
- ◆ Exogen: phase of active shedding of club hair between telogen and anagen
  - ➔ Lose about 100 hairs/day
- ◆ Kenogen: subphase of telogen in which no shaft is present
- o Hair and hormones
  - ◆ Estrogens prolong anagen
  - ◆ Thyroxine promotes growth
  - ◆ Corticosteroids retard anagen onset
  - ◆ Hair follicle converts testosterone to dihydrotestosterone locally via 5-α-reductase
    - ➔ Inhibitors of 5-α-reductase are used in androgenetic alopecia: dutasteride (5-α-reductase I, II, III) and finasteride (5-α-reductase II and III)
- o Color of hair 2° to hair melanocytes in **anagen** bulb/matrix (**melanin unit = 1 melanocyte: 5 keratinocytes**; melanocytes only produce pigment in anagen phase!)
  - ◆ Eumelanin (brown/black hair pigment) versus pheomelanin (red/blonde hair pigment)
- o **Hair follicle stem cells** reside in **bulge** and contribute to hair cycling, **tissue regeneration**, and wound healing; follicular melanocytes can migrate to interfollicular areas in disease states (e.g., vitiligo) to assist with repigmentation
  - ◆ As with interfollicular stem cells in the basal layer of skin, also produce transient amplifying cells with restricted mitotic capacity
- o **Disulfide bonding** via cysteine residues determines **curliness of hair:** these bonds are broken when hair is straightened, but subsequently reform with time
- ▪ Nail
  - o Appendageal structure important for protection and function of fingertips, for proper function of the feet, ability to scratch, and esthetic appearance
  - o Plate is composed of keratin-producing onychocytes
  - o Important anatomic structures: Table 1.7
  - o Growth rate
    - ◆ Fingernails: **2 to 3 mm/month** (~6 months to grow out)
    - ◆ Toenails: **1 mm/month** (~12 months to grow out)

1.2 EMBRYOLOGY

- See Table 1.8 for summary
- Skin structures derived from two of three primary germ layers
  - ▪ Ectoderm: epidermis, adnexal structures, Merkel cells, melanocytes (neural crest), and nerves (neuroectoderm)
  - ▪ Mesoderm: fibroblasts, LCs, vessels, and inflammatory cells
- Skin stem cell biology
  - ▪ Epidermal stem cells responsible for maintenance, repair, and renewal of epidermis
  - ▪ Keratinocyte stem cells located within the **bulge region** of the hair follicle and at the **base of rete ridges** of interfollicular epidermis
  - ▪ Complete renewal of epidermis every 40 to 56 weeks
  - ▪ Stem cells are multipotent with unlimited capacity to divide
  - ▪ Asymmetric division gives rise to transient amplifying cells, which divide rapidly to produce terminally differentiated cells

1.3 WOUND HEALING

- Three phases: inflammatory, proliferative, and remodeling (Fig. 1.7)
  - ▪ Inflammatory phase (starts within the first 6–8 hours, and can last 3–4 days):
    - o Clot formation and coagulation are initial steps
      - ◆ **Platelets come to the site of wound first** → release various factors (ADP, clotting factors, PDGF, EGF, fibrinogen, fibronectin, TGF-α, and TGF-β), some of which are chemotactic for platelets, fibroblasts, and immune cells; interact with fibrin
      - ◆ **Fibrin** (first ECM component deposited) and **fibronectin** (helps provide a matrix for fibroblasts to rebuild) are essential to the process of clotting and coagulation (see Fig. 1.4C)
        - ➔ Important to remember that the clot must be cleared (by plasminogen/plasmin and metalloproteinases) for appropriate scar healing

Table 1.7 Nail Anatomy

Nail Location	Description
Proximal nail fold	Superficial layer continuous with skin, deep layer continuous with nail matrix
Eponychium (cuticle)	Located between nail plate and nail matrix; acts as seal against the environment
Nail matrix	At the proximal end of nail unit, generates the plate. **Proximal matrix→ superficial portion of nail plate; distal matrix → ventral portion of plate.** Melanocytes found in nail matrix
Lunula (distal nail matrix)	Junction between matrix and bed
Nail plate	Hard, functional unit of nail, composed primarily of keratins; strong attachment to nail bed
Nail bed	Extends from lunula to onychodermal band. Provides support for nail plate. **Very minimal contribution to nail plate synthesis**
Onychodermal band	Red/pink transverse band marking end of bed
Hyponychium	Continuous with ventral edge of free nail plate and distal fingertip skin
Lateral nail folds	Guide growth of nail plate

Table 1.8 Major Cutaneous Embryologic Events

	Epidermis	Basement Membrane, Dermis, Subcutis	Appendages
*During the **first trimester**, the foundation is laid with migration of future epidermal residents into epidermis, subdivision of dermis from epidermis, basic subdivisions of the epidermis, and anlagon (=rudimentary form) of appendages are demarcated in the embryo.*			
5 weeks	Periderm and inner basal epidermal layer form		
8 weeks	Rudimentary epidermal stratification	Fibroblasts begin to appear at 6–8 weeks	
9–12 weeks	Cells from neuroectoderm/neural crest and bone marrow migrate to epidermis **(Melanocytes, Langerhans cells, Merkel cells)** **Melanocyte migration guided by KIT/KIT ligand**	9 weeks: Distinct border between dermis and epidermis (dermoepidermal junction present) Primordial vasculature formed	Primordial follicles of scalp, eyebrows, upper lip and chin–spreads caudally and ventrally; epidermal placodes (derived from ectoderm) induce underlying dermal papilla formation (derived from mesoderm) Nail beds demarcated (8–10 weeks) Eccrine gland anlage form on palms and soles (10 weeks)
*In the transition from first to **second trimester**, cells and appendages begin to **function** rudimentarily.*			
12–18 weeks	Melanin production begins.	16 weeks: initial fat formation in subcutis 20 weeks: mature thickness of dermis and dermal ridges present	Proximal nail folds form (12 weeks), nail plate formed (17 weeks) Eccrine primordia bud down, glands begin to develop (14–16 weeks)
*The **end of the second trimester** reveals a fully-stratified epidermis, fully functional melanocytes, cycling hairs, fully grown nail plates, and functioning eccrine glands on volar surfaces.*			
18–24 weeks	Melanocytes proliferate and become fully functional/able to transfer melanosomes to keratinocytes (16–20 weeks)		Hair canal fully formed Nail plate covers nail bed (by week 20) 22 weeks: apocrine glands form and eccrine glands on trunk form Eccrine glands and ducts of volar skin are mature and functioning Sebaceous gland formation parallels hair follicle development (derived from outer root sheath)
24–28 weeks	Keratinocytes terminally differentiate and epidermis fully stratifies.		Hair cycling (anagen, catagen, telogen) initiates; **sonic hedgehog** is an important molecule for telogen to anagen transition.

- Vasodilation caused by histamine, prostaglandins, complement, and kinins
- **Influx of neutrophils in first 48 hours** (fibrinogen/fibrin products, C5a, and other cytokines chemoattract neutrophils)
  - Involved in clearance of bacteria and debridement
- **Macrophages** arrive next → they are the cell type that is **ABSOLUTELY REQUIRED** for wound healing!!!
  - Phagocytose/debride tissue/organisms and set the stage for the proliferative stage (via secretion of growth factors → ↑ fibroblasts and ECM development)

- Proliferative phase (starts around day 5–7 and may last up to 1 month):
  - Initiated by fibrinogenic growth factors (PDGF, TGF-α/β, FGF, and others) released by macrophages
    - Fibrinogenic growth factors drive fibroblasts to proliferate and to produce ECM components
    - As the wound matures, these fibrinogenic growth factor levels return to baseline. In pathologic conditions such as **hypertrophic scars and keloids**, persistent up-regulation and activation of **TGF-β signaling** is observed.
  - Re-epithelialization begins within 24 hours, and is mediated by EGF, KGF, IGF-1, and other growth factors released by fibroblasts, platelets, and keratinocytes
    - **Keratinocytes** from sites adjacent to the wound **leapfrog** over each other (lateral mobilization 2° to breakdown of desmosomes) → Re-epithelialization
      - ➔ Collagenase produced by monocytes also helps with keratinocyte migration
  - Formation of granulation tissue (macrophages, fibroblasts, and vessels) at 3 to 5 days, and deposition of ECM scaffolding for repair (see Fig. 1.4D)
    - **Fibronectin needed for granulation tissue formation → replaced by collagen III and ultimately collagen I**
  - Fibroplasia at 3 to 14 days—deposition of collagen and other ECM components by fibroblasts (migrate about 2 days after wound creation; rely on fibronectin framework for migration/travel)
    - **Wound contraction mediated by myofibroblasts (maximal at 1–2 weeks**; these cells contain actin microfilaments)
  - Neovascularization/angiogenesis—mediated by VEGF, TGF-β, angiogenin, and other molecules
    - Starts in first week of wound healing
- Remodeling (starts at 3–4 weeks and can take 1 year):
  - Scar matrix formation (via fibroblast production of collagen/fibronectin/hyaluronic acid), and

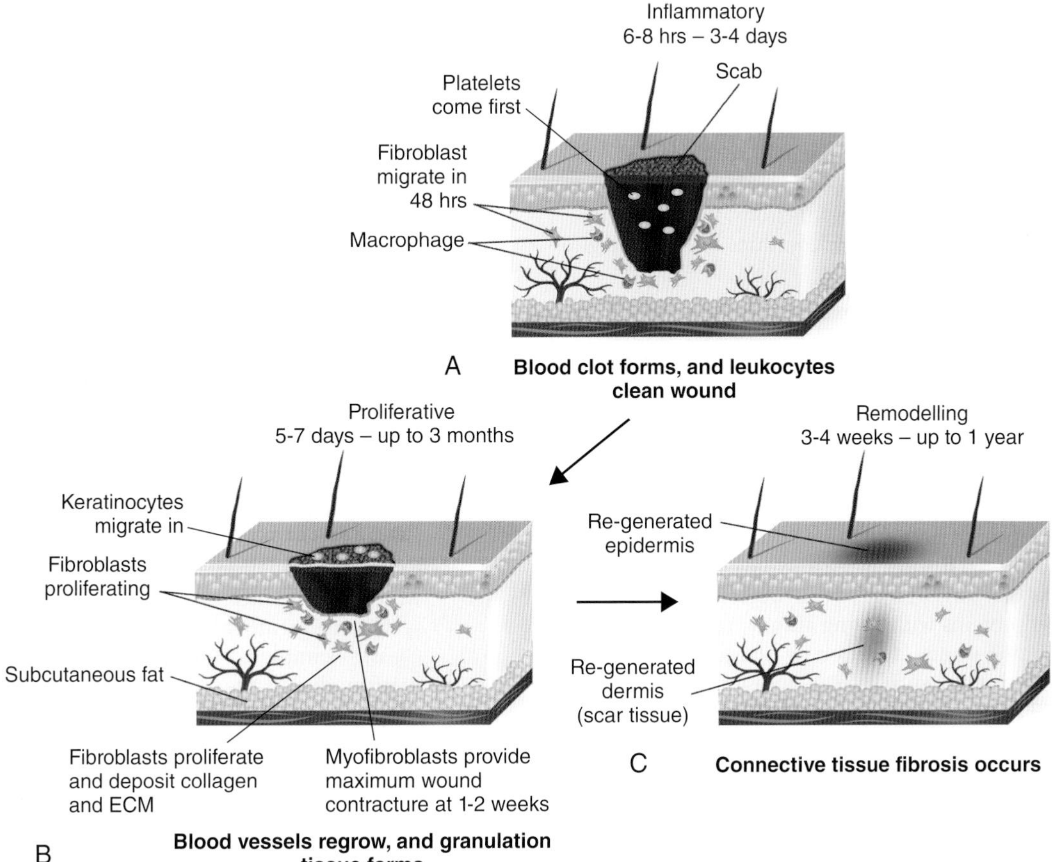

Fig. 1.7 Three phases of cutaneous wound healing. (A) Inflammatory phase: platelets help form clot, neutrophils and macrophages clean the wound; macrophages secrete growth factors to stimulate fibroblasts. (B) Proliferation phase: granulation tissue forms, Re-epithelialization begins, wound contracts. (C) Remodeling: scar matrix formation. *ECM,* Extracellular matrix. (Modified from Ramazan E. Advances in fabric structures for wound care. In: Rajendran S. *Advanced Textiles for Wound Care*, 2nd ed. Philadelphia: Elsevier; 2019.)

regression of granulation tissue (endothelial cells are first to undergo apoptosis and macrophages are last); collagen remodeling

- Scar strength (High-yield!)
  - 1 week: up to 5%
  - 3 weeks: 20%
  - 3 months: 50%
  - 1 year: 80%

1.4 GENETICS

Basic cell biology of genome

- DNA (deoxyribonucleic acid): molecule composed of nucleic acids, encoding heritable information. Composed of a sense and antisense strand.
  - Intron: non-coding nucleotide sequence on DNA (and its corresponding RNA) that is not translated and is typically removed prior to translation via splicing. Introns of varying size and number are found intervening between exons of a gene (Introns intervene).
  - Exon: coding nucleotide sequence on DNA (and its corresponding RNA) that will be translated into final peptide (Exons are expressed).
- RNA (ribonucleic acid): molecule composed of nucleic acids, regulating protein synthesis. Many types of RNAs, some are noted below:
  - RNAs involved in protein synthesis
    - Messenger RNA (mRNA): acts as template for translation of genetic code into protein. RNA polymerase transcribes DNA at a locus into a single-stranded mRNA
    - Transfer RNA (tRNA): facilitates translation by acting as an adaptor molecule to bring correct amino acid to matching nucleotide triplet (codon) on the mRNA
    - Ribosomal RNA (rRNA): acts as a ribozyme within ribosomes to catalyze the peptide bond between amino acids
  - Regulatory RNAs
    - Short interfering RNA (siRNA)—short, double-stranded RNA (21–23 nucleotides long) that acts to downregulate gene expression via the RNA interference (RNAi) pathway in a process known as "gene silencing." In this pathway, siRNAs, along with the RNA-induced silencing complex (RISC), target specific complementary mRNAs for degradation
    - MicroRNA (miRNA) – similar to siRNAs, miRNAs are short RNA sequences (19-25 nucleotides) that downregulate gene expression via RISC. The major

differences are that that miRNA binds imperfectly to targets (thus is less specific than siRNA in its targets) and that miRNA inhibits mRNA translation.
  - RNA Aptamer- single-stranded RNA that folds into complex 3-dimensional structure that is able to bind to target protein with strong affinity
- RNA therapies
  With the wide range of RNA functions, the therapeutic potential of RNAs is wide. Below, three broad strategies are briefly described.
  - Encoding proteins – **mRNAs** are used therapeutically to instruct host cells to produce proteins of interest. This strategy is being explored/utilized to produce protein replacement therapy, to produce cancer vaccines, and to produce infectious disease vaccines such as the **Moderna and Pfizer Covid-19 vaccines.**
  - Regulating nucleic acids – siRNAs or miRNAs are used to direct the cells RNAi pathway to prevent translation of harmful mRNA, as may be seen in depositional disorders (eg amyoid).
  - RNAs that target proteins – RNA Aptamers bind to target proteins with strong affinity, typically inhibiting protein function by occluding key sites on the protein, such as seen with inhibition of VEGF in macular degeneration **(Pegaptinib)**.

Inheritance patterns

- Genetic basis of diseases can be straightforward, a single-gene defect (epidermolysis bullosa), polygenic, or only partially genetic (diabetes and psoriasis). Examination of family tree and its affected individuals can help predict the risk of future offspring to be affected.
- Mendelian inheritance is based upon straightforward, single-gene inheritance that follows the laws of segregation and independent assortment (Table 1.9)
- Modifying factors and non-Mendelian inheritance
  - Incomplete or reduced penetrance: not all individuals with disease genotype will manifest the disease. Penetrance is an all-or-nothing phenomenon (complete or incomplete). Incomplete penetrance leads to the phenomenon whereby the disease is observed to "skip a generation." The degree of penetrance refers to the probability of an individual with the disease genotype to manifest the disease (in contrast to variable expression)
    - Penetrance can be age-related. Examples include androgenetic alopecia (increased degree of penetrance later in life), and Hailey-Hailey disease and Darier's disease (complete penetrance after a certain age)
  - Variable expression: variation in severity of the symptoms of disease that manifest
    - Darier's disease and NF1 have variable expression (broad range of severity)
    - Genetic anticipation: a type of variable expression in which severity increases and age of onset of symptoms is earlier with each successive generation. Classic example is Huntington's disease.
  - Mosaicism: due to alteration of DNA during embryonic development (post-zygotic mutation)
    - In skin, mosaic expression follows lines of Blaschko
    - If mutation affects gametes (germline mosaicism), then mutation may be inherited by offspring. Example: Mosaic KRT1 or KRT10 mutation → nevi with epidermolytic hyperkeratosis. If offspring inherits this mutation, offspring may manifest full expression of KRT1 or KRT10 mutation → epidermolytic ichthyosis.
  - Loss of heterozygosity: occurs when presence of single WT allele maintains normal function of gene, and subsequently a single mutation ("single hit") on the

Table 1.9 Mendelian Patterns of Inheritance

Pattern	Parents Affected	Gender Affected	Transmission	Recurrence Risk	Risk Factors
Autosomal recessive	No (carriers), unless parent carries two mutated copies (affected)	Both equally	Disease seen in siblings of proband, not in parents or offspring Usually only in one generation	1 in 4	Consanguinity, isolated population (e.g., geographically, linguistically)
Autosomal dominant	Yes[a]	Both equally	Disease seen in successive generations	1 in 2	*De novo* mutations
X-linked recessive	Mother a "carrier"[a]	Males have the "complete" disease Female "carriers" may have mild manifestations (e.g., in a mosaic pattern)[b]	No male-to-male transmission (but all daughters of an affected male are "carriers")	1 in 2 male children born to a female "carrier" will be affected (and 1 in 2 of her female children will be carriers)	*De novo* mutations
X-linked dominant	Yes[a]	Predominantly females if lethal in males during embryonic development; otherwise milder in females (often with a mosaic pattern of skin lesions) and more severe in males	Affected males have: (1) no affected sons; and (2) all daughters affected No male-to-male transmission	1 in 2 children born to affected female; may spontaneously abort male fetuses if "male-lethal" condition	*De novo* mutations

[a]*Unless the proband has a* de novo *mutation and is therefore the first generation affected.*
[b]*Does not represent a "pure" X-linked recessive disorder if there are manifestations in female "carriers."*
From DeStefano GM, Christiano AM. Basic principles of genetics. In: Bolognia JL, Schaffer JV, Cerroni L, eds. Dermatology. *4th ed. Philadelphia: Elsevier; 2018:844–858.*

WT allele causes a complete loss of function gene. Important in context of certain tumor suppressor genes (TSGs), where individuals heterozygous for the TSG are more susceptible to forming tumors. Examples: Gorlin syndrome, hereditary leiomyomatosis.
- Mitochondrial inheritance: both males and females may be affected, but only passed to offspring via maternal lineage.

1.5 ULTRAVIOLET LIGHT

Ultraviolet light (Fig. 1.8)

- Ultraviolet light (UV) is made up of:
  - Vacuum UVC (10–200 nm)
  - UVC (200–280 nm)
  - UVB (280–320 nm)
  - UVA (320–400 nm) → divided into UVAII (320–340 nm) and UVAI (340–400 nm)
- Solar radiation is made up of approximately 50% visible light, 40% infrared, and 9% UVR
  - **UVA is present consistently from sunrise to sunset, whereas UVB peaks midday**
  - UVB is 1000 times more erythemogenic than UVA
    - **UVB signature mutation = C → T** at pyrimidine dimer sites (also may see CC → TT)
    - UVA contributes to mutations via reactive oxygen species (ROS)
  - Whereas UVA > UVB contributes to immediate pigment darkening (redistribution of existing melanin), primarily UVB leads to erythema, burning, delayed melanogenesis (i.e., tanning) and thickening of the stratum corneum
  - Depth of UV penetration varies by wavelength; **UVA (longer wavelength) penetrates deeper** into dermis than UVB (shorter wavelength) (Fig. 1.9)
- Light has properties of both waves and photons
- For light to have a cutaneous effect, it must be absorbed by a chromophore of the epidermis (nucleic acid, protein, urocanic acid, and melanin) or dermis (hemoglobin and porphyrins)
- **Absorption spectrum**: the portion of the electromagnetic (EM) spectrum that is absorbed by a particular molecule or chromophore

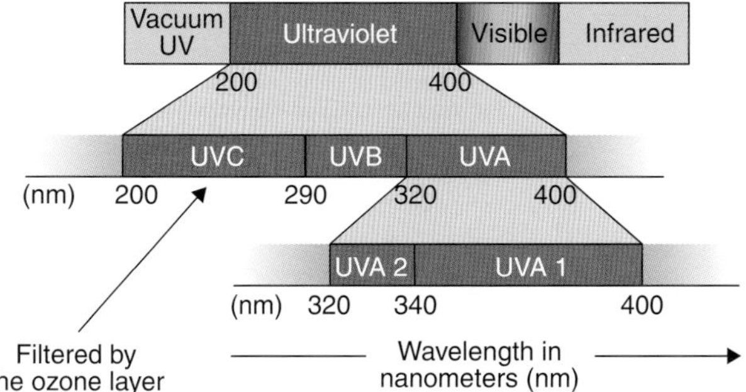

Fig. 1.8 Electromagnetic spectrum. *UV,* Ultraviolet. (From Hönigsmann H. Skin diseases in Europe. Photodermatology. *Eur J Dermatol*. 2009;19(6):658–662.)

- **Action spectrum**: the portion of the EM spectrum that produces a particular effect
- **Vitamin D**: UVB converts **provitamin** D3 (7-dehydrocholesterol) to **previtamin** D3
  - Previtamin D3 is isomerized in the peripheral circulation to vitamin D3
  - **Vitamin D3 is converted to 25 hydroxyvitamin D3 in the liver** (this is what we measure to assess vitamin D stores)
  - 25(OH) D3 is converted **to its active form 1,25-hydroxyvitamin D3 in the kidneys**
  - 90% of vitamin D produced in this manner, 10% from dietary intake

Minimal erythema dose

- Minimal erythema dose (MED) is the minimal amount of a particular UVR that leads to erythema of the exposed skin 16 to 24 hours after exposure
- MEDs are important to determine the appropriate starting dose of phototherapy
- Sun protection factor (SPF) measures the degree of protection an agent confers against UV-induced erythema

Important definitions

- Irradiance/power (watts) is the intensity of UVR to which a patient is exposed
- Exposure time (seconds) is the length of time a patient undergoes UVR treatment
- The dose (J/cm^2) is the amount of light energy a patient is exposed to
  - These three values are important for the formula: **dose (J/cm^2) = irradiance ($J/s.cm^2$) × exposure time (s)**

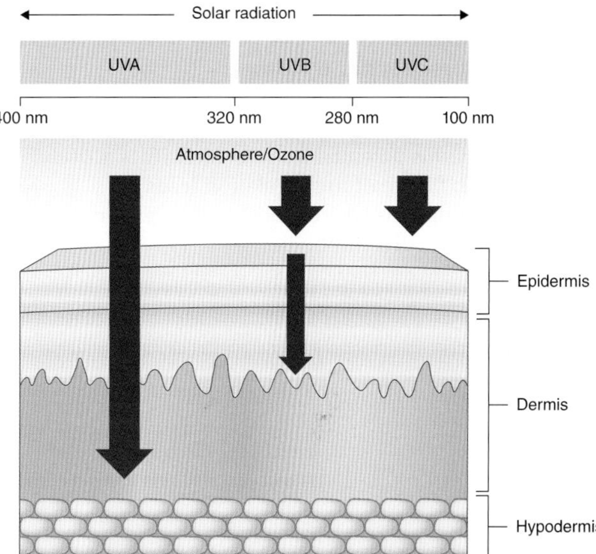

Fig. 1.9 Ultraviolet (UV) penetration into the layers of the skin. (From Pérez-Sánchez A, Barrajón-Catalán E, Herranz-López M, Micol V. Nutraceuticals for skin care: a comprehensive review of human clinical studies. *Nutrients*. 2018;10(4):403. This figure was created using Servier Medical Art [https://smart.servier.com/], licensed under the Creative Commons Attribution 3.0 Unported License [www.creativecommons.org/licenses/by/3.0/].)

1.6 IMMUNOLOGY

1.6.1 Innate versus adaptive immunity (Table 1.10)

Innate immunity

- Provides initial defense against epithelial breach and infectious threats, but with **no memory response**; recognizes **foreign antigens only** (does not recognize self-antigens)
  - Responses may be heightened by repeat microbial encounters (trained immunity), but does **not** possess capacity for true immunologic antigen-specific memory
- Relies on pattern recognition receptors, such as **toll-like receptors (TLRs)** and **NOD-like receptors (NLRs)**, that are expressed by many cell types and recognize conserved structures among microorganisms, that is, pathogen-associated molecular patterns (PAMPS) or damage-associated molecular patterns (DAMPS)
- Central cellular players: phagocytes, DCs, natural killer (NK) cells, mast cells, eosinophils, basophils, and innate lymphoid cells (ILCs)
- Key acellular components include the complement system and antimicrobial peptides (Cathelicidins, defensins, etc)

Adaptive immunity

- Lag phase before activation, maturation and proliferation of lymphocytes (B and T cells) in response to specific antigens
- Key lymphocyte subsets include $CD4^+$ T cells, $CD8^+$ T cells, gamma-delta T cells, NK T cells and B cells
- Primary response to a new antigen leads to gene rearrangement of T-cell and B-cell receptors which optimize the ability to bind and recognize that antigen upon future exposure
- Secondary response is quicker and larger due to presence of these "memory" lymphocyte populations that facilitate a robust antigen-specific response
- The T-cell and B-cell receptors **have the potential to recognize both foreign and self-antigens**
  - Normally this potential for self-reactivity is actively regulated; failure of this regulation leads to autoimmune disease (often defined by presence of many self-reactive antibodies)

1.6.2 Immunologic Mediators

Cytokines

- Cytokines bind to cellular receptors → activate or inhibit downstream signaling pathways → modulate proliferation, function, and/or differentiation of target cells (Table 1.11)
- Signaling downstream of several cytokine receptors (e.g., IFNα, IFNγ, IL-4, IL-6, IL-22, IL-12/23, IL-31) relies on the **JAK-STAT signaling pathway**. Genetic associations with STAT pathway mutations have been reported in **atopic dermatitis, psoriasis, and lupus**. Thus, JAK-inhibitors such as **tofacitinib and ruxolitinib** have therapeutic potential in treatment of various inflammatory skin diseases
  - Write: Tyrosine kinase 2 (TYK2) pairs with JAK1 or JAK2 to mediate cytokine pathways; deucravacitinib is an oral TYK2 inhibitor used for psoriasis
- A specific subset of cytokines called chemokines mediate recruitment/migration of immune cells in tissues. These will be further discussed later in this chapter

Pattern recognition receptors

- <u>Toll-Like Receptors (TLRs; Table 1.12):</u> recognize conserved molecules expressed by microbes (PAMPs) or damaged cells (DAMPs)
  - TLRs are expressed by immune cells as well as keratinocytes; APCs express the greatest number and widest variety
  - Some TLRs are expressed on the cell surface and others intracellularly in endosomes
  - Binding of TLRs by their ligand results in increased expression of type-1 interferons (to promote antiviral defense) and **activation of NFκB** which stimulates the adaptive immune response via expression of cytokines, chemokines, endothelial adhesion molecules, and co-stimulatory molecules
  - All TLRs except TLR3 use the **Myd88 signaling pathway** following activation; TLR3 signals through the adaptor protein TRIF; TLR4 can signal through either pathway
  - IRF5 functions downstream of Myd88 to promote type 1 interferon production in response to endosomal

Table 1.10 Features of Innate and Adaptive Immunity

	Innate	Adaptive
Characteristics		
Specificity	For molecules shared by groups of related microbes and molecules produced by damaged cells	For microbial and non-microbial antigens
Diversity	Limited; recognition molecules encoded by inherited (germline) genes	Very large; receptor genes are formed by somatic recombination of gene segments in lymphocytes
Memory	None or limited	Yes
Nonreactivity to self	Yes	Yes
Components		
Cellular and chemical barriers	Skin, mucosal epithelia; antimicrobial peptides	Lymphocytes in epithelia; antibodies secreted at epithelial surfaces
Blood proteins	Complement, various lectins and agglutins	Antibodies
Cells	Phagocytes (macrophages, neutrophils), dendritic cells, natural killer cells, mast cells, innates lymphoid cells	Lymphocytes

Table 1.11 Major Cytokines

Cytokine	Immune System Source	Principal Effects
IL-1α, IL-1β	Macrophages, keratinocytes	Increased production of acute phase proteins, **fever**, lymphocyte activation (Th17 differentiation), macrophage activation, ↑ leukocyte/endothelial adhesion; levels increased in autoinflammatory diseases such as DIRA; signaling inhibited by IL-1 receptor antagonist, of which **anakinra** is a modified form
IL-2	T cells	Proliferation of T, B, and NK cells; **T-cell differentiation** into memory and effector cells; at high doses, promotes NK and effector T cells (rationale for use as melanoma adjuvant therapy); at low doses promotes Treg function
IL-4	CD4+ T cells (Th2, Tfh), mast cells	**Isotype switching to IgE** upon stimulation of B cells; ↑ **Th2 proliferation** and differentiation, alterative activation of macrophages; SNPs in IL-4, IL-5, IL-13, and IL-31 (among others) **associated with atopic dermatitis**; **dupilumab blocks IL4Rα (shared receptor with IL-13)**
IL-5	CD4+ T cells (Th2), group 2 ILCs	**Eosinophil activator**, B-cell activation, ↑ IgA secretion
IL-6	T cells, macrophages, endothelial cells	Stimulates acute phase protein synthesis, B-cell antibody production and Th17 differentiation
IL-8	Monocytes, T cells, keratinocytes	Chemokine → neutrophil chemotaxis
IL-10	Tregs, macrophages	**Inhibition** of macrophages/dendritic cells; ↓ **expression of IL-12/Th1 response**, co-stimulatory molecules, and class II MHC
IL-12	Macrophages, dendritic cells	Facilitates **Th1 differentiation**; ↑ IFN-γ production and enhanced cytotoxic activity of NK cells; composed of **p40** and **p35** subunits (Note: IL-23 also has p40 subunit, but it is paired with p19; **ustekinumab** targets shared p40 subunit, while tildrakizumab-asmn specifically targets IL-23 via p19)
IL-13	Th2 cells, group 2 ILCs, mast cells, NKT cells	B cells isotype switching to IgE; alternate activation of macrophages: SNPs in IL4Rα, IL5Rα, and IL13Rα confer AD risk
IL-15	Macrophages	NK-cell differentiation; survival of **memory CD8+ T cells**
IL-17A/ IL-17F	Th17 cells, group 3 ILCs	Increased cytokine and chemokine production by keratinocytes and macrophages → key role in **psoriasis** pathogenesis and anti-fungal defense; secukinumab and ixekizumab are monoclonal antibodies to IL-17A
IL-18	Monocytes, macrophages, dendritic cells, keratinocytes, fibroblasts	Promotes IFN-γ production by T cells and NK cells, neutrophil activation, and monocyte production of GM-CSF, TNF and IL-1β
IL-22	CD4+ cells (may co-produce IL-17)	Promotes **keratinocyte proliferation** and hyperplasia, promotes AMP production
IL-23	Dendritic cells, macrophages	Promotes **Th17 proliferation and differentiation** → key role in **psoriasis**; composed of **p40** and **p19** subunits (Note: IL-12 also has p40 subunit, but it is paired with p35; **ustekinumab** targets shared p40 subunit, while **tildrakizumab-asmn** specifically targets IL-23 via p19) SNPs in IL23R, IL-23A and IL-12B (shared subunit of IL-12/IL-23) associated with psoriasis
IL-31	T cells (especially Th2), innate cells, keratinocytes	Key role in pruritus; receptor IL-31RA signals through JAK/STAT pathway
IL-36	Keratinocytes	Activates keratinocytes and dendritic cells; promotes Th1/Th17; **increased in pustular psoriasis (spesolimab in an IL-36 receptor antibody used in pustular psoriasis) and psoriatic arthritis**
TGFβ	T cells (especially Tregs), macrophages	Promotes fibroblast collagen synthesis, inhibits T- and B- cell proliferation and effector functions, inhibits macrophage activation
TNF-α	**Macrophages**, mast cells, NK cells, T cells, and others	Activation of macrophages and T and B lymphocytes, ↑ **proinflammatory cytokine production**, leukocyte/endothelial cell adhesion, cachexia, pyrexia, induction of acute phase proteins, ↑ MHC class I production
IFN-α/β	Plasmacytoid dendritic cells (both), macrophages (α), fibroblasts (β)	Activation of antiviral/antitumor state (antiproliferative), ↑ MHC class I expression, NK-cell activation
IFN-γ	T cells (Th1, CD8), NK cells	MHC class I and II induction on various cell types, **macrophage activation** and cytokine synthesis, **Th1 differentiation**
GM-CSF	T cells, macrophages	Maturation of granulocytes and monocytes, activation of macrophages
TSLP	**Keratinocytes**, mast cells, some myeloid cells	**Th2 differentiation,** activation of dendritic cells, eosinophils and mast cells SNPs associated with atopic dermatitis

DIRA, *Deficiency of interleukin-1 receptor antagonist;* GM-CSF, *granulocyte colony-stimulating factor;* IFN, *interferon;* IL, *interleukin;* ILCs, *innate lymphoid cells;* MHC, *major histocompatibility complex;* NK cells, *natural killer cells;* SNP, *single nucleotide polymorphisms;* TGF, *transforming growth factor;* TNF, *tumor necrosis factor;* TSLP, *thymic stromal lymphopoietin.*
Modified from Abbas AK, Lichtman AH, Pillai S. Cellular and Molecular Immunology. *9th ed. Philadelphia: Elsevier; 2018.*

TLRs; **activating SNPs in IRF5 are a/w systemic lupus erythematosus (SLE)**

- <u>NOD-like receptors (NLRs)</u>: a family of more than 20 cytosolic proteins, many of which recognize PAMPs/DAMPs; well-known NLRs include NOD1 (SNP mutations increase psoriasis risk) and **NOD2 (mutated in Blau syndrome)**, both of which lead to NFκB activation, and **NLRP3** (aka **cryopyrin/CIAS**; mutated in **cryopyrin-associated periodic syndrome**); mutations in **NLRP1 (a/w vitiligo)**
- Note that mutations which **augment NFκB** and related signaling are a/w **psoriasis** (i.e., REL, TNIP1, TNFAIP3, NFKBIA, CARD14, TRAF31P3), whereas those which **diminish NFκB signaling, (i.e., hypomorphic alleles of CARD11)** are a/w **atopic dermatitis**

Table 1.12 Toll-Like Receptors

Receptor	Ligand/Key Facts
TLR1	Bacterial lipopeptides (especially gram-negative and mycobacterial)
TLR2	Bacterial lipopeptides, lipoteichoic acid on gram-positive bacteria; peptidoglycan (activated by ***Propionibacterium acnes***); can dimerize with TLR1 and TLR6.
TLR3[a]	Viral dsRNA
TLR4	Bacterial **lipopolysaccharide (LPS)**
TLR5	Bacterial flagellin
TLR6	Bacterial lipopeptides
TLR7[a]	Viral ssRNA/synthetic ligand **imiquimod activates IFN-γ production**
TLR8[a]	Viral ssRNA
TLR9[a]	Unmethylated CpG DNA (bacterial)

[a]*Denotes endosomal localization.*
Modified from Male D, Peebles RS Jr, Male V. Mechanisms of innate immunity. In: Immunology. *9th ed. Philadelphia: Elsevier; 2021:46–53.*

Antimicrobial proteins (AMPs)

- AMPs are produced by keratinocytes, sebocytes, sweat glands, and innate immune cells in skin
- They contribute to host defense via direct killing of microbes (collectively they target both gram-positive and gram-negative bacteria. fungi, viruses, and protozoa)
- **Cathelicidins (LL37) and β-defensins** are the two most abundant families of AMPs in skin (others include S100 proteins and RNAses)
- These small cationic peptides are produced constitutively by keratinocytes
- Their main mechanism of microbial killing is **non-enzymatic membrane disruption**
- LL37 binding of host DNA also activates TLR9, which leads to production of IFNα/β and Th17 activation, thereby further augmenting host defense
- **TLR2 and 1,25-OH vitamin D3** are both important in regulating the production of skin AMPs
- LL37 and β-defensins are expressed at relatively low levels in healthy skin but **significantly upregulated in psoriasis and rosacea; by comparison, upregulation of AMPs is partially suppressed in atopic dermatitis**

The complement system

- Consists of small proteins found freely in blood or on cell membranes, which are usually present in an inactive state as zymogens
- Most complement proteins are synthesized in the liver and also are acute phase reactants
- Upon activation, they acquire protease activity that facilitates cleavage or activation of subsequent protein(s) in the complement cascade, thereby amplifying the response
- Stable activation is only achieved after attachment to microbes, antibodies, or dying cells
- Normal host cells possess proteins that inhibit complement activation
  - Thus, full functioning of the complement system is usually restricted to the cell surface of microbes or sites where antibodies are bound to antigens
- Complement has a number of important functions
  - **Direct lysis** of bacteria
  - **Opsonization** of bacteria (complement binds to an organism and augments phagocytosis)
  - **Chemotaxis of innate immune cells**
  - Clearing of immune complexes (hence, complement deficiency syndromes are a/w increased risk of lupus)
  - Activating immune responses
  - Anaphylaxis
- **Three complement pathways:**
  - **Classical pathway: activated by antibodies** (IgM and IgG, **except IgG4**) bound to antigen
  - **Alternative pathway: activated by microbial cell surface structures** without antibodies
  - **Lectin pathway: activated by mannose-binding lectin** which attaches to carbohydrates on the surface of microbes
- Although they differ in early activation events, all three pathways converge on the central event of **C3 cleavage by C3 convertase** and generation of the biologically active molecule C3b
- Likewise, following cleavage of C5, all three pathways are identical in the final steps which assemble **C5b to C9 into the membrane attack complex (MAC),** which creates transmembrane pore in cell surfaces to facilitate lysis/death (Fig. 1.10)
- Key molecules involved in the three complement pathways as well as those that regulate their activity are listed in Table 1.13.

1.6.3 Cells of significance

B Cells

- B cells are formed from pluripotent progenitor stem cells in the bone marrow
- Located in the lymphoid follicle of lymph node
- Main function is **antibody/immunoglobulin production** and **differentiation into plasma cells** (requires surface immunoglobulin receptors to bind antigen)
- **B-cells isotype switch (can switch from one antibody class to another) if they interact with T-helper cells (IgM to IgG, IGA, or IgE)**; isotype is determined by the heavy chain
- B cells can also present antigen on major histocompatibility complex (MHC) class II to CD4$^+$ T cells (following recognition and binding of the antigen to B-cell receptor and subsequent endocytosis)
- **Initial exposure** to antigen leads to a primary immune response:
  - Has lower antibody production (**typically IgM** with a lower-affinity antibody)
  - Some B cells differentiate into memory B cells or plasma cells
- **Subsequent exposure** leads to a secondary immune response:
  - **Memory B cells** more rapidly develop into plasma cells
  - ↑ **High-affinity antibody** production (IgA, IgE, and IgG)
  - ↑ **Isotype switching** in the presence of T-helper cells, CD40 ligand, and other cytokines

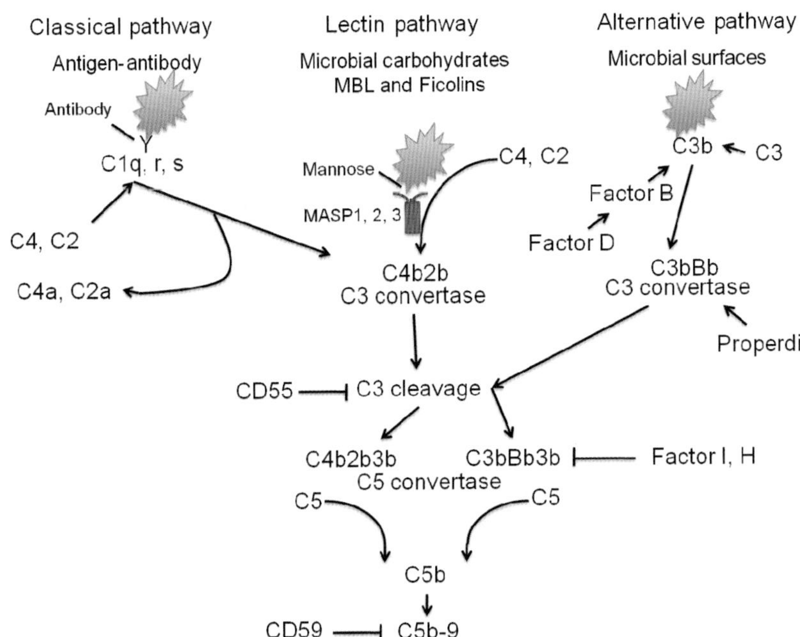

Fig. 1.10 Complement activation pathways. The classical complement cascade is activated by antibody bound to microbial surfaces, which is a binding site for the C1 complex. The alternative pathway is activated by the binding of spontaneously generated C3b to microbial surfaces. Microbial bound C3b binds factor B, which is converted to factor Bb, forming C3 convertase. The lectin pathway is activated by the binding of mannose-binding lectin *(MBL)* to mannose residues on microbial surfaces. MBL binds MBL-associated serine proteases *(MASP)*, which bind and cleave C4 and C2, forming C3 convertase. (From McDonald DR, Levy O. Innate immunity. In: Rich RR, Fleisher TA, Shearer WT, Schroeder HW Jr, Frew AJ, Weyand CM, eds. *Clinical Immunology: Principles and Practice*. 5th ed. Philadelphia: Elsevier; 2019.)

- **B cell markers/receptors**: FC receptor, MHC class II, various complement receptors, **CD19**, **CD20 (target of rituximab)**, CD79a
- BCL2 is an anti-apoptotic molecule which provides a survival advantage for malignant B cells; BCL6 is a transcription factor that generally represses pathways within B cells to help regulate the germinal center response; both are used as immunohistochemical markers of healthy germinal center B cells as well as certain types of B-cell lymphomas
- Antibody structure has two identical heavy and two identical light chains with variable and constant domains that are connected by disulfide bonds. The **variable region (Fab) has a unique/specific antigen-binding domain.** The constant region (Fc) interacts with cell surface Fc receptors on various immune cells (e.g., phagocytes, NK cells, mast cells) → binding of Fc by Fc receptors promotes phagocytosis of Ig-coated particles and cellular activation or degranulation (e.g., FcεRI binding of IgE on mast cells) (Fig. 1.11, Table 1.14). Of note, papain cleaves antibody into two Fab fragments and one Fc fragment

T cells (majority of lymphocytes)

- Derived from the bone marrow, but mature in the **thymus**; reside in paracortex of lymph nodes
- T cells are divided into CD4$^+$ T-helper cells (Th1, Th2, Th17, Tfh, and Treg) and CD8$^+$ cytotoxic T cells; minor populations include γδ T cells and NK T cells (Table 1.15)
- CD4$^+$ T cells recognize **extracellular** antigens presented by a **professional APC** on **MHC class II**
- CD8$^+$ T cells recognize **intracellular** antigens presented by **any nucleated cell** on **MHC class I**
- Activation of naïve T cells requires both recognition of antigen (signal 1) and co-stimulation (signal 2) → this leads to proliferation and differentiation that is further influenced via specific cytokines provided by the APC or other cells
- **Signal 1**: T-cell receptor recognizes its cognate antigen complexed with MHC class I/II molecules on a professional or non-professional APC (see 1.6.4 Major Histocompatibility Complex)
- **Signal 2**: For successful activation of T cells, **co-stimulation via a secondary receptor is required;** in the absence of this, T cells become anergic; signal 2 can alternatively be inhibitory, shutting down activation of the T cell (Fig. 1.12)
  - **CD28** on T cell binds to **CD80 (B7-1)** or **CD86 (B7-2)** on APCs → stimulation
  - **CD2** on T cells binds to **LFA-3** on APCs → stimulation
  - **LFA-1** on T cells binds to **ICAM-1** on APCs → stimulation
  - **CD40L** on T cell binds to CD40 on APCs or phagocytes → stimulation
  - **CTLA-4** on T cell (often a Treg) binds to B7-1 and B7-2 on APCs → inhibition
  - **PD-1** on T cell binds to PDL-1 on APCs (or tumor cells) → inhibition
  - Clinical relevance: blocking these inhibitory pathways is the rationale behind cancer immunotherapies that enable greater T-cell activation and antitumor activity in melanoma and other malignancies, for example, **pembrolizumab** and **nivolumab** block PD-1, **ipilimumab** blocks the CTLA-4 (Fig. 1.13)
- IL-2 is produced after T-cell activation and leads to proliferation of antigen-specific T cells; Tregs can provide a sink for IL-2 via the high-affinity receptor CD25 to limit effector cell activation
- PTPN22 is a tyrosine kinase involved downstream of TCR activation; mutations in PTPN22 are a/w autoimmune skin diseases such as lupus and vitiligo
- Clonal expansion of the responding T cells during the primary response is followed by contraction of this

Table 1.13 Important Players in the Complement System

Name	Pathway	Key Function(s)
C1	Classical	Initiates classical pathway activation
C1q	Classical	Binds to Fc portion of antibody (IgM or IgG [IgG3 > IgG1 > IgG2; IgG4 does NOT activate classical complement pathway]) that has bound antigen; can also bind apoptotic cells and cationic surfaces. Deficiency most strongly associated with lupus
C1r	Classical	Serine protease, cleaves and activates C1s
C1s	Classical	Serine protease, cleaves C4 and C2 → **C3 convertase** (C4b/C2b)
C2	Classical/Lectin	C2b (formerly referred to as C2a) is serine protease that contributes enzymatic activity to C3 and C5 convertases Most common deficiency; association with SLE of early onset with more extensive skin involvement but mild systemic disease course
C3	All	Cleaved by C3 convertase into C3a and C3b **C3a is an anaphylatoxin** stimulating inflammation **C3b is an opsonin.** It binds to pathogens → phagocytosis
C3a	All	**C3a is an anaphylatoxin** stimulating inflammation
C3b	All	**C3b is an opsonin**. It binds to microbial pathogens facilitating **phagocytosis.** It is also a component of **C3 convertase (in alternative pathway, C3 convertase is stabilized by properidin; X-linked deficiency in properidin confers susceptibility to fulminant meningococcal disease)** In all pathways, it is part of C5 convertase
C3 convertase	All	Cleaves C3 into C3a and C3b In classical/lectin pathways: composed of C4b/C2b In alternative pathway: composed of C3b and Bb
C4	Classical/Lectin	C4**b binds to** surface of microbe or cells where antibody is bound or complement is activated C4**b binds** C2 for cleavage by C1s **C4a is an anaphylatoxin** stimulating inflammation Defect in C4A/B both associated with lupus
C5	All	C5b initiates assembly of MAC **C5a is an anaphylatoxin** stimulating inflammation
C5 convertase	All	Assembly of C3b + C4b2b. Cleaves C5 into C5a and C5b.
C5b-C9	All	Components of membrane attack complex (MAC); defects associated with infection by encapsulated organisms (*Neisseria*, pneumococcus)
Mannose-binding lectin (MBL), ficolins	Lectin	Agglutinin, opsonin, complement fixing. MBL activates the lectin pathway: binds to cell surface polysaccharides (via pattern recognition) on microbes → cleavage of C2 and C4.
MASP1-3	Lectin	Homology to C1r/C1s in classical pathway; form complex with lectins, collectins or ficolins; serial activation eventually leads to cleavage of C4
C1 esterase inhibitor (C1 inh)	Regulatory role in classical pathway	Binds to C1r and C1s to dissociate them from C1q; **defects associated with hereditary angioedema**
Factor B	Alternative	Cleaved by factor D, producing Ba and Bb. Bb is the active subunit, a serine protease, that joins C3b to form C3 convertase
Factor D	Alternative	Cleaves factor B
C4-binding protein, factor I, factor H, membrane cofactor protein, decay-accelerating factor	Regulatory role	Limit activity of key molecules above (especially C3b and C4b) by displacement (which disassembles convertase complexes) or cleavage. For example, factor H inhibits formation of C3 convertase.

Data from Abbas AK, Lichtman AH, Pillai S. Effector mechanisms of humoral immunity. In: Cellular and Molecular Immunology. *9th ed. Philadelphia: Elsevier; 2018:275–298.*

population and indefinite persistence of memory T cells; these cells:
- Respond more rapidly to antigen stimulation than naïve cells
- Memory T cells in the skin consist of both recirculating memory T cells (Ccr7$^+$, L-selectin$^{+/-}$) and tissue-resident memory T cells (CCR7^{neg}, L-selectin^{neg}, CD69$^+$, CD103$^{+/-}$)

- Activation of a specific CD4$^+$ helper response often has the effect of suppressing another, that is, Th1 suppresses Th2/Th17, Th17 suppresses Th2 (**mutations in STAT3 lead to hyperactivation of Th2 in Job/Hyper IgE syndrome**)
- CD4$^+$ and CD8$^+$ T cells play a critical role in **cell-mediated immunity**, which provides defense against intracellular threats (invasive bacteria, viruses, cancer), in contrast to humoral immunity, in which antibodies help fight extracellular threats. Both CD4$^+$ Th1 and CD8$^+$ T cells help to activate phagocytes via IFNγ production and CD40L. CD8$^+$ T cells, that is, cytotoxic T lymphocytes, kill infected/cancerous cells.
- Leukocyte extravasation through vascular endothelium:
  - **Selectins** bind carbohydrates to facilitate first step of leukocyte "rolling" (i.e., P and E selectin expressed on the endothelium bind to CLA glycoprotein on immune cells; mutations in GDP fucose transport, needed to

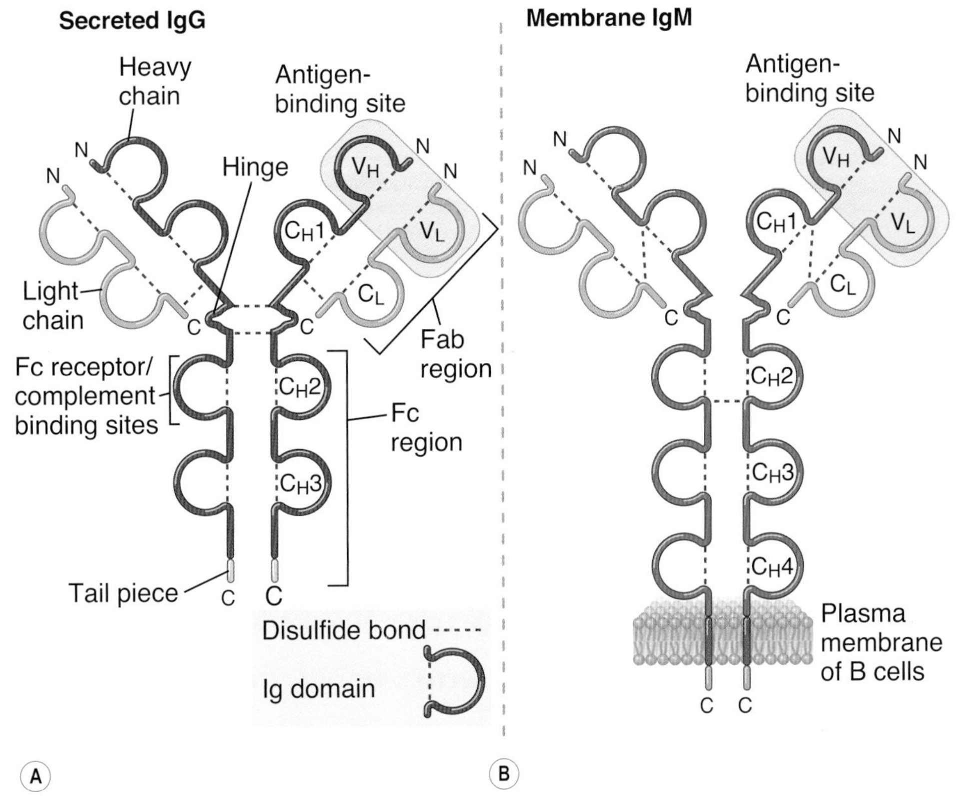

Fig. 1.11 Structure of an antibody molecule. (A) Schematic diagram of a secreted IgG molecule. The **antigen-binding sites are formed by the juxtaposition of V_L and V_H domains.** The heavy chain C regions end in tail pieces. The **locations of complement- and Fc receptor-binding sites within the heavy chain constant regions are approximations.** (B) Schematic diagram of a membrane-bound IgM molecule on the surface of a B lymphocyte. The IgM molecule has one more C-domain than IgG has, and the membrane form of the antibody has C-terminal transmembrane and cytoplasmic portions that anchor the molecule in the plasma membrane. (From Abbas A, Lichtman AH, Pillai S. Antibodies and antigens. In: *Cellular and Molecular Immunology*. 9th ed. Philadelphia: Elsevier; 2018. Courtesy of Dr. Alex McPherson, University of California, Irvine.)

Table 1.14 Classes of Immunoglobulins

Isotype	IgM	IgD	IgG	IgE	IgA
Structure	**Pentamer**	Monomer	Monomer	Monomer	Monomer, dimer
Complement activation	**Strong**	No	**Yes, except IgG4**	No	Weak
Bacterial toxin neutralization	Yes	No	Yes	No	Yes
Antiviral activity	No	No	Yes	No	Yes
Binding to mast cells and basophils	No	No	No	**Yes** (→ release of mediators)	No
Additional properties	**First antibody in primary immune response; Naïve B cell antigen receptor**	B-cell antigen receptor	Antibody-dependent cell cytotoxicity; opsonization for phagocytosis; Feedback inhibition of B cell activation; **Only antibody that crosses the placenta**	**Mast cell degranulation (immediate hypersensitivity), eosinophil-mediated helminthic responses**	Active as dimer on epithelial/**mucosal surfaces**

Modified from Actor JK. Elsevier's Integrated Review: Immunology and Microbiology. *2nd ed. Philadelphia: Elsevier; 2012.*

express ligands for these selectins on neutrophils, lead to **type 2 leukocyte adhesion deficiency**)

- **Integrins** covalently bind various ligands to promote attachment between cells or to ECM; their ligand affinity is increased by chemokines and antigen recognition (**LFA-1** on T cells binds to **ICAM-1** on activated endothelium to promote next step in extravasation; mutations in subunit of LFA lead to **type 1 leukocyte adhesion deficiency**)
- **Chemokines** are a subfamily of cytokines that facilitate leukocyte movement from blood and within tissues (Table 1.16).

Table 1.15 Key T Lymphocyte Subsets

Lymphocyte Type (Defining Transcription Factor, if Applicable)	Key Cytokines and/or Effector Molecules	Principal Target Cells	Major Immune Effect	Microbial Target/ Role in Host Defense	Role in Disease
CD4+ Th1 (Tbet, STAT1, STAT4)	**IFN-γ, and IL-12** stimulate Th1 differentiation; Th1 cells produce IL-2, IFN-γ (downregulates Th2 pathway), IL-12 and TNF-α	Macrophages	Macrophage activation and phagocytosis; IgG2 and IgG3 class switching → complement activation	Intracellular pathogens	**Cell-mediated immunity,** autoimmunity; chronic inflammation (i.e., tuberculoid leprosy, cutaneous leishmaniasis, sarcoidosis, **delayed-type hypersensitivity**; CTCL, psoriasis)
CD4+ Th2 (GATA3, STAT6)	IL4 stimulates Th2 proliferation by activating STAT6 and GATA 3; Th2 cells produce IL-4, IL-5, IL-6, IL-10 (suppresses Th1 response), IL-13	Eosinophils, mast cells	Activation of **eosinophils** via **IL-5** and (indirectly) of mast cells via IgE cross-linking; alternative macrophage activation; IgE and IgG4 class switching in B cells	Helminths	Important in normal **humoral immunity**. Excessive response in allergy (i.e., **atopic dermatitis**, **lepromatous** leprosy, Sézary, disseminated leishmaniasis)
CD4+ Th17 (RORγT/ STAT3)	IL-16, IL-17, IL-22, IL-23, IL-36, TNF-α	**Neutrophils**	Neutrophil recruitment and activation; increase AMPs, barrier function	Extracellular bacteria and fungi	Autoimmunity; inflammation (i.e., **psoriasis**, allergic contact dermatitis)
CD4+ Tfh (Bcl6)	IL-21	B cells	Antibody production	Extracellular pathogens	Autoimmunity (autoantibodies)
CD4+ Treg (FOXP3)	IL-10, **CD25**, CTLA4	Effector lymphocytes and innate immune cells	**Suppress Th1** system via IL-10	Limiting tissue damage by other cell types	Mutations in Foxp3 lead to **autoimmunity (IPEX syndrome);** SNPs related to Treg function associated with **vitiligo and AA**
CD8+ CTL	Granzyme, perforin, Fas ligand, IFN-γ; TNFα	Infected cells, opsonized cells (recognize intracellular antigens presented on MHC class I)	Killing (cytotoxicity) via **perforin** (perforates cell) & **granzyme** (enters cytoplasm) → apoptosis. Can also kill cells via **Fas ligand**, which binds to Fas on target cell.	Intracellular pathogens, cancer	Autoimmunity; inflammation (vitiligo; checkpoint blockade therapy); CD8 lymphomas are highly aggressive
γ/δ T cell	IL-17	Neutrophils	Suppress Th1 system via IL-10	Extracellular bacteria and fungi	Enriched in leprosy and cutaneous leishmaniasis; **lymphomas of γ/δ types are highly aggressive**
NK T cells	IFN-γ, IL-4		Recognize lipid antigens presented by CD1 molecules; provide B cell help	Myocobacteria and other lipid-rich pathogens	May contribute to UV-induced immunosuppresion

IFN, interferon; *IL*, interleukin; *CTCL*, cutaneous T cell lymphoma; *AMPs*, antimicrobial peptides; *SNPs*, single nucleotide polymorphisms; *AA*, alopecia areata; *MHC*, major histocompatibility complex; *TNF*, tumor necrosis factor; *UV*, ultraviolet; *IPEX*, Immune dysregulation, polyendocrinopathy, enteropathy, X-linked
Data from Abbas AK, Lichtman AH, Pillai S. Differentiation and functions of CD4+ effector T cells. In: Cellular and Molecular Immunology. *9th ed. Philadelphia: Elsevier; 2018:225–242.*

- Chemokines implicated in atopic dermatitis: **CCL5/CCL11** (Eos/Th2), **CCL17**, **CCL18**, CCL22, CCL26; in certain settings (e.g., chronic lesions, Asian cohorts) CCL20 (Th17), and CXCL9/10 (Th1)
- Chemokines implicated in psoriasis: CCL17, **CCL20** (Th17), **CXCL1/8** (Neuts), **CXCL9/10** (Th1), CX3CL1 (Th1)
- Chemokines implicated in vitiligo: CCL5, CXCL8, **CXCL9/10** (Th1/CD8)
- Chemokines implicated in alopecia areata: CXCL1 (Neuts), **CXCL9/10** (Th1/CD8)

Innate lymphoid cells

- Bone marrow–derived cells share similar morphology to lymphocytes but **lack T-cell receptors**; thought to function mainly through cytokine secretion
- Three major subsets: ILC1, ILC2, ILC3 (somewhat analogous to Th1, Th2, and Th17 subsets)
  - ILC1: express Tbet transcription factor; secrete IFNγ; contribute to viral defense
  - ILC2: express GATA3 transcription factor; secrete IL-5, IL-13; defend against helminths, contribute to allergic inflammation
  - ILC3: express RORγt transcription factor; secrete IL-17, IL-22; may be increased in psoriasis

NK cells

- Key component of the **innate immune system**
- Like ILCs, they share lymphocyte morphology and originate from a common bone marrow precursor but lack T-cell receptors
- Cell surface markers include CD2, **CD56**, and CD16

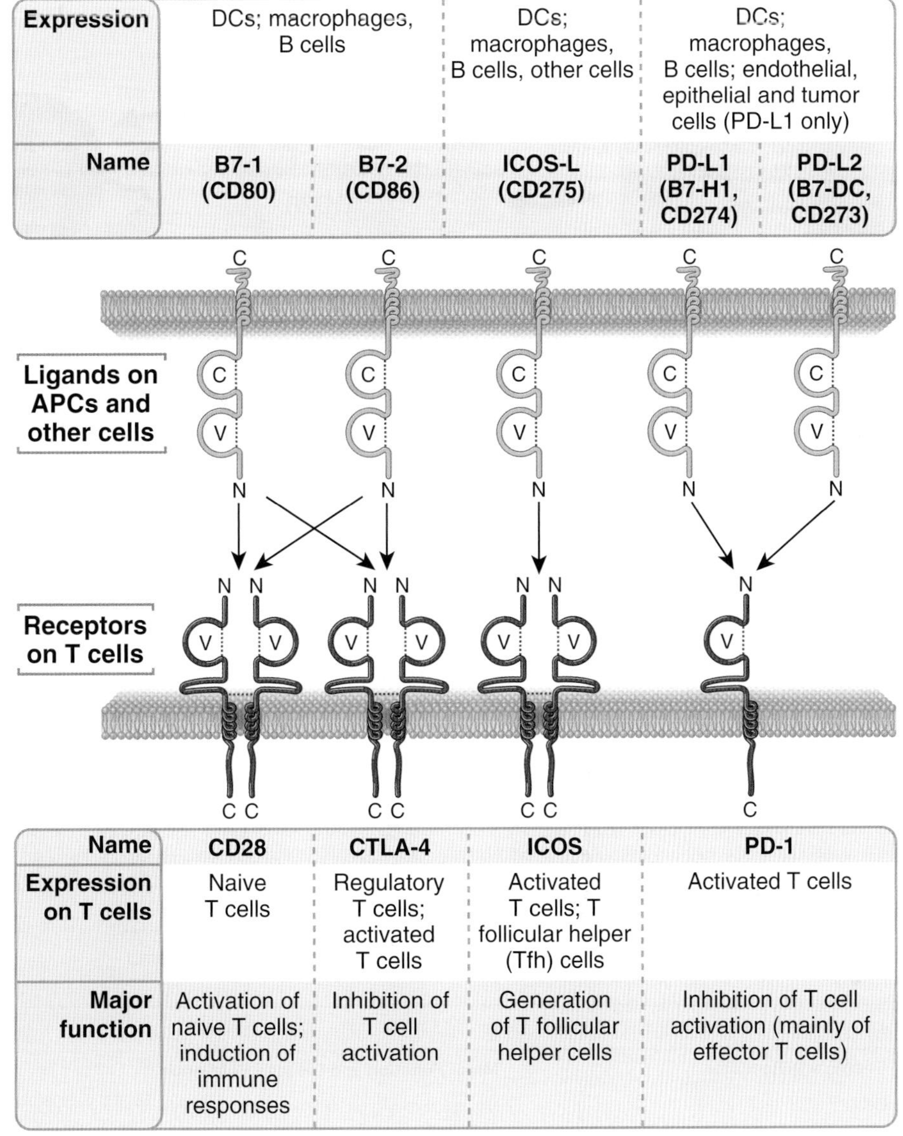

Fig. 1.12 The major members of the B7 and CD28 families. The known B7 family ligands are expressed on antigen presenting cells *(APCs)* (dendritic cells *[DCs]*, macrophages, and B cells), and CD28 family receptors are expressed mainly on T cells. Different CD28 family members stimulate or inhibit different stages and types of T-cell responses. (From Abbas A, Lichtman AH, Pillai S. Activation of T lymphocytes. In: *Cellular and Molecular Immunology*. 9th ed. Philadelphia: Elsevier; 2018.)

- Identify infected (viral) or tumor cells that have decreased MHC I surface expression via a group of surface receptors (CD16, NKp44/46, NKG2D, and others)
- NK cells destroy target cells via **perforin/granzymes** in a manner analogous to CD8$^+$ T cells
- They also work synergistically with macrophages by **secreting IFNγ that enhances macrophage phagocytic capacity**
- NK cells are activated by IL-12, IL-15, and type I interferons
- STAT4 is a key transcription factor involved in response to IL-12 and type 1 interferon in NK and Th1 cells; **SNPs in STAT4 are a/w early-onset lupus with increased risk of stroke and nephritis**

Mononuclear phagocytes

- Monocytes (in bloodstream) differentiate into macrophages (in tissue)
- Tissue-resident macrophages constitute another subset derived from hematopoietic precursors that seed the skin during fetal life
- Derived from a common CD34+ progenitor cell in the bone marrow
- Cell markers: CD11a/b/c, CD6, Fc receptor for IgG, and MHC II (for antigen presentation)
- Primary function is to ingest/destroy microbes, apoptotic cells and debris
- After ingestion of these targets into phagosomes, they fuse with lysosomes to form phagolysosomes, in which reactive oxygen/nitrogen species and proteolytic enzymes contribute to destruction and death
- Other functions include:
  - Cytokine production → modulation of inflammation
  - Tissue remodeling, **wound healing** (absolutely required), and coagulation
  - Antigen presentation

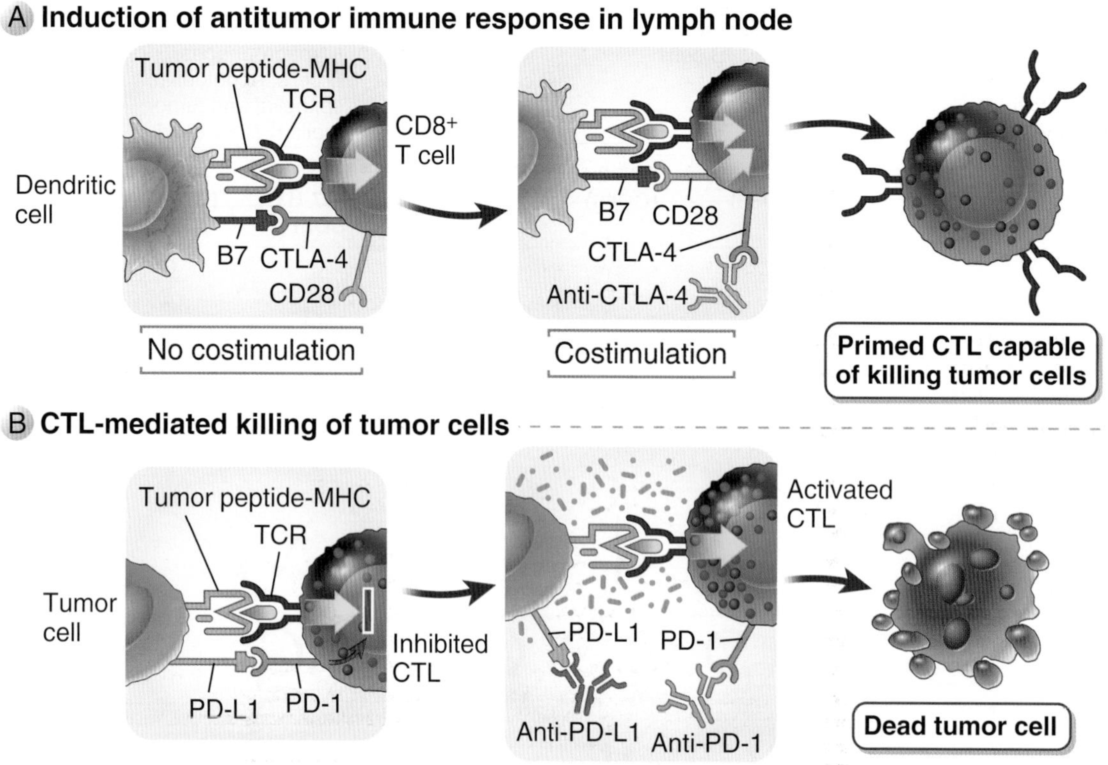

Fig. 1.13 Checkpoint blockade. Tumor patients often mount ineffective T-cell responses to their tumors because of the upregulation of inhibitory receptors such as CTLA-4 and PD-1 on the tumor-specific T cells, and expression of the ligand PD-L1 on the tumor cells. Blocking anti-CTLA4 antibodies (A) or anti-PD-1 or anti-PD-L1 antibodies (B) are highly effective in treating several types of advanced tumors, by releasing the inhibition of tumor-specific T cells by these molecules. Anti-CTLA-4 may work by blocking CTLA-4 on effector T cells (shown) or on Tregs. (From Abbas A, Lichtman AH, Pillai S. Immunity to tumors. In: *Cellular and Molecular Immunology*. 9th ed. Philadelphia: Elsevier; 2018.)

Table 1.16 Dermatologically Relevant Chemokines

Chemokine	Chemokine Receptor	Major Function and Disease Relevance
CCL2	CCR2	Mixed leukocyte recruitment; especially inflammatory monocytes **(involved in wound healing)**
CCL4	CCR5	T cell, dendritic cell, monocyte, and NK recruitment
CCL5 (RANTES)	CCR1, CCR3, CCR5	Mixed leukocyte recruitment, notably **eosinophils;** SNPs associated with **atopic dermatitis**
CCL11 (eotaxin-1)	CCR3 (preferentially expressed on eosinophils)	**Eosinophil**, basophil, and **Th2** recruitment
CCL17	CCR4	**T cells;** elevated in **psoriasis and atopic dermatitis**
CCL18		**T cells;** elevated in atopic dermatitis
CCL19/CCL21	CCR7	T cell and dendritic cell migration from skin to lymph nodes **(CCR7 is a marker of central memory T cells)**
CCL20	CCR6	Recruitment of Th17 cells; role in **psoriasis**
CCL22	CCR4	NK cell, **T-cell** recruitment
CCL26		T cells; elevated in atopic dermatitis
CCL27	CCR10	T-cell recruitment to skin
CXCL1	CXCR2	Neutrophil recruitment
CXCL8	CRCR1. CXCR2	Neutrophil recruitment; role in **psoriasis**
CXCL9, CXCL10	**CXCR3**	Effector **T-cell** recruitment; **especially Th1**
CXCL12	CXCR4	B-cell migration into lymph nodes
CXCL13	CXCR5	B-cell migration to lymph nodes; T follicular helper cell migration into lymph node follicles
CXCL16	CXCR6	Effector **T-cell** recruitment; **especially Th1**
CX3CL1	CX3CR1	T-cell, NK-cell and monocyte recruitment

Modified from Abbas AK, Lichtman AH, Pillai S. Leukocyte circulation and migration into tissues. In: Cellular and Molecular Immunology. *9th ed. Philadelphia: Elsevier; 2018:39–56.*

Langerhans cells

- Embryonically seeded tissue-resident macrophage population residing in the epidermis
- Compared with other macrophages, they are poorly phagocytic and instead function as **professional APCs** (following antigen uptake, they cross the BMZ with help of MMP-9, move to the lymph nodes where MHC-bound antigen is presented to T cells, which are then activated)
- Dependent on TGF-β1 and macrophage colony-stimulating factor receptor ligands for development and retention in epidermis
- LCs usually not visualized during routine histologic analysis, and on electron microscopy have rod-shaped organelles (**Birbeck granules**)
- **Langerin is a very sensitive and specific immunohistochemical marker** for LCs, because it stains receptors found on Birbeck granules; **CD1a** is also a fairly specific marker
- LCs are S100+, langerin (CD207)+, vimentin+, and CD1a+; adhere to keratinocytes via E-cadherin

Dendritic cells

- **Professional APCs** that play a central role in initiating T-cell response
- Activated by cytokines and direct TLR sensing of PAMPs which increase their function
- Derived from bone marrow–derived myeloid precursors
- One subset called plasmacytoid DCs reside primarily in blood and produce type I interferon upon activation; not found in healthy skin, but **may play a role in psoriasis and lupus**

Mast cells

- Differentiate in tissues, for example, skin, from bone marrow–derived progenitor cells expressing **CD34/c-kit/CD13**
  - Also stain with Giemsa, toluidine blue, and Leder
- Express high levels of **c-kit receptor (CD117)** and its ligand, **stem cell factor**, which are critical for the differentiation, survival, and proliferation of mast cells
- Typically located in papillary dermis
- Important in **immediate-type hypersensitivity reactions** (e.g., anaphylaxis, urticaria, and angioedema)
- Express high levels of FcεRI (high-affinity receptor for IgE)
- Mast cell degranulation triggers: **cross-linking of FcεRI by binding to IgE**, anti-FcεRI antibodies, stem cell factor, neuropeptides (e.g., substance P), drugs (opiates, aspirin, vancomycin, curare, and polymyxin B), C5a anaphylatoxin, and radiocontrast media
- Mast cell mediators are listed in Table 1.17

Eosinophils

- Bone marrow–derived granulocytes with important role in defense against parasitic/helminth infections and in allergic disease
- **IL-5 produced by Th2 and type 2 ILC cells promotes eosinophil activation and recruitment**
- Weakly phagocytic, instead upon activation they release granule contents that promote helminth killing and also contribute to tissue damage (Table 1.18)

Table 1.17 Mast Cell Mediators

Mediator		Function
Preformed and stored in granules	**Histamine**	Vasodilation, smooth muscle cell contraction, tissue edema via vascular permeability
	Heparin	Anticoagulant, controls function of other mediators
	Tryptase	Production of C3a and bradykinin, increased fibroblast proliferation
	Chymase	Increased mucous secretion
	Cathepsin G	Protease
	Carboxypeptidase	Protease
Major lipid mediators: **newly formed**	**Prostaglandin D_2**	Vasodilation, bronchoconstriction, leukocyte chemotaxis
	Leukotrienes C_4, D_4, E_4	Bronchoconstriction, dendritic cell recruitment and activation
	Platelet-activating factor	Vasodilation
Cytokines: newly formed	IL-3, IL-4, IL-5, IL-6, IL-8, IL-13, TNF-α	See cytokine section (includes mast cell proliferation, IgE production, mucus secretion and eosinophil activation)

Modified from Metcalfe DD. Mastocytosis. In: Burks AW, Holgate ST, O'Hehir RE, et al., eds. Middleton's Allergy: Principles and Practice. *9th ed. Philadelphia: Elsevier; 2020:1216–1227.*

Table 1.18 Eosinophil Mediators

Mediator		Function
Preformed and stored in granules	**Major basic protein**, eosinophil cationic protein	Toxic to helminths, bacteria, host cells
	Eosinophil peroxidase, lysosomal hydroxylases, lysophospholipase	Degradation of helminthic and protozoan cell walls; tissue damage/ remodeling
Major lipid mediators: **newly formed**	Leukotrienes C_4, D_4, E_4	Bronchoconstriction, mucus secretion, increased vascular permeability
Cytokines: newly formed	IL-3, IL-5, IL-8, IL-10, RANTES, MIP-1α, eotaxin	See cytokine section (includes eosinophil production/activation, and chemotaxis of leukocytes)

Modified from Abbas AK, Lichtman AH, Pillai S. Allergy. In: Cellular and Molecular Immunology. *9th ed. Philadelphia: Elsevier; 2018:437–457.*

Neutrophils

- Highly abundant; short-lived, produced in the bone marrow
- First to arrive at sites of acute inflammation (**chemotactic factors include c5a, IL-8, LTB4, kallikrein**)
- Destroy microbial pathogens (**phagocytosis** followed by oxidation [via ROS] → death)
- Extrude nuclear contents to form neutrophil extracellular traps (NETosis); **overactive in certain autoimmune diseases, for example, lupus**

- Contain four granule types, two most significant are:
  - **Primary granules** (azurophilic) containing defensins, cathelicidins, cathepsins, myeloperoxidase (along with NADPH oxidase, **creates ROS** → oxidation of engulfed organisms → death; of note, defect in NADPH oxidase → chronic granulomatous disease and negative nitroblue tetrazolium test [cannot turn color from yellow to blue])
  - **Secondary granules** (specific) most abundant, contain lysozyme, elastase, collagenase

1.6.4 Major histocompatibility complex

- MHC locus in humans is known as the human leukocyte antigen (HLA) locus
- The MHC locus is found on **chromosome 6**, and its key role is to present antigen to T cells
- Divided into three classes: MHC class I, MHC class II, and MHC class III (encodes for complement molecules)
- Typically, T cells only recognize peptides in the presence of MHC molecules
- MHC genes are co-dominantly expressed
- During immune activation, the expression of MHC genes is increased in response to the surrounding cytokine milieu
- MHC class I molecules: present **endogenous antigens** (peptides) to **CD8$^+$ T cells** and have the **ability to induce apoptosis** in both virus-infected and tumor cells
  - MHC class I is expressed on **all nucleated cells**
  - Peptide size bound by MHC class I is 8 to 10 residues
  - **Intracellular proteins** are processed by proteasomes into cytosolic peptides that are transported to the endoplasmic reticulum, followed by binding to MHC class I on the surface
  - Three main MHC I loci: HLA-A, **HLA-B (most variable class I)**, and HLA-Cw
  - Subunits encoded by these loci bind to β_2-microglobulin to produce a heterodimer
- MHC class II molecules present **exogenous** antigens (peptides) to **CD4$^+$ T cells**
  - Expressed on **APCs** (i.e., monocytes, macrophages, DCs, B cells, and activated T cells)
    - Not expressed on plasma cells
  - Peptide size bound by MHC class I is 10 to 34 residues
  - Endocytosis of **extracellular antigens** into vesicles where the antigens are processed, peptides loaded on MHC class II molecules, and expressed on the surface
  - Three main MHC II loci:
    - HLA-DP: α-chain encoded by HLA-DPA1 locus, β-chain by HLA-DPB1 locus
    - HLA-DQ: α-chain encoded by HLA-DQA1 locus, β-chain by HLA-DQB1 locus
    - HLA-DR: α-chain encoded by HLA-DRA locus, 4 β-chains (three possible per person) encoded by **HLA-DRB1** (most variable class II locus), HLA-DRB3, HLA-DRB4, HLA-DRB5 loci
- The old system of MHC nomenclature was based on antibody typing where antigens were assigned letters and numbers (e.g., HLA-DQ3); a more recent system includes a number after the loci to provide more information about the specific allele and loci (e.g., HLA-B*6801)
  - Where possible, both are listed below
  - **MHC-associated diseases:** (note prevalence of certain alleles in autoimmune conditions)
    - Alopecia areata (AA): HLA-DQ3 (DQB1*03)
    - AA totalis/universalis: HLA-DQ7 (DQB1*0301) and **HLA-DR4 (DRB1*0401)**
    - Lupus (SCLE and SLE): **HLA-DR3** (DRB1*0306)
    - Psoriasis: **HLA-Cw6** (Cw*06) **especially early onset**
    - Psoriatic and reactive arthritis: HLA-B27 (B*27)
    - Behçet's disease: **HLA-B51** (B*51) 80% of Asian patients, 15% of Caucasians
    - Lepromatous leprosy: HLA-DQ1 (DQB1*06(11,12)), tuberculoid leprosy: HLA-DR2 (DRB1*108), **HLA-DR3** (DRB1*0306)
    - Pemphigoid gestationis: **HLA-DR3** (DRB1*0306) and **HLA-DR4** (DRB1*04)
    - Pemphigus vulgaris: **HLA-DR4** (DRB1*04) and HLA-DR8 (DQB1*0302) in Caucasians; HLA-DR14 (DRB1*14) and HLA-DQ3 (DQB1*0503) in Asians
    - Dermatitis herpetiformis: **HLA-DQ2** (DQB1*02)
    - HCV-associated oral lichen planus: HLA-DR6 (DRB1*13/14)
    - Vitiligo: HLA-A2 (A*02); **HLA-DR4** (DRB1*04)

1.7 LABORATORY TECHNIQUES

1.7.1 Tissue acquisition and processing

- Direct assays on human skin specimens are rapidly advancing our understanding of pathogenesis of many skin diseases
- Skin samples are usually obtained through biopsy or excision, although other research techniques can be performed on cells obtained via epidermal tape stripping, skin surface swabs, or blood samples (e.g., those looking for circulating antibodies, genomic DNA)
- To perform these studies, proper processing of the skin tissue is required. The first decision point is whether the tissue will be transferred freshly to the laboratory for immediate processing, frozen for later processing, or formalin fixed (as for traditional pathology samples). The rationale for each of these strategies depends on the intended assay (Fig. 1.14).
- To investigate a specific subset of cells, isolation of the target population is sometimes achieved by laser microdissection (using a laser and microscope to cut a small section of frozen/fixed tissue from a slide) or fluorescence-activated cell sorting, where the whole tissue is digested into a single-cell suspensions which is stained with fluorescent antibodies and then "sorted" for cells of interest that express the correct markers as detected by flow cytometry)

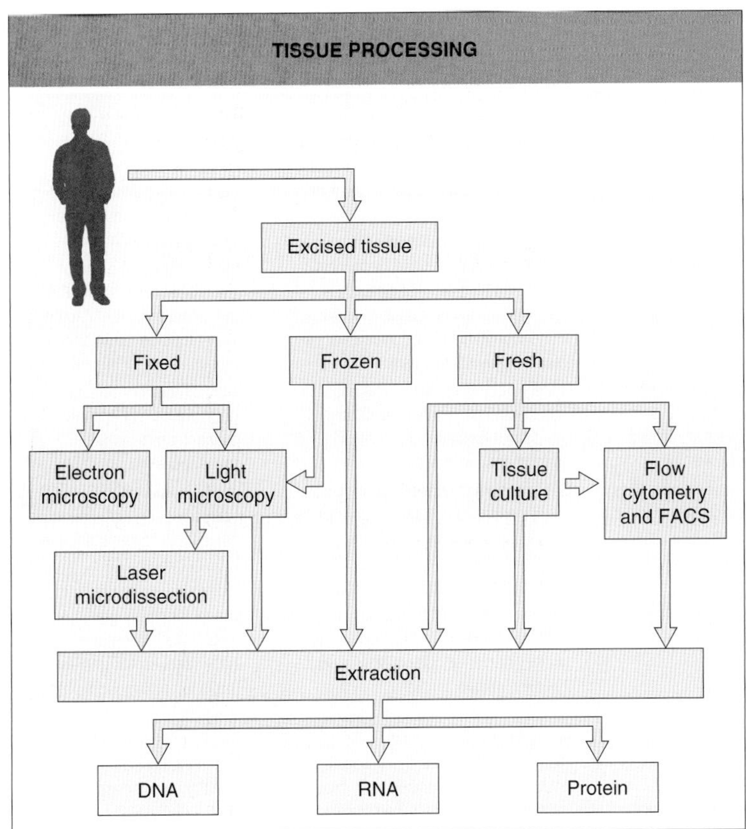

Fig. 1.14 Tissue processing. A tissue sample can be processed in various ways for the analysis of DNA, RNA, or protein. *FACS*, Flow-assisted cell sorting. (From Darling TN. Molecular biology. In: Bolognia JL, Schaffer JV, Cerroni L, eds. *Dermatology*. 4th ed. Philadelphia: Elsevier; 2018:66–80.)

1.7.2 Specific techniques of interest (Table 1.19)

Polymerase chain reaction (PCR)

- Used to amplify a specific piece of DNA from sample, for example, genomic DNA, specific cell type (Fig. 1.15); following PCR, DNA product can then be examined by gel electrophoresis to determine its size or sent for sequencing to determine the content of the region between the two primers
- Applications: testing for a gene mutation (can detect a deletion/insertion by examining PCR product size; need mutation-specific primers; needs to be sent for sequencing to detect SNPs/substitutions)
- Variations: quantitative PCR (qPCR) is an adaptation designed to measure the relative copy number of a specific segment of DNA between samples; here a special machine can measure the amount of PCR product at the end of each PCR cycle (i.e., as in Fig. 1.15B). The higher the amount of that DNA type in the sample, the earlier the cycle at which the product can be detected.

Quantitative reverse transcriptase PCR (qRT-PCR)

- In contrast to qPCR, the target starting template is RNA rather than dsDNA. This allows one to determine the relative level of gene expression/transcription by measuring the amount of mRNA for that gene in a given sample or set of samples. First a polymerase and primer set is used to generate dsDNA complementary (cDNA) to the RNA template. Often the primers will anneal to the poly(A) 3′ end of mRNA. DNA is more stable and can then be subjected to qPCR technique as above to measure the relative amount of RNA in original sample.

16S ribosomal RNA (rRNA) sequencing

- Portions of the 16S rRNA gene are conserved across all bacteria such that universal primers can be designed to amplify this region of DNA from mixed/complex samples. This PCR product can then be sequenced and variability in specific regions of the 16S gene used to identify the types of bacteria present in the sample, that is, taxonomic classification (Fig. 1.16).
- Benefits: can be performed non-invasively from skin swabs or sebum samples; provides significant information about the types of bacteria present in a clinical sample; does not require cultivation/culturing of microbes
- Limitations: does not distinguish live from dead bacteria (both are detected), can determine relative amounts of bacteria between samples but not absolute quantities, reference databases for making taxonomic assignments based on 16S sequence are still incomplete and depending on the region of gene amplified there can be misassignments or failure to assign, cannot distinguish cause from effect in terms of relationship to disease
- Adaptations: 18S sequencing, analogous analysis for fungal communities

Table 1.19 Specific Laboratory Techniques of Interest

Method	Purpose	Benefits	Limitations	Applications
Polymerase chain reaction (PCR)	Amplify a specific piece of DNA	Rapid, sensitive, inexpensive	Contamination by small amount of foreign DNA can confound results; need to know enough about DNA target to design specific primers	Amplification of a specific region (gene) in genome; other methods can then be used to identify alterations in intervening sequence
Quantitative reverse transcriptase PCR (qRT-PCR)	Determine relative gene expression by measuring the amount of mRNA for a specific gene between samples	Rapid, sensitive, inexpensive	Contamination of cDNA with genomic DNA can lead to false detection of genes that are not actually expressed/transcribed; isolation of high-quality RNA requires fresh or specifically stored tissue	Determine relative expression of a gene of interest across a set of samples, e.g., IL-17 from skin biopsies from different diseases
16S rRNA sequencing	Determine types of bacteria present in a sample	Can be performed on non-invasive samples, e.g., skin swabs; does not require culturing of microbes	Does not distinguish live vs. dead bacteria; not highly quantitative; does not examine content of microbial genomes	Determination of relative abundance of bacteria present on healthy vs. diseased skin
Sanger DNA sequencing	Determine oligonucleotide sequence of a DNA sample	Fairly rapid; can contiguously sequence several hundred DNA bases	Still somewhat expensive on a per sample basis; requires high-quality DNA; difficulty with G/C-rich regions of DNA; requires primers complementary to DNA template	Determine genetic sequence, i.e., of a specific gene to determine if there is a mutation
Next-generation DNA sequencing	Determine oligonucleotide sequence of a DNA sample	Cheaper and higher throughput	Difficulty with highly repetitive regions of DNA, large genome assembly from shorter sequences fragments can introduce errors	Screen for many gene-associated mutations at once; search for genetic basis for poorly understood disease
RNA sequencing	Determine level of expression of many genes in parallel	Looks broadly at transcriptional landscape within a tissue sample; no prior knowledge of gene sequence required	Somewhat costly, mostly still used for research rather than diagnostic purposes; fresh or specially frozen tissue is usually required; lowly expressed genes may not be detected depending on depth of sequencing	Broadly profile level of expression of all genes in healthy vs. diseased skin
RNA microarray	Determine relative level of expression of many genes in parallel	Looks broadly at transcriptional landscape within a tissue sample	Looks at many (100s–1000s) but not all genes; requires lots of high-quality RNA to ensure good hybridization; lowly expressed genes may not be detected, assays relative vs. absolute level of gene expression	Broadly profile level of expression of *many* genes in healthy vs. diseased skin
Fluorescence *in situ* hybridization (FISH)	Visualize large chromosomal abnormalities	Can be performed on formalin-fixed tissue, can select specific areas of tissue to test (i.e., tumor vs. normal skin), requires only 20–30 visualized cells	Probe design requires knowledge of likely abnormalities, processing/interpretation not standardized across labs; technical issues may arise such as incomplete hybridization or non-specific binding	Assist in distinguishing melanocytic nevi with atypical features from melanoma
Comparative genomic hybridization (CGH)	Visualize large chromosomal abnormalities	Typically assays a larger genomic region than does FISH	Assays a population of cells so changes in a subset (<30–50%) may be not be detected; more expensive and longer turnaround time than FISH because cells are microdissected	Assist in distinguishing melanocytic nevi with atypical features from melanoma
T-cell receptor (TCR) gene rearrangement	Detection of clonal populations of T cells using DNA extraction, PCR of TCR gene(s) and size detection on a gel	Can detect clones of malignant T cells that lack variability present in mixed healthy cell populations	Can have false-negative and false-positive results; good adjunct assay but cannot be used alone for basis of a diagnosis	Detection of malignant clones in CTCL
Immunofluorescence staining (direct)	Localize specific antigens using fluorescent primary antibodies	Very helpful for diagnosis of autoimmune skin conditions	Requires fresh tissue; qualitative rather than quantitative	DIF for IgG in pemphigus or lupus
Immunofluorescence staining (indirect)	Localize specific antigens using fluorescent secondary antibodies	Can be used to detect antibodies and other factors circulating in serum	Not widely available, not very standardized across labs, not highly quantitative	Detection of circulating auto-antibodies in cicatricial pemphigoid pemphigus or lupus
Immunohistochemistry (IHC)	Localize specific antigens in tissue sections	Can be performed on FFPE tissue, wide variety of different target antigens that can be detected and studied	Non-standardized across laboratories, not all antigens equally preserved during fixation/processing steps, less sensitive and specific than PCR-based diagnostics	Identification of plasmacytoid dendritic cells (stain positive for CD123) in tissue sections of cutaneous lupus

Table 1.19 Specific Laboratory Techniques of Interest—cont'd

Method	Purpose	Benefits	Limitations	Applications
Enzyme-linked immunosorbent assay (ELISA)	Technique to detect and quantify peptides, protein or antibodies in serum	Fast, can be somewhat standardized, more quantitative than IIF, may be cheaper and easier than western blot	Requires knowledge of substance to be detected.	Detection and quantification of circulating anti-dsg3 antibodies in patients with pemphigus vulgaris
Western blot	Detects and measures size and amount of a protein	Can detect amount of a given protein in a sample, determine its size and conformation	Requires a specific and sensitive antibody to the protein of interest, proteins may be degraded during extraction	Measurement of epidermal proteins and their enzymatic processing
Mass spectrometry	Analysis of all proteins present in a sample	Highly sensitive	Very expensive and technically difficult and time consuming, more qualitative than quantitative	May have future diagnostic application where ability to detect small amounts of a peptide is required

Data from Bolognia JL, Schaffer JV, Cerroni L, eds. Dermatology. *4th ed. Philadelphia: Elsevier; 2018; Jo JH, Kennedy EA, Kong HH. Research techniques made simple: bacterial 16S ribosomal RNA gene sequencing in cutaneous research.* J Invest Dermatol. *2016;136(3):e23–27; Grada A, Weibrecht K. Next-generation sequencing: methodology and application.* J Invest Dermatol. *2013;133(8):e11; Chen AYY, Chen A. Fluorescence* in situ *hybridization.* J Invest Dermatol. *2013;133(5):e8; Schacht V, Kern JS. Basics of immunochemistry.* J Invest Dermatol. *2015;135(3):1–4; Odell ID, Cook D. Immunofluorescence techniques.* J Invest Dermatol. *2013;133(1):e4; Chitgopeker P, Sahni D. T-cell receptor gene rearrangment detection in suspected cases of cutaneous T-cell lymphoma.* J Invest Dermatol. *2014;134(4):1–5.*

- Alternative approaches: whole-genome shotgun sequencing broadly examines the sequence of all DNA in a sample, both microbial and host; advantages here are that functional genes in microbial genomes are assays which might provide insight into potential function; limitations include both cost and depth of sequencing required to adequately assay microbial DNA which is a small percent (< 1%) of most skin samples

DNA sequencing

- Determination of a DNA sequence can help inform the likelihood of disease based on presence or absence of specific gene mutations or variants
- In first generation, chain termination (Sanger) sequencing an oligonucleotide primer (as used in PCR above) hybridizes to the target DNA and a polymerase starts to synthesize a complementary strand until a fluorescent nucleotide analog (e.g., ddATP instead of dATP) is instead incorporated and terminates the chain extension; gel electrophoresis is then used to separate the synthesized strands of varying length and a detector is used to determine the order of the sequence (Fig. 1.17)
- In next-generation sequencing, DNA is sheared into smaller pieces which are then ligated to adapter sequences which help anchor the DNA in the machine and can be used to identify samples later during data download and analysis; these "DNA libraries" are then amplified and sequenced by synthesis, meaning that the existing DNA fragments serve as a template and complementary nucleotides are incorporated by introducing these sequentially one by one into the machine; identity and order of the nucleotides incorporated is recorded either by fluorescent signal or pH change (Fig. 1.18)
- Although sequencing is most often still applied in the realm of research rather than routine diagnosis, its rapidly decreasing cost is leading to its increasing use for clinical purposes

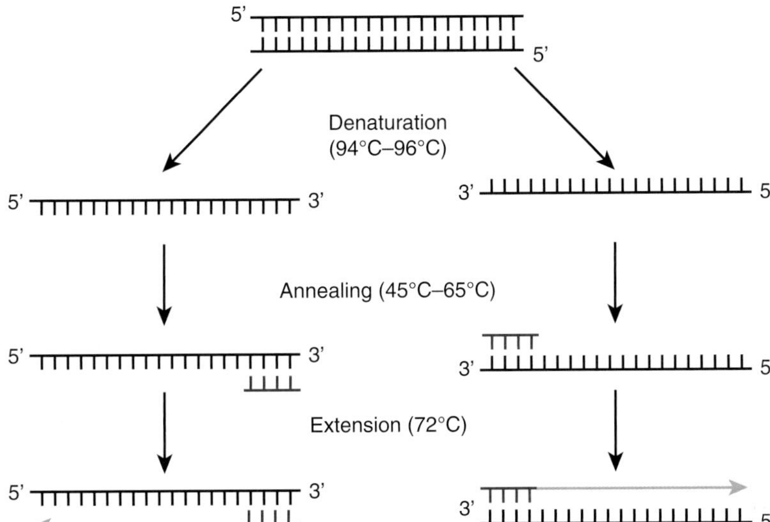

Fig. 1.15 First cycle of polymerase chain reaction. During the denaturation step, DNA is heated to above 90°C and the two strands of the DNA target sequence separate. The temperature of the reaction is then cooled to 45°C–65°C and primers anneal to their complementary sequence in the template DNA. In the extension step, the reaction is heated to 72°C to allow the DNA polymerase to synthesize a new DNA strand complementary to the template strand. (From Jalali M, Zaborowska J, Jalali M. The polymerase chain reaction: PCR, qPCR, and RT-PCR. In: Jalali M, Saldanha FYL, Jalali M. *Basic Science Methods for Clinical Researchers.* Philadelphia: Elsevier; 2017:1–18.)

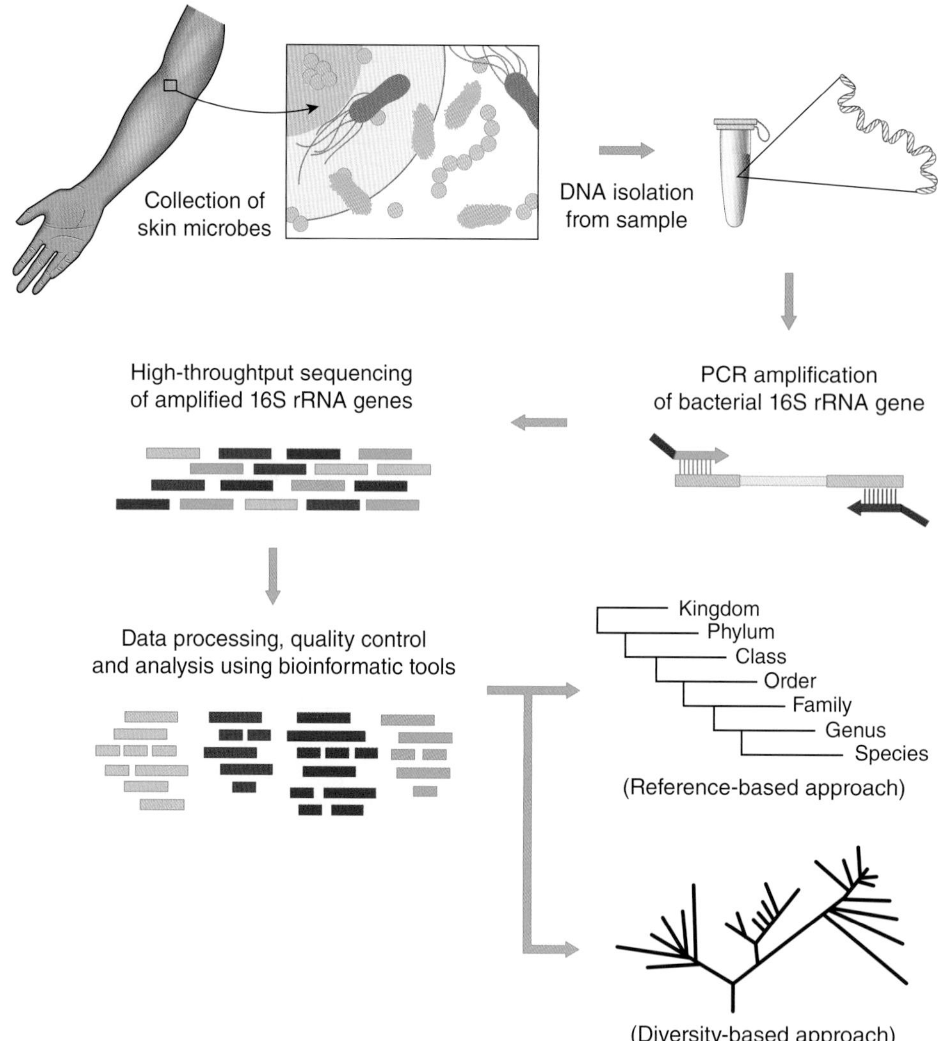

Fig. 1.16 Schematic illustration of basic workflow for skin 16S rRNA gene-based sequencing. (From Jo JH, Kennedy EA, Kong HH. Research techniques made simple: bacterial 16S ribosomal RNA gene sequencing in cutaneous research. *J Invest Dermatol*. 2016;136(3):e23–27; Adapted and modified with permission from Kong HH: Skin microbiome: genomics-based insights into the diversity and role of skin microbes. *Trends Mol Med*. 2011;17(6):320–328.)

- Variations: whole-exome sequencing helps to further reduce the costs of sequencing by focusing only 1%–2% of the genome that encodes for protein, where mutations disproportionately contribute to disease. Note: this will miss mutations in non-coding regions and enhancers/promoters/RNAs that also contribute to disease in some instances

RNA sequencing

- RNA sequencing (RNAseq) is a method of broadly assaying the number and identification of mRNAs in a sample to better understand which genes are actively being transcribed and thus (likely) expressed at the protein level. Just as DNA sequencing expands the breath of focus from one gene (as in a single qPCR reaction) to all potential genes, RNAseq does the same for mRNA. As with qRT-PCR, the first steps involve generation of a cDNA library for mRNA. This is then sequenced by next-generation methods as described above.
- Variations/alternatives: prior to next-generation sequencing, RNA microarrays were more commonly used for a similar purpose. This method is based instead on designing a panel of probes to genes of interest on a chip/array and then visualizing the extent to which nucleic acids within a sample bind to these probes.

Fluorescence in situ hybridization (FISH)

- FISH is designed to *visualize* the location of specific genetic sequences. The method involves hybridization of labeled probes to DNA in a tissue sample, that is, on a sectioned slide. Each bound probe (appearing as a dot) identifies a single copy of the target DNA sequence. Nuclei with two copies will have two dots. It is best used to identify large chromosomal changes (copy number variations), that is,

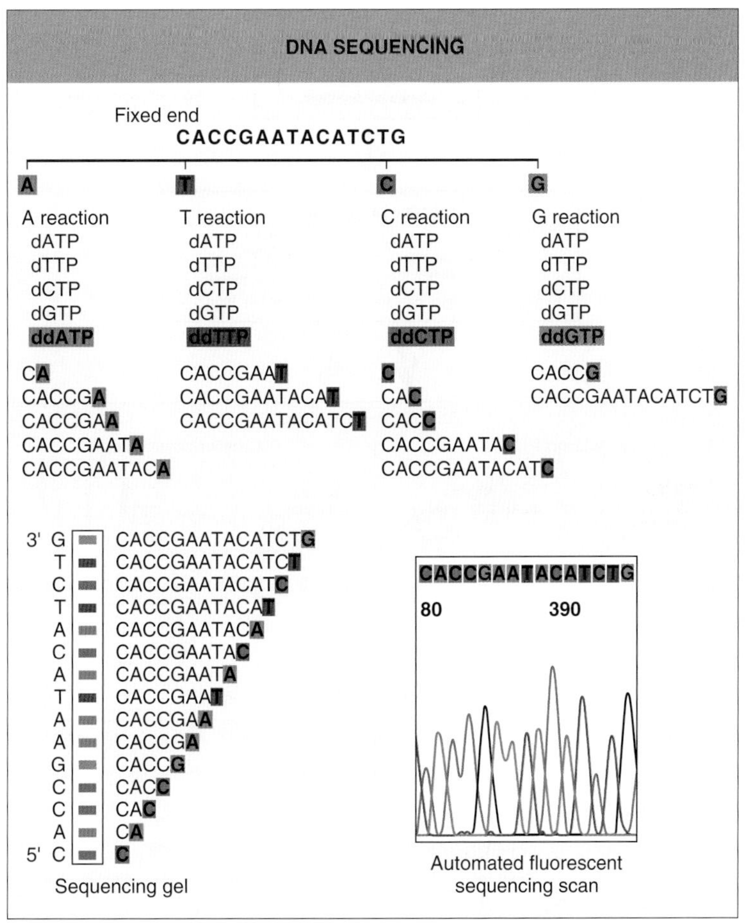

Fig. 1.17 Sanger DNA sequencing. An oligonucleotide primer hybridizes to the DNA to be sequenced and DNA polymerase synthesizes a second complementary strand. The synthesis of the second strand is interrupted randomly by the incorporation of fluorescent nucleotide analogs (ddATP, ddGTP, ddCTP, ddTTP). The DNA fragments containing this final nucleotide analog can be identified because each of the four ddNTPs is labeled with a different color fluorochrome. Gel electrophoresis is used to separate the different sizes of DNA fragments. The different-length DNA strands terminating with different fluorochrome-labeled nucleotide analogs pass a fluorescence detector and indicate the order of the DNA sequence. (From Darling TN. Molecular biology. In: Bolognia JL, Schaffer JV, Cerroni L, eds. *Dermatology*. 4th ed. Philadelphia: Elsevier; 2018:66–80.)t

deletions, amplifications, translocations. While classically used for prenatal diagnosis, its central role in dermatology is in identifying genomic aberrations diagnostic of certain skin malignancies, most often melanoma. A commercially available four-probe FISH assay reportedly has > 85% sensitivity and > 95% specificity in distinguishing melanoma from melanocytic nevi. More recently, researchers designed an 11-probe panel to assist in the diagnosis of cutaneous T cell lymphoma (CTCL) with leukemic involvement, by examination of peripheral blood.

- FISH is best used as a supplementary diagnostic tool to traditional histopathology
- Variations/alternatives: microarray-based comparative genomic hybridization which can more broadly interrogate copy number aberrations across the whole genome but has other limitations

Immunofluorescence (IF)

- In IF, fluorescently labeled antibodies are incubated with a sample (tissue biopsy or serum) to allow binding to specific antigens and binding is then assayed microscopically
- Direct IF (DIF) detects and localizes antigens in the skin. In dermatology, DIF is most often used to detect autoantibody-antigen complexes deposited in the skin as a result of autoimmune skin disease. Here the fluorescently labeled antibodies are designed to bind to patient's own autoantibodies (IgA, IgG, IgM) or complement (C3). DIF must be performed on fresh tissue that is transported in ammonium sulfate–containing media to preserve autoantibody-antigen complexes. Other applications of DIF include detection of infectious organisms by incubating with labeled primary antibodies against the suspected microbe
- Indirect IF (IIF) is used to detect circulating autoantibodies in a patient's serum. First, the sample is incubated with an unlabeled primary antibody designed to bind the target molecule, then it is incubated with a labeled secondary antibody directed against the Fc portion of the primary antibody. This two-step process makes IIF more complicated and time-consuming but also more sensitive than some

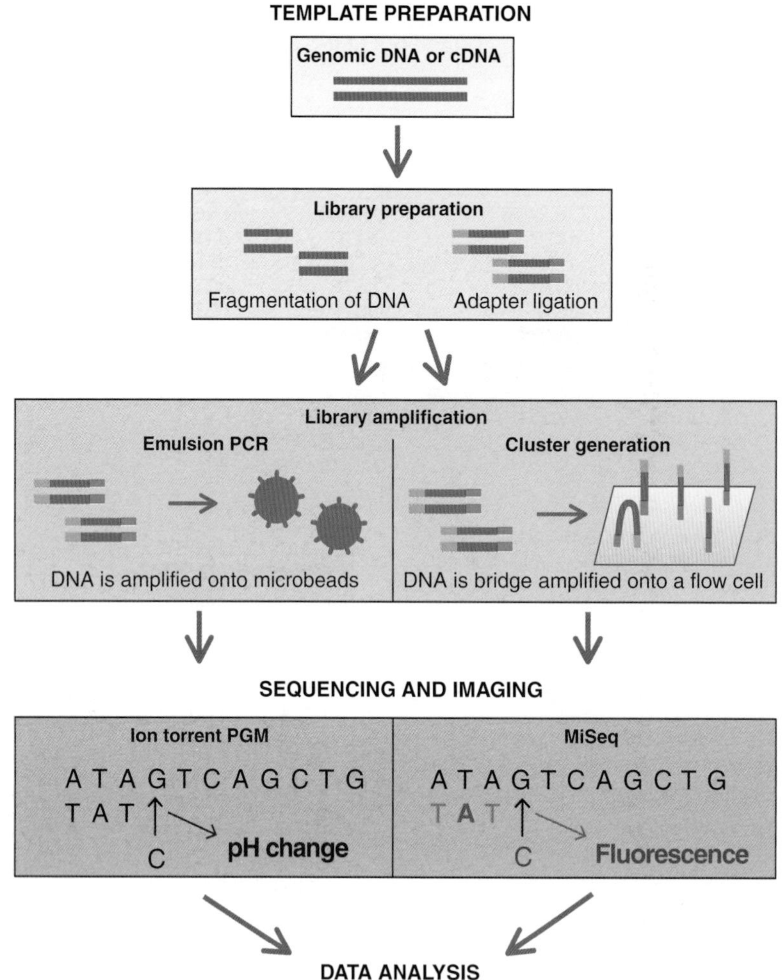

Fig. 1.18 Next-generation sequencing methodology. Although specific processes vary based on the sequencing platform, this figure depicts the major steps involved in next-generation sequencing. (From Grada A, Weibrecht K. Next-generation sequencing: methodology and application. *J Invest Dermatol*. 2013;133(8):e11.)

other assays. In dermatology, we more commonly think of a variation of IIF used to detect circulating autoantibody. Here, serum is incubated with slide sections of a foreign tissue known to consistently bind the antibody of interest (e.g., monkey esophagus for anti-desmoglein antibodies), a labeled secondary antibody directed against the Fc portion of the autoantibody is then added and the fluorescence pattern interpreted by microscopy.

Immunohistochemistry (IHC)

- IHC is used to localize specific molecules/antigens in formalin-fixed, paraffin-embedded (FFPE) tissue based on binding of a specific antibody to that target and visualizing where and to what extent that binding occurs. Because formalin fixation reversibly compromises antigenicity of epitopes to a certain extent, after tissue sectioning these are "retrieved" or "unmasked" usually by heating the slide in a buffered solution. The tissue section is then incubated with the antibody/ies of interest and these patterns are then visualized (Fig. 1.19) and interpreted by the pathologist. IHC is used extensively in dermatopathology to identify cell types within a tissue section.
- IHC is also commonly used on **fresh frozen tissue during Mohs surgery** for melanoma (Melan-A), poorly-differentiated keratinocyte carcinomas (CK5/6), and EMPD (CK7).

Enzyme-linked immunosorbent assay (ELISA)

- ELISA is a test to detect and measure levels of peptides, protein, or antibodies from a sample in the form of a liquid suspension (i.e., cannot be performed on whole tissue without further processing). It is most often used to detect levels of circulating proteins or antibodies. When detecting antibodies, the target antigen is bound to the bottom of wells in a plate and the sample incubated so that if antibodies to that antigen are present they will bind to the antigen. A secondary antibody directed at the Fc portion of the autoantibody bound to an enzyme is then added. Finally, a substrate for the enzyme is added (often resulting in generation of a colored product that

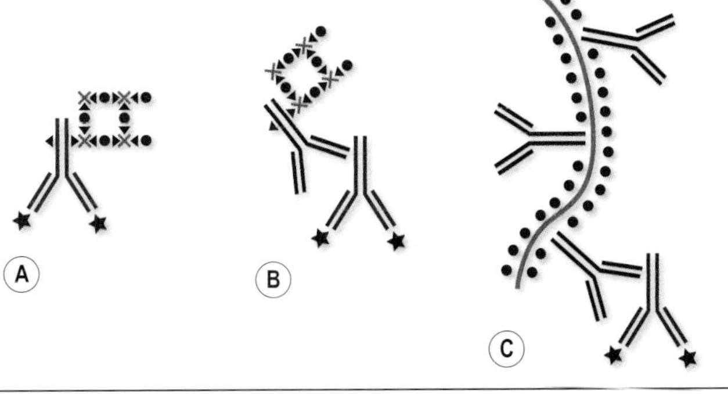

Fig. 1.19 Schematic diagram of immunohistochemical techniques. (A) Direct method: the antigen-specific primary antibody is biotin labeled. Biotin binds to avidin/streptavidin. Color visualization is achieved through enzymatic reaction of horseradish peroxidase/alkaline phosphatase. (B) Indirect method: the antigen-specific primary antibody is unlabeled. The secondary, biotin-labeled antibody binds to primary antibody. Visualization is achieved accordingly through avidin/streptavidin and peroxidase/alkaline phosphatase complexes. The indirect method increases versatility because unlabeled primary antibodies can be used. (C) Indirect method with polymer chain detection system. Biotin and avidin/streptavidin are replaced by a labeled polymer chain, allowing for increased sensitivity and specificity. (From Schacht V, Kern JS. Basics of immunochemistry. *J Invest Dermatol*. 2015;135(3):1–4.)

can be quantified by a plate reader) and the level of autoantibody measured.

- Variations/alternatives: IIF (see above) is an alternative to this method, and Western blot is another way to detect proteins in a sample. In this method, the antigen is run on a gel and precipitated on a membrane; binding of the antibody is then visualized similarly to ELISA. Western blot is somewhat less quantitative than ELISA but can provide information about the size of an antigen and conformation in the sample. Mass spectrometry is a technique used mostly in research to measure the precise size of the mass of proteins or peptides. Usually the proteins are first separated by electrophoresis to simplify the sample. Mass spectrometry is then performed by ionizing the peptides and then measuring the time of flight of these charged ions. By calculating the peptide mass/charge ratio, the sequence of the peptide can then be identified.

1.7.3 Cellular engineering and gene therapy

- Skin's accessibility provides a unique opportunity for therapies that aim to restore or repair skin structure and function via genetic manipulation. This approach, historically termed "gene therapy," is now encompassed under the umbrella of genetic and cellular engineering.
- Although these approaches remain in the research stage, there are already case reports of successful treatment of genetically based diseases such as **epidermolysis bullosa**
- Due to risks and challenges involved in genetically manipulating cells *in vivo* (e.g., requirement of injecting material to transform cells, limited durability of gene expression, and oncogenic potential), most approaches rely on harvesting cells from a patient, genetically manipulating them *ex vivo* and then re-delivering them as therapy. This can be done in theory for keratinocytes, induced pluripotent stem (iPS) cells, and immune cells among other types. For keratinocytes, cells are often differentiated *in vitro* to more closely resemble a functional epidermis before grafting back onto the patient.
- In cases where a gene is mutated or absent, the usual strategy is to transform cells with a viral or non-viral vector that contains a functional copy of the gene. The DNA transposon *Sleeping Beauty* is an example of a non-viral vector that will incorporate randomly into the genome. However, it could do so at an inopportune location, activating a proto-oncogene. Viral vectors include self-inactivating lentiviral and gamma retroviral vectors. Limitations of these include broad tropism for many cell types, limited DNA packaging capacity and immunogenicity (i.e., development of an immune response against elements of the viral DNA; an immune response to the corrected protein is a potential caveat to any approach).
- An alternative approach to providing a second functional copy of a gene is to repair it in its endogenous location in the genome. More recently developed technologies, in particular CRISPR/cas (Fig. 1.20), but also zinc-finger nucleases and transcription activator-like effector nucleases, have enabled this by being able to introduce double-stranded DNA breaks in a specific location flanking the gene of interest. If a copy of the gene with the correct sequence and flanking DNA outside the area of the induced breaks is then provided via a plasmid, the gene is then repaired via homologous recombination.
- Finally, in situations where production of an aberrant protein has a dominant-negative effect, the better approach might be to suppress expression of the gene via elimination of mRNA. Here, there are also various options as outlined in Fig. 1.21

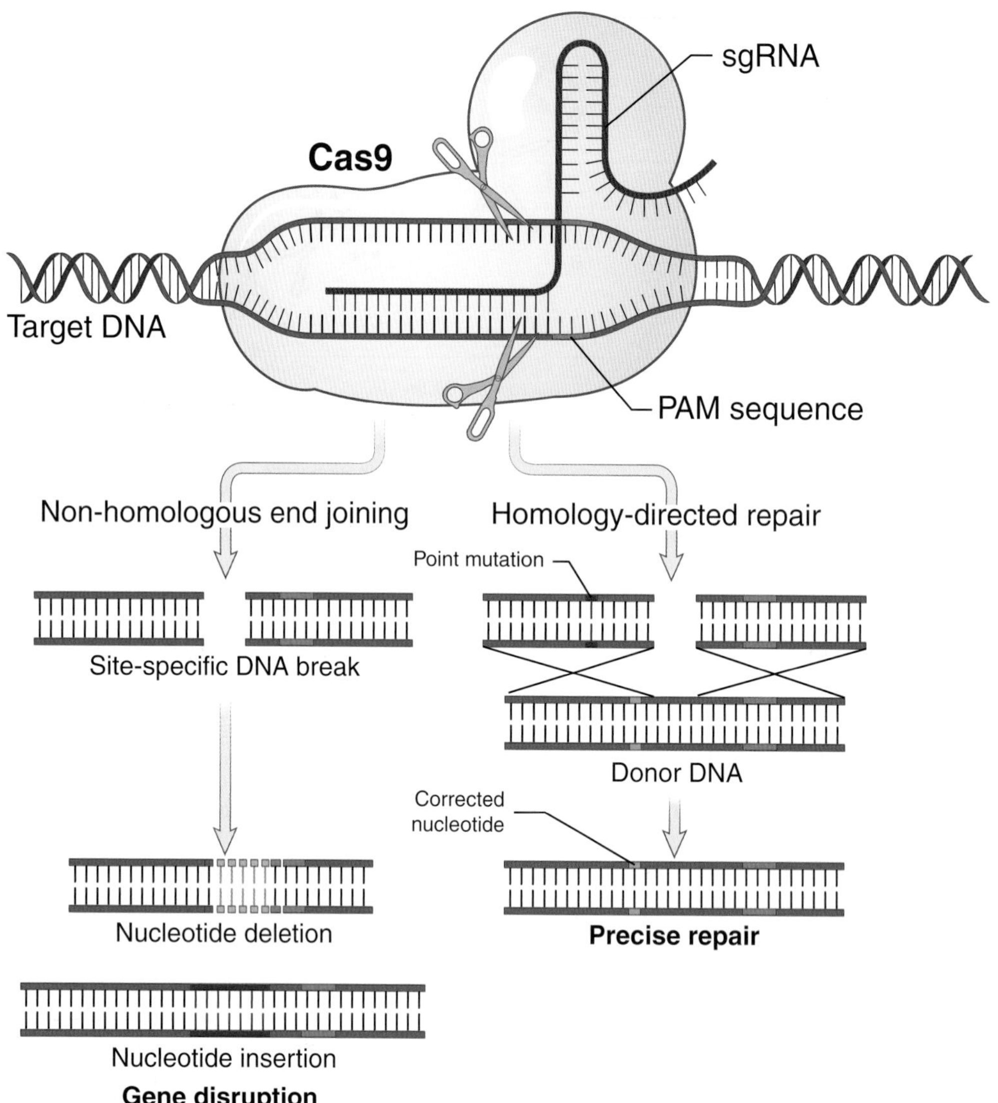

Fig. 1.20 Clustered regularly interspaced palindromic repeats (CRISPR)-induced nonhomologous end-joining (NHEJ) and homology-directed repair (HDR). Upon CRISPR-associated protein 9 *(Cas9)*-induced DNA double-stranded break (DSB), the cell repairs the DSB by either NHEJ or HDR. In NHEJ, random nucleotide insertions and deletions occur as the cell ligates the DNA DSB, resulting in gene disruption. In HDR, the DSB is repaired using an externally supplied homologous DNA as a template for copying. The nucleotide sequence of the donor template is copied into the targeted site, resulting in a directed precise repair. *PAM,* Protospacer adjacent motif; *sgRNA,* single-guide RNA. (From Guitart JR Jr, Johnson JL, Chien WW. Research techniques made simple: the application of CRISPR-Cas9 and genome editing in investigative dermatology. *J Invest Dermatol.* 2016;136(9):e87–e93; Adapted and modified from Savić N, Schwank G. Advances in therapeutic CRISPR/Cas9 genome editing. *Transl Res.* 2016;168:15–21.)

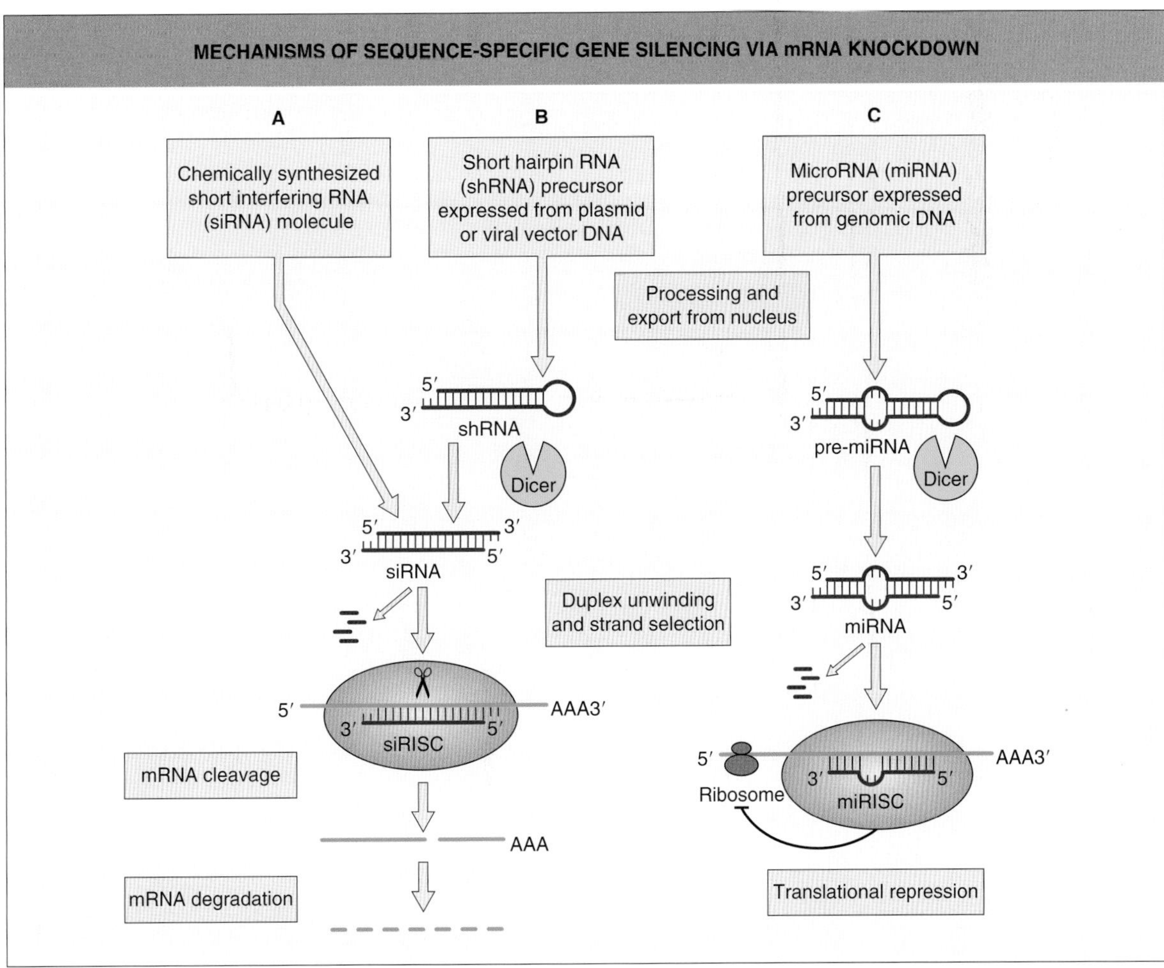

Fig. 1.21 Mechanisms of sequence-specific gene silencing via mRNA knockdown. (A) Short (small) interfering RNA *(siRNA)* is unwound and the "guide" antisense strand incorporated into an RNA-induced silencing complex *(RISC)* that degrades a specific target mRNA sequence. Processing short hairpin RNA *(shRNA)*; (B) and pre-microRNA *(miRNA)*; (C) by the Dicer enzyme can generate siRNA and miRNA, respectively. (C) Endogenously produced miRNA regulates up to a third of human genes and tends to have less complementarity with target mRNA; it recruits RISC proteins and typically inhibits mRNA translation (rather than decreasing mRNA levels). (From Darling TN. Molecular biology. In: Bolognia JL, Schaffer JV, Cerroni L, eds. *Dermatology*. 4th ed. Philadelphia: Elsevier; 2018:66–80.)

2 Dermatopharmacology

Alexander Maley and Ali Alikhan

CONTENTS LIST

2.1 ANTIHISTAMINES
2.2 RETINOIDS
2.3 CORTICOSTEROIDS
2.4 IMMUNOMODULATORY AGENTS
2.5 ONCOLOGIC AGENTS IN DERMATOLOGY
2.6 ANTIMICROBIAL AGENTS
2.7 PHOTOTHERAPY
2.8 MISCELLANEOUS AGENTS
2.9 DRUG INTERACTIONS AND THE CYTOCHROME P-450 SYSTEM
2.10 DRUG REACTIONS

2.1 ANTIHISTAMINES

Mechanism of action

- Histamine is released by mast cells and is a mediator of inflammation when bound to its receptor
- The primary function of histamine is to stimulate local blood vessels and nerves, producing vasodilatation and pruritus
  - H_1 receptors are found in the skin
  - H_1 and H_2 antihistamines are inverse agonists (downregulate constitutively activated state of receptor) or antagonists at histamine receptors

Important facts

- Treatment of choice for mast cell disease, urticaria, and angioedema
- 2014 atopic dermatitis guidelines do not recommend use in atopic dermatitis outside of short-term use for sleep loss

First-generation H_1 antihistamines

- Adverse effects (AEs): **sedation**, impaired cognitive function (from lipophilicity; cross blood-brain barrier, risk factor for dementia), and **anticholinergic effects** (dry mouth, constipation, dysuria, tachycardia, and blurred vision)
- Diphenhydramine: topical formulation → limited efficacy, can cause contact dermatitis; safe in pregnancy
- Cyproheptadine: interferes with hypothalamic function → may ↑ appetite and retard growth in children
- Promethazine: used for allergies and urticaria, but may cause respiratory depression (do not use in patients < 2 years), tissue damage, extrapyramidal symptoms, and neuroleptic malignant syndrome
- Chlorpheniramine: historically safe in pregnancy
- Hydroxyzine: strong affinity for muscarinic receptors, high risk in patients aged > 65 years

Second-generation H_1 antihistamines

- **Less sedating** (because of ↓ ability to cross blood-brain barrier) and **lack anticholinergic effects**
- More selective for histamine receptors over muscarinic receptors
- 2018 urticaria guidelines recommend over first-generation antihistamines for the treatment of urticaria
- Recommended treatment in pregnancy and lactation
- Fexofenadine: active metabolite of the prodrug terfenadine (which was withdrawn because of Q-T prolongation and torsades de pointes); not metabolized by the liver and excreted unchanged
- Loratadine: ↓ dose in patients with hepatic or renal impairment
- Cetirizine: carboxylic acid metabolite of hydroxyzine; **both can cause systemic contact dermatitis due to ethylenediamine**; >10% get drowsiness (most sedating of second-generation antihistamines); ↓ dose in patients with hepatic or renal impairment
- Levocetirizine: active metabolite and R-enantiomer of cetirizine; suppresses histamine wheal better than desloratidine and fexofenadine
- Desloratadine: active metabolite of loratadine, more potent than loratadine in suppressing histamine wheal

Other antihistamines

- Doxepin: **tricyclic antidepressant (TCA)** with **H_1 and H_2** antihistamine activity; effective in urticaria and psychiatric patients with neurotic excoriations; available orally and topically (5% cream—can cause allergic contact dermatitis, and sedation via absorption)
  - Much higher affinity for histamine receptors than most antihistamines
  - Therapeutic effect longer lasting than diphenhydramine and hydroxyzine because of long half-life (thus QHS dosing)
  - Sedation is most common AE; others include anticholinergic and orthostatic hypotension
  - Do not give with other antidepressants, or in severe heart disease (risk of heart block)
  - Can ↓ seizure threshold
  - Can induce manic episodes in patients with manic-depressive disorder; black box warning for suicidality (since it is an antidepressant)

2.2 RETINOIDS (TABLES 2.1 AND 2.2)

Introduction

- Retinoids are derived from vitamin A
- Three interconvertible forms: retinol (alcohol), retinal (aldehyde), and retinoic acid (acid)
  - Retinoic acid is the active metabolite
- Stored in the liver as retinol
- Retinol is transported in plasma by binding to a complex of retinol-binding protein and transthyretin

Mechanism

- Binds cytosolic retinoid-binding protein → transported to the nucleus → binds intracellular nuclear receptors
- Binds to two families of nuclear receptors: retinoic acid receptors (RARs) and retinoid X receptors (RXRs)
  - Each receptor family contains three isotypes (α, β, and γ)
  - RARs are homodimers, whereas RXRs can form heterodimers with other nuclear receptors: vitamin D, thyroid hormone, and peroxisome proliferator-activated receptors
  - The major receptors in keratinocytes are RXR-α and RAR-γ (most abundant in skin)
    - Photoaging → ↓ RXR-α and RAR-γ
- Binding to RAR/RXR affects various genes and transcription factors that are involved in many functions (cellular proliferation, differentiation, embryonic development, cellular cohesiveness, and inflammatory effects)
  - Inhibits AP1 and NF-IL-6, which are important in proliferation and inflammatory responses
  - **Inhibits toll-like receptor 2**, which is an activator of inflammatory cytokine responses
  - ↓ Tumorigenesis and induces apoptosis
  - Antikeratinization (downregulates K6 and K16)
  - ↑ Stratum corneum thickness, epidermal hyperplasia, correction of atypia, dispersion of melanin granules,

Table 2.1 Topical Retinoids

Retinoid	Generation	Systemic Absorption (% Dose)	Timing of Improvement	Nuclear Receptor Profile	Uses/Treatment Indications	Miscellaneous
Tretinoin (all-*trans*-RA)	First (nonaromatic)	1%–2% in normal skin	8–12 weeks	All RAR	Acne, fine lines and wrinkles, hyperpigmentation	**Inactivated by UV →** apply at night **Oxidized by benzoyl peroxide**
Alitretinoin (9-*cis*-RA)	First	Not measurable	4–8 weeks	All RAR and RXR	**Kaposi sarcoma**	**"AL(L)** itretinoin binds **ALL** forms (RARs and RXR) of receptors"
Adapalene	Third (poly aromatic)	Trace amounts	8–12 weeks	RAR-β/γ > α	Acne, fine lines and wrinkles, hyperpigmentation	**Light stable**
Tazarotene	Third	<5% in normal skin	8–12 weeks	RAR-β/γ > α	Acne, fine lines and wrinkles, hyperpigmentation and plaque psoriasis	**Teratogenic**
Bexarotene	Third	Trace amounts	20 weeks	All RXR	**CTCL** patch/plaque stage	"be**X**arotene = R**X**R" Teratogenic
Trifarotene	Fourth	Not measured, no changes in lab results	8–12 weeks, significant reduction seen by 2 weeks	RAR-γ – selective	Acne	Selectivity for γ receptor results in less irritation
Retinol	Precursor of retinoic acid		8–12 weeks		Cosmeceutical product, photoaging, and hyperpigmentation	
Retinaldehyde	Precursor of retinoic acid		8–12 weeks		Cosmeceutical product, photoaging, and hyperpigmentation	

CTCL, *Cutaneous T-cell lymphoma;* RAR, *retinoic acid receptor;* RXR, *retinoic X receptor;* UV, *ultraviolet.*

Table 2.2 Systemic Retinoids

Retinoid	Generation	Half-Life	Metabolism	Excretion	Nuclear Receptor Profile	Uses/Treatment[a]	Miscellaneous
Tretinoin (ATRA or all-*trans*-RA)	First (nonaromatic)	1 hour	Hepatic	Bile, urine	All RAR	Acute promyelocytic leukemia	**Treats acute promyelocytic leukemia (APML)**
Isotretinoin (13-*cis*-RA)	First	20 hours	Hepatic, metabolizes to tretinoin	Bile, urine	None	Severe acne, treatment-resistant moderate acne Usual dose: 0.5–2 mg/kg/day Goal cumulative dose: 120–220 mg/kg for severe acne Take with a fatty meal (lipophilic), formulation of isotretinoin with lidose OK to take on empty stomach Women must have 2 negative pregnancy tests prior to initiating; requires 2 forms of contraception for 1 month before, during and 1 month after cessation of therapy (abstinence is an alternative)	**Only retinoid to affect sebum production so *Cutibacterium acnes* unable to thrive** **Avoid with tetracyclines (↑ risk of pseudotumor cerebri)** All patients must enroll in iPLEDGE for pregnancy prevention Stop before LASIK → risk of dry eye ASDS guidelines state do not need to delay superficial chemical peel, superficial dermabrasion, non-ablative laser. Fully ablative laser should be avoided for 6 months
Etretinate	Second (monoaromatic)	120 days	Hepatic, metabolizes to acitretin	Bile, urine	None	No longer available	50 times more lipophilic than acitretin → long elimination half-life
Acitretin	Second	2 days	Hepatic, re-esterification to etretinate by alcohol	Bile, urine	None	Psoriasis (pustular, erythrodermic, severe and recalcitrant plaque) Can be combined with PUVA (Re-PUVA); acitretin is given 10–14 days prior to starting PUVA, which accelerates the response Usual dose: 25–50 mg/day	**Must avoid pregnancy 3 years after therapy** **Must avoid concurrent alcohol use** (alcohol → conversion to etretinate → increased half-life and increased teratogenicity)
Bexarotene	Third (polyaromatic)	7–9 hours	Hepatic	Hepato-biliary	All RXR	CTCL resistant to at least one systemic therapy Usual starting dose is 75 mg/day up to 300 mg/day Response to treatment takes up to 6 months	**Central hypothyroidism,** leukopenia, ↑ TG **Avoid gemfibrozil** (worsens hyper-TG) "beXarotene = RXR"

[a]*Other off-label uses include: disorders of keratinization (ichthyosis,* ***pityriasis rubra pilaris,*** *keratoderma, acantholytic disorders),* ***chemoprophylaxis*** *of premalignant and malignant skin cancers (typically acitretin; nevoid basal cell carcinoma syndrome, xeroderma pigmentosum, and transplant patients).*

ASDS, *American Society for Dermatologic Surgery;* CTCL, *cutaneous T-cell lymphoma;* PUVA, *psoralen plus ultraviolet light A;* RAR, *retinoic acid receptor;* RXR, *retinoic X receptor;* TG, *triglyceride.*

↓ melanosome transfer to keratinocytes, ↑ dermal collagen I, ↑ papillary dermal elastic fibers, ↑ hyaluronic acid, ↓ matrix metalloproteinases, and ↓ angiogenesis
- **Inhibits ornithine decarboxylase**
- ↑ TH1 cytokines and ↓ TH2 cytokines (helpful in cutaneous T-cell lymphoma [CTCL])

Adverse effects of retinoids

Mucocutaneous

- Topical retinoids: dermatitis, exfoliation, and photosensitivity
- Systemic retinoids: **cheilitis (#1 AE)**, thirst, dry nasal mucosa, epistaxis, xerosis, xerophthalmia, palmoplantar peeling, **photosensitivity**, exacerbation of eczema, ***Staphylococcus aureus*** colonization in isotretinoin patients (75%–90%; as a result of dryness of the nasal mucosa), **telogen effluvium**, hair kinking, nail fragility/paronychia, **pyogenic granulomas**, **eruptive xanthomas**, delayed wound healing/keloid scar formation, and sticky sensation (palms and soles)

Systemic

- Myalgias, arthralgias, anorexia, nausea, diarrhea, abdominal pain, headache, **pseudotumor cerebri** (if used in conjunction w/ tetracyclines), fatigue, reduced night vision, hepatitis, **pancreatitis** secondary to **hypertriglyceridemia,** rarely bone toxicity (**diffuse idiopathic skeletal hyperostosis**; more common with acitretin), calcification of tendons and ligaments, and premature epiphyseal closure
- Meta-analyses have refuted the development of depression and inflammatory bowel disease
- Hyperlipidemia/hypertriglyceridemia: most common laboratory abnormality; highest risk w/ bexarotene; discontinue if fasting triglycerides **> 800 mg/dL** because of a pancreatitis risk
- Elevated liver function tests: usually transient; more frequent with acitretin than with isotretinoin or bexarotene; consider discontinuation if >3X upper limit of normal
- Central hypothyroidism (↓ TSH and T4): occurs in 80% on bexarotene; start low-dose levothyroxine in all patients
- Leukopenia (neutropenia) and agranulocytosis: most common with bexarotene
- Note: the antiretroviral drug indinavir has retinoid-like AEs

Teratogenicity

- 50%–60% of isotretinoin-exposed pregnancies result in "healthy-appearing" births (lack obvious retinoid embryopathy)
  - However, ↓ **mental function** becomes apparent in majority of these children over time: 30% have gross intellectual disability and 60% have mild-moderate mental deficits
- Most common AEs in pregnant patients exposed to isotretinoin:
  - Spontaneous abortion (20%)
  - Retinoid embryopathy (18%–28%): craniofacial, cardiac, CNS, and thymic abnormalities

Specific features of retinoid embryopathy:

- **Craniofacial:** microtia, cleft palate, mircophthalmia, hypertelorism, dysmorphic facies, and ear abnormalities
- **CNS:** microcephaly, hydrocephalus, CNVII palsy, and cortical and cerebellar defects
- **CV:** cardiac septal defects, tetralogy of Fallot, transposition of great vessels, and aortic arch hypoplasia
- **Thymic:** thymic aplasia/ectopia
- Note: no risk of retinoid embryopathy reported in male partners taking retinoids.

Contraindications

- Absolute: pregnancy, women contemplating pregnancy, noncompliance with contraception, breastfeeding, hypersensitivity to parabens (some capsules may contain parabens)
- Relative: leukopenia, moderate-to-severe hypercholesterolemia or hypertriglyceridemia, significant hepatic or renal dysfunction, and hypothyroidism (bexarotene)

Interactions

- Oral retinoids are lipophilic → **fatty meals ↑ bioavailability**
- Avoid vitamin A supplements (hypervitaminosis A)
- Methotrexate (MTX) → increased liver toxicity
- **Alcohol** + **acitretin** → conversion of acitretin to etretinate (longer half-life → increased teratogenicity)
- **Isotretinoin** + **tetracyclines** → **pseudotumor cerebri**
- **Bexarotene** + **gemfibrozil** → bexarotene is metabolized by cytochrome P-450 3A4; avoid with gemfibrozil as it inhibits 3A4 → ↑ plasma levels of bexarotene → **severe hypertriglyceridemia**
  - Treatment of ↑ **LDL**: **statin** (may use any except simvastatin, because it interacts with 3A4)
  - Treatment of ↑ **triglycerides**: **fenofibrate** and/or omega 3

2.3 CORTICOSTEROIDS

Pharmacology key points (Table 2.3)

- Basic structure = three hexane rings and one pentane ring—modifications to this structure result in various corticosteroids (CS; e.g., addition of 1,2 double bond to hydrocortisone → prednisone)
- CS used in dermatology achieve their **desired effects via glucocorticoid** activity; **mineralocorticoid (MC) effects are never desirable** (sodium and water retention, hypertension [HTN])
  - Short-acting (hydrocortisone and cortisone): ↓ **glucocorticoid,** ↑ MC activity
  - Intermediate-acting (prednisone, prednisolone, methylprednisolone, and triamcinolone): ↑ **glucocorticoid** and ↓ **MC** activity
  - Long-acting (dexamethasone and betamethasone): ↑↑ **glucocorticoid, no MC** activity
- Glucocorticoid receptor **binds to CS in the cytoplasm → translocates to nucleus** → binds nuclear DNA to act as transcription factor → altered gene regulation/ transcription

Table 2.3 Pharmacology Key Concepts: Systemic Corticosteroids

Corticosteroid	Equivalent Dose (mg)	Glucocorticoid Potency[a]	Mineralocorticoid Potency	Plasma Half-Life (minutes)	Biologic Half-Life (hours)
Short-acting					
Cortisone	25	0.8	2 +	30–90	8–12
Cortisol (hydrocortisone)	20	1	2 +	60–120	8–12
Intermediate-acting					
Prednisone	5	4	1 +	60	24–36
Prednisolone	5	4	1 +	115–212	24–36
Methylprednisolone	4	5	0	180	24–36
Triamcinolone	4	5	0	78–188	24–36
Long-acting					
Dexamethasone	0.75	20–30	0	100–300	36–54
Betamethasone	0.6–0.75	20–30	0	100–300	36–54

[a]Glucocorticoid potency is expressed in a relative scale without specific units of measure; this relative potency number is inversely related to the equivalent dose in the first column.
From Wolverton S. Comprehensive Dermatologic Drug Therapy. 3rd ed. Philadelphia: Elsevier; 2012.

- Cortisol-binding globulin (CBG) is main carrier protein—steroid that is bound to CBG is inactive and unbound steroid (free fraction) is active
  - ↑ CBG: estrogen therapy, pregnancy, and hyperthyroidism → ↓ CS free fraction
  - ↓ CBG: hypothyroidism, liver disease, renal disease, and obesity → ↑ CS free fraction
- 11β-**hydroxysteroid dehydrogenase** in liver converts steroids to active forms:
  - Cortisone (inactive form) → cortisol (aka hydrocortisone, active form)
  - Prednisone (inactive form) → prednisolone (active form)
  - **Liver disease can impair conversion** → preferable to **give active forms** of steroids in this setting (e.g., prednisolone instead of prednisone)
- Mechanism of action (MoA) via immunosuppressive and anti-inflammatory effects, primarily via cytokine alterations (e.g., ↓ proinflammatory cytokines and ↑ anti-inflammatory cytokines)
  - Decreased: NF-κB, AP-1, phospholipase A2, eicosanoids (e.g., leukotrienes, prostaglandins, 12-HETE, and 15-HETE), COX-2, activity of all types of WBCs, fibroblast activity, and prostaglandin production
  - Increased: IL-10 (major downregulator of cell-mediated immunity), anti-inflammatory proteins (e.g., vasocortin, lipocortins, and vasoregulin), and ↑ apoptosis of lymphocytes and eosinophils
  - Major effects on **cellular immunity** (> humoral immunity) and cell trafficking
- Physiologic CS = 5 to 7.5 mg/day of prednisone
  - Serum cortisol peaks between 6 and 8 a.m.

Adverse effects (systemic)

Hypothalamic-pituitary-adrenal (HPA) axis suppression (Box 2.1)

- Resulting from **systemic steroids** > topical CS
- Hypothalamus releases corticotropin-releasing factor (CRH) → anterior pituitary releases adrenocorticotropic hormone (**ACTH**) → adrenal glands release **cortisol**
- **HPA axis** (CRH → ACTH → cortisol) is **suppressed** by use of exogenous CS
  - Hypothalamus: first to be suppressed, but quickest to recover
  - Adrenals: last to be suppressed, but **slowest to recover**
- **MC axis** (renin-angiotensin-aldosterone) is **NOT suppressed** by exogenous CS used in dermatology → true adrenal (Addisonian) crisis does not occur because of the preserved MC axis function
- Exogenous adrenal insufficiency (HPA axis suppression) typically seen in patients taking pharmacologic CS doses for **≥3 to 4 weeks**
- Risk factors:
  - **Abrupt cessation** of CS (taper if CS course is > 4 weeks)
  - Major stressor (surgery, trauma, or illness)
  - Divided dosing (BID or TID)
  - Daily dose given at any time other than the morning
- **Alternate-day (QOD)** dosing → ↓ **risk** of nearly all major complications
  - ↓ Risk of: HPA axis suppression, growth suppression, HTN, opportunistic infections, and electrolyte disturbances
  - Does **not** lower risk of: **cataracts** or **osteoporosis**
- Exogenous adrenal insufficiency most commonly presents as **steroid withdrawal syndrome:** arthralgias, myalgias, mood changes, headache, fatigue, and anorexia/nausea/vomiting; **no change in serum cortisol level**, but rather ↓ available intracellular CS

Box 2.1 Layman's Explanation of Exogenous Adrenal Insufficiency

If you keep giving a person systemic steroids with glucocorticoid (cortisol-like) effects, their adrenal glands become "lazy" and stop making endogenous cortisol → over time, the adrenals become shrunken/atrophic, and can no longer produce adequate cortisol; immediately upon cessation of systemic steroid administration → "exogenous adrenal insufficiency" as a result of insufficient cortisol → may appear to be steroid withdrawal syndrome (most common), or very rarely, adrenal (Addisonian[a]) crisis.

[a]Of note, the mineralocorticoid axis (renin-angiotensin-aldosterone) is almost NEVER suppressed in "exogenous adrenal insufficiency" → almost never get true adrenal (Addisonian) crisis with hypotension, coma.

Glucocorticoid effects

- Hyperglycemia and increased appetite/weight gain

Mineralocorticoid effects (tend to occur with CS with high MC effect)

- As a result of "aldosterone-like" activity of some CS
- HTN, congestive heart failure (CHF), weight gain, and hypokalemia

Lipid effects

- Hypertriglyceridemia (may result in acute pancreatitis), cushingoid changes, menstrual irregularity, and lipodystrophy (**moon face, buffalo hump, and central obesity**)

Pediatric effects

- Growth impairment (as a result of ↓ growth hormone and IGF-1 production)
- ↓ risk with QOD dosing

Musculoskeletal/vascular effects

- **Osteoporosis: QOD dosing does NOT ↓ risk**; consider calcium + vitamin D and/or bisphosphonates, teriparatide, nasal calcitonin; **greatest reduction in bone mass occurs in first 6 months**; ↑ fracture risk in postmenopausal women; **greatest absolute loss of bone mass occurs in young men** (they have highest baseline bone mass)
- Osteonecrosis: usually at least 2- to 3-month courses; proximal femur most common
  - Imaging test of choice: **MRI**
- Hypocalcemia
- Venous thromboembolism

Gastrointestinal effects

- Bowel perforation, peptic ulcer disease (mainly if total dose ≥ 1 g, H_2 antagonists or proton pump inhibitors can help), fatty liver changes, esophageal reflux, and nausea/vomiting

Ocular effects

- **Cataracts (risk does NOT change with QOD dosing)**, glaucoma, infections, and refraction changes

Psychiatric changes

- Psychosis, hypomania, insomnia, agitation, and depression

Neurologic effects

- Pseudotumor cerebri, seizures, epidural lipomatosis, and peripheral neuropathy

Opportunistic infections

- Tuberculosis (TB) reactivation, deep fungi, prolonged herpes virus infections, and *Pneumocystis jiroveci* pneumonia
- **↓ risk with QOD dosing**

Muscular effects

- Myopathy (proximal lower extremity weakness) and muscular atrophy

Cutaneous effects

- **↓ wound healing, striae, atrophy, telangiectasias, steroid acne**, purpura, infections (staphylococcal, herpes virus), telogen effluvium, hirsutism, generalized pustular psoriasis (upon drug withdrawal), perioral dermatitis, contact dermatitis, and hypopigmentation

Contraindications

- Systemic fungal infections, herpes simplex keratitis, and steroid allergy

Pregnancy

- **Likely safe for short** courses—high dose may result in intrauterine growth retardation and inhibition of endogenous corticosteroid production

Clinical use

- Inflammatory dermatoses (atopic and allergic contact dermatitis, urticaria, connective tissue disorders, vasculitides, neutrophilic dermatoses, autoimmune blistering disease, papulosquamous dermatoses, drug reactions): commonly dosed at 0.5 to 2 mg/kg/day
  - A steroid-sparing immunosuppressive drug is often used concurrently for chronic inflammatory disease
- Toxicodendron dermatitis: short steroid taper → ↑ likelihood of rebound flare; best option is a 3-week tapering course starting at about 1 mg/kg daily
- Note: oral CS ↓ acute pain in herpes zoster, but likely do not prevent postherpetic neuralgia
- Longer duration of treatment = ↑ AE risk
- **Divided dose regimens** are **more effective**, but have a **higher risk of AEs** than single-dose regimens (best taken in AM to simulate body's diurnal variation of cortisol production)
- QOD dosing: the anti-inflammatory effects of CS last longer than the HPA axis suppressive effects → QOD dosing helps maintain control of disease activity after course with daily CS

Intramuscular CS

- Unique AEs: **cold abscesses**, subcutaneous fat atrophy, crystal deposition, menstrual irregularities, and purpura
- Main advantages (vs. oral CS): **compliance**, can be given in setting of nausea/vomiting
- Main disadvantages (vs. oral CS): **↑ HPA axis suppression** because levels are constant throughout the day (↑ frequency of intramuscular [IM] injections → ↑ risk of HPA axis suppression), and less ability to precisely taper
  - Per Wolverton, do not use long-acting IM CS (such as triamcinolone) >3 to 4 times/year

Pulse IV CS

- Generally 0.5 to 1 g of methylprednisolone intravenously (IV) over ≥1 hour × 5 consecutive days

- Indications: systemic vasculitis, systemic lupus erythematosus (SLE), pyoderma gangrenosum, and bullous pemphigoid
- AEs: sudden cardiac death, atrial fibrillation, anaphylaxis, electrolyte shifts, and seizures

Intralesional CS

- Typically triamcinolone acetonide 2 to 40 mg/mL, depending on disorder/location/thickness of lesion
- Used for prurigo nodularis, keloids, alopecia areata, discoid lupus, and lichen planopilaris
- AEs: **atrophy** (inject in dermis!) and hypopigmentation

Topical CS (Table 2.4)

- Of note, more potent topical steroids (e.g., clobetasol) and those in more highly absorbed bases (e.g., gels and ointments) are more likely to cause adverse cutaneous effects
  - Potency based off of vasoconstriction assay
  - Risk of HPA suppression is low with topical steroids
  - Can develop contact dermatitis to topical steroids (see Chapter 3.2)
- One fingertip unit = 0.5 g of topical steroids and covers 2% body surface area
- Wet wrap therapy—topical steroid covered by a wetted layer of bandages, followed by a dry outside layer → occludes topical steroid for increased penetration and absorption
  - Use with high-potency steroids has the potential for HPA axis suppression

Monitoring

Consider monitoring:

- Fasting glucose levels, blood pressure lipids, weight, height/weight for children, **DEXA** scans (T score < −2.5 = osteoporosis), **MRI** if pain in hip/shoulder/knee (osteonecrosis), and slit-lamp examination q6–12 months
- Screening for infectious disease (TB, hepatitis, HIV)
- Tests to evaluate adrenal insufficiency
  - **AM cortisol**: primary screening tool, >10 mcg/dL = good basal adrenal function
  - **24-hour urine free cortisol**: more accurate test for basal adrenal function (advantage); main disadvantage is patient compliance with 24-hour urine collection
  - **ACTH stimulation**: most commonly used provocative test for adrenal function; check basal cortisol level →

Table 2.4 Potency of Topical Steroids

Class	Drug	Dosage Form(s)	Strength (%)
I. Very high potency	Augmented betamethasone dipropionate	Ointment	0.05
	Clobetasol propionate	Cream, foam, ointment	0.05
	Diflorasone diacetate	Ointment	0.05
	Halobetasol propionate	Cream, ointment	0.05
II. High potency	Amcinonide	Cream, lotion, ointment	0.1
	Augmented betamethasone dipropionate	Cream	0.05
	Betamethasone dipropionate	Cream, foam, ointment, solution	0.05
	Desoximetasone	Cream, ointment	0.25
	Desoximetasone	Gel	0.05
	Diflorasone diacetate	Cream	0.05
	Fluocinonide	Cream, gel, ointment, solution	0.05
	Halcinonide	Cream, ointment	0.1
	Mometasone furoate	Ointment	0.1
	Triamcinolone acetonide	Cream, ointment	0.5
III-IV. Medium potency	Betamethasone valerate	Cream, foam, lotion, ointment	0.1
	Clocortolone pivalate	Cream	0.1
	Desoximetasone	Cream	0.05
	Fluocinolone acetonide	Cream, ointment	0.025
	Flurandrenolide	Cream, ointment	0.05
	Fluticasone propionate	Cream	0.05
	Fluticasone propionate	Ointment	0.005
	Mometasone furoate	Cream	0.1
	Triamcinolone acetonide	Cream, ointment	0.1
V. Lower-medium potency	Hydrocortisone butyrate	Cream, ointment, solution	0.1
	Hydrocortisone probutate	Cream	0.1
	Hydrocortisone valerate	Cream, ointment	0.2
	Prednicarbate	Cream	0.1
VI. Low potency	Alclometasone dipropionate	Cream, ointment	0.05
	Desonide	Cream, gel, foam, ointment	0.05
	Fluocinolone acetonide	Cream, solution	0.01
VII. Lowest potency	Dexamethasone	Cream	0.1
	Hydrocortisone	Cream, lotion, ointment, solution	0.25, 0.5, 1
	Hydrocortisone acetate	Cream, ointment	0.5–1

From Eichenfield LF, Tom WL, Berger TG, et al. Guidelines of care for the management of atopic dermatitis: section 2. Management and treatment of atopic dermatitis with topical therapies. J Am Acad Dermatol. *2014;71(1):116–132.*

then inject ACTH → check cortisol levels at 30 and 60 minutes
  - Others: insulin hypoglycemia, metyrapone, and CRH

2.4 IMMUNOMODULATORY AGENTS

Apremilast and other PDE-4 inhibitors

- Intracellular phosphodiesterase-4 (PDE-4) inhibitor
  - PDE-4 hydrolyzes cAMP (an intracellular messenger which regulates inflammation) to AMP
  - Inhibiting PDE-4 → ↑ cAMP → ↓ IFN-γ, TNF-α, IL-23, and ↑ IL-10 (anti-inflammatory mediator)
- Food and Drug Administration (FDA) approved for psoriasis, psoriatic arthritis, and Behçet's disease
- AEs: diarrhea, nausea, weight loss, depression (1%)
- Dose halved in patients with severe renal impairment
- No laboratory monitoring required
  - No reports of TB or malignancy
- **Crisaborole** (FDA approved for atopic dermatitis in patients aged 3+ months) and **roflumilast** (FDA approved for psoriasis in patients aged 12+ years) are topical PDE-4 inhibitors
  - Crisaborole AEs: application site pain (burning, stinging); roflumilast AEs (diarrhea, headache)

Janus Kinase (JAK) and Tyro sine Kinase 2 (TYK2) inhibitors

Mechanism of action

- Regulates intracellular signaling via the JAK STAT pathway (Fig. 2.1); inhibits gene transcription/growth factor signaling pathways and cytokine production
- There are 4 JAK proteins (JAK1-3, TYK2) and 7 STAT proteins (STAT1-4, 5A, 5B, 6)

Agents used in dermatology

- Tofacitinib: JAK 1 and 3 inhibitor; FDA approved for rheumatoid arthritis and psoriatic arthritis
- Ruxolitinib: JAK 1 and 2 inhibitor; 1.5% cream FDA approved for atopic dermatitis and non-segmental vitiligo; max of 60 g/wk, tx area < 20% BSA for atopic dermatitis and < 10% for vitiligo
- Upadacitinib: JAK 1 inhibitor; FDA approved for moderate to severe atopic dermatitis [12 years and older], psoriatic arthritis and rheumatoid arthritis
- Abrocitinib: JAK 1 inhibitor; FDA approved for moderate to severe atopic dermatitis in adults
- Baricitinib: JAK 1 and 2 inhibitor; FDA approved for severe alopecia areata and rheumatoid arthritis in adults
- Deucravactinib: TYK2 inhibitor; FDA approved for moderate to severe psoriasis in adults

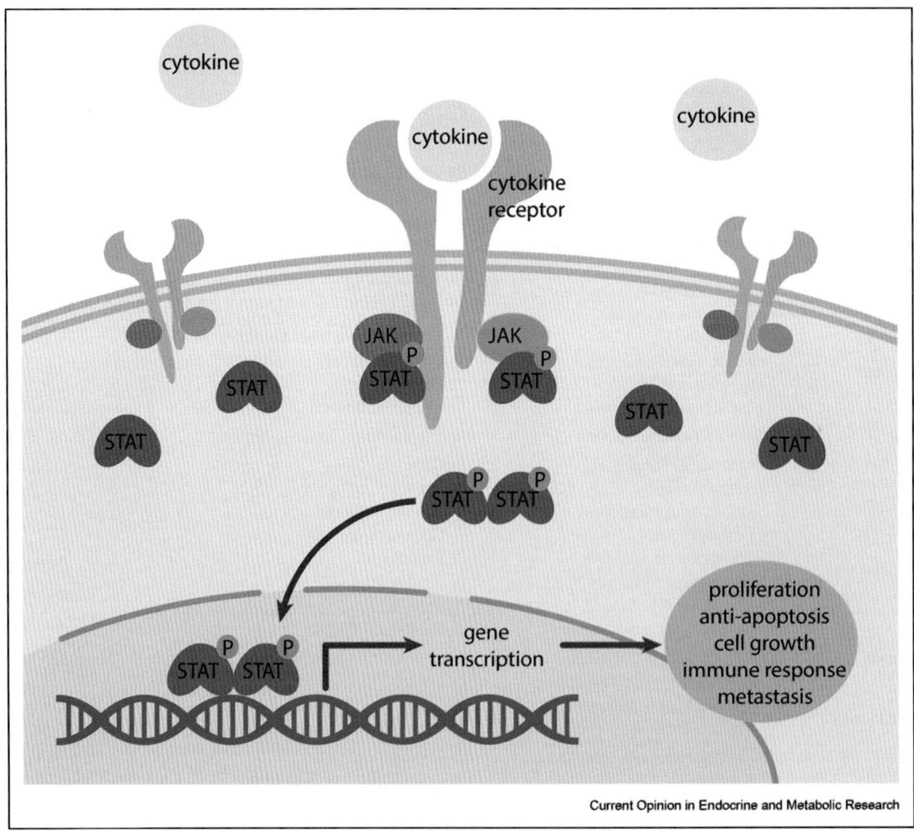

Fig. 2.1 Upon cytokine binding to their receptors, Janus kinase (JAK) family members are recruited and activated through tyrosine-phosphorylation of their cytoplasmic domains, which results in phosphorylation of signal transducer and activator of transcription (STAT). STAT heterodimers and homodimers translocate to the nucleus and bind to DNA sequences at the promoter regions of genes that regulate cell proliferation, differentiation, and apoptosis. (From Canesin G, Krzyzanowska A, Hellsten R, Bjartell A. Cytokines and Janus kinase/signal transducer and activator of transcription signaling in prostate cancer: overview and therapeutic opportunities. Curr Opin Endocr Metab Res. 2020;10:36-42.)

Adverse effects

- Common: upper respiratory infections, diarrhea/nausea, headaches, increases in cholesterol/LFTs/CPK/Cre, herpes simplex/zoster, acne
- Serious: cardiovascular death/event risk, severe infections (e.g. TB, invasive fungal infections, viral reactivation), malignancy (e.g. lymphoproliferative disorders, lung cancer, non-melanoma skin cancer), thromboembolism (e.g. DVT, pulmonary embolism, arterial thrombosis), GI perforation, neutropenia/lymphopenia/anemia
- Major adverse cardiovascular death/event and thromboembolism risk higher in those over 50 years with at least 1 risk factor
- Deucravacitinib does not carry black box warnings like the other JAK inhibitors; when used appropriately, topical ruxolitinib appears to be quite safe

Laboratory monitoring

- Monitoring depends of specific medication but includes TB testing (baseline), hepatitis panel (baseline), pregnancy testing (baseline; if appropriate), lipid panel, LFTs, Cr/eGFR, CBC w/ differential

Azathioprine

Mechanism of action (Fig. 2.2)

- Azathioprine's **active metabolite, 6-TG (thioguanine)**, is produced by the hypoxanthine guanine phosphoribosyltransferase (HPRT) pathway and shares similarities with endogenous purines → incorporated into DNA and RNA (S-phase of replication) → inhibits purine metabolism and cell division (particularly in fast-growing cells that do not have a salvage pathway, like lymphocytes)
- Xanthine oxidase and **thiopurine methyltransferase** (TPMT) convert azathioprine into inactive metabolites
  - ↓ activity of **TPMT** (measured by allele activity) or ↓ **xanthine oxidase** (as a result of **allopurinol** or **febuxostat**) → ↑ azathioprine levels → ↑ risk of **life-threatening myelosuppression**
  - ACE inhibitors, sulfasalazine, and concomitant use of folate antagonists also increases risk of myelosuppression
  - Azathioprine may decrease anticoagulant effects of warfarin and reverse neuromuscular blockade
- Diminishes T-cell function > antibody production by B cells

Adverse effects

- Leukopenia (correlates with low TPMT activity)
- Cutaneous squamous cell carcinoma (SCC) and lymphoma (controversial)
- Infection (particularly human papilloma virus [HPV], herpes simplex virus [HSV])
- Teratogenicity
- **Hypersensitivity syndrome**: occurs within the first **4 weeks** of therapy; fever, nausea, vomiting, diarrhea,

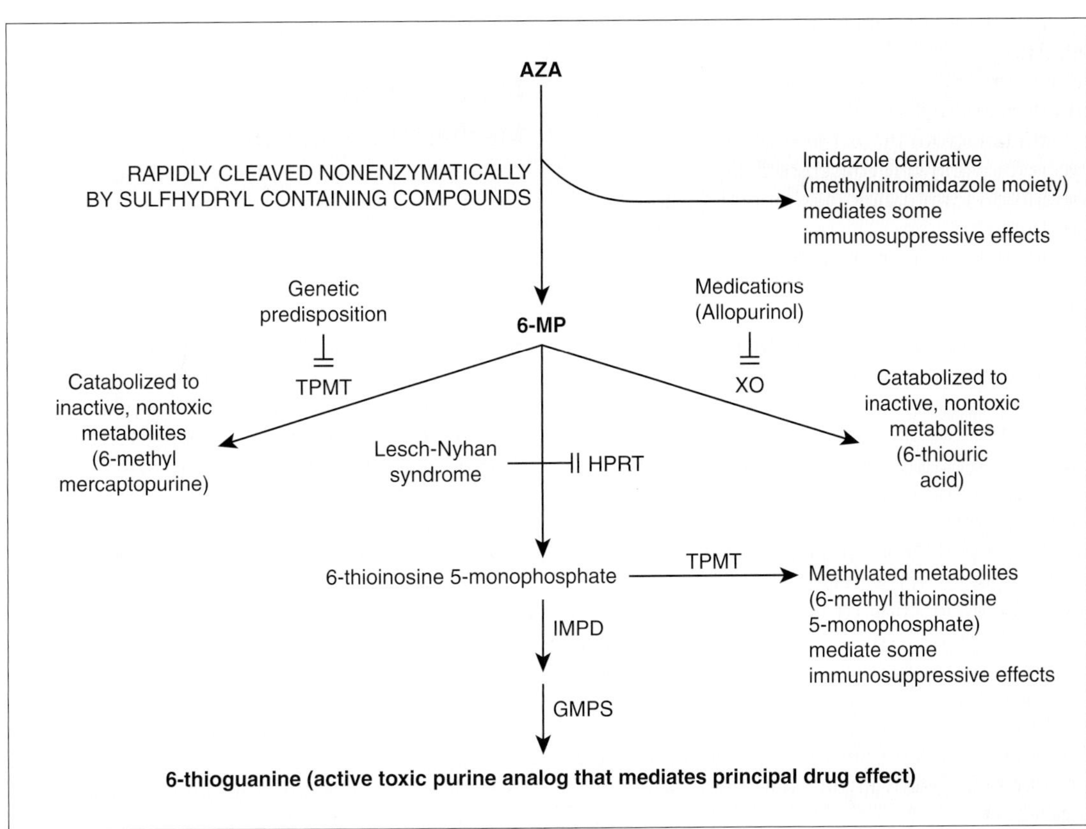

Fig. 2.2 Azathioprine metabolism. *6-MP*, 6-Mercaptopurine; *AZA*, azathioprine; *GMPS*, Guanosine monophosphate synthetase; *HPRT*, hypoxanthine guanine phosphoribosyltransferase; *IMPD*, Inosine monophosphate dehydrogenase; *TPMT*, thiopurine methyltransferase; *XO*, xanthine oxidase. (Redrawn from Patel AA, Swerlick RA, McCall CO. Azathioprine in dermatology: the past, the present, and the future. *J Am Acad Dermatol*. 2006;55[3]:369–389.)

arthralgia, and malaise → hypotension, shock; resolves with discontinuation
  - Skin manifestations may mimic neutrophilic dermatosis
- Gastrointestinal (GI) AEs—**most common AEs**—nausea, vomiting, diarrhea, gastritis, and pancreatitis
- Hepatoxicity is rare
- If given with TNF-α inhibitor → ↑ risk of **hepatosplenic T-cell lymphoma** in patients with inflammatory bowel disease

Important monitoring points

- TPMT assay before starting therapy (homozygous TPMT deficiency is a contraindication to therapy)
- Monitor CBC, comprehensive metabolic panel (CMP; with LFTs) every 2 weeks for 2 months, then every 2–3 months
- Skin exams due to SCC and lymphoma risk

Cyclosporine

Mechanism of action

- Forms a complex with cyclophilin, which inhibits calcineurin—an intracellular enzyme—which in turn reduces the activity of nuclear factor of activated T cells/ NFAT-1(transcribes various cytokines, such as IL-2)
- ↓ **IL-2 production** → ↓ CD4 and CD8 T-cell activation

Important pharmacology points

- Rapid onset of action; cyclosporine should ideally be gradually tapered while an alternative therapy is instituted to prevent flaring
- Microemulsion formulation more easily absorbed
- **Maximum dermatologic dose** = **5 mg/kg** daily and can be used continuously for up to 1 year according to the FDA (2 years for worldwide consensus data)
  - Microemulsion formulation maximum dermatologic dose = 4 mg/kg
- Bioavailability determined by CYP450

Indications

- FDA approved for psoriasis but used off-label for various inflammatory and autoimmune dermatoses

Adverse effects

- Contraindicated in patients with uncontrolled HTN, renal disease, serious infections, and in those with a previous history of malignancy
- **Nephrotoxicity** and **HTN** are the two most notable AEs, which are dose- and duration-dependent
  - 2° to vascular dysfunction (renal vasoconstriction) and tubular dysfunction
  - Irreversible kidney damage is avoided if patients receive **dermatologic doses** (2.5–5 mg/kg daily), have **dose adjusted when creatinine increases by 30%** from baseline, and use cyclosporine for **no longer than 1 year**
  - HTN can be managed by medication rather than by dose reduction
    - **Prescription of choice** = **calcium channel blockers (CCBs;** e.g., nifedipine or isradipine)—vasodilate renal arterioles and do not alter cyclosporine serum levels
- ↑ **risk of nonmelanoma skin cancer (NMSC)** in psoriasis patients, especially those who have history of psoralen plus ultraviolet light A (PUVA)
  - Risk of other malignancies, such as lymphoma, is unclear
- **Hyperlipidemia** not uncommon—dietary changes and ↑ physical activity should be recommended
- ↑ risk of **myopathy when taken with statins**
- Other AEs include: **hypertrichosis**, **gingival hyperplasia**, myalgia, neurologic AEs (paresthesia, tremors), malaise, **hyperuricemia** (can precipitate gout), **hypomagnesemia**, and **hyperkalemia**

Important monitoring points

- Recheck creatinine level if ↑ by > 30% from baseline on two separate readings 2 weeks apart → if remains elevated above 30%, ↓ dose by at least 1 mg/kg for 4 weeks, then:
  - If the creatinine level drops back down to < 30% above baseline, can continue therapy
  - If the creatinine level remains elevated, then discontinue therapy; if it returns to within 10% of baseline, cyclosporine can be resumed at a lower dose
  - If at any time the creatinine level increases by ≥ 50% above baseline, discontinue therapy until the level returns to baseline
- Blood pressure, blood urea nitrogen (BUN), and creatinine levels should be measured at baseline, weeks 2, 4, 6, and 8, and then monthly
- Baseline CBC, CMP (including uric acid, Mg^{++}, K^{+}), urinalysis (UA), lipid profile—recheck monthly
- Regular dental care
- No risk of teratogenicity in pregnancy

Methotrexate

Mechanism of action

- Binds dihydrofolate reductase with greater affinity than folic acid → **prevents conversion of dihydrofolate to tetrahydrofolate** (a necessary cofactor of purine synthesis) → inhibition of cell division (S phase specific)

Important pharmacology points

- The inhibition of dihydrofolate reductase may be bypassed by **leucovorin (folinic acid)** or thymidine
  - Folinic acid: naturally occurring folate (vitamin B_9) used for rescue of high-dose MTX AEs (pancytopenia)
- **Folic acid** (synthetic) and folinic acid (naturally occurring): ↓ **MTX-induced AEs**
  - ↓ GI AEs by 26% (nausea, vomiting, and abdominal pain)
  - ↓ risk of LFT abnormalities by 76%
  - ↓ risk of pancytopenia
  - ↑ ability to tolerate MTX (↓ MTX discontinuation rate for any reason)
- Folic acid supplementation likely has minimal impact on MTX efficacy
- MTX-induced hepatic fibrosis—liver biopsy is gold standard
  - Risk factors (significant alcohol consumption, abnormal LFTs, hepatitis, genetic liver disease, diabetes mellitus [DM], obesity, hyperlipidemia, exposure to hepatotoxins)—liver biopsy indicated after 1 to 1.5 g of MTX

- American College of Rheumatology guidelines: no risk factors—liver biopsy indicated when:
  - 5/9 LFTs elevated in a 12-month period (LFTs checked q3–4 months)
  - 3.5 to 4.0 g total cumulative dosage
- Other tests for liver toxicity: magnetic resonance elastography, vibration-controlled transient elastography, algorithm-based serologic testing, and the amino terminus of type III procollagen peptide assay (PIIIP)

Indications and contraindications

- FDA approved for psoriasis and mycosis fungoides (MF)
- Off-label dermatologic uses include: pemphigus, pemphigoid, autoimmune connective tissue diseases, sarcoidosis, vasculitis, and other inflammatory dermatoses
- **Absolute contraindications:** pregnancy (teratogenic, abortifacient), alcoholism, immunodeficiency syndromes, chronic liver disease, severe hematologic abnormalities, and lactation
  - Contraception required after completion: 3 months (M), one ovulatory cycle (F)
- Relative contraindications: ↓ renal function, hepatic disease, metabolic disease (i.e., obesity or DM), childbearing age, active infectious disease or history of potentially serious infection that could reactivate, and malignancy

Adverse effects

- Rarely reported to cause acute pneumonitis, which is idiosyncratic and can be life-threatening if MTX is not stopped, and pulmonary fibrosis (even less common)
  - Routine radiography or pulmonary function studies, without symptoms to suggest pneumonitis, are not helpful in preventing lung toxicity
- **Pancytopenia**, which can be life-threatening, usually **occurs early** (initial 4–6 weeks) in therapy and may be idiosyncratic
  - Risk factors: old age, poor renal function, and lack of folic acid supplementation
- No data that patients with psoriasis and taking MTX have ↑risk of malignancy such as lymphoma
- **GI AEs are common** (nausea/anorexia > diarrhea, vomiting, and ulcerative stomatitis)
- MTX has been reported to accumulate in renal tubules and cause renal toxicity when given at high doses for chemotherapy
- Increased serum levels due to decreased renal function can result in skin necrosis, including **epidermal necrosis limited to psoriatic plaques**
- Other AEs: alopecia, headaches, fatigue, dizziness, accelerated **nodule development in patients with rheumatoid arthritis** (RA; similar to rheumatoid nodules, but smaller and classically on fingers) and **phototoxicity** (including **UV and radiation "recall reactions"**)
- ↑ risk of **myelosuppression** when co-administered with agents that inhibit folic acid metabolism (e.g., **trimethoprim, sulfonamides, and dapsone**) or increase MTX levels by displacing MTX from bound plasma proteins (tetracyclines, phenytoin, phenothiazines, **sulfonamides**, **NSAIDs**, and salicylates)

Important monitoring points

- Viral hepatitis panel and TB at baseline; CBC w/ differential, LFTs, BUN/creatinine at baseline, then monthly for several months, decreasing frequency to q3–4 months
- May repeat CBC after 1 week to check for bone marrow suppression

Mycophenolate mofetil

Mechanism of action

- Binds and **inhibits inosine monophosphate dehydrogenase**—a key enzyme for the *de novo* synthesis of purines—which is essential in activated lymphocytes which cannot use purine salvage

Important pharmacology points

- **Requires gastric acidity** for cleavage into its active state (antacids and proton pump inhibitors ↓ serum levels)
- Dermatologic doses range from 2 to 3 g divided in twice-daily doses

Indications

- FDA approved for renal, cardiac, and liver allograft rejection prevention, but used off-label in various autoimmune and inflammatory dermatoses (e.g., atopic dermatitis, pemphigus, lupus, etc.)

Adverse effects

- Absolute contraindications: pregnancy (teratogen) and drug allergy
- Relative contraindications: lactation (may be excreted in breast milk), peptic ulcer disease, hepatic or renal disease (may require dose adjustment), drugs that interfere with enterohepatic circulation (e.g., cholestyramine), and concomitant administration with azathioprine (↑ risk of bone marrow toxicity)
- **Risk of carcinogenesis** (lymphoma and lymphoproliferative malignancies) shown in transplant population (who usually had several immunosuppressive medications given concomitantly)—unknown whether this holds true in dermatologic patients and whether there is increased risk of NMSC
- **Most common AEs = diarrhea, abdominal pain, nausea, and vomiting**
- Associated with a form of neutrophil dysplasia termed pseudo-Pelger- Huët anomaly, which is characterized by nuclear hypolobulation with a left shift—this may predict the development of neutropenia

Monitoring guidelines

- CBC/differential, CMP (w/ LFTs) at baseline, then q2–4 weeks after initiating treatment or dose escalation, and then q2–3 months once the dose is stable
- Baseline hepatitis B and C panel, TB screen

Cytotoxic agents

Hydroxyurea

- Impairs DNA synthesis through inhibition of ribonucleotide diphosphate reductase; hypomethylates DNA resulting in altered gene expression

- FDA approved for SCC of head and neck
- Dermatologic uses are mainly off-label for treatment of polycythemia vera, Sweet's syndrome, erythromelalgia, and hypereosinophilic syndrome
- Severe anemia, thrombocytopenia, and leukopenia are relative contraindications
- **Most common AE: megaloblastic anemia** (myelosuppression)
- Can cause **dermatomyositis-like eruption**, lichenoid drug eruption resembling GVHD, **leg ulcers**, alopecia, photosensitivity, radiation recall, and **hyperpigmentation of the skin and nails**

Cyclophosphamide

- An **alkylating agent** (exerts its effect by directly damaging DNA via cross-linking)
  - Nitrogen mustard derivative
  - Aldophosphamide, one of its metabolites, is cleaved intracellularly into acrolein and enhances cellular damage by depleting glutathione store
- FDA approved for the treatment of MF (advanced disease)
- Off-label dermatologic uses: severe immunobullous disease (e.g., **ocular cicatricial pemphigoid**), severe systemic vasculitides, neutrophilic dermatoses, and autoimmune connective tissue diseases
- **Hemorrhagic cystitis** occurs in 5%–41% as a result of acrolein (prevented by adequate hydration as well as mesna, which binds acrolein in the bladder and reduces irritation)
  - ↑ **risk of transitional cell carcinoma** of the bladder, non-Hodgkin's lymphoma, leukemia, and SCC (in transplant and oncology patients)
  - Monitoring: periodic urine analysis with cytologic examination
- Nausea and vomiting are the most common AEs and can be decreased by co-administering with ondansetron and dexamethasone
- ↑ **risk of infertility**: amenorrhea (27%–60%); premature ovarian failure (up to 80%)
- Cutaneous AEs: permanent pigmented band on the teeth, **anagen effluvium**, and **hyperpigmentation of skin and nails**

Chlorambucil

- Alkylating agent that directly damages DNA via cross-linking
- Rare off-label dermatologic uses: necrobiotic xanthogranuloma (shown to be effective and safe in a retrospective review of 48 cases), pyoderma gangrenosum, and immunobullous and connective tissue disease
- Allergy to nitrogen mustard is a contraindication
- Epileptogenic and mood-altering potential
- Other AEs: nausea, vomiting, azoospermia, amenorrhea, pulmonary fibrosis, hepatotoxicity, bone marrow suppression, and oral ulcers

Antimalarial agents

- Include hydroxychloroquine (HCQ), chloroquine (CQ), and quinacrine (off the market in the United States, but still available in compounding pharmacies)

Mechanism of action

- Unknown, thought to work via several different proposed mechanisms:
  - **Inhibit UV-induced cutaneous reactions** by binding to DNA and inhibiting superoxide production
  - Raise intracytoplasmic pH and stabilize lysosomes → ↓ ability of macrophages to express MHC complex antigens on cell surface (↓ antigen presentation, inflammation)
  - Reduce lysosomal size and impair chemotaxis
  - Block toll-like receptors
  - Inhibit platelet aggregation and adhesion (antithrombotic)

Important pharmacology points

- CQ and HCQ have long half-lives and steady-state concentration is attained at 3 to 4 months, which explains the long treatment duration required to achieve clinical benefit
- **Quinacrine may be added to HCQ or CQ for ↑ therapeutic effect**
- CQ and HCQ should **not** be given together

Indications

- FDA approved for lupus, malaria, and RA
- Off-label dermatologic uses: particularly useful in disorders with significant lymphocytic infiltrates (polymorphous light eruptions, lymphocytic infiltrate of Jessner, lupus panniculitis, and discoid lupus erythematosus [LE]), GVHD, sarcoid
- **Low (twice-weekly) dosing used in porphyria cutanea tarda (PCT)**

Adverse effects

- Possibly safe in pregnancy with debatable risks (CQ > HCQ)
- Absolute contraindications: hypersensitivity to the drug (may have cross-reaction between CQ and HCQ); continued use is contraindicated in patients who develop **retinopathy**
- Relative contraindications include severe blood dyscrasias, significant hepatic dysfunction, significant neurologic disorders, retinal or visual field changes, pregnancy and lactation (however, some suggest that the risk of discontinuing treatment in pregnancy in patients with SLE outweighs the risk of toxicity to the fetus), and psoriasis
- CQ is contraindicated in patients with myasthenia gravis
- **Mucocutaneous drug reactions:**
  - Affinity for melanin (skin and retina)—absorbs UV light
  - Yellow pigmentation of the skin (quinacrine)
  - Lichenoid drug eruption
  - Morbilliform hypersensitivity eruption; may also present as erythroderma or Stevens-Johnsons syndrome (SJS)
    - **Risk is much greater in dermatomyositis (31%) than lupus (3%)**
  - Psoriasis exacerbation (CQ in particular)
  - **Bluish-gray to black hyperpigmentation** in 10% to 30% of patients treated for ≥ 4 months typically affecting the **shins** (clinically indistinguishable from type II minocycline hyperpigmentation), face, and palate
  - Hair hypopigmentation (CQ)

- **Nail hyperpigmentation**
- Ophthalmologic toxicity includes corneal deposits (keratopathy), neuromuscular eye toxicity (ciliary body dysfunction), and retinopathy (maculopathy)
  - Premaculopathy is reversible, but bull's eye retinopathy is **irreversible**
  - **Ocular toxicity is NOT seen in quinacrine therapy**
  - Additive risk of retinal toxicity when CQ and HCQ combined
- Current eye monitoring recommendations from American Academy of Ophthalmology:
  - Maximum daily dose of HCQ < 5.0 mg/kg real weight
  - Fundus examination **within first year** of starting therapy
  - Annual screening **after 5 years** of treatment (some patients, such as the elderly, may require more frequent examinations)
- GI AEs (CQ > HCQ): most common reason for early reduction or D/C of treatment
- Restlessness, excitement, confusion, and seizures (usually in patients on higher-than-recommended doses)
- Rare, but potentially fatal, bone marrow toxicity has been reported with quinacrine and agranulocytosis with CQ
- **Hemolysis in the glucose-6-phoshate dehydrogenase (G6PD)-deficient population** is mainly a concern for 8-aminoquinoline and primaquine, but not for usual doses of HCQ and CQ
  - G6PD testing is not necessary for HCQ, CQ, and quinacrine given low risk of hemolysis with therapeutic doses

Dapsone

Mechanism of action

- **Inhibits myeloperoxidase** → ↓ oxidative damage to normal tissue in various **neutrophilic dermatoses** (affects eosinophils and monocytes to a lesser extent)
- Also ↓ hydrogen peroxide and hydroxyl radical levels
- It may also ↓ chemotaxis of neutrophils, although this has not been demonstrated in therapeutic doses

Important pharmacology points

- Dapsone undergoes significant enterohepatic recirculation, thus remaining in the circulation 30 days after a single dose
- Hemolysis has been demonstrated in nursing infants of mothers taking dapsone. No harmful *in utero* developmental effects are demonstrated when taken during pregnancy, but theoretical risk of neonatal hyperbilirubinemia
- There is significant variability both in individual rates of acetylation (not clinically relevant) and hydroxylation. The hydroxylamine metabolite dapsone hydroxylamine (DDS-NOH) is responsible for hematologic AEs.

Indications

- FDA-approved indications are **dermatitis herpetiformis** and leprosy
- Off-label dermatologic uses are numerous and include various **neutrophilic dermatoses** (linear IgA dermatosis, bullous SLE, erythema elevatum diutinum, pyoderma gangrenosum, Sweet's syndrome, neutrophilic urticaria, subcorneal pustular dermatosis/IgA pemphigus, and Behçet's disease), and vasculitides
  - Most patients treated with dapsone for **dermatitis herpetiformis rapidly respond within 24 to 36 hours**

Adverse effects

- Cross-reactivity between dapsone and sulfapyridine, or other sulfonamide-type drugs, is rare
- Greater care should be taken in patients with increased risk of developing hematologic, cardiovascular, or pulmonary AEs (patients with **G6PD deficiency**; significant cardiopulmonary, liver, or renal disease)
- **Hemolytic anemia** and **methemoglobinemia:** dose-related and **occurs in ALL individuals** to some degree (related to oxidative stress from N-hydroxy metabolites)
  - ↑ methemoglobin → ↓ oxygen-carrying capacity → may exacerbate preexisting cardiopulmonary disease
  - Can cause a falsely low hemoglobin A1c
  - Cimetidine decreases the risk of methemoglobinemia without affecting dapsone's plasma level
  - Vitamin E may also provide small amount of protection against methemoglobinemia
  - Methemoglobinemia emergency → use **methylene blue**
  - Worsening of methemoglobinemia has been shown intra- and postoperatively after both local amide and general anesthetic; vitamin C can be used when this occurs
- **Agranulocytosis**, the most serious **idiosyncratic** reaction to dapsone, occurs between 3 and 12 weeks and may manifest as fever, pharyngitis, and occasionally sepsis
  - Most recover quickly after cessation of dapsone; may consider giving G-CSF
- **Peripheral neuropathy** (predominantly **distal motor**) + some degree of sensory involvement; may present as wasting of hand muscles; reversible if detected early
- Nausea, gastritis, reversible cholestasis and hepatitis, and hypersensitivity syndrome (typically after 3–12 weeks of therapy) have also been reported

Important monitoring points

- **Baseline G6PD level** (lower levels may preclude patient from receiving medication, or require ↓ dose)
- CBC w/ differential, LFTs, renal function tests, and UA at baseline
- Must monitor CBC very closely during "high-risk window" for agranulocytosis: CBC weekly for 4 weeks, then every 2 weeks until 3 months into treatment (agranulocytosis is most common in first 12 weeks of treatment)
- After 3 months, continue checking renal function, LFTs, and UA q3–4 months
- Methemoglobin levels are needed if there is clinical suspicion of decreased oxygen circulation or anemia

Biologics (Fig. 2.3, Table 2.5)

TNF-α inhibitors

Etanercept

- Fully human dimeric fusion protein (TNF-receptor linked to Fc portion of IgG) that binds both TNF-α (soluble and membrane-bound) and TNF-β
- Subcutaneous

Infliximab

- Chimeric monoclonal IgG antibody binding TNF-α (targets soluble and transmembrane TNF receptor)
- Intravenous

Adalimumab

- Fully human monoclonal IgG antibody against transmembrane TNF receptor
- Subcutaneous

Certolizumab pegol

- PEGylated TNF-α inhibitor—attachment of PEG polymers delays metabolism and increases half-life
- Lacks an IgG Fc region—limits transfer through the placenta and decreases teratogenic potential during pregnancy
- Subcutaneous

Golimumab

- Human monoclonal IgG antibody against soluble and transmembrane TNF
- Subcutaneous

Indications

- FDA approved for plaque psoriasis and psoriatic arthritis; adalimumab approved for hidradenitis suppurativa
- Golimumab approved for psoriatic arthritis but not psoriasis
- Etanercept approved for pediatric psoriasis age > 4

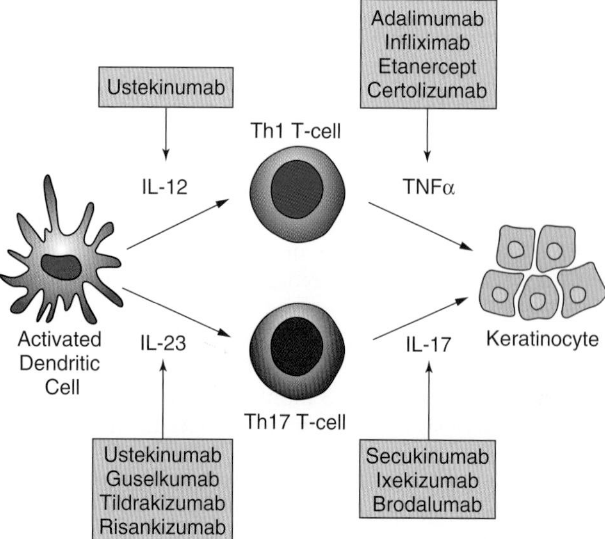

Fig. 2.3 Mechanism of action of biologic drugs for psoriasis. *IL*, Interleukin; *TNF*, tumor necrosis factor

Adverse effects

- **Injection site reactions: etanercept** (14%) > adalimumab (3.2%)
  - For etanercept, these are believed to be most pronounced during the second injection and usually improve after 1 month of therapy (hypothesized to be caused by delayed-type hypersensitivity). Treatment is to change to a new injection site
- Infliximab commonly causes infusion reactions (20%):
  - Nausea, headache, flushing, dyspnea, injection site infiltration, and taste perversion
  - ↓ **infusion rate** and **premedication** may help
  - Epinephrine and systemic CS are given for serious reactions (less than 1% of treated patients) including hypotension, chest pain, dyspnea, anaphylaxis, and convulsions
- Multiple case series report patients on TNF-inhibitors developing various **demyelinating diseases** (e.g., multiple sclerosis, Guillain-Barré syndrome, and optic neuritis)
- **Development of psoriasis, palmoplantar pustulosis, connective tissue disease (+ANA, lupus, DM) and cutaneous vasculitis have been reported with all TNF inhibitors**
  - Highest risk of drug-induced lupus with infliximab; treatment is withdrawal of drug
- Malignancy risk, particularly **lymphoma** and possibly skin cancer, may be increased in patients treated with biologic agents
  - **Hepatosplenic T-cell lymphoma** (fatal) has been reported in patients on TNF inhibitor + azathioprine
- ↑ risk of TB (primary infection and reactivation), invasive fungal infections, and opportunistic infections like **legionella** and **listeria**
  - Contraindicated if patient has active infection
  - Screening test for TB before starting treatment
- Conflicting evidence exists as to whether TNF inhibitors may increase risk of developing or exacerbating **CHF** → should be used w/ caution in at-risk population **(particularly infliximab)**
- **Reactivation of hepatitis B**
  - TNF inhibitors are thought to be safe in hepatitis C, HIV
- **Neutralizing anti-drug antibodies** usually form before week 24 of treatment and interfere with the biologic agent's binding activity → ↓ **decrease efficacy**
  - Studies show that anti-drug antibodies directed against infliximab (5.4%–43.6%) and adalimumab (6%–45%) → ↓efficacy and serum levels; effect not seen with etanercept
  - Co-administration with MTX may → ↓ rates of antibody formation

Ustekinumab

- Fully human monoclonal IgG1 antibody directed against the common **p40 subunit of IL-12 and IL-23**
  - IL-12: activates TH_1; IL-23: activates TH_{17}
  - Ustekinumab may work better in patients with HLA-C*06:02
- FDA approved for adults and pediatric patients aged > 6 years with psoriasis and psoriatic arthritis
- URIs are the most frequently reported AEs; also increased risk of infections, including TB reactivation, fungal disease, and viral illnesses

Table 2.5 Mechanism of Action, Efficacy, and Dosing of Agents for Psoriasis

Drug	Mechanism of Action	Effectiveness at 10–16 weeks[a]	Administration	Dosing
Etanercept	TNF-α receptor antagonist	PASI 75 - 40 PASI 90 -18 PASI 100 - 4	Subcutaneous	50 mg twice weekly for 12 weeks, then 50 mg once weekly
Adalimumab	Human monoclonal anti-TNF-α antibody	PASI 75 -70 PASI 90 - 44 PASI 100 - 17	Subcutaneous	80 mg initial dose, then 40 mg every 2 weeks, starting 1 week after initial dose
Infliximab	Chimeric TNF-α antibody	PASI 75 - 80 PASI 90 - 57 PASI 100 - 27	Intravenous	5 mg/kg at week 0, 2, and 6, then every 8 weeks
Certolizumab	PEGylated human monoclonal anti-TNF-α antibody	PASI 75 - 71 PASI 90 - 46 PASI 100 - 18	Subcutaneous	400 mg at week 0, 2, and 4, then 200 mg every other week or 400 mg every 4 weeks
Secukinumab	IL-17A monoclonal antibody	PASI 75 - 83 PASI 90 - 61 PASI 100 - 30	Subcutaneous	300 mg at week 0, 1, 2, 3, and 4,followed by 300 mg every 4 weeks
Ixekizumab	IL-17A monoclonal antibody	PASI 75 - 89 PASI 90 - 71 PASI 100 - 40	Subcutaneous	160 mg at week 0, then 80 mg at week 2, 4, 6, 8, 10, 12, then 80 mg every 4 weeks
Brodalumab	IL17 receptor monoclonal antibody	PASI 75 - 89 PASI 90 - 71 PASI 100 - 40	Subcutaneous	210 mg at week 0, 1, and 2, then every 2 weeks
Ustekinumab	IL-12/-23 monoclonal antibody	PASI 75 - 79 PASI 90 - 44 PASI 100 - 18	Subcutaneous	45 mg (≤100 kg) or 90 mg (>100 kg) at week 0 and 4, then every 12 weeks
Guselkumab	IL-23 monoclonal antibody	PASI 75 - 87 PASI 90 - 71 PASI 100 - 39	Subcutaneous	100 mg at week 0, week 4, and then every 8 weeks
Tildrakizumab	IL-23 monoclonal antibody	PASI 75 - 63 PASI 90 - 37 PASI 100 - 13	Subcutaneous	100 mg at week 0 and 4, and then every 12 weeks
Risankizumab	IL-23 monoclonal antibody	PASI 75 - 89 PASI 90 - 71 PASI 100 - 40	Subcutaneous	150 mg at week 0 and 4, and then every 12 weeks
Apremilast	PDE-4 inhibitor	PASI 75 - 31 PASI 90 - 12 PASI 100 - 2	Oral	30 mg PO BID after 5-day titrating starter dose
Methotrexate	Antimetabolite, inhibits dihydrofolate reductase	PASI 75 - 44 PASI 90 - 21 PASI 100 - 5	Oral or subcutaneous injection	12–15 mg weekly
Acitretin	Retinoid	PASI 75 - 20 PASI 90 - 6 PASI 100 - 1	Oral	25–50 mg daily
Cyclosporine	Inhibits IL-2	PASI 75 - 44 PASI 90 - 20 PASI 100 - 5	Oral	2.5–5 mg/kg/day
Deucravacitinib	TYK2 inhibitor	PASI 75 - 53 PASI 90 - 27 PASI 100 - 10	Oral	6 mg daily

IL, *Interleukin;* PASI, *Psoriasis Area and Severity Index;* PDE-4, *phosphodiesterase-4;* TNF, *tumor necrosis factor.*
[a]*Data from Armstrong AW, Puig L, Joshi A, et al. Comparison of biologics and oral treatments for plaque psoriasis: a meta-analysis.* JAMA Dermatol. *2020;156(3):258–269.*

   - Long-term safety data did not show increased risk of infection and malignancy (excluding skin cancer)
- Two cases of reversible posterior leukoencephalopathy syndrome reported

IL-23 inhibitors

- Guselkumab, risankizumab, and tildrakizumab selectively bind the p19 subunit of IL-23, preventing its interation with IL-23 receptor
- FDA approved for psoriasis; guselkumab and risankizumab also approved for psoriatic arthritis
- AEs: URI, injection site reaction (lower risk than TNF-α inhibitors), arthralgia, GI AEs, HSV infections, tinea

IL-17 inhibitors

- Ixekizumab and secukinumab neutralize IL-17A
- Brodalumab antagonizes the IL-17 receptor
- FDA approved for psoriasis and psoriatic arthritis (except brodalumab); ixekizumab and secukinumab approved for pediatric patients aged > 6 years
- Most commonly reported AE = nasopharyngitis

- Other common AEs include URI, injection site reactions, and headache; candidiasis and herpes infections have also been reported
- **Can worsen inflammatory bowel disease**
- Brodalumab associated with **suicidality**

Spesolimab

- Monoclonal IL-36 receptor (IL1RL2/IL1RAP) antibody
- FDA approved for generalized pustular psoriasis flares (administered as single 900 mg IV dose; can repeat one week later)
- AEs: infusion site reactions, infections (e.g. UTI, herpes simplex, cellulitis), DRESS, Guillain-Barre syndrome

Rituximab

- **Chimeric IgG** monoclonal antibody targeting the B-cell surface antigen **(CD20)**
  - **Binds B cells but not plasma cells (do not express CD20)**
  - Kills B cells through multiple mechanisms: apoptosis, activation of the complement cascade, antibody-dependent cell-mediated cytotoxicity and antibody-dependent phagocytosis
- FDA approved for **pemphigus vulgaris**, granulomatosis with polyangiitis and microscopic polyangiitis; used off-label for other autoimmune blistering diseases
- Depletion of B cells occurs within 2 to 3 weeks of initial treatment with sustained depletion for an average of 6 months; B-cell numbers return to normal within the first year of treatment
- Relative contraindication in patients with history of bronchospasm, hypotension, or angioedema
- Common AEs include: **infusion reactions** (generally mild and occur with the first infusion), HTN, nausea, URI, arthralgia, pyrexia, and pruritus
  - Patients with history of cardiac or pulmonary conditions should be more closely monitored as they are susceptible to severe infusion reactions
- Serious AEs: hepatitis B virus reactivation, progressive multifocal leukoencephalopathy, SJS/toxic epidermal necrolysis (TEN), serious infection, hepatic failure, and myelosuppression

IL-1 inhibitors

- Canakinumab (human anti-IL-1β mAB), anakinra (IL-1 receptor antagonist), rilonacept (fusion protein behaving like a soluble decoy receptor binding IL-1α and IL-1β), and gevokizumab (humanized anti-IL-1β mAB)
- Anakinra is FDA approved for moderate to severe RA that has failed other disease-modifying treatments
- Off-label uses in dermatology: pyoderma gangrenosum, pyogenic arthritis, pyoderma gangrenosum and acne (PAPA) syndrome, hidradenitis suppurativa, lamellar ichthyosis, Sweet's syndrome, panniculitis, **Muckle-Wells syndrome and other autoinflammatory syndromes (e.g., Schnitzler syndrome)**, and synovitis, acne, pustulosis, hyperostosis, osteitis (SAPHO) syndrome
- Risk of TB reactivation appears to be lower in IL-1 inhibitors than in TNF-α agents, although more studies are needed
- Most common AEs are injection site reactions; **important to monitor absolute neutrophil count** as neutropenia can occur
- IL-1 inhibitors should not be initiated in patients with active infections

Omalizumab

- **Monoclonal anti-IgE antibody** → ↓ IgE levels and ↓ IgE receptors on mast cells and basophils
- FDA approved for asthma and chronic idiopathic urticaria
- AEs: **anaphylaxis**, malignancy, and injection site reaction
  - Unmasking of Churg-Strauss syndrome in patients with underlying eosinophilic disorder

Dupilumab

- IL-4 receptor antagonist, blocks signaling from both IL-4 and IL-13
  - Key mediators of the TH_2 pathway
- FDA approved for atopic dermatitis for ages ≥ 6 months and **prurigo nodularis** in adults
- AEs: **conjunctivitis and keratitis**, hypersensitivity/injection site reactions

Lebrikizumab and tralokinumab

- Monocolonal anti-IL-13 antibodies
- Tralokinumab approved for atopic dermatitis, lebrikzumab under investigation
- Appear to have lower conjunctivitis risk than dupilumab and better dosing regimens

Nemolizumab

- IL-31 receptor antagonist
- Effective against itch in atopic dermatitis and prurigo nodularis, under investigation

2.5 ONCOLOGIC AGENTS IN DERMATOLOGY (FIG. 2.4)

Vismodegib and sonidegib

- Patched (PTCH) tumor suppressor gene is a receptor for sonic hedgehog; PTCH inhibits smoothened in the absence of sonic hedgehog
- Vismodegib and sonedigib target sonic hedgehog pathway by **inhibiting smoothened** → SUFU stays bound to GLI → GLI1/2 transcription factors stay inactive → inhibition of transcription of target genes
  - Ineffective in nevoid BCC syndrome (Gorlin) patients with SUFU gene mutations (5%)
  - Itraconazole also inhibits hedgehog pathway through smoothed and GLI
- Used for metastatic and locally advanced basal cell carcinoma (BCC), as well as those unamenable to

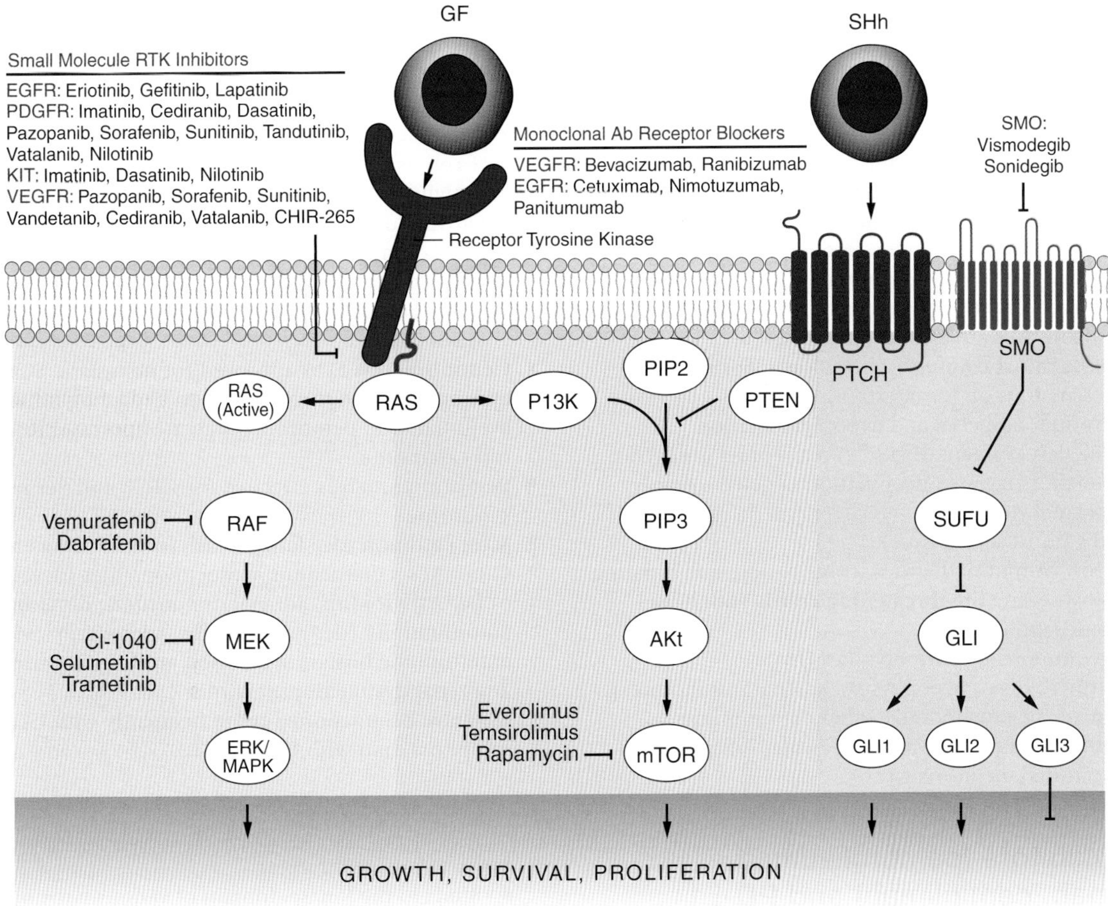

Fig. 2.4 Molecular signaling pathways. Targeted agents listed are meant to be representative and are not intended to be all-inclusive for targeted agent families. *GF*, Growth factor; *RTK*, receptor tyrosine kinase; *SHh*, sonic hedgehog; *SMO*, smoothened. (Modified from Macdonald JB, Macdonald B, Golitz LE, LoRusso P, Sekulic A. Cutaneous adverse effects of targeted therapies. *J Am Acad Dermatol*. 2015;72[2]:221–236.)

surgery/radiation; may be used in patients with nevoid BCC syndrome
- AEs: **muscle spasms, alopecia, dysgeusia**, fatigue, nausea, anorexia, and diarrhea
- Teratogenic, hedgehog pathway regulates fetal development—contraceptives required for 24 months (F) and 3 months (M) post-treatment

BRAF inhibitors (vemurafenib, encorafenib, and dabrafenib)

- BRAF: serine/threonine signal transduction kinase important to the **MAPK pathway**, which regulates cell division
- The most common genetic mutation in **melanoma** is V600E mutation (valine replaced by glutamic acid at amino acid position number 600) of BRAF proto-oncogene; BRAF inhibitors target this mutation and can increase survival rates in late stage melanoma
- Cutaneous reactions are most common AE:
  - Exanthematous rash—papulopustular on face, torso, and arms
  - Keratotic lesions
    - **SCC and keratoacanthoma due to paradoxical MAP kinase activation keratinocytes** (blocked by addition of a MEK inhibitor)
    - Verrucous keratosis, warts: most common skin lesion
  - **Keratosis pilaris-like eruption**
  - Photosensitivity, alopecia, and hyperkeratotic hand-foot reaction
  - May change preexisting nevi, with possible risk of **melanoma**
    - BRAF blockade in **wild-type melanoma** may accelerate cellular proliferation
- Noncutaneous AEs: arthralgias, panniculitis, nausea, diarrhea, fatigue, QT prolongation, and retinal vein thrombosis

MEK inhibitors (trametinib, cobimetinib, binimetinib)

- **Inhibit MEK1/2** of the MAPK pathway
- Can be used as monotherapy or in combination with BRAF inhibitors for late stage **melanoma**
  - Combination improves efficacy and decreases toxicity
  - ↓ SCC risk when MEK inhibitor added to BRAF inhibitor
- AEs: morbilliform eruption, papulopustular eruption, GI AEs most common (diarrhea, nausea, and vomiting), hypoalbuminemia, dysgeusia, xerostomia, cardiomyopathy, interstitial lung disease, and retinal vein occlusion

Ipilimumab

- Fully human monoclonal antibody that binds and inhibits cytotoxic T-lymphocyte-associated antigen 4 (**CTLA-4**) → ↑ T-cell activation against tumor cells (Fig. 2.4)
  - Two signals used for T-cell activation: (1) MHC-TCR and (2) CD28-B7; CTLA-4 competes with CD28 for B7 binding; CTLA4 is an inhibitor receptor which downregulates the immune response
- Used to treat metastatic **melanoma**
- AEs are called **immune-related adverse events**:
  - Cutaneous AEs are most common (24%)
    - **Rash (most common)**: maculopapular or eczematous on trunk/extremities
    - Pruritus, alopecia, and hypopigmentation
    - The development of vitiligo may confer a survival benefit (suggests inflammation targeted towards melanocytes)
  - GI AEs (most severe issue)
    - Most common: diarrhea, constipation, and bloating
    - Most severe: **life-threatening colitis** with bowel perforation
  - Less common: endocrinopathies (hypo/hyperthyroidism, hypophysitis, adrenal insufficiency), hepatoxicity, pneumonitis, other autoimmune conditions (myositis, vasculitis, ocular inflammation, myocarditis), neurotoxicity

PD-1 inhibitors (pembrolizumab, nivolumab, cemiplimab) and PD-L1 inhibitors (avelumab, atezolizumab)

- PD-1 is an immune checkpoint receptor expressed by activated T cells (see Fig. 2.5)
  - Normally functions as a "brake" on the immune response
  - PD-1 on activated T cells binds to its ligands PD1-L1 (B7-H1) and PD1-L2 (B7-DC), which are expressed on tumor cells → deactivation of T cells → loss of immune response against tumor
  - **Monoclonal antibodies that target PD-1** → prevent T-cell deactivation → ↑ immune-mediated tumoricidal activity
- Approved for **metastatic melanoma**
  - Efficacy improved when used in combination with ipilimumab: 5-year overall survival rate of ipilimumab + nivolumab is 52%; main disadvantage = ↑ immune-mediated AEs
- **Cemiplimab** is FDA approved for metastatic SCC, advanced BCC not responsive to hedgehog inhibitors; avelumab and pembrolizumab are approved for Merkel cell carcinoma
- Pembrolizumab is effective for CTCL and Sézary syndrome
- Most common AEs: fatigue, rash (pruritic drug eruption)
- Other AEs: enterocolitis, endocrinopathies (development of DM2 thyroiditis, adrenal dysfunction) development of autoimmunity (dermatomyositis, scleroderma, vitiligo, autoimmune blistering disease), arthralgia, neuropathy, and renal dysfunction/nephritis
- AEs have been reported more frequently with CTLA-4 inhibitors than with PD-1/PD-L1

Imatinib mesylate

- Tyrosine kinase inhibitor
  - Binds to the kinase domain of various tyrosine kinases (e.g., Bcr-Abl, c-Kit receptor [CD117], and platelet-derived growth factor receptor [PDGFR])
- Dermatologic applications: melanoma, myeloproliferative hypereosinophilic syndrome, and **dermatofibrosarcoma protuberans**
- Cutaneous reactions are common

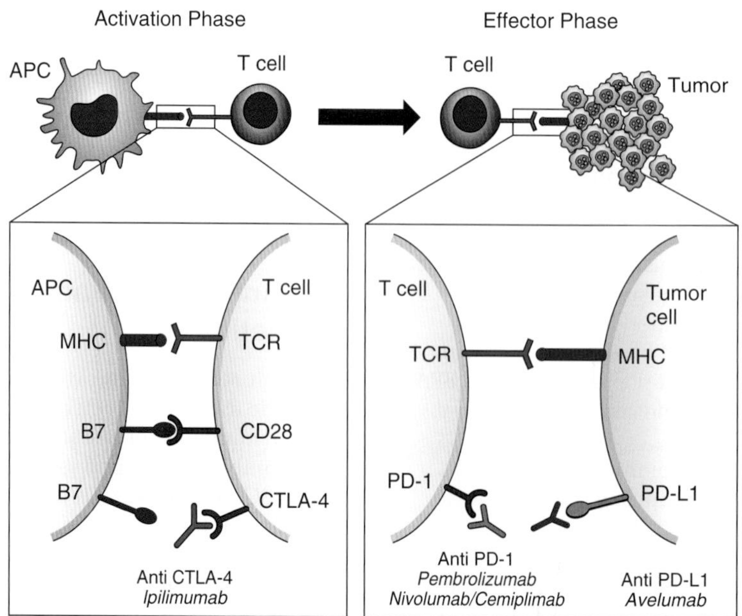

Fig. 2.5 Mechanism of action of immune checkpoint inhibitors.

- Most common: superficial edema (**periorbital edema**)
- Second most common: **rash** (maculopapular, nonspecific)
- Other AEs: **hypopigmentation/depigmentation** (via inhibition of c-Kit pathway, which is involved in melanocyte activation), hyperpigmentation (less common), lichenoid eruptions (oral and mucosal), and photosensitivity

Ibrutinib

- Selective inhibitor of Bruton's tyrosine kinase, an enzyme required for activation of pathways necessary for B-cell trafficking, chemotaxis, and adhesion
- FDA approved for chronic GVHD
- AEs: thrombocytopenia, anemia, infection

Talimogene

- Engineered oncolytic herpes virus that replicates within cancer cells, destroying them
- FDA approved for injection directly into metastatic melanoma lesions
- AEs: fatigue, fever, nausea, flu-like symptoms

Mechlorethamine hydrochloride

- A nitrogen mustard alkylating agent used for patch/plaque MF; **contact dermatitis** is the most common AE, but anaphylaxis and SCC development are the most concerning
- Carmustine is also an alkylating agent used for patch/plaque MF; it can cause severe local reactions and myelosuppression

Brentuximab vedotin

- **Anti-CD-30 monoclonal antibody used for advanced CTCL**; also used for Hodgkin lymphoma and **ALCL**
- Most common AE is **peripheral neuropathy**; other AEs include fatigue and nausea

Mogamulizumab

- **Antibody against CCR4** (expressed on malignant T cells) used for relapsed or refractory CTCL
- AEs: infusion-related skin eruption, nausea/diarrhea, thrombocytopenia, dysgeusia, and elevated creatinine.
  - May increase risk of GVHD in allogenic stem cell transplant recipients

Romidepsin and vorinostat

- **Histone deacetylase inhibitors** used for relapsed or refractory CTCL
- AEs: EKG changes, electrolyte abnormalities, nausea/dysgeusia, anemia, thrombocytopenia

Topical agents for acitinic keratoses (AKs) and NMSC (Table 2.6)

- 2019 NEJM randomized trial for facial AKs showed 5-fluorouracil > imiquimod > methyl aminolevulinate photodynamic therapy > ingenol mebutate

2.6 ANTIMICROBIAL AGENTS

Topical antibacterial agents

Bacitracin

- Made by *Bacillus subtilis*
- Bactericidal
- Binds to C55-prenol pyrophosphatase → disruption of bacterial cell wall peptidoglycan synthesis

Table 2.6 Topical Treatments for Actinic Keratoses and Non-Melanoma Skin Cancer

	Mechanism of Action	FDA-Approved Indications	Adverse Effects
5-Fluorouracil	Antimetabolite/pyrimidine analog which binds to **thymidylate synthase** (normally converts deoxyuridine → thymidine), and results in ↓ DNA synthesis	AKs, and superficial BCCs (5% strength only)	Local reactions (e.g., erythema, blistering, necrosis, erosions, and burning) Dihydropyrimidine dehydrogenase deficiency can lead to severe toxicity
Imiquimod	Activator of **toll-like receptors 7 and 8** → activation of NF-κB transcription factor → ↑ cytokines/chemokines (e.g., **TNF-α and IFN-γ**) → innate/acquired immune pathway stimulation → antitumor and antiviral activity Also anti-angiogenic, proapoptotic, and ↑ lymphatic transport of immune cells/factors → tumor destruction	AKs, superficial BCCs (5% strength only), and genital/perianal warts	Local reactions similar to 5-fluorouracil **Flu-like or GI symptoms** (especially if larger areas treated), and psoriasis exacerbation
Diclofenac	↓ Cyclooxygenase enzymes → ↑apoptosis	AKs	Mild irritation, rare photosensitivity/photocontact dermatitis; avoid in patients with NSAID hypersensitivity and known bleeding diatheses Pregnancy category B
Ingenol mebutate	Induces rapid cellular death (within hours) via mitochondrial swelling/plasma membrane disruption, neutrophil-mediated antibody dependent cytotoxicity; intense inflammatory response (within days) via protein kinase C activation	AKs	Local reactions (erythema, scaling, and crusting), which are worse on days 4–7
Tirbanibulin	Microtubule inhibitor	AKs on face or scalp	Local skin reaction, pruritus, pain

AKs, *Actinic keratosis;* BCC, *basal cell carcinoma;* FDA, *Food and Drug Administration;* GI, *gastrointestinal;* IFN, *interferon;* NF-kB, *nuclear factor-kB;* TNF, *tumor necrosis factor.*

- Activity against *Neisseria* and gram positives (GPs); poor activity compared with gram negatives (GNs)
- Commonly causes **allergic contact dermatitis** (especially common in patients with stasis dermatitis/ulcers)

Polymyxin B

- Made by *Bacillus polymyxa* and *B. subtilis*
- Bactericidal
- ↑ Cell membrane permeability via detergent-like phospholipid interaction
- Activity against GNs (e.g., ***Pseudomonas***)

Neomycin

- Aminoglycoside made by *Streptomyces fradiae*
- Binds 30s subunit of bacterial ribosomal RNA → ↓ protein synthesis
- Activity against GPs and GNs
- Can be combined with bacitracin and polymyxin B (e.g., Neosporin)
- **Common contact allergen**, like bacitracin (**co-react w/ each other**); allergy more common in those w/ stasis dermatitis and when applied to ulcers; possibility of ototoxicity/nephrotoxicity but very rare

Mupirocin

- Made by *Pseudomonas fluorescens*
- Binds to bacterial isoleucyl tRNA synthetase → ↓ RNA/ protein synthesis
- Activity against methicillin-resistant *S. aureus* (**MRSA;** can ↓ nasal carriage) and *Streptococcus pyogenes*; resistance has been reported
- Not effective against *Pseudomonas* (made by *Pseudomonas*)

Retapamulin

- Pleuromutilin made by *Clitopilus scyphoides*
- Binds to L3 protein on 50S subunit of bacterial ribosome → ↓ protein synthesis
- Activity against MRSA, *S. pyogenes*, and anaerobes; FDA approved for impetigo to methicillin-susceptible *S. aureus* (MSSA) and *S. pyogenes*
- Can cause contact dermatitis

Gentamicin

- Aminoglycoside made by *Micromonospora purpurea*
- Binds to bacterial 30s ribosomal subunit → ↓ protein synthesis
- Activity against GPs and GNs (e.g., ***Pseudomonas***)

Silver sulfadiazine

- Binds bacterial DNA → ↓ DNA synthesis; also disrupts cell walls and membranes
- Activity against GPs and GNs, including MRSA and *Pseudomonas aeruginosa*
- May cross-react with sulfonamides; pregnancy category B
- Used extensively for **burn wounds**
- Rare AEs include: **hemolysis** in G6PD patients, **methemoglobinemia**, renal insufficiency, **argyria**, leukopenia, and unmasking porphyria

Iodoquinol

- Quinolone derivative with high iodine concentration
- Activity against GPs and GNs and dermatophytes/yeasts

Benzoyl peroxide

- Broad-spectrum antibacterial agent that functions via strong oxidizing properties (good vs. *Cutibacterium acnes*)—**no bacterial resistance reported to date**
- Used for acne (alone and in combination with topical antibiotics and retinoids); has keratolytic properties
- When used with certain formulations of tretinoin, can → oxidation/degradation of retinoid agent
- Most common AE is local irritation; can bleach hair/fabric

Metronidazole

- Nitroimidazole that disrupts DNA synthesis
- Activity against protozoa and anaerobes; not active against *C. acnes*, staphylococcus, streptococcus, fungi, or *Demodex*
- Used primarily for rosacea (anti-inflammatory properties)

Azelaic acid

- Dicarboxylic acid that disrupts mitochondrial respiration, ↓ DNA synthesis (especially in abnormal melanocytes), and ↓ reactive oxygen species (ROS) production
- Also competitively **inhibits tyrosinase → ↓ pigmentation**
- Activity against *C. acnes;* used in acne and rosacea (including perioral dermatitis)
- May be used in acne and hyperpigmentation disorders (e.g., melasma and pregnancy-induced hypertension [PIH])
- Safe in pregnancy

Sodium sulfacetamide

- Activity against *C. acnes*
- Inhibits bacterial dihydropteroate synthetase (prevents conversion of PABA → folic acid) → ↓ nucleic acid/ protein
- Used in acne and rosacea as a combination agent with or without precipitated sulfur

Systemic antibacterial agents

Penicillins

- MoA: β-lactam ring binds to bacterial enzyme DD-transpeptidase → **inhibits formation of peptidoglycan cross-links in the bacterial cell wall** → cell wall breakdown
- Many are susceptible to β-lactamases
- Generations
  - First: dicloxacillin, oxacillin
    - Good for GP cocci, like MSSA
  - Second: aminopenicillins (ampicillin and amoxicillin)
    - GN bacilli and GP cocci
    - Amoxicillin has fewer GI AEs
    - **Ampicillin + mononucleosis/allopurinol/ lymphocytic leukemia → generalized morbilliform itchy eruption** starting 1 week after antibiotic initiation
    - May be associated with allergic reactions
  - Third and fourth: carboxypenicillins (carbenicillin) and ureidopenicillins (piperacillin)
    - **Antipseudomonal** activity
  - Combination β-lactam + β-lactamase inhibitor
    - Amoxicillin-clavulanate, ampicillin-sulbactam (IV), ticarcillin-clavulanate (IV), and piperacillin-tazobactam (IV)

- β-lactamase inhibitors inhibit β-lactamase → allows the β-lactam antibiotic to function—helpful in MSSA, *Haemophilus, Klebsiella, Escherichia coli, Proteus,* and *Bacteroides fragilis* infections
- Good for polymicrobial infections (e.g., **amoxicillin-clavulanate is the treatment of choice for animal or human bites**; ticarcillin-clavulanate good for **diabetic foot ulcers** and burn wounds)
- Ticarcillin/piperacillin → hypernatremia, ↑ LFTs, neutropenia, and ↑ bleeding times
- ↑ risk of cholestatic injury with amoxicillin/clavulanate

- Good for various common streptococci (treat β-hemolytic streptococci for at least 10 days to prevent possible rheumatic fever) and MSSA skin infections (e.g., erysipelas, cellulitis, impetigo, folliculitis, furunculosis, and ecthyma)
- Other uses include staphyloccal scalded skin syndrome (**IV nafcillin**), syphilis (**IM injection of penicillin G**), erysipeloid, cutaneous anthrax, Lyme disease, and leptospirosis
- AEs: hypersensitivity reactions (common association; **2% of cephalosporin [CSN]-allergic patients are penicillin [PCN]-allergic**), GI AEs (common), hematologic AEs, shore nails (dicloxacillin), onychomadesis/photo-onycholysis (cloxacillin), interstitial nephritis (very rare), and acute generalized exanthematous pustulosis (AGEP)
- **Probenecid prolongs renal excretion** → ↑ PCN levels (also can ↑ CSN levels)

Cephalosporins

- MoA similar to PCNs as structure is β-lactam ring + six-membered dihydrothiazine ring
- Resistant to β-lactamases
- Generations
  - First: cefadroxil and cephalexin
    - Best for GP cocci, but not good for MRSA or PCN-resistant *Streptococcus pneumonia*
  - Second: cefaclor and cefuroxime
    - More GN activity and less GP activity
    - Good for *Haemophilus influenzae, Moraxella catarrhalis, Neisseria meningitidis,* and *Neisseria gonorrhoeae*
    - Cephamycins (cefoxitin and cefotetan) are good for *B. fragilis*
  - Third: cefixime, cefdinir, cefotaxime, ceftazidime, cefpodoxime, and ceftriaxone
    - Good GN activity, but not GP activity
    - Some good for *P. aeruginosa* (i.e., ceftazidime)
    - Good for soft tissue abscesses and diabetic foot ulcers
  - Fourth: cefepime (IV)
    - Broad coverage—MSSA, nonenterococcal streptococci, and GNs (including *P. aeruginosa*)
  - Fifth: ceftaroline (IV)
    - MRSA *S. pyogenes, Streptococcus agalactiae, E. coli, K. pneumoniae,* and *K. oxytoca.*
    - Acute bacterial skin and soft tissue infections
- Oral cephalosporins used frequently in dermatology for uncomplicated skin and soft tissue infections; may need IV agents for complicated cellulitis or necrotizing fasciitis
- AEs: GI symptoms (most common), hypersensitivity reactions (**cross-reactivity in ≈ 5%–10% of PCN-allergic patients**), *Candida* infections, hematologic AEs (e.g., hemolytic anemia—cefotetan most common), ↑ LFTs, **serum sickness-like reaction (cefaclor)**, Jarisch-Herxheimer reaction (in Lyme disease patients receiving cefuroxime axetil), disulfiram-like reaction (cefotetan), and **AGEP**
- **Do not give w/ aminoglycosides → ↑ risk of nephrotoxicity**

Vancomycin

- MoA: tricyclic glycopeptide that inhibits bacterial cell wall synthesis
- Only works for GP organisms—most important use in dermatology is against MRSA skin and soft tissue infections
- AEs: vancomycin infusion (hypersensitivity) reaction, **linear IgA bullous dermatosis (LABD;** most common cause of drug-induced LABD; as a result of IgA antibodies to LAD285 and **IgA/IgG to BP180**), hearing loss (patients with renal failure), and nephrotoxicity (if given with aminoglycosides)

Macrolides

- MoA: bind to 50S subunit of bacterial ribosome → ↓ protein synthesis; also has anti-inflammatory properties
- Good for GPs, except MRSA and enterococcus—used in dermatology for skin and soft tissue infections
  - Erythromycin
    - Not used as commonly because of ↑ resistance (particularly *S. aureus*) and GI AEs
    - Some indications include: erythrasma/pitted keratolysis, anthrax, erysipeloid, chancroid, and lymphogranuloma venereum (LGV)
    - May be used for acne, rosacea, and pityriasis rosea
    - **Potent CYP3A4 inhibitor** (e.g., monitor use of warfarin, mexiletine, theophylline, and statins [↑ rhabdomyolysis])
    - AEs: **GI symptoms** (most common and dose-limiting), ototoxicity/hear loss, QT prolongation/torsades de pointes (worse when given with terfenadine, astemizole, cisapride, and certain quinolones), and hypersensitivity reactions; erythromycin estolate in pregnancy may → hepatotoxicity (intrahepatic cholestasis) in mother; possible association of cardiovascular malformation and pyloric stenosis if fetus exposed *in utero*
  - Azithromycin
    - Better than erythromycin for GPs (→ often used as second-line prophylactic antibiotic in dermatology surgery for PCN/CSN-allergic patients); has some GN activity (*E. coli, N. gonorrhoeae, Haemophilus ducreyi,* and *Chlamydia trachomatis*)
    - Activity against *Pasteurella multocida* (animal bites), *Eikenella corrodens* (human bites), and atypical mycobacteria, *Treponema pallidum, Borrelia burgdorferi* **(if doxycyline contraindicated),** *Toxoplasma gondii,* and *Klebsiella granulomatis* (granuloma inguinale)
    - Has been used for acne

- AEs: deafness, angioedema, photosensitivity, hypersensitivity, and contact dermatitis; antacids can ↓ absorption
- Clarithromycin
  - Better than erythromycin for GPs
  - CYP3A4 inhibitor (less potent than erythromycin)
  - Has activity against some GNs, atypical mycobacteria (good activity against *Mycobacterium. leprae*), *T. pallidum*, *B. burgdorferi*, and *T. gondii*
  - AEs: metallic/bitter taste, fixed drug eruption, leukocytolcastic vasculitis (LCV), and hypersensitivity reactions; contraindicated in renal dysfunction

Fluoroquinolones

- MoA: inhibits DNA gyrase (bacterial topoisomerase II) +/– topoisomerase IV → DNA fragmentation
  - DNA gyrase is predominant target in GN, whereas topoisomerase IV is target in GP
- First- and second-generation quinolones (ciprofloxacin, ofloxacin, and nalidixic acid): only target DNA gyrase (topoisomerase II) → only effective against GN
- Third- and fourth-generation quinolones (levofloxacin, moxifloxacin, sparfloxacin, and gatifloxacin): target both topoisomerase forms (IV > II) → ↑ GP coverage and ↓ bacterial resistance; slightly ↓ efficacy against GN
- Ozenoxacin—topical non-fluorinated quinolone for treatment of impetigo
- Delafloxacin—new fluroquinolone with unique structural and chemical characteristics; increased potency against GPs
- Good for GNs, like *P. aeruginosa* (especially ciprofloxacin); may be used with some GPs like *S. aureus* and *S. pyogenes* (primarily third- and fourth-generation quinolones); ciprofloxacin is the treatment of choice for **cutaneous anthrax** (*B. anthracis*); various fluoroquinolones effective for mycobacterial infections
- Generally excreted renally, except for moxifloxacin
- Used in dermatology to treat GN skin and soft tissue infections, some GP skin/soft tissue infections, GN toe web-space infections, diabetic foot ulcers, and GN folliculitis
- AEs: GI symptoms (#1), CNS AEs (headache, dizziness, seizures, psychosis, and depression), **tendinitis/tendon rupture**, hypersensitivity (especially ciprofloxacin), and **photosensitivity/photo-onycholysis (lomefloxacin, enoxacin, and sparfloxacin >> ciprofloxacin > norfloxacin > ofloxacin >> levofloxacin)**
  - Photosensitivity is from the **UVA spectrum** (and visible spectrum for sparfloxacin)
  - **Levofloxacin** NOT associated with photosensitivity
- Administration with divalent cations (calcium, magnesium, aluminum, and zinc) → ↓ absorption
- CYP1A2 inhibitors (caution with warfarin, theophylline, caffeine, anti-arrhythmics [↑ QT/torsades], zileuton, and beta blockers); also caution with cyclosporine (in setting of organ transplant, can → ↑ creatinine levels)

Tetracyclines

- MoA: binds 30s subunit of bacterial ribosome → ↓ protein synthesis; anti-inflammatory properties (e.g., inhibits multiple matrix metalloproteinases, neutrophil migration, and ↓ innate cytokines)
- Main uses in dermatology: acne, perioral dermatitis, rosacea, bullous pemphigoid, confluent and reticulated papillomatosis **(CARP; minocycline)**, cutaneous sarcoidosis/other **granulomatous diseases (minocycline)**, acne keloidalis nuchae, PLEVA/PLC, and **acneiform eruptions 2° to epidermal growth factor receptor (EGFR) inhibitors**
  - Sarecycline—narrow-spectrum tetracycline developed for acne only; limited activity against bowel flora, less GI upset, less photosensitivity
- Also useful for various GP and GN skin infections, including **MRSA** (doxycycline and minocycline) and those caused by *Chlamydia* spp. (**doxycycline is the treatment of choice in LGV**), *Rickettsia* spp. (**doxycycline is the treatment of choice for rickettsial and rickettsial-like infections**—Rocky Mountain spotted fever (RMSF), rickettsialpox, Q fever, trench fever, and ehrlichiosis), *Mycoplasma* spp., atypical mycobacteria, spirochetes (syphilis [if patient is PCN-allergic], and **Lyme disease—doxycycline is the treatment of choice in early disease**)
  - **Subantimicrobial doses**, (<50 mg, or extended release) **effective for rosacea and acne**, and **do NOT ↑ bacterial resistance**; may also have ↓ rate of vaginal candidiasis
  - Bacterial resistance via ribosomal protection and/or drug efflux
  - Lipophilic (**minocycline** > doxycycline > tetracycline)
  - **Food decreases absorption**, more so in tetracycline than in doxycycline or minocycline
  - Various **metallic cations** (e.g., calcium, iron, zinc, magnesium, bismuth, and aluminum) can ↓ **absorption via chelation** (tetracycline > doxycycline > minocycline)
    - Found in products like antacids, laxatives, dairy, and supplements
- AEs: **GI symptoms** (esophagitis, nausea, and abdominal pain; most common with doxycycline, but less so with enteric-coated form), acute vestibular AEs (dizziness and vertigo; usually with minocycline), benign intracranial HTN/**pseudotumor cerebri** (usually minocycline; ↑ risk if given w/ isotretinoin), **photosensitivity/photo-onycholysis (demeclocycline > doxycycline > tetracycline > minocycline)**, hyperpigmentation of skin/nail beds/teeth/mucous membranes/bone (minocycline), vaginal candidiasis, **GN acne/folliculitis**, serum sickness-like reactions (minocycline), drug-induced Sweet's syndrome (minocycline), autoimmune hepatitis (minocycline), DRESS/DHS (minocycline), lupus-like syndrome (minocycline; usually ANA+, may be anti-histone + or –), and cutaneous PAN/vasculitis (minocycline; pANCA+)
  - Minocycline hyperpigmentation types:
    - Type 1: Blue-gray in sites of **facial** scarring—stains for iron and melanin
    - Type 2: Blue-gray on **shins** and/or forearms—stains for iron and melanin
    - Type 3: **Diffuse** muddy brown on **sun-exposed skin**—stains melanin only; represents a low-grade phototoxic eruption with PIH

- Tetracyclines are **unsafe** in pregnancy → affect fetal teeth/ bones
- Do not give to **patients under 8 years old → tooth discoloration**
  - Tetracycline and minocycline can also induce **adult-onset tooth pigmentation**
    - Severe rickettsioses (**RMSF**) are the **exception** for treating children with tetracyclines
- Tetracyclines excreted renally, **except** doxycycline (mainly via GI tract—so can be used in renal failure)

Rifampin

- MoA: binds β-subunit of bacterial **DNA-dependent RNA polymerase** → ↓ RNA/protein synthesis
- Effective against various mycobacteria (e.g., *Mycobacterium tuberculosis, M. leprae,* and *Mycobacterium marinum*) and some other GP and GN organisms (e.g., staphylococcus)
  - Single-agent rifampin is an effective treatment agent for latent TB; also used in combination with other antimicrobials due to rapid development of resistance
- **Major CYP450 inducer** → ↑ drug clearance/↓ efficacy (e.g., oral contraceptive pills **[OCPs]**, warfarin, azoles, CCBs, statins, and cyclosporine)
- Dermatologic uses: mycobacterial infections (part of multidrug therapy), *Bartonella* infections (e.g., cat-scratch disease and bacillary angiomatosis), MRSA/MSSA, rhinoscleroma, and cutaneous leishmaniasis; also used in **combination with clindamycin for hidradenitis suppurativa**
- AEs: **orange-red discoloration of body fluids**, CNS (headache and drowsiness), GI symptoms, development of rifampin-dependent antibodies (can → anaphylaxis, flu-like symptoms, renal failure, and hemolytic anemia), hepatotoxicity (especially w/ isoniazid), DVTs, pulmonary fibrosis, ocular AEs, **worsening of porphyria (induces δ-aminolevulinic acid [(ALA] synthase)**, and possible hemorrhagic disease of the newborn and mother in pregnancy

Trimethoprim-sulfamethoxazole (TMP-SMX; cotrimoxazole)

- **Dihydrofolate reductase inhibitor (trimethoprim) + dihydropteroate synthase inhibitor (sulfamethoxazole)** → ↓ tetrahydrofolic acid → ↓ bacterial nucleic acid/ protein synthesis
- Effective against various GP cocci (e.g., MRSA, *Enterococcus faecalis,* and *S. pyogenes*), *H. influenzae, P. jirovecii, Nocardia* spp., *Chlamydia,* and various GNs
- Dermatologic uses: acne, hidradenitis suppurativa, **granuloma inguinale**, actinomycetoma, cat-scratch disease, and chronic melioidosis (*Burkholderia pseudomallei*)
- Caution in patients w/ renal insufficiency as it is primarily renally cleared
- AEs: most commonly GI and CNS, but also antibiotic-associated colitis, hypersensitivity reactions (cutaneous eruptions much more common in HIV patients; TMP-SMX accounts for 30% of SJS/TEN cases), hematologic AEs (agranulocytosis, thrombocytopenia, folate deficiency + megaloblastic anemia, neutropenia, and hemolytic anemia in patients w/ G6PD deficiency)
- May not be safe in pregnancy—sulfamethoxazole can result in jaundice, hemolytic anemia, and kernicterus of baby if taken in third trimester
- Can ↑ dapsone levels, ↑ **hematologic toxicity in patients taking MTX (both ↓ tetrahydrofolate)**, ↑ renal toxicity in patients taking cyclosporine, ↑ K+ in patients on ACEIs/ARBs

Clindamycin

- Lincosamide that binds to **50S** subunit of bacterial ribosomal RNA → ↓ ribosomal translocation/protein synthesis
- Effective against GP cocci (e.g., *Staphylococcus* spp. and *Streptococcus* spp.) and anaerobes (*Bacteroides* spp. and *Clostridium perfringens*), but not usually GNs (except *Capnocytophaga canimorsus*)
  - **"D zone" test** helps determine whether inducible resistance is present in an erythromycin-resistant, clindamycin-sensitive organism (bacteria with *erm* gene)
- Dermatologic uses: skin and soft tissue infections (e.g., staphylococci, MRSA, and MSSA), including some deep soft tissue infections (e.g., streptococcal myositis, *C. perfringens* infection, and diabetic foot ulcers); acne; hidradenitis suppurativa (with rifampin)
- AEs: **antibiotic-associated colitis**, rashes, and rare bone marrow suppression may ↑ neuromuscular blocking

Carbapenems

- MoA: similar to other beta-lactam antibiotics but differs by addition of a double bond to the 5-membered ring of the penicillin nucleus and the substitution of a sulfur atom by a carbon atom
- Agents include imipenem (formulated with cilastin to protect kidney against nephrotoxicity), ertapenem, doripenem, meropenem; all are administered parenterally
- Good for multidrug-resistant bacterial infections, and have a broad spectrum of activity (GN bacteria, GP bacteria, aerobes and anaerobes)
- Typically not highly active against MRSA and CNS but can be used in mixed flora infections (e.g. decubitus ulcer/ diabetic foot ulcer) and skin/soft-tissue infections resistant to other agents; **imipenem also used in acute flares of severe hidradenitis suppurativa**
- AEs: may have cross sensitivity in those with PCN allergies, **seizures (imipenem > meropenem)**, nausea/ vomiting, LFT elevation, leukopenia, severe allergic reactions, hypersensitivity reactions, *Clostridium difficile* colitis

Linezolid

- MoA: binds 23S portion of 50S ribosomal subunit of bacteria
- Good for skin infections caused by staphylococcus (including MRSA) and streptococcus
- Typically not first line, but good for resistant cases

- AEs: myelosuppression in 2%, serotonin syndrome (if given with serotonergic drugs like selective serotonin reuptake inhibitors [SSRIs], monoamine oxidase inhibitor, and tricyclics), and optic/peripheral neuropathy

Quinupristin and dalfopristin

- MoA: diffuses through bacterial cell wall and binds 50S ribosomal subunit sites → ↓ protein synthesis
- Used in complicated skin and soft tissue infections caused by GPs (e.g., MRSA and vancomycin-resistant enterococci [VRE])
- AEs: anaphylaxis, angioedema, and ↑ bilirubin
- Potent CYP3A4 inhibitor

Daptomycin

- MoA: depolarizes bacterial cell membrane → cell death
- Good for complicated skin and soft tissue infections caused by GPs (e.g., MRSA, VRE, and linezolid-resistant GPs)
- AEs: neuropathy, myopathy (check CPKs; caution w/ statins), eosinophilic pneumonia, and nephrotoxicity

Others

- Some new antibiotics for complicated skin infections include: telavancin, tigecycline, tedizolid, ozenoxacin, ceftaroline fosamil, omadacycline, dalbavancin, and oritavancin

Antiviral agents

Acyclovir

- Guanosine analog that requires:
  - Phosphorylation first by herpes-specific thymidine kinase → acyclovir monophosphate
  - Subsequent phosphorylation by human cellular GMP kinase and other cellular kinases → acyclovir triphosphate
    - At this stage, it competes with deoxyguanosine triphosphate as a substrate for viral DNA polymerase → incorporates into viral DNA → **chain terminates** and ↓ viral duplication
- Penciclovir also works in this fashion
- Valacyclovir and famciclovir are prodrugs of (and converted to) acyclovir and penciclovir, respectively, so they are also dependent on these enzymes and pathways
- Topical and systemic forms available; considered safe in pregnancy
  - Topical form only approved for HSV, not varicella zoster virus (VZV)
- Dermatologic uses: HSV infections, VZV, and recurrent erythema multiforme (EM) 2° to HSV
  - Consider suppressive doses in HSV patients if more than six outbreaks per year
  - IV form used in cases of disseminated HSV/VZV, eczema herpeticum, and in immunosuppressed patients
- Low rate of AEs and interactions:
  - IV infusions rarely associated with renal impairment (2° to **crystalline nephropathy**)
  - Zidovudine (AZT) + acyclovir can → drowsiness/ lethargy
  - Probenecid → ↑ bioavailability and ↓ renal clearance
- If **viral resistance** occurs (via mutations in thymidine kinase, or less commonly in DNA polymerase) → use **foscarnet** or **cidofovir**
  - Patients resistant to acyclovir will also be resistant to valacyclovir, famciclovir, and penciclovir

Valacyclovir

- Prodrug of acyclovir with greater bioavailability (almost as much as IV acyclovir); oral and topical forms
- Same uses as acyclovir with excellent AE profile and easier dosing
  - Rarely can cause **TTP/HUS in HIV patients**

Famciclovir and penciclovir

- Famciclovir is a prodrug of penciclovir
  - Famciclovir is available orally, but penciclovir only available topically
  - Penciclovir triphosphate has significantly longer half-life than acyclovir triphosphate
  - Famciclovir has even better bioavailability than valacyclovir
  - Famciclovir and valacyclovir more effective at ↓ VZV pain than acyclovir
  - Indications:
    - Famciclovir: same indications as acyclovir/ valacyclovir
    - Penciclovir: herpes labialis only

Cidofovir

- Nucleoside phosphate analog of deoxycytidine monophosphate effective in HPV, HSV, cytomegalovirus (CMV) retinitis ("Cidofovir = **CMV**"), orf, and molluscum
  - Must be phosphorylated twice, to cidofovir diphosphate, in order to be active
  - **Does NOT require viral thymidine kinase**
  - Once active, acts as a competitive inhibitor and alternate substrate for viral DNA polymerases → incorporates into DNA strand → blockage/termination of DNA synthesis
- IV and topical forms available (topicals are not commercially available, however)
- AEs: nephrotoxicity (most common), neutropenia, alopecia, uveitis/iritis, and cardiomyopathy

Foscarnet

- A pyrophosphate analog that binds to pyrophosphate-binding site on viral DNA polymerase → inhibition of pyrophosphate cleavage from deoxyadenosine triphosphate → disruption of DNA elongation
- **Treatment of choice for acyclovir-resistant HSV** (does not require same enzymes as acyclovir and penciclovir); also used to treat CMV retinitis and CMV skin infection in HIV patients
- AEs: **penile erosions**, thrombophlebitis, nephrotoxicity, seizures, and electrolyte disturbances

Bleomycin

- Chemotherapeutic agent that can be used intralesionally for warts

- MoA: binds DNA → single strand breaks → ↓ protein synthesis → ↑ apoptosis/necrosis of keratinocytes
- AEs: **injection pain**, **Raynaud's** phenomenon, loss of nail plate/**nail dystrophy**, and **flagellate hyperpigmentation**

Podophyllin resin and podophyllotoxin

- Podophyllin administered in office and its derivative podophyllotxin administered at home by patient
  - podophyllotxin is safer—fewer mutagens
- Antimitotic agent that **binds tubulin** → cell cycle arrest in metaphase
- FDA approved for genital warts
- AEs are typically local (contraindicated in pregnancy—teratogenic)

Cantharidin

- Blistering agent (comes from blister beetle/**Spanish fly,** ***Lytta vesicatoria***)
- MoA: disrupts desmosomes → intraepidermal acantholysis → bullae
- Applied in office under occlusion for warts/molluscum; washed off at home 4 hours later
- AEs: pain from blister and **ring wart** formation

Sinecatechins

- Green tea (*Camellia sinensis*)-derived polyphenol epigallocatechin gallate → apoptosis, inhibition of telomerase, and an antioxidant effect on cells
- Approved for genital/perianal warts; AEs are local (e.g., pain, itch, and swelling)

5-Fluorouracil and imiquimod (discussed in section 2.5)

Antifungal agents

I. Azoles

- MoA: inhibit 14α demethylase (catalyzes conversion of lanosterol to ergosterol) → ↓ ergosterol → ↓ cell membrane synthesis, ↑ membrane rigidity/permeability, growth inhibition, and cell death

Itraconazole

- Metabolized mainly in liver (CYP3A4); **absorption enhanced in an acidic environment**
- FDA-approved indications: dermatophyte onychomycosis (200 mg BID once a week for 2 months for fingernails and 200 mg daily for 12 weeks for toenails), oropharyngeal/esophageal candidiasis, **blastomycosis, histoplasmosis**, and aspergillosis refractory to amphotericin B
- Off-label dermatologic uses: other tinea infections, Candida infections, extensive tinea versicolor (for very short courses or even single doses), and nondermatophyte/saprophytic onychomycosis.
- Contraindications:
  - Ventricular dysfunction and **CHF**
  - Active liver disease or h/o liver toxicity with other drugs
  - Concurrent use of certain drugs metabolized via **CYP3A4 (e.g., pimozide, quinidine, and cisapride)** as it is a CYP3A4 inhibitory
  - Concurrent use with **levomethadyl**, **dofetilide**, **statins**, **midazolam**, **triazolam**, **nisoldipine**, and **ergot alkaloids**
- Common AEs: GI (e.g., nausea, vomiting, and abdominal pain), cutaneous (e.g., rash—more common if also using immunosuppressive meds), neurologic (e.g., headache), edema, ↑ LFTs, rhinitis, and fever
- Rarer AEs: hearing loss, peripheral neuropathy, CV events (e.g., **CHF**), dysgeusia, pancreatitis, hepatotoxicity, neutropenia/leukopenia, pulmonary edema, and hypokalemia

Fluconazole

- Very little hepatic metabolism; pregnancy category D
- **Unlike itraconazole, absorption not dependent on food or gastric pH**
- FDA approved for vaginal/oropharyngeal/esophageal candidiasis and cryptococcal meningitis
- Off-label dermatologic uses: tinea infections, systemic *Candida* infections, cutaneous candidiasis, coccidioidal meningitis, and onychomycosis due to dermatophyte and non-dermatophyte (e.g. *Scopulariopsis* and *Candida*) (150–300 mg once a week for 6–9 months in fingernails and 12–18 months in toenails)
- Contraindications:
  - **Potent CYP2C9 inhibitor** - caution with substrates
  - Do NOT administer with pimozide, quinidine, cisapride, **erythromycin**, terfenadine, astemizole, voriconazole, or statins
- Common AEs: GI (e.g., nausea and abdominal pain), skin rash, and headache
- Rare AEs: CV events (e.g., torsades), cholestasis/hepatocellular damage/liver failure, severe skin reactions, seizures, leukopenia/thrombocytopenia, dysgeusia, and hyperlipidemia

Ketoconazole

- Systemic form not commonly used because of the associated high rate of **hepatic toxicity**
- FDA approved for tinea corporis/cruris/pedis/capitis, chronic mucocutaneous candidiasis, vaginal and cutaneous candidiasis, chromoblastomycosis, blastomycosis, histoplasmosis, coccidioidomycosis, and paracoccidioidomycosis
- Topical uses: tinea infections, cutaneous candidiasis, tinea versicolor, and seborrheic dermatitis
- Do NOT administer with **cisapride, terfenadine, or astemizole**, as interaction can → serious CV events like **↑ QT syndrome**
- AEs (systemic form only): GI symptoms, idiosyncratic adrenal suppression, pruritus, and urticaria

Voriconazole

- New generation of azoles used primarily for serious, invasive fungal infections in immunosuppressed hosts (invasive aspergillosis, *Candida* infections, and *Fusarium* infections)
- Unique AEs: **severe phototoxicity** (including **pseudoporphyria**, and **xeroderma pigmentosum [XP]-like changes**) and ↑ **risk SCC**, visual disturbances (e.g.,

blurriness), hepatotoxicity, GI issues, and QT prolongation

Posaconazole

- Triazole anifungal (similar to itraconazole), used for invasive *Aspergillus* and *Candida* infections in immunocompromised patients
- AE: fever, diarrhea/nausea/vomiting, CYP3A4 inhibitor, LFT elevations

Miconazole, clotrimazole, and econazole

- Topical azoles active against various dermatophytes, *Malassezia furfur*, and *Candida albicans*
- Good for tinea infections, tinea versicolor, and cutaneous candidiasis

Efinaconazole

- Solution triazole for onychomycosis—daily 48-week course 15%–20% complete cure; AEs: ingrown toenail, application site dermatitis

Luliconazole

- Once-daily 1% cream used for cutaneous dermatophyte infections
- Other topical antifungals good for cutaneous dermatophyte infections and possibly cutaneous *Candida* infections include oxiconazole, sulconazole, and sertaconazole

II. Allylamines/benzylamines

- MoA: inhibit squalene epoxidase (catalyzes conversion of squalene to lanosterol) → ↓ cell membrane synthesis

Terbinafine

- Oral and topical formulations
- Metabolized mainly in liver—do NOT give in active liver disease; also do not give if CrCl ≤ 50 mL/min
- FDA approved for dermatophyte onychomycosis and tinea capitis (granule formulation)
- Off-label dermatologic uses (systemic formulation): other tinea infections, subcutaneous/systemic mycoses (e.g., histoplasmosis and chromoblastomycosis), and other types of onychomycosis (good for *Aspergillus*, but not *Candida*)
- Topical formulation: utility limited to superficial dermatophyte infections
  - More effective than clotrimazole and oxiconazole for tinea pedis
- **6-week 250 mg/day course for fingernail onychomycosis and 12-week 250 mg/day course for toenail onychomycosis** (clinical cure ≈ 60%–70%)
- Tinea capitis:
  - Highly effective against **endothrix** organisms (most commonly *Trichophyton tonsurans*)
  - Less effective against **ectothrix** organisms like ***Microsporum canis*** **(griseofulvin preferred)**
- Most common AEs: GI (e.g., diarrhea), cutaneous (e.g., rash), headache, and ↑ LFT
- Rarer AEs: **taste/smell disturbance**, severe skin reactions (e.g., SJS/TEN), visual disturbance, **hepatobiliary dysfunction/hepatitis/liver failure (idiosyncratic)**, hematologic abnormalities (e.g., neutropenia or thrombocytopenia), rhabdomyolysis, **depression, exacerbation of SLE, drug-induced subacute cutaneous lupus (SCLE)**
- **Inhibits CYP2D6**, so exercise caution if giving with CYP2D6 substrates (e.g., doxepin or amitriptyline)

Naftifine

- Topical effective for dermatophyte infections primarily (may be more effective than azoles in treatment of cutaneous dermatophytoses)

Butenafine

- Benzylamine class topical antifungal effective in cutaneous dermatophyte infections, tinea versicolor, and cutaneous candidal infections

III. Griseofulvin

- MoA: **interferes with tubulin** → inhibition of mitosis; binds to keratin in keratin precursor cells → resistance to fungal infections
- FDA approved for dermatophyte onychomycosis and tinea corporis/cruris/pedis/capitis
  - **More effective than terbinafine in tinea capitis caused by *Microsporum* (e.g., *M. canis*)**
- AEs: GI disturbance and headache are most common; fixed drug eruption, photosensitivity, and exfoliative dermatitis; can instigate or worsen porphyria and lupus

IV. Ciclopirox olamine

- MoA: disrupts fungal cell membrane transport of important molecules, ↓ cell membrane integrity, inhibits cellular respiratory enzymes, and blocks important enzymatic cofactors
- Topical cutaneous dermatophyte infections, *Malassezia* spp., tinea versicolor, cutaneous candidiasis, and onychomycosis (in lacquer form)
  - Ciclopirox and topical azoles are superior to allylamine/benzylamine drugs for *Candida*

V. Selenium sulfide

- Topical cytostatic effect on epithelium, diminishing the formation rate of the stratum corneum—treats tinea versicolor, seborrheic dermatitis of scalp, and CARP

VI. Nystatin

- Polyene topical agent that binds *Candida* cell membrane sterols → ↑ permeability → cell death
- Used for cutaneous/mucosal *Candida* infections

VII. Echinocandins (caspofungin, micafungin, and anidulafungin)

- MoA: inhibit β-(1,3)-D-glucan synthase → ↓ glucan production → disrupt cell wall synthesis

- Used primarily in invasive *Candida* infections and invasive aspergillosis (second line)
- Unique AEs: facial swelling (caspofungin), ↑ alkaline phosphatase (caspofungin), hypokalemia (caspofungin), and hematuria/proteinuria (caspofungin)

VIII. Tavaborole

- Novel oxaborole; inhibits protein synthesis enzyme cytosolic leucyl-transfer RNA synthetase
- Topical solution for onychomycosis; complete cure rate = 6.5%

Antiparasitic agents (Tables 2.7 and 2.8)

- Interesting facts about drugs not in the tables: benzyl benzoate may → disulfiram-like reaction; precipitated sulfur is safe in pregnant women and children under 2 months of age with scabies; permethrin is safe in pregnant women and children over 2 months of age; topical thiabendazole compound may be helpful for cutaneous larva migrans

2.7 PHOTOTHERAPY

- Divided into ultraviolet A **(UVA) (320–400 nm)** and ultraviolet B **(UVB) (280–320 nm)** modalities
- Doses of light determined by skin type usually or 70% of minimum erythema dose (MED; lowest dose that results in minimally visual erythema) and increased as tolerated each visit up to a maximum dose

Table 2.7 Systemic Antiparasitic Treatments

Agent	Mechanism	Uses	Adverse Effects (AEs)
Ivermectin	Binds **glutamate-gated chloride ion channels** of parasite nerve/muscle cells → ↑ membrane permeability → hyper-polarization → death Of note, resistance can occur due to SNPs of P-glycoprotein-like protein	FDA: onchocerciasis, intestinal strongyloidiasis (secondary to *Strongyloides stercoralis*), rosacea (topical) Off-label: scabies (0.2 mg/kg/dose po q1wk × 2 doses), cutaneous larva migrans, and pediculosis	Commonly rashes, pruritus, fever, and lymphadenopathy (less with scabies infection) Rarely death and encephalopathy when used in patients with loiasis **Mazzotti reactions** = rash/systemic symptoms/ocular reactions; occurs in patients with onchocerciasis → doxycycline helps reduce these reactions
Albendazole	Stops **tubulin polymerization** → immobilization and death of parasite	FDA: neurocysticercosis and hydatid disease Off-label: *Ascaris lumbricoides, Trichuris trichiura, Enterobius vermicularis, Ancylostoma duodenale* and *Necator americanus* (hookworms), *Taenia, Strongyloides stercoralis, Giardia,* scabies	Bone marrow suppression (↑ risk if patient has liver disease), aplastic anemia, agranulocytosis, hepatotoxicity, GI AEs, rash May ↑ theophylline levels Resistance higher in patients with HTLV-1 infection
Thiobendazole	Inhibits **fumarate reductase**	FDA: strongyloides, cutaneous larva migrans, and visceral larva migrans Off-label: trichinosis, uncinariasis, *Necator, Ancylostoma,* trichuriasis, and ascariasis	Hepatotoxicity, GI AEs, CNS AEs, SJS May ↑ theophylline levels

CNS, *Central nervous system;* FDA, *Food and Drug Administration;* GI, *gastrointestinal;* HTLV-1, *human T-lymphotropic virus type 1;* SJS, *Stevens-Johnsons syndrome;* SNPs, *single nucleotide polymorphisms.*

Table 2.8 Topical Antiparasitic Treatments

Agent	Mechanism	Uses	Adverse Effects (AEs)
Permethrin	Related to pyrethrins, which come from flowers of genus ***Compositae*** Disables sodium transport channels on the cell membranes of arthropods → paralysis	Scabies (5% cream is the treatment of choice; neck down application—2 overnight applications separated by 1 week) and *Pediculosis capitis* (1% cream rinse)	Local irritation, rare neurotoxicity (numbness, tingling, tremors, and at high exposures, paralysis and seizures)
Malathion	Organophosphate that inhibits acetylcholinesterase in arthropods → neuromuscular paralysis	*P. capitis* (0.5% lotion; most effective treatment in the United States; treatment of choice in children ≥ 6 years old)	Local irritation Potentially **flammable** Malodorous If ingested → symptoms of **organophosphate poisoning**/↓ cholinesterase
Spinosad	Instigates arthropod motor neurons → paralysis	*P. capitis* (very rapid effect: 10-minute application)	Local irritation
Lindane	Organochlorine → ↓ neurotransmission → arthropod respiratory/muscular paralysis	Scabies and *P. capitis*	**Seizures** if ingested or multiple applications Aplastic anemia, leukemia
Abametapir	Metalloproteinase inhibitor	*P. capitis* in patients aged 6 months or older	Local irritation
Crotamiton	Mechanism unknown but is toxic to scabies mites and has anti-pruritic effects	Scabies (10% cream or lotion; neck down application once and then again in 24 hours with no shower till 48 hours after the initial application)	Local reaction; frequent treatment failure

UVA modalities

Psoralen plus UVA (PUVA)

- Photochemical reaction between psoralen (**8-methoxypsoralen** usually) and UVA
  - Psoralen (0.4–0.6 mg/kg 1–2 hours before UVA) can be administered orally or topically
    - Of note, before UV exposure, **psoralen intercalates into DNA**
    - Photoactivated psoralen molecules form 3,4 or 4′,5′ cyclobutane monofunctional adducts to pyrimidines in DNA → **inter-strand DNA cross-link** → ↓ DNA synthesis/cell cycle arrest
    - PUVA → selective immunosuppression, selective cytotoxicity (via production of ROS and free radicals), and melanocyte stimulation
    - Psoralens ideally taken under fasting conditions, because food slows absorption
    - Absorption and bioavailability vary widely with 8-methoxypsoralen
    - Metabolized by liver
    - Used in many inflammatory dermatoses including atopic dermatitis, psoriasis, vitiligo, CTCL, photodermatoses (using desensitization protocols), GVHD, and lichen planus
    - AEs include: nausea/vomiting (food may help), **phototoxic reactions** (e.g., symptomatic erythema and pruritus), hepatic toxicity, bronchoconstriction, HSV recurrences, cardiovascular stress, CNS disturbances, photoaging, melanoma, and **NMSC (SCC >> BCC**; usually if ≥ 250 treatments), and ocular issues (e.g., **cataracts**)
    - UV-opaque goggles and face/genital protection in unit; UV-opaque glasses after exposure until sunset, along with photoprotection
    - Contraindications: lactation and photosensitizing skin disorders (LE, albinism, porphyria, XP); autoimmune blistering disease has been induced by PUVA)
  - Treatments administered two to three times per week initially till mostly clear, then a maintenance schedule where radiation dose is kept the same and visit frequency slowly decreased (even to one treatment a month), then stopped
  - Safe in combination with other treatments (e.g., topicals, MTX, acitretin, and UVB)

UVA-1 (340–400 nm)

- Treatments can be low, medium, or high dose
- Dose based on MED as sensitivity to UVA-1 can vary greatly between people
- Not many centers in the United States have UVA-1 units and not necessarily superior to PUVA and/or NB-UVB
- Various skin disorders including SLE (low dose), scleroderma/other sclerodermoid skin conditions (need at least 30 treatments), atopic dermatitis, and MF
- AEs include erythema in the short-term; no long-term studies for AEs

UVB modalities

- MoA: ↓ DNA synthesis (i.e., in psoriatic epidermis) and ↑ **p53** → cell cycle arrest/keratinocyte apoptosis; ↓ proinflammatory cytokines, ↓ **Langerhans cells in skin**
- **Narrowband UVB (311–313 nm)**
  - Treatments given three times a week initially (based on skin type or 70% MED) and increased by 10%–15% each treatment; may have to adjust the dose based on erythema severity
  - UV-opaque goggles during treatment and covering face/genitals
  - AEs: skin reactions (e.g., erythema or pruritus), mucosal reactions (recurrent herpes labialis, or blepharitis), exacerbation of SLE and blistering disorders. No significant risk of skin malignancy
  - Used in psoriasis (most commonly prescribed phototherapy), vitiligo, MF (patch and plaque), atopic dermatitis, photodermatoses (using desensitization protocols), and pruritus (idiopathic and secondary)
  - Similar contraindications to PUVA
- **Broadband UVB**—280–320 nm; more convenient in darker-skinned individuals than NB-UVB (shorter treatment times), but largely has been replaced by NB-UVB
- **Excimer laser—308 nm**; high-intensity treatment with higher efficacy than standard NB-UVB for treating smaller surface areas (<2 cm^2; e.g., in psoriasis and vitiligo)

Extracorporeal photochemotherapy

- Pheresis via venous catheter in arm vein → blood cells separated into leukocyte-rich buffy coat and RBCs (returned back to patient) → 8-methoxypsoralen added to leukocytes → UVA radiation → reinfusion (net gain of 500 mL of fluid, but initially 200 to 400 mL are pheresed)
  - Usually 2-day cycle every 4 weeks and slow weaning after desired response
- Various effects on immune system, including T cells (e.g., apoptosis of activated T cells, induction of regulatory T cells/immunologic tolerance), cytokines (e.g., favors immunoregulatory cytokines), and dendritic cells (↓#)
- Effective in **CTCL** (selectively targets lymphoma cells; can be used in combination with other treatments) and other dermatoses (e.g., scleroderma, **chronic GVHD**, nephrogenic systemic fibrosis, and pemphigus)
- **Contraindicated in severe cardiac disease** (because of difficulty in handling added fluid volume); caution in patients with low BP, hematocrit, and CHF
- AEs: nausea, photosensitivity, hypotension, CHF, and tachycardia

Photodynamic therapy (PDT)

- Activation of topical photosensitizer by light
  - **Aminolevulinic acid (ALA):** activated by **blue light** (Blu-U device); no need for occlusion
  - **Methyl aminolevulinate (MAL):** activated by **red light** (Aktilite) and is more lipophilic; **occlusion recommended**
  - These photosensitizers are ultimately converted to **protoporphyrin IX** within cells → activated to a higher energy state (along with production of ROS, including singlet O_2) primarily with light ≈ **410-417 nm (Soret band, blue)**, but also has other peaks **(e.g., 635 nm,**

red) → localize by mitochondria → necrosis/apoptosis of malignant cells
  - **Neoplastic cells accumulate more porphyrins than normal cells**—thus PDT effective in actinic keratoses and NMSCs
  - Of note, **protoporphyrin IX** is also elevated in the inherited condition, **protoporphyria**
  - In acne, targets sebaceous glands and *C. acnes*, which accumulates porphyrins (light alone is effective in acne +/− photosensitizer)
- Only FDA-approved indication is actinic keratosis (≈90% response on individual lesions), but also used in BCC, SCCIS, acne, photoaging, hidradenitis, and MF
- Technique: (1) skin cleansed (acetone for ALA and gentle curette debridement of scale/crust for MAL); (2) photosensitizer applied; (3) incubation time (3–4 hours for MAL, 1–4 hours for ALA); (4) light exposure (37 J/cm^2 for MAL: 7–9 minutes, 10 J/cm^2 for ALA: 16 minutes); and (5) retreat in 7 days for MAL and 1 to 2 months for ALA if needed
- Protective eyewear during procedure and avoid sunlight for 48 hours
- AEs: phototoxic reactions/photosensitivity, hypo-/hyperpigmentation, hypersensitivity to photosensitizer, pain, systemic absorption, and inflammation (edema, blistering, and crusting)

2.8 MISCELLANEOUS AGENTS

Sunscreens

- Sun protection factor (SPF) = MED of protected skin divided by MED of unprotected skin
  - UVB is 1000× more effective at causing erythema than UVA
  - SPF of 15 blocks 93% of erythematous radiation, while SPF 30 blocks 97%
  - 2 g/cm^2 of sunscreen applied in phototesting, but real-life application thickness is lower which reduces effective SPF
- Broad spectrum = UVA + UVB protection
  - UVA—tanning, photoaging
  - UVB—erythema and DNA damage via pyrimdine dimer formation
- Water resistant = SPF value after 40 or 80 minutes of water immersion is the same as the value before immersion
- **Chemical absorbers**: aromatic compounds that **absorb** radiation and convert it into longer, lower-energy wavelengths
  - UVB: para-aminobenzoic acid (PABA), padimate O, octinoxate, cinoxate, octisalate, homosalate, trolamine salicylate, octocrylene, ensulizole
    - PABA—most potent UVB agent; associated with contact dermatitis, skin staining; has largely been replaced by other agents
  - UVA: oxybenzone, sulisobenzone, dioxybenzone, meradimate, avobenzone, ecamsule
    - Oxybenzone—**contact dermatitis, photoallergy**
    - Avobenzone—**photolabile**, combined with other agents to prevent degradation
- **Physical blockers**: chemically inert compounds that **reflect/scatter** radiation
  - Zinc oxide and titanium dioxide
  - More broad-spectrum coverage (UVA, UVB, and visible light) → better for patients with photosensitivity disorders
  - Do not cause contact dermatitis; micronized formulations decrease visible light scatter, absorb UV light and offer improved cosmetic application
- AEs: irritation, contact urticaria, irritant contact dermatitis, **allergic and photoallergic contact dermatitis (oxybenzone** is #1 culprit; **cinnamates** and **PABA** also common), photosensitivity, and may ↓vitamin D synthesis
- Concurrent administration of DEET (insect repellant) and oxybenzone may increase absorption of both agents and reduce SPF
- Dihydroxyacetone (found in sunless tanning products) has only SPF 4 protection
- Window glass absorbs UVB but NOT UVA

Insect repellants (Table 2.9)

Topical cosmetic agents

Bimatoprost

- **Prostaglandin analog** that is approved for eyelash hypotrichosis (↑ length, thickness, and pigment); AEs include periorbital skin pigmentation, **iris hyperpigmentation** (more common in glaucoma treatment), and ocular irritation

Brimonidine and oxymetazoline

- Topical alpha-adrenergic agonists for treatment of facial redness in rosacea; ophthalmic oxymetazoline solution is approved for acquired ptosis
- AEs: contact dermatitis, **rebound erythema** (more so with brimonidine)

Eflornithine

- Binds/inhibits **ornithine decarboxylase**; used in treatment of female facial hirsutism; **acne** is the most common AE

Hydroquinone

- Lightens skin color via active reduction of pigment production (i.e., auto-oxidation of melanin, tyrosinase, and phenol oxidases into various reactive substances); **competes with tyrosine as substrate for tyrosinase**; production of ROS → melanocyte damage
  - Dermatitis is most common AE; most concerning AEs are **paradoxical hyperpigmentation** or **exogenous ochronosis** (usually at higher concentrations for longer time periods); reversible nail discoloration can occur
  - Other bleaching agents: monobenzyl ether of hydroquinone (potent; used for permanent depigmentation of normal skin in severe vitiligo), kojic acid, and mequinol

Psychiatric agents

- For a thorough discussion of the subject, we recommend *Journal of the American Academy of Dermatology* 2017;76(5):795–808

Table 2.9 Insect Repellants

Insect Repellent Compound	Available Concentration/ Average Duration	Efficacy Against Mosquitoes and Ticks	Adverse Effects/Special Considerations
Synthetic			
DEET	5%–100%/5 hours @ 24%	Mosquitoes and ticks **Most efficacious insect repellant**	Urticaria, vesiculobullous skin necrosis at 50%–75% concentration, anaphylaxis, cardiovascular (hypotension, bradycardia), neurologic (lethargy, confusion, headaches, ataxia, disorientation, seizures, tremors)/sunscreen and topical retinoids may increase risk of toxicity. **Decreases efficacy of sunscreen.** May cause fabric and plastic degradation. Not recommended for age < 2 months
Picaridin	7%–20%/8–10 hours @ 20%	Mosquitoes and ticks	Minor skin irritation/odorless, non-sticky, no harm to clothing or plastics
IR3535	7.5%–19.7%/2–3 hours	Mosquitoes and ticks	Eye irritation/odorless, biodegradable
Natural			
Oil of lemon eucalyptus	10%–40%/6 hours	Mosquitoes	Minor skin irritation
Oil of citronella	0.5%–20%/2 hours	Mosquitoes	Eye and minor skin irritation
Catnip oil	7%–15%/7 hours	Mosquitoes	N/A
2-Undecanone	1%–2%/5 hours	Mosquitoes and ticks	N/A
Only clothing applied			
Permethrin	0.5%/6 weeks or re-apply after 6 washings	Mosquitoes and ticks	Eye and skin irritation, neurologic (numbness, tingling, tremors, and at high exposures, paralysis and seizures)/ both an insect repellant and an insecticide

From Nguyen QD, Vu MN, Hebert AA. Insect repellents: an updated review for the clinician. J Am Acad Dermatol. *2018;S0190-9622(18)32824-X.*

- Some classic uses in dermatology include:
  - SSRIs for obsessive compulsive disorders, trichotillomania, excoriation disorder; associated with increased suicidal ideation; other AEs include weight changes, nausea, insomnia and reduced libido
  - **Mirtazapine** for idiopathic pruritus; AEs: weight gain and sedation
  - **Doxepin** for depressed patients with neurotic excoriations
  - Pimozide (low doses of 3–5 mg/day) for **delusions of parasitosis**
    - Antipsychotic (potent centrally acting dopamine receptor antagonist)
    - AEs include: **extrapyramidal AEs** (tardive dyskinesia—may be irreversible with long-term use, withdrawal dyskinesia, and akathisia), and cardiac effects (e.g., **arrhythmias** from a **prolonged QT interval**)—not typically seen with low doses
  - Atypical antipsychotics (e.g., risperidone, olanzapine, and quetiapine) for delusions of parasitosis
    - Dopamine (D2) and serotonin receptor antagonists
    - Significantly ↓ the risk of extrapyramidal AEs (vs. pimozide)
  - Amitriptyline for nonspecific cutaneous sensations, such as burning/stinging/pain
    - Works as analgesic in this scenario
    - AEs are anticholinergic, cardiac, sedative, and orthostatic hypotension (use low doses)

Antiandrogens and androgen inhibitors

Spironolactone

- MoA: **antiandrogen**; **blocks androgen receptor** → ↓ androgen production; aldosterone antagonist = diuretic properties
- Dermatologic uses: hirsutism, acne, and androgenetic alopecia
- AEs: **hyperkalemia** (typically in patients with renal insufficiency; do not give with agents that ↑ K+ [like TMP-SMX]), **gynecomastia**/breast pain, **menstrual irregularities**, dizziness, and agranulocytosis (rare); data does **NOT** indicate increased risk of estrogen-dependent malignancies
- Theoretical risk of feminization of male fetuses if taken during pregnancy (observed only in animal studies)

Finasteride and dutasteride

- MoA: finasteride is **type II and III 5-α reductase inhibitor** (of note, 5-α reductase converts testosterone to dihydrotestosterone [DHT]) and dutasteride inhibits **type I, II, and III 5-α reductase**
- Dermatologic uses: androgenetic alopecia (dutasteride more effective than finasteride), hirsutism, and hidradenitis suppurativa
- AEs: **sexual** (↓ libido, impotence, and abnormal ejaculation), gynecomastia, ↓ PSA, ↓ overall risk of prostate cancer, and a possible slight ↑ **high-grade prostate cancer** and breast cancer; **teratogenic** (if pregnant female is exposed), depression
  - A large randomized controlled trial found: ↓ overall risk of prostate cancer, ↓ low-grade prostate cancer, and slight ↑ high-grade prostate cancer (3.5% vs. 3.0%; RR = 1.17); no difference in mortality between the finasteride and placebo groups

Combination oral contraceptive pills

- MoA: contains both an estrogen and progestin component, inhibits gonadotropin-releasing hormone which prevents ovulation. For treatment of acne,

mechanism is based on antiandrogenic properties: decreases androgen production at the ovary, increases sex hormone–binding globulin (decreases free testosterone), and reduces 5-α reductase activity.
- FDA approved for acne: ethinyl estradiol/norgestimate, ethinyl estradiol/norethindrone, acetate/ferrous fumarate, ethinyl estradiol/drospirenone, and ethinyl estradiol/drospirenone/levomefolate
- AEs: thromboembolism, stroke (increased risk in age > 35, cigarette smoking), potential increased risk of breast and cervical cancer, decreased bone mass

Clascoterone
- MoA: topical androgen receptor inhibitor that competes with DHT for binding androgen receptors within the sebaceous glands and hair follicles
- FDA approved for acne in ages 12 and older

Vitamin D_3 analogs
Calcipotriene and calcitriol
- MoA: product binds to vitamin D receptors → drug-receptor complex + RXR-α binds to DNA at vitamin D response elements → ↓ keratinocyte proliferation/epidermal differentiation, ↓ IL-2/IL-6/IFN-γ/GM-CSF, ↓ NK-cell and cytotoxic T-cell activity, ↑ involucrin/transglutaminase → enhanced cornified envelope formation
- Dermatologic uses: FDA approved for psoriasis, but used in morphea and vitiligo; can be used in combination with 5-fluorouracil BID × 4 days for actinic keratoses
- AEs: **hypercalcemia** (uncommon), irritation (most common), and mild photosensitivity

Attenuated androgens
Danazol and stanozolol
- MoA: complex, but involves ↑ production of various proteins by the liver, including various clotting factors, inhibitor of first component of complement (C1 INH), fibrinolytic proteins
- Dermatologic uses: **hereditary angioedema (FDA approved)**, cryofibrinogenemia, **lipodermatosclerosis**, and livedoid vasculitis
- AEs: **hormonal-related AEs** (hirsutism, deeper voice, alopecia, acne, and menstrual irregularities), muscle cramps, **myalgias, myopathy (in patients on statins)**, hematuria/hemorrhagic cystitis, insulin resistance, headaches, worsening HTN and CHF (drugs retain sodium), hyperlipidemia, and hepatic AEs (jaundice and liver tumors)
- Contraindicated in childhood and pregnancy

Agents used for anti-inflammatory properties
Clofazimine
- Riminophenazine dye used for **antibiotic** (i.e., antimycobacterial, especially multibacillary leprosy and erythema nodosum leprosum) and **anti-inflammatory** (e.g., SLE, pyoderma gangrenosum, **erythema dyschromicum perstans**, and discoid LE) purposes
- AEs: reversible **orange-brown skin and body fluid** discoloration, xerosis, and crystal deposition in organs → enteropathy/splenic infarction/eosinophilic enteritis/cardiac dysrhythmia

Colchicine
- MoA: **binds tubulin dimers** in leukocytes → mitotic arrest in metaphase and ↓ chemotaxis
- Dermatologic uses: familial Mediterranean fever (treatment of choice), neutrophilic dermatoses (e.g., Behcet's disease), **cutaneous small vessel vasculitis**, autoimmune connective tissue disorders, and gout
- AEs: GI AEs (e.g., **cramping, diarrhea**, and abdominal pain, which can → discontinuation); rarely **bone marrow suppression, neuropathy**, and myopathy

Nicotinamide (vitamin B_3)
- MoA: inhibits PARP-1 → ↓ NF-κB transcription → ↓ leukocyte chemotaxis; ↓ lysosomal enzyme release; stabilizes leukocytes by inhibiting PDE → immunomodulation; ↓ lymphocytic transformation/antibody production; ↓ mast cell degranulation
- Dermatologic uses: **pellagra, autoimmune bullous disorders** (in combination w/ tetracyclines), **NMSC chemoprevention**
- AEs: occasional GI complaints; niacin causes flushing, but nicotinamide does not

Pentoxifylline
- Phosphodiesterase inhibitor that:
  - ↑ **Erythrocyte/leukocyte deformability**
  - ↓ **Platelet aggregation**
  - ↓ TNF-α
  - ↓ Neutrophil adhesion
- Used in Raynaud's, **livedoid vasculopathy**, necrobiosis lipoidica, **venous ulcers**, and **lipodermatosclerosis**
- AEs are primarily GI; decrease dose in renal dysfunction

Potassium iodide
- MoA: unknown, likely anti-inflammatory (especially toward neutrophils)
- Dermatologic uses: **sporotrichosis, erythema nodosum**, and **erythema induratum**
- AEs: **hypothyroidism** (with chronic high-dose treatment, mainly in patients with preexisting thyroid issues), chronic iodine intoxication, skin eruptions (e.g., **iododerma**, acneiform, dermatitis, and vascular), GI AEs (most common), "iodism" (metallic taste, sore/burning mouth, and headache), and **exacerbation of dermatitis herpetiformis**
- Check for thyroid disorders before starting medication; do not give large doses during pregnancy (can → goiter/hypothyroidism in fetus)

Tapinarof
- MOA: non-steroidal topical aryl hyrocarbon receptor agonist which decreases IL-17 expression
- FDA approved for plaque psoriasis
- AEs: folliculitis and contact dermatitis

Thalidomide

- MoA: immunomodulatory and antiangiogenic; exact MoA unknown
  - Anti-inflammatory effects: inhibits TNF-α and IFN-γ, ↓ IL-12 production, ↓ helper T cells, ↑ suppressor T cells
- Dermatologic uses: **erythema nodosum leprosum (FDA approved)**, HIV-related disorders, LE, GVHD, **prurigo nodularis** (due to neural effects), and neutrophilic dermatoses (e.g., Behcet's disease)
- AEs: **teratogenic** (category X—most common defect is **phocomelia**), peripheral **neuropathy** (proximal muscle weakness + distal painful paresthesias/sensory loss), **venous thrombosis**, hypersensitivity reaction (more common in patients with HIV), **sedation/drowsiness (most common)**, constipation, and various drug interactions

Topical calcineurin inhibitors

Pimecrolimus and tacrolimus

- MoA: **bind to FK506-binding protein** forming a complex → complex binds to enzyme calcineurin → prevention of calcineurin from dephosphorylating transcription factor NFAT-1 → ↓transcription of cytokine IL-2 → ↓T-cell activation/proliferation
- Dermatologic uses: atopic dermatitis (FDA approved), lichen planus, vitiligo, psoriasis, cutaneous lupus, and Zoon balanitis
- AEs: **black box warning for malignancy** (likely extremely low, if any, true risk); be aware of **high levels of absorption in Netherton syndrome**; burning sensation with initial use of tacrolimus

Intravenous immunoglobulin (IVIG)

- Comes from purified plasma of more than 1000 donors; contains supraphysiologic IgG primarily
- MoA:
  - ↓ antibody production
  - ↓ complement activation
  - Neutralization of pathogenic antibodies and bacterial superantigens
  - Binds various immune receptors → immunomodulation
  - ↓ TNF-α and other proinflammatory cytokines
  - Antioxidant
  - Blocks Fc receptors
  - ↓ T-cell activation through various pathways
  - ↑ regulatory T cells
  - Contains anti-Fas receptor antibodies → ↓ keratinocyte apoptosis
  - ↓ migration of immune cells to target tissues
- Dose: varies, but generally 1 cycle = 2 g/kg total, divided into three doses, with one dose given on each of the 3 consecutive days; usually spaced 2 to 4 weeks apart until clinical remission, then ↑ intervals thereafter
- Dermatologic uses: autoimmune blistering disorders, **dermatomyositis**, **SJS/TEN**, **Kawasaki disease**, SLE, chronic autoimmune urticaria, scleroderma, and livedoid vasculopathy
- AEs: **infusion-related AEs** (e.g., headache, myalgia, flushing, fever, and wheezing; pretreatment with antihistamines/NSAIDs/CS may help), **fluid overload** (i.e., in cardiac failure and renal failure patients), **aseptic meningitis**, thromboembolic events (e.g., MI and stroke; as a result of ↑ serum viscosity), and dyshidrotic hand eczema; contraindicated in patients with *thimerosal* sensitivity
  - **Screen for immunoglobulin levels before treatment—patients with IgA deficiency may develop anaphylaxis with treatment**
  - Excipients in IVIG may cause renal failure (i.e., sucrose, glycine, proline)

Agents for hyperhidrosis

Glycopyrrolate

- Anticholinergic agent used orally or topically for hyperhidrosis
- MoA: blocks acetylcholine's effects on sweat glands
- AEs include **anticholinergic effects** (e.g., dry mouth, blurred vision, urinary retention), seizures (rare), and hyperthermia (rare)
- Caution with TCAs, atenolol, and digoxin

Oxybutynin

- Anticholinergic agent
- Approved for overactive bladder but can be used for hyperhidrosis
- AEs: anticholinergic effects

Botulinum toxin

- MoA: neurotoxin which binds to SNARE complex on the presynaptic terminal resulting in blockade of acetylcholine release
- FDA approved for axillary hyperhidrosis

Aluminum chloride

- Aluminum salt applied topically plugs the distal acrosyringium, blocking the output of sweat
- AE: dermatitis, irritation

2.9 DRUG INTERACTIONS AND THE CYTOCHROME P-450 SYSTEM

- This is a very brief review of drug interactions, mainly as they relate to cytochrome P-450 (CYP) system

Key points

- CYP enzymes metabolize endogenous and exogenous compounds (e.g., drugs)
- Most commonly located in the **endoplasmic reticulum of hepatocytes**
- Divided into families and subfamilies based on genetic similarity
- Defects in CYP genes can → altered drug metabolism (e.g., CYP2D6 mutations may → poor tolerance to doxepin)

- Substrate drugs = drugs metabolized by a certain CYP isoform
  - If given with a drug that **inhibits** the CYP → ↓ clearance of substrate drug → ↑ levels of substrate drug and possible toxicity
    - In this scenario, may need ↓ dose of substrate drug
  - If given with a drug that **induces** the CYP → ↑ clearance of substrate drug → ↓ levels of substrate drug and ↓ therapeutic effect
    - In this scenario, may need ↑ dose of substrate drug

Specific CYP isoforms

CYP1A2

- Substrates: theophylline/caffeine, **warfarin**, and pimozide
- Inhibitors: **fluoroquinolones**, **macrolides** (e.g., **erythromycin**), and ketoconazole
- Inducers: phenytoin, barbiturates, rifampin, and cigarette smoke

CYP2C9

- Substrates: **phenytoin**, sulfonamides, **warfarin**, fluvastatin, **abrocitinib**, and losartan
- Inhibitors: **fluconazole** and TMP-SMX
- Inducers: carbamazepine and rifampin

CYP2D6

- Accounts for one-fourth of all drug metabolism
- Substrates: TCAs (e.g., **doxepin** and amitriptyline), **metoprolol/propranolol**, antidysrhythmics (e.g., encainide and propafenone), antipsychotics (e.g., clozapine and pimozide)
- Inhibitors: **SSRIs** (e.g., fluoxetine and sertraline), pimozide, and **terbinafine**
- Inducers: carbamazepine, phenytoin, and rifampin

CYP3A4 (most relevant to dermatologists)

- Accounts for **up to 50%** of all drug metabolism
- Substrates: many!—**warfarin**, carbamazepine, doxepin, sertraline, antidysrhythmics (e.g., amiodarone, digoxin, and quinidine), CCBs (e.g., diltiazem and **nifedipine**), chemotherapy (e.g., doxorubicin, vinblastine, and cyclophosphamide), **H1 antihistamines**, **HMG CoA reductase inhibitors** (lovastatin and simvastatin), **OCPs/estrogens**, **cyclosporine**, **tacrolimus**, CS, dapsone, **pimozide**, benzodiazepines, **protease inhibitors**, **tofacitinib**, upadactinib, and colchicine
- Inhibitors: **azole** antifungals (e.g., ketoconazole and itraconazole), **clarithromycin/erythromycin**, metronidazole, protease inhibitors, SSRIs (e.g., sertraline), **grapefruit juice**, cimetidine, and CCBs
  - Important examples: itraconazole given with cyclosporine → toxicity; same idea if itraconazole given w/ warfarin (→ ↑ anticoagulant potential/INR) or lovastatin (→ rhabdomyolysis)
  - Azithromycin is NOT a CYP3A4 or -1A2 inhibitor like other macrolides
- Inducers: **rifampin**, **griseofulvin**, **anticonvulsants** (e.g., phenytoin and carbamazepine), dexamethasone, efavirenz, nevirapine, and **St. John's wort**
  - E.g., rifampin given with OCPs → failure of OCPs

Classic CYP mnemonics

- Queen Barbara's Phenny—she refuses greasy carbs and alcohol chronically
  - Inducers: quinidine, barbiturates, phenytoin, rifampin, griseofulvin, carbamazepine, chronic alcohol intake
- PICK EGS
  - Inhibitors: protease inhibitors, isoniazid, cimetidine, ketoconazole, erythromycin, grapefruit juice, sulfonamides

2.10 DRUG REACTIONS

- Cutaneous drug eruptions (CDEs) are one of the most common adverse drug reactions; occur in up to 1% of patients receiving systemic meds
  - Highest risk medications (% on medication that develop rash): **aminopenicillins** (up to 8%) > **anticonvulsants** (5%) > **TMP-SMX** (4%) > **NSAIDs** (0.5%)
- CDEs are divided into **simple** (no visceral/systemic involvement) and **complex** (systemic involvement)
  - 2% of all CDEs are SCARs (severe cutaneous adverse reactions = SJS/TEN, DRESS/DHS, AGEP, anaphylaxis, anticoagulant-induced skin necrosis, and generalized fixed drug eruption)
    - SCARs are seen in 1/1000 hospitalized patients
- Three most common morphologies: **morbilliform** (>92%) > urticarial (6%) > vasculitis (2%)
- Pathophysiology: immunologically mediated (Table 2.10) (drugs act as haptens inducing immunologic response) or non-immunologic (overdose, pharmacologic AEs, cumulative toxicity, delayed toxicity, drug-drug interactions, alterations in metabolism, and exacerbation of existing disease)
  - Patch testing may be useful in identifying the responsible drug in some immunologic reactions such as fixed drug eruption, AGEP, or symmetrical drug-related intertriginous and flexural exanthema (SDRIFE)
- **HIV(+) patients have ↑↑ incidence of CDEs**
  - Highest risk when CD4 count is 100 to 400/mm^3
  - Most common: **TMP-SMX** (rash in 40% of HIV patients), dapsone, β-lactams, **nevirapine**, **abacavir**, and anticonvulsants

Table 2.10 Immunologic Drug Reactions

Type	Mechanism	Examples
Type I	IgE-dependent	**Urticaria**, angioedema, anaphylaxis
Type II	Cytotoxic (due to antibodies directed against fixed antigens)	Drug-induced thrombocytopenia
Type III	Immune complex–dependent	Serum sickness, **vasculitis**, some urticarias
Type IV	Delayed-type/cell-mediated	**Morbilliform**, fixed drug, lichenoid drug, SJS/TEN

SJS/TEN, *Stevens-Johnsons syndrome/toxic epidermal necrolysis.*

Morbilliform (aka exanthematous or maculopapular drug eruption)

- **Most common drug reaction** affecting skin; mechanism = cell-mediated hypersensitivity; onset typically **7–14 days after drug initiation**
- Most common culprit drugs: **β-lactams** (PCNs and CSNs), **TMP-SMX**, **anticonvulsants**, and **allopurinol**
- Viral infections ↑ incidence of drug reactions:
  - **Ampicillin** in patients w/ **EBV**-mononucleosis → rash in ~100% of children and up to 70% adults
  - Up to 40% of **AIDS** patients get rash to **TMP-SMX**
- Rash starts w/ red-pink macules/papules in groin/axilla → later, symmetrically distributed red macules, papules, and urticarial-like lesions on the trunk and upper extremities → confluent over time; significant pruritus (helps distinguish from viral exanthema); spares mucous membranes; eruption subsides 1 to 2 weeks after drug cessation
  - Features concerning for SCAR: **facial edema** or peripheral **eosinophilia** (DRESS); **mucosal involvement** or **dusky/painful skin** (early SJS/TEN)
- Histopathology: mild basal vacuolar and spongiotic changes with a few necrotic keratinocytes (50%), superficial to mid dermal perivascular lymphohistiocytic infiltrate with some eosinophils
- Rx: supportive, with topical steroids and anti-pruritics; stop drug usually, but may attempt to **"treat through"** if drug is essential (very low rate of progression to SJS/TEN)

Urticaria, angioedema, and anaphylaxis

- See Chapter 3.9

Fixed drug eruption/Stevens-Johnson syndrome/toxic epidermal necrolysis

- See Chapter 3.3

Drug-induced hypersensitivity syndrome/drug reaction with eosinophilia and systemic symptoms (DIHS/DRESS)

- Severe systemic drug reaction with **10% mortality**
- Develops **2–6 weeks** after initiation of drug (**later** than other drug reactions)
- Most common symptoms = **fever** (85%) and **morbilliform skin eruption** (75%); also see lymphadenopathy, arthralgias (> arthritis), **multiorgan involvement** (Table 2.11) (**liver** most common [primary cause of mortality in DRESS], followed by kidney), peripheral **eosinophilia** (>1500 absolute eosinophils), mononucleosis-like **atypical lymphocytosis**
  - RegiSCAR criteria can be helpful (Table 2.12)
- Rash starts on **face** and **upper trunk/extremities**; appears morbilliform at onset → becomes **edematous (facial edema** is classic early clue), with follicular accentuation +/− tense vesicles/bullae, pustules, and purpuric lesions
- Systemic involvement can persist after drug withdrawal

Table 2.11 Visceral Involvement in Drug-Induced Hypersensitivity Syndromes

Medication	Clinical Abnormality
Allopurinol	Renal
Ampicillin	Cardiac
Carbamazepine	Renal
Dapsone	Hepatic and renal
Minocycline	Hepatic, pulmonary, and cardiac
Phenytoin	Hepatic

From Husain Z, Reddy BY, Schwartz RA. DRESS syndrome: part I. Clinical perspectives. J Am Acad Dermatol. *2013;68(5):693.e1–14, quiz 706–708.*

- Late sequelae: **thyroiditis/Graves' syndrome**, SIADH, myocarditis and diabetes; 10%–20% mortality
- Risk factors:
  - Genetic polymorphisms in drug metabolism: inability to detoxify **arene oxide** metabolites (aromatic anticonvulsants: phenobarbital, phenytoin, and carbamazepine) or **slow acetylator** (sulfonamides)
  - HLA-A*3101 (Northern Europeans on carbamazepine), HLA-B-5801 (Han Chinese on allopurinol)
  - Possible role for viral reactivation (HHV-6 or EBV > HHV-7, CMV)
- Most common meds: **aromatic anticonvulsants** (phenytoin, carbamazepine, and phenobarbital; **all cross-react**), lamotrigine (when co-administered with valproate), **sulfonamides, minocycline, dapsone, allopurinol, contrast media, allopurinol, abacavir, and nevirapine**
- DIHS variants:
  - <u>Anticonvulsant hypersensitivity syndrome</u>: ↑ risk if cannot detoxify **arene oxide** metabolites; liver involvement in 70%; less common to have kidney, lung, or heart involvement; switch to **valproic acid** or **levetiracetam** instead of aromatic anticonvulsants
  - <u>Allopurinol hypersensitivity syndrome</u>: usually seen in patients with **renal failure**; ↑↑ risk for Han Chinese with HLA-B-5801; liver involvement in 70%; **kidney** in up to 80%; also a/w **pancreatitis** and **diabetes**; rare to have lung or lymph node involvement; 25% mortality
  - <u>Sulfonamide hypersensitivity syndrome</u>: ↑ risk if **slow acetylator**
  - <u>Dapsone hypersensitivity syndrome</u>: concomitant **hemolysis and methemoglobinemia** common (due to dapsone effect) → ↑ bilirubin → **icterus**; lymphadenopathy in 80%; **lacks eosinophilia**; liver involvement can be fatal; ↑ risk in Chinese with HLA-B*13:01
  - <u>Minocycline hypersensitivity syndrome</u>: typically seen in **young adults** undergoing acne treatment; F > M; a/w **glutathione S-transferase deficiency**; strong a/w **interstitial eosinophilic pneumonia; liver involvement** in 75%; renal involvement in up to 20%
- Treatment: discontinue medication, supportive care, and **systemic steroids**
  - **Relapse common if steroids tapered too rapidly** → usually give for weeks to months
  - Use **valproic acid** or **levetiracetam** in place of aromatic anticonvulsants

Table 2.12 RegiSCAR Criteria for Drug-Induced Hypersensitivity Syndrome/ Drug Reaction With Eosinophilia and Systemic Symptoms (DRESS)

	No	Yes	Unknown
Fever ≥ 38.5°C	−1	0	−1
Enlarged lymph nodes (≥2 sites, >1 cm)	0	1	0
Atypical lymphocytes	0	1	0
Eosinophilia	0	—	0
0.7–1.499 × 10^9/L or 10%–19.9%	–	1	—
≥1.5 × 10^9/L or ≥20%	—	2	—
Skin rash	0	–	0
Extent > 50%	0	1	0
At least 2 of edema, infiltration, purpura, scaling	−1	1	0
Biopsy suggesting DRESS	−1	0	0
Internal organ involved	0	—	0
1	—	1	—
≥2	—	2	—
Resolution in > 15 days	−1	0	−1
At least three biological investigations performed and negative to exclude alternative	0	1	0

Final score: <2, no case; 2–3, possible case; 4–5, probable case; >5, definite case.

Acute generalized exanthematous pustulosis (AGEP)

- Acute, febrile pustular drug eruption that mimics von Zumbusch pustular psoriasis; occurs rapidly (<**4 days**) after drug administration
- Presents with **high fever** and small (<5 mm) non-follicular, **sterile pustules** arising on the background of edematous red skin; most commonly begins on **face and intertriginous sites** → generalizes within hours
  - 50% of patients have purpuric or EM-like lesions, mucosal involvement, **edema of hands/face**, or bullae → these findings help differentiate from pustular psoriasis
  - ↑↑↑ WBC count with peripheral **neutrophilia** +/− eosinophilia, **hypocalcemia**, and renal insufficiency
- **Patch test positive** in majority (50%–60%)
- Most common drugs: β-**lactam** (PCNs and CSNs) and **macrolide antibiotics** > **CCBs** (diltiazem most common) and antimalarials. Other causes: **mercury** exposure, radiocontrast, or enterovirus
- Histopathology: subcorneal and **intraepidermal spongiform pustules with neutrophils**, prominent superficial dermal edema, and perivascular mixed inflammatory infiltrate with neutrophils and eosinophils
  - Presence of **edema and eosinophils**, and lack of significant acanthosis helps differentiate from pustular psoriasis
- Rx: stop drug, supportive therapy with topical steroids and antipyretics

Photosensitive drug reactions

- Due to exogenous photosensitizing agents (meds); may be either phototoxic (most common) or photoallergic
- Phototoxic: common and predictable; occurs in **anyone** who receives enough drug and UVR; most commonly due to **systemic** meds
  - Mechanism: direct interaction between UVR (**UVA most common)** and drug/drug metabolites → free radicals → damage to skin cells
  - Presents with painful **exaggerated sunburn**-like eruption +/− blistering within **hours** → heals with **hyperpigmentation**
  - Histopathology (same as sunburn): necrotic keratinocytes (**"sunburn cells"**), dermal edema, minimal dermal inflammation, and vasodilation
  - Most common drugs: **tetracyclines** (demeclocycline > doxycycline > TCN »> minocycline), NSAIDs (naproxen and piroxicam), **fluoroquinolones**, amiodarone, **psoralens**, phenazothiazines (chlorpromazine and prochlorperazine), **voriconazole (XP-like presentation w/ ↑↑ risk of aggressive SCC**, eruptive lentigines, premature aging, and early death), St. John's wort, EGFR inhibitors, RAF inhibitors, **HCTZ**, imipramine
  - Clinical variants:
    - Pseudoporphyria
      - Causes: NSAIDs (**naproxen is #1**), thiazides, **voriconazole**, furosemide, TCNs, nalidixic acid, and tanning bed exposure; may also occur in hemodialysis patients
      - Skin findings similar to PCT, but **lacks hypertrichosis**, **sclerodermoid features**, and **hyperpigmentation**
      - Normal porphyrin studies
      - Histology/DIF: similar to PCT
    - Photoonycholysis (**psoralens and TCNs**)
    - Slate gray hyperpigmentation (**amiodarone, TCAs**, and diltiazem)
    - Photolichenoid eruptions (**HCTZ** and **NSAIDs** most commonly)
    - UV recall (**MTX**)
    - Phytophotodermatitis (**furocoumarin**-containing plants = parsley, celery, lime, fig, and yarrow)
- Photoallergic: less common, but more chronic than phototoxic; idiosyncratic; only occurs in **sensitized** patients (delayed-type hypersensitivity); often persists after withdrawal of medication; most commonly due to **topical** photoallergens
  - Mechanism: cell-mediated hypersensitivity; UVR (**especially UVA**) induces chemical change in drug → becomes photoallergen; **requires sensitization** with **7- to 10-day incubation** period
  - Presents with itchy, eczematous to lichenoid eruption on sun-exposed areas initially → later spreads to non-sun-exposed sites; less likely to be bullous than phototoxic reactions
  - Histopathology: spongiotic dermatitis, superficial perivascular inflammation with eosinophils
  - Most common drugs: sunscreens containing **oxybenzone** (benzophenone-3) > fragrances (6-methyl coumarin, **musk ambrette**, and sandalwood oil), NSAIDs (**piroxicam** [patch positive to thimerosal] and **ketoprofen**), griseofulvin, quinidine/quinine, sulfonamides, and quinolones
  - Diagnosis confirmed by **photopatch testing** (utilizing UVA)

Drug-induced pigmentary changes

- Hyperpigmentation:
  - May be localized or generalized; often **photodistributed**
  - Arises by many mechanisms, including: (1) drug/drug metabolite deposition; (2) induction of melanin production; (3) post-inflammatory changes due to photosensitive eruptions
  - Often a/w **melanonychia** (longitudinal, diffuse, or transverse) and/or **oral pigmentation**
  - Most common drugs: **minocycline**, chemotherapeutics, and **AZT**, **antimalarials**, and heavy metals
  - Usually reversible, but may take months to years
- Hypopigmentation:
  - Most frequently due to **topical medications**, but also seen with **tyrosine kinase inhibitors (imatinib** most commonly; due to inhibition of KIT receptor inhibition, which is involved in melanogenesis)
  - May be a/w lightening of hair
  - Most common agents: **(1) phenols/catechols** (includes hydroquinone, monobenzyl ether of hydroquinone, various phenol derivatives, and p-cresol); **(2) sulfhydryls** (includes methimazole); and **(3) miscellaneous drugs** (PPD, CS, azelaic acid, benzyl alcohol, **tyrosine kinase inhibitors**, mercurials, arsenic, thiotepa, and physostigmine)
  - **Reversible, except monobenzyl ether of hydroquinone** (permanent depigmentation at application site and distant skin)

Bullous drug reactions, lichenoid drug eruptions, drug-induced connective tissue disease

- See Chapter 3.3–3.5

Other drug eruptions

- See Table 2.13

Table 2.13 Drug Eruptions Not Covered Elsewhere

Drug/Reaction	Clinicopathologic Features	Most Common Drugs
Skin necrososis		
Coumadin-induced skin necrosis	Rare, life-threatening reaction; **begins 2–5 days after drug initiation, when protein C levels at nadir**; ↑ risk in patients with pre-existing protein C deficiency (hereditary or acquired); initially p/w painful red plaques → **hemorrhagic bullae, ulcers on fatty areas** (breast, buttocks, thighs); Rx: stop warfarin, give vitamin K, heparin, and IV infusions of protein C; **histology: non-inflammatory thrombotic vasculopathy** (multiple fibrin thrombi in dermal/SQ vessels), lacks LCV	Coumadin (occurs in 1/10,000 patients)
Heparin-induced skin necrosis (heparin-induced thrombocytopenia with thrombosis syndrome)	Systemic syndrome that p/w ↓ **PLT levels, thrombosis and cutaneous necrosis**; mechanism = **autoantibodies against heparin/platelet factor 4 complexes** → bound antibodies lead to PLT aggregation and consumption → thrombocytopenia and clotting (due to PLT aggregates); histology: thrombotic vasculopathy with PLT aggregates (usually not easily seen on H&E); Rx: stop heparin, start direct thrombin inhibitor or factor Xa inhibitor	Unfractionated heparin (> fractionated LMWH)
Drug-induced hyperpigmentation		
Amiodarone	Up to **60%** of all patients treated for >3–6 months will develop hyperpigmentation; most commonly p/w **phototoxic eruption** (erythema) of **face** (>other photo-exposed areas) → a smaller subset of cases develop **slate-gray** discoloration; most common after **long-term** use of amiodarone; hyperpigmentation **fades slowly** after drug d/c; histology: unique appearing **yellow-brown** granules of **lipofuscin (Fontana Masson[+])** in macrophages in perivascular distribution; EM shows **lipid-like lysosomal inclusions** (unique!)	
Anti-psychotics and anti-depressants	Progressive **blue-gray** hyperpigmentation in **photo-exposed** skin; histology: refractile golden brown granules (**Fontana Masson+**, Perls negative) in macrophages in perivascular distribution	**Phenazothiazines** (thioridazine, chlorpromazine, promethazine), **TCAs**
Antimalarials	**Hyperpigmentation occurs in 25**% of patients taking antimalarials; does **not** fully resolve after drug d/c; histology: deposition of **drug-melanin complexes (Fontana Masson+)** and **hemosiderin (Perls+)** in dermis Chloroquine/hydroxychloroquine: blue-black to gray hyperpigmentation on **pretibial area** (most common presentation, looks identical to **type II minocycline** hyperpigmentation of shins) > face, oral mucosa (subungual and hard palate), sclera Quinacrine: diffuse **yellow-brown** discoloration of skin and eyes (mimics jaundice)	Chloroquine, hydroxychloroquine, quinacrine
AZT (zidovudine)	**Widespread mucocutaneous hyperpigmentation** (reversible) with accentuation in **photo-exposed** sites and sites of friction; frequent **longitudinal melanonychia** (> transverse or diffuse); histology: dermal melanophages, ↑melanin in keratinocytes	

Table 2.13 Drug Eruptions Not Covered Elsewhere—cont'd

Drug/Reaction	Clinicopathologic Features	Most Common Drugs
Chemotherapy	BCNU (carmustine) and nitrogen mustard (mechlorethamine): hyperpigmentation at **sites of topical application**; ↑melanocytes and melanin in keratinocytes Bleomycin (IV or IL): linear or **flagellate** hyperpigmented patches on **trunk;** hyperpigmentation of palmar creases and skin overlying joints; may be a/w minor trauma/**scratching**; transverse melanonychia; **sclerodermoid** changes; ↑melanin in keratinocytes but normal # melanocytes Busulfan: Addison's-like generalized hyperpigmentation +/– **pulmonary fibrosis**; ↑ melanin in keratinocytes + dermal melanophages Cyclophosphamide: diffuse mucocutaneous hyperpigmentation or localized hyperpigmentation in nails, teeth, palms/soles; resolves within 12 months Ifosfamide: related to cyclophosphamide—hyperpigmentation of flexural areas, hands, feet, scrotum, and under occlusive dressings (**like thiotepa**) 5-FU: **phototoxic** dermatitis followed by hyperpigmentation (following systemic 5-FU) or **serpentine hyperpigmentation overlying veins** that were infused; histology: necrotic k'cytes, pigment incontinence, ↑melanin in basal k'cytes Hydroxyurea: early **lichenoid/DM-like** eruption overlying joints → PIH at involved sites; melanonychia, lunula hyperpigmentation Imatinib: generalized or localized **depigmentation** (40%; due to blockade of c-KIT) Sunitinib: depigmentation of hair and yellowing of skin MTX: **phototoxic dermatitis** → PIH Dactinomycin: reversible hyperpigmention of face (> generalized) Doxorubicin: hyperpigmentation on skin of **dorsal hands/joints**, palmar creases, oral mucosa and soles; transverse melanonychia; ↑ melanocytes and melanin in k'cytes	
Clofazimine	Most commonly seen in setting of **leprosy** treatment; similar to minocycline, may have **diffuse** (**red-brown** color of skin and **conjunctivae**) or **lesional** hyperpigmentation (**blue-gray** discoloration of **face, sites of inflammation**); histology: birefringent red crystals of clofazimine seen in perivascular distribution on fresh frozen tissue only (routine H&E fails to demonstrate)	
Diltiazem	Occurs in **dark-skinned** patients (Fitzpatrick IV-VI); ↑risk in **African Americans**; slate-gray discoloration on **photo-exposed** skin with reticular or perifollicular pattern; histology: lichenoid dermatitis with melanophages	
Heavy metals	Arsenic: hyperpigmentation patches with superimposed **"raindrops" of hypopigmentation**; most commonly **intertriginous** sites, **palms/soles**, pressure points; occurs up to **20 years after** exposure (strongly dose-dependent); **PPK** and **SCC** arise after hyperpigmentation stage; histology: deposits of arsenic in dermis and epidermis + ↑ melanin in keratinocytes Bismuth: generalized blue-gray discoloration on head/neck, dorsal hands, oral mucosal; histology: dermal bismuth deposits Gold (chrysiasis): **permanent blue-gray hyperpigmentation** on **face** (**pericoular** #1) and other sun-exposed sites; histology: gold deposits in macrophages in perivascular/peri-eccrine distribution; particles have orange-red birefringence on polarized light; **does not bind to BMZ or eccrine membrana propria** (distinguishes from argyria) Iron: arises after injection of iron, use of **Monsel's** solution (ferric subsulfate), post-sclerotherapy, or in setting of chronic stasis or PPD; histology: dermal hemosiderin **(+Perls)** deposits on collagen fibers and in macrophages Lead: **lead lines** (on gingival margins); histology: subepithelial lead deposits Mercury: Topical mercury ointments (no longer used) lead to slate-gray discoloration; histology: **huge deposits** (300 μm) of brown-black mercury granules within macrophages in superficial dermis Mercury ingestion (due to teething powders for babies) → **acrodynia** (acral sites are dusky red and painful) Accidental implantation (broken thermometers) → sclerosing granulomatous nodules Silver (argyria): **diffuse slate-gray pigmentation**, with accentuation in **photo-exposed** areas; due to silver in alternative meds/**elixirs** and **silver sulfdiazine** on burn wounds; +/-scleral and nail hyperpigmentation; histology: deposits of silver bound to **BMZ and membrana propria of eccrine glands** (best seen with darkfield microscopy)	
Hydroquinone	Two mechanisms: irritant contact dermatitis (→PIH), or **exogenous ochronosis**; histology: exogenous ochronosis demonstrates **yellow-brown, banana-like** deposits in dermis; hyperpigmentation fades after drug d/c	
Imatinib	Gingival and tooth hyperpigmentation; melanonychia (diffuse); **HYPOpigmentatation** of skin Of note, also a/w **periorbital edema**	

Continued

Table 2.13 Drug Eruptions Not Covered Elsewhere—cont'd		
Drug/Reaction	**Clinicopathologic Features**	**Most Common Drugs**
Minocycline	Typically after **long-term** use, since dose related (except type I); 40% get hyperpigmentation within 1 year; **oral mucosae**, **sclerae**, **nails**, **bones**, **cartilaginous sites (ear)**, and **teeth** may also be affected; typically fades slowly after drug d/c; may treat with Q-switched lasers Type 1: focal blue-black hyperpigmentation at **sites of inflammation or scars** (esp. acne); not dose-related; Histology: dermal deposits of drug complexes with **iron/hemosiderin (Perls+)** Type 2: circumscribed blue-gray **"bruise-like"** hyperpigmentation of **pretibial area** and arms; Histology: dermal deposits are drug complexes with both iron/hemosiderin **(Perls+)** and melanin (**Fontana Masson+)** Type 3: diffuse **brown** hyperpigmentation of **sun-exposed** areas; due to low-grade phototoxic dermatitis; ↑ melanin in basal keratinocytes, dermal melanophages/melanin **(Fontana Masson+)**	Boards Factoid: fetal exposure to TCN class stains the teeth at different locations: **M**inocycline = **M**idportion TCN = gingival one-third
OCPs	p/w **melasma** +/− **nipple hyperpigmentation** and darkening of nevi; histology: ↑ melanocyte #, ↑ melanin production	
Prostaglandin analogs	**Periocular hyperpigmentation**, eyelash hypertrichosis, and **iris hyperpigmentation** may follow use of glaucoma meds; self-resolve upon drug d/c	Prostaglandin F-2α analogs **(bimatoprost, latanoprost)**
Psoralens	May be **diffuse** (systemic PUVA) or **focal** hyperpigmentation (topical PUVA or phytophotodermatitis due to psoralen-containing plants); histology: ↑ melanin in k'cytes, dermal melanophages	
Chemotherapy-related drug reactions		
Toxic erythema of chemotherapy (TEC)	Umbrella term that encompasses a variety of clinical variants of chemotherapy-induced CDEs; chemotherapeutics concentrate into eccrine glands → **direct toxic effect** on **eccrine glands** (> epidermis) leads to rash; all variants of TEC have **overlapping clinical features (acral dysesthesia**, **red swollen hands**, **morbilliform** eruption on trunk, **prominent desquamation)** and similar histologic features (epidermal dysmaturation, scattered necrotic k'cytes and eccrine glandular cells, squamous metaplasia of eccrine glands); starts **days-months** after drug initiation; Rx: supportive care TEC variants: eccrine squamous syringometaplasia, **neutrophilic eccrine hidradenitis** (patients with AML on cytarabine > daunorubicin, neutrophils infiltrating the eccrine gland secretory coils and epithelial necrosis on histopathology—can be lymphocytic if neutropenic), palmoplantar erythrodysesthesia/hand-foot syndrome/acral erythema, **Ara-C ears** (swelling and erythema of ears), pseudocellulitis (Gemcitabine)	Most common: **Cytarabine/Ara-C (#1)**, **taxanes** (atypical hand/foot syndrome with red plaques on dorsal hands/Achilles tendon/malleoli, nail toxicity +/− paronychia), **anthracyclines** (doxo/dauno/idarubicin), **5-FU** Others: capecitabine (5-FU prodrug), MTX, busulfan, cisplatin, cyclophosphamide, gemcitabine, topotecan
Hand-foot skin reaction (HFSR)	Clinically similar to acral erythema variant of TEC but less severe acral dysesthesia and hand swelling; classic feature is **prominent hyperkeratotic plaques** on areas of friction; Rx: tazorac, 40% urea and efudex (treats hyperkeratosis)	**Multi-kinase inhibitors** (sorafenib, sunitinib, VEGF inhibitors)
Radiation enhancement and recall	Radiation enhancement: doxorubicin, hydroxyurea, taxanes, 5-FU, etoposide, gemcitabine, MTX Radiation recall: **MTX**, other chemotherapeutics, high dose IFN-α, simvastatin Sunburn recall: **MTX**	**MTX** (radiation recall) is most important for boards
Photosensitivity	Phototoxic eruption on sun-exposed areas	**5-FU** (and 5-FU prodrugs), **MTX**, **hydroxyurea**, docetaxel, dacarbazine
Alopecia	**Anagen effluvium** is one of most common side effects of most chemotherapies; **scalp** most commonly (> eyebrows, axillary, pubic hairs); **reversible**; hairs may re-grow curly	Reversible alopecia: most chemotherapeutics Irreversible alopecia: **busulfan**, docetaxel Cooling the skin may help prevent alopecia
Mucositis	Oral and GI tract most frequently affected mucosal sites (**stomatitis** most common, 40%); may be severe and dose-limiting; mainly due to direct toxic effect on rapidly-dividing mucosal epithelial cells; **starts within first week**; resolves within 3 weeks; Rx: oral hygiene, antimicrobials to ↓ secondary infections (*Candida*, HSV), **palifermin** (keratinocyte growth factor)	Most chemotherapeutic agents
Extravasation reactions	Ulcerations and/or indurated red plaques at sites of chemotherapy **leakage** from infusion	**5-FU, anthracyclines** (doxo + daunorubicin), carmustine, vinblastine, vincristine (of note, can also cause peripheral neuropathy), mitomycin C
Chemotherapy recall	Tender sterile inflammatory nodules at sites of previous chemotherapy drug leakage or prior infusion sites	5-FU, mitomycin C, paclitaxel, anthracyclines
Nail hyperpigmentation (melanonychia)	Longitudinal, transverse or generalized melanonychia	**Doxorubicin (#1)**, **5-FU**, cyclophosphamide, hydroxyurea, bleomycin
Inflammation of AKs	AKs become inflamed	**5-FU** (and 5-FU prodrugs)
Inflammation of DSAP	DSAP lesions become inflamed	**5-FU** (and 5-FU prodrugs), taxanes
Inflammation of SKs	Seborrheic keratoses become inflamed	Cytarabine, taxanes

Table 2.13 Drug Eruptions Not Covered Elsewhere—cont'd

Drug/Reaction	Clinicopathologic Features	Most Common Drugs
Important reactions to specific agents (**Boards Favorite!**)	Serpentine supravenous hyperpigmentation (overlying infused veins): **5-FU** Onycholysis (painful and hemorrhagic) with dorsal acral erythema: **taxanes** Exudative hyponychial dermatitis: combination of **docetaxel** and **capecitabine** (setting of breast cancer) Lower extremity/foot ulceration: **hydroxyurea** Dermatomyositis-like eruption: **hydroxyurea** Necrosis of psoriatic plaques: high-dose **MTX** (seen in setting of pre-existing psoriasis) Alternating dark and light bands of hair ("flag sign"): **MTX** Oral leukoplakia resembling flat warts: **palifermin** Flushing: **asparaginase**, high-dose BCNU Urticaria: asparaginase Acquired cutaneous adherence/"sticky skin syndrome:" combination of **doxorubicin** + **ketoconazole** Sclerodermoid reaction (lower extremities most common): **taxanes** Palmoplantar hyperkeratosis: **capecitabine** Flagellate hyperpigmentation: **bleomycin** > docetaxel Raynaud's syndrome +/− digital necrosis: **bleomycin** Acral sclerosis: **bleomycin** Hyperpigmentation of occluded skin: **thiotepa** (seen in 80% of pediatric patients; starts as diffuse erythema → resolves with hyperpigmentation)	
Interferon reactions	Vasculopathy, necrosis, psoriasis exacerbation, **cutaneous sarcoid**	
IL-2 reactions	Granulomatous eruption, lobular panniculitis, **capillary leak syndrome**	
EGFR inhibitors	**Papulopustular eruption** (treat with topical steroids/oral tetracyclines), xerosis, hair changes (kinky hair, **trichomegaly**, hirsutism, alopecia), mucositis, nail changes (paronychia, onychloysis, PG like lesions, brittle nails, photosensitivity)	Cetuximab, panitumumab, erlotinib, gefitinib, lapatinib, canertinib, vandetanib
KIT and BCR-ABL inhibitors	**Edema,** morbfilliform eruption, **hypopigmentation**	Imatinib, nilotinib, dasatinib
Anti-angiogenesis (VEGF/VEGFR) inhibitors	Mucocutaneous hemorrhage, impaired wound healing	Bevacizumab, ranibizumab
Tyrosine kinase inhibitors	**Yellow skin pigmentation (sunitinib), hand-foot skin reaction, PPK**, **acral/facial erythema**, **SCCs**, **KAs**, fingernail splinter hemorrhages, facial edema, depigmentation of the hair (sunitinib), **wart-like squamoproliferative lesions**, scalp pruritus, flushing, alopecia, stomatitis, KP-like eruption, nipple hyperkeratosis	Sorafenib, Sunitinib
RAF inhibitors	Rash, **squamoproliferative lesions** (SCC/KA, warts), melanocytic nevi, **melanoma,** KP like reaction, hand-foot reaction, photsensitvity, panniculitis	Vemurafenib, dabrafenib. Addition of MEK inhibitor results in less adverse effects
MEK inhibitors	Morbilliform eruption, papulopustular eruption, xerosis, paronychia	Selumetinib, trametinib
mTOR inhibitors	Stomatitis, rash	Rapamycin, everolimus, everolimus
Immunomodulators	**Vitiligo (favorable response to therapy)**, rash, pruritus	Ipilimumab—CTLA 4 inhibitor Nivolumab, pembrolizumab, cemiplimab, avelumab—PD-1/PD-L1 inhibitor
Injection site reactions		
Corticosteroids	Dermal and **SQ fat atrophy, vascular ectasias**, hypopigmentation	Triamcinolone
Cosmetic dermal fillers (HA, silicone)	Swelling, **granulomas**, dermal sclerosis	
Embolia cutis medicamentosa (Nicolau syndrome)	May occur with virtually **any intramuscular**-injected med; due to **vascular thrombosis** from periarterial injection; p/w **severe pain, ischemia, and pallor of injection site within minutes** → progresses to purple, livedoid plaques with dendritic borders, then **ulcerates**; Rx: supportive surgery if severe necrosis (amputation may be required)	Wide variety of meds (NSAIDs, vaccines, antibiotics, corticosteroids, IFN, Depo-Provera, local anesthetics)
Glatiramer acetate	Immunomodulator (SQ injection) used in the treatment of multiple sclerosis; p/w dermal fibrosis, panniculitis/SQ atrophy, vasospasm	
Heparin/LMWH	Necrosis, ecchymosis, calcinosis cutis	
Vaccines containing aluminum	**Granulomatous nodules**	
Vitamin B12	Pruritus, indurated morpheaform plaques	
Vitamin K	Red annular plaques, or **Texier's disease** (indurated/morpheaform plaques)	
Other drug reactions		
Alopecia	Drug-induced alopecia is non-scarring, diffuse, and reversible; two main types: Telogen effluvium: **delayed** (2–4 months after starting med) diffuse non-scarring alopecia Anagen effluvium: **rapid** (within 2 weeks of starting med) diffuse non-scarring alopecia; due to rapid cessation of cell division (mitoses) within hair matrix	Telogen effluvium: **Heparin**, **β-blockers**, **IFN**, **lithium**, **retinoids**, OCP discontinuation, antidepressants, anticonvulsants, ACE inhibitors, colchicine, NSAIDs Anagen effluvium: **Chemotherapy**, **heavy metals** (arsenic, gold, thallium, bismuth)

Continued

Table 2.13 Drug Eruptions Not Covered Elsewhere—cont'd

Drug/Reaction	Clinicopathologic Features	Most Common Drugs
Bromoderma and iododerma	**Acneiform lesions**, papulopustules, nodules, **vegetating lesions** simulating *Pemphigus vegetans* or blastomycosis; clear or hemorrhagic blisters (iododerma > others); skin lesions usually appear after chronic exposure; histology: **PEH with intraepidermal neutrophilic microabscesses** and dense dermal neutrophilic inflammation (need bug stains to r/o deep fungal)	Bromide, iodine-containing radiocontrast, iodine-containing drugs (amiodarone, SSKI, iodine nutritional supplements, povidone-iodine)
Discoloration other than melanin	See nail section, Chapter 3.25	**Minocycline**, **antimalarials**, gold
Drug-induced Sweet syndrome (acute febrile neutrophilic dermatosis)	Fever, neutrophilia, painful erythematous plaques on face and upper extremities	**GM-CSF,** pegfilgrastim, retinoids, antibiotics, azathioprine
Flagellate eruptions	**Bleomycin:** urticarial initially → later becomes hyperpigmented; occurs at sites of scratching **Raw shiitake mushroom** ingestion: more urticarial than bleomycin Other causes: adult onset Still's disease, **dermatomyositis**, docetaxel	
Gingival hypertrophy	Typically occurs in first year of drug; starts in **interdental papillae** of the **front teeth**, on labial side → may progress to involve rest of teeth with multinodular overgrowth of gums; **spares edentulous areas**; degree of hyperplasia strongly correlated with **poor oral hygiene**; histology: excess buildup of otherwise normal gum tissue; Rx: strict oral hygiene, drug d/c, surgical removal if all else fails	**Phenytoin** (**most common**, 50%) > **nifedipine** (25%) and **cyclosporine** (25%) Less common: other anticonvulsants, other CCBs, lithium, amphetamines, OCPs
Ischemic changes	Raynaud's, digital ischemia	**β-blockers, bleomycin**
Melanonychia	See nail section, Chapter 3.25	**Chemotherapeutic agents** (doxorubicin, 5-FU), zidovudine (**AZT**), **psoralens**
Mucositis	p/w **buccal** and **tongue** erosions and ulcerations; **foscarnet may give penile ulcerations**	Mostly due to **chemotherapy** or **immunosuppressive** drugs (5-FU, MTX, doxorubicin)
Paronychia and periungual pyogenic granulomas	See nail section, Chapter 3.25	**Retinoids (isotretinoin)**, HAART drugs (**indinavir**, efavirenz, lamivudine), **EGFR inhibitors**, MTX, sirolimus, capecitabine
Pseudolymphoma (cutaneous lymphoid hyperplasia)	Medication leads to immune dysregulation → aberrant proliferation of **polyclonal** B- and/or T-lymphocytes, hypergammaglobulinemia; p/w **solitary** or multiple grouped (> widespread) firm red to **plum-colored** plaques and nodules lacking surface changes; most commonly affects "upper half of body:" **face**, **neck**, **upper extremities**, **upper trunk**; +/– **lymphadenopathy**; Rx: self-resolving; subsides within weeks of drug d/c Histology: <u>T-cell pseudolymphoma</u>: resembles MF with band-like lymphoid infiltrate at DEJ, epidermotopism and lymphocytic atypia (cerebriform nuclei); usually **polyclonal** (but occasionally clonal → use clinical judgment to DDx from MF) <u>B-cell pseudolymphoma</u>: dense dermal **mixed infiltrate** (lymphocytes > eosinophils, plasma cells) with **Grenz zone**; dermal infiltrate is organized as multiple **large blue nodules (follicles)** throughout the dermis and superficial fat +/– pale-appearing **germinal centers** (with **tingible body macrophages**) within the follicles; a **mantle zone** of normal-appearing lymphocytes surrounds the follicles (unlike true B-cell lymphoma); **mixture of κ and γ** seen on IHC; **never see clonality by IGH** gene rearrangement	**Anticonvulsants** (phenytoin, phenobarbital, carbamazepine, lamotrigine), **neuroleptics** (promethazine, chlorpromazine), **ARBs**, imatinib, antibiotics (TMP-SMX, CSNs), antidepressants, antihistamines, β-blockers, CCBs, statins, NSAIDs, benzodiazepines Other common causes: **Arthropod** bite/infestation, ***Borrelia***, **tattoo reaction**, HSV, HIV, **post-zoster** (dermatomal), vaccinations (hepatitis A and B)
Radiation-induced EM	Has a **very specific clinical scenario—**occurs when phenytoin is given to neurosurgical patients undergoing whole brain radiation; p/w edema and red discoloration on **head at radiation ports** → develops into EM or SJS-like lesions within 2 days and **spreads downward** +/– mucosal involvement; histology: same as EM or SJS	**Phenytoin** + **radiation**
Serum sickness eruption	Morbilliform-urticarial plaques or **vasculitis**; fever, **arthralgias**, arthritis, lymphadenopathy, **renal disease**, **hypocomplementemia**, **circulating immune complexes**; due to administration of **non-human proteins**; histology: LCV	**Anti-thymocyte globulin**, infliximab
Serum sickness-like eruption	**Morbilliform to urticarial** eruption that starts 1–3 weeks after drug initiation; most commonly affects **children**; **edema of face/hands/feet**; +/– arthralgias, arthritis, lymphadenopathy, fever; **lacks many elements of true serum sickness** (vasculitis, renal disease, hypocomplementemia, circulating immune complexes); self-limited Treatment options: long-acting H1-antihistamines +/– H2 antihistamine, NSAIDs, systemic steroids	**Cefaclor (#1)** > other β-lactams, NSAIDs, minocycline, phenytoin True serum sickness is due to non-human proteins
Symmetrical drug-related intertriginous and flexural exanthem (SDRIFE, "baboon syndrome")	**Symmetric** well-defined red plaques in **anogenital area** +/– other intertriginous/flexural sites after administration of **systemic medication** (may be either first or repeated exposure); lack systemic symptoms (Note: SDRIFE and "baboon syndrome" variant of systemic ACD have similar clinical presentations and both have been termed "baboon syndrome")	**β-Lactams** (aminopenicillins and CSNs), **radiocontrast**, other antibiotics Patch test (+)
Vancomycin infusion (hypersensitivity) reaction	Appears within 10 minutes of drug infusion; p/w **flushing** of **posterior neck** +/– face, upper trunk with associated pruritus and **hypotension** +/– angioedema; due to non-immunologic mast cell degranulation; Rx: ↓ rate of infusion, pretreat with antihistamines	**Vancomycin** (rate-related infusion reaction)

Data from Tables 21.15, 21.16, 26.18 in Valeyrie-Allanore L, Obeid G, Revuz J. Drug reactions. In: Bolognia JL, Schaffer JV, Cerroni, L, eds. Dermatology. *4th ed. Philadelphia: Elsevier; 2018. p. 348–375.*

3 General Dermatology

Christopher Sayed, Ali Alikhan, Olayemi Sokumbi, Anand Rajpara, and Julia S. Lehman

CONTENTS LIST

3.1 PAPULOSQUAMOUS DERMATOSES
3.2 ECZEMATOUS DERMATOSES
3.3 INTERFACE DERMATITIS
3.4 BLISTERING DISEASES
3.5 CONNECTIVE TISSUE DISEASES (CTD) AND SCLEROSING DERMOPATHIES
3.6 GRANULOMATOUS/HISTIOCYTIC DISORDERS
3.7 MONOCLONAL GAMMOPATHIES OF DERMATOLOGIC INTEREST
3.8 XANTHOMAS
3.9 URTICARIA AND ANGIOEDEMA
3.10 NEUTROPHILIC DERMATOSES
3.11 EOSINOPHILIC DISORDERS
3.12 FIGURATE ERYTHEMAS
3.13 FOLLICULAR AND ECCRINE/APOCRINE DISORDERS
3.14 DRUG REACTIONS
3.15 PHOTODERMATOSES AND OTHER PHYSICAL DERMATOSES
3.16 AMYLOIDOSES
3.17 NEURODERMATOLOGY AND PSYCHODERMATOLOGY
3.18 PALMOPLANTAR KERATODERMAS
3.19 NUTRITIONAL DISORDERS IN DERMATOLOGY
3.20 DEPOSITIONAL AND CALCIFICATION DISORDERS NOT DISCUSSED ELSEWHERE
3.21 ULCERS
3.22 VASCULITIDES, VASCULOPATHIES, AND OTHER VASCULAR DISORDERS
3.23 PANNICULITIDES AND LIPODYSTROPHIES
3.24 DERMATOSES OF PREGNANCY
3.25 HAIR, NAIL, AND MUCOSAL DISORDERS
3.26 PIGMENTARY DISORDERS

3.1 PAPULOSQUAMOUS DERMATOSES

Psoriasis

Epidemiology

- 2% worldwide prevalence
- Psoriatic arthritis (PsA) in 25%–30% (cutaneous manifestations usually precede PsA onset)
- Peaks at **20** to **30** years and **50** to **60** years

Pathogenesis (Fig. 3.1)

- Genetic factors (family history, twin studies) important
  - Psoriasis susceptibility regions, PSORS1–9: **PSORS1** (chromosome 6p and contains *HLA-Cw6* allele) is **most important**
  - PSORS1 in 50% of patients
- Important HLA associations in psoriasis:
  - **HLA-Cw6 (strongest association)**: 10-15X ↑ risk
    - Positive in **90% of early-onset psoriasis**, 50% of late onset (vs. 7% of control population)

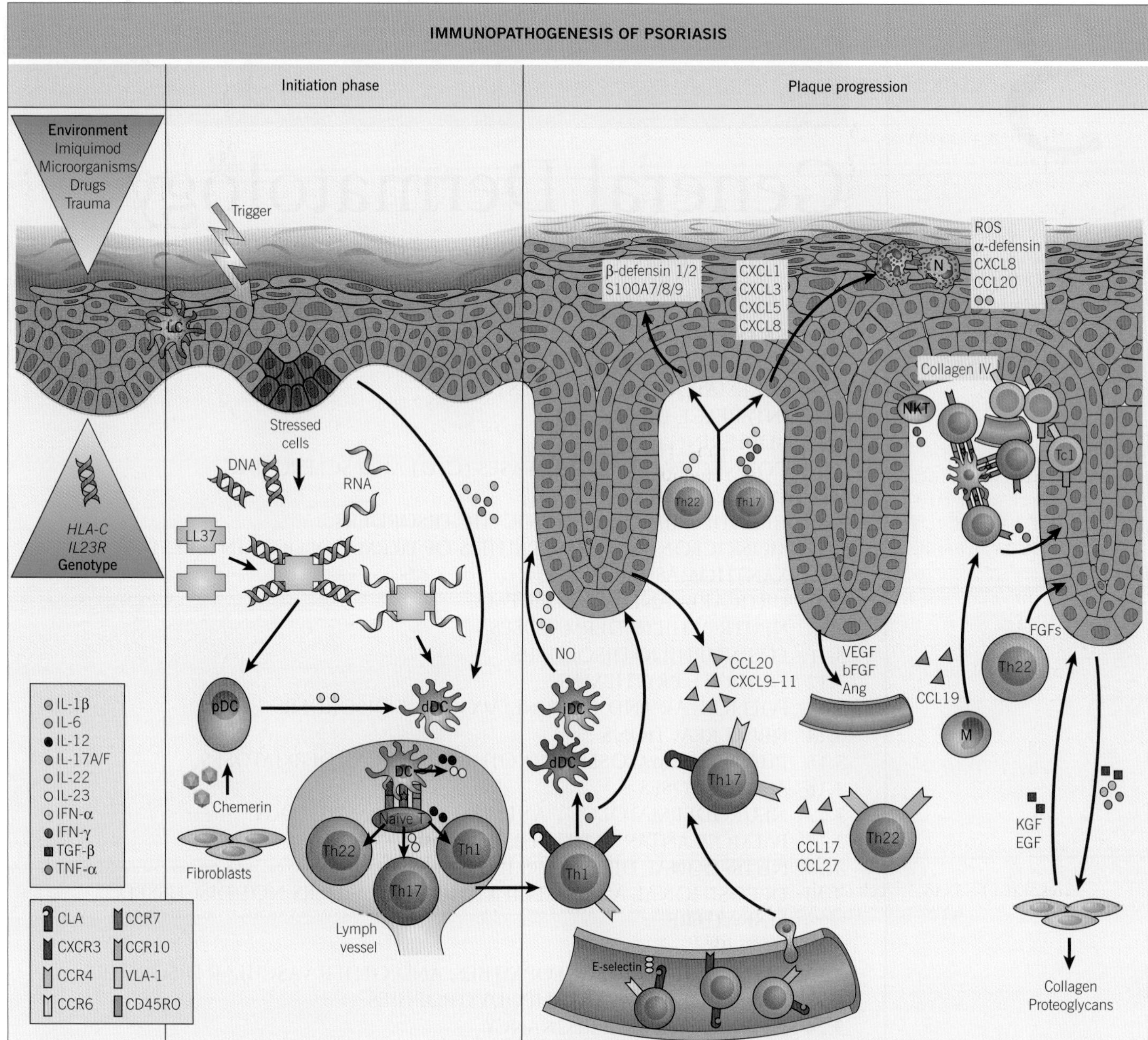

Fig. 3.1 Immunopathogenesis of psoriasis. The occurrence of **triggering environmental factors in genetically predisposed individuals**, carrying susceptibility alleles of psoriasis-associated genes, results in disease development. During the initiation phase, **stressed keratinocytes can release self DNA and RNA**, which form complexes with the cathelicidin LL37 that then **induce interferon-α *(IFN-α)* production** by plasmacytoid dendritic cells (*pDCs*; recruited into the skin via fibroblast-released chemerin), **thereby activating dermal DCs *(dDCs)***. Keratinocyte-derived **interleukin-1β (IL-1β), IL-6, and tumor necrosis factor-α *(TNF-α)* also contribute** to the activation of dDCs. **Activated dDCs then migrate to the skin-draining lymph nodes** to present an as-yet-unknown antigen (either of self or of microbial origin) to naive T cells and (via secretion of different types of cytokines by DCs) **promote their differentiation into T helper 1 *(Th1)*, Th17, and Th22 cells**. Th1 cells (expressing cutaneous lymphocyte antigen *[CLA]*, CXC-chemokine receptor 3 [CXCR3] and CC-chemokine receptor 4 *[CCR4]*), Th17 cells (expressing CLA, CCR4 and CCR6), and Th22 cells (expressing CCR4 and CCR10) **migrate via lymphatic and blood vessels into psoriatic dermis**, attracted by the keratinocyte-derived chemokines CCL20, CXCL9–11, and CCL17; this ultimately leads to the formation of a psoriatic plaque. **Th1 cells release IFN-γ and TNF-α**, which amplify the inflammatory cascade, acting on keratinocytes and dDCs. **Th17 cells secrete IL-17A and IL-17F (and also IFN-γ and IL-22) which stimulate keratinocyte proliferation** and the release of β-defensin 1/2, S100A7/8/9, and the neutrophil-recruiting chemokines CXCL1, CXCL3, CXCL5, and CXCL8. Neutrophils *(N)* infiltrate the stratum corneum and produce reactive oxygen species *(ROS)* and α-defensin with antimicrobial activity, as well as CXCL8, IL-6, and CCL20. **Th22 cells secrete IL-22**, which induces further release of keratinocyte-derived T-cell–recruiting chemokines. Moreover **inflammatory DCs *(iDCs)* produce IL-23**, nitric oxide *(NO)* radicals, and TNF-α, whereas natural killer T cells *(NKT)* release TNF-α and IFN-γ. Keratinocytes also release vascular endothelial growth factor (VEGF), basic fibroblast growth factor *(bFGF)*, and angiopoietin *(Ang)*, thereby promoting neoangiogenesis. Macrophage (M)-derived chemokine CCL19 promotes clustering of Th cells expressing chemokine receptor CCR7 with DCs in the proximity of blood vessels and further T-cell activation. At the dermal–epidermal junction, memory CD8+ cytotoxic T cells *(Tc1)* expressing very-late antigen-1 *(VLA-1)* bind to collagen IV, allowing entry into the epidermis and contributing to disease pathogenesis by releasing both Th1 and Th17 cytokines. Cross-talk between keratinocytes producing TNF-α, IL-1β, and transforming growth factor-β *(TGF-β)* and fibroblasts, which in turn release keratinocyte growth factor *(KGF)*, epidermal growth factor *(EGF)*, and TGF-β. Th22 cells releasing FGFs possibly contribute to tissue reorganization and deposition of the extracellular matrix (e.g., collagen, proteoglycans). *LC*, Langerhans cell. (Courtesy of Dr. Paola DiMeglio. From van de Kerkhof PCM, Nestlé FO. Psoriasis. In: Bolognia JL, Jorizzo JL, Schaffer JV. *Dermatology*. 4th ed. Philadelphia: Elsevier; 2017:135–156.)

- Strongest HLA risk factor for early-onset disease (Cw6 > B57, DR7)
- Also strongly a/w **guttate** psoriasis (74%)
  - **HLA-B27**: sacroiliitis-associated psoriasis, PsA, and pustular psoriasis
  - **HLA-B13** and **HLA-B17**: guttate and erythrodermic psoriasis
  - HLA-B8, Bw35, Cw7, and DR3: palmoplantar pustulosis
- Immunologic factors:
  - T-cell disorder, primarily: CD8+ in epidermis and mix of CD4+/CD8+ in dermis (α1β1 integrin [VLA-1] on psoriatic T cells interacts w/ collagen IV in Basement membrane → T-cell epidermal penetration)
    - Primarily memory T cells with cutaneous lymphocyte antigen (CLA) and chemokine receptors (e.g., CCR4, CCR6); also some natural killer (NK) T-cell involvement
    - Increased: Th1 cytokines (e.g., interferon-γ [IFN-γ], IL-2 [interleukin-2], IL-12), IL-1, IL-6, and tumor necrosis factor-α (TNF-α)
    - Decreased: **IL-10**
    - **IL-23 (from dendritic cells [DCs]) → Th17 cell stimulation → IL-17 and IL-22 release →** dermal inflammation and keratinocyte replication
  - ↑ Dendritic cells in psoriatic skin
  - **↑ CXCL8 → neutrophil chemotaxis** (spongiform pustules of Kogoj and microabscess of Munro)
  - Vascular endothelial growth factor (VEGF) → angiogenesis
  - Keratinocytes secrete **antimicrobial proteins (hBD1-2, cathelicidin LL37**, and SLP1), IL-1, IL-6, IL-8, and TNF-α; also express toll-like receptors (TLRs)
  - STAT-3 expression → keratinocyte proliferation
- Triggering factors:
  - External: trauma (**Koebner phenomenon**/isomorphic response)—1- to 3-week lag time
  - Systemic: infections (**streptococcal pharyngitis #1**), HIV, endocrine factors (e.g., **hypocalcemia** in generalized pustular psoriasis and **pregnancy** in impetigo herpetiformis), stress, **drugs (lithium**, IFNs, **β-blockers**, antimalarials, **TNF-α inhibitors**, and **corticosteroid [CS] tapers** in pustular psoriasis), alcohol consumption, smoking, and obesity
    - Latency period between drug initiation and skin eruption varies:
      - Short latency (<4 weeks): terbinafine, NSAIDs
      - Intermediate latency (4–12 weeks): antimalarials, angiotensin-converting enzyme (ACE) inhibitors
      - Long latency (>12 weeks): β-blockers, lithium
    - **TNF-α inhibitors** (adalimumab and infliximab most commonly) may → plaque psoriasis and/or palmoplantar pustulosis

Clinical features

- Chronic plaque psoriasis (most common)
  - Symmetric, well-defined red papules and plaques w/ prominent white scale
  - Most common sites: scalp, elbows, knees, presacrum, hands, feet, and genitalia
- Guttate psoriasis: children and adolescents; drop-like lesions measuring 2 to 6 mm; symmetric distribution; favors trunk and proximal extremities
  - Triggers: **group A *Strep* infection (oropharynx or perianal)** or upper respiratory infection (URI; 1–3 weeks prior to onset)
  - 40% progress to plaque-type
- Erythrodermic psoriasis: generalized erythema and scale (>90% body surface area [BSA])
  - Triggers: poor management decisions most common (e.g., abrupt withdrawal of systemic steroids)
- Generalized pustular psoriasis:
  - **Pustular psoriasis of pregnancy** (impetigo herpetiformis): pregnancy-associated; begins in flexures then generalizes w/ toxicity; early delivery recommended
  - von Zumbusch: rapid and generalized, painful skin, fever, **leukocytosis**, **hypoalbuminemia**, and malaise; a/w **hypocalcemia** (risk factor)
  - Inherited autoinflammatory disorders (e.g., deficiency of IL-1 receptor antagonist, deficiency of IL-36 receptor antagonist, CARD14-mediated pustular psoriasis, ADAM17 deletion) may resemble generalized pustular psoriasis
- Palmoplantar pustulosis: pustules and yellow-brown macules localized to palms/soles; has a chronic course
  - May be a/w sterile inflammatory bone lesions (synovitis, acne, pustulosis, hyperostosis, osteitis **[SAPHO] syndrome**)
- Acrodermatitis continua of Hallopeau: "**lakes of pus**" on distal fingers, toes, and nail beds → scale, crust, and **nail shedding**
- Site-specific types
  - Scalp: can coexist w/ seborrheic dermatitis; may advance to edge of face, retroauricular areas, and upper neck
    - Psoriasis is **#1 cause of pityriasis amiantacea**
  - Inverse: shiny pink-red, **well-defined** thin plaques w/ fissuring
    - Axillae, inguinal crease, intergluteal cleft, inframammary region, and retroauricular folds
  - Oral: annulus migrans (presents like geographic tongue, seen in pustular psoriasis)
  - Nail: **fingernails** > toenails (vs. opposite pattern in onychomycosis)
    - Nail psoriasis has ↑ risk of PsA
    - **Proximal matrix → pits (small parakeratotic foci)**
    - **Distal matrix** → leukonychia and loss of transparency; subungual hyperkeratosis
    - **Nail bed → oil spots, salmon patches**, splinter hemorrhages, **onycholysis**, and subungual hyperkeratosis
- PsA: affects up to **30%** of psoriasis patients (correlated w/ skin severity and nail involvement)
  - Typically rheumatoid factor **(RF)-negative** ("seronegative")
  - Classic early symptom = **morning joint stiffness** lasting > 1 hour
  - **Vast majority have nail changes** +/– tendon/ligament involvement (**enthesopathy/enthesitis**)
  - Strong genetic predisposition (**50% HLA-B27+**)
  - Treatment options: biologics (TNF-α inhibitors, IL-17 inhibitors [excluding brodalumab], ustekinumab , IL-23 inhibitors [excluding tildrakizumab], abatacept [fusion

protein of CTLA-4 and IgG1, which binds B7-1 (CD80) and B7-2 (CD86), preventing co-stimulatory signal and T cell activation]), methotrexate (MTX; not FDA approved), apremilast, cyclosporine (not FDA approved), sulfasalazine (not FDA approved), and tofacitinib
- Five distinct PsA patterns:
  - **Oligoarthritis** w/ swelling and tenosynovitis of hands **(60%–70%)**: affects distal interphalangeal **(DIP) +** proximal interphalangeal **(PIP)** joints of hand and feet (may → "sausage digit") +/− large joint involvement; **spares metacarpophalangeal joints (MCP;** vs. rheumatoid arthritis [RA])
  - Asymmetric DIP involvement + nail changes (16%): exclusively affects DIP → **"sausage digit,"** nail damage
  - RA-like (15%): symmetric polyarthritis of **small and medium** joints (PIP, MCP, wrist, ankle, and elbow); hard to DDx from RA and **may be RF+**
  - Ankylosing spondylitis (5%): axial arthritis +/− sacroiliac, knee, and peripheral joint involvement; M > F, **usually HLA-B27+,** a/w inflammatory bowel disease (IBD) and uveitis
  - Arthritis mutilans (5%): least common, most severe (osteolysis of phalanges/metacarpals → short, wide, and soft digits w/ **"telescoping phenomenon"**)
- Comorbidities
  - ↓ Risk of allergic diseases
  - **↓ Risk of superinfection (due to ↑ antimicrobial peptides)**, but ↑ risk of onychomycosis and *Candida* (in inverse psoriasis)
  - Possible ↑ risk of lymphoma
  - **↑ Risk of cardiovascular diseases**, hyperlipidemia (HLD), hypertension (HTN), diabetes mellitus, non-alcoholic steatohepatitis, and metabolic syndrome
    - Systemic psoriasis treatments may ↓ risk
  - Asymmetric anterior uveitis (15% of juvenile psoriasis)

Histopathology

- Mature plaques:
  - **Confluent parakeratosis**
  - **Regular acanthosis** w/ elongated rete ridges
  - Thinning of suprapapillary plates
  - ↓ or absent stratum granulosum
  - Dilated capillaries in dermal papillae
  - Micropustules of **Kogoj** (stratum spinosum) and microabscesses of **Munro** (stratum corneum [SC])
    - Mnemonic: "Marilyn Munro is always on **top** (higher in epidermis)"
- Guttate:
  - Milder acanthosis, spongiosis, foci of intraepidermal neutrophils, **mounded parakeratosis,** ↓ granular layer
  - Thin, tortuous capillaries in papillary dermis
  - Mixed perivascular infiltrate w/ scattered neutrophils
- Pustular:
  - Large clusters of neutrophils in upper epidermis

Treatment

- Topical treatments: may be used alone for mild psoriasis
  - CS: **first line for mild-moderate** psoriasis
  - Anthralin: second line
  - Vitamin D3 analogs: typically used in conjunction w/ topical CS
  - Topical retinoids: tazarotene
  - Miscellaneous: salicylic acid, coal tar, tapinarof (aryl hydrocarbon receptor-modulating agent; safe in senstivie areas), roflumilast (PDE-4 inhibitor) and topical calcineurin inhibitors (TCIs; especially facial and flexural)
- Phototherapy: **first line in moderate-severe** psoriasis
  - **Narrowband ultraviolet B (NB-UVB; 311–313 nm)**: highly effective, ↓ risk of secondary nonmelanoma skin cancer relative to broadband ultraviolet B (BB-UVB) and psoralen plus ultraviolet light A (PUVA)
  - BB-UVB: more effective than NB-UVB for **guttate psoriasis flares**
  - Excimer laser (308 nm): useful for limited/localized disease
  - PUVA: topical for limited areas; oral for more generalized disease
  - Goeckerman regimen: combination of crude coal tar and BB-UVB
- Systemic therapy: moderate-severe psoriasis
  - Apremilast: phosphodiesterase-4 [PDE-4] inhibitor
  - MTX
  - Cyclosporine: **do not use > 1 year**; ↑ risk of squamous cell carcinoma (SCC; particularly in a/w PUVA); do NOT use with acitretin
  - Systemic retinoids: acitretin is the only systemic retinoid used in psoriasis; **monotherapy effective in erythrodermic and pustular psoriasis**; combination w/ phototherapy (Re-PUVA) effective for plaque psoriasis
  - Biologics
    - TNF-α inhibitors: infliximab, etanercept, certolizumab, and adalimumab
    - **IL-12/-23 inhibitor**: ustekinumab
    - **IL-23 inhibitors**: guselkumab, tildrakizumab, risankizumab
    - **IL-17 inhibitors**: secukinumab, brodalumab, ixekizumab
  - Deucravacitinib: TYK2 inhibitor

Prognosis/clinical course

- Depends on the type; often chronic
- Spontaneous remission in ≤ 35%

Additional boards factoids

- **Woronoff ring**: pale blanching ring around psoriatic lesions
- **Auspitz sign**: scraping of psoriasis scale → pinpoint bleeding (due to dilated capillaries and suprapapillary plate thinning)
- Treatment of choice (ToC) for psoriasis subtypes:
  - Pustular (von Zumbusch): **acitretin** (>cyclosporine, MTX, and biologics)
  - Impetigo herpetiformis: **early delivery**, prednisone
  - Guttate: **BB-UVB** at erythemogenic doses (>NB-UVB)
  - Erythrodermic: **cyclosporine**, infliximab, and acitretin

Pityriasis rubra pilaris (PRP)

Pathogenesis/epidemiology

- Bimodal age distribution: first and sixth decade
- Most cases are acquired (of note, COVID-19 vaccine/infection and EBV may be possible triggers), some familial forms
- Dominantly inherited form of PRP a/w gain of function mutation in *CARD14* gene (aka PSORS2)

Clinical features

- Classically begins on head/neck → progresses caudally
- Most important features:
  - **Scalp erythema** w/ fine, diffuse scaling
  - Folliculocentric keratotic papules on erythematous base ("**nutmeg-grater**" papules)
    - Papules coalesce into **orange to salmon-colored** plaques w/ **"islands of sparing"** on trunk and extremities → can progress to erythroderma w/ exfoliation
  - **Orange-red waxy keratoderma** of palms/soles **("sandal-like PPK")** w/ fissures
  - Thick, yellow-brown nails w/ subungual debris; **lacks nail pits (vs. psoriasis)!**
- **Six distinct subtypes** (Fig. 3.2)
  - **Type 1** (55%, classic adult): **most common form**, rapid onset of classic PRP features, good prognosis (80% resolve within 3 years)
  - Type 2 (5%, atypical adult): slow onset, **ichthyosiform** leg lesions + **keratoderma w/ coarse and lamellated scale** +/− **alopecia**; chronic course
  - Type 3 (10%, classic juvenile): same presentation/course as type 1; peaks in adolescence and first 2 years of life
  - **Type 4 (25%,** circumscribed juvenile): **most common form in children** (Fig. 3.3); only focal/**localized** form of PRP; p/w follicular papules and erythema on elbows and knees; prepubertal onset; variable course
  - Type 5 (5%, atypical juvenile): first few years of life, PRP + **sclerodermoid changes** of hands/feet; chronic; familial forms of PRP (e.g., *CARD14* mutations) present with this type

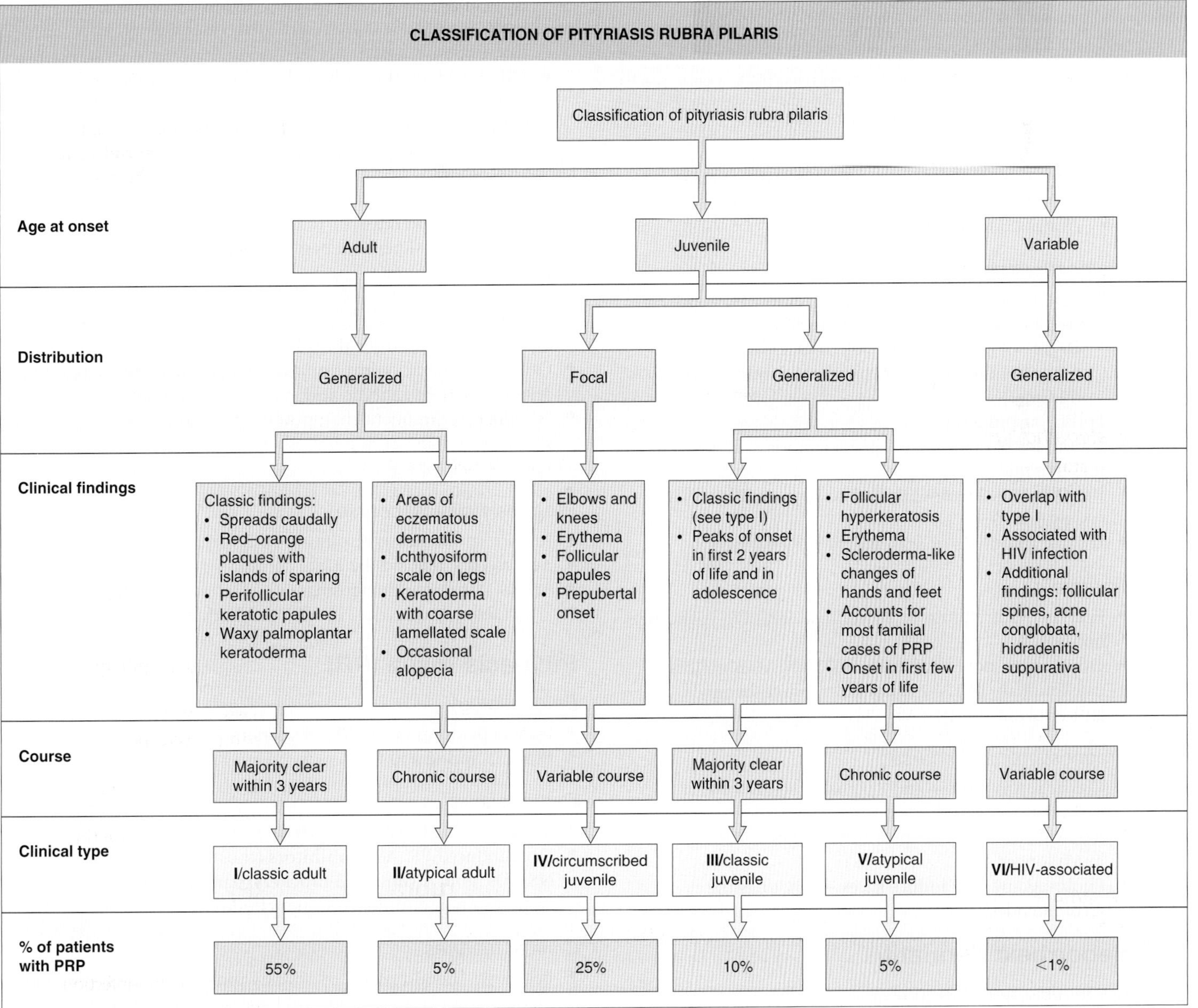

Fig. 3.2 Classification of pityriasis rubra pilaris *(PRP)*. Type VI PRP is also referred to as HIV-associated follicular syndrome. (From Wood GS, Reizner GT. Other papulosquamous disorders. In: Bolognia JL, Schaffer JV, Cerroni L. *Dermatology*. 4th ed. Philadelphia: Elsevier; 2018:161–174.)

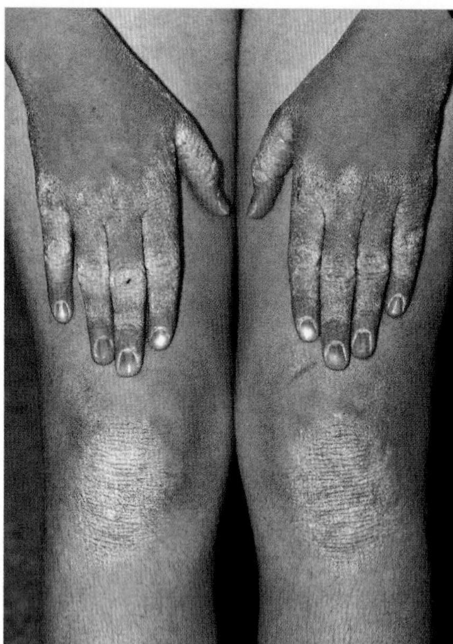

Fig. 3.3 Circumscribed juvenile (type IV) pityriasis rubra pilaris. (From Hogan PA, Langley RGB. Papulosquamous diseases. In: Schachner LA, Hansen RC. *Pediatric Dermatology*. 4th ed. London: Elsevier; 2011:901–951.)

- Type 6 (<1%): generalized PRP in **HIV** patients w/ hidradenitis suppurativa, acne conglobata, and elongated follicular spines

Histopathology

- Alternating vertical and horizontal orthohyper- and parakeratosis (**"checkerboard pattern"**)
  - Degree of hyperkeratosis (often massive!) is out of proportion to degree of epidermal acanthosis (fairly minimal)
- **Follicular plugging**
- **"Shoulder parakeratosis"** (parakeratosis at edges of hair follicle orifice)
- Irregular acanthosis w/ thickened suprapapillary plates (vs. psoriasis)
- Focal acantholysis or acantholytic dyskeratosis

Treatment

- First line: isotretinoin or **acitretin**; alitretinoin is another option
- Others: high-dose vitamin A, MTX, TNF-α inhibitors, ustekinumab, IL-17/-23 inhibitors, phototherapy; antiretrovirals for type VI

Prognosis/clinical course

- Classic forms (type 1 and 3) reliably self-resolve in 3–5 years
- Atypical and circumscribed forms (types 2, 4, 5, 6) persist much longer
- Phototherapy may induce flares → phototesting recommended

Seborrheic dermatitis

Epidemiology/pathogenesis

- Peaks in fourth to sixth decades, but occurs in all ages; M > F
- Multifactorial etiology
  - ↑ ***Malassezia furfur*** in cutaneous lesions
  - Sebum composition altered (↑ triglycerides/cholesterol; ↓ squalene and free fatty acids [FFAs])
  - Immune dysregulation (some cases)

Clinical features

- Pediatric:
  - Erythematous, scaly, sometimes pruritic rash affecting "seborrheic" areas (scalp, face, postauricular, presternal, and intertriginous areas)
  - Infants often present w/ **"cradle cap"** (greasy yellow scales adherent to scalp)
  - Erythematous, scaly, macerated plaques in body creases (anterior neck crease, axillae, groin, and popliteal fossae)
- Adolescent/adult:
  - Well-defined, pink-yellow patches w/ **"greasy" scale** in highly sebaceous areas (scalp, eyebrows, nasolabial folds, forehead, ears/retroauricular, central chest, and intertriginous areas)
  - Often itchy (particularly scalp)
  - Dandruff (pityriasis simplex capillitii)—mild form on scalp

Histopathology

- Irregular to psoriasiform acanthosis, **spongiosis**, **"shoulder parakeratosis,"** focal neutrophils in the cornified layer, superficial perivascular/perifollicular lymphocytic infiltrate

Treatment

- **Gold standard = topical azoles**
- Other options: ciclopirox, topical CS, TCIs, pyrithione zinc, selenium sulfide, salicylic acid, and coal tar shampoos
- "Cradle cap": frequent shampooing (antiseborrheic shampoos), baby or mineral oil, brushing/combing, and low-potency topical CS

Prognosis/clinical course

- Infants: spontaneous resolution by 8 to 12 months
- Adolescents: tends to be more chronic
- Adults: chronic and relapsing
- ↑ Incidence and severity in **HIV and Parkinson's**

Pityriasis rosea (PR)

Epidemiology

- Female predominance; **10–35 years**
- Peaks in spring and fall

Pathogenesis

- Possibly viral (**HHV-7 and HHV-6**)
- Drug-induced PR: **ACE inhibitors** (most common), NSAIDs, **gold**, bismuth, **β-blockers**, barbiturates, isotretinoin, metronidazole, and clonidine

Clinical features

- Begins w/ **"herald patch"** = solitary pink, enlarging plaque w/ fine central scale and larger **trailing collarette** of scale; favors trunk

- Diffuse eruption (begins hours to weeks later): oval patches/plaques on trunk and proximal extremities
  - Lesions appear similar to "herald patch," but smaller
  - Vertical axes oriented along Langer's lines (**"Christmas tree pattern"**)
  - 25% experience significant pruritus
- **Atypical PR**: term utilized when rash has unusual features, including:
  - Inverse PR pattern: prominent involvement of **intertriginous** sites, or more prominent involvement of **limbs** (>trunk)
  - Papular, vesicular, or targetoid morphology
    - PR is often more papular and extensive in African American children
  - Oral involvement (e.g., ulceration)
- Drug-induced PR-like eruptions: ↑ inflammation/pruritus, lacks herald patch; older patient population

Histopathology

- **Nonadherent thin mounds of parakeratosis** (vs. thicker, adherent mounds in guttate psoriasis), **spongiosis**, perivascular lymphohistiocytic infiltrate, and **RBC extravasation**

Treatment

- Not required; symptomatic treatment w/ topical CS, antipruritic lotions
- **Oral erythromycin** hastens clearance; NB-UVB for tough cases

Prognosis/clinical course

- Self-limited (6–8 weeks)
- Drug-induced PR-like eruptions resolve rapidly (<2 weeks) after discontinuing drug

Intertriginous/axillary granular parakeratosis

- **Adult women** > infants (diaper area)
- Pruritic, keratotic red-brown papules and plaques in intertriginous areas (**axillae > inguinal, inframammary**)
- Possible defect in filaggrin metabolism → retention of keratohyalin granules in SC
  - Alternative theories: irritant dermatitis, reaction to deodorants/antiperspirants
- Histology: characteristic thickened eosinophilic SC w/ prominent **parakeratosis and retained keratohyalin granules**; vascular ectasia (Fig. 3.4)
- Can be chronic/recurrent
- Rx: topicals (CS, vitamin D analogs, keratolytics, and antifungals), destructive (cryotherapy), and systemic (isotretinoin, antifungals)

Erythroderma

Epidemiology

- M > F, average age = 50 yo

Clinical features

- Erythema and scale involving more than **90% BSA**
- Not a defined entity, but rather a clinical presentation of various disorders (Box 3.1), characterized by:
  - **Pruritus** (>**90%** of cases, especially atopic dermatitis [AD] or Sézary); lichenification (>30%); dyspigmentation (>50%); PPK (30%); nail changes (40%, typically "shiny nails")
  - Other skin findings: ***Staphylococcus aureus* colonization**, eruptive seborrheic keratoses, ectropion, and conjunctivitis
  - Systemic findings: **peripheral lymphadenopathy** (#1 extracutaneous finding), hepatomegaly (20%), pedal/pretibial edema (50%), tachycardia (40%), thermoregulatory disturbances (hyperthermia > hypothermia), hypermetabolism, and anemia
- Primary (erythema involves whole skin surface in days to weeks) versus secondary (generalization of localized skin disease)

Box 3.1 Causes of Erythroderma (SCALP-ID mnemonic)

S Sézary syndrome, Seborrheic dermatitis, Scabies
C CTCL, Contact dermatitis, Chronic actinic dermatitis
A Atopic dermatitis
L Leukemia/lymphoma, Lichen planus, LCH
P Psoriasis, PRP, Pemphigus/pemphigoid, Paraneoplastic
I Infection (HIV, SSSS), Idiopathic, Ichthyoses, Immunodeficiencies
D Drug reactions, Dermatitis

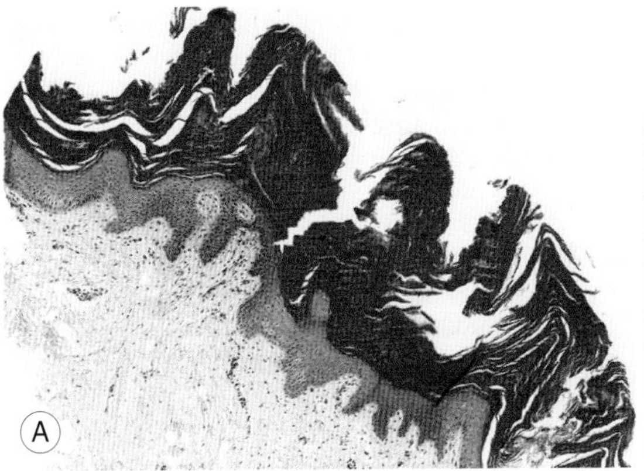

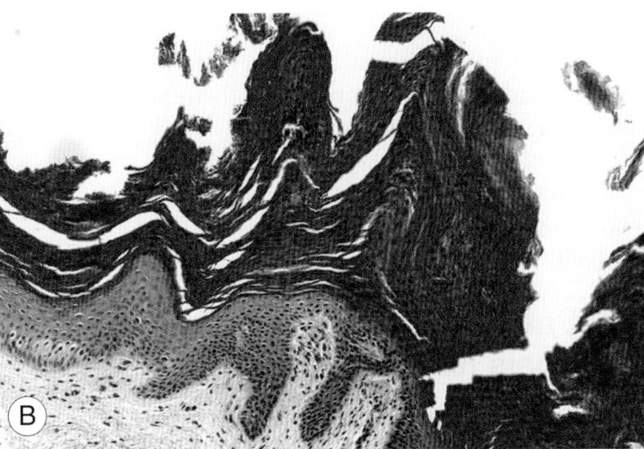

Fig. 3.4 (A) and (B) Axillary granular parakeratosis. Marked, compact parakeratosis with small bluish granules within the stratum corneum representing keratohyalin granules. (Courtesy of Olayemi Sokumbi, MD.)

- Causes:
  - **Psoriasis (most common cause** in healthy patients):
    - Usually preceded by typical plaques
    - 25% are idiopathic; less scaly than typical psoriasis lesions
    - Erythroderma is usually **due to drug withdrawal** (steroid, MTX, or cyclosporine A)
    - Nails w/ characteristic psoriasis findings
    - Histologically, changes of early psoriasis seen
  - Atopic dermatitis:
    - Typically have atopic history
    - Severe pruritus and lichenification
    - ↑ Serum IgE and eosinophilia
  - Drug reactions:
    - Most common cause in **HIV patients** (40% vs. 23% in non-HIV patients)
    - Lesions may become purpuric in the ankles and feet
    - Shorter duration than other erythrodermas (resolves 2–6 weeks after drug withdrawal, except in DRESS)
    - Most common drugs: **allopurinol**, **sulfa** (TMP-SMX, dapsone), **antiepileptics**, isoniazid (INH), minocycline, and **highly active antiretroviral therapy (HAART)**
  - Idiopathic erythroderma: elderly men w/ relapsing course
    - Lymphadenopathy (≈70%), PPK, and peripheral edema seen frequently
  - Cutaneous T-cell lymphoma (CTCL) (Sézary and erythrodermic mycosis fungoides [MF]):
    - **Sézary**: primary erythroderma; T-cell clone in blood plus one of the following: (1) ≥ 1000 Sézary cells/μL; (2) CD4:CD8 ratio of ≥ 10:1; or (3) ↑ percentage of CD4+ cells w/ abnormal phenotype (loss of CD7 or CD26)
    - **Erythrodermic MF**: secondary erythroderma; due to progression from classic MF patches/plaques
  - Less common causes: **PRP** (salmon-orange color, follicular keratotic papules on extensors, islands of sparing), **graft-versus-host disease (GVHD)**, paraneoplastic erythroderma (**usually lymphomas**), papuloerythroderma of Ofuji, **chronic actinic dermatitis**, bullous dermatoses, and ichthyoses (congenital ichtyiosiform erythroderma/non-bullous congenitcal ichthyosiform erythroderma, epidermolytic ichthyosis/bullous congenital ichthyosiform erythroderma, Netherton syndrome)

Treatment

- Initial management: nutritional assessment, fluid and electrolyte correction; prevention of hypothermia; treatment of secondary infections
- Tailor treatment to underlying condition: sedating antihistamines, topical and/or systemic steroids (caution when tapering; may need systemic steroids in drug reactions and idiopathic presentation), wet dressings, and emollients

Confluent and reticulated papillomatosis (CARP)

- Starts at puberty; F > M; Blacks > Whites
- Unknown etiology
- Red or brown, rough, keratotic, slightly raised papules that first appear in **intermammary region** → spreads outward and forms reticulated pattern (Fig. 3.5) laterally

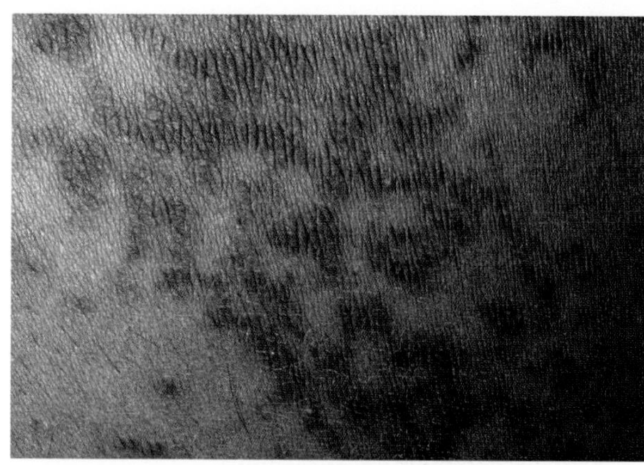

Fig. 3.5 Confluent and reticulated papillomatosis. Multiple hyperpigmented papules that are confluent centrally and assume a reticulated pattern laterally. (From James WD, Elston DM, McMahon PJ. Pityriasis rosea, pityriasis rubra pilaris, and other papulosquamous and hyperkeratotic diseases. In: *Andrews' Diseases of the Skin: Clinical Atlas*. Philadelphia: Elsevier; 2018:139–151.)

- Histology: **acanthosis nigricans-like** (hyperkeratosis, acanthosis, and papillomatosis)
- **ToC**: **minocycline** 100 mg BID × 6 weeks (effective in 50%)
  - Other options: oral retinoids, oral antibiotics, or topical antifungals
- **Pseudoatrophoderma colli**: variant that occurs on neck; appears as vertically oriented hyperpigmented papillomatous lesions w/ wrinkling; also responsive to minocycline

3.2 ECZEMATOUS DERMATOSES

Atopic dermatitis (AD)

Epidemiology

- Part of **atopic triad**: AD (often first manifestation), allergic rhinitis, and asthma
- More common in **high-income and urban areas** (exposure to pollutants and lack of exposure to infectious agents may → AD development)
- Affects 25% of children, 3% of adults; increasing in prevalence
- Subsets:
  - **Early onset (most common):** arises by 1 to 2 yo, 50% have allergen-specific IgE antibodies, 60% resolve by 12 yo
  - Late onset: arises after puberty
  - Senile onset: arises after 60 yo
- Onset: 50%–60% by first year of life (often 3–6 months), 90%–95% by 5 yo

Pathogenesis (Fig. 3.6)

- Complex interaction of epidermal barrier dysfunction, immune dysregulation, and microbiome alteration (e.g., AD skin significantly more likely to be colonized by *S. aureus*)
- Genetic factors are important
  - Twin studies (monozygotic > dizygotic concordance) and family history (high probability that one or both parents are atopic)

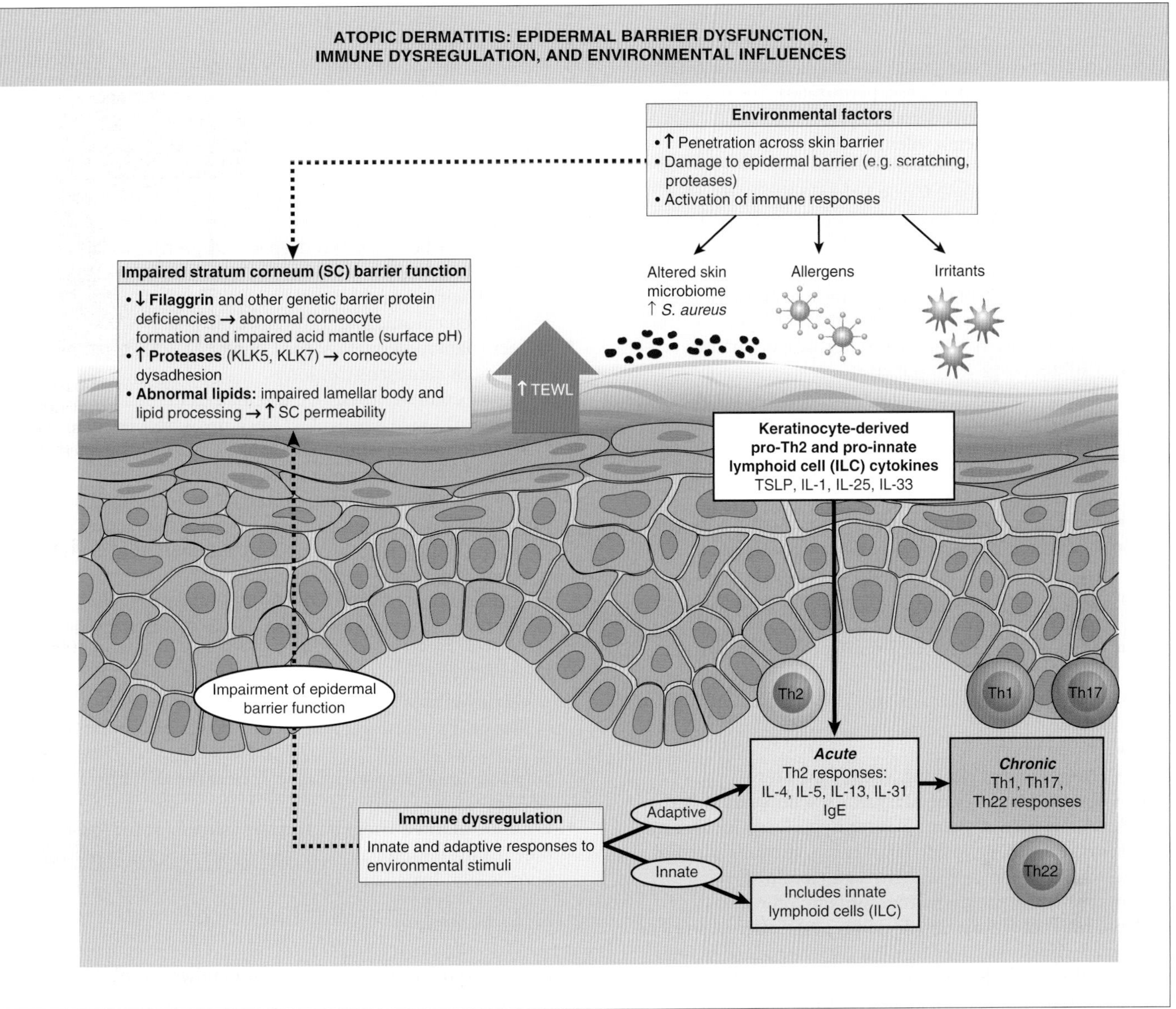

Fig. 3.6 Atopic dermatitis results from defects in epidermal barrier function, immune dysregulation, and environmental influences. *KLK*, Kallikrein; *TEWL*, transepidermal water loss; *TSLP*, thymic stromal lymphopoietin. (Courtesy of Harvey Lui, MD. From McAleer MA, O'Regan GM, Irvine, AD. Atopic dermatitis. In: Bolognia JL, Schaffer JV, Cerroni L. *Dermatology*. 4th ed. Philadelphia: Elsevier; 2018:208–227.)

- Genes encoding epidermal proteins (e.g., FLG and SPINK)
    - **Filaggrin (FLG) mutations** (loss of function) cause alterations in epidermal barrier (e.g., terminal differentiation, ↓epidermal barrier proteins, abnormal lipid organization); **strongest genetic risk factor a/w AD development**; a/w **severe disease, early-onset AD that continues to adulthood, hand dermatitis, food allergy**
    - **SPINK5** (encoding serine protease inhibitor LEKT1) mutations → barrier alterations as well due to Dsg1 degradation
    - Barrier dysfunction causes **transepidermal water loss** and xerosis, allowing penetration of allergens/irritants
- ↑ Transcription of genes encoding immunologic proteins (TLR2, FCER1A, and DEFB1) and cytokines (**Th2** > Th1 [especially **IL-4, IL-5, IL-10, and IL-13**]); Th2 cytokines → ↓ filaggrin, loricrin, involucrin; ↑ IL-31 (important in pruritus) and ↑ IL-17
    - Acute AD: **Th2 predominance** w/ eosinophilia, ↑ IgE production, and ↓ cutaneous antimicrobial peptides (e.g., β-defensin 2/3)
    - Chronic AD: **Th1** (and Th22) **predominance** w/ ↑ IL-1, IFN-γ
- Mediators of itch
    - Histamines less important than neuropeptides, proteases, kinins, and certain cytokines

Clinical features

- Clinical criteria
    - Essential: pruritus
    - Plus ≥3 of the following:
        - History of xerosis

  - Personal history of allergic rhinitis or asthma
  - Onset < 2 yo
  - History of skin crease involvement (antecubital, popliteal, ankle, neck, periorbital)
  - Visible flexural dermatitis
- Acute form: erythema, edema, vesicles, oozing, and crusting
- Subacute and chronic forms: lichenification, papules, nodules, and excoriations
- Pediatric AD
  - Infantile (birth to 6 months of age)
    - Acute presentation and clinical features
    - Favors face, scalp, and **extensor** surfaces
    - May have overlap with seborrheic dermatitis
  - Childhood (2 yo to puberty)
    - Clinical manifestations more chronic in nature, though acute flares may occur
    - Favors **flexures**
    - **Diffuse xerosis** becomes more prominent
- Adolescent/adult AD (>12 yo)
  - **Lichenified plaques** > weeping eczematous lesions
  - Prominent involvement of **flexures**, face, neck (retroauricular), upper arms, back, acral sites
  - AD beginning during childhood is a/w more severe, treatment-resistant disease as adults
  - May manifest as isolated prurigo nodularis, hand or eyelid dermatitis
- Senile AD: marked xerosis rather than typical AD lesions
- Pruritus
  - Worse in evening
  - Triggers: wool clothing, sweat, and stress
- **Associated features of AD:** xerosis, **ichthyosis vulgaris, keratosis pilaris, palmoplantar hyperlinearity, Dennie-Morgan lines,** periorbital darkening, circumoral pallor, anterior neck folds, Hertoghe sign (diminished lateral eyebrows), **white dermatographism**, follicular prominence (favors darker skin types), "**allergic shiners**" (gray infraorbital discoloration), and exaggerated linear nasal crease ("**allergic salute**")
  - Children have ↑ incidence of: **pityriasis alba** (hypopigmentation seen on face/neck; more common in **darker skin types** and more visible after sun exposure), lichen spinulosis, nummular dermatitis, dyshidrotic eczema, and juvenile plantar dermatosis
- Infectious complications: secondary to impaired barrier function and immunologic factors
  - Bacterial: impetiginization w/ ***S. aureus*** > *Streptococcus pyogenes*
  - Viral: **eczema herpeticum**, molluscum dermatitis, and **eczema vaccinatum** (seen w/ smallpox vaccination)
- Ocular complications: **atopic keratoconjunctivitis** (adults), vernal keratoconjunctivitis (children, warm climates), **posterior subcapsular cataracts**, **keratoconus** (elongation of the cornea), and retinal detachment
- Comorbidities: asthma, allergic rhinitis, food allergies, alopecia areata, urticaria, depression, anxiety, osteoporosis, bone fractures, skin infections

Regional variants

- Ear: erythema/scaling/fissuring under earlobe and retroauricular region
- Eyelid: lichenification of periorbital skin
- Nipple dermatitis
- Frictional lichenoid eruption: occurs during spring and summer in boys on the **elbows**/knees/dorsal hands (clusters of small 1–2 mm lichenoid papules)
- Hand: may be **intrinsic** (atopic, psoriasis, dyshidrotic, hyperkeratotic), **extrinsic** (irritant or water exposure, or allergic), or **infectious** (tinea, *S. aureus*) in nature
  - Dyshidrotic eczema on lateral fingers and palms: "**tapioca-like,**" firm and deep-seated pruritic vesicles
    - Pathogenesis is multifactorial (irritant, atopic, and allergic contact)
    - Often chronic and recurrent/relapsing
- Diaper (napkin dermatitis; see Chapter 4)
- Id reactions (autosensitization)
  - Classic example: a vesicular eczematous id reaction of the hands arising in a patient w/ **tinea pedis**; secondary id reaction resolves when underlying dermatosis is treated
- Juvenile plantar dermatosis (see Chapter 4)
- Lip (cheilitis sicca): **irritant contact dermatitis** (ICD; including "**lip-licker's eczema**") > allergic contact dermatitis (ACD; **fragrance mix most commonly**) > AD > eczema of unknown cause
  - Worse in winter; vermilion lip most affected
- Head and neck: occurs post-puberty, *Malassezia* may aggravate

Histopathology

- Acute: **prominent spongiosis**, intraepidermal vesicles/bullae, and perivascular lymphohistiocytic inflammation w/ eosinophils
- Subacute: **milder spongiosis w/ ↑ acanthosis**; lacks vesicles
- Chronic: **marked irregular to psoriasiform acanthosis** (key feature), minimal to no spongiosis, +/– dermal fibrosis, and hyperkeratosis

Laboratory testing

- IgE not typically helpful
- In some patients, identification of allergens via fluorescence enzyme immunoassays, radioallergosorbent (RAST) testing, skin prick testing, and atopy patch testing may be warranted
- Consider testing for food hypersensitivity (eggs, milk, peanuts, soy, and wheat) in children with severe/refractory AD and reliable history of immediate reaction, or worsening dermatitis after ingestion of specific food
  - **Food allergy** most commonly causes a **type I** immediate hypersensitivity reaction
  - 10%–15% of children with severe AD have coexistent food allergies
- Consider testing for aeroallergens (dust mites, pollen, animal dander, and fungi) in teens/adults w/ severe or refractory AD on exposed skin surfaces
  - ↑ Incidence of airborne allergy w/ ↑ age

Treatment

- Review 2022-2023 atopic dermatitis guidelines published in the *Journal of the American Academy of Dermatology*
- Education regarding emollients, short lukewarm baths w/ minimal soap, bleach baths (especially if history of skin infection), and wet dressings +/– topical steroids

- Avoid **irritants**: overheating, wool, sweating, saliva, harsh soaps, fabric softeners, bubble baths, and smoke
- Treatment ladder that ranges from topical treatments (steroids, ruxolitinib, crisaborole, and calcineurin inhibitors) to light therapy (NB-UVB > BB-UVB, UVA1, and PUVA) to systemics (steroids, cyclosporine, azathioprine [AZA], mycophenolate mofetil [MMF], MTX, tacrolimus, dupilumab [anti-IL-4/-13 mab → reduces Th2 response], tralokinumab [anti-IL-13 mab]) depending on severity
  - **Topical CS are mainstay**
  - May experience rebound flares after short courses of systemic steroids
  - **Sedative antihistamines** as adjunctive treatment for itch
  - Treat secondary infections (AD skin has ↓ antimicrobial peptides and a compromised barrier → ↑ infection risk)
- **Primary prevention via breastfeeding** or formulas w/ hydrolyzed milk products for the first 4 to 6 months of life is protective in high-risk AD patients
  - Prenatal, followed by postnatal **probiotic supplementation**, and postnatal prebiotic supplementation, may ↓ risk of AD
    - Prebiotics = non-digestible plant fibers/oligosaccharides that help nourish "good gut bacteria"
- If true IgE-mediated allergy → practice avoidance or undergo allergen-specific immunotherapy through allergist

Prognosis/clinical course

- AD tends to clear in most children by puberty
  - **Classic teaching: 75% resolve by adolescence** (however, new study suggests that only 50% remit by early adulthood)
- If disease persists beyond childhood → tends to be chronic

Asteatotic dermatitis (Eczema craquelé)

- Typically > 60 yo; worse in winter
- In elderly, ↓ **natural moisturizing factor** → ↓ water-binding capacity → when humidity is low in winter, get skin dehydration/**xerosis** → scaling, cracking, and dermatitis
- Xerotic skin w/ fine cracking (resembles **"cracked porcelain"** → hence ***eczema craquelé***), erythema and scale +/- oozing, and crusting
- Pruritic; favors **lower legs**
- Histology: xerosis (compact SC) + spongiotic dermatitis
- Rx: emollients to treat xerosis/prevent flares (applied immediately after bathing); avoid aggravating factors; topical CS and TCIs for flares

Nummular dermatitis

- Associated factors: external irritants, venous HTN, infection, atopy, and xerosis
- **Round or coin-shaped** ("nummular") pink plaques on **extremities**; **very pruritic**; can have acute (eczematous) or chronic (lichenified) appearance; tends to be more recalcitrant
  - Secondary *Staphylococcus* infection common
- Histology: subacute-chronic spongiotic dermatitis
- Rx: **mid- to high-potency topical steroids** (ointments preferable to creams), TCIs, and phototherapy; good skin care w/ emollients

Progesterone dermatitis

- Cyclic flares of dermatitis during the **luteal phase** of menstrual cycle (starts **1 week before menses** → resolves a few days after menses)
- Variable morphology (urticarial, vesicles, and oral erosions)
- Diagnostic test = **intradermal injection of progesterone** → skin reaction
- Rx = **oral contraceptive pills (OCPs)** or tamoxifen to inhibit ovulation
- **Estrogen dermatitis** (chronic w/ exacerbations just prior to menses; Rx = tamoxifen) is major DDx → intradermal estrone test distinguishes

Contact dermatitis

Epidemiology

- ICD (80%) > ACD (20%)
- Occupations most affected:
  - Manufacturing/mining (United Kingdom)
  - Agricultural workers (United States)
- Most common causes of ACD:
  - **Nickel** (worldwide)
  - **Poison ivy** (United States)
- ICD is the most common form of occupational skin disease
  - Petrochemical, rubber, plastic, metal, and automotive industries
  - Causes: soaps > wet work > petroleum products > cutting oils > coolants
- Infants, elderly, and those w/ AD have ↑ risk, due to ↑ penetration of contactants

Pathogenesis

- ICD: **direct damage of keratinocytes** by irritant; **not immune-mediated**, does NOT require previous sensitization
  - Acute ICD: strong irritants (acids/bases) → direct cytotoxic damage to keratinocytes
  - Chronic ICD (more common): repetitive use of mild irritants (soap/water) → over time removes lipid and water-retaining substances of keratinocytes → ↑ transepidermal water loss, ↑ epidermal turnover, inflammation
  - Frictional irritants: repeated rubbing, vibration, and pressure
  - Cold temperature, low humidity → ↑ permeability to irritants
  - Occlusion/maceration/↑ humidity may → ↑ permeability of water-soluble compounds
- ACD: immune-mediated, **delayed-type (type IV) hypersensitivity, initial sensitization** to allergen is required
  - Sensitization can occur with just a few exposures, or after years of exposure
  - Subsequent **reexposure** to allergen → T-cell mediated release of cytokines/chemotactic factors → eczema **within 48 hours**

- Only need exposure once every 3 weeks to keep allergic reaction going
- Cross-reactions and co-reactions can occur:
  - Cross-reaction: sensitization to one compound results in sensitization to compounds w/ a **similar chemical structure** (e.g., **poison ivy and mango peel**; neomycin and gentamicin)
  - Co-reaction: sensitization to two chemicals simultaneously because they are **contacted/used together**, but otherwise allergy to one would not result in allergy to the other (e.g., nickel and cobalt; **neomycin and bacitracin**)

Clinical features

Irritant contact dermatitis

- Clinical presentation variable; **burning** may be more common than itch
- **Hands most common** site of involvement; face is #2
- Ranges from acute ICD with vesiculation/necrosis that has more clearly defined margins to chronic ICD w/ dryness, scaling, lichenification, and fissuring
- Pustular/acneiform irritant ICD: metals, croton oil, **mineral oils**, tars, greases, cutting and metal working fluids, and naphthalenes
- Airborne ICD: resembles photoallergic reaction, but **involves upper eyelids, philtrum, and submental region**
- Phytophotodermatitis: **furocoumarins + light (UVA; 320–400 nm)** → erythema +/– blistering (24–72 hours postcontact) followed by **hyperpigmentation** (1–2 weeks later)
  - Berloque dermatitis: pigmentation of neck/trunk/arms from **cologne** application containing **bergamot oil** (bergapten = 5-methoxypsoralens; a furocoumarin)
- Can have concomitant ulceration, folliculitis, miliaria, pigmentary alterations, alopecia, and urticaria

Allergic contact dermatitis

- Acute: erythema/edema/papules/**oozing/vesiculation**; sharp demarcation between normal and involved skin
- Subacute: ↑ **acanthosis**, ↑ **crusting**/scaling, and ↓ vesiculation
- Chronic: **marked lichenification**/fissuring/scaling, **no vesicles**, **less well-defined** than acute, and may spread beyond site of exposure
- Distribution depends on exposure:
  - **Linear** streaks on extremities: **rhus** (poison ivy/poison oak/poison sumac)
  - Fingertips in florists: flowers (**tulips** #1)
  - Scalp is fairly resistant to allergens → often only the surrounding skin is involved (neck, cheeks, and postauricular)
    - Allergens: hair products (especially dyes), perms, and rinse-off products (shampoo)
  - Perioral/baboon syndrome: flavorings, foods, cosmetics, shellac, meds, and sunscreens
  - Periocular/eyelid:
    - Nail products (**tosylamide >** acrylates, formaldehyde, resin, glutaraldehyde, and benzalkonium chloride)
    - Cosmetics (false eyelashes, adhesives, mascara, rubber sponges for make-up, and eye-shadow)
    - Other allergens: **gold (rings)**, other metals, volatile gases, fragrances/balsam of Peru, **aminoglycosides** (e.g., neomycin, gentamycin), sodium metabisulfite (excipient in topical antibiotics), anesthetics, timolol, thimerosal, surfactants, and preservatives
  - Lips: **gallates**, dyes, flavorings, sunscreens, and **propolis**
  - Earlobe: **nickel**
  - Neck: fragrances and hair products
  - Wrist: chromates (leather)
  - Hands: gloves (latex, rubber [thiuram], and acrylates in medical gloves)
  - Clothing dermatitis: **spares the folds (axillary vault)** and is **accentuated where clothing fits tightly** (waistline); most common allergens:
    - Fabric finishers (i.e., antiwrinkle and stain repellant): **formaldehyde and formaldehyde releasers**
    - Dyes (**disperse blue dyes 106 and 124**)
    - Rubber (bleached underwear → bleaching causes release of carbamates)
  - Cosmetics dermatitis: commonly on face/neck; **fragrances are #1 cause**, preservatives are second most common
  - Perianal: lidocaine and preservatives (e.g., methylchloroisothiozolinone/methyisothiozolinone [MCI/MI])
  - Shoe dermatitis: **spares toe webs**, begins on base of great toe and spreads over the dorsal surface (plantar surfaces generally spared)
    - Causes: adhesives (**colophony**, p-tert-butylphenol formaldehyde resin), rubber and rubber accelerators (**mercaptobenzothiazole**), leather (**chromates**), and dyes
  - Ulcers: **bacitracin, neomycin, and lanolin**
  - Oral stomatitis: dental fillings (**mercury/gold/amalgam** → **lichenoid** reaction), epoxy resins, and **flavoring** (mint/cinnamon)
  - Airborne ACD: usually from plants (***Compositae* = #1 cause**), but other chemicals also implicated
  - Systemic ACD: diffuse dermatitis due to systemic allergen (e.g., systemic dermatitis from IV aminophylline in patients w/ ethylenediamine sensitivity)
- Occupational ACD: **rubber** > nickel > epoxy and other resins > aromatic amines
- Adhesives
  - Most tape reactions are ICD
  - ACD to tape: rubber, resins, and acrylates

Histopathology

- ICD: mild spongiosis, **scattered necrotic keratinocytes**, and mild perivascular inflammation
- ACD: **spongiotic dermatitis** (may be acute/subacute/chronic, depending on stage), more prominent dermal inflammation
  - Versus ICD: ↑ spongiosis, ↑ dermal inflammation w/ eosinophils, and lacks necrotic keratinocytes

Laboratory testing

- **Patch testing will confirm diagnosis of ACD**
  - Tailor the examined allergens to patient; NEVER apply unknown product during patch testing (can cause

severe reaction/burn); determine <u>relevance</u> of any positive reaction
  - Patches applied to upper back area free of dermatitis on day 0; patches removed at 48 hours (day 2); reactions recorded day 2 (first reading) and days 3–7 (second reading, usually 96 hours)
    - Reactions that **fade** between first and second readings = **irritant**
    - Reactions that **continue or develop** between first and second readings = **allergic**
    - **Delayed positive patch tests** (arise after 7 days) can be seen with: **gold**, neomycin, dodecyl gallate, palladium, *p*-phenylenediamine, and **CS**
    - Gold can cause a persistent positive reaction at the site of patch testing
  - TRUE test: currently 3 panels of 12 allergens each (www.truetest.com)
    - Not as complete as comprehensive patch testing
- Repeat open application test (ROAT): use if patient cannot do patch test, or to confirm patch test results
  - Apply product to single clear area of BID for 1 to 2 weeks → monitor for reaction
- Material safety data sheets (MSDS) and workplace visit can help determine what workers are handling

Specific contactants

Irritant contact dermatitis

- <u>Fiberglass dermatitis</u>
  - Injury via skin penetration → pruritus/tinging → pink papules
  - Rx: talcum powder
- <u>Bodily fluids</u> (e.g., **saliva, urine, feces**) and water
  - Rx: provide barrier protection (e.g., **zinc oxide** paste, improved hygiene)
- <u>Alkalis</u>
  - Strong alkalis are corrosive: dissolve keratin and penetrate deeply → **worse reactions than acids**
  - Ca/Na/K hydroxides; ammonia; lye
  - Soap, detergent, bleaches, and depilatories
  - Treatment: apply weak acid (vinegar or lemon juice)
- <u>Acids</u>
  - Powerful acids are corrosive and weaker ones are astringent (a compound that shrinks or constricts tissues)
  - Sulfuric acid
    - Causes severe burns, produces brownish staining
    - Brass and iron workers, battery makers, jewelers, weapon of vitriol attacks ("acid throwers")
  - Nitric acid
    - Distinctive burns with yellow discoloration
    - Explosives, fertilizer
  - Hydrofluoric acid
    - Penetrates very deeply due to low dissociation rate → **severe damage to bones**, nerves; **exquisitely painful**; symptoms may be delayed for up to 24 hours
    - Used for dissolving/etching glass in semiconductor industry
    - Rx: neutralize w/ **calcium gluconate** gel, seek emergency care
  - Hydrochloric acid
    - Superficial burn → produces blisters
  - Oxalic acid
    - Paresthesia of fingertips; cyanosis; gangrene
  - Phenol
    - Used in cosmetic peels
    - Produces **white eschar** and temporary anesthesia; systemic absorption → **glomerulonephritis and arrhythmias**
    - **Neutralized by 65% ethyl or isopropyl alcohol**
- <u>Plants</u>
  - May cause non-immunologic contact urticaria (CU), irritant dermatitis (mechanical or chemical), phytophotodermatitis, and ACD (discussed in Allergic Contact Dermatitis section)
  - **Non-immunologic CU**:
    - Urticaceae family (nettle family): ***Urtica dioica***
      - Sharp hairs on plants contain toxins (**histamine, serotonin, and acetylcholine**) → rapid edema, pruritus, and burning
  - **Mechanical ICD:**
    - *Opuntia* spp. (**prickly pear**)
      - Causes **glochid dermatitis**: mechanical ICD as a result of larger spines or smaller glochids (collections of short barbed hairs) that cause penetrating injuries → inoculation of ***Clostridium tetani, S. aureus,*** *Sporothrix schenckii,* **and atypical mycobacteria**
      - Remove larger pieces w/ tweezers; use glue and gauze for smaller pieces
  - **Chemical ICD (Boards favorite!):**
    - Bromelin
      - *Ananas comosus* (**pineapples**)
    - Calcium oxalate
      - Family Amaryllidaceae/Liliaceae
        - **Daffodil** (*Narcissus* spp.), hyacinth, and tulip bulbs
        - Most common cause of ICD in florists, "daffodil itch"
      - Family Araceae
        - **Dumb cane** (*Dieffenbachia*; house plant)
      - *A. comosus*
        - Pineapple (also contains bromelin)
    - Capsaicin
      - Family **Solanaceae**
        - Hot peppers
        - Neutralized with acetic acid (vinegar) or antacids
    - Phorbol esters
      - Family Euphorbiaceae
        - **Croton plant, spurges**, and poinsettias
        - Also contains diterpenes (**latex**)
        - May cause temporary blindness
    - Protoanemonin/**ranunculin**
      - Family Ranunculaceae
        - **Buttercups** and marigolds
        - Classic **linear vesicles** like phytophotodermatitis, but NO hyperpigmentation afterward
    - Thiocyanates
      - Family **Alliaceae**
        - Garlic
      - Family Brassicaceae
        - Black mustard, radish

- **Phytophotodermatitis**
  - Caused by **furocoumarins** in plants + **UVA light (320–400 nm)** (Fig. 3.7)
  - Apiaceae/Umbelliferae
    - **Hogweed** (*Heracleum*), cow parsley, and wild chervil: **"strimmer dermatitis"** after weed whacking
    - **Parsley**, **parsnips**, **celery**, and carrots: "harvester's dermatitis" in gardeners
    - Flowers easily identified as they are clustered on a stalk and arise from a single point (mnemonic: "**Ap**iaceae/**Umb**elliferae phytophotodermatitis = **Ape** holding an **Umbrella**-looking plant to stay protected from **sun**")
  - Rutaceae
    - **Citrus** (lemon, lime, grapefruit), rue
    - *Citrus bergamia* (bergamot orange): causes **berloque dermatitis**
    - *Pelea anisata* **(Hawaiian leis)**
    - Common cause in **bartenders** and spring breakers
    - "**Mexican beer dermatitis**:" phytophotodermatitis variant that may be widespread rather than linear, due to aerosolization of lime-beer mixture
  - Moraceae
    - Fig and fig leaves
    - Mulberry
  - Fabaceae (legumes):
    - Bavachi/scurf pea (used as vitiligo treatment)
    - **Balsam of Peru** (*Myroxylon balsamum*, *Myroxylon pereiae*)

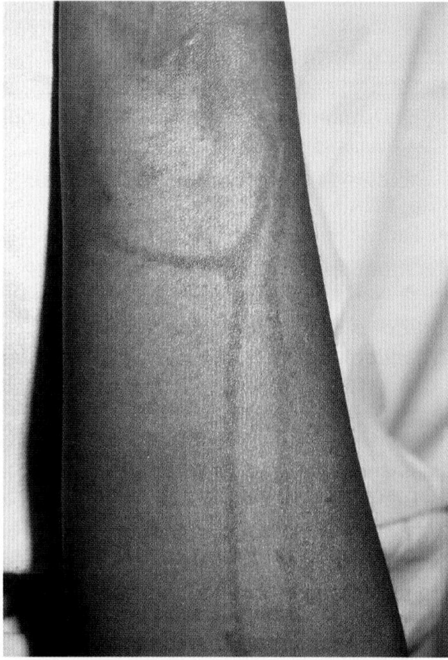

Fig. 3.7 Phytophotodermatitis; the patient had rinsed her hair with lime juice in Mexico. (From James WD, Berger TG, Elston DM. Dermatoses resulting from physical factors. In: *Andrews' Diseases of the Skin*. 11th ed. Philadelphia: Elsevier. 2011:18–44.)

Allergic contact dermatitis

- Specific allergens involved in ACD (Table 3.1)
- ACD due to plants (Table 3.2)
  - Rhus dermatitis: **Anacardiaceae** family, ***Toxicodendron*** species
    - Allergen: **urushiol** (an oleoresin)
      - Sensitizing ingredient: **pentadecylcatechol**
    - Poison ivy/poison oak/poison sumac
      - Contained in leaves, stems, and roots
    - Direct contact (plant/fingers) → linear/streaky erythematous vesicles/bullae
    - Indirect contact (pet/burning plant) → diffuse
    - **Black lacquer/spot dermatitis**: sap from *Toxicodendron* species turns black w/ oxidation in stratum corneum
  - Asteraceae (Compositae; daisy/sunflower family): causes **airborne ACD**
    - Unlike photosensitive dermatitis, involves **eyelids/ melolabial folds/submental**/retroauricular sulci/ antecubital fossae
    - Classically affects middle-aged men
    - Worse in summer, resolves in winter
  - Essential oils: cinnamon oil (cassia), eucalyptus oil, and citrus peel
  - Exotic hardwoods (cocobolo/rosewood): can cause erythema multiforme (EM)-like reaction
  - Foods: variety of vegetables, fruits, and spices can cause ACD
  - Photoallergic contact dermatitis
    - Allergen + light (usually **UVA**) → dermatitis via immune mechanisms

Treatment

- Gold standard is education and avoidance of allergen/irritant
- Additional treatments similar to other dermatitides
- For ICD, many cases resolve spontaneously due to "hardening" phenomenon
- After acute ACD exposure (i.e., poison ivy), whole area/ body should be first washed with water, then soap can be considered; systemic CS over **3 weeks** are very effective

Stasis dermatitis

- Incompetent valves of lower extremities → venous HTN → capillary distention and leak → extravasation of fluid, plasma proteins, and erythrocytes → edema, **hemosiderin** deposition, fibrosis, ulceration, inflammation, and microangiopathy
- **Contact sensitization** (often from topical products [i.e., neomycin] or medicaments), irritant factors, and superinfection may complicate the picture
- **Pitting edema and hemosiderin deposits** over distal third of leg, scaling, inflammation, and pruritus or tenderness; skin changes **often begin on medial ankle**; can become lichenified from rubbing
- A/w **Lipodermatosclerosis** (stasis panniculitis; "**inverted wine bottle**" appearance w/ tight circular cuff over distal calf from chronic inflammation → adherent skin/subcutaneous tissue/fascia; may need danazol or pentoxifylline treatment)
- Atrophie blanche and ulceration from venous changes can occur **(typically medial supramalleolar region)**

Table 3.1 High-Yield Allergic Contact Dermatitis (ACD) Allergens

Metals and metal salts	
Pure metals generally do not cause sensitivity; metals in salts more often cause reactions	
Nickel	**Most common positive patch test** (relevance ≈50%) Sources: jewelry (white gold, 14-carat gold), buckles, belts, cell phones, buttons, zippers, clothing hooks, musical instruments, keys, doorknobs, European coins, and cement Direct relationship between nickel allergy and number of pierced sites Nickel in foods: cocoa, licorice, margarine, peanuts, brown lentils, walnuts, almonds, hazelnuts, and beans Nickel testing: **dimethylglyoxime** in 10% ammonia test (turns pink in presence of nickel) Safe metals for pts w/ nickel allergy: titanium, platinum, and sterling silver
Chromates	Sources: dyes **(green felt fabric on pool table)**, yellow-green pigment (tattoos/cosmetics), **leather (shoe dermatitis), cement**, matches, and crude oils (engine/aircraft workers and photographers) Cross-reacts w/ nickel and cobalt
Cobalt	Sources: metal products, cosmetics, dyes (**blue-green dyes**, paint, tattoos), **glass/pottery, cement**, vitamin B12 injections (can lead to intractable hand dermatitis), and artificial joints **Poral reaction:** irritant reaction w/ purpuric pores Cross-reacts w/ nickel and chromate Cobalt testing: **1-Nitroso-2-naphthol-3, 6-disulfonic acid disodium salt** can be used to detect trace cobalt in items
Mercury	Common cause of **oral lichenoid reaction** (mercury amalgams) Sources: **amalgams** (dentistry), insecticides, industry (glues and starch pastes), felt hat workers, etching/artwork, and furs
Gold	Common cause of **oral lichenoid reactions** and **eyelid dermatitis** Sources: jewelry (hand/facial/eyelid dermatitis) and amalgams/fillings Most frequent cause of **persistently positive patch test reactions** Cross-reacts w/ nickel and cobalt
Aluminum	Sources: sunscreen, cosmetics, dental restorations, food, vaccines, immunotherapy Aluminum hydroxide is the most allergenic aluminum salt
Rubber and rubber additives	
Sources: shoes, gloves, adhesives, elastic (if bleached), pacifiers, cosmetic applicators, latex (gloves, balloons, condoms), swim goggles, tires, fungicides (thiurams), and neoprene (synthetic rubber)	
Latex	Derived from *Hevea brasiliensis* sap Far more likely to cause **immunologic contact urticaria** (type I hypersensitivity reaction) than type IV delayed-type hypersensitivity reaction Risk factors: **healthcare profession, spina bifida** Latex **cross-reacts w/ "BACK Passion"** (Bananas, Avocado, Chestnut, Kiwi, PASSION fruit)
Thiuram (tetramethylthiuram disulfide)	Most common **glove allergy** and most common allergen in healthcare workers **Cross-reacts with disulfiram**
Carba mix/carbamates	Released from **bleached elastic**; perform use-test (patch test often false negative)
Mercaptobenzothiazole (MBT)	#1 cause of **allergic shoe dermatitis**
Black rubber mix	Found in heavy-duty rubber products (tires, rubber balls) May cause purpuric reaction
Dialkyl thioureas (neoprene)	**Wetsuit dermatitis** and allergy to goggles
p-phenylenediamine (PPD)	Sources: hair dye, black henna (temporary tattoos), **black rubber** (rubber vulcanization, antioxidant), photograph development, photocopies, printer ink, other darkly colored cosmetics **Rubber workers** p/w eczema of **hands**, wrists, forearms, eyelids, nose
Adhesives	
Substances used for gluing things together	
Rosin (colophony and abietic acid)	Uses: de-epilation waxes, adhesives, painting, chewing gum, **violin** and other musical instruments
p-tert-butylphenol formaldehyde resin (PTBP)	Used for **gluing together leather products** (watchbands, leather handbags, shoes) Can cause depigmentation
Epoxy resin (bisphenol A)	Encountered in: **PVC and plastic materials,** electrical insulation, paint, artists, sculptors, glues Only produce ACD when in their liquid (non-cured, monomeric) state → fully polymerized product is non-sensitizing
Cyanoacrylates	Used for different purposes, depending on specific type **Ethyl cyanoacrylate**: KrazyGlue; used to glue-on **artificial nails**; is more toxic to skin than butyl- and octyl cyanoacrylates → not used for skin Butyl cyanoacrylate (GluStitch): sutureless skin closures Octyl cyanoacrylate (Dermabond): sutureless skin closures
Methacrylate	Very hard, rigid **plastic**; may also be used as adhesive in orthopedic and dental prostheses; **isobornyl acrylate** is found in glucose sensors and insulin pumps Uses: artificial nail **plates**, hard contact lenses, adhesive ("bone cement") for **artificial joints**, **dental prostheses**, dental sealant **Diffuses through rubber and polyvinyl gloves → paresthesias**
Preservatives	
Added to anything with water in order to prevent spoilage; most commonly found in personal care products and cosmetics	
Formaldehyde	Frequent sensitizer, but decreased cosmetic use recently (formaldehyde releasers now more commonly used) Found everywhere—meds, textiles/clothing, paints, embalming process, and paper—but most notably **wrinkle-free clothing** **100% cotton or cotton/synthetic fiber blends have most formaldehyde** **Polyester has least formaldehyde of any textile**

Continued

Table 3.1 High-Yield Allergic Contact Dermatitis (ACD) Allergens—cont'd

Formaldehyde-releasing preservatives (chemical compounds that slowly release formaldehyde)	Formaldehyde-releasing preservatives are #2 cause overall of cosmetic-related ACD (fragrances are #1) **Quaternium-15 (Dowicil 200)**: found in soaps, shampoos, moisturizers; **#1 preservative sensitizer** in the United States **Imidazolidinyl urea** Diazolidinyl urea DMDM hydantoin
Kathon CG (methychloroisothiazolinone/ methylisothiazolinone (MCI/MI)	Found in **wet wipes** → common cause of **perianal ACD** Also present in Eucerin and other personal care products
Parabens	Preservative in topical medications, antiperspirants Cross-reacts with **PPPASTA family** (**P**ara-aminosalicylic acid, **P**ABA, **P**PD, **A**zo dyes, **S**ulfonamides, **T**hiazides, ester **A**nesthetics
Thimerosal (ethyl mercury)	Mercury-containing preservative in **vaccines**, **eye-drop solutions**, cosmetics, and nasal sprays **Positive thimerosal patch test almost never relevant!** → ok to give vaccines even w/ positive patch test **Cross-reacts with piroxicam and mercury**
Other preservatives	2-bromo-nitropropane-1,3-diol (Bronopol) Euxyl K 400 (methyldibromoglutaronitrile) Benzylkonium chloride Triclosan Benzyl alcohol Tea tree oil
Vehicles, emollients, and emulsifiers	
Propylene glycol	Vehicle base in many creams and lotions Also in **ECG and lubricant** jelly, **antifreeze**, **brake fluid**, food dyes/flavorings
Cocamidopropyl betaine	Non-ionic **surfactant** found in **shampoo**, soaps Derived from coconut oil
Ethylenediamine	Found in topical steroid and antifungal creams (**Mycolog**) Cross-reacts w/ **aminophylline** and hydroxyzine → can develop systemic ACD if allergic and receive aminophylline!
Lanolin	Used in emollients Allergen is **wax-wool alcohol** (derived from sheep) Allergy common among **leg ulcer** pts Cross-reacts w/ **Aquaphor** and Eucerin
Propolis	Made by **bees** from resinous exudates of plants Most notable for **ACD of lips** (lip balms)
Alkyl glucosides	Gentle eco-friendly surfactants used in cosmetic and household products Found in many hypoallergenic, sensitive skin products, as well as sunscreen ingredient Tinosorb M
Fragrances ***Fragrance allergy is #1 cause of all cosmetic-related ACD****; almost all cosmetics contain fragrance; "fragrance free" ≠ no fragrance (still may have masking fragrances!); fragrances are used for* ***cologne, perfumes, food flavoring****; patch test to* ***balsam of Peru + fragrance mix detects 90%*** *of fragrance allergies*	
Fragrance mix	Patch test to mixtures of eight fragrances (cinnamic alcohol, cinnamic aldehyde, amyl cinnamic alcohol, eugenol, isoeugenol, geraniol, hydroxycitronellal, oak moss absolute) Rash typically limited to face, hands, arms, and tongue Cross-reaction w/ propolis, colophony, turpentine
Balsam of Peru	Derived from ***Myroxylon pereirea*** tree Detects 50% of fragrance-related ACD
Hair products	
p-phenylenediamine (PPD)	Potent sensitizer! Sources: **hair dye**, **black henna (temporary tattoos)**, **black rubber** (rubber vulcanization, antioxidant), **photograph** development, photocopies, printer ink, and other darkly colored cosmetics **Hairdressers**, photographers, rubber workers: eczema of **hands**, wrists, forearms, eyelids, nose Clients who get hair dyed: scalp and hairline dermatitis **Beard dermatitis** in those who dye their beards Note: **natural henna** (*Lawsonia inermis*) is a traditional red-brown dye used in South Asian cultures; **does not commonly cause ACD**
Perms	Alkaline (home) perm: **ammonium thioglycolate** (rare sensitizer, more likely to cause ICD than ACD) Acid (professional/salon) perm: **glyceryl monothioglycolate** (allergen); a common sensitizer, remains in hair shaft for >3 months, penetrates rubber and vinyl gloves Neutral perm: cysteamine hydrochloride (uncommon sensitizer)
Hair bleach (contains ammonium persulfate and peroxides)	**Ammonium persulfate** → **contact urticaria** reaction and generalized histamine reaction
Nail products	
Tosylamide (toluene-sulfonamide) formaldehyde resin	**Nail lacquer**/polish Very common cause of **eyelid**, neck, and **finger/periungual dermatitis**
Artificial nails	Ethyl cyanoacrylate: KrazyGlue; used to **glue-on** artificial nails **Methacrylate**: rigid plastic material, forms artificial (acrylic) **nail plates**
Medications	
Transdermal patches	Clonidine has highest rate of sensitization
Antihistamines	Doxepin > diphenhydramine

Table 3.1 High-Yield Allergic Contact Dermatitis (ACD) Allergens—cont'd

Anesthetics (**esters** » amides)	Esters = **one "i"** = **benzocaine** (#1 sensitizer; used for **hemorrhoids**, toothaches, and sore throats), procaine, tetracaine **Esters cross-react w/ "PPPASTA" family** (**P**PD, **P**ABA, **P**ara-aminosalicylic acid, **A**zo dyes, **S**ulfonamides, **T**hiazides, ester **A**nesthetics) Amides = two **'i's'** = dibucaine, lidocaine, mepivacaine, and prilocaine Cross-reactivity: occurs for drugs within each class, but rarely between classes
Antibiotics (Neomycin, Bacitracin, Polymyxin)	Late reactions on patch testing (day 7) Risk factors: use on **chronic leg ulcers**, chronic otitis externa, postoperative application Co-reactions may occur with all, but most common with **neomycin** and **bacitracin** Cross-reactions: **neomycin and aminoglycosides** (gentamicin, tobramycin, kanamycin)
Corticosteroids	Grouped into categories based on allergenic potential. Each group with standardized screening allergen for patch testing: • Group A (screening agent = **Tixocortol pivalate**): **most frequently allergenic**; includes hydrocortisone, prednisone, prednisolone, and methylprednisolone • Class B (screening agent = **Budesonide**): includes triamcinolone, desonide, fluocinolone, fluocinonide, halocinonide, and hydrocortisone butyrate • Class C (screening agent = **Betamethasone**): **least allergenic**; includes betamethasone, desoximetasone, dexamethasone, and flucortisone • Class D (screening agent = **Hydrocortisone-17-butyrate**): includes mometasone, aclomethasone, betamethasone valerate, and clobetasol ▪ Class B and D cross-react with each other ▪ On patch testing, positive test may be an allergenic ring at edge of patch test site (steroid suppresses allergic response in center) ▪ **Delayed reading important!**
Nitrogen mustard/ mechlorethamine	ACD occurs in **66% w/ aqueous** solution, but < **5% w/ ointment**
Sunscreens	**Oxybenzone** (UVA): **most common** sunscreen allergen PABA/padimate O (UVB): no longer commonly used; **PABA cross-reacts w/ other "PPPASTA" allergens** (**P**PD, **P**ABA, **P**ara-aminosalicylic acid, **A**zo dyes, **S**ulfonamides, **T**hiazides, ester **A**nesthetics) Zinc oxide and titanium dioxide (physical sun blockers): do NOT cause ACD
Miscellaneous allergens	
Disperse blue dyes	Disperse blue dyes **106 and 124** are best screening agents Spares axillary vault
Dimethylfumarate	Antifungal agent used to prevent mold growth in **leather couches ("Chinese sofa dermatitis") and shoes**
Glutaraldehyde	Chemical antiseptic used to sterilize surgical instruments
Acetophenone azine	Potent allergen in shin pads and athletic footwear

Table 3.2 Allergic Contact Dermatitis Due to Plants

Family	Sensitizer	Sources	Cross-Reaction
Anacardiacea (*Toxicodendron* genus)	Pentadecylcatechol in oleoresin (urushiol)	Poison ivy/poison oak/poison sumac	**Japanese lacquer tree; cashew** nut (nutshell); **mango** rind/leaves/sap; Indian marking nut; **ginkgo** (fruit pulp); Brazilian pepper tree
Alstromeriaceae	Tuloposide or tulipalin A	Peruvian lily (Alstromeria) favors dominant hand	
Liliceae	Tulipalin A/B	Tulip bulb (favors dominant hand, usually first/second fingertips), asparagus, hyacinth	
Parmelia	d-usnic acid	Lichens	
Pinaceae	Colophony (abietic acid)	*Pinus palustris* (pine) tree	Balsam of Peru, turpentine, colophony, benzoin, wood tars, spices
Asteraceae (Compositae)	Sesquiterpene lactone	Ragweed, **dandelion**, pyrethrum, mugwort, **chrysanthemum** (dominant hand), weeds, feverfew, artichoke, daisy, **sunflower**, endive, arnica, marigold, chamomile	Permethrin
Alliaceae	Diallyl disulfide	Onions, garlic **(non-dominant hand w/ hyperkeratosis/fissuring of thumb, index, and middle finger tips)**, chive	
Primulaceae	Primin	Primrose (dominant hand)	
Myrtaceae	D-limonene	Tea tree oil/malaeuca oil	

- Histology: spongiotic dermatitis, **lobular capillary hyperplasia** +/− fibrin cuffing, **hemosiderin**, and **fibrosis** of dermis and subcutaenous fat septae (later stages)
- Rx: manage venous HTN w/ **compression stockings** and elevation; diosmiplex 630 mg may help (↓ leukocyte activation, VEGF expression, TNF-α)
- For dermatitic component: emollients/topical steroids

Autosensitization (Id reaction and disseminated eczema)

- Secondary eczematous lesions develop in sites distant from primary exposure site (usually ACD +/− stasis dermatitis [>60% w/ **contact dermatitis and stasis dermatitis develop id reactions**]; can also occur in **tinea pedis**)

- Disseminated lesions appear days to weeks after primary lesion
- Eczema tends to be ill-defined and symmetric, often occurring in analogous anatomical sites (e.g., palms, soles, extremities)
- Pathogenesis unknown but possibly related to:
    - Hematogenous dissemination of allergens
    - ↓ Sensitization threshold in distant skin sites after primary inflammation
    - Circulating activated memory T cells
- Rx: topical steroids, systemic antihistamines, treatment of any underlying causes

Contact urticaria (CU)

Epidemiology

- Most frequently seen in healthcare workers, food handlers (e.g., bakers, agricultural workers, butchers), hairdressers, dental assistants
- Risk factors: **atopy**, hand dermatitis, and allergy to fruits (kiwi, avocado, banana, and melon)

Pathogenesis

- Immunologic CU: mediated by allergen-specific IgE on mast cells → mediator release (e.g., histamine); since **IgE-mediated**, can be **a/w anaphylaxis**
- **Raw vegetables/meats**: **potato** (**#1**, often a/w asthmatic response), celery (more likely to cause anaphylaxis), raw meat, fish, and shellfish
    - Latex:
        - Most common in **healthcare workers** (up to 10% incidence)
        - Increased risk in **spina bifida patients** and atopics
        - Type I reaction to latex is much more common than type IV (delayed-type hypersensitivity)
        - Symptoms include itching and swelling of hands within minutes of applying gloves → resolves within 1 hour; chronic exposure may → chronic hand eczema
        - **Aerosolized glove powder** or mucosal exposure may induce **anaphylaxis**
        - 50% have **cross-reaction** w/ **"BACK Passion"** (**B**ananas, **A**vocado, **C**hestnuts, **K**iwi, **Passion** fruit)
        - Other causes: henna, **ammonium persulfate** (hair bleach), and **bacitracin** (may lead to anaphylactic reactions when applied to chronic leg ulcers)
    - Flour/grain/feed and cow dander are other culprits
- Non-immunologic CU: more common, occurs in any exposed individual, and **much lower risk of anaphylaxis**; due to prostaglandin release primarily
    - **Urticaceae/stinging nettles (#1)**, euphorbiaceae (spurge nettle), caterpillars, and jellyfish
        - Agents lead to direct release of histamine, acetylcholine, and serotonin
    - Other causes: dimethyl sulfoxide (**DMSO**), sorbic acid, benzoic acid, and cinnamic aldehyde
- Protein contact dermatitis: dermatitic reaction to protein-containing products in foods/animal products; reactions both allergic (type I and/or type IV) and non-allergic

Clinical features

- Pruritic cutaneous urticaria (wheal and flare) within 1 hour of exposure (3–5 minutes for stinging nettles); resolves in 24 hours
    - Oral allergy syndrome = mucosal CU (type of immunologic CU)
- Foods are common cause of CU; can get cross-reactions between foods and other topical/aeroallergens:
    - Birch pollen allergy a/w CU to various fruits/vegetables (apples, pears, and cherries)

Laboratory testing

- Standard closed patch testing method is ineffective → use **open patch test** instead
    - Open patch test: apply substance to forearm and wait 30 minutes for wheal and flare response; if no response, can wait 30 minutes longer
    - Open patch testing is superior to prick, scratch, and intradermal testing as these can lead to anaphylaxis
- RAST testing detects 75% of latex allergies

Treatment

- Varies depending on severity: avoidance and **antihistamines (most cases)**, systemic steroids (generalized urticaria or asthmatic reactions), and epinephrine + supportive care (anaphylaxis)

3.3 INTERFACE DERMATITIS

Vacuolar interface dermatitis

Autoimmune connective tissue disease (AICTD)

Discussed in Section 3.5

Erythema multiforme (EM)

Epidemiology

- Predominantly young adults (M ≈ F) in spring and fall

Pathogenesis

- **90% of cases are caused by infection:**
    - Herpes simplex virus (**HSV1** > HSV2) infection by far **most common trigger**
        - Herpes-associated EM (HAEM) is #1 cause of **EM minor (von Hebra's disease)**
        - Herpes labialis outbreak most commonly precedes EM by 1 to 3 weeks
    - ***Mycoplasma pneumoniae***: severe **mucous membrane** involvement (simulates Stevens-Johnson syndrome [SJS]) and atypical papular target lesions; most common cause of **EM major**
- Less common causes:
    - *Histoplasma capsulatum:* commonly have **concomitant erythema nodosum (EN)**
    - Drug-induced (<10%): NSAIDs, antibiotics, sulfonamides, antiepileptics, and TNF-α inhibitors
    - Other: radiation-induced, idiopathic, and chronic oral EM

Clinical features

- Abrupt onset of numerous symmetric, fixed red macules → papules → "target" lesions (mixture of typical targets and papular atypical targets)
- Typical target (classic primary lesion of EM):
  - **Three zones**: dusky, vesicular or necrotic center; elevated, edematous pale surrounding ring; outer rim of macular erythema
  - Well-demarcated
  - Favors **face and distal extremities** (upper extremities > lower extremities; dorsal hands and forearms most common) (Fig. 3.8)
- Papular (elevated) atypical target:
  - Only two zones, but is **palpable**
  - Ill-defined peripheral border
    - Important clinical pearl: **macular** (non-palpable, non-elevated) atypical targets are seen in **SJS/toxic epidermal necrolysis (TEN), but not EM!**
- Presence of elevated/papular target lesions and acrofacial distribution allow for reliable distinction from SJS/TEN
- **EM minor**: target lesions w/ minimal mucosal involvement and no systemic symptoms
- **EM major**: target lesions w/ **severe** mucosal involvement and **systemic symptoms** (fever, arthralgias)
  - Buccal mucosa and lips most common mucosal sites (>ocular, genital)
  - Primary mucosal lesions are raised targets → rapidly become painful erosions
- Oral EM (clinical variant): middle-aged women w/ recurrent disease limited primarily to oral cavity

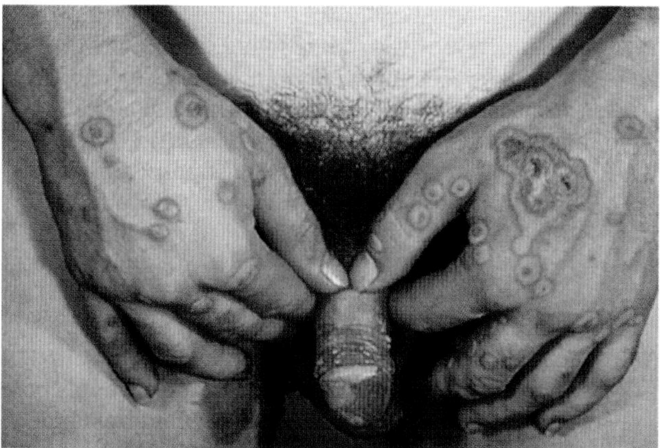

Fig. 3.8 Erythema multiforme involving the dorsal hands and penis. (From James WD, Elston DM, Treat JR, Rosenbach MA, Neuhaus IM. Erythema and urticaria. In: *Andrews' Diseases of the Skin*. 13th ed. Philadelphia: Elsevier; 2020:140–156.)

Histopathology

- Individual keratinocyte apoptosis scattered throughout **all levels** of epidermis, **prominent basal vacuolar change**, spongiosis w/ lymphocyte exocytosis, moderately dense superficial dermal perivascular lymphohistiocytic infiltrate (Fig. 3.9), and **absent/rare eosinophils** (vs. SJS/TEN)
  - Versus SJS/TEN: ↑↑ dermal inflammation, ↓ epidermal necrosis, and ↓ eosinophils

Laboratory testing

- **80% have detectable HSV DNA by PCR** in early erythematous papules or outer rim of targets

Treatment

- Most cases: symptomatic treatment (e.g., topical steroids)
- Severe cases: consider systemic steroids or immunosuppressants
- **HSV prophylaxis to prevent future outbreaks**
  - Antiviral prophylaxis (valacyclovir 1 g/day or famcyclovir 250 mg/day): ↓ frequency and duration of recurrence in 90% of HAEM cases

Prognosis/clinical course

- Acute onset of lesions over 24 hours → eruption fully developed by 72 hours → self-resolves w/o sequelae w/ in 2 weeks
  - **Exceptions: EM major w/ severe mucosal involvement** → persists for up to 6 weeks and may be a/w ocular complications (if proper eye care not instituted)

Stevens-Johnson syndrome (SJS), and toxic epidermal necrolysis (TEN, Lyell's syndrome)

Epidemiology

- Overall incidence of SJS/TEN = 5 cases/million people annually

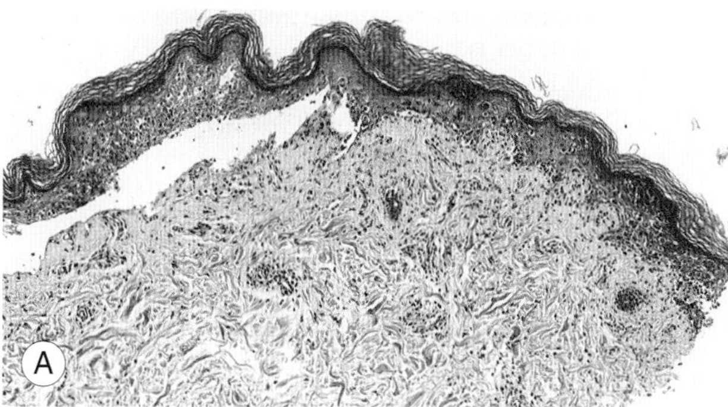

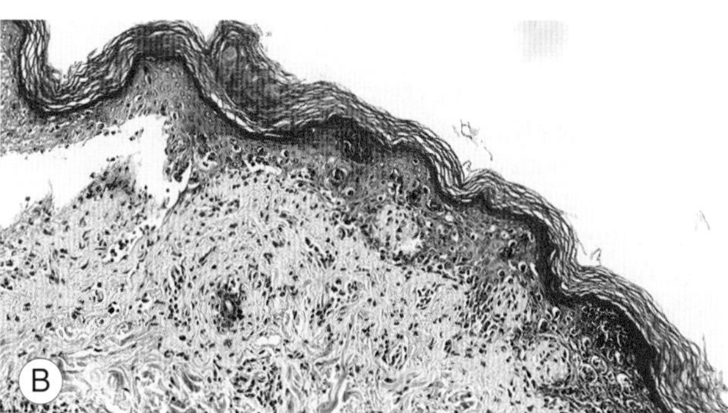

Fig. 3.9 (A) and (B) Histopathologic features of erythema multiforme. Early lesion—focal sites of apoptosis of keratinocytes with an interface dermatitis and vacuolar degeneration of the basal layer. A perivascular lymphocytic infiltrate is also present. (Courtesy of Olayemi Sokumbi, MD.)

- F > M; **elderly more frequently affected**
- Groups with ↑ risk of SJS/TEN:
  - Slow acetylator genotypes
  - **HLA-B*1502** (Asians and East Indians exposed to carbamazepine; up to 220-fold ↑ risk)
  - **HLA-A*3101** (Europeans exposed to carbamazepine)
  - **HLA-B*5701** (abacavir)
  - **HLA-B*5801** (Han Chinese exposed to allopurinol)
  - HLA-DQB1*0601 (White patients with SJS + ocular complications)
  - **AIDS patients** (1000-fold ↑ risk)
    - Markedly ↑ risk of SJS/TEN in **HIV patients** due to loss of skin-protective CD4+/CD25+/regulatory T cells
  - Patients undergoing radiotherapy + anticonvulsant therapy

Pathogenesis

- Exact mechanism still being elucidated, but the key players are known:
  - Drug
    - Binds to MHC I complex or other intracellular peptides → forms antigen recognized by cytotoxic CD8+ T cells → downstream proapoptotic effects
  - Granulysin
    - Currently felt to be the **major mediator of apoptosis** in SJS/TEN
    - Found in cytotoxic granules of CD8+ T cells, NK/T cells, and NK cells
    - Secreted granulysin directly damages target keratinocytes → apoptosis
    - Serologic tests for **granulysin** (80% sensitivity and 95% specificity) and high-mobility group protein B1 (**HMGB1**) have been shown to differentiate SJS/TEN from ordinary morbilliform drug eruptions
  - **FasL (CD95L)**
    - Transmembrane protein of TNF family, found on cytotoxic T cells, NK cells, and keratinocytes
    - FasL binds to the Fas death receptor (CD95/Apo-1) on target keratinocytes → **FasL-Fas complex** leads to activation of **caspases** → **apoptosis**
  - Granzyme B and perforin
    - Activated cytotoxic CD8+ T cells exocytose granzyme B and perforin → molecules poke holes in target cell and activate caspases → apoptosis
- **SJS/TEN is almost always drug-induced**
  - Typically occurs 5 to 28 days after initiation of medication
  - Occurs later with anticonvulsants (within first 2 months)
  - Even within the same class, drugs with longer half-lives are more likely to cause drug reactions and fatal outcomes than drugs with short half-lives
  - Most common culprit drugs:
    - **Allopurinol**
    - **Anticonvulsants**
      - **Lamotrigine**, **carbamazepine**, **phenytoin**, **phenobarbital**, clobazam
      - Risk highest in first 2 months
      - Valproic acid does NOT cross-react w/ others
      - Lamotrigine does not cross-react w/ aromatic anticonvulsants
    - Antibiotics (**sulfonamides** > β-lactams, cephalosporins, minocycline, quinolones, and antifungals)
      - Sulfonamide antibiotics do NOT cross-react w/ non-antibiotic sulfonamides (e.g., hydrochlorothiazide [HCTZ] and hypoglycemic agents)
    - Oxicam NSAIDs
    - **Sulfasalazine**
    - Non-nucleoside reverse transcriptase inhibitors (**nevirapine**, **abacavir**, efavirenz, and etravirine)
    - Other notable causes:
      - *M. pneumoniae* (aka *M. pneumoniae*-associated mucositis; mainly seen in children; may also cause EM major), contrast medium, dengue virus, and cytomegalovirus

Clinical features

- **SJS and TEN** are two intimately related, potentially life-threatening adverse drug reactions that **differ only in their degrees of severity**, as determined by degree of epidermal detachment (% BSA):
  - SJS: <10%
  - SJS/TEN overlap: 10%–30%
  - **TEN: >30%**
- Skin findings preceded by **prodrome** (fever, malaise, anorexia, and rhinorrhea) → **atypical targetoid <u>macules</u>**, mucocutaneous erythema, and skin pain → **dusky plaques** w/ full-thickness sloughing
- **Mucosal involvement** almost always present (92%–100% of SJS; ~100% of TEN)
  - Erosions and erythema of oral/ocular/genital mucosae
  - Photophobia and painful urination
  - <u>Eye and genital care is essential</u> for preventing adverse sequelae
  - **Respiratory involvement in 25%** (e.g., hypoxemia, bronchial hypersecretion, dyspnea)
- Characteristic cutaneous lesional morphology:
  - Poorly demarcated erythematous to **dusky macules** of variable size and shape
    - Macules commonly become confluent (TEN > SJS/TEN overlap > SJS)
  - **Flat/macular atypical targets** (macules w/ central dusky hue)
    - Resemble target lesions of EM, but lack three concentric rings and are **flat** (non-palpable)
    - **SJS/TEN lacks raised targets** (vs. EM)!
- **Lesions appear first on trunk** → spreads to neck/face, proximal upper extremities
  - Unlike EM, distal extremities are largely spared
  - Early lesions are erythematous, dusky or purpuric macules, or flat atypical targets of varying size and shape → macules rapidly coalesce → hours to days later full-thickness necrosis ensues → dusky red macules develop a gray hue → flaccid blisters develop with positive **Nikolsky** and **Asboe-Hansen** signs (Fig. 3.10)
    - (+) Nikolsky sign: **tangential pressure** induces dermal-epidermal cleavage
    - (+) Asboe-Hansen sign: **vertical pressure** (applied to top of a bulla) results in extension of blister onto adjacent previously unblistered skin

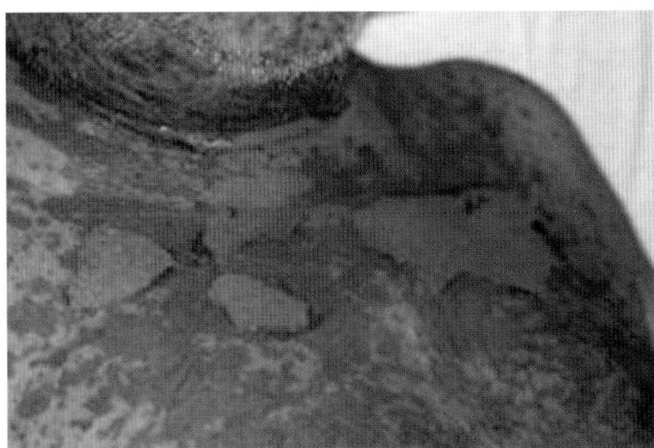

Fig. 3.10 Toxic epidermal necrolysis. Patient with denudation of the epidermis in sheets resembling wet cigar paper. Note the widespread involvement of the trunk. (From Schwartz RA, McDonough PH, Lee BW. Toxic epidermal necrolysis: Part I. Introduction, history, classification, clinical features, systemic manifestations, etiology, and immunopathogenesis. *J Am Acad Dermatol*. 2013;69[2]:173.e1–e13, quiz 185–186.)

Histopathology

- Early: individual apoptotic keratinocytes scattered about all layers of epidermis; scant dermal lymphohistiocytic infiltrate w/ **eosinophils**
- Later: **confluent full-thickness epidermal necrosis,** subepidermal blister (due to diffuse keratinocyte necrosis); scant dermal lymphohistiocytic infiltrate w/ **eosinophils**

Laboratory testing

- **SCORTEN system** relies on seven parameters (Tables 3.3 and 3.4):
  - Serum bicarbonate (<20 mmol/L) is the **#1 most important risk factor for mortality**

Table 3.3 SCORTEN Criteria

Finding	0 Points	1 Point
Age (years)	<40	>40
Associated malignancy	No	Yes
Heart rate (beats/min)	<120	>120
Serum BUN (mg/dL)	<27	>27
Detached or compromised body surface (%)	<10	>10
Serum bicarbonate (mEq/L)	>20	<20
Serum glucose (mg/dL)	<250	>250

Table 3.4 SCORTEN-Predicted Mortality Rates

# of Points	Mortality Rate (%)
0	1
1	4
2	12
3	32
4	62
5	85
6	95
7	99

  - **Mnemonic**: TAMEBUG (**t**achycardia, **a**ge, **m**alignancy, **e**pidermal loss > 10%, **b**icarbonate, **u**rea, **g**lucose)
- Check chest X-ray (CXR), bacterial/fungal swabs of lesional skin, complete blood count (CBC), erythrocyte sedimentation rate (ESR) < C-reactive protein (CRP), comprehensive metabolic panel, *Mycoplasma* serology, coagulation studies

Treatment

- Prevention is ideal
  - FDA recommends **routine screening for HLA-B*1502 in East Asian patients** prior to giving carbamazepine, and screening for HLA-B*5701 in all potential abacavir patients prior to treatment
- Early Dx is critical!
  - **Prognosis correlated w/ rapidity of drug discontinuation**
  - Drug timeline: typically **medication started 5 to 28 days prior** (as early as 2 days with reexposure)
- Initiate intensive supportive skin regimen (e.g., regularly cleanse wounds, apply greasy emollients/topical antimicrobials, **DO NOT** remove detached epidermis, use nonadherent dressings [e.g., Telfa, Mepitel] in denuded areas and foam dressings in exudative areas; **ICU or burn setting** if extensive epidermal detachment), nutritional (e.g., nasogastric feeding if needed)/fluid (e.g., peripheral venous access)/electrolyte support, possibly urinary catheter if genitourinary (GU) involvement, oral care (e.g., anti-inflammatory/antiseptic oral rinse)
- Data for systemic treatment is mixed: **intravenous immunoglobulin (IVIG), cyclosporine, systemic CS, etanercept**
- **Ophthalmology** consult as **ocular damage from corneal scarring** is a disabling complication
- Urology/gynecology consults if GU involvement; intensivist/pulmonologist if respiratory symptoms
- Drug list should be aggressively minimized; especially **avoid drugs w/ long half-lives**

Prognosis/clinical course

- **Ocular sequelae** are most common complication (up to 80%)
  - Dry eye syndrome (most common), entropion, symblepharon, blindness, scarring, and persistent erosions
- Other sequelae: phimosis, vaginal synechiae, nail dystrophy/loss, hair loss, and eruptive nevi
- Mortality:
  - SJS: <5%
  - **TEN: 30%** (reported range: 25%–50%)
    - SCORTEN must be performed during hospital days 1 (**within first 24 hours**) and 3 to maximize predictive value
    - Rapid withdrawal of causative agent ↓ risk of death by 30% per day
    - **Death is most commonly due to infection** (*S. aureus* and *Pseudomonas*)
      - Other causes: transepidermal fluid loss, electrolyte imbalance, inhibition of insulin secretion, and insulin resistance
      - Wood lamp can be used to identify *Pseudomonas* fluorescence

Pityriasis lichenoides

- Pityriasis lichenoides et varioliformis acuta (PLEVA; acute) and pityriasis lichenoides chronica (PLC; chronic) represent two ends of a disease spectrum; both are characterized by **recurrent crops of self-resolving lesions**
- Etiology unclear; may represent response to infections/drugs, or may represent a low-grade T-cell lymphoproliferative disorder
- PLEVA (Fig. 3.11)
  - Rapid onset of widespread (**trunk, buttock, and proximal extremities** > other sites) pink papules → evolves into vesicular, ulceronecrotic, purpuric, and crusted papules → **heals w/ varioliform scars**
    - **Febrile ulceronecrotic Mucha-Habermann disease** (PLEVA variant): severe form w/ high fever, constitutional symptoms, lymphadenopathy, arthritis, mucosal, pulmonary, and GI involvement; a/w ↑ TNF-α levels
- PLC
  - Widespread, red-brown, scaly papules and plaques
  - Resolves w/ **hypopigmentation**
  - Persists longer than PLEVA
  - Adults: PLC > PLEVA

Histology

- PLEVA: Parakeratosis, Lichenoid infiltrate, Extravasation of erythrocytes, **V**-shaped dermal lymphocytic infiltrate, Acute epidermal changes (dyskeratosis, ulceration, neutrophilic scale crust)
- PLC: similar changes as PLEVA, but **much more subtle**—mild parakeratosis, milder vacuolar interface w/ fewer necrotic keratinocytes, milder RBC extravasation, and less dermal inflammatory infiltrate; almost never ulcerates
- Both have **strict absence of eosinophils!**
- **CD8+ T cells** predominate within infiltrate → helps distinguish from majority of other conditions in DDx

Treatment/clinical course

- First line: topical steroids, phototherapy, and systemic antibiotics (**erythromycin**, azithromycin, and tetracyclines)
- Severe forms: MTX, cyclosporine, and IVIG
- Distribution is the best predictor for speed of disease resolution: **diffuse distribution is fastest to resolve** (average 11 months) > central distribution > peripheral distribution (slowest resolution; average 33 months)

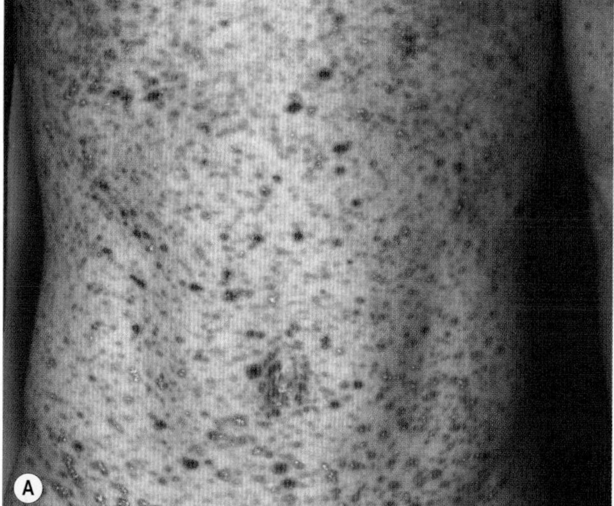

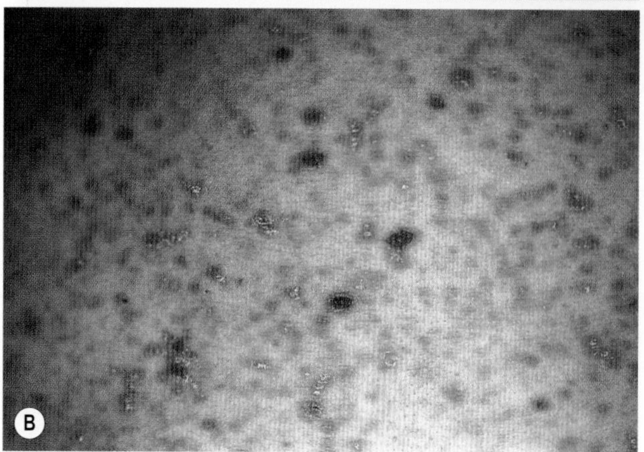

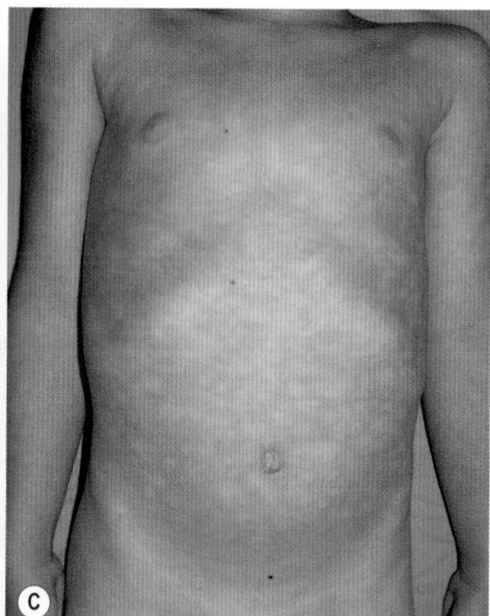

Fig. 3.11 (A) The polymorphic eruption of pityriasis lichenoides; note the mixture of acute (crusted) and chronic (scaly) lesions. (B) Higher power of (A). (C) Postinflammatory hypopigmentation associated with pityriasis lichenoides. (Courtesy of A. Torrelo, MD. From Hogan PA, Langley RGB. Papulosquamous diseases. In: Schachner LA, Hansen RC. *Pediatric Dermatology*. 4th ed. London: Elsevier; 2011:901–951.)

Fixed drug eruption (FDE)

Pathogenesis

- Most common causative meds:
  - **Sulfonamides** (75% of cases; #1 cause on **genitalia**)
  - NSAIDs (especially **naproxen** and other pyrazolone derivatives), predilection for **lips**
  - **Tetracyclines**
  - **Phenolphthalein** (previously in **laxatives**; now less common because it has been removed)
  - Others: barbiturates, aspirin (ASA), OCPs, and carbamazepine
- Non-pigmented FDE (clinical variant)
  - **Pseudoephedrine** (classic cause)
  - Others: NSAIDs, acetaminophen, and tetrahydrozoline (eye drops)

Clinical features

- Most commonly affects **oral and genital mucosa (#1 sites)**, face, and hands/feet
- **Initial episode**: develops **1–2 weeks** after administration of causative drug
- **Subsequent episodes:** eruption recurs at same site **very rapidly** after reexposure (30 minutes to 8 hours)
- **If medications are continued may → generalized FDE**
  - Generalized FDE may have mucosal involvement (difficult to distinguish from EM or SJS)
- Well-demarcated, edematous plaques w/ erythematous-violaceous hue
- Epidermal damage from interface reaction commonly → **central dusky hue, bulla, or erosion**
- Lesions self-resolve over 1 to 2 weeks, w/ prominent **postinflammatory hyperpigmentation**
- Clinical variants:
  - Non-pigmenting FDE
    - Most commonly due to **pseudoephedrine**
    - Very large, tender, "juicy red" plaques
  - Linear FDE: sometimes confused w/ linear lichen planus (LP)
  - Vulvar FDE: symmetrical erosive vulvitis on labia minora/majora and perineum
  - Generalized bullous FDE (GBFDE): significant overlap with SJS/TEN

Histopathology

- **EM-like vacuolar interface** changes w/ scattered apoptotic keratinocytes in all layers of epidermis, moderately brisk superficial to mid dermal perivascular lymphohistiocytic infiltrate w/ **admixed eosinophils and neutrophils**, **↑↑ dermal melanophages** within papillary and reticular dermis (deeper than other interface processes)
  - Versus EM: "dirtier" inflammatory infiltrate (admixed eosinophils and neutrophils), deeper pigment deposition
  - Versus SJS/TEN: ↑ inflammation, ↑ lymphocyte exocytosis, ↓ necrosis, and ↑ pigment incontinence

Laboratory testing

- Patch testing **within a site of prior involvement** may be used to identify culprit medication

Prognosis/clinical course

- Benign; self-resolves in days to few weeks if causative med is discontinued
- Exception: GBFDE may have mortality rate comparable to SJS/TEN (up to 22%)
- Occasionally, a "refractory period" after drug exposure occurs → thus, FDE does not necessarily occur every time implicated medication is administered

Graft- versus- host disease (GVHD)

Epidemiology

- Frequent (>50%) complication of **allogeneic hematopoietic stem cell transplant (HSCT)** → severe skin disease and ↑ mortality
- Less commonly occurs in setting of:
  - Transfusion of non-irradiated blood products to immunocompromised hosts
  - Maternal-fetal transmission
  - Solid organ transplantation (**small intestine** > liver > kidney > heart)
- Single **most important predictor** of developing GVHD after HSCT is **HLA compatibility**
  - ↑ Frequency of GVHD largely due to ↑ use of matched **unrelated** donor (MUD) transplants over past few decades → MUD transplants have ↑ rate of minor HLA mismatch compared with matched related donors (70% vs. 40%)
- Other risk factors for GVHD:
  - Female donor (especially multiparous women) w/ male recipient
  - Older age
  - Stem cell source
    - Risk of GVHD: **peripheral blood (PB-HSCT) >** bone marrow > cord blood
      - ↑ popularity of PB-HSCTs due to ease of collection, but there is ↑ GVHD risk
  - Myeloablative preconditioning regimen (↑ acute GVHD [aGVHD] risk due to host tissue damage)
    - Alternatively, non-myeloablative/reduced-intensity conditioning regimens → ↓ conditioning-related toxicities (better tolerability in elderly) and ↓ risk of aGVHD, but may also delay the onset to beyond the classic ≤100-day period → ↑ incidence of "delayed-onset aGVHD"
- **Skin is most commonly affected organ** in all forms of GVHD (≈80% aGVHD)

Pathogenesis

- aGVHD:
  - HSCT conditioning regimen damages host tissues → activation of host antigen-presenting cells (APCs) → host APCs bind altered host proteins/neo-antigens → donor lymphocytes recognize altered host protein-APC complex → **donor lymphocytes proliferate and target host tissue** in skin, GI tract, and liver
- Chronic GVHD (cGVHD):
  - Molecular pathogenesis still unclear
  - May involve interaction of B cells and T cells
    - Rituximab (anti-CD20 antibody) helpful in some cases of cGVHD

- Early cGVHD (↑ IFN-γ, IL-2Rα, Treg cells) versus late cGVHD (B-cell activation, ↑ TLR9) versus chronic lichenoid GVHD (↑ Th1/Th17)

Clinical features

- aGVHD:
  - Traditionally defined as starting within **first 100 days** after transplant
    - Time period now felt to be arbitrary and not essential for diagnosis
  - Typically starts 2 to 6 weeks (**peak at day 30**) after HSCT
  - Initially p/w morbilliform eruption
    - First sites affected: **acral** sites (hands, feet, ears) and upper trunk
    - Early clues to diagnosis:
      - **Acral erythema**
      - **Violaceous hue on ear**
      - **Follicular/peri-eccrine erythema** (darker punctate lesions help distinguish from simple morbilliform eruptions)
  - Rash may progress to confluent erythematous plaques (SJS/TEN-like)
  - **GI tract and liver involvement** usually accompany skin findings
  - Clinical staging based on three factors:
    - Skin: severity assessed by **% BSA**
    - GI: severity assessed by **volume of diarrhea** (and severe abdominal pain)
    - Liver: severity assessed by degree of **bilirubin** elevation
- cGVHD:
  - Traditionally defined **as starting ≥ 100 days** (average: 120 days) after transplant
    - Time period is now felt to be arbitrary and not essential for diagnosis
  - Preceded by aGVHD in 50%
    - Occurs *de novo* in 50%
  - cGVHD affects a greater variety of organ systems (nearly any organ)
    - Classified as non-sclerotic cGVHD or sclerotic cGVHD
  - **Non-sclerotic cGVHD**:
    - Often, but not always, precedes sclerotic cGVHD phase
    - Most common presentation is **lichenoid** eruption (80% of cases of cGVHD): coalescent, slightly scaly, violaceous-to-pink papules arranged in reticulate pattern (Fig. 3.12)
      - Most common sites: dorsal hands/feet, forearms, and trunks
    - Other morphologies of non-sclerotic cGVHD: **AD-like**, psoriasiform, poikilodermatous, lupus-like, and keratosis pilaris-like
  - **Sclerotic cGVHD**: encompasses multiple morphologies
    - Lichen sclerosis-like (generally upper back)
    - **Sclerodermoid**/morphea-like plaques (generally areas of pressure/prior injury)
      - Unlike true scleroderma, the distribution is more patchy and lacks classic features of scleroderma (bird facies, puffy/indurated hands, and sclerodactyly)
    - Eosinophilic fasciitis (EF)-like
    - Mucosal involvement common (oral looks like LP; vaginal scarring may occur)
    - Nail involvement may occur (e.g., dorsal pterygium, anonychia)

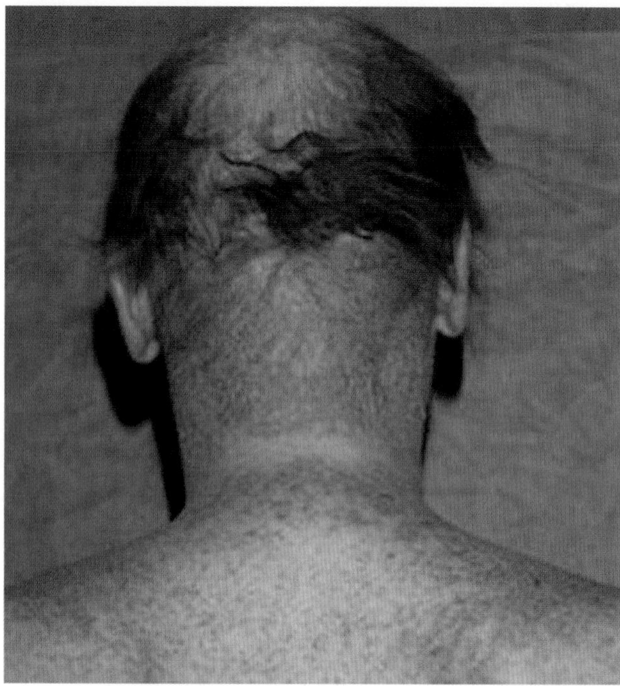

Fig. 3.12 Chronic graft-versus-host disease (GVHD). Epidermal GVHD characterized by lichen planus-like changes on the posterior surface of the neck and upper aspect of the back. (From Hymes SR, Alousi AM, Cowen EW. Graft-versus-host disease: part I. Pathogenesis and clinical manifestations of graft-versus-host disease. *J Am Acad Dermatol*. 2012;66[4]:515.e1–e18, quiz 533–534.)

Histopathology

- aGVHD: **basal vacuolar interface**, +/− keratinocyte necrosis (seen only in grade 2 and higher), sparse superficial perivascular lymphohistiocytic infiltrate
  - **Apoptotic cells in adnexal structures** (hair follicles and sweat ducts): very helpful clue to distinguish from simple drug eruptions!
  - Background of **epidermal dysmaturation** (resembles bowenoid AK or chemotherapy effect): almost always present, useful clue
- cGVHD: variable; the two most common patterns are:
  - **Lichenoid**: moderately dense perivascular to band-like lymphohistiocytic infiltrate w/ vacuolar or lichenoid interface changes and keratinocyte apoptosis; degree of lichenoid inflammation is typically less dense than in classic LP
  - **Sclerotic**: dermal sclerosis, +/− subcutaneous and fascial fibrosis, may see overlying vacuolar or lichenoid interface

Laboratory testing

- aGVHD: **bilirubin and diarrhea** volume

- cGVHD: **MRI** can detect fasciitis (may eliminate need for fascial biopsy)

Treatment

- Prophylaxis improves survival
  - Most common prophylactic regimens: MTX + cyclosporine or tacrolimus
- aGVHD:
  - Limited GVHD (skin only): topical steroids, TCIs, and phototherapy
  - Most cases (skin + internal involvement): **systemic CS** (1 mg/kg BID) **are first-line** treatment (added to existing immunosuppressive regimen)
    - Systemic steroids achieve durable response in only 50% of patients
    - **Mortality rate for steroid-refractory cases = 70%**
- cGVHD
  - Very difficult to treat
  - First line: topical + **systemic CS** added to immunosuppressive regimen
    - Only 50% respond
  - Second line: no option shown to be reliably effective
    - Extracorporeal photopheresis (ECP), PUVA/UVA1/UVB, imatinib, hydroxychloroquine, rituximab, MMF, acitretin

Prognosis/clinical course

- aGVHD: mortality = 30%–50% if moderate-severe disease (70% if steroid refractory)
- cGVHD: most common cause of death is infection
- Maraviroc (CCR5 inhibitor) decreases incidence of visceral GVHD by blocking CCR5-mediated CD8+ T-cell recruitment to liver and gut → may be useful for patients at high risk for GVHD
  - Does not ↓ incidence of skin GVHD
- **Ibrutinib** (inhibitor of Bruton's tyrosine kinase on B lymphocytes) approved for treatment of cGVHD

Lichenoid interface dermatitis

Lichen planus (LP)

Epidemiology

- Cutaneous LP affects ≤ 1% of adults; oral LP affects 4% of adults
- Most common in **middle-aged adults** (peak onset: 40–50 yo); F > M

Pathogenesis

- **Various triggers** (viral, contact allergens, drugs, or idiopathic) → basal keratinocytes express altered self-antigens on cell surface → **CD8+ cytotoxic T cells** target basal keratinocytes → **lower level (basal) keratinocyte apoptosis** and basement membrane permeability → further CD8+ T-cell inflow → further basal keratinocyte apoptosis (loop); ↑IL-1α, IL-6, IL-8, IFN-γ, TNF-α, VEGF, TGF-β1, caspase-3, Bcl-2, Brn2, **CXCL9**, **CXCL10**, **CXCL11**; **genetic loci (HLA-A5, HLA-A3, HLA-B7, HLA-DR1)**
  - Viral
    - **Hepatitis C virus**
      - Implicated in subset of **oral ulcerative/erosive LP**
      - a/w LP in Asia, South America, Europe, Middle East, but failed to detect an association in North America
    - Hepatitis B (vaccine): a/w oral LP, and bullous LP in children (an otherwise uncommon presentation)
  - Contact allergens (**mercury amalgam**, copper, and **gold**)
    - A/w Oral LP
    - **95% improve** w/ removal of sensitizing metal
    - Even w/ negative patch test, 75% clear when metal is removed (may be related to irritant effects)
  - Drugs
    - **HCTZ, β-blockers, ACE inhibitors, antimalarials, gold** salts, TNF-α inhibitors, NSAIDs, penicillamine, and quinidine
  - Psychological: depression, anxiety
  - Environmental: radiotherapy, dimethylfumarate, methacrylic acid esters

Clinical features

- Inflammatory disease of the skin, hair, nails, and mucous membranes
- Pruritic, Purple-violaceous Polygonal, flat-topped Papules
  - Papules may be umbilicated
  - **Wickham's striae** and small gray-white puncta
  - **Koebnerization** very common
- Most common sites: **oral mucosa (#1 site)**, **ventral wrists/forearms**, dorsal hands, shins, genitalia, presacral area, and neck
  - **Oral mucosa involved in 75%** of all cases (only site of involvement in 15%–25% of cases); **only 10% of patients who have oral LP subsequently develop cutaneous LP**
- Although LP is pruritic, rarely see excoriations or impetiginization
- Multiple clinical variants (Table 3.5)

Histopathology

- All clinical variants have similar histology
- Classic features: orthohyperkeratosis, **wedge-shaped hypergranulosis**, irregular acanthosis w/ **"saw-toothed" rete** ridges, vacuolar degeneration of the basal layer, **apoptotic keratinocytes confined to the basal layer** of epidermis with some falling into superficial dermis (**cytoid/civatte/colloid bodies**), and superficial dermal band-like **("lichenoid") lymphocytic infiltrate**
- Lacks eosinophils
  - **Exceptions**: drug-induced LP and hypertrophic LP
- Lacks parakeratosis
  - **Exceptions**: drug-induced LP and oral LP
- Dyskeratotic keratinocytes are NOT present in higher levels of epidermis (spinous and granular layers) → differentiates from EM, FDE, and SJS/TEN (all have suprabasilar keratinocyte apoptosis)
  - **Exceptions**: drug-induced LP
- Deep dermal and peri-eccrine/perifollicular inflammation is not seen → differentiates from discoid lupus erythematosus (DLE) and lichen striatus
  - **Exceptions**: drug-induced LP

Table 3.5 Key Features of Lichen Planus (LP) Variants	
Acute (exanthematous) LP	Rapid onset of disseminated lesions; heals with PIH; rapidly self-resolves (3–9 months)
Actinic LP (LP subtropicus)	Most common in **Middle Eastern and Indian patients** (also Africans); young adults or children; onset in spring or summer on **sun-exposed sites** (face, forehead > dorsal UE, neck, intertriginous sites); comprised of discoid papules/plaques (hyperpigmented focus with hypopigmented rim) or melasma-like patches (less common)
Annular LP	Usually asymptomatic; annular plaques with raised violaceous-white edge with central clearing; resembles GA but is scaly; **axilla** is most common site, followed by **penis**
Atrophic LP	Enlarging small violaceous, annular plaques with centrally depressed/atrophic, hyperpigmented area; clinically resembles early morphea or LS&A; **legs** most common site
Bullous LP	Blisters develop on longstanding LP lesions due to extensive epidermal damage **(expanded Max-Joseph spaces)**
Drug-induced LP (lichenoid drug eruption)	In comparison with idiopathic LP: **patients typically 10 years older** (mid 60s); often spares "classic LP sites;" lesions **more generalized** and more **eczematous or psoriasiform** than classic morphology; **Wickham's striae absent**; **frequently photodistributed** (esp. HCTZ)—various drugs have spectrum of activity in UVB range; **spares mucous membranes**; histology: like LP but frequently has parakeratosis, deeper infiltrate, **eosinophils**, apoptotic keratinocytes in higher levels of epidermis; **average latency period of 12 months** after initial medication exposure; delayed resolution (months) Culprits: ACE inhibitors, antimalarials, β-blockers, gold, lithium, mercury amalgam, allopurinol, anticonvulsants, antiretovirals, NSAIDs, penicillamine, carbamazepine, diltiazem, thiazide diuretics, quinidine, TNF-α inhibitors
Genital LP	Men: **annular LP** on glans penis Women: vulvar LP is most commonly **erosive** and 70% have concomitant vaginal involvement; often a/w oral involvement ("**vulvovaginal-gingival syndrome**:" protracted course with scarring, chronic pain, dyspareunia, and ↑ nail involvement)
Hypertrophic LP (aka LP verrucosus)	Extremely pruritic, thick, scaly plaques; most commonly on **dorsal feet/shins**, wrists; symmetric; lasts longer (avg. duration 6 years); may → **multiple keratoacanthomas** or follicular-based **SCCs**; biopsy may show **many eosinophils**
Inverse LP	**Axilla** > inguinal and inframammary folds > antecubital and popliteal fossae; poorly defined **hyperpigmentation** usually present (thus may overlap with LP pigmentosus)
Linear LP	Refers to lesions that appear spontaneously (not due to koebnorization) in a **Blaschkoid** distribution; favors younger patients (20–30 yo); likely due to somatic mosaicism
Oral LP	Over half of patients with cutaneous LP have oral involvement <u>Reticular LP:</u> **most common**; lacy white raised linear lines; usually asymptomatic; most commonly on **bilateral buccal mucosa** > gingivae > tongue > lips <u>Atrophic, erosive, and bullous oral LP:</u> more painful, F > M; must check for esophageal and genital involvement; may progress to SCC (1%–2%)
Nail LP	Seen in 10% of LP patients; usually affects several nails; classic findings = **longitudinal ridging**, **lateral thinning**, **fissuring**, and **dorsal pterygium**; kids lack these other nail findings but may present as **20-nail dystrophy** (rare in adults)
LP/LE overlap	Acral sites with bullae, ulceration, nail loss, and pain; overlapping features of lupus and LP seen clinically and on H&E/DIF
Palmoplantar LP	Commonly ulcerative (esp. on soles); occurs in 30–40 yo age group; extremely painful and recalcitrant to therapy; usually with typical LP elsewhere
LP pemphigoides	Vesicobullous lesions occur anywhere on skin (most commonly on uninvolved skin) due to **circulating IgG antibodies against BPAG2** (180-kD antigen, type XVII collagen); occurs weeks to months after onset of LP; pathogenesis: LP damages epidermis → exposes hidden antigens that are recognized by T cells
LP pigmentosus	**Skin types 3 and 4**; brown or slate gray macules on **sun-exposed face, neck, and flexures**; lacks preceding erythema and minimally pruritic; evolves into reticulate hyperpigmented patches; classic LP lesions in only 20%; occurs later in life (30–40 yo) than ashy dermatosis (childhood to late 20s); discussed further in Section 3.26
Lichen planopilaris (LPP; follicular LP)	**Perifollicular hyperkeratosis** with narrow violaceous rim on scalp (> other hair-bearing areas) → scarring hair loss; **frontal fibrosing alopecia**: variant in elderly women along the frontal hairline
Graham-Little-Piccardi-Lasseur syndrome	Variant of LPP; classic triad = **non-scarring pubic and axillary hair loss** w/ disseminated spiny **follicular papules** (KP-like), cutaneous or mucosal LP, and scarring **alopecia** on scalp

- Minimal lymphocyte exocytosis (vs. lichen striatus and PLEVA/PLC)
- DIF: **"shaggy" fibrinogen along the basement membrane zone (BMZ)**; colloid bodies stain with IgM (>IgA, IgG, C3)

Laboratory testing

- Patch testing to metals in patients w/ oral LP may be helpful

Treatment

- First, rule out lichenoid drug eruption (biopsy **NOT** a reliable distinguishing test → need careful drug history)
  - Lichenoid drug eruptions may persist for several months after drug discontinuation
- Once drug-induced LP has been ruled out, there are multiple treatment options:
  - **CS (first line)**: topical (medium to high potency; occlusion for nail LP), intralesional (good for hypertrophic LP and nail LP), and systemic (for more severe forms; 30–60 mg/day up to 4–6 weeks)
  - TCIs (both pimecrolimus and tacrolimus): effective for oral LP; topical calcipotriol is another option
  - MTX: useful for generalized LP (>90% response rate)
  - Acitretin (30 mg/day): effective in recalcitrant LP (64% have significant improvement); alitretinoin may be useful in nail LP
  - Metronidazole: generalized LP (79% effective)

- Hydroxychloroquine: mainly used for lichen planopilaris (LPP)/frontal fibrosing alopecia
- Oral cyclosporine (recalcitrant cases)
- Phototherapy (NB-UVB—52% effective in generalized LP; UVA1; PUVA)
- Other options: AZA, sulfasalazine, griseofulvin, thalidomide, biologics, MMF, apremilast

Prognosis/clinical course

- Duration depends on the type of LP variant
- **Most forms of LP resolve in 1–2 years** (60% by 1 year)
- **Oral** (especially ulcerative/erosive), **hypertrophic**, and **nail LP are chronic**
  - Ulcerative oral LP very rarely resolves
  - Conjunctival and esophageal involvement are particularly worrisome
- ↑ **SCC risk** in hypertrophic LP, oral (**ulcerative/erosive** type > erythematous/atrophic > reticular), and vulvovaginal LP

Keratosis lichenoides chronica (KLC)

- Symmetric eruption on the **extremities and trunk** comprises **violaceous keratotic papules** coalescing into plaques w/ **linear to reticular** arrangement
- **Classic clue**: greasy, sebopsoriasis-like centrofacial plaques
- Nails and scalp may be involved
- Typically chronic and progressive; no effective treatment
- **Histologic** and direct immunofluorescence (DIF) findings are identical to LP

Erythema dyschromicum perstans (Ashy dermatosis)

- Asymptomatic, symmetric eruption of upper trunk, neck, and proximal extremities
- Preferentially affects **Latin Americans** (HLA-DL4 may be a risk factor)
- Characterized by slow onset of **slate gray-brown** or gray-blue, oval macules and patches w/ erythematous rim
- Histology: subtle basal vacuolar change (usually only discernable at active inflammatory edge), **numerous dermal melanophages**, +/– band-like dermal lymphocytic infiltrate (sparse)
- DIF identical to LP
- Course: 70% of kids resolve within 2 to 3 years; adults typically more persistent
- Treatment: **clofazimine (ToC)**, dapsone, phototherapy/laser, and LP treatments

Lichenoid keratosis (benign lichenoid keratosis [BLK], LP-like keratosis)

- 85% occur between 35 to 65 years of age; F > M
- Usually due to inflammation of a lentigo, seborrheic keratosis or actinic keratosis
- Solitary, **pink or red-brown**, scaly, 0.5 to 1.5 cm papules; lesions often confused for basal cell carcinoma (BCC)
- Most common sites: **forearm, upper chest** > shins (women), and other sun damaged sites
- Histology: similar to LP, but often has **eosinophils**, **spongiosis**, **parakeratosis**, and less wedge-shaped hypergranulosis than LP; often see intact SK/lentigo/AK on the periphery
- DIF: like LP
- No treatment necessary
- **Caution**: 1% of "BLKs" may demonstrate regressing melanoma *in situ* on deeper sections!

Lichen nitidus

- More common in **children and young adults**
- Multiple/grouped **pinpoint, uniform**, discrete, shiny, flat-topped or umbilicated, flesh-colored papules (Fig. 3.13)
  - Tend to be hypopigmented in dark-skinned patients
  - **Koebnerization** common
- Favored sites: **genitalia**, **lower abdomen**, dorsal hands, flexor wrists, and inner thighs
  - Oral, nail, and palm/sole involvement uncommon
- Histology: classic "**ball and claw**" appearance
  - Well-circumscribed, superficial dermal inflammatory nodule (**lymphocytes, histiocytes, and giant cells [GCs]**) surrounded by two to three hyperplastic epidermal rete ridges that "clasp the dermal infiltrate"
  - Infiltrate is more "mixed" than LP (GCs and CD1a+ Langerhans cells)
  - **Interface changes** (vacuolar-lichenoid)
  - **Atrophic overlying epidermis** w/ loss of granular layer +/– parakeratotic cap
- Majority (60%–70%) resolve spontaneously within 1 year
- Has been a/w Crohn's disease, Down syndrome, congenital megacolon, AD
- Treatment often just symptomatic: topical steroids, TCIs, and phototherapy
- DDx:
  - **Lichen spinulosis**: follicular hyperkeratotic papules w/ **central keratotic spine** on neck, buttocks, abdomen, and upper arms
  - **Disseminate and recurrent infundibulofolliculitis**: pruritic follicular-based eruption of **trunk, neck, and arms**; almost exclusively affects young **Black** adults, often hx of AD; worsened by hot and humid environments; Rx = UVR or oral retinoids

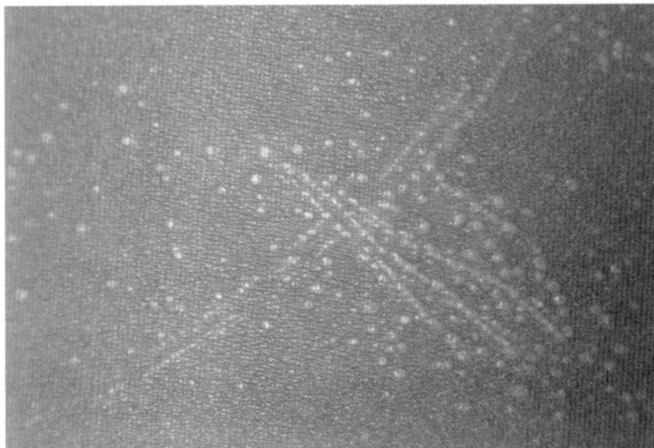

Fig. 3.13 Isomorphic phenomenon in child with lichen nitidus. (From Weston WL, Lane AT, Morelli JG. Papulosquamous disorders. In: *Color Textbook of Pediatric Dermatology*. 4th ed. Philadelphia: Elsevier; 2007:149–180.)

Lichen striatus

- F > M (average age = 4yo)
- 50% of affected children are atopic
- ↑ Incidence in spring and summer
- Typically asymptomatic 2 to 4 mm pink or hypopigmented scaly papules, **linear/Blaschkoid** distribution
  - **Extremities** » face, trunk, buttocks
  - **Nail dystrophy** may occur if a digit is affected
- Treatments: topical steroids and TCIs
- Resolves spontaneously in 3 to 24 months

Lichen sclerosus (LS; lichen sclerosus et atrophicus [LS&A], and balanitis xerotica obliterans [BXO])

Epidemiology

- **F > M**; Caucasians > non-Caucasians
- Any age, but has **bimodal** peaks:
  - Major peak = 40–50 yo **postmenopausal females**
  - Second peak = prepubertal girls (8–13 yo)
- A/w Autoimmune diseases (especially in women)
  - Most common: **autoimmune thyroid** disease (15%)
  - Others: pernicious anemia, **localized scleroderma/ morphea** (6%), psoriasis, AD (in boys), vitiligo
- Most commonly affects male and female **anogenital region (85%)**
- Extragenital LS&A accounts for only 15%
- Male penile involvement = BXO
  - Common cause of **phimosis**

Pathogenesis

- Unclear, but thought to be genetic predisposition and associated with **HLA-DQ7**, HLA-DR11, HLA-DR12
- 80% of patients have circulating **IgG autoantibodies against extracellular matrix protein 1 (ECM-1)**
  - ECM-1 = glycoprotein involved in regulation of BMZ integrity, collagen fibril assembly, and other functions; of note, ECM-1 is mutated in lipoid proteinosis
- Hormonal factors: predominance in postmenopausal women, resolution in pregnancy, and ↑ OCP use in patients
- **Men circumcised early in life rarely develop BXO**

Clinical features

- Classic lesions: **sclerotic**, **ivory-white**, atrophic, and flat-topped papules coalescing into plaques
  - **Follicular plugging** more prominent in extragenital LS&A
- **Genital LS&A is usually symptomatic** (itching, pain, and burning), whereas extragenital LS&A is typically asymptomatic
- Unlike LP, LS&A very rarely affects oral cavity or vagina
- <u>Genital LS&A (85% of cases)</u>:
  - Most commonly affects vulvar and perianal area with classic "**figure-of-8**" pattern in women (rarely see perianal involvement in men)
  - Pruritus and/or soreness is typical (often severe) → dysuria, **constipation (especially in kids**; related to pain with defecation), dyspareunia, and discharge
  - Disease evolution: starts as well-demarcated, thin erythematous plaques that may have focal superficial erosions → **epidermal atrophy**, **dermal scarring**, **hypopigmentation**, dermal hemorrhage/bruising, and fissures → **fusion of labia minora to majora**, **obliteration of clitoral hood**, and narrowing of vaginal introitus
  - Males: **glans penis** (most commonly), but also prepuce and coronal sulcus with atrophic ivory plaques, scars, and erosions → can develop **phimosis** if uncircumcised
  - **Purpuric/ecchymotic** areas in anogenital LS&A are often misdiagnosed as sexual abuse
  - ↑ **risk of SCC** in patients w/ genital LS&A (5% risk)
  - Koebnerization possible
- <u>Extragenital LS&A (15% of cases)</u>:
  - Usually asymptomatic
  - Most common sites: **upper trunk/neck**, proximal upper extremities, and flexor wrists
  - Disease evolution: begins as polygonal blue-white shiny papules → coalesce into sclerotic plaques with **ivory white** color → **follicular plugging**, telangiectasias, and bruising

Histopathology (Fig. 3.14)

- Compact orthohyperkeratosis, follicular plugging, epidermal atrophy with mild vacuolar interface changes, and **papillary dermal edema or homogenization** w/ underlying **lichenoid lymphocytic infiltrate**
  - Mnemonic: **"Red, white, and blue sign"** = orthohyperkeratotic SC (**pink-red**), hyalinized/ edematous papillary dermis (**pale/white**), and band-like lymphocytic infiltrate (**blue band**)

Treatment

- First line: **ultra-potent topical steroids** (e.g., clobetasol) in adults and children
  - Safe even if used long-term
- Second line: TCIs (e.g., tacrolimus)

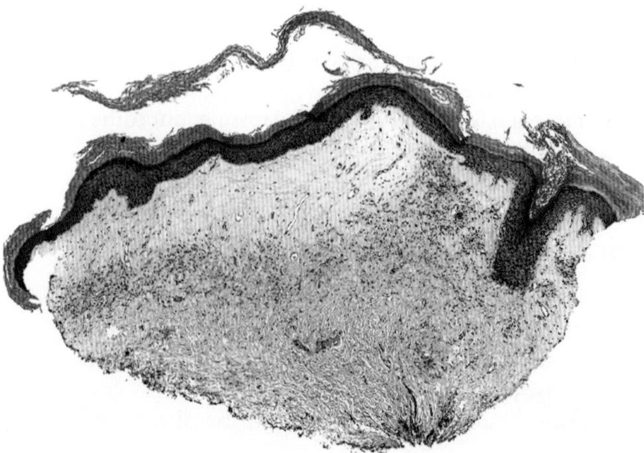

Fig. 3.14 Lichen sclerosis. (Courtesy of Olayemi Sokumbi, MD.)

- Consider circumcision in males not responding to topicals (**ToC in males w/ phimosis**)
- Refractory cases: acitretin, CO_2 laser, PUVA/UVA1, systemic immunosuppressants

Prognosis/clinical course

- May resolve spontaneously in childhood (especially in puberty for girls), but relapsing course in adults
- **Up to 50% of all vulvar SCCs occur in setting of LS&A!!!**
- Estimated 5% risk of genital LS&A progressing to SCC
  - Vulvar SCC in setting of LS&A has recently been shown to be distinct from human papillomavirus-induced vulvar SCC
    - Much higher risk of developing invasive disease (33% vs. 5.7%)
    - SCC due to LS&A may be difficult to diagnose histologically because it is well-differentiated → mistaken for reactive epidermal hyperplasia
- Up to 55% of penile SCC is a/w LS&A

3.4 BLISTERING DISEASES

Pemphigus disease family

- In normal tissue, epithelial cells are held together by two major types of junctions:
  - **Adherens junctions**: classic cadherins (calcium-dependent adherins; E-, P-, and N-cadherins) are transmembrane proteins that bind to the armadillo family intracytoplasmic plaque proteins (β-catenin, plakoglobin) → bind to intracytoplasmic α-catenin → anchor bundles of actin microfilaments → mediate **quick but weak cellular adhesion**
  - **Desmosomes**: desmosomal cadherins (calcium-dependent adherins; **desmogleins** and **desmocollins**) are transmembrane proteins that bind to the armadillo family intracytoplasmic plaque proteins (plakophilin and plakoglobin) → bind to intracytoplasmic **plakins** (desmoplakin 1 and 2, BPAG1, plectin, envoplakin, and periplakin) → anchors keratin intermediate filaments → mediate **slow but strong cellular adhesion** (Box 3.2)
- In various forms of pemphigus, autoantibodies (IgG or IgA) interfere w/ various proteins in **desmosomal** complex → loss of connection between adjacent epithelial cells → acantholysis at various mucocutaneous sites/levels
  - Desmoglein 1: expressed in **all levels** of the epidermis (**top > bottom**)
    - **Dsg1 can compensate for Dsg3 loss in skin** → therefore, if only Dsg3 is targeted by autoantibodies (as in pemphigus vulgaris [PV]), the skin remains intact
    - Dsg1 has no significant role in mucosal epithelial adhesion→ CANNOT compensate for Dsg3 loss in mucosa → if Dsg3 function is lost (as in PV), mucosal blisters ensue (Box 3.3)
  - Desmoglein 3: expressed mostly in **lower portion** of epidermis and **throughout mucosal epithelium**
    - Dsg3 CANNOT compensate for Dsg1 loss in superficial epidermis → if Dsg1 is targeted (as in pemphigus foliaceus [PF] and mucocutaneous PV), the skin develops blisters
    - Dsg3 is the major desmoglein involved in **mucosal** epithelial adhesion
  - Desmoglein 4: important role in **hair follicles**
    - Dsg4 is mutated in autosomal recessive localized hypotrichosis and also **autosomal recessive monilethrix**

Box 3.2 Boards Factoid

Plakoglobin is an armadillo protein that is present in **both desmosomes and adherens junctions**; it can substitute for β-catenin in the latter

Box 3.3 Boards Factoids

Dsg1 is cleaved by *Staphylococcus aureus* exfoliatoxins (bullous impetigo, SSSS)

Dsg1 mutation (autosomal dominant) is present in striate PPK 1 (of note, desmoplakin is mutated in striate PPK 2, and keratin 1 in striate PPK 3; all are part of the desmosome complex)

Pemphigus vulgaris (PV)

Epidemiology

- **Most common form of pemphigus** in most parts of the world (PV:PF ~3:1)
- M = F; 50 to 60 yo
- **Jewish** ancestry a/w 10× ↑ incidence
- May be a/w other autoimmune diseases: **myasthenia gravis, thymoma, and autoimmune thyroiditis**

Pathogenesis

- Autoantibodies to **Dsg3** (mucosal-dominant pemphigus) or both **Dsg1 and Dsg3** (mucocutaneous pemphigus)
- In **neonates of mothers w/ PV**, maternal IgG autoantibodies against Dsg3 cross placenta → transient blistering in infant
  - Does not occur in mothers with PF, because neonatal skin has same Dsg expression pattern as **adult mucosa** (i.e., Dsg1 loss can be compensated for by Dsg3 expression)

Clinical features

- All patients have painful **mucosal erosions** (most common sites = **buccal** and **palatine** mucosa of the oropharynx) w/ irregular borders and different shapes and sizes
  - Other sites: esophagus (sloughing/cast formation), conjunctiva, nasal mucosa, vagina, penis, and anus
- **Skin involvement (50%)**: flaccid vesicles/bullae (Fig. 3.15), positive **Nikolsky** and **Asboe-Hansen** signs → bullae easily rupture, erode, and form crust
  - Heals without scarring
  - Widespread denudation may result in death from fluid imbalance or secondary infection
- **Pemphigus vegetans**: vegetative variant of PV affecting **intertriginous areas** (> scalp and face)
  - Reactive phenomenon to friction

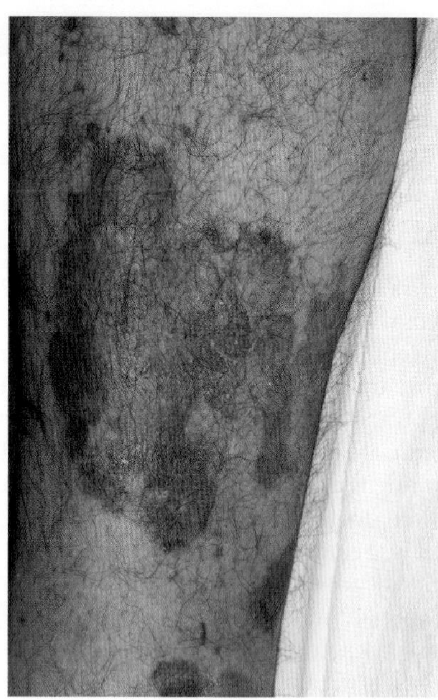

Fig. 3.15 Flaccid blisters and erosion as a result of a ruptured bulla in a patient with pemphigus foliaceus. (Courtesy of Julia S. Lehman, MD.)

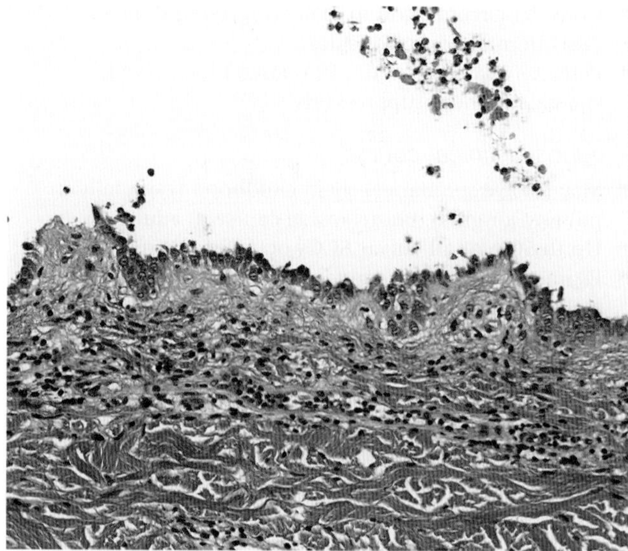

Fig. 3.16 Histopathology of pemphigus vulgaris. Blisters in the skin show suprabasilar acantholysis. Attachment of the basal cells to the basement membrane via hemidesmosomes leads to the "tombstone" appearance. (Courtesy of Julia S. Lehman, MD.)

Box 3.4 Best Indirect Immunofluorescence Substrates for Pemphigus Variants

Pemphigus foliaceus: Guinea pig esophagus
Pemphigus vulgaris: Monkey esophagus
Paraneoplastic pemphigus: Rat bladder

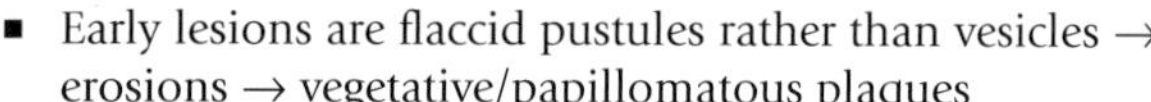

  - Early lesions are flaccid pustules rather than vesicles → erosions → vegetative/papillomatous plaques
  - Histology: pseudoepitheliomatous hyperplasia, **intraepidermal eosinophilic abscesses**, and suprabasilar acantholysis (often subtle)

Histopathology

- **Eosinophilic spongiosis** (earliest finding) → later, see classic findings of **suprabasilar acantholysis** without keratinocyte necrosis, "**tombstoning**" (vertically oriented basilar keratinocytes attached to BMZ, but not surrounding keratinocytes), and individual **rounded-up (acantholytic) keratinocytes** within blister cavity (Fig. 3.16); **hair follicles extensively involved**
  - Versus Hailey-Hailey (the main histologic DDx): pemphigus has prominent **acantholysis of hair follicles**, ↑ eosinophils, lacks "dilapidated brick wall" appearance (i.e., lacks diffuse acantholysis in upper layers of epidermis), and **lacks epidermal hyperplasia**
  - Versus herpetic infection: pemphigus lacks viral cytopathic changes (multinucleation, margination of chromatin, nuclear molding) but can have concomitant herpetic superinfection

Laboratory testing

- **DIF**: most reliable test (~100%); perilesional biopsy; assesses patient's **skin** for *in vivo* bound IgG; characteristic intercellular "**chicken wire**" staining with IgG +/- C3; lower epidermis most strongly involved
- **Indirect immunofluorescence (IIF)**: assesses patient's **serum** for circulating IgG autoantibodies (80%–90%); **monkey esophagus** is best substrate (Box 3.4); **levels correlate w/ disease activity** → useful for monitoring
- Immunoprecipitation and immunoblotting: detect target antigens of specific molecular weights via protein electrophoresis; distinguish between pemphigus types more accurately than DIF or IIF but is not readily available commercially
- Enzyme-linked immunosorbent assay (ELISA): assesses patient's **serum** for circulating IgG autoantibodies (both Dsg1 and Dsg3); **levels correlate w/ disease activity** → useful for monitoring; can **distinguish between pemphigus types** though clinical correlation is required

Treatment

- First line (moderate to severe pemphigus): **rituximab** or oral steroids (**1 mg/kg/day**) + steroid-sparing immunosuppressive (AZA or MMF)
  - Tetracyclines + nicotinamide may be sufficient for very mild cases
- Potent topical steroids can be effective
- Plasmapheresis and/or IVIG may be useful for rapid control of severe disease
- Monitor treatment response clinically +/- **IIF or ELISA levels**

Pemphigus foliaceus (PF)

- Second most common form of pemphigus*; milder
  - *Exceptions: **Brazil** (17:1 PF:PV), Tunisia (4:1), Finland (2:1)
- Important clinical variants:
  - **Fogo selvagem**: endemic variant of PF with identical clinical and histologic features; highest incidence in

rural Brazilian towns within 10 miles of rivers rich in **black flies** (*Simulium* spp); affects **children and young adults** (vs. middle-aged to elderly in typical PF)
  - **Pemphigus erythematosus** (Senear-Usher syndrome): lupus/PF overlap; localized to **malar** region of face and other seborrheic areas; DIF shows intercellular pemphigus pattern + **granular to linear IgG and C3 along BMZ** (lupus pattern)
    - Positive antinuclear antibody (ANA) test in 30%
    - Rx: sun protection, steroids +/− dapsone
- Pathogenesis: autoantibodies to **Dsg1** (IgG4 subclass)
- Clinical presentation:
  - Subacute onset of well-demarcated, transient, **impetigo-like crusted erosions** on an erythematous base
  - Favors **seborrheic distribution** (face, scalp, central upper trunk) (Fig. 3.17)
  - Blisters are so superficial and fragile that usually only eroded/crusted lesions or plaques with "cornflake" scale are seen
  - (+) Nikolsky sign
  - **Lacks mucosal involvement**
  - Not severely ill; **low mortality**
- Histopathology: eosinophilic spongiosis (early) → **subcorneal acantholysis (granular layer** » midlevel epidermis) w/ acantholytic single cells in the roof or floor of blister cavity; +/− neutrophils and eosinophils in blister cavity
  - PF, pemphigus erythematosus, staphylococcal scalded skin syndrome (SSSS), and bullous impetigo all show nearly identical findings on H&E staining
- **DIF**: same as PV, but upper epidermis most intensely involved
  - Unique exception: pemphigus erythematosus shows intercellular pemphigus pattern + **granular to linear IgG and C3 along BMZ** (lupus pattern)
- **IIF**: same appearance as PV; **guinea pig esophagus** is best substrate (see Box 3.4)
- Must differentiate from drug-induced PF and other pemphigus variants (Table 3.6)

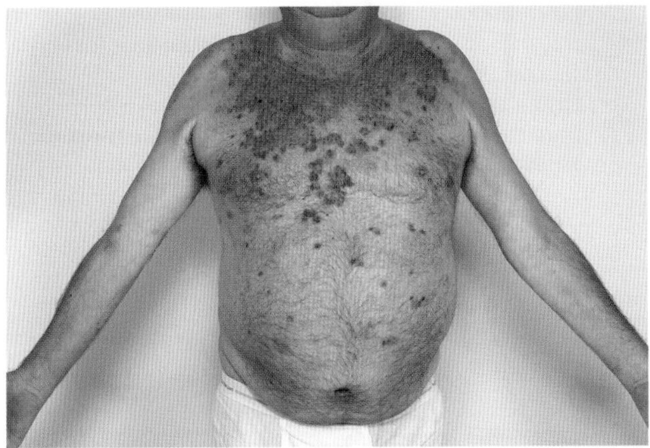

Fig. 3.17 Pemphigus foliaceus. Scaly, crusted erosions widely distributed in a seborrheic distribution on the chest. (Courtesy of Julia S. Lehman, MD.)

Table 3.6 Pemphigus Variants

Pemphigus herpetiformis	Variant of PF (>PV) that clinically **resembles DH**; p/w pruritic urticarial plaques and small, DH-like vesicles in herpetiform arrangement; histopathology: **minimal to no acantholysis**; eosinophilic spongiosis and subcorneal pustules; DIF: same as PF; antigen: **Dsg1** > Dsg3; chronic, but not severe; may evolve into classic PF (>PV)
IgA pemphigus	May affect patients of any age; p/w pruritic flaccid vesicles/**pustules in annular/circinate pattern** with central crusting; most common on **axillae**, **groin**; no mucosal involvement; no significant morbidity; DIF+ in 100% (by definition); IIF+ with IgA conjugate in 50%; **may be a/w IgA gammopathy** (and possibly multiple myeloma and inflammatory bowel disease); **ToC = Dapsone** (#1; resolution within 48 hours), sulfapyridine, steroids **Subcorneal pustular dermatosis type:** clinically and histologically indistinguishable from Sneddon-Wilkinson → need DIF/IIF; DIF shows intercellular IgA staining in upper epidermis; target antigen = **Desmocollin 1**; histopathology: subcorneal neutrophilic pustule; acantholysis not usually present **Intraepidermal neutrophilic type**: characteristic **"sunflower-like"** arrangement of vesicopustules; DIF: IgA intercellular staining throughout entire epidermis; target antigen = **Dsg1/Dsg3;** histopathology: suprabasilar neutrophilic pustule in lower-mid epidermis +/− mild acantholysis
Drug-induced pemphigus	Typically has **PF-like presentation** (4:1, PF:PV); most commonly induced by thiol (sulfhydryl)-containing drugs (>non-thiols) **Thiols** (may cause acantholysis directly): **penicillamine** (50%), **ACE inhibitors** (captopril > enalapril, lisinopril), ARBs **Non-thiol** (acantholysis via immune mechanisms, more likely to cause PV-like presentation): β-lactams, gold, CCBs, β-blockers, piroxicam, rifampin

- Rx: systemic steroids +/− dapsone (widespread disease); superpotent topical steroids (localized disease)
- Like PV, may be a/w other autoimmune diseases

Paraneoplastic pemphigus (PNP)/ paraneoplastic autoimmune multiorgan syndrome (PAMS)

- **Multisystemic**, erosive, **paraneoplastic syndrome** a/w various underlying neoplasms (one third undiagnosed at time of PNP onset):
  - **Non-Hodgkin lymphoma** (40%) > **chronic lymphocytic leukemia (CLL**; 20%) > **Castleman** disease (15% overall, **#1 cause in children**) > **thymoma** (6%; myasthenia gravis is frequently associated) > Waldenström macroglobulinemia (1%)
  - Solid organ tumors in 15% (9% with epithelial origin [e.g., breast, colon] and 6% with sarcomas)
- Autoantibodies against nearly all components of desmosome:
  - **Entire plakin family**: desmoplakin 1 and 3, BPAG1, plectin, periplakin, envoplakin, and A2ML1
  - Desmogleins: **Dsg1** and **Dsg3**
- Mucosal involvement is severe:

- **Severe stomatitis** w/ extension onto vermillion is the **earliest, most common,** and **most persistent** sign
- Severe scarring conjunctivitis (ophthalmologic evaluation is essential); esophageal, genital, and nasopharyngeal lesions also common
- Skin findings are polymorphous:
  - Most commonly pemphigus-like or **lichenoid** (most common chronic presentation)
    - Other presentations: pemphigoid-like, EM-like
  - **Palms/soles/nails** frequently affected (unlike PV)
- Histopathology: polymorphous, just like the clinical presentation (**overlap between PV, LP, and EM findings**):
  - Suprabasilar acantholysis, vacuolar or lichenoid interface dermatitis w/ necrotic keratinocytes (not seen in PV), and far fewer eosinophils than PV
- DIF: IgG and C3 deposited in **intercellular** spaces and **linearly along BMZ**; lichenoid tissue reaction (cytoids with IgG, IgM, IgA, C3, and shaggy BMZ deposition with fibrinogen) is seen frequently
- IIF shows cell surface deposition of IgG on transitional cells of **rat bladder (best substrate)**
- Immunoprecipitation/immunoblotting detecting anti-periplakin IgG and anti-envoplakin IgG = most sensitive/specific for diagnosis
- Treatment:
  - **Excision of benign neoplasms** (thymomas and localized Castleman) → resolution within 6 to 18 months
  - PNP a/w **malignant processes** is highly recalcitrant
    - Attempt to treat underlying malignancy
    - Poor prognosis (**90% mortality rate**)
    - Most common causes of death = **infection (#1)**, underlying **malignancy and bronchiolitis obliterans** (detect w/ pulmonary function tests [PFTs] » high-resolution computed tomography [CT])
  - Medical treatment: high-dose steroids + steroid-sparing immunosuppressants (MMF, AZA, cyclosporine) often required, though minimizing immunosuppression important; treatment may be tailored to patient's malignant comorbidity (e.g., rituximab, MTX, alemtuzumab); IVIG is another option and can help with bronchiolitis obliterans

Autoimmune subepidermal blistering diseases

- Subepidermal bullae result from autoantibodies directed against components of the BMZ
- Sites of damage: (1) basal keratinocyte (and its hemidesmosomal plaques); (2) lamina lucida; (3) lamina densa; and (4) sublamina densa
- Know the location and interactions of various components of BMZ (Fig. 3.18) and (Table 3.7)

Bullous pemphigoid (BP; pemphigoid)

Epidemiology

- **Most common** autoimmune blistering disorder
- Usually **chronic**; may be a/w significant morbidity and elevated mortality compared with age-matched patients without BP

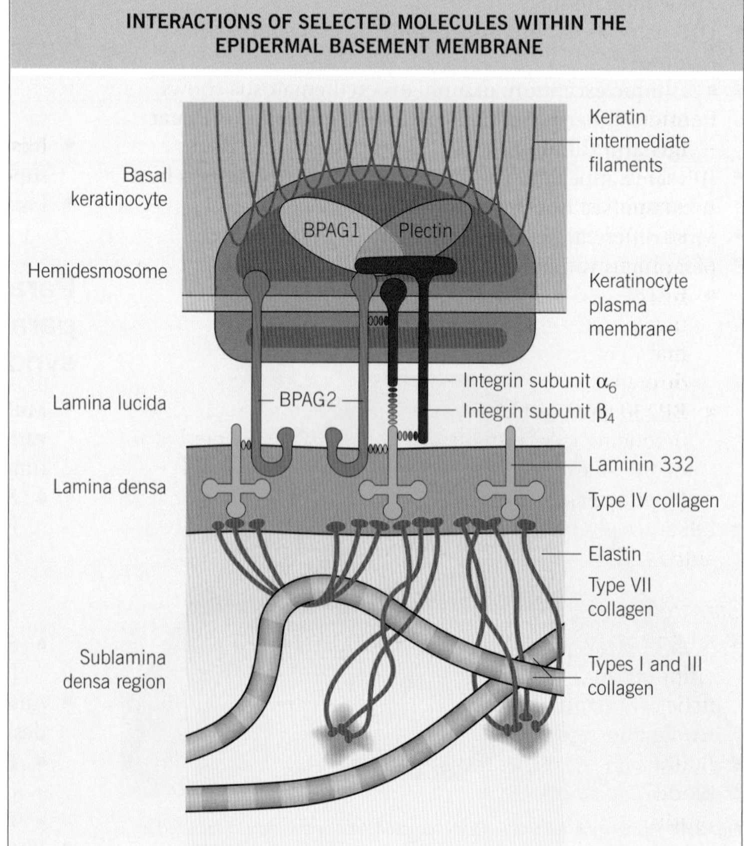

Fig. 3.18 Interactions of selected molecules within the epidermal basement membrane. These interactions promote epidermal adhesion and also play a key role in a number of dermatologic diseases. Important molecular interactions include those between: (1) plakin family members, BPAG1 and plectin, with keratin intermediate filaments; (2) the former with BPAG2 and integrin $\alpha6\beta4$ (specifically, the large cytoplasmic domain of integrin subunit $\beta4$); (3) the cytoplasmic domains of BPAG2 and integrin subunit $\beta4$; (4) the extracellular domains of BPAG2 and integrin subunit $\alpha6$ as well as laminin 332 (formerly laminin 5); (5) integrin $\alpha6\beta4$ in hemidesmosomes and laminin 332 in the lamina densa; (6) laminin 332 and type VII collagen and; (7) type VII collagen with type IV collagen, fibronectin, and type I collagen in the sublamina densa region. (From Yancey KB. The biology of the basement membrane. In: Bolognia JL, Schaffer JV, Cerroni L. *Dermatology*. 4th ed. Philadelphia: Elsevier; 2018:483–493.)

Table 3.7 Subepidermal Blistering Disease Characteristics

Disease	Antigen	Size (kDa)	DIF	Salt-Split Skin IIF
Bullous pemphigoid	BPAG1 (plakin)	230	**Linear C3 and IgG** along BMZ in **"n-serrated"** pattern	Epidermal
	BPAG2 (collagen XVII)	**180**		
Pemphigoid gestationis	BPAG2 (collagen XVII)	180	**Linear C3 > >> IgG** along BMZ	Epidermal
Linear IgA bullous dermatosis (LABD)	**LAD-1 (120 kD** cleaved portion of BPAG2) **LABD97 (97 kD** cleaved portion of LAD-1)	120 → **97**	Linear IgA +/– C3 along BMZ	Epidermal (IgA)
Mucous membrane pemphigoid (classic form)	BPAG2 **(C-terminus)**	180	Linear IgG and C3 along BMZ	Epidermal, mixed (epidermal and dermal, but stronger staining on epidermal side)
Ocular-predominant MMP	**β_4 integrin**	NA	Linear IgG and C3 along BMZ	Epidermal, mixed (epidermal and dermal but stronger staining on epidermal side)
Anti-epiligrin MMP	**Laminin 332**	400-440	Linear IgG and C3 along BMZ	Dermal
p200 pemphigoid	Laminin γ1	200	Linear IgG and C3 along BMZ	Dermal
p105 pemphigoid	NA	105	Linear IgG and C3 along BMZ	Dermal
Epidermolysis bullosa acquisita	**Type VII collagen** (anchoring fibrils)	290	**Linear IgG > C3** along BMZ in **"u-serrated"** pattern	Dermal
Bullous systemic lupus erythematosus	**Type VII collagen** (anchoring fibrils)	290	**Granular to linear** staining w/ **multiple reactants** (IgG, IgA, IgM, C3)	Dermal
Porphyria cutanea tarda	NA	NA	**Linear IgG (>IgM), C3 and fibrinogen** along BMZ and **around superficial vessels**	Negative

BMZ, *Basement membrane zone; DIF, direct immunofluorescence; IIF, indirect immunofluorescence.*

- **Elderly** (>**60 yo**, mean 75–81 yo) most commonly affected
  - Drug-induced BP may affect younger age groups
- Slight male predominance
- a/w HLA-DQB*0301 (Caucasians)

Pathogenesis

- IgG (IgG1 and IgG4) autoantibodies bind **hemidesmosomal proteins** → complement activation → eosinophil and neutrophil recruitment to tissues → release of matrix metalloproteinases, proteases, and neutrophil elastase → degradation of ECM proteins → subepidermal blister
- Most important target antigens:
  - **BP180** (BPAG2, type XVII collagen): 180-kD transmembrane protein; **primary mediator** of BP; main pathogenic target = non-collagenous **NC16A domain**
  - **BP230** (BPAG1): 230-kD cytoplasmic plaque protein belonging to **plakin** family; **not the primary mediator of BP** → antibodies arise as secondary phenomenon ("epitope spreading")
- IgE a/w early urticarial phase of BP and IgE autoantibodies to type XVII collagen have been detected

Clinical features

- Non-bullous phase (early): persistent, polymorphous eruption; may p/w isolated intense pruritus or **fixed urticarial papules/plaques** (often annular); usually affects **trunk**, **abdomen**, and **flexural extremities**
- Bullous phase: **tense**, fluid-filled vesicles/bullae (clear > blood-tinged) arising on **urticarial background**; intense pruritus; **trunk**, **abdomen**, and **flexural extremities** most common; bullae rupture to leave erosions and crusted areas; **oral involvement (10%–30%)** may occur, but much less common than PV; other mucosal sites less commonly affected; **peripheral eosinophilia (50%)**
- Pemphigoid variants: Table 3.8

Histopathology

- Urticarial phase: **eosinophilic spongiosis** w/ eosinophils lining up at dermoepidermal junction (DEJ) and scattered in superficial dermis, vacuoles at DEJ (represents early blister formation)
- Bullous phase (Fig. 3.19) **subepidermal split** w/ numerous **eosinophils in blister cavity**, dense dermal lymphoeosinophilic inflammation
  - May see **flame figures** at any phase

Laboratory testing

- **DIF (most sensitive)**: **skin test** for ***in vivo*** bound antibodies; substrate = biopsy from erythema next to, but not involving, blister **(perilesional)**
  - **Linear C3 (n-serrated pattern)** (~100%) and **IgG** (>90%) located along DEJ
- **Salt-split skin DIF**: modified DIF study that allows for **localization** of *in vivo* bound antibodies
  - Technique: first use 1 M NaCl to split the biopsied skin specimen at lamina lucida → examine w/ DIF for *in vivo* bound antibodies → determine to which side of blister (roof vs. floor) the antibodies are bound
  - Enables differentiation of **BP ("roof staining")** from "floor staining" blistering diseases (mainly epidermolysis bullosa acquisita [EBA])
  - Examination of **serration pattern (n-serrated vs. u-serrated)** on standard DIF can be used in lieu of this technique (Box 3.5)

Table 3.8 Pemphigoid Variants	
Pemphigoid vegetans	Vegetative plaques in **intertriginous** areas
Infantile/childhood pemphigoid	Frequently p/w **acral bullae** → generalizes; ↑ **facial/genital** involvement; clinically indistinguishable from childhood LABD/CBDC → need DIF/IIF
Pemphigoid nodularis	Clinically resembles prurigo nodularis; typically lacks bullae
Lichen planus (LP) pemphigoides	**LP/BP overlap** syndrome w/circulating antibodies against BP180; p/w LP-like papules/plaques and tense bullae arising on skin unaffected by LP
Pemphigoid gestationis (gestational pemphigoid, herpes gestationis)	Abrupt onset; **any trimester (second and third most common)**, immediately **postpartum**, or a/w trophoblastic tumors (**choriocarcinoma**, hydatidiform mole); starts as urticarial/vesicular plaques on trunk, abdomen, **umbilicus** → rapidly generalizes; **75% flare at time of delivery**; **anti-HLA antibodies (~100%)**; strongly a/w **HLA-DR3 (70%)**, **DR4 (50%)**, or both (45%); DIF: **linear C3 (100%) > linear IgG (30%)**; IIF: only positive in 30%; **ELISA for BP180-NC16A** is best serum test; ↑ risk of **premature delivery** and small-for-gestational-age neonates; **neonates may develop transient blistering** (10%); **recurs** in subsequent pregnancies; a/w **Graves' disease** and anti-thyroid antibodies; Rx: systemic steroids
Localized pemphigoid	Pretibial, peristomal, vulvar, umbilical, distal portion of amputated limb ("stump pemphigoid"), radiotherapy sites, paralyzed limbs
Drug-induced pemphigoid	**Furosemide (#1)**, **checkpoint inhibitors, dipeptidyl peptidase 4 (DPP-4) inhibitors, ACE inhibitors**, **cephalosporins**, **β-lactams**, **D-penicillamine**, sulfasalazine, NSAIDs, neuroleptics, gold, SSKI, bumetanide, phototherapy Mnemonic: "**F**at **A**bdomens **C**overed **B**y **P**emphigoid = **F**urosemide, **A**CE-inhibitors, **C**ephalosporins, **β**-lactams, **P**enicillamine"
Anti-p200 pemphigoid	Most often p/w classic BP eruption (>DH, eczematous presentations); head and mucous membranes more frequently involved; often **a/w psoriasis**; target antigen: **laminin γ1**; salt-split skin: IgG binding to **dermal** side
Anti-p105 pemphigoid	Extensive blistering and denudation on both mucous membranes and skin, resembling **SJS/TEN** ("p105 = TEN"); target antigen: 105-kDa protein; salt-split skin: IgG binding to **dermal** side

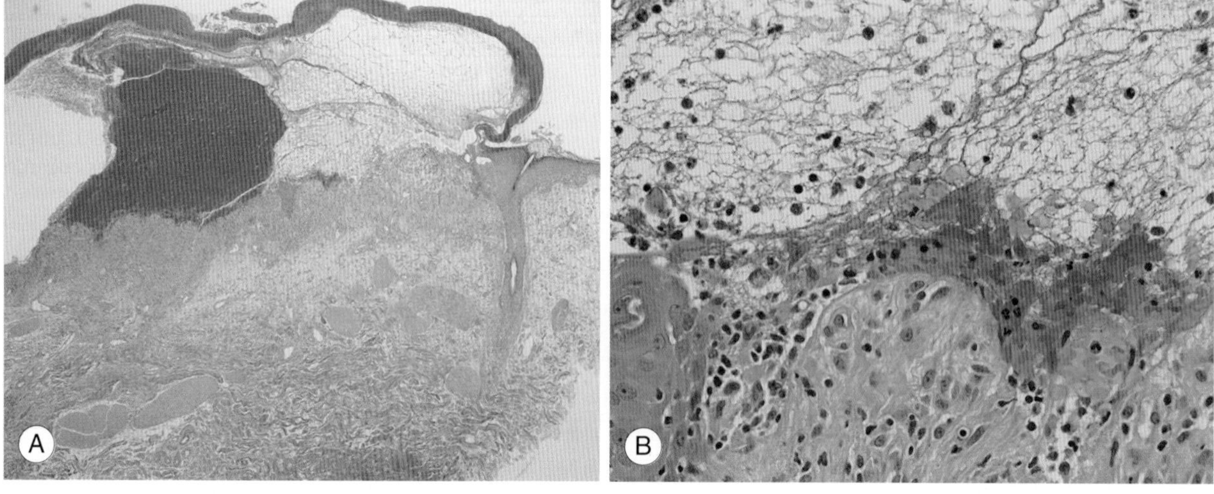

Fig. 3.19 Bullous pemphigoid—histopathologic features. (A) Subepidermal blister which contains fibrin, eosinophils, and mononuclear cells. (B) Higher power of (A) highlighting numerous eosinophils in the blister space. (Courtesy of Julia S. Lehman, MD.)

Box 3.5 Serration Patterns in Subepidermal Blistering Diseases

n-serrated linear DIF pattern: bullous pemphigoid (including anti-p200), linear IgA

u-serrated linear DIF pattern: epidermolysis bullosa acquisita

- IIF (60%–80% sensitive): **serum test** for circulating anti-BMZ IgG; substrate = salt-split normal human skin (not patient's skin); allows for **localization** of antigens targeted by circulating autoantibodies
  - Serum from BP patients → **epidermal (roof) staining** (vs. EBA = dermal/floor staining)
  - IIF levels do **NOT** correlate well w/ BP disease activity (unlike IIF for PV)
- ELISA (80%–90% sensitive): **serum test** for detecting circulating antibodies to BP180 and BP230
  - ELISA levels (both IgG and IgE) correlate w/ BP disease activity → useful for monitoring response to treatment along with clinical parameters

Treatment

- First line (moderate to severe pemphigoid): **systemic steroids + steroid-sparing immunosuppressives** (MMF, MTX, AZA) or application of superpotent topical steroids (high risk of skin atrophy)
- Other treatment options:
  - Tetracycline class + nicotinamide (mild disease)
  - Dapsone (mucosal-predominant BP)
  - IVIG, plasma exchange, rituximab, and omalizumab can be considered in recalcitrant cases

Prognosis/clinical course

- Tends to be chronic, w/ significant morbidity and variably reported mortality (10%–40% in first year)

- ↑ **ELISA** levels and/or **positive DIF** at time of therapy cessation → **high chance of relapse**

Mucous membrane pemphigoid (MMP; cicatricial pemphigoid)

Epidemiology

- Rare, chronic disease of **elderly** (60–80 yo)
- F > M

Pathogenesis

- Autoreactive IgG antibodies directed against various antigens in **anchoring filament zone** (vs. hemidesmosomal plaque in conventional BP)
- Three well-defined subgroups:
  - Anti-epiligrin MMP: target = **laminin 332 (laminin 5, epiligrin)**; salt-split skin shows **dermal deposition of IgG**; strongly a/w underlying **solid organ malignancy** (#1 = adenocarcinoma of the upper aerodigestive tract)
  - Ocular MMP: target = β_4 **subunit** of $\alpha_6\beta_4$ integrin (**boards clue: "β" sideways looks like eyeglasses**); nearly exclusive ocular involvement
  - Anti-BP antigen MMP: target = BP180 (**C-terminus**); skin and mucosal involvement

Clinical features

- Chronic disease characterized by predominant involvement of **mucosae (> skin)** w/ **scarring**; all mucosal sites susceptible, but **oral** (85%) and **conjunctival mucosa** are most common (Fig. 3.20)
  - **Oral (#1 site)**: gingiva, buccal mucosa, and palate (> tongue, lips); p/w erythema and erosions of gingiva **(desquamative gingivitis)**, painful chronic erosions (especially palate), and rarely blisters
  - **Conjunctiva (#2 site)**: bilateral > unilateral; begins as non-specific conjunctivitis → subepithelial conjunctival fibrosis → **symblepharon** (adhesion of bulbar and palpebral conjunctivae), **trichiasis** (inward facing eyelashes), entropion, **ectropion**, and xerosis → trauma induces corneal neovascularization, ulceration, and **blindness**
  - **Other mucosal**: nasopharyngeal/upper aerodigestive tract (epistaxis and airway obstruction); laryngeal (hoarseness, life-threatening stenosis); esophageal (dysphagia and strictures); anogenital (strictures and obliteration of orifices)
  - **Skin involvement** (25%): fewer lesions, different distribution and morphology than conventional BP
    - Most common sites: **scalp/face/neck** and upper trunk
    - Erythematous plaques and recurrent blisters/ erosions → heal w/ **atrophic scars** (not seen in BP)
- **Brunsting-Perry variant**: lesions limited to **head/neck** → **scarring alopecia**; no mucosal involvement

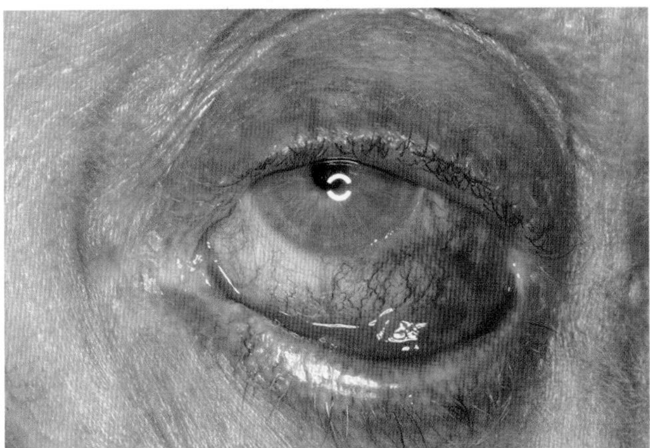

Fig. 3.20 Scarring ocular disease in a patient with cicatricial pemphigoid. (Courtesy of Julia S. Lehman, MD.)

Histopathology

- Similar to BP except has fewer eosinophils (mostly lymphocytes and plasma cells) and ↑ dermal fibrosis/ scarring

Laboratory testing

- DIF: **most reliable** test (80%–95% sensitive) → linear IgG, IgA, and/or C3 along BMZ; may require multiple biopsies for DIF to increase test sensitivity
- IIF: only a minority (20%–30%) have detectable circulating antibodies (low titers)
- Salt-split skin: mixed epidermal/dermal or epidermal deposition with IgG for most patients with MMP **(anti-epiligrin [anti-laminin 332] MMP = dermal/floor staining)**

Treatment

- Mild-moderate oropharyngeal and cutaneous disease: **dapsone** (first line; may also help in mild ocular disease) + potent topical/IL steroids; other options include:
  - Tetracyclines + nicotinamide
  - Short courses of oral steroids
- Severe or progressive ocular disease: **cyclophosphamide** (ToC) + systemic steroids or steroid-sparing **immunosuppressive (MMF**, AZA, or rituximab)
  - IVIG and TNF-α inhibitors are other options for severe disease
  - Surgical correction of severe ocular scarring may only be attempted AFTER disease controlled!

Prognosis/clinical course

- Chronic, disfiguring, and blindness-inducing (most common concern), but rarely fatal

Linear IgA bullous dermatosis/chronic bullous disease of childhood (LABD/ CBDC)

- Rare autoimmune subepidermal blistering disease defined by linear IgA deposition along BMZ
- Affects elderly adults (average > 60 yo; termed **LABD**) and preschool-aged children (average age: 4 yo; termed **CBDC**)
  - **Adult-onset LABD is typically drug-induced → vancomycin (most common)** > penicillin/ cephalosporin, captopril (> other ACE inhibitors), NSAIDs > phenytoin, sulfonamides > many others (e.g., furosemide and lithium)
- Pathogenesis: **IgA autoantibodies** directed against two related antigens, both derived from BPAG2:
  - **LAD-1** (120 kD cleaved portion of BP180 antigen)
  - **LABD97** (97 kD cleaved portion of LAD-1)

- Clinical presentation
  - Tense vesicles/bullae and urticarial plaques in an **annular, polycyclic, or herpetiform ("crown of jewels")** arrangement (Fig. 3.21)
  - Most common sites: flexures of **lower trunk/thigh/groin/buttocks**, and face (kids)
  - Vesiculopustules located at peripheral/expanding edge of plaques (helpful clue)
  - +/- mucosal involvement resembling MMP
  - Drug-induced LABD may have a TEN-like or morbilliform appearance → need biopsy and DIF
- Histopathology (cannot reliably distinguish from other neutrophil-rich subepidermal blistering conditions, such as dermatitis herpetiformis [DH], bullous LE, neutrophil-rich EBA → need DIF):
  - Early urticarial lesions: **neutrophils diffusely lined up along BMZ** w/ basal vacuolar change (represents early epidermal separation) +/- neutrophilic papillitis
  - Fully developed bullae: subepidermal blister w/ neutrophils in blister cavity and in superficial dermis +/- neutrophilic papillitis
- DIF: **linear IgA** along BMZ
- IIF with IgA conjugate (+ in 65%): usually stains **epidermal side/roof** on salt-split skin
- Rx: **dapsone (ToC)** or sulfapyridine
  - Oral steroids and immunosuppressants can be added in refractory cases (uncommon)
- Usually undergoes spontaneous remission within a few years

Epidermolysis bullosa acquisita

- Very rare, **acquired** subepidermal bullous disease
- Most commonly **adults**
- ↑ Incidence in East Asians and African Americans
- Associated diseases: **Crohn's disease/IBD (most common**; 25%–50%) > multiple myeloma, SLE, RA, diabetes, and thyroiditis
- Autoantigen: **IgG autoantibodies** against **NC1 domain of type VII collagen** (major component of **anchoring fibrils**, located in lamina densa/sublamina densa)
- MHC class II HLA-DR2 association

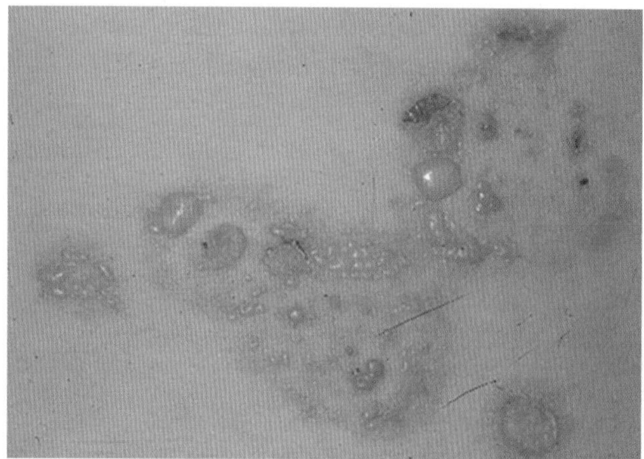

Fig. 3.21 Linear IgA bullous dermatosis. (Courtesy of Julia S. Lehman, MD.)

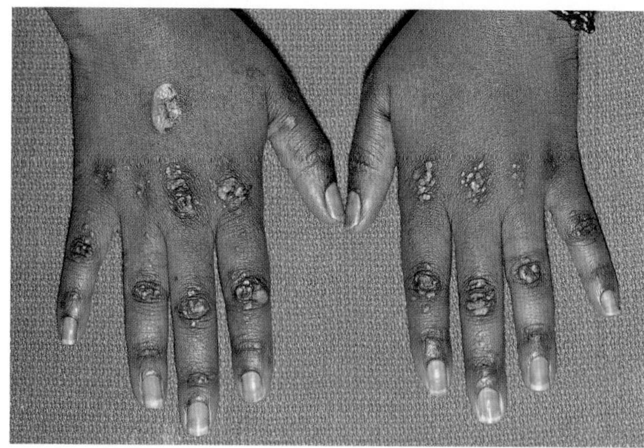

Fig. 3.22 Epidermolysis bullosa acquisita. (From James WD, Berger TG, Elston DM, Neuhaus IM.Chronic blistering dermatoses. In: *Andrews' Diseases of the Skin*, ed 12. Philadelphia: Elsevier; 2016, pp 451–470.)

- Two distinct clinical patterns:
  - Classic mechanobullous EBA (Fig. 3.22): mimics dystrophic EB; p/w **non-inflammatory** bullae (often hemorrhagic) and erosions on **acral/trauma-prone sites** (elbows, knees, and dorsal hands/feet) → may result in **"mitten" deformities** of the hands, syndactyly, and nail dystrophy/loss; bullous lesions **heal w/ atrophic scars, milia**, and dyspigmentation; scalp involved in 20% (→ scarring alopecia); histopathology: **cell-poor subepidermal blister**
  - Inflammatory (BP-like) EBA: **clinically indistinguishable from BP**; p/w widespread vesicles and bullae affecting same sites as BP; lesions may heal **without classic scarring or milia** seen in mechanobullous form; may closely mimic MMP with erosions/vesicles in mouth, eyes, larynx, and esophagus → same complications; histopathology: neutrophil- or eosinophil-rich subepidermal blister → **must differentiate from other entities via DIF serration pattern, salt-split skin DIF, IIF, immunoblotting, or ELISA**
- DIF: perilesional skin shows a **linear band of IgG (>linear C3) (u-serrated** pattern) along BMZ
  - Pattern is opposite of BP (linear C3 > linear IgG; n-serrated pattern)
- IIF: circulating antibodies only detectable in 50%
- Salt-split skin IIF: dermal (floor) deposition of IgG
- Rx: **often resistant to treatment**; may try systemic steroids, immunosuppressants, cyclophosphamide, colchicine, dapsone, IVIG, rituximab, or photopheresis

Bullous systemic lupus erythematosus

- See Section 3.5 Connective Tissue Diseases and Sclerosing Dermopathies

Dermatitis herpetiformis (Duhring disease)

Epidemiology

- **Northern Europeans** most commonly affected; rare in patients of African or Asian descent

- Average age of onset = **30** to **40 yo**, but children and elderly may also be affected
- M > F
- Over **97% of DH** and celiac disease (CD) patients have one or both of the following HLA II alleles:
  - **HLA-DQ2 (90%)**
  - HLA-DQ8 (7%)
- Strongly a/w other autoimmune diseases: **Hashimoto** thyroiditis (most common; >50%) > insulin-dependent diabetes mellitus (IDDM) > **pernicious anemia** » Addison's, alopecia areata (AA), myasthenia gravis, vitiligo, and SLE

Pathogenesis

- **Gluten** is a grain protein found in **wheat, rye, and barley**
  - NOT in oats, rice, or corn
- **Gliadin** (antigenic component of gluten): soluble by-product of gluten
- **TTG2**: transglutaminase protein present in **GI lamina** propria; anti-TTG2 IgA antibodies responsible only for **gut** involvement (not skin) in DH and CD
- **TTG3** (epidermal transglutaminase): present in **epidermis** and dermal papillae; anti-TTG3 IgA antibodies responsible for **skin** involvement in DH
- Pathogenesis: ingestion of gluten-containing grains → gluten broken down into gliadin inside GI lumen → gliadin transported across GI mucosa to lamina propria → TTG2 in lamina propria deamidates gliadin → deamidated gliadin forms a covalent bond w/ TTG2 → **TTG2-gliadin complex is a neoantigen** recognized by HLA-DQ2 (or HLA-DQ8) on APCs → specific Th and B cells activated → production of IgA autoantibodies against TTG2 or TTG2-gliadin complex → IgA antibodies bind to TTG2 complexes in lamina propria → neutrophil recruitment, damage to intestinal villi → enteropathy and villous atrophy → later, **epitope spreading** results in IgA autoantibodies against **epidermal transglutaminase (TTG3)** → circulating **anti-TTG3 IgA binds locally to TTG3 within dermal papillae** → neutrophils recruited to dermal papillae ("neutrophilic papillitis") → release elastase and MMPs → subepidermal blister most prominent above papillae

Clinical features

- Extremely itchy **herpetiform vesicles** arising on urticarial plaques
  - Vesicles rupture easily → **excoriations** usually the only finding on exam
- Classic distribution (most helpful clue): symmetric **extensor extremities**, **buttocks**, knees, and back/neck (> face/scalp) (Fig. 3.23)
  - Hemorrhagic/petechial palmoplantar lesions (useful clue)
- Only **20%** of patients w/ DH have **symptomatic** GI disease, but >**90%** have some degree of gluten-sensitive enteropathy on GI biopsy

Histopathology

- Ideally, biopsy an early blister for H&E: **subepidermal bulla** (most pronounced above dermal papillae), **neutrophilic papillitis** (neutrophils "stuffing" dermal papillae).
- In reality, often indistinguishable from LABD, but for Boards purposes, DH has less confluent dermal neutrophilic inflammation, and blisters are more localized to dermal papillae.

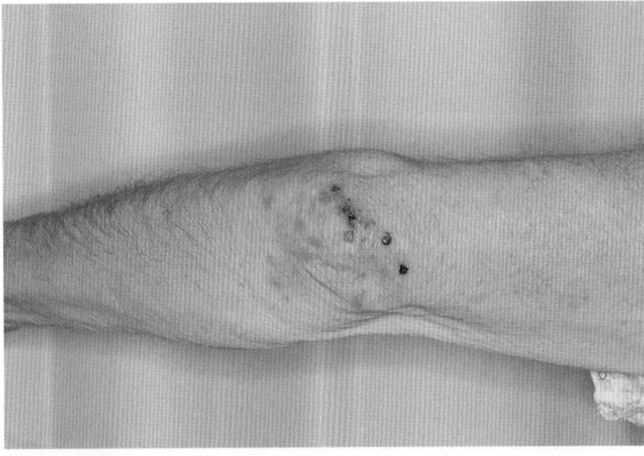

Fig. 3.23 Erosions on an urticarial base on the elbow of a patient with dermatitis herpetiformis. (Courtesy of Julia S. Lehman, MD.)

Laboratory testing

- DIF: **granular IgA deposits** in dermal papillae (90%)
  - Other pattern (10%): granular IgA deposition along BMZ
  - Ideal biopsy site for DIF: **1 cm away from blister**
- Serologic tests:
  - **Tissue transglutaminase antibodies (ELISA) are often positive**
  - **Antiendomysial** antibodies (IIF on monkey esophagus with IgA) may be positive in DH (80%) and CD (>95%)
  - Anti-gliadin antibodies may also be positive, but have high false (+) rates

Treatment

- **Dapsone (ToC):** controls skin disease very rapidly (<48–72 hours); **no effect on GI disease/lymphoma risk; check for G6PD deficiency before initiating**
  - If dapsone not tolerated, use sulfapyridine (good second-line agent w/ ↓ risk of hemolysis)
- **Gluten-free diet**: **controls both skin and GI disease**; is only way to ↓ **risk of GI lymphoma** (mucosa-associated lymphoid tissue [MALT]-lymphoma)
- **Avoid iodide** (ingestion or topically) since may → DH exacerbation

Prognosis/clinical course

- Lifelong (90%), waxing and waning

Comparative DIF images

- PV (Fig. 3.24)—epidermis stained in chicken-wire pattern; strongest in lower epidermis (vs. PF)
- PF (Fig. 3.25)—chicken-wire pattern evident diffusely in epidermis (upper epidermis > lower epidermis)
- BP versus EBA (Figs. 3.26 and 3.27)

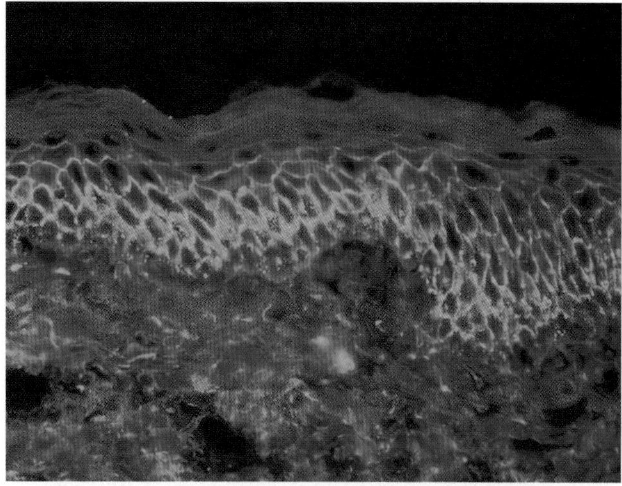

Fig. 3.24 DIF of pemphigus vulgaris with IgG deposition predominantly in the lower epidermis. (Courtesy of Kerith Spicknall, MD.)

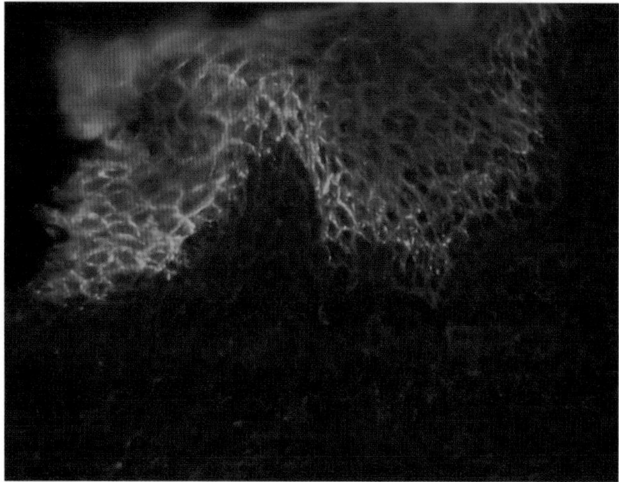

Fig. 3.25 DIF of pemphigus foliaceus with C3 deposition throughout the epidermis, but more intensely in the superficial layers. (Courtesy of Dr. Derek Marsee, Diagnostic Pathology Medical Group.)

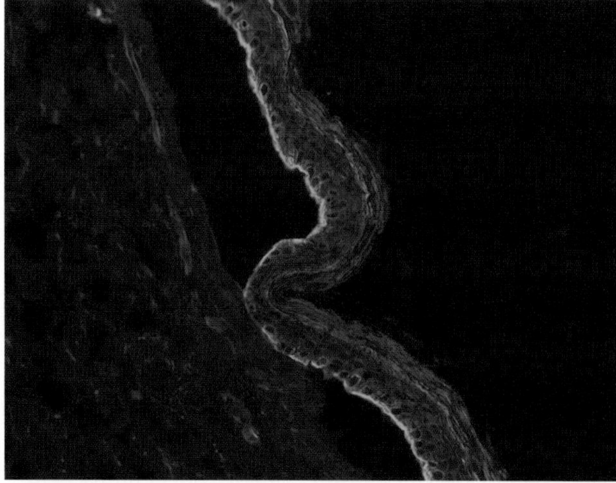

Fig. 3.26 Circulating IgG autoantibodies from bullous pemphigoid patients bind to the epidermal side (roof) of the salt-induced split.

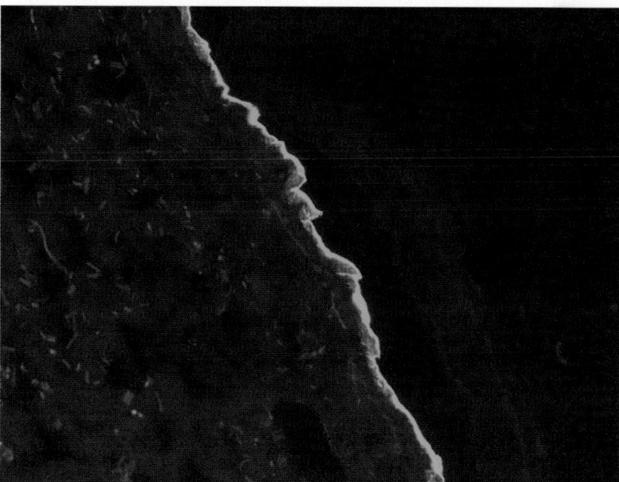

Fig. 3.27 IgG autoantibodies from patients with epidermolysis bullosa acquisita, anti-p200 pemphigoid, and certain types of mucous membrane pemphigoid (e.g., antibodies against laminin 5/332) bind to the dermal side (floor) of the blister.

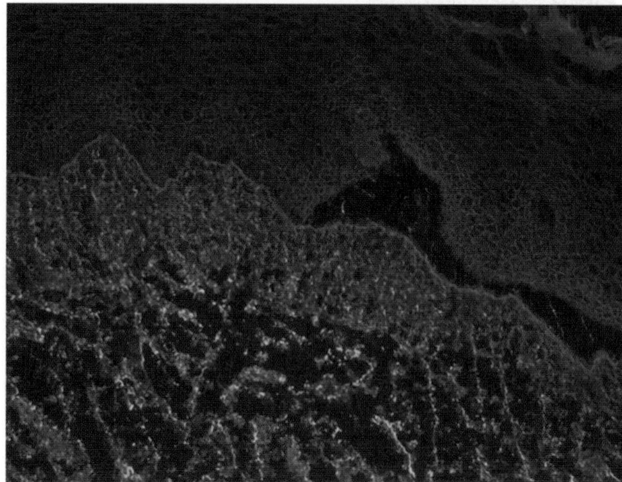

Fig. 3.28 Direct immunofluorescence specimen of a patient with paraneoplastic pemphigus, showing both cell-surface deposition on keratinocytes and basement membrane zone deposition with IgG. (Courtesy of Julia S. Lehman, MD.)

- PNP—pemphigus erythematosus looks similar (Fig. 3.28)
- DH (Fig. 3.29) versus LABD (Fig. 3.30)
- Porphyria cutanea tarda (PCT; Fig. 3.31)

Inherited blistering diseases

Epidermolysis bullosa (see Chapter 4)

Darier disease (Keratosis follicularis)

- **Autosomal dominant**; complete penetrance, variable expressivity
- Peak age of onset = **puberty** (70% prior to 20 yo)
- Chronic course, without spontaneous remission
- Mutation: *ATP2A2* (encodes **SERCA2** = calcium ATPase of endoplasmic reticulum) → defective Ca^{2+} sequestration into ER → impaired synthesis and folding

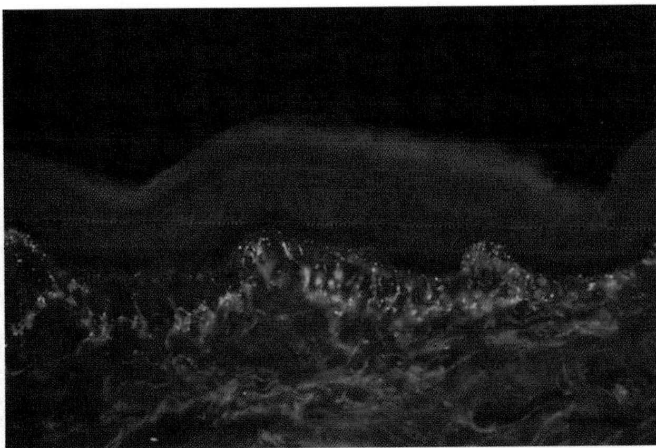

Fig. 3.29 Dermatitis herpetiformis. Granular IgA deposition along the dermal–epidermal junction, with stippling in the dermal papillae. (Courtesy of Julia S. Lehman, MD.)

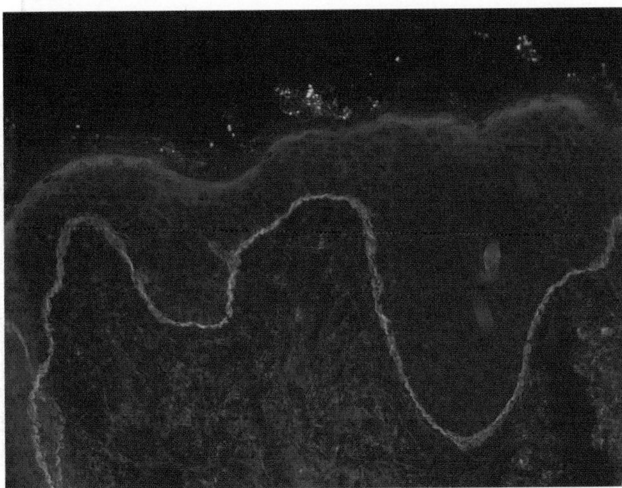

Fig. 3.30 Linear IgA bullous dermatosis—direct immunofluorescence. A linear pattern of IgA deposition is present within perilesional skin. (Courtesy of Julia S. Lehman, MD.)

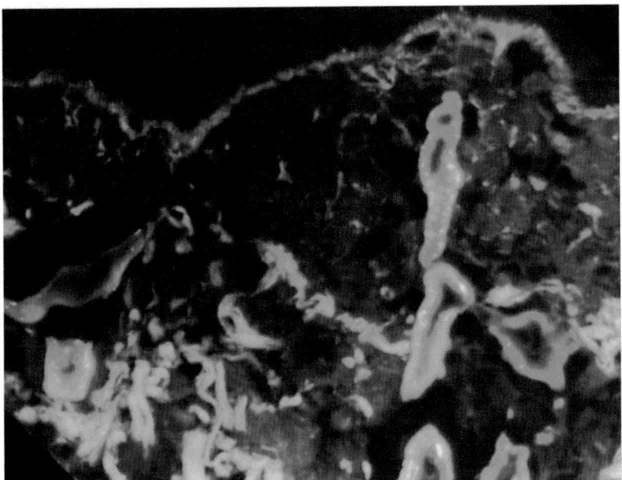

Fig. 3.31 Homogeneous staining of C5b-9, accompanied by concomitant granular deposition within the microvasculature of this patient with underlying porphyria cutanea tarda. (Direct immunofluorescence; original magnification: ×1000). (From Vasil KE, Magro CM. Cutaneous vascular deposition of C5b-9 and its role as a diagnostic adjunct in the setting of diabetes mellitus and porphyria cutanea tarda. *J Am Acad Dermatol*. 2007;56[1]:96–104.)

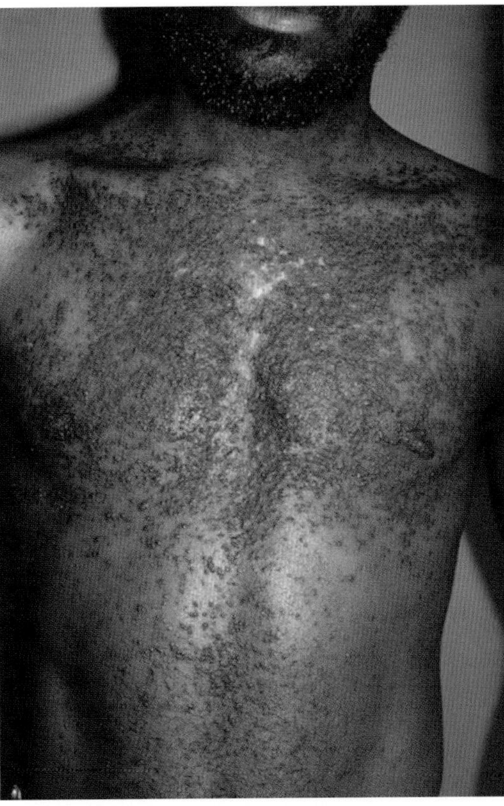

Fig. 3.32 Darier disease. Typical seborrheic distribution of brown, keratotic papules. (Courtesy of Dr. Lawrence Lieblich, MD.)

of cell adhesion proteins → keratinocyte acantholysis and apoptosis

- Malodorous, warty, crusted, and red-brown papules/plaques in seborrheic distribution (Fig. 3.32); often see **keratotic palmar papules/pits; longitudinal red and white alternating nail streaks** w/ distal **"V-shaped" notching;** 50% have **oral cobblestoning** (hard palate most common)
- Segmental Darier disease
  - Type 1 (most common): Blaschkoid streaks of Darier lesions; post-zygotic *ATP2A2* mutation
  - Type 2: generalized Darier w/ focal areas of severe involvement; heterozygous germline mutation + postzygotic loss of other allele
- Prone to secondary infections (**Kaposi varicelliform eruption** can be particularly serious)
- ↑ Incidence of **epilepsy**, intellectual impairment, **bipolar disorder**, and depression
- Histopathology: papillomatous epidermal hyperplasia w/ **epidermal acantholysis and dyskeratosis** (corps ronds and grains)
  - Corps ronds: large, **round**, acantholytic keratinocytes w/ dark nuclei surrounded by a bright pink rim of condensed keratin; located mostly in **spinous layer**
  - Corps grains: **flattened** cells composed of bright pink condensed keratin and a very thin dark nuclear remnant (looks like parakeratotic nucleus); located mostly in stratum corneum
- Rx: **systemic retinoids (>90% effective)**, topical steroids and retinoids, and topical antimicrobials to ↓ odor

Hailey-Hailey disease (Familial benign chronic pemphigus)

- **Autosomal dominant**; complete penetrance, variable expressivity
- **Wider range of onset age than Darier** (teens to 20 yo mostly, but may arise later)
- Mutation: *ATP2C1* (encodes hSPCA1, a Ca^{2+} ATPase of the Golgi apparatus) → defective Ca^{2+} sequestration into golgi → impaired processing of proteins involved in cell-cell adhesion → acantholysis
- Most commonly affects **intertriginous** sites (lateral neck, inframammary, **axillae**, **groin**, and perianal)
- Subtle, flaccid vesicle on normal or inflamed skin → ruptures to give **macerated, eroded plaques** (Fig. 3.33), often w/ circinate shape
- **No mucosal involvement** (unlike Darier)
- Prone to secondary infections (**Kaposi varicelliform eruption** can be most serious)
- Histopathology: **psoriasiform hyperplasia** (differentiates from pemphigus) w/ **diffuse acantholysis** (resembling a **"dilapidated brick wall"**); fewer dyskeratotic keratinocytes than Darier
- Rx: topical steroids; **procedural intervention** (e.g., CO_2 laser ablation) is very effective
  - Retinoids not nearly as effective as in Darier

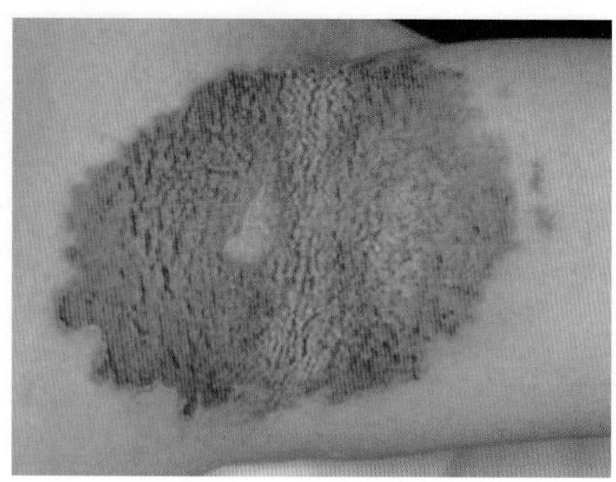

Fig. 3.33 A 47-year-old patient with axillary Hailey-Hailey disease. (From Pretel-Irazabal M, Lera-Imbuluzqueta JM, España-Alonso A. Carbon dioxide laser treatment in Hailey-Hailey disease: a series of 8 patients. *Actas Dermosifiliogr*. 2013;104[4]:325–333.)

Other blistering diseases

- Multiple non-immunobullous and non-inherited diseases may cause blistering
- Clinicopathologic correlation is often needed for accurate diagnosis
- See Tables 3.9 and 3.10

Table 3.9 Other Blistering Disorders

Disease	Clinical Setting	Clinical Presentation	Blister Location
Bullous diabeticorum	Longstanding diabetics w/ peripheral neuropathy, retinopathy, or nephropathy	p/w sudden eruption of **tense**, **non-inflammatory**, clear fluid-filled vesicles/bullae, 0.5 to several cm, on **feet** (>lower legs > hands > forearms); histopathology: **cell-poor subepidermal blister**; DIF negative; Rx: spontaneous resolution in 2–6 weeks; may aspirate if uncomfortable	Subepidermal
Coma blister	Coma due to meds (**barbiturates** > **benzos**, alcohol, opioids), or non–drug-induced coma	**Tense blisters** arising on **sites of pressure** 48–72 hours after loss of consciousness; blisters due to pressure-induced necrosis; histopathology: cell-poor subepidermal blister w/ **basophilic sweat gland necrosis** +/– epidermal necrosis; DIF negative; Rx: heals spontaneously in 1–2 weeks	Subepidermal
Friction blisters	New pair of **ill-fitting shoes**; sports or military involvement	Very common in **young**, **physically active**, repetitive friction; initially red macules at site of friction → painful **intraepidermal blisters** w/ blood-tinged fluid; histopathology: pauci-inflammatory **blister just under granular layer**; DIF negative; Rx: heals spontaneously; may drain to relieve pressure	Intraepidermal
Bullous small vessel vasculitis	Pts w/ small vessel vasculitis (cutaneous or systemic), often IgA vasculitis	LCV w/superimposed hemorrhagic vesicles and bullae, usually on **distal extremities** → may ulcerate; histopathology: **LCV or IgA vasculitis w/ subepidermal edema/bullae** and often epidermal necrosis	Subepidermal
Bullous drug eruptions	Pts receiving meds, often with polypharmacy	See Table 3.10	See Table 3.10
Bullous arthropod assault	Most common in children or pts with **hematologic malignancy** (**CLL** > mantle cell lymphoma, NK/T-cell lymphoma)	**Grouped pruritic papules** w/ central blistering; may have persistent papulonodules (persistent arthropod assault); **pts w/ lymphoma may have reaction in absence of definitive insect bite ("bug bite-like reactions")**; histopathology: eosinophilic spongiosis, **superficial and deep perivascular/periadnexal lympho-eosinophilic inflammation** (+/– flame figures), superficial dermal edema; Rx: topical steroids, oral antihistamines	**Intraepidermal** > subepidermal blister (may occur if dermal edema severe)
Delayed postburn/postgraft blisters	Blisters at sites of prior trauma (burns, graft site)	Tense vesicles/bullae appearing weeks to months (avg. 37 days) after original wound has completely healed; **due to fragility of new DEJ**; histopathology: cell-poor subepidermal blister with dermal fibrosis and angioplasia; negative DIF; Rx: spontaneous resolution	Subepidermal
Edema blisters	Anasarca or acute exacerbation of chronic edema	**Tense** blisters in edematous dependent sites (**distal LE**, **feet** most common); histopathology: cell-poor subepidermal bullae with massive dermal edema and epidermal spongiosis; Rx: treat underlying edema, compression wraps	Subepidermal

PUVA-induced acrobullous dermatosis is the rapid occurence of tense bullae on distal extremities due to PUVA damage to the epidermodermal cohesion + friction/trauma.

Modified from Mascaró JM Jr. Other vesiculobullous diseases. In: Bolognia JL, Jorizzo JL, Schaffer JV. Dermatology. *3rd ed. Philadelphia: Elsevier; 2012:515–522.*

Table 3.10 Bullous Drug Eruptions

Disease	Characteristic Features	Commonly Implicated Drugs
Fixed drug eruption	Sharply circumscribed **erythematous to dusky** violaceous patches Central blisters or erosions may appear Often resolves with **postinflammatory hyperpigmentation** Recurrence at same location(s) following drug reexposure	**Sulfonamides, NSAIDs, tetracyclines**, barbiturates, aspirin, acetaminophen (paracetamol), metronidazole, phenolphthalein
Stevens–Johnson syndrome (SJS), toxic epidermal necrolysis (TEN)	Prodrome of fever and **painful skin** Areas of dusky erythema associated with epidermal detachment (varying from <10% [SJS] to >30% [TEN]) Mucosal involvement	NSAIDs, antibiotics (sulfonamides and β-lactams), anticonvulsants, allopurinol
Drug-induced autoimmune blistering diseases	Primarily linear IgA bullous dermatosis, pemphigus, bullous pemphigoid Diagnosis based on histologic findings, immunofluorescence studies, and drug history	Linear IgA bullous dermatosis: **vancomycin** > β-lactams, captopril, NSAIDs Pemphigus: **penicillamine, captopril**, β-lactams, gold Bullous pemphigoid: diuretics (especially **furosemide**), antibiotics, dipeptidyl peptidase 4 inhibitors, checkpoint inhibitors; PUVA can rarely induce BP
Drug-induced pseudoporphyria	Eruption resembles porphyria cutanea tarda clinically and microscopically Porphyrin determinations are within normal limits	NSAIDs (especially **naproxen**), nalidixic acid, thiazides, furosemide, tetracyclines
Acute generalized exanthematous pustulosis	Acute onset, usually occurring within 2 days of drug exposure Areas of erythema studded with pustules; occasionally vesicles Fever, malaise, leukocytosis	**β-Lactams**, macrolides, pristinamycin, terbinafine, calcium channel blockers (diltiazem), hydroxychloroquine, carbamazepine, acetaminophen, metronidazole
Phototoxic drug eruptions	Limited to sun-exposed areas Resembles exaggerated sunburn Necrotic keratinocytes are seen on biopsy	**Tetracyclines** (especially doxycycline), **quinolones, psoralens**, NSAIDs, diuretics
Bromoderma and iododerma	**Acneiform lesions**, papulopustules, nodules, or even **vegetative lesions** simulating pemphigus vegetans Clear or hemorrhagic blisters can develop (more common in iododerma)	Bromides, iodine-containing drugs (e.g., amiodarone), radiographic contrast media
Palmoplantar erythrodysesthesia (acral variant of toxic erythema of chemotherapy)	Painful erythema develops primarily on the palms, soles and digits following chemotherapy administration The skin becomes edematous, its color changes to dark red or violet, and blisters and erosions may develop	**Cytarabine**, doxorubicin, capecitabine, 5-fluorouracil (especially prolonged infusions), multi-kinase inhibitors (e.g., sorafenib, sunitinib), busulfan, taxanes, clofarabine, pralatrexate

Occasionally, eczematous drug reactions (e.g., secondary to warfarin, calcium channel blockers) and systemic contact dermatitis can be papulovesicular; patients with drug reaction eosinophilia and systemic symptoms (DRESS)/drug-induced hypersensitivity syndrome (DIHS) can also develop vesicles.
Modified from Mascaró JM Jr. Other vesiculobullous diseases. In: Bolognia JL, Schaffer JV, Cerroni L. Dermatology. 4th ed. Philadelphia: Elsevier; 2018:554-561.

3.5 CONNECTIVE TISSUE DISEASE (CTD) AND SCLEROSING DERMOPATHIES

Connective tissue disease laboratory studies

Antinuclear antibodies (ANA)

- ANAs are autoantibodies that target various nuclear antigens:
  - Extractable nuclear antigens (ENAs):
    - **Ro/SSA**: most strongly a/w Sjögren's syndrome (SjS; 70%) and neonatal lupus (~100%), but also present in subacute cutaneous lupus erythematosus (SCLE; 75%–90%) and SLE (50%)
    - **La/SSB**: most strongly a/w SjS (40%), but also in SCLE
    - **Scl-70** (DNA topoisomerase I): most strongly a/w diffuse systemic sclerosis (SSc; 60%)
    - **Jo-1** (histidyl tRNA synthetase): Dermatomyositis/polymyositis (DM/PM) with antisynthetase syndrome
    - **Smith (Sm)**: highly specific for SLE (only 10%–30% sensitive)
    - **RNP (U1 RNP)**: very high titers correlate with mixed connective tissue disease (**MCTD; 100%**); lower titers in SLE
  - Non-ENA targets:
    - Double-stranded DNA **(dsDNA)**: highly specific for SLE (60% sensitive), a/w lupus nephritis, correlates with lupus band test (LBT) from sun-protected skin
    - **Histone**: most a/w drug-induced SLE (95%)
    - **Centromere**: a/w CREST (80%)

- ANAs may be detected by ELISA (newer, cheaper method) or IIF (older but more sensitive method; substrate is Hep2 cancer cell line)
  - Despite its limitations, the classic IIF ANA test still remains the most efficient screening test for systemic AICTD
  - ELISA studies useful for identifying specific antigenic targets → helpful in serologically narrowing the diagnosis between CTDs
- ANA titer = highest dilution of patient's serum that still produces fluorescence (considered **positive if > 1:40**)
- Range of ANAs in "healthy" individuals
  - ≥1:40 (20%–30%)
  - ≥1:80 (10%–12%)
  - ≥1:160 (5%)
  - ≥1:320 (3%)
- Rates of ANA positivity:
  - **SLE: 99%**
    - Less than 1% of SLE patients have negative ANA by IIF → highly unlikely to get false (-) result by current testing methods!
  - SSc: 90%
  - SjS: 70%
  - DM/PM: 40%–65%
- Common ANA IIF patterns (and corresponding antigenic targets by ELISA):
  - Homogenous (aka "diffuse"): anti-dsDNA and anti-histone antibodies
    - A/w SLE and **drug-induced SLE**
  - Peripheral (aka "rim"): dsDNA
    - A/w **SLE**
  - Speckled (aka "particulate"): Ro/SSA, La/SSB, U1RNP, Smith, RNA polymerases, and Scl-70
    - Non-specific but may be a/w SjS and MCTD
  - Nucleolar: RNA processing molecules (**fibrillarin/ U3RNP**), anti-PM/Scl
    - A/w **SSc**, PM-SSc overlap
  - **Centromere** (aka "discrete speckled"): anti-centromere antibodies
    - Specific for **CREST**
- Know the autoantibody associations for each AI-CTD (Table 3.11)

Lupus band test (LBT)

- Granular continuous band of immunoglobulin deposits (**IgM >** IgG > IgA) and complement (C3) at DEJ in lesioned and non-lesioned skin of sun-exposed or sun-protected sites in **patients w/ SLE** visualized via DIF

Table 3.11 High-Yield Autoantibodies in Connective Tissue Diseases

Target	Prevalence (%)	Molecular Specificity	Key Association
Lupus erythematosus (listed prevalence is for SLE)			
ANA	99	N/A	Most sensitive serologic test for SLE → most common IIF pattern in SLE = **homogenous, peripheral** **SCLE positive in 60%–80%** (speckled/particulate IIF) **DLE positive in 5%–25%**
ssDNA	70	Denatured DNA	**Risk for developing SLE in DLE patients**; also seen in linear morphea
C1q	60	C1q component of complement	Severe SLE, **hypocomplementemic urticarial vasculitis** syndrome
dsDNA	60	Double-stranded (native) DNA	**Highly specific test for SLE**; a/w **LE nephritis** → useful for monitoring nephritis activity
U1RNP	50 **(low titers)**	Splicesome RNP	Overlapping features with other AI-CTDs; **high titers in MCTD (100%)**
Ro/SSA	50	hYRNP	**Neonatal LE/congenital heart block (99%)**; **SCLE** (75%–90%); primary SjS (70%); **a/w photosensitivity**
La/SSB	20	hYRNP	SCLE (30%–40%); SjS (40%); occurs in conjunction with SSA/Ro
Cardiolipin	50	Cardiolipin (phospholipid)	**Antiphospholipid syndrome in SLE**: recurrent abortions, thrombocytopenia, hypercoagulable state, livedo reticularis, leg ulcers, acral infarction, hemorrhagic cutaneous necrosis
Histone	40	Histones	**Drug-induced SLE**
Smith (Sm)	10–30	Splicesome RNP	**Highly specific for SLE**; higher prevalence in African Americans and Asians (30%–40%)
β2 glycoprotein 1	25	Cofactor for cardiolipin	High risk of thrombosis in SLE; primary antiphospholipid syndrome
rRNP	7–15 (40% in Asians)	Ribosomal P proteins	Highly specific for SLE; a/w **neuropsychiatric LE**
Ku	10	DNA repair complex	Overlap syndromes with DM/PM and SSc
PCNA	50	Component of multiprotein complexes involved in cellular prolifertion	
DM/PM			
ANA	40	N/A	Most common IIF patterns: **speckled**, **nucleolar**
p155 (TIF1-γ)	18–23 (adults) 18–35 (juvenile DM)	Transcriptional intermediary factor 1-γ (tumor suppressor protein)	**Clinically amyopathic/hypomyopathic DM**; **cancer-associated classic DM (adults only)**; GI involvement; severe cutaneous disease w/ heliotrope rash/V sign/Gottron papules, **psoriasiform plaques**, **ovoid palatal patches**, palmar hyperkeratosis, "red on white patches" (atrophic hypopigmented patches w/ telangiectasias) **Younger age of onset in kids**

Table 3.11 High-Yield Autoantibodies in Connective Tissue Diseases—cont'd

Target	Prevalence (%)	Molecular Specificity	Key Association
p140 (NXP-2)	15 (adults) 20–25 (juvenile DM)	Nuclear matrix protein (MORC family CW-type zinc finger 3 [MORC3])	Adults: **a/w malignancy,** subcutaneous edema and calcinosis; 80% of all cancer-related DM has autoantibodies to **NXP-2 or TIF1-γ** Juvenile: severe muscle disease, GI bleeding (vasculopathy), calcinosis
Aminoacyl tRNA synthetases	Up to 20	tRNA synthetases	**Anti-synthetase syndrome** (myositis, **mechanic's hands**, arthritis, Raynaud phenomenon, **severe ILD [worse with non-Jo1 antibodies]**)
Anti-Jo1	Jo1 (20)		
Anti-PL7	PL7 (5)		
Anti-PL12	PL12 (3)		
EJ/OJ	EJ/OJ (<1)		
Mi-2	4–35 (adults) 4–10 (juvenile DM)	**Helicase**	**Classic DM skin findings** (e.g., shawl sign, Gottron papules, etc.), mild muscle disease; **good response** to treatment
MDA5/ CADM-140	10–30 (adults) 7–50 (juvenile DM)	MDA5	**CADM w/rapidly progressive ILD** (adults and kids); distinctive skin findings (**skin ulcers** [MCP/IP joints, elbows, knees, nail folds]**, oral ulcers**, **painful palmar papules**, lateral digit hyperkeratosis/scaling, nonscarring diffuse alopecia, panniculitis); arthritis, fever, hand swelling
SRP	5	Signal recognition particle	Fulminant DM/PM (severe muscle weakness) with **cardiac involvement, poor prognosis**
Ku	3	DNA repair complex	DM overlap syndromes with SLE, Sjögren's, or SSc
SAE	8	Post-translational modification	Adults: strong HLA associations, severe skin disease, progressive muscle disease, a/w hydroxychloroquine drug eruptions Juvenile: severe skin disease BUT minimal muscle disease
Systemic sclerosis			
ANA	95	N/A	Most common patterns: speckled, nucleolar, **centromere (CREST)**
Centromere	30 (PSSc) 80 (CREST)	CENP-B	Most specific for **CREST**, a/w pulmonary HTN
DNA topoisomerase I (formerly Scl-70)	60 (PSSc) 15 (CREST)	DNA topoisomerase I	Most strongly a/w progressive systemic sclerosus (**PSSc**) with pulmonary fibrosis and **poorer prognosis**
RNA polymerases (I and III)	45 (PSSc) 6 (CREST)	RNA polymerase I/ III	High levels correlate w/ **severe skin involvement (diffuse) and renal crisis** in PSSc; a/w internal malignancy (breast cancer #1)
Fibrillarin (U3RNP)	5 (overall)	U3RNP	a/w internal organ involvement
MMP1 and MMP3	50 (overall) 70 (PSSc) 33% (CREST)	Degrade ECM proteins	
Calpastatin	25 (overall)	Endogenous inhibitor of calcium-dependent protease, calpain	
Morphea			
ANA	40	NA	N/A
Topoisomerase IIα	75	Topo Iiα	Not used clinically
ssDNA	50	NA	Most prevalent in **linear morphea**, correlates w/ disease severity/activity
Histones	35	Histones	Most prevalent in **linear and generalized morphea,** correlates w/ disease severity/activity
Fibrillin-1	30	Fibrillin-1 (component of ECM)	Rarely positive in PSSc or CREST
Rheumatoid arthritis			
Rheumatoid factor	80	Fc portion of IgG	Low levels: very non-specific, may be seen in other AI-CTDs, infections, liver dz, sarcoid, systemic vasculitides High levels: a/w **severe**, **crippling**, **erosive RA** and extra-articular manifestations of RA (systemic vasculitis, neuropathy); may also have high levels in **mixed cryoglobulinemia** (types II and III) secondary to Hep C infection
Cyclic citrullinated proteins	70	CCP proteins in skin (filaggrin) and joints	a/w **Severe RA**; also a predictor for development of RA
Sjögren's syndrome			
α-Fodrin	70	Actin-binding protein (involved in secretion)	**Most specific** antibody for SjS
Ro/SSA	60–70	hyRNP	Also important in neonatal LE (~99%) and SCLE (may be a/w photosensitivity)
La/SSB	20–40	hyRNP	Seen in same contexts as Ro/SSA; almost never positive if Ro/SSA is negative
Mixed connective tissue disease (MCTD)			
U1RNP	100 (by definition)	Splicesome RNP	Low titer positivity can be seen in SLE

LE, *lupus erythematosus*; SCLE, *subacute lupus erythematosus*; RA, *rheumatoid arthritis;* SjS, *Sjogren syndrome;* AI-CTDs, autoimmune connective tissue, diseases; PSSc, progressive systemic sclerosus; ECm, extracellular membrane; HTN, *hypertension;* DM, *dermatomyositis;* PM, *polymyositis;* SSc, *systemic sclerosus.*
Modified from Dutz JP, Jacobe HT, Sontheimer RD, Saxton-Daniels S. Autoimmune connective tissue diseases. In: Bolognia JL, Schaffer JV, Cerroni L. Dermatology. *4th ed. Philadelphia: Elsevier; 2018:649–661.*

- Three different types of LBTs exist:
  - Lesional LBT
    - High sensitivity in patients w/ SLE
    - LBT may also be positive in patients with chronic cutaneous lupus erythematosus (CCLE; 60%–80%)
    - Helpful in differentiating from other rashes in non-SLE patients
      - Can see false (+) LBT in rosacea, telangiectasias, and polymorphous light eruption (PMLE) → band is usually weaker in intensity and more focal/interrupted
    - Positive LBT seen in < 5% of DM
    - **↑ # of immunoreactants → ↑ specificity for SLE**
  - Sun-exposed, non-lesional skin (shoulder, proximal extensor forearm)
    - Positive in 70%–80% of SLE
    - Useful in making diagnosis of SLE in patients without skin lesions
    - 25% of people without SLE will demonstrate a weak interrupted linear and granular DEJ deposition of IgM and Clq (less frequently IgG, IgA, and C3), which usually does not meet criteria for a positive LBT
  - Sun-protected, non-lesional skin (medial flexor forearm, medial upper arm, and buttocks)
    - Positive in 35%–55% of SLE
    - Useful for measuring disease activity and assessing prognosis
    - **Correlates with anti-dsDNA autoantibodies** → a/w severe extracutaneous disease including renal disease

Lupus erythematosus

- There are three major **"specific"** cutaneous manifestations of lupus: acute (ACLE), subacute (SCLE), and chronic (CCLE) (Fig. 3.34)
  - These three cutaneous manifestations are not mutually exclusive→ patients may have more than one cutaneous morphology at any given time
  - **Every form of cutaneous lupus may be** seen in the setting of **SLE** or as an **isolated cutaneous** disease
  - Degree of association with SLE varies by cutaneous subtype (Table 3.12)
- **All patients with "specific" cutaneous lesions of lupus should be evaluated for systemic disease** (SLE) via clinical exam, H&E, DIF, and serologic studies
- In addition, multiple **"non-specific"** cutaneous lesions may be seen in lupus (discussed in SLE section)

Chronic cutaneous lupus erythematosus (CCLE)

Epidemiology

- Female predominance
- **DLE accounts for the majority of CCLE**
  - 40%–70% of SLE patients will have discoid lesions
  - However, only **5%–20% of patients with DLE progress to SLE**
    - 5% for patients w/ head-only involvement
    - 20% for patients w/ diffuse involvement
    - Majority of DLE patients who progress to SLE do so within first 5 years; younger age, high ANA titer, skin type V/VI may also increase progression risk
  - **African Americans** more commonly affected w/ DLE

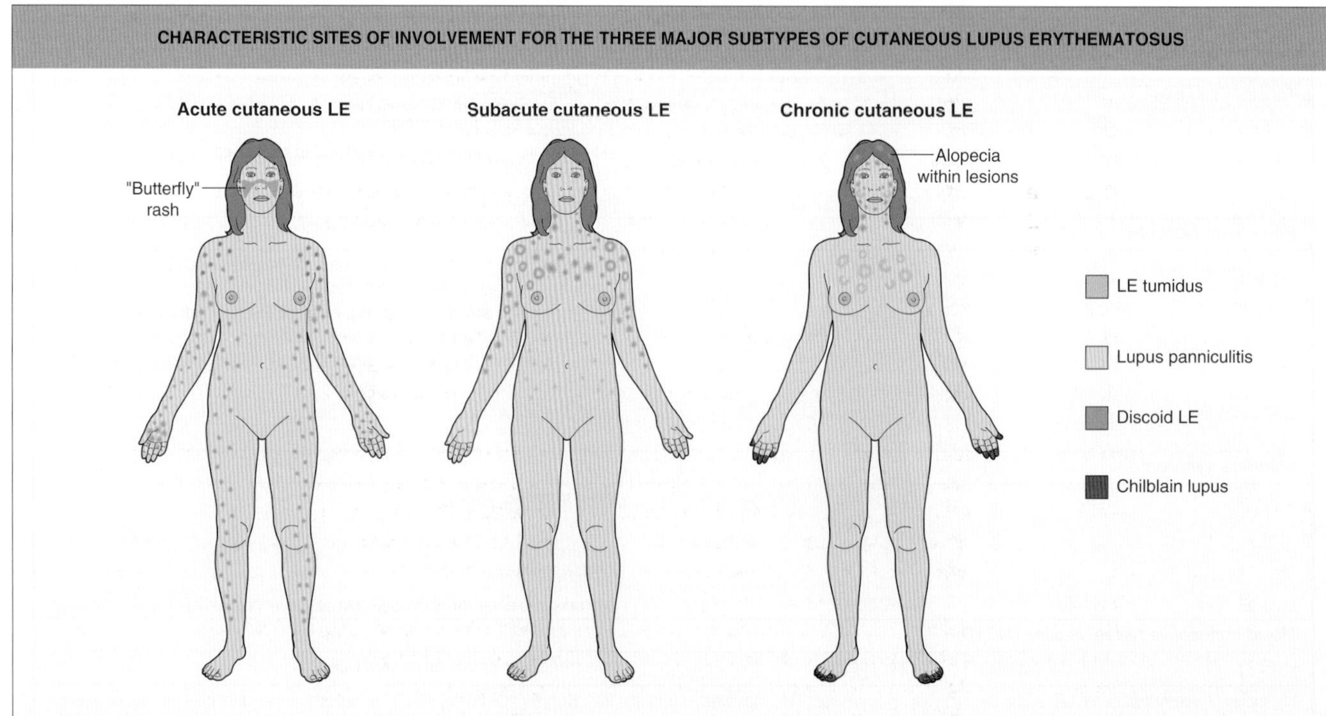

Fig. 3.34 Characteristic sites of involvement for the three major forms of cutaneous lupus erythematosus *(LE)*. (From Lee LA, Werth VP. Lupus erythematosus. In: Bolognia JL, Schaffer JV, Cerroni L. *Dermatology*. 4th ed. Philadelphia: Elsevier; 2018:662–680.)

Table 3.12 Different Forms of Cutaneous Lupus and Their Association With Systemic Lupus Erythematosus (SLE)

Type of Cutaneous Lupus	Association With SLE
• Acute cutaneous lupus erythematosus (ACLE)	++++
• Subacute cutaneous lupus erythematosus (SCLE)	++
• Chronic cutaneous lupus erythematosus (CCLE)	
Localized DLE (head and neck)	+
Widespread/disseminated DLE	++
Hypertrophic DLE	+
Lupus erythematosus tumidus (LET)	+/–
Lupus panniculitis	+
Chilblain lupus	++
• Other variants	
Bullous eruption of SLE	++++
Rowell's syndrome	++ to +++

Modified from Lee LA, Werth VP. Lupus erythematosus. In: Bolognia JL, Jorizzo JL, Schaffer JV. Dermatology. *4th ed. Philadelphia: Elsevier; 2017:615–629.*

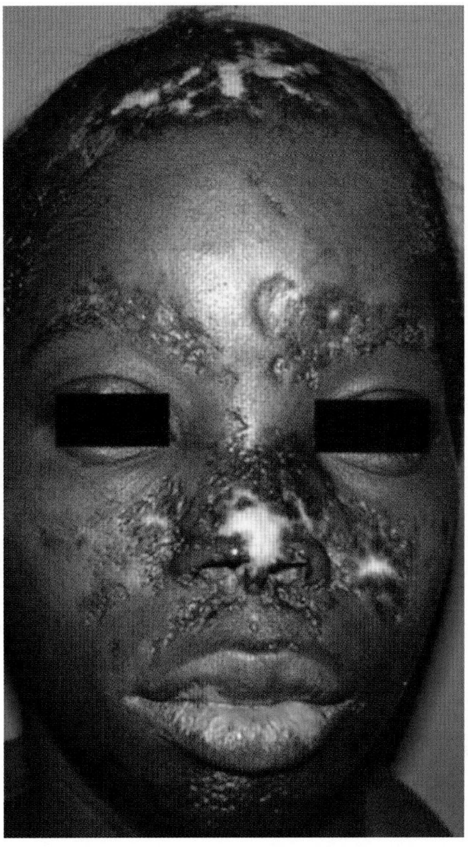

Fig. 3.35 Extensive scarring from discoid lupus erythematosus. (From James WD, Elston DM, Treat JR, Rosenbach MA, Neuhaus IM. Connective tissue diseases. In: *Andrews' Diseases of the Skin*. 13th ed. Philadelphia: Elsevier; 2020:157–183.)

Pathogenesis

- UVR (UVB > UVA) has role in lesional development
- Type I IFN signature w/ CD4+ T-helper 1 (Th1) cells and CD8+ cytotoxic T-cell recruitment and activation
- Tobacco:
  - Smoking is a risk factor for DLE
  - Stopping may help resolve recalcitrant lesions
- Genetic predisposition (multiple genes—e.g., *TYK2, IRF5, CTLA4*); *TREX1* mutations a/w familial chilblain lupus

CCLE clinical subtypes

1. Discoid LE
- Most common form of CCLE
- Begin w/ red macules or plaques → later develop scale, **atrophy, and scarring**, w/ **central hypopigmentation and peripheral hyperpigmentation** (more apparent in darker-skinned patients) (Fig. 3.35)
- Langue du chat (cat's tongue): **carpet "tack-like" spines** on undersurface of scale
- Typical locations: **face, scalp** (cicatricial alopecia), and ears (esp. **conchal bowl)**
  - Occasionally occurs in photoprotected sites, but rare to see discoid lesions below the neck unless lesions above the neck are also present
  - 25% have mucosal involvement (lips, conjunctiva, nasal mucosa, genitals)
- ANA (+) in 5%–25%
- DLE variants:
  - Localized DLE
    - Above neck only
  - Widespread DLE
    - Above and below neck
    - **Stronger association w/ SLE**, more likely to have serologic abnormalities
  - Childhood DLE
    - Higher rate of progression to SLE

2. Hypertrophic (verrucous) LE
- Thick, hyperkeratotic and verrucous scaling plaques w/ indurated border
- ↑ **Risk SCC** (akin to hypertrophic LP)
- Typical locations: **extensor forearms** > face, and upper trunk (sun-exposed sites)
  - Favors **upper half of body** (vs. hypertrophic LP = lower half)
- Usually accompanies typical discoid lesions

3. Chilblain LE
- Red or dusky purple papules/plaques on **fingertips, rims of ears**, calves, and heels
- Chronic relapsing course
- Precipitated by cold, but often **persists year-round** (vs. non-lupus-associated chilblains)

4. Tumid lupus erythematosus
- Edematous, indurated, erythematous, often **annular** plaques without epidermal involvement (Fig. 3.36), lesions resolve without scarring or atrophy
  - Plaques may have central clearing
- Typical locations: **face and trunk**
- Responds well to antimalarials
- Considered to be on a clinical spectrum w/ Jessner's and reticular erythematous mucinosis (REM), with similar findings on histology

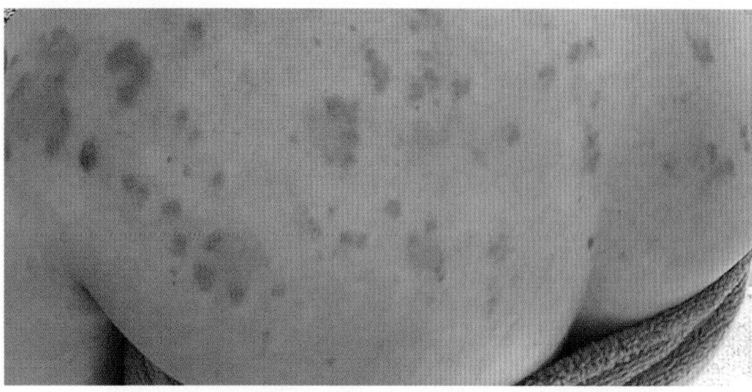

Fig. 3.36 Lupus erythematosus tumidus. Annular pink plaques on the back. (Courtesy Dr. Heather Holahan, University of North Carolina, Department of Dermatology.)

- Differentiating tumid LE versus Jessner's versus REM:
  - Jessner's: similar clinical appearance, but has CD8+ predominant infiltrate w/ ↓ mucin
  - REM is histologically identical to tumid LE, but is morphologically distinctive (erythematous macules and papules or plaques on mid back/chest in a reticular pattern)

5. LE panniculitis/profundus

- Indurated, non-tender, subcutaneous nodules or plaques that **heal w/ atrophy** (depressed scarring of fatty areas)
- Overlying skin often normal, but may have **discoid changes** (if DLE lesions above panniculitis plaques = **lupus profundus**)
- Typical locations: face, **upper arms**, **upper trunk**, breasts, buttocks, and thighs
- Antimalarials effective
- **15% a/w SLE** (panniculitis may be first sign)

6. DLE-LP overlap

- Coexisting DLE and LP w/ overlap lesions
- Palmoplantar involvement is characteristic
- DDx: LP-like rash can also occur in SLE patients on antimalarials

7. Mucosal LE

- Does not include non-lupus specific mucosal ulcers a/w SLE
- Most commonly seen in conjunction w/ cutaneous DLE
- Lesions:
  - Classic plaque with central erythema and surrounding white keratotic border, usually on hard palate
  - Discoid lesions most commonly on the lip
- Typical locations: buccal mucosa, hard palate, and vermillion lip (lower > upper)
- ↑ Risk SCC
- Presence of ulceration → a/w ↑ risk for systemic involvement

Laboratory testing

- (+/−) ANA, leukopenia, and ↑ ESR
  - **Serologic abnormalities more common in patients w/ widespread DLE**

Histopathology

- DLE
  - H&E: compact othrohyperkeratosis, **vacuolar interface** dermatitis w/ necrotic keratinocytes and pigment incontinence, **epidermal atrophy, BMZ thickening, follicular plugging**, superficial and **deep** perivascular/periadnexal lymphohistiocytic inflammation with plasma cells, **CD123+ plasmacytoid dendritic cells** (helpful in distinguishing lupus from most lymphomas and other inflammatory diseases), and **mucin** deposition (Fig. 3.37)
    - Lacks eosinophils
  - DIF
    - LBT(+) on lesional skin in 75%; ideal to choose lesion that has been present for a few months or more
      - More likely to be positive on head/neck and extremities compared with trunk
- Hypertrophic (verrucous) LE
  - Similar histologic features as DLE but w/ greater orthohyperkeratosis and **endophytic buds of hyperplastic follicular epithelium** (> interfollicular epidermal hyperplasia)
    - Pseudoepitheliomatous hyperplasia is **often mistaken for SCC**

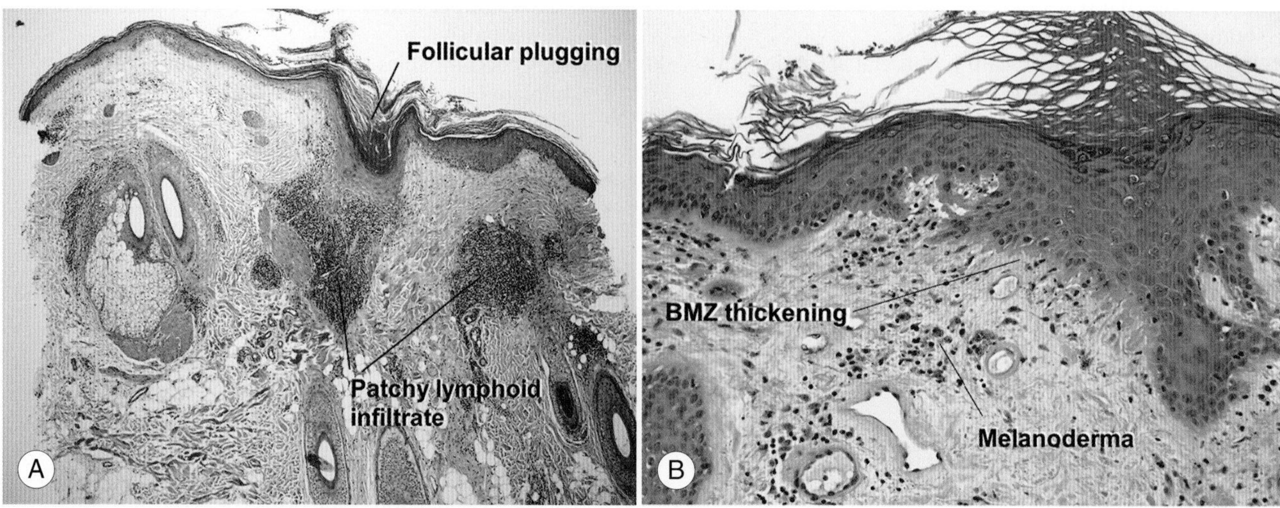

Fig. 3.37 (A) and (B) Discoid lupus erythematosus histology. Note focal interface dermatitis, dense perivascular/periadnexal lymphoid infiltrates, and thickened basement membrane zone *(BMZ)*. (From Elston DM: Interface dermatitis. In: Elston DM, Ferringer T, eds. *Dermatopathology*. 3rd ed. Philadelphia: Elsevier, 2019:132–152.)

- Chilblain LE
  - Demonstrates features of both chilblains (papillary edema, perivascular and dermal lymphohistiocytic infiltration) and DLE
  - DIF: (+) LBT
- Tumid LE
  - **No significant epidermal changes** (e.g., lacks follicular plugging, vacuolar interface, and BMZ thickening)
  - Shares characteristic dermal features of DLE:
    - Perivascular and periadnexal lymphoid aggregates in upper and lower dermis, with clusters of CD123+ plasmacytoid dendritic cells
    - **Massive mucin deposition** (more than classic DLE; amount rivals that seen in DM)
  - Histologically similar to REM and Jessner's, except Jessner's has CD8+ predominant infiltrate and lacks mucin
  - DIF: (+) LBT in 50%
- LE panniculitis
  - May have histologic findings of overlying DLE (if DLE epidermal and dermal changes present = lupus profundus)
  - Dermal mucin deposition
  - Subcutaneous findings:
    - Lymphocytic lobular panniculitis
    - Hyaline (**"waxy pink"**) fat necrosis
    - Nodular lymphoid aggregates, with clusters of **CD123+ plasmacytoid dendritic cells**
    - Fat lobules may be rimmed by lymphocytes
      - **Important to differentiate from subcutaneous T-cell lymphoma:** atypical cells, lacks dermal lymphoid nodules, lacks CD123+ plasmacytoid dendritic cells (helpful IHC stain), lacks mucin
  - DIF: (+) LBT in 35%–70%
- DLE-LP overlap
  - Typical lesions of LE or LP will demonstrate H&E and DIF findings for that condition
  - Overlap lesions may show features typical for both
- Mucosal LE
  - Hyperkeratosis, atrophy of rete pegs, vacuolar-to-lichenoid interface dermatitis; superficial and deep perivascular lymphocytic infiltrate
  - DIF: (+) LBT

Treatment

- Treatment algorithm: (Fig. 3.38)

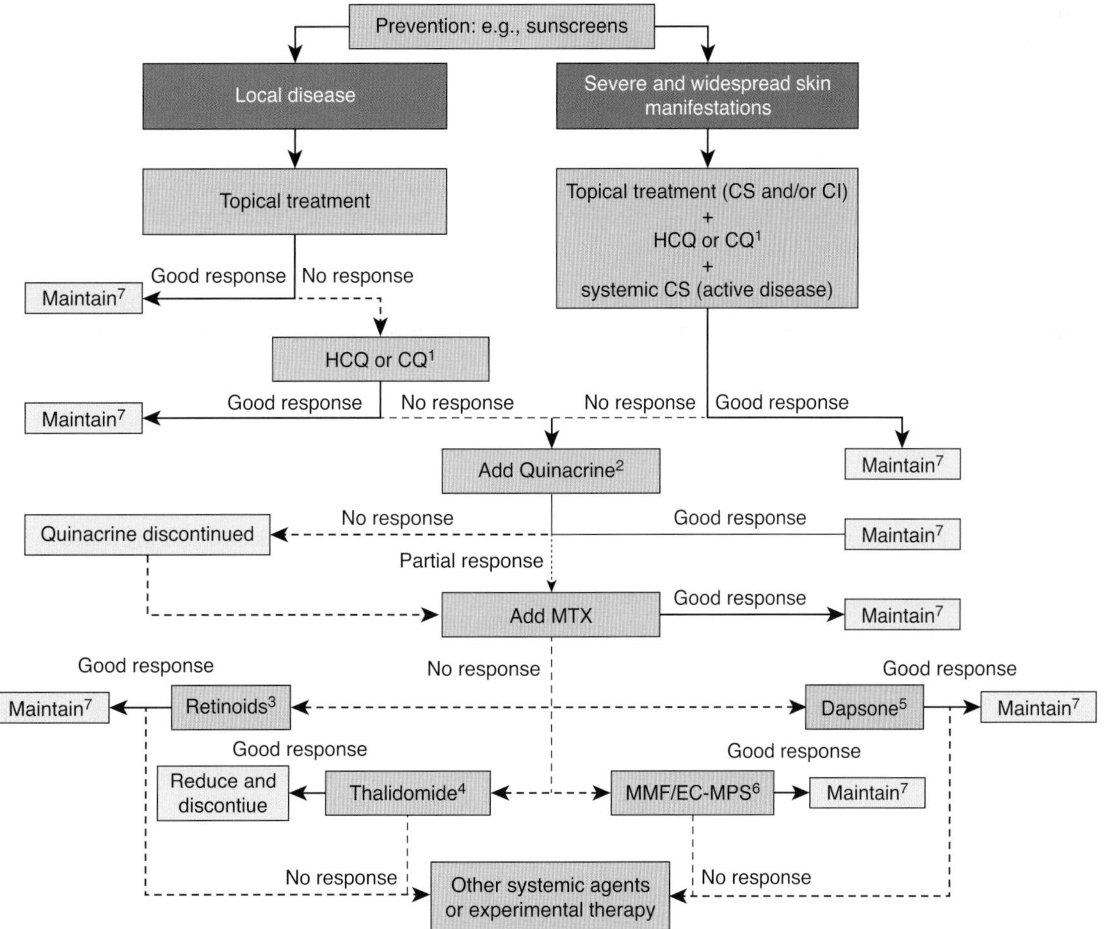

Fig. 3.38 Cutaneous lupus erythematosus (CLE): update of therapeutic options. Algorithm of treatment for CLE. Topical agents include topical steroids, calcineurin inhibitors, and retinoids. Consider retinoids earlier for discoid lupus-lichen planus overlap. Thalidomide is used at 50 to 100 mg daily for clearing and 25 to 50 mg daily-twice weekly for maintenance; lenalidomide works similarly but without the peripheral neuropathy of thalidomide. *CI*, Calcineurin inhibitor; *CQ*, chloroquine; *CS*, corticosteroids; *EC-MPS*, mycophenolate sodium; *HCQ*, hydroxychloroquine; *MMF*, mycophenolate mofetil; *MTX*, methotrexate. (From Kuhn A, Ruland V, Bonsmann G. Cutaneous lupus erythematosus: update of therapeutic options part I. *J Am Acad Dermatol*. 2011;65[6]:e179–e193.)

Prognosis/clinical course

- 5%–20% progress to SLE (typically within first 5 years after diagnosis)
- ↑ **Risk of progression w/ widespread DLE and childhood DLE**

Subacute cutaneous lupus erythematosus

Epidemiology

- **Female** predominance (4:1)
- More common in whites (vs. DLE)
- 30%–50% of patients w/ SCLE lesions will eventually meet criteria for SLE, but most usually only have mild disease

Pathogenesis

- Proposed mechanism: UVR-induced apoptosis → apoptotic bodies containing high levels of nuclear antigens (e.g., Ro, La, DNA) + reduced clearance of apoptotic cells (particularly in complement deficiency-related LE) → loss of immune tolerance → release of proinflammatory cytokines and production of ANAs, most importantly anti-Ro/SSA autoantibodies
- Genetic associations:
  - **HLA-B8** (strongest association), **HLA-DR3**, and others
  - Hereditary C2 and C4 deficiencies
- Antibodies
  - **Anti-Ro/SSA** (75%–90%)—of note, SSA plays role in cell survival after ultraviolet radiation and regulates inflammation
    - Thought to be **pathogenic in SCLE**
    - May cause clinical overlap w/ SjS
- Complement
  - SCLE is a/w **complement deficiencies**, especially deficiencies in the **early intrinsic pathway** (C1q/r/s, C2, and C4)

Clinical features

- Often has a chronic, relapsing course
- **Photosensitivity** prominent in 50%
- Two clinical variants:
  - Papulosquamous SCLE: psoriasiform plaques (Fig. 3.39)
  - Annular SCLE: scaly polycyclic annular plaques with central clearing
- Typical locations: sun-exposed areas **of lateral face (central face spared)**, neck, **V-chest**, and **upper back**/extremities
- Often heals w/ hypopigmentation, but **no scarring**
- May have clinical overlap w/ SjS (both have Ro/SSA autoantibodies)
- Systemic manifestations are common, but **only 30%–50% fully meet criteria for SLE**
  - **Arthritis/arthralgias** = most common systemic finding (up to 70%)

Laboratory testing

- Antibodies
  - **Anti-Ro/SSA** (75%–90%)

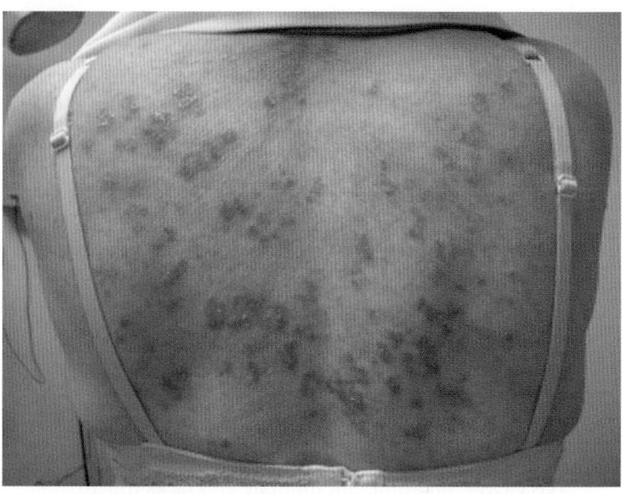

Fig. 3.39 Subacute cutaneous lupus erythematosus, papulosquamous. Psoriasiform lesions coalesce to form retiform arrays. (From Okon LG, Werth VP. Cutaneous lupus erythematosus: diagnosis and treatment. *Best Pract Res Clin Rheumatol*. 2013;27[3]:391–404.)

  - Anti-La (30%–40%)
  - ANA (60%–80%; usually in a speckled/particulate pattern)
- Other
  - Leukopenia (20%)

Histopathology

- Compact hyperkeratosis, prominent **epidermal atrophy, vacuolar interface** dermatitis w/ pigment incontinence, BMZ thickening, PV/PA lymphoid aggregates (limited to superficial dermis) w/ scattered plasma cells, clusters of CD123+ plasmacytoid dendritic cells, and **mucin** deposition
  - Lacks eosinophils and follicular plugging
- DIF:
  - Granular particulate IgG/IgM within the epidermis
  - (+) LBT in 60%–85% (usually not as thick or intensely stained as in DLE)

Treatments

- First line: **antimalarials and sun protection**
- Recalcitrant: may require other immunosuppressive meds

Drug-induced SCLE (DI-SCLE)

- **Skin always involved!**
- **Rare to have systemic involvement**
- **Photosensitive** papulosquamous eruption (often **psoriasiform to lichenoid**) w/ annular plaques on upper body and extensor upper extremities
- Antibodies: **anti-Ro/SSA (80%)**, anti-La/SSB
- Hundreds of drugs have now been implicated in DI-SCLE:
  - Most common: **HCTZ**, **terbinafine**, **TNF-α inhibitors** (may also cause drug-induced SLE), proton pump inhibitors (**PPI**), calcium channel blockers (**CCBs**), anti-epileptic agents, taxanes, griseofulvin
  - Less common: ACE inhibitors, β-blockers, statins, antihistamines, IFN-α and IFN-β, NSAIDs

SCLE-like syndromes

Neonatal lupus erythematosus (NLE)

- Epidemiology
  - **Female predominance** for NLE of skin (3:1) and cardiac NLE (2:1)
- Pathogenesis
  - Result of transplacental passage of maternal autoantibodies, most importantly **anti-Ro/SSA (99%)**
    - Autoantibodies can result in heart block requiring pacemaker
    - Unselected women w/ anti-Ro/SSA antibodies → 1%–2% risk of having child w/ NLE
    - Women w/ SLE or another defined CTD with anti-Ro/SSA antibodies → 15% risk having a child w/ NLE
    - Women who have a **prior child w/ NLE → 25% risk of NLE in subsequent children**
- Clinical features
  - Cutaneous findings:
    - Lesions arise within first weeks of life but usually not present at birth
    - Skin lesions (similar to adults w/ SCLE but more prominent facial involvement):
      - Photosensitivity
      - Periorbital erythema = **"raccoon eyes"**
      - **Annular, polycyclic erythematous plaques** w/ central clearing and raised red border, fine scale, typically located on scalp, neck, or face
      - Non-scarring
      - **Resolves w/ dyspigmentation and telangiectasias**
  - Systemic findings:
    - **Cardiac** (70% overall have some cardiac abnormality; **30–40% have congenital third-degree heart block**)
      - Heart block is **almost always present by birth**, developing *in utero* between 16 and 24 weeks gestation
      - Usually p/w **bradycardia and irreversible complete heart block (third degree)**
        - ➔ Occasionally p/w first- or second-degree heart block → may progress to complete heart block
    - Hepatobiliary disease (50%)
      - P/w transient conjugated hyperbilirubinemia in first weeks of life, or transient elevations of aminotransferases
    - Hematologic abnormalities
      - Thrombocytopenia
      - Neutropenia, lymphopenia, and hemolytic anemia
  - Mother
    - **50% of women with a child w/ NLE are asymptomatic at time of child's birth**
      - Half of mothers who are initially asymptomatic later develop SjS or SLE
- Histology
  - Same as SCLE
  - DIF: (+) LBT in 50%
- Laboratory testing
  - Autoantibodies
    - **Anti-Ro/SSA antibodies (99%)**
    - Anti-La/SSB and anti-U1RNP antibodies may be found in combination with anti-Ro/SSA antibodies (rarely present alone)
  - ↑ LFTs
  - Hematologic cytopenias (mainly thrombocytopenia)
- Treatment
  - Skin disease
    - Sun protection + topical CS
  - Cardiac disease
    - <u>*In utero*</u>:
      - **Prenatal systemic CS** may ↓ risk of developing congenital heart block
        - ➔ Does not decrease rate of cutaneous NLE, however
      - **Hydroxychloroquine throughout pregnancy** → ↓ risk of a child w/ cardiac NLE for women w/ SLE and anti-Ro/SSA (+) women with a previous child affected by NLE
    - <u>Neonatal</u>:
      - Once complete heart block occurs, it is **irreversible**
      - **Pacemaker** required for heart block in two thirds of patients w/ cardiac NLE
  - Hematologic and LFT abnormalities
    - Usually no treatment needed
- Prognosis/clinical course
  - Children with NLE may be at ↑ risk of developing SLE or autoimmunity later in life
  - Skin disease
    - Lesions **resolve without scarring** by ~6 months (as maternal antibodies clear from neonatal circulation)
    - **Residual atrophy, dyspigmentation, and telangiectasias** persist for months to years
  - Cardiac disease
    - Low-grade AV blocks are reversible and sometimes normalize without therapy
    - **Complete (third-degree) heart block is irreversible**
    - Cardiac NLE has **20%–30% mortality rate**
  - Hematologic and LFT abnormalities
    - Transient with spontaneous resolution within 4 to 6 months

Complement deficiencies

- Epidemiology
  - <u>Primary C2 deficiency</u>
    - **Most common** hereditary complement disorder
    - Only 10%–20% with homozygous C2 deficiency will develop SLE (**low risk**)
      - Since C2 deficiency is more common than other early complement deficiencies, it is the **most common cause of complement deficiency-associated SLE**
  - <u>Primary C1q and C4 deficiencies</u>
    - Homozygous deficiencies are **very rare**, but are associated with a **very high risk** of developing autoimmune disease
    - **SLE risk** with homozygous mutations: **C1q (~90%) > C1r/s > C4 > C2 (10%–20%)**

- Pathogenesis
  - UV-damaged apoptotic keratinocytes express autoantigens (esp. Ro/SSA) on cell surface
  - Early components of complement normally help clear out these apoptotic keratinocytes
  - **Deficiencies in early components (C1, C4, C2)** of classic complement pathway → **impaired phagocytic clearance** of apoptotic bodies containing high levels of autoantigens → loss of immune tolerance and autoantibody-mediated inflammation
- Clinical
  - Deficiency of any early classical complement component (C1, C2, C4) a/w ↑ **risk for SLE and infections w/ encapsulated bacteria**
  - C2 deficiency-associated SLE (**most common but least severe**):
    - Adult onset (average 30 yo)
    - F > M
    - SLE w/ less severe systemic disease (e.g., mild or absent renal disease)
    - Prominent photosensitivity and SCLE lesions
    - ↑ Bacterial infections w/ encapsulated bacteria, especially *Streptococcus pneumonia*
  - C1q/r/s and C4 deficiency-associated SLE (less common but more severe)
    - Childhood onset
    - **Severe, recalcitrant renal disease**
    - Photosensitivity with CCLE or SCLE
    - Palmoplantar keratoses (C4 deficiency only)
    - ↑ Risk of infection with encapsulated bacteria and candida
  - Anti-C1q autoantibodies (acquired)
    - Arise in 30%–50% of SLE patients, **a/w lupus nephritis**
    - Seen in ~100% of patients w/ **hypocomplementemic urticarial vasculitis (HUV)**
- Laboratory findings
  - Low or absent ANA titers
  - Anti-Ro/SSA antibodies in majority
  - ↓ **Complement levels (screening test is CH50**, which is markedly decreased)

Acute cutaneous lupus erythematosus (ACLE)

- 60% of SLE patients develop a malar rash
- Of the three major cutaneous lupus subtypes, **ACLE is most strongly a/w SLE**
- Classically p/w localized **(malar) erythema** = **"butterfly rash"** (Fig. 3.40); a **transient** eruption following sun exposure lasting hours to weeks
  - Classically involves the nasal bridge and bilateral malar eminence, **sparing the melolabial folds** (in contrast to facial erythema of DM), but may also involve the forehead, periorbital areas, and sides of neck
  - Morphology ranges from mild erythema to edematous lesions
  - Lesions may develop scaling, papules, erosions, **poikiloderma**, atrophy, or dyspigmentation that can help distinguish it from other facial rashes
  - Malar discoid lesions do not count as a "butterfly rash"
- Butterfly rash may occasionally be accompanied by a more generalized photodistributed eruption involving the **V-neck**, **upper back**, **extremities**, and dorsal hands, **classically sparing the knuckles** (in contrast to the confluent macular violaceous erythema [CMVE] of DM)

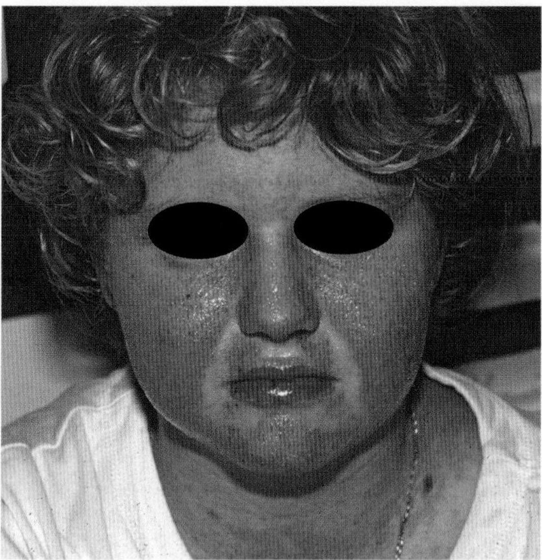

Fig. 3.40 Patient with severe acute lupus erythematosus, with marked erythema in a photodistribution. (From the William Weston Collection, Aurora, CO. In: Fitzpatrick JE, High WA, Kyle WL. *Urgent Care Dermatology: Symptom-Based Diagnosis*. Philadelphia: Elsevier; 2018.)

- Histopathology: vacuolar interface dermatitis, dermal edema, and **sparse** perivascular lymphocytic infiltrate limited to upper dermis
  - Lacks follicular plugging and other dermal changes
- DIF: (+) LBT
- Laboratory tests: **ACLE is highly a/w SLE → perform same lab studies as in SLE** to search for end-organ damage
- Treatment: skin lesions of ACLE respond to treatment for systemic symptoms; for recalcitrant skin disease, refer to treatment algorithm presented in DLE section
  - Cutaneous flares tend to correlate w/ systemic disease activity

Other rare cutaneous lupus variants

Bullous SLE

- Epidemiology
  - Female predominance
  - Predominately **African Americans**
- Pathogenesis
  - Antibodies against NC1 and NC2 domains of **type VII collagen (same as EBA)**
  - a/w HLA-DR2
- Clinical
  - By definition, **patients must meet American College of Rheumatology criteria for diagnosis of SLE** in order to term it "bullous SLE"
  - Widespread, symmetric eruption of **tense, subepidermal bullae** on erythematous-to-urticarial base (Fig. 3.41)
  - Involves both sun-exposed and non-exposed areas
  - Typical locations: face, neck, upper trunk, and proximal extremities
    - Mucosal involvement is common
  - Systemic symptoms same as SLE

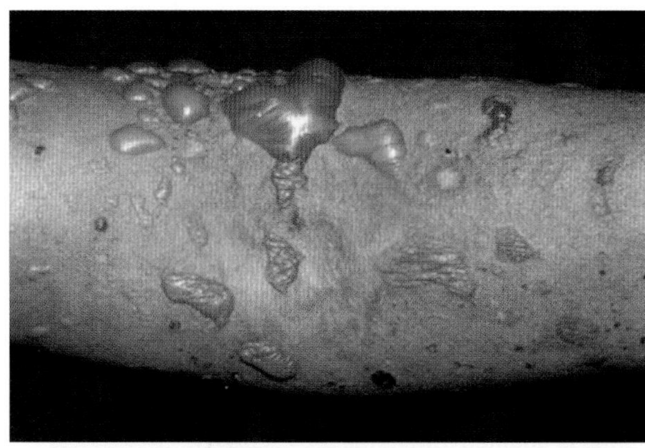

Fig. 3.41 Bullous lupus erythematosus. (From James WD, Elston DM, Treat JR, Rosenbach MA, Neuhaus IM. Connective tissue diseases. In: *Andrews' Diseases of the Skin*. 13th ed. Philadelphia: Elsevier; 2020:157–183.)

- Histopathology
  - **Subepidermal bulla with neutrophils at DEJ** and in dermal papillae
  - DIF: multiple immunoreactants **(IgG, C3, IgA, IgM) present in granular pattern along BMZ, along with linear deposition of IgG and/or C3**
- Laboratory testing
  - Salt-split skin IIF: **dermal deposition with IgG**
  - ELISA: autoantibodies to collagen VII
  - **ANA (+) in ~100%**
    - Frequently positive for dsDNA, Sm, Ro/SSA, and La/SSB
  - Also, perform standard labs as per SLE to search for end-organ damage; 50% of cases a/w lupus nephritis
- Treatment
  - **Dapsone (ToC)** → dramatic response within 1 to 2 days
    - Differentiates bullous SLE from EBA!
  - Immunosuppressant meds may be needed for recalcitrant disease
- Prognosis/clinical course
  - Often a/w systemic lupus flare
  - Lesions of bullous LE respond dramatically to dapsone with cessation of new lesions and healing over a few days

Rowell's syndrome

- Targetoid lesions clinically resembling EM, arising in setting of ACLE, SCLE, or DLE; **typically Ro/SSA (+)**

Toxic epidermal necrolysis-like lupus erythematosus

- Triggered by excessive UV exposure in patients with preexisting ACLE or SCLE

Systemic lupus erythematosus (SLE)

Epidemiology

- 80% of SLE patients will have skin findings
  - ACLE is the cutaneous phenotype most strongly a/w systemic lupus (71%; 60% with malar rash), but patients with any form of cutaneous lupus may develop SLE
  - Also, patients with SLE may have any combination of the various forms of cutaneous lupus
- Female predominance
- **African Americans have a 4× ↑ incidence**, earlier age of onset, and higher mortality

Pathogenesis

- UV → ↑ IL-1, IFN-γ, TNF-α, and AMPs, as well as NETosis; other major cytokines: B-lymphocyte stimulator (BLyS), IL-6, IL-17, IL-18
  - UV → CCL5 and CXCL8 → ↑WBC and adhesion molecules/endothelial cell activation
- ↑ IFN in lupus for various reasons → ↑CXCL9 and CXCL10 and dendritic cells (may present keratinocyte-derived antigens to CD8+ T cells; produce more IFN)
- CXCL9 and CXCL10 → ↑CXCR3(+) CD4+ and CD8+ T cells and immature plasmacytoid dendritic cells = interface lichenoid reaction
- Genetics
  - Strong genetic component
  - Susceptibility loci conferring the highest risk for SLE:
    - Genes encoding **early complement components**—C1Q, C2, C4B, C4A; ITGAM (cellular adhesion, immune complex clearance)
    - Innate immunity (TREX1, TYK2, IRF5, STAT4 [also apoptosis])
    - B- and T-cell function (HLA-DR, CTLA4, PTPN22, STAT4)
- Environmental triggers: **sunlight** (UVB > UVA), **cigarettes**, infections, vitamin D deficiency, estrogen

Clinical

- SLE diagnostic criteria (ACR criteria for SLE)
  - Need to satisfy **four items** (at least one clinical and one immunologic item) <u>OR</u> have biopsy-proven nephritis compatible w/ SLE in the presence of ANA or anti-dsDNA antibodies (Fig. 3.42)
- Cutaneous manifestations of SLE
  - <u>**Lupus-specific skin findings**</u>:
    - ACLE
    - SCLE
    - CCLE (11%)
    - Rowell's syndrome
    - TEN-like LE
    - Bullous SLE
  - <u>**Non-specific skin findings suggestive of SLE**</u>:
    - Diffuse non-scarring alopecia (31%)
    - Periungal telangiectasias and erythema
      - Dermoscopy: **"wandering" dilated glomeruloid loops** (in contrast, DM and SSc both have symmetric dilation and dropout of vessels; Osler-Weber-Rendu has ectasia of half of the capillary loop)
    - Non-specific mucosal ulcers (26%)
    - Vasculitis:
      - **Leukocytoclastic vasculitis (LCV**; most common)
      - Urticarial vasculitis (especially **HUV**)
      - Polyarteritis nodosa (PAN)-like lesions
      - **Palisaded neutrophilic granulomatous dermatitis (PNGD)**/interstitial granulomatous dermatitis and arthritis (IGDA)
    - Cutaneous signs of antiphospholipid syndrome (APLS):
      - Livedo reticularis (10%); LR + ischemic strokes = **Sneddon syndrome**

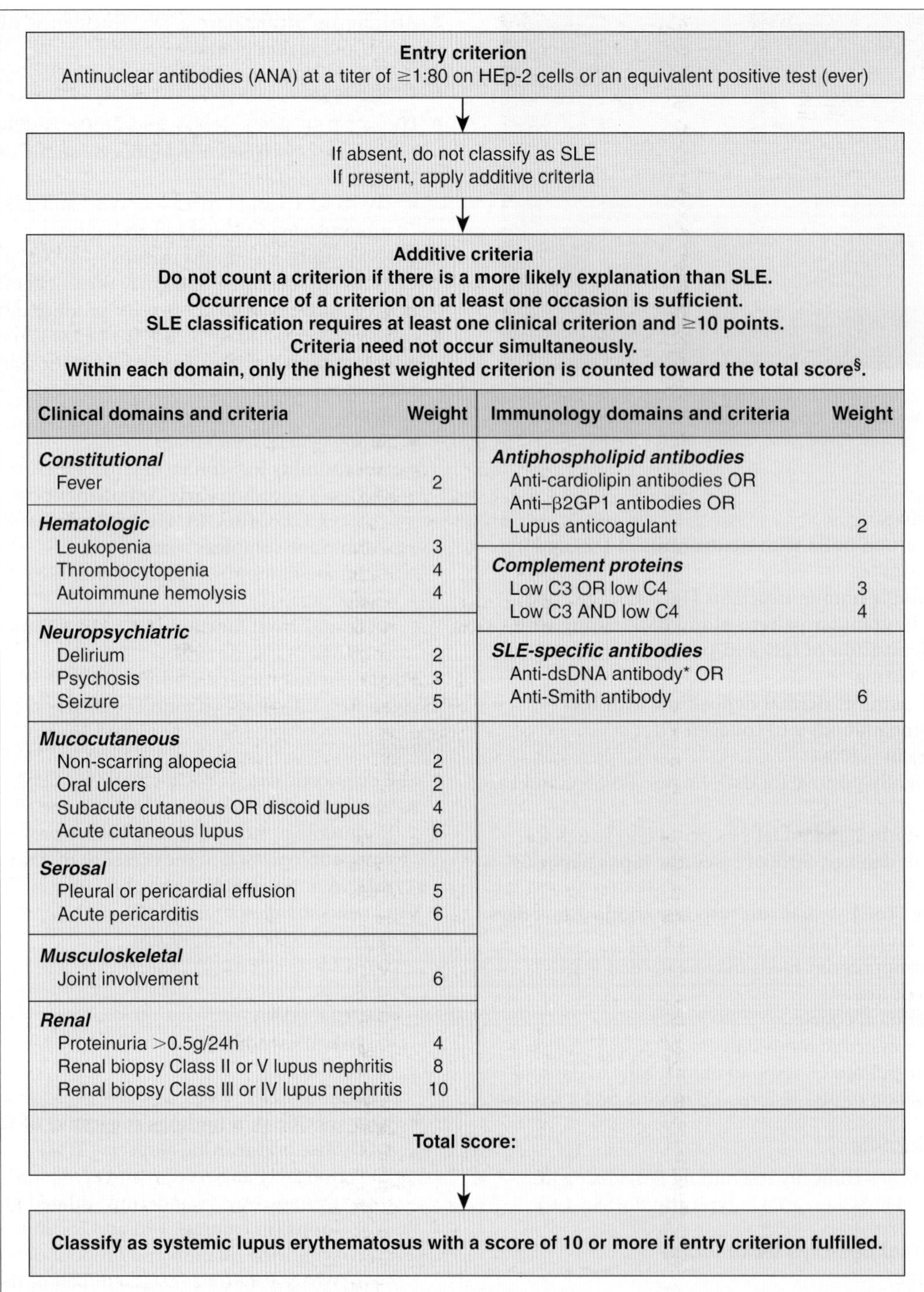

Entry criterion
Antinuclear antibodies (ANA) at a titer of ≥1:80 on HEp-2 cells or an equivalent positive test (ever)

↓

If absent, do not classify as SLE
If present, apply additive criteria

↓

Additive criteria
Do not count a criterion if there is a more likely explanation than SLE.
Occurrence of a criterion on at least one occasion is sufficient.
SLE classification requires at least one clinical criterion and ≥10 points.
Criteria need not occur simultaneously.
Within each domain, only the highest weighted criterion is counted toward the total score§.

Clinical domains and criteria	Weight	Immunology domains and criteria	Weight
Constitutional		***Antiphospholipid antibodies***	
Fever	2	Anti-cardiolipin antibodies OR	
Hematologic		Anti–β2GP1 antibodies OR	
Leukopenia	3	Lupus anticoagulant	2
Thrombocytopenia	4	***Complement proteins***	
Autoimmune hemolysis	4	Low C3 OR low C4	3
Neuropsychiatric		Low C3 AND low C4	4
Delirium	2	***SLE-specific antibodies***	
Psychosis	3	Anti-dsDNA antibody* OR	
Seizure	5	Anti-Smith antibody	6
Mucocutaneous			
Non-scarring alopecia	2		
Oral ulcers	2		
Subacute cutaneous OR discoid lupus	4		
Acute cutaneous lupus	6		
Serosal			
Pleural or pericardial effusion	5		
Acute pericarditis	6		
Musculoskeletal			
Joint involvement	6		
Renal			
Proteinuria >0.5g/24h	4		
Renal biopsy Class II or V lupus nephritis	8		
Renal biopsy Class III or IV lupus nephritis	10		

Total score:

↓

Classify as systemic lupus erythematosus with a score of 10 or more if entry criterion fulfilled.

Fig. 3.42 Classification criteria for systemic lupus erythematosus *(SLE)*. Of note, neurological disease occurs in 18% of SLE patients, serositis in 19%, leukopenia in 35%, thrombocytopenia in 16%, APLS in 10%, lymphadenopathy in 9%, autoimmune hemolytic anemia in 3%, fever in 31%, and arthritis in 85%. *Anti-β2GPI*, Anti-β2 glycoprotein I; *anti-dsDNA*, anti-double-stranded DNA. *, In an assay with ≥ 90% specificity against relevant disease controls. §, additional criteria items within the same domain will not be counted. (From Aringer M, Costenbader K, Daikh D, et al. 2019 European League against Rheumatism/American College of Rheumatology classification criteria for systemic lupus erythematosus. *Arthritis Rheumatol*. 2019;71[9]:1400–1412.)

- Atrophie blanche-like lesions
- **Degos-like lesions**
- Ulcerations
- Purpura fulminans and retiform purpura due to catastrophic APLS

- **Papulonodular mucinosis**
  - Highly a/w SLE (75% of cases)!
  - Asymptomatic skin-colored to red papules w/ central depression and pigmentation; favors V-neck, upper chest/back, and upper extremities

- Others:
  - Secondary Raynaud phenomenon (37%), **multiple eruptive dermatofibromas**, palmar erythema, Sweet-like neutrophilic dermatosis, calcinosis cutis
- SLE and pregnancy
  - Course may be stable, worsen, or improve
  - Patients w/ lupus nephritis are at ↑ risk of complications
  - Postpartum period is highest risk
  - Fetal complications
    - Preterm birth
    - Preeclampsia, especially w/ lupus nephritis
    - Anti-cardiolipin antibodies → ↑ **risk of fetal loss**
    - **NLE** in patients w/ **anti-Ro/SSA** and anti-La/SSB
  - Management in pregnancy
    - Continuation of hydroxychloroquine and low-dose steroids
    - Consider AZA
    - Anticoagulation for APLS

Histopathology

- Please refer to sections on types of lupus-specific skin lesions

Laboratory testing

- Routine labs: ↑ inflammatory markers (ESR and CRP), hemolytic anemia (Coombs positive), leukopenia or lymphopenia, thrombocytopenia, proteinuria, and hematuria
- Complement abnormalities: ↓ **total complement levels (CH50)**, **autoantibodies against C1q** (a/w severe **SLE nephritis** and HUV)
- Serologies:
  - **ANA (99%)**
  - Anti-ssDNA antibodies
    - Neither sensitive nor specific for SLE
  - **Anti-dsDNA (60%)**
    - Not sensitive, but **highly specific** (95%) for SLE
    - Useful in **monitoring** disease activity (esp. **lupus nephritis)**
    - Correlates strongly w/ **LBT from sun-protected skin**
    - Likely contribute to pathogenesis of disease
  - **Anti-Smith antibodies** (10%–30%)
    - Not sensitive, but **highly specific** for SLE
  - Anti-U1RNP (50%)
    - Lower titers in SLE than in MCTD (most important association)
  - Anti-Ro/SSA antibodies (50%)
  - Anti-histone antibodies
    - **Drug-induced SLE** (>95%)
  - Anti-RNP (ribosomal P) antibodies
    - High specificity but low sensitivity for SLE
    - a/w **Neuropsychiatric SLE**
    - Not currently used in clinical practice
  - Antiphospholipid antibodies
    - Anti-β2-glycoprotein IgM/IgG/IgA
    - Anti-anticardiolipin IgM/IgG/IgA
    - Lupus anticoagulant activity

Treatment

- Photoprotection in all patients
- Mild active disease (no life-threatening visceral organ involvement): **hydroxychloroquine** (≤5 mg/kg/day actual body weight) +/− NSAIDs; chloroquine if not working; can add quinacrine to either
- Moderate-severe active disease lacking renal involvement: prednisone + steroid-sparing agent (AZA, MTX, MMF, **belimumab** [monoclonal human antibody that inactivates BLyS causing apoptosis and inhibition of B-cell maturation], anifrolumab)
- Severe active disease w/ renal (or other organ) involvement: **prednisone (high dose)** versus IV solumedrol + **cyclophosphamide** or MMF (depending on nephritis class)
- Moderate-severe recalcitrant disease: rituximab, belimumab, volvosporin

Prognosis/clinical course

- Childhood onset has a higher risk of lupus nephritis and mortality
- 10-year survival: ~90%
- Most common causes of death:
  - First 5 years: inflammatory lesions of SLE and infection
  - Beyond 5 years: arterial (e.g., MI) and venous (i.e., deep venous thrombosis/pulmonary embolism) **thromboses**
    - ↑ Risk of thrombosis w/ anticardiolipin antibodies and OCPs

Drug-induced SLE (DI-SLE)

- Lupus-like syndrome related to continuous drug exposure (**usually > 1 year after drug initiation**) that typically resolves within 4 to 6 weeks of discontinuation of offending drug
- Serologically characterized by **(+) anti-histone antibodies (>95%)** and **(−) dsDNA** autoantibodies
  - Positivity for ANAs may persist for up to 12 months, even in absence of clinical symptoms!
- Patients generally do not meet ACR criteria for SLE
- DI-SLE typically **lacks skin findings** and has milder systemic involvement **(lacks renal and CNS findings)** than idiopathic SLE
- Most common clinical findings:
  - **Arthritis/arthralgia (90%)**
  - Myalgia (50%)
  - Serositis (pericarditis, pleuritic)
  - Fever and weight loss
- Most important implicated drugs:
  - High risk: **procainamide, hydralazine**
    - a/w **slow acetylators**
  - Medium and low risk: quinidine, **methyldopa, INH**, chlorpromazine, **D-penicillamine**, propylthiouracil, PUVA, **minocycline, TNF-α inhibitors** (infliximab and etanercept > adalimumab), interferon
    - D-penicillamine may "unmask" true SLE
    - **Minocycline differs from classic DI-SLE:**
      - Often negative for anti-histone antibodies
      - **(+) antineutrophil cytoplasmic antibody (ANCA)** against myeloperoxidase (MPO) or elastase
    - **TNF-α inhibitors differ from classic DI-SLE:**
      - Anti-dsDNA antibodies frequently positive (> anti-histone)
      - ↑↑↑ **Skin involvement** (malar rash, photosensitivity, SCLE and DLE lesions)

Lupus-related diseases

Jessner's lymphocytic infiltrate of skin

- Epidemiology
  - Primarily middle-aged adults with no sex predilection
- Pathogenesis
  - Photosensitive eruption
  - Possibly a variant of LE, on a spectrum w/ tumid LE and REM
- Clinical
  - Red papules or plaques (often **annular w/ central clearing**) (Fig. 3.43)
  - Absent epidermal changes
  - Typical locations: **head, neck, and upper back**
  - Duration: weeks to months
  - No systemic manifestations
- Histopathology
  - Similar to tumid LE and REM, but with a predominance of suppressor **CD8+ T cells** and **↓ mucin**
  - Absent interface dermatitis
  - Superficial and **deep dense PV/PA lymphocytic infiltrate**
  - DIF: negative
- Laboratory testing
  - No associated laboratory abnormalities
- Treatment: sun protection, antimalarials
- Prognosis/clinical course: resolves spontaneously without sequelae

Reticular erythematous mucinosis

- Middle-aged females often w/ **history of tanning bed use**
- Likely variant of LE, on spectrum w/ tumid LE
- P/w persistent, **photoaggravated** (UVA and UVB) eruption consisting of erythematous papules or plaques on **middle of chest/back**, typically in a reticular configuration
- Exacerbating factors: OCPs, menses, pregnancy, heat, and sweating
- Histopathology: same as tumid lupus; DIF negative (most cases)

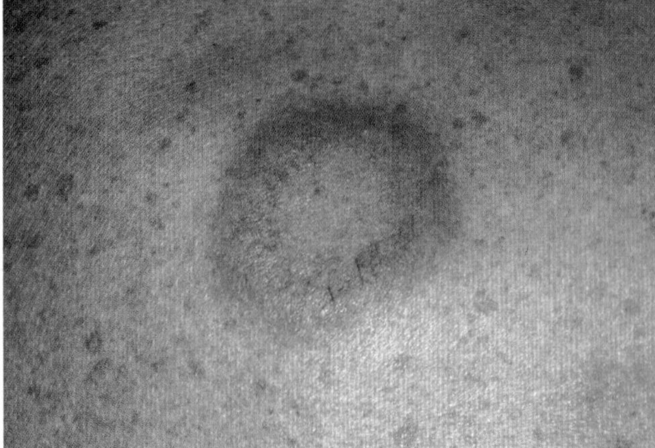

Fig. 3.43 Lymphocytic infiltrate of Jessner. Annular erythematous plaque on the trunk. (From James WD, Elston DM, McMahon PJ. Cutaneous lymphoid hyperplasia, cutaneous T-cell lymphoma, other malignant lymphomas, and allied diseases. In: *Andrews' Diseases of the Skin Clinical Atlas*. Philadelphia: Elsevier; 2018:501–516.)

- Laboratory testing: no associated laboratory abnormalities
- Treatment: sun protection, resolution within 4 to 8 weeks w/ antimalarials

Other autoimmune connective tissue diseases and sclerosing dermopathies

Dermatomyositis (DM)

Epidemiology

- Female predominance (2:1); African Americans > Caucasians
- **Bimodal peaks**: childhood (4–14 years) and adulthood (40–60 years)
  - ~25% of adult-onset patients have underlying malignancy
  - Juvenile dermatomyositis (JDM) is **not** associated with malignancy

Pathogenesis

- Evidence of issues with humoral immunity (**B-cell autoantibody;** e.g., myositis-specific autoantibodies) and cellular immunity/apoptosis (e.g., CD8+ lymphocytes in skin and muscle); both environmental and genetic factors contribute to development of disease
- Genetic predisposition:
  - Polymorphisms in various HLA alleles (e.g., HLA-DR3 and HLA-B8 with JDM, HLA-DR52 with anti-Jo-1 antibodies)
  - TNF-α308A polymorphism (a/w JDM) → ↑ thrombospondin-1 (a potent anti-angiogenic factor) → ↑ occlusion of capillaries
- Environmental factors (e.g., **malignancy**, UV, viral infections, drugs) trigger a humoral autoimmune process in genetically susceptible individuals → differences in the specific autoantibodies account for the different clinical manifestations
  - 80% of patients with **cancer-associated DM** have antibodies against **TIF-1γ** (p155) or **NXP-2** (p140)
  - Drug-induced dermatomyositis: **hydroxyurea (most common, >50%), statins**, TNF-α inhibitors, checkpoint inhibitors (ipilimumab), D-penicillamine, cyclophosphamide, BCG vaccine, NSAIDs
    - Drug-induced DM is separated into two groups:
      - <u>Hydroxyurea-induced DM</u>: much longer latency period **(average 60 months)** after drug initiation; **myositis never seen** (0%); only 16% have (+) ANA
      - <u>Non-hydroxyurea–induced DM</u>: occurs within 2 months after drug initiation; **80% have muscle weakness/myositis**; ANA usually (+) (54%)
      - Both groups have pathognomonic skin lesions of DM (heliotrope rash, Gottron's papules), and may have (+) ANA
      - Both forms resolve within 1 to 2 months of discontinuation

Clinical features

- <u>Muscle disease (no longer required for diagnosis!)</u>:
  - Slowly progressive, **symmetric proximal muscle weakness (extensors > flexors)**
    - Biopsies = perifascicular atrophy

        - Generally **lacks muscle pain** (myalgias)
        - Typically affects **quadraceps, triceps**, shoulders, hip girdle, and neck flexors → **difficulty walking up stairs**, standing up from sitting position, or **brushing hair**
        - Esophageal/oropharyngeal muscles → dysphagia, aspiration pneumonia
        - Cardiac disease (common)
            - Mostly subclinical EKG abnormalities
            - Clinically overt disease (congestive heart failure, complete heart block, myocarditis, dangerous arrhythmias, and coronary artery disease) is rare but life-threating
        - Diaphragm weakness (rare but life-threatening)
- Classic skin findings:
    - **Gottron's papules (pathognomonic)**
        - Lichenoid papules **overlying knuckles** (> other extensor joints) (Fig. 3.44)
        - Less common than Gottron's sign (macular erythema overlying joints)
    - Symmetric confluent macular violaceous erythema (CMVE)
        - Facial erythema w/ **malar involvement, usually involving the melolabial folds** (vs. nasolabial sparing in lupus)
        - Eyelids = **heliotrope sign** +/− periorbital edema
            - Arises as a result of inflammation of underlying orbicularis oculi muscle, NOT the skin!
        - Overlying joints = **Gottron's sign**
            - Elbows, knees, DIP, PIP, and MCP joints
        - Overlying extensor tendons of hands and forearms = linear extensor erythema

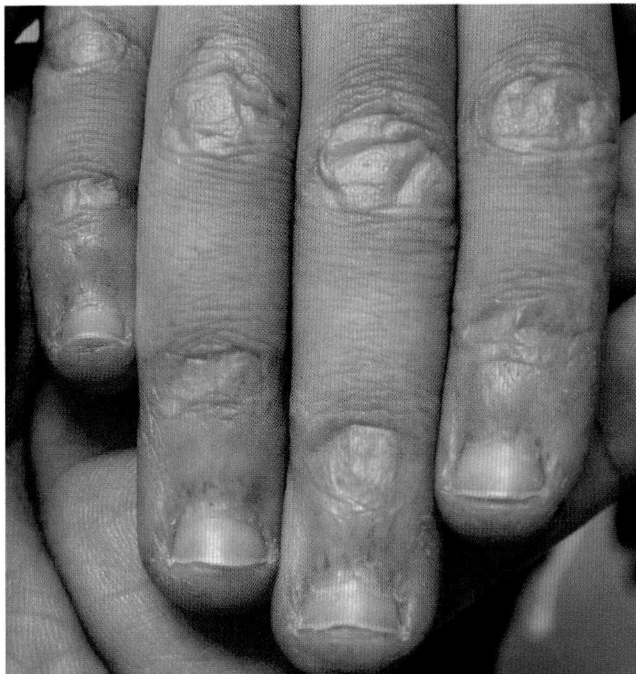

Fig. 3.44 Gottron's papules of dermatomyositis. Classic skin lesions over the distal and proximal interphalangeal joints with coalescence of pink–violet lichenoid papules. (From James WD, Elston DM, Treat JR, Rosenbach MA, Neuhaus IM. Connective tissue diseases. In: *Andrews' Diseases of the Skin*, 13th ed. Philadelphia: Elsevier; 2020:157–183.)

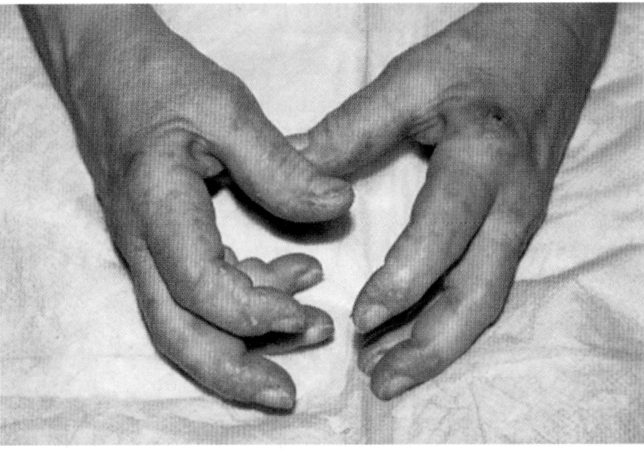

Fig. 3.45 "Mechanic's hands" in dermatomyositis. (From James WD, Elston DM, Treat JR, Rosenbach MA, Neuhaus IM. Connective tissue diseases. In: *Andrews' Diseases of the Skin*. 13th ed. Philadelphia: Elsevier; 2020:157–183.)

        - Photodistributed CMVE or **poikiloderma** (hyperpigmentation, hypopigmentation, telangiectasias, and atrophy)
        - Chest ("V-neck sign"), upper back ("Shawl sign"), lateral thigh ("Holster sign")
- Other common skin findings:
    - **Mechanic's hands**
        - Rough, hyperkeratosis and fissuring of the lateral and palmar side of fingers, usually more radial digits involved (Fig. 3.45)
        - Strongly a/w anti-MDA5 antibodies and **anti-synthetase syndrome**
    - Nail changes
        - **"Ragged" cuticles**
        - Proximal nailfold w/ **dilated capillary loops** alternating with areas of **vessel dropout** (Fig. 3.46)
        - Periungual erythema
    - Pruritus—often severe (especially on scalp)
    - Psoriasiform scalp dermatitis and non-scarring alopecia
- Less common skin findings:
    - Calcinosis cutis

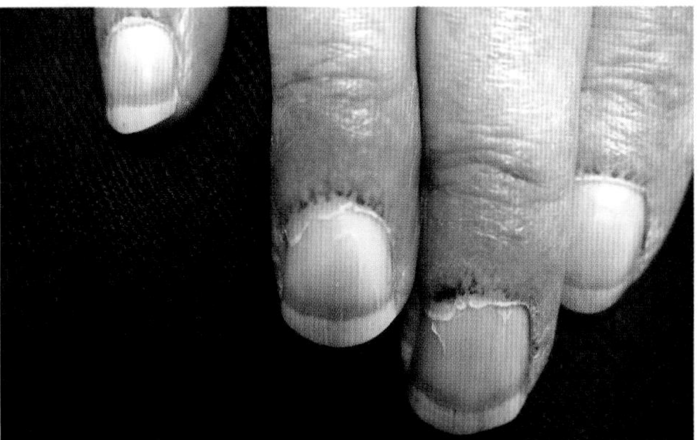

Fig. 3.46 Cuticular hypertrophy, splinter hemorrhages, and periungual telangiectasias in a patient with dermatomyositis. (From Vleugels RA, Callen JP. Dermatomyositis. In: Callen JP, Jorizzo JL, Bolognia JL, Piette WW, Zone JJ. *Dermatological Signs of Internal Disease.* 4th ed. Philadelphia: Elsevier; 2009:11–19.)

- Much more common in JDM (25%–70%) than adults (<20%)
  - a/w anti-p140 (NXP-2) autoantibodies in JDM
- Favors elbows, knees, and buttocks
- a/w fingertip ulcers, pain, loss of function, and prolonged course

- Palmar papules
  - Erythematous palmar papules or macules +/− overlying hyperkeratosis/ulceration; **painful** (unlike Gottron's papules)
  - a/w **anti-CADM-140/MDA-5** antibodies
- Clinical features overlapping w/ PRP (Wong-type dermatomyositis, more common in Asians, follicular hyperkeratosis)
- **Vasculitis (never a good sign!)**: more common in JDM
  - In adults → a/w **malignancy**
  - JDM w/ severe systemic vasculitis = **Banker variant JDM**
    - Cutaneous **ulcerations**, muscle infarction, GI involvement (hemorrhage, ulceration, perforation), **widespread calcinosis**, and a **severe course** w/ poor response to therapy
- Others: **flagellate erythema** (a/w anti-Mi2 antibodies), panniculitis (a/w anti-MDA5 antibodies), lipodystrophy, hypertrichosis, Raynaud phenomenon (a/w antisynthetase syndrome), oral mucosal changes (a/w anti-TIF1 antibodies), necrotic/ulcerative lesions (due to cutaneous vasculopathy; **anti-MDA5 antibodies**), and erythroderma (a/w malignancy)

- Other common (non-muscular) systemic findings:
  - Pulmonary disease (15%–65%)
    - p/w diffuse **interstitial lung disease** (ILD) of varying severity
    - Rapidly progressive ILD → a/w **anti-synthetase** and **anti-CADM-140/MDA5** autoantibodies
  - GI involvement (up to 37% of JDM cases): dysphagia, dysmotility, GI infraction
  - Arthralgia and/or non-erosive arthritis

Classification (Box 3.6)

- Adult-onset DM
  - Classic DM
    - Slowly progressive symmetric, proximal muscle weakness w/ classic skin findings
  - CADM (amyopathic or hypomyopathic)
    - Classic skin findings **without clinical muscle** disease
    - a/w **CADM-140 (MDA5)** and **TIF1-γ (p155)** autoantibodies
      - When a/w CADM-140 → **rapidly progressive ILD**
  - Cancer-associated myositis (CAM)
    - May p/w classic DM or CADM
    - Associated with: ↑ **age** (fifth to sixth decades most common), **rapid disease onset, skin necrosis,** periungal erythema, markedly elevated ESR or CK, lack of antisynthetase syndrome features, and lack of Raynaud phenomenon
    - Boards Fodder: **TIF1-γ (p155)** or **NXP-2 (p140) autoantibodies** are present in 80% of all cancer-associated DM!
    - Most common cancers:
      - **Ovarian** (classic exam answer!) and **GI** (colon > other) cancer are overrepresented
      - Nasopharyngeal carcinoma overrepresented in Asians
      - Others: breast, lung, pancreatic, and non-Hodgkin's lymphoma
    - Timing:
      - Malignancy may be discovered before, after, or at the same time as the diagnosis of DM
      - Cancers diagnosed before DM precede diagnosis by ≤ 2 years
      - **Most cancers are detected within 1–2 years** of DM diagnosis
      - **Risk for most cancers returns to normal 3 years after diagnosis** (exceptions = pancreatic and colorectal cancers → risk remains elevated beyond 5 years)
  - **Antisynthetase syndrome**
    - Antisynthetase autoantibodies (**Jo-1**, PL-7, PL-12, OJ, EJ)
    - Acute disease onset
    - Constitutional symptoms
    - Raynaud phenomenon
    - **Mechanics hands**
    - Non-erosive arthritis
    - **ILD**
  - DM overlap syndromes
    - Definition: DM + other CTD
    - Autoantibodies suggestive of overlap
      - Anti-U1-RNP = mixed CTD
      - Anti-Ku = PM overlapping with either SLE, SjS, or scleroderma
      - Anti-PM/Scl (PM-1) = DM/PM + scleroderma ("sclerodermatomyositis")
- Juvenile DM
  - DM in patients < 16 yo (average 7 yo); F > M (2–5:1)
  - **JDM is not a/w ↑risk malignancy!**
  - Important autoantibodies in JDM (some antibodies may have different associations in kids vs. adults):
    - Anti-CADM-140 (MDA5) → a/w ILD in kids
    - **Anti-p140 (NXP-2)** → a/w **calcinosis and contractures** in kids but NO increase in malignancy
  - Variants:
    - **Classic JDM (Brunsting variant):**
      - Most common (90%)
      - Gradual onset of classic skin and muscle disease

Box 3.6 Dermatomyositis (DM) Classification

Adult-onset DM

- Classic DM
- Cancer-associated myositis (CAM)
- DM overlap syndrome
- Clinically amyopathic DM (CADM)
  - Amyopathic DM
  - Hypomyopathic DM

Juvenile DM

- Classic DM
- Clinically amyopathic DM (CADM)
  - Amyopathic DM
  - Hypomyopathic DM

- ♦ **Frequent calcinosis cutis** → favors sites of trauma (fingers, elbows, knees, and buttocks); may ulcerate
- ♦ CS responsive
- o **Vasculopathic/ulcerative JDM (Banker variant):**
  - ♦ Fortunately rare (<10%)
  - ♦ Rapid onset of severe muscle disease
  - ♦ Severe vasculitis w/ cutaneous ulcerations, LR, severe periungal capillary alterations, muscle infarction; GI ulceration, pneumatosis, and perforation
  - ♦ Recalcitrant to CS therapy, **poor prognosis**

Histopathology

- **Subtle** vacuolar interface w/ rare scattered necrotic keratinocytes (much less keratinocyte death compared to other interface dermatitides), epidermal atrophy, ↑ **BMZ** material, **sparse** PV/PA lymphocytic inflammation, and **massive dermal mucin** deposition
- DIF (non-specific): granular deposition of immunoglobulins and C3 at DEJ (50%) and on colloid bodies

Laboratory testing

- (+) ANA (40%)
- ↑↑ Muscle enzymes (**CK, aldolase**)
  - ▪ CK is a more sensitive marker of muscle involvement in DM, but there can be a discordant elevation in aldolase w/ normal CK levels
- Electromyography (EMG)
- Imaging: MRI or contrast-induced ultrasound
- Muscle biopsy (gold standard)
- Myositis-specific autoantibodies (see Table 3.11)
- If anti-MDA5 antibody (+)—PFTs, DLCO, high resolution CT scan
- If high risk for malignancy—detailed screening, whole body imaging, EGD/colonoscopy

Treatment

- <u>Skin-limited disease</u>:
  - ▪ First line: photoprotection, topical CS and calcineurin inhibitors +/− antimalarials
    - o Caution w/ antimalarials → ↓ efficacy and ↑ risk of cutaneous drug eruptions in DM, relative to lupus
  - ▪ Second line: MTX (high dose, fast onset), MMF (high dose, helps with ILD), IVIG, cyclosporine, rituximab (particularly in severe skin disease w/ ulceration)
  - ▪ Calcinosis cutis: **diltiazem**, surgical excision; early aggressive treatment of JDM → ↓ risk calcinosis cutis
  - ▪ Disease monitoring:
    - o Re-check muscle enzymes and clinical exam q2–3 months → if muscle disease arises → initiate systemic steroids
    - o Physical exams q4–6 months to screen for malignancy for the first 2–3 years after diagnosis
- <u>Skin + muscle disease</u>
  - ▪ First line: **systemic CS**, MTX, and AZA
  - ▪ Second line: **IVIG** (increased risk of thromboembolic events), MMF, cyclosporine, cyclophosphamide, rituximab

Prognosis/clinical course

- Adult DM
  - ▪ **Most common causes of death** = malignancy, ischemic heart disease, and pulmonary complications
- JDM
  - ▪ Prior to the availability of CS, JDM had poor prognosis: one third of children died, one third had a progressive crippling course, and one third had chronically active disease
  - ▪ With CS therapy, **most have favorable outcomes** with minimal to no sequelae
  - ▪ Delayed or inadequate CS therapy = important predictor of poor outcome and chronic course

Sjögren's syndrome

Epidemiology

- Mean age of onset: 30–50 yo
- **Strong female predominance** (F:M = 9:1)
- One-third with extraglandular disease
- May be primary or secondary to other CTDs (RA, SLE, SSc)

Pathogenesis

- Lymphocytic infiltration of exocrine glands **(lacrimal and salivary glands)** → apoptosis, autoantibodies, metalloproteinases, cytokines → gland dysfunction/impaired secretion
- Frequently a/w **anti-Ro/SSA** (60%–70%) and **anti-La/SSB** (20%–40%) antibodies
  - ▪ (+) autoantibodies a/w ↓ age of onset and ↑ risk of extraglandular disease
- Germline abnormality of TNFAIP3 → ↑ risk of antigen-driven **B-cell lymphomas**

Clinical

- ACR diagnostic criteria
  - ▪ In individuals with signs/symptoms suggestive of SjS, a score of at least 4 is required for diagnosis:
    - o Anti-SSA/Ro (+) (3 points)
    - o Positive labial salivary gland biopsy (3 points)
    - o Ocular staining score ≥ 5, Schirmer ≤ 5 mm/5 min, unstimulated whole saliva flow rate ≤ 0.1 ml/min (each of these is 1 point)

Symptoms and signs

- <u>Mucous membranes</u>
  - ▪ **Mucosal xerosis occurs later in disease course after > 50% of glands destroyed**, so early disease may present with only non-specific symptoms of fatigue, arthralgias, and myalgias
  - ▪ **Xerophthalmia (aka keratoconjunctivitis sicca):**
    - o Due to involvement of lacrimal gland
    - o Symptoms: dry eyes, pain, photophobia, or foreign body sensation
    - o Complications: keratitis, corneal ulceration, and recurrent infections
    - o Signs of impaired lacrimal gland function (uncommonly performed)
      - ♦ **Schirmer test:** Whatman paper wick fold over lower eye (tear film migrates < 5 mm in 5 minutes = positive test)

- Tear film stability test, fluorescein clearance test, Rose Bengal test (measures quality of ocular surface epithelium)
- **Xerostomia:**
  - Due to involvement of major (parotid and submandibular) and minor salivary glands
  - Symptoms: **dry mouth**, sore/burning mouth/lips, dysphagia, and transient bilateral or unilateral **swelling of parotid** and submandibular glands
    - If persistent swelling → consider workup for lymphoma
  - Complications: perlèche, thrush, dental caries, and severe gastroesophageal reflux disease (GERD)
  - Tests for impaired salivary gland function/flow rate: salivary gland scintigraphy, sialometry or parotid sialography (uncommonly performed)
- Vaginal xerosis
  - Symptoms: dyspareunia, dryness, and burning
  - Complication: bacterial and *Candida* overgrowth

- Skin
  - Xerosis/pruritus
    - **Most common skin finding (≈50%)**
  - **Vasculitis (most important skin finding** due to associated complications; affects ≈10%)
    - May present as small to large vessel vasculitis (any size)
      - **Classic LCV** of lower extremities = most common presentation
      - Cryoglobulinemic vasculitis = second most common presentation
      - Urticarial vasculitis (either hypo- or normocomplementemic) = third most common
      - PAN-like subcutaneous nodules and ulcers (rare)
    - Vasculitis is a/w:
      - **Systemic involvement** (arthritis, peripheral neuropathy, Raynaud phenomenon, and renal involvement)
      - Positive serology (**anti-Ro/SSA**, ANA, and RF)
      - ↑ ESR
      - **B-cell lymphoma**
      - **↑ Hospitalization/↑ mortality**
  - Annular erythema of SjS
    - **Indicates less systemic involvement/better prognosis**
    - Clinically similar to SCLE (SCLE has more epidermal changes and ↑ lupus band (+) on DIF); mostly in Japanese
  - Raynaud phenomenon **(typically mild)**
  - **Localized cutaneous nodular amyloidosis** (skin and lungs)
  - Purpura with capillaritis on histology
  - Waldenström's hypergammaglobulinemic purpura
  - EN
  - LR
- Systemic
  - Neurologic
    - Neuropathy: distal, symmetric, painful sensory or sensorimotor polyneuropathy (most common)
    - Other: memory loss, hearing loss, and Devic syndrome (aka neuromyelitis optica; variant of MS with optic neuritis and transverse myelitis)
  - Arthritis
    - Usually polyarticular, chronic progressive
    - May be asymmetric
    - Ankles and knees most commonly involved
  - **Lymphomas (most severe complication)**
    - 19-fold ↑ risk of **non-Hodgkin lymphomas**, predominately extranodal marginal zone B-cell lymphomas (aka **MALT**), usually involving organs in which SjS is most active, such as **major salivary glands (most common)**
  - Glomerulonephritis
  - Pulmonary (e.g., tracheobronchial sicca), cardiac (e.g., pericarditis, congenital heart block), endocrinologic (e.g., Hashimoto thyroiditis), GI (e.g., dysphagia, GERD)
  - Pregnancy
    - ↑ **Risk of NLE** in mothers with anti-Ro/SSA antibodies

Histopathology

- Salivary gland histology
  - Presence of focal lymphocytic sialoadenitis with two or more dense aggregates of 50+ lymphocytes per 4 mm of glandular tissue
  - A mixture of T cells and B cells with a normal CD4:CD8 ratio

Laboratory testing

- Autoantibodies:
  - **Anti-fodrin** (70%), most sensitive and specific test
  - **Anti-Ro/SSA** (60%–70%)
  - Anti-La/SSB (20%–40%)
- Other: ↑ ESR/CRP, polyclonal hypergammaglobulinemia, monoclonal gammopathy of undetermined significance (MGUS), ↓ C3/C4, anemia, leukopenia, thrombocytopenia, and mixed cryoglobulinemia

Treatment

- Treatment primarily symptomatic
  - Xerophthalmia
    - Preservative-free artificial tears during the day
    - Lubricating ointments at night
    - Punctae occlusion: plugs placed in the lacrimal puncta to ↑ accumulation of tear film
    - Cyclosporine (0.05%) eye drops BID for moderate to severe dry eyes; tacrolimus aqueous suspension also an option
  - Xerostomia
    - Artificial saliva (not usually tolerated well)
    - Frequent water ingestion
    - For patients with residual salivary gland function
      - Salivary stimulants (e.g., acid-free and sugar-free gum containing xylitol and sorbitol)
      - Sialagogue therapy: pilocarpine and cevimeline
    - Meticulous dental hygiene and fluoride treatments to prevent dental caries
    - Avoid alcohol, smoking, and low pH drinks (e.g., soda)
  - Xerosis—liberal use of emollients
- Immunosuppressants (hydroxychloroquine, steroids (low-dose), MTX, AZA, MMF, leflunomide) only used for

refractory cutaneous manifestations and severe extraglandular systemic involvement
  - Rituximab may be considered for refractory cases

Prognosis/clinical course

- On average, mortality rate similar to general population, but is 2–3 × higher in patients with extraglandular disease
- **Adverse prognostic factors a/w ↑ mortality:** hypocomplementemia, cryoglobulinemia, vasculitis, and **lymphoproliferative diseases**

Relapsing polychondritis

Epidemiology

- Age of onset 20–60 yo; M = F
- A/w second autoimmune disease in 30%

Pathogenesis

- Intermittent episodes of inflammation of articular and non-articular cartilage → chondrolysis and structural collapse
- Autoantibody titers against **type II collagen** correlate w/ disease activity, but are only present in 30%–50% of patients
- a/w **HLA-DR4**

Clinical

- Diagnostic criteria: three of six criteria required for diagnosis
  - Recurrent chondritis of both auricles (90%)
    - Presenting sign in 25%
    - Bright red, swollen, tender cartilaginous portion of ears, and **sparing earlobes**
    - Recurrent episodes leading to floppy **("cauliflower") ears** (Fig. 3.47)
    - May lead to conductive **hearing loss** due to collapse and edema of external auditory canal
  - Chondritis of nasal cartilages (70%)
    - Nasal congestion, rhinorrhea, crusting, epistaxis, ↓ sense of smell
    - May lead to **saddle nose deformity** (more common in females and younger patients)
  - Non-erosive inflammatory polyarthritis (50%–75%)
    - Episodic, migratory, asymmetric, non-erosive oligo- or polyarthritis, typically effecting knees, wrists, MCPs, and PIPs
    - Peripheral arthritis has worse prognosis
    - Other joints involved:
      - Costochondritis
      - Sternoclavicular and sternomanubrial joints
  - Inflammation of ocular structures (65%)
    - Any part of eye affected → conjunctivitis, corneal ulcers, scleritis, iritis, or uveitis
  - Chondritis of respiratory tract (laryngeal/tracheal/bronchial cartilages)
    - **Hoarseness**, **wheezing**, coughing, dyspnea, and subglottic strictures
    - May → airway collapse/obstruction and ↑ risk of **pneumonia (#1 cause of mortality)**
  - Cochlear and/or vestibular damage
    - Neurosensory hearing loss, tinnitus, and vertigo

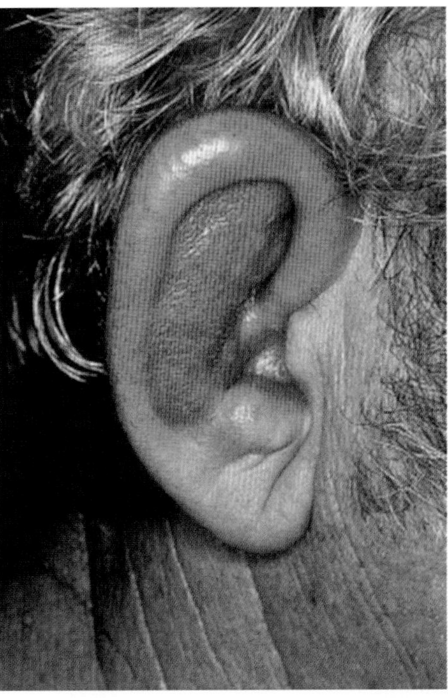

Fig. 3.47 Relapsing polychondritis characteristically involves cartilaginous portions of the ear but spares the lobe. (From James WD, Elston DM, Treat JR, Rosenbach MA, Neuhaus IM. Connective tissue diseases. In: *Andrews' Diseases of the Skin*. 13th ed. Philadelphia: Elsevier; 2020:157–183.)

- Other clinical findings
  - Cardiovascular
    - Valvulopathy: usually mitral or aortic valve regurgitation
    - Vasculitis
      - Portends worse prognosis (**#2 cause of mortality**)
      - Ranges from cutaneous small vessel vasculitis (CSVV) to large vessel vasculitis w/ aneurysmal dilation, most commonly involving abdominal and thoracic aorta
  - Non-specific skin/mucosal findings (35%)
    - Aphthous ulcers, EN
- Associated with:
  - Other autoimmune diseases
    - **MAGIC syndrome** (Mouth And Genital ulcers with Inflamed Cartilage) = **Behçet's disease + relapsing polychondritis**
  - Hematologic malignancies, most commonly myelodysplastic syndrome (MDS)

Histopathology

- Early: cartilaginous neutrophilic infiltrate
- Later: lymphoplasmacytic infiltrates with replacement of cartilage by granulation tissue and fibrosis

Laboratory testing

- Normochromic/normocytic anemia (a/w worse prognosis), ↑ ESR/CRP, mild leukocytosis, ↑ Creatinine/blood urea nitrogen (Cr/BUN) and microscopic hematuria (if vasculitis affects kidneys)

Treatment

- **First line**: **prednisone** (0.5–1 mg/kg/day, or higher if systemic involvement)
  - Adjunct: NSAIDs, colchicine and dapsone for fever, auricular chondritis, and arthralgias
- Immunosuppressive agents have variable response (MTX most effective)

Prognosis/clinical course

- In the past was a/w high morbidity and mortality
- Currently, w/ treatment, survival rates are > 95% at 8 years
- **Chronic course w/ acute flares** lasting days to weeks → destruction of cartilage and collapse of supported structures
- **Most common causes of death = infection #1 (pneumonia) >** systemic vasculitis > large artery aneurysm dissection or rupture, airway collapse, renal failure, and malignancy
- Poor prognostic factors: anemia, saddle nose deformity, arthritis, and vasculitis

Mixed connective tissue disease (MCTD)

Epidemiology

- Strong female predominance (9:1)
- Majority present in second to fourth decades

Pathogenesis

- CTD characterized by overlapping features of two or more of the following: SLE, PM/DM, scleroderma, or RA
- **Anti-U1RNP** (high titers) antibodies thought to play pathogenic role
- a/w **HLA-DR4**

Clinical

- Three classification criteria for MCTD have been published, but **no current consensus**
- **Most common constellation**: Raynaud phenomenon, esophageal dysfunction, swollen fingers/hands ("sausage digits"), arthralgias/arthritis, and inflammatory myopathy
- Clinical findings
  - Scleroderma-like findings:
    - Raynaud phenomenon (~100%): **earliest** and most common sign; can develop digital infarcts and gangrene
    - Esophageal dysmotility (85%)
    - Edema of hands, sausage digits
    - Sclerodactyly
    - Periungal telangiectasias w/ dropout areas
    - Pulmonary HTN (25%) = most serious complication of MCTD → accounts for 40% of MCTD deaths
    - Pulmonary fibrosis (usually mild)
    - Notably, do **NOT** see diffuse sclerodermoid involvement of face, trunk, and proximal extremities
  - DM-like findings:
    - Inflammatory myopathy +/− poikilodermatous areas on upper trunk and proximal extremities
    - Do NOT usually see DM-specific signs (Gottron's papules, heliotrope, psoriasiform scalp dermatitis)
  - Lupus-like findings: DLE, SCLE, or ACLE-like skin lesions
  - Other findings: **arthralgias/arthritis** (50%–70%), serositis (pleuritic, pericarditis, myocarditis), neurologic findings, cytopenias (30%–40%), APLS, glomerulonephritis

Histopathology

- Varies depending on type of skin lesion biopsied

Laboratory testing

- (+) ANA with **speckled nuclear pattern**
- **High-titer anti-U1RNP autoantibodies** (serologic hallmark)
  - Lacks anti-dsDNA, Smith antibodies, and hypocomplementemia → helps differentiate from SLE
- ↑ ESR
- Cytopenias (e.g., anemia, leukopenia)
- Antiphospholipid autoantibodies

Treatment

- First line: prednisone
- Adjuncts: NSAIDs, antimalarials, PPIs (for GERD), sildenafil (for Raynaud)
  - Lupus, RA, and DM-like features are more likely to be steroid-responsive compared with scleroderma-like features (e.g., sclerodactyly, Raynaud, and pulmonary HTN)
- **MTX** is first line for severe arthritis, but should be used with caution due to **frequent pulmonary fibrosis in MCTD patients**

Prognosis/clinical course

- Good response to CS therapy → favorable prognosis
- 40% evolve into one of the six diffuse CTDs
  - Presence of **anti-dsDNA** → a/w evolution into **SLE**
  - Presence of esophageal hypomotility/dilation or sclerodactyly → a/w evolution into SSc
- Survival rates
  - 5-year survival: 98%; 10-year survival: 88%
  - Mortality is due to: **pulmonary artery HTN (40%)** > acute cardiovascular events, thrombotic thrombocytopenic purpura (TTP)/hemolytic uremic syndrome (HUS) > infections

Rheumatoid arthritis

Epidemiology

- 1%–3% US adult population
- Female predominance (3:1)
- Peak onset between 30 and 55 yo
- a/w HLA-DR1 and HLA-DR4

Pathogenesis

- Self-reactive CD4+ T cells produce Th1 and Th17 cytokines → promotes inflammation, stimulates synovial macrophages and fibroblasts to produce proinflammatory cytokines (e.g., TNF-α, IL-1, and IL-6) and proteases that break down cartilage and activate B cells to differentiate into plasma cells → downstream effects:
  - **RANKL** (expressed by stromal cells, synovial fibroblasts, and T cells) binds RANK on osteoclasts → **bone erosion**

- **RF and anti-cyclic citrullinated protein (CCP) antibodies** form immune complexes inside joints → activates complement cascade

- Majority of **cutaneous findings are due to neutrophil-mediated damage** (as a result of complement activation)
- Genetics:
  - PTPN22 gene
    - Encodes a lymphoid-specific protein tyrosine phosphatase, in which a gain of function polymorphism results in selection of autoreactive T cells and B cells (confers susceptibility to RA, juvenile idiopathic arthritis [JIA], and other CTDs)
  - HLA-DRB1
    - ↑ Propensity to develop autoantibodies against CCPs
      - CCPs are proteins located within skin and joints!

Clinical

- 2010 ACR/EULAR diagnostic criteria: requires score ≥ 6 points (out of 10 total possible points) for definite diagnosis
  - Joint involvement: swollen or tender joint, which may be confirmed by imaging ("large joints" = shoulders, elbows, hips, knees, and ankles; "small joints" = MCP, PIP, second to fifth metatarsophalangeal joint [MTP], thumb interphalangeal joint, and wrists joints with exclusion of DIP, first MTP, and first carpometacarpal joints)
    - One large joint (0 points)
    - 2 to 10 large joints (1 point)
    - 1 to 3 small joints (with or without involvement of large joints) (2 points)
    - 4 to 10 small joints (with or without involvement of large joints) (3 points)
    - More than 10 joints (at least one small joint) (5 points)
  - Serology:
    - Negative RF *and* negative CCP (0 points)
    - Low positive RF (≤ three times upper limit of normal) or low positive anti-CCP antibody (≤ three times upper limit of normal) (2 points)
    - High positive RF (> three times upper limit of normal) or high positive anti-CCP antibody (> three times upper limit of normal) (3 points)
  - Acute phase reactants:
    - Normal CRP *and* normal ESR (0 points)
    - Abnormal CRP or abnormal ESR (1 point)
  - Duration of symptoms
    - Shorter than 6 weeks (0 points)
    - ≥6 weeks (1 point)
- Skin findings:
  - Rheumatoid nodules (20%–30%)
    - Usually occurs in female patients w/ **high-titer RF**
    - Firm, non-tender papules/nodules **over bony prominences** (especially extensor forearms, dorsal hands, elbows), but can occur anywhere including visceral organs (Fig. 3.48)
    - Nodules located in dermis, subcutaneous tissue, or attached to periarticular capsule or tendons → may lead to tendon rupture

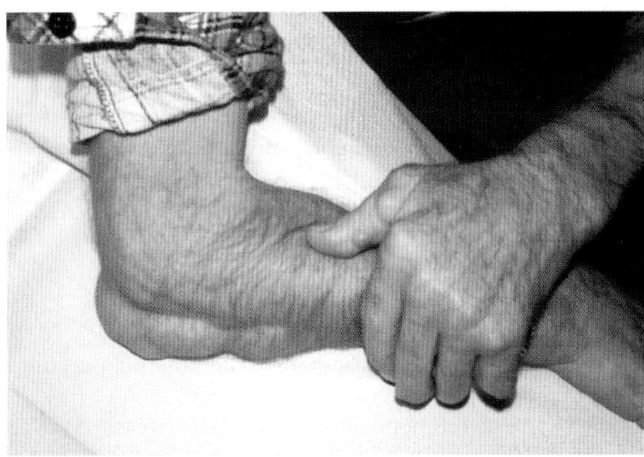

Fig. 3.48 Rheumatoid nodules. Large rheumatoid nodules are seen in a classic location along the extensor surface of the forearm and in the olecranon bursa. (From McInnes I, O'Dell JR. Rheumatoid arthritis. In: Goldman L, Schafer AI. *Goldman-Cecil Medicine*. 26th ed. Philadelphia: Elsevier; 2020:1709–1718.)

    - Resolve spontaneously or with RA improvement
    - **Rheumatoid nodulosis**: disease variant where patients p/w multiple ulcerative nodules and **high RF, but in absence of active joint disease**
    - **Therapy-induced rheumatoid nodulosis**
      - Occurs in patients w/ preexisting RA, classically **following initiation of MTX** (termed MTX-induced accelerated nodulosis = "MAIN")
        - ➔ More recently described following initiation of TNF-α inhibitors
      - **p/w acute onset** of numerous symmetrically grouped rheumatoid nodules; often **painful** (unlike normal rheumatoid nodules)
      - Typical locations: fingers, helix of ears, soles of feet, penis, chest, and surgical incision sites
  - Rheumatoid vasculitis
    - Late complication arising in patients w/ **history** of severe erosive RA (but joint disease is now burnt-out), **high-titer RF** and rheumatoid nodules
    - CSVV or PAN-like eruption w/ **systemic vasculitis** (neuropathies, alveolitis, carditis, cerebral infarction)
    - a/w **high mortality (up to 40%)** → must **refer to rheumatology for aggressive treatment** (cyclophosphamide + systemic steroids)
  - Bywaters' lesions
    - Purpuric papules usually on digital pulp; demonstrates LCV histologically
    - Not a/w systemic vasculitis of other organs (vs. rheumatoid vasculitis)
  - Superficial ulcerating necrobiosis (aka rheumatoid necrobiosis)
    - Atrophic, shiny, telangiectatic, yellow plaques w/ red-brown edges resembling necrobiosis lipoidica diabeticorum (NLD) w/ ulceration
    - Typically numerous lesions on **bilateral lower extremities**
    - Occurs in patients with **severe RA w/ high-titer RF** and rheumatoid nodules

- Neutrophilic dermatoses
  - Erythema elevatum diutinum
  - Sweet's syndrome
  - Pyoderma gangrenosum (PG)
  - **Rheumatoid neutrophilic dermatitis/dermatosis**
    - Persistent urticarial red papules/plaques symmetrically distributed on extensor forearms and hands
    - Histology: neutrophilic urticaria (or occasionally Sweet's-like)
  - MTX-induced papular eruption
    - Erythematous urticarial papules and plaques on buttocks and proximal extremities
    - Arise during treatment of disease flares w/ MTX
  - **PNGD**
    - Symmetrically distributed eroded, umbilicated papules overlying joints (elbows, knees, and knuckles)
    - May represent earliest phases of rheumatoid nodules
  - **IGDA**
    - Annular red-violaceous plaques on trunk and intertriginous areas, sometimes with "**rope sign**" (red flesh-colored cords extending down flanks or back)

Histopathology

- Rheumatoid nodules
  - Early lesions (resembles PNGD and IGDA): interstitial granulomatous or neutrophilic infiltrate +/− LCV (Fig. 3.49)
  - Later (well-developed lesions): **large palisading granulomas** surrounding degenerated **eosinophilic** connective tissue ("necrobiosis") and **fibrin** in deep dermis or subcutaneous tissue, often w/ **neutrophilic debris** (helps DDx from GA)
- Rheumatoid vasculitis: histologic features correlate w/ clinical morphology → may see palpable purpura or PAN-like changes
  - DIF: strong IgM and C3 in small and medium-sized vessels (vs. weaker and limited- to medium-sized vessels in classic PAN)

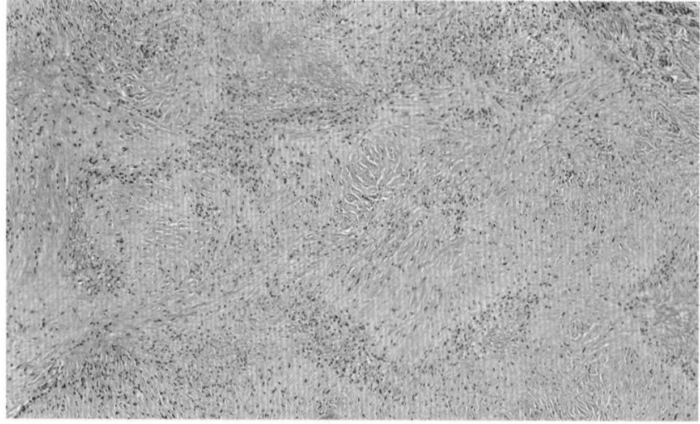

Fig. 3.49 Rheumatoid nodule—histologic features. A large irregular area of necrobiosis surrounded by a palisade of histiocytes. (Courtesy of Olayemi Sokumbi, MD.)

Laboratory findings

- **(+) RF** (sensitivity 80%, specificity 85%)
- **Anti-CCP** (sensitivity 70%, specificity 95%)

Treatment

- Arthritis
  - **Glucocorticoids** (rapid disease control before onset of efficacy of disease-modifying anti-rheumatic drugs [**DMARDs**])
    - Non-biologic DMARDs (first line): **MTX**, sulfasalazine, hydroxychloroquine, leflunomide, JAK inhibitors (e.g. tofacitinib, baricitinib, upadacitinib)
    - Biologic DMARDs (second line): TNF-α inhibitors, abatacept, tocilizumab/sarilumab (IL-6R inhibitor), rituximab, anakinra
  - NSAIDs used as adjunct to DMARDs
- Rheumatoid nodules
  - **Do not respond to treatment for arthritis** → consider intralesional CS (↓ size) or excision (but recurrences common)
- Neutrophilic dermatoses: oral CS, dapsone, colchicine
- Rheumatoid vasculitis
  - Mild-to-moderate: AZA, MMF
  - Severe: IV methylprednisolone, followed by prednisone +/− cyclophosphamide +/− plasmapheresis

Prognosis/clinical course

- Majority have chronic progressive disease activity that waxes and wanes over time
- A few patients may exhibit an aggressive form of rapidly progressive and erosive arthritis
- Mortality rate 2× higher than general population → most common causes of death = ischemic heart disease (most common) and infection
- Poor prognostic factors: extraarticular disease, low functional capacity, low socioeconomic status, low education, and chronic prednisone use

Additional boards factoids

- **Felty syndrome**: **seropositive RA** characterized by neutropenia, splenomegaly, and refractory **leg ulcers** (may resemble PG)
  - a/w ↑ Risk of lymphomas/leukemias
  - Rx: G-CSF and/or **splenectomy**

Systemic-onset juvenile idiopathic arthritis (Still's disease)

Epidemiology

- Still's disease is one of many forms of JIA (20% of JIA), but the **other forms of JIA rarely have skin findings**
  - Other forms of JIA (will not be discussed further):
    - RF(−) polyarthritis (5%): favors small joints (hands and feet); usually non-erosive; RF(−) and ANA(−)
    - RF(+) Polyarthritis (15%): favors small joints (hands and feet); usually erosive; shares same features as adult RA → **rheumatoid nodules**, RF(+) in 100%, ANA(+)
    - Oligo/pauciarticular arthritis (60%): most common form of JIA; favors knees; divided into two types → type I [most common subtype; onset = 1–8 yo;

uveitis in 50%; ANA(+), RF(−)]; type II [onset = 9–16 yo; strongly a/w HLA-B27; RF(−), ANA(−)]
  - Other rare forms: enthesitis-related arthritis (a/w HLA-B27), PsA (ANA-negative, a/w anterior uveitis)
- JIA is the **most common rheumatologic disease in childhood**
- Still's has no gender predilection (M = F); in contrast, all other forms of JIA have female predominance
- By definition, onset ≤ 16 yo (mean age = 6 yo)

Pathogenesis

- Best classified as an **autoinflammatory syndrome** (disorder of innate immune system), rather than autoimmune disease (disorder of adaptive immune system)
  - Inflammasome activation and/or aberrant **caspase-1** alternative secretory pathway (↑S100A8/9/12) → ↑ **IL-1 production** (as well as IL-6 and TNF-α)
  - Up to three-fold increased risk of JIA in kids exposed to multiple courses of antibiotics

Clinical

- Diagnostic criteria:
  - **High episodic fevers** (>38.9 °C) daily for ≥ 2 weeks and documented to be quotidian for ≥ 3 days
    - Classically arises in late afternoon to early evening
  - Plus one of the following features:
    - **Transient evanescent, salmon pink, blanching eruption** (90%): typically arises in late afternoon/evening (**corresponds w/ fever spikes**); p/w generalized distribution (favors axilla and waist); **Koebnerization** w/ linear lesions (Fig. 3.50)
      - Less common skin findings: **persistent papules and plaques**, periorbital edema, rheumatoid nodule-like lesions
    - Generalized lymphadenopathy
    - Hepatomegaly/splenomegaly
    - Serositis (pericarditis, pleuritis, and peritonitis)
    - Symmetric polyarthritis > oligoarthritis; erosive in 20%

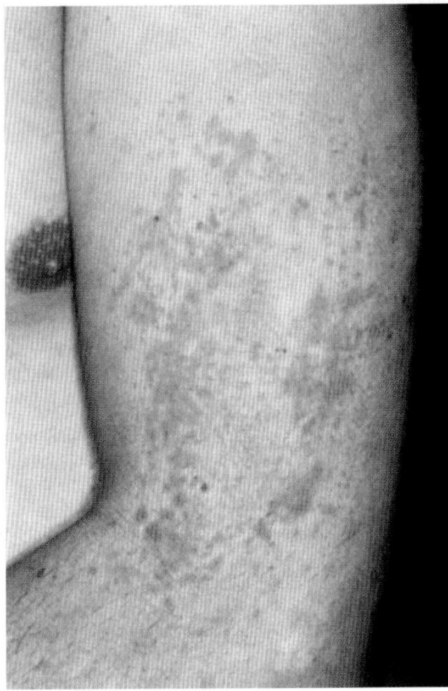

Fig. 3.50 Evanescent eruption of Still's disease. (From James WD, Berger TG, Elston DM, Neuhaus IM. Connective tissue diseases. In: *Andrews' Diseases of the Skin*. 12th ed. Philadelphia: Elsevier; 2016:153–178.)

Histopathology

- Two types of cutaneous lesions, each w/ distinctive features:
  - Evanescent transient exanthem: edema of superficial dermis, superficial, perivascular, and interstitial **neutrophilic infiltrate** (denser and more neutrophil-predominant than urticaria) in **absence of vasculitis**
  - Persistent papules/plaques: same as above + **parakeratosis, superficially scattered necrotic keratinocytes**

Laboratory testing

- Leukocytosis, anemia, and thrombocytosis
- ↑ **ESR/CRP**
- ↑↑↑ **Ferritin** (extremely high)
- RF-negative (>95%)
- ANA-negative (>95%)

Treatment

- Mild disease: **NSAIDs** +/− hydroxychloroquine
- Moderate or severe disease: **systemic steroids** +/− steroid-sparing immunosuppressants (MTX, TNF-α inhibitors, AZA, leflunomide, thalidomide)
- Biologic agents targeting **IL-1 receptor** (e.g., **anakinra**, rilonacept, canakinumab) and IL-6 receptor (e.g., **tocilizumab**) have demonstrated efficacy; consider HSCT in refractory disease

Prognosis/clinical course

- Arthritis resolves completely in 50%
  - Other 50% have a chronic course w/ persistent arthritis and systemic complications
  - Extensive arthritis or symptoms lasting > 6 months → a/w poorer prognosis
- 5% develop **macrophage activation syndrome** (MAS; life-threatening)
  - Highly activated immunologic state → hemophagocytosis and cytokine overproduction
  - Characterized by pancytopenia, coagulopathy, hepatic dysfunction, and neurologic complications
  - Requires treatment w/ high-dose systemic CS/other immunosuppressants

Adult-onset Still's disease

Epidemiology

- Vast majority < 30 yo
- Slight female predominance

Pathogenesis

- Possibly triggered by an infectious agent (e.g., *Yersinia enterocolitica*)
- a /w numerous HLA groups (B17, B18, B35, DR2)

Clinical

- **Prodrome of flu-like illness w/ sore throat**, constitutional symptoms, **high fever**, arthralgias, and myalgias, occurring daily

- **Fever usually > 39 °C w/ spiking pattern** (late afternoon to early evening)
- Skin manifestations
  - **Salmon patch exanthema** (asymptomatic and transient/evanescent)
    - Occurs concomitantly with fever spikes
    - Typical location: trunk/extremities and sites of pressure with koebnerization
  - Violaceous to reddish-brown, scaly, **persistent papules and plaques** (50%)
- Systemic manifestations
  - Arthralgias/arthritis (65%–100%; usually oligoarthritis)
    - Typically involves knees, wrists, and ankles symmetrically
    - **Carpal ankylosis (characteristic feature):** limited range of motion with minimal pain
  - Hepatosplenomegaly
- Complications
  - MAS (15%) → life-threatening!

Histopathology

- Same as systemic-onset JIA (classic Still's disease)

Laboratory findings

- Negative ANA and RF
- Anemia, leukocytosis (neutrophilic predominance), and thrombocytosis common
- ↑ **ESR/CRP**
- ↑↑↑ Ferritin
  - Levels correlate w/ disease activity
  - A/w Chronic pattern of disease, recurrent flares, and poor prognosis
- Laboratory abnormalities a/w MAS

Treatment

- Majority require **systemic steroids** (prednisone 40–60 mg/d)
  - May add steroid-sparing agent (MTX = first choice; cyclosporine)
- Anakinra (better for systemic inflammation), tocilizumab, infliximab (better for arthritis) are options

Prognosis/clinical course

- Usually benign, non-fatal course, w/ low mortality (3%–10%)
- Deaths due to infections, acute respiratory distress syndrome, and multiple organ failure from MAS and thrombotic microangiopathy

Morphea (Localized scleroderma)

Epidemiology

- Two thirds of cases present in childhood
- F > M (2.6:1)
  - Exception: linear morphea has no sex predilection
- Frequencies of various morphea types:
  - Plaque (>50%): **most common subtype in adults**
  - Linear (20%): most common subtype in **children**
  - Generalized (13%)
  - Morphea profunda (11%)

Pathogenesis

- Genetic predisposition + environmental trigger → vascular injury (e.g., decreased capillary density, endothelial injury) → inflammation → profibrotic Th2 cytokines (IL-4, IL-6, and **TGF-β**) → fibroblast proliferation and collagen deposition
- Environmental triggers: trauma, radiation, medications (e.g., bleomycin, bromocriptine, and D-penicillamine), and *Borrelia* spp. (Europe and Japan mainly; **a/w *Borrelia* *afzelii* and *Borrelia garinii***)

Clinical features

- Clinical subtypes
  - Plaque morphea (most common form overall, and in adults)
    - Begin as erythematous to violaceous patches on **trunk and proximal extremities** → evolves into indurated **hyperpigmented or ivory plaques**; plaques often **hairless and anhidrotic**, w/ prominent follicular orifices
    - May have surrounding **lilac-violaceous inflammatory rim** (indicates persistent activity) (Fig. 3.51)
    - Often develops in areas of pressure
  - Guttate morphea
    - Multiple, small chalk white, flat or slightly depressed macules; only minimally indurated
    - Appears similar to guttate LS&A, but lacks follicular plugging and epidermal atrophy
    - Typical locations: upper half of trunk
  - Linear morphea
    - Important because **a/w significant morbidity** (esp. in kids)
    - Morphology similar to plaque morphea, but with **linear distribution**, often following Blaschko's lines
    - Most common sites: **lower extremities (#1)** > upper extremities > head, trunk
    - **May involve deeper structures (muscle, fascia, and bone)**
      - **Melorheostosis** = roughening long bone surfaces underlying area of linear morphea (also Buschke-Ollendorff syndrome) that resembles wax dripping down the side of a candle on X-ray

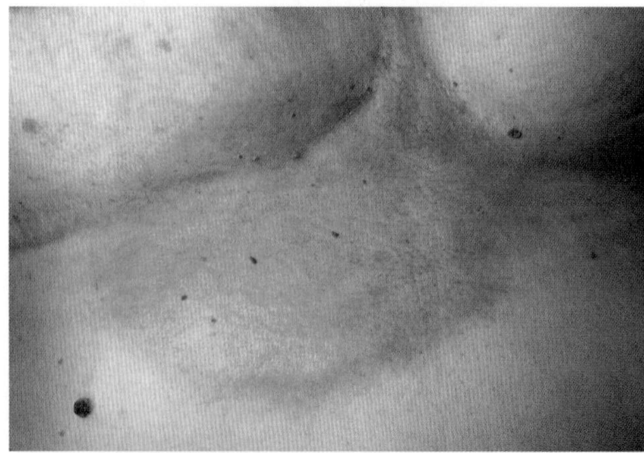

Fig. 3.51 Morphea. A single or few oval areas of non-pitting erythema and edema typically appear on the trunk. A violaceous border (lilac ring) surrounds the indurated area. The center of the lesion then develops smooth, ivory-colored hairless or hyperpigmented plaques, and the ability to sweat is lost. (From Dinulos JGH. Connective tissue diseases. In: *Habif's Clinical Dermatology: A Color Guide to Diagnosis and Therapy*. 7th ed. Philadelphia: Elsevier; 2021:669–712.)

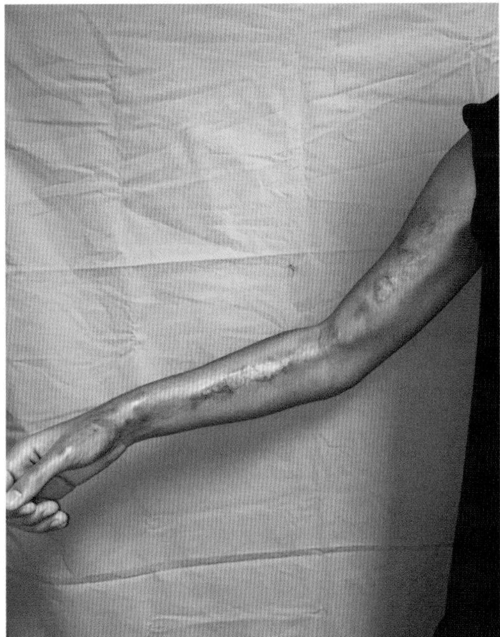

Fig. 3.52 Linear morphea of the arm with extensive induration, hypoplasia, and flexion contracture. (From Morris MS, Matcuk G, DeClerk BK, Arkfeld D, Stevanovic M. Linear morphea with inflammatory myositis. *J Hand Surg*. 2020; 45[8]:782.e1–782.e5.)

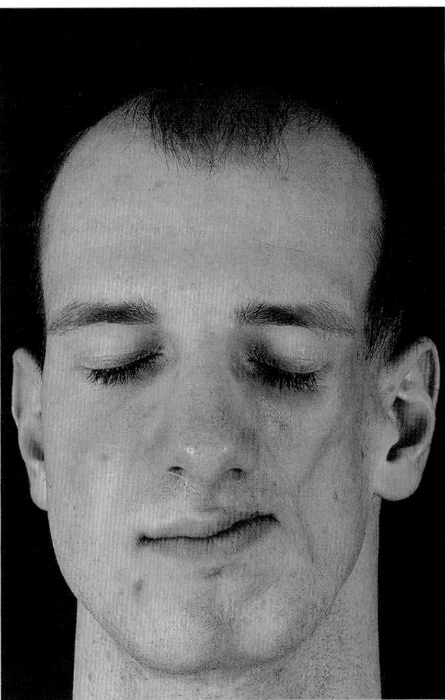

Fig. 3.53 Parry-Romberg syndrome. Marked atrophy of subcutaneous structures, including bone. (From Sommer A, Gambichler T, Bacharach-Buhles M, von Rothenburg T, Altmeyer P, Kreuter A. Clinical and serological characteristics of progressive facial hemiatrophy: a case series of 12 patients. *J Am Acad Dermatol*. 2006;54[2]:227–233.)

- Anti-ssDNA autoantibodies common
- Typical locations: extremities and trunk
- Complications: **undergrowth of limbs (permanent!)** (Fig. 3.52), deformity, **joint restriction/contractures** (risk highest if plaques extend over joints), and arthralgias
- Head/neck subtypes of linear morphea:
  - **En coup de sabre:**
    - ➔ Indented appearance of frontal, frontoparietal, or parasagittal forehead or scalp
  - **Parry-Romberg syndrome** (aka progressive hemifacial atrophy)
    - ➔ Unilateral atrophy of face involving dermis, subcutaneous tissue, muscle, and bone (Figs. 3.53 and 3.54)
    - ➔ May have associated epilepsy, exophthalmos, headache, trigeminal neuralgia, myopathy of the eye muscles, cerebral atrophy, white matter hyperintensity, alopecia
  - Children with head/neck morphea should have regular ophthalmologic examinations to monitor for asymptomatic ocular involvement

- <u>Atrophoderma of Pasini and Pierini</u>
  - Large (up to 20 cm) brownish-gray hyperpigmented oval, atrophic, well-demarcated plaques w/ **sharp sloping borders ("cliff drop")**
  - Typical location: trunk/upper arms of young females (typically second to third decades)
  - Begins as a persistent single lesion with additional lesions forming over time
  - Histology: ↓↓ **dermal thickness** compared with normal skin
    - Biopsy should contain affected skin and adjacent normal skin to show "cliff drop"

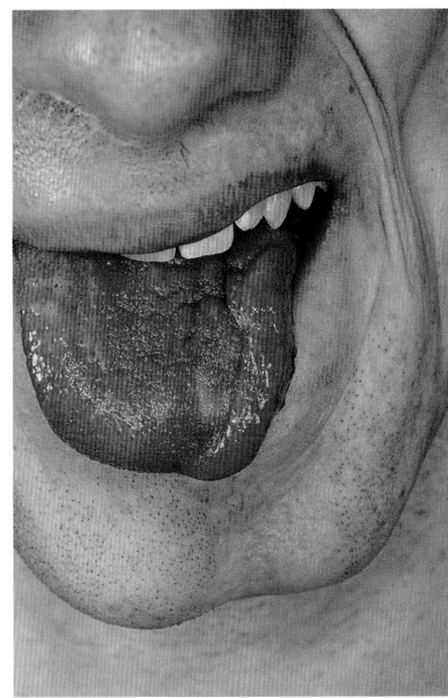

Fig. 3.54 Hemiatrophy of the tongue. (From Sommer A, Gambichler T, Bacharach-Buhles M, von Rothenburg T, Altmeyer P, Kreuter A. Clinical and serological characteristics of progressive facial hemiatrophy: a case series of 12 patients. *J Am Acad Dermatol*. 2006;54[2]:227–233.)

  - Variant:
    - **Linear atrophoderma of Moulin**: linear form of atrophoderma that is chronic but non-progressive with benign course; less induration and pigmentary changes compared with other types of morphea

- Generalized morphea
  - Widespread indurated plaques that expand to involve entire trunk and extremities → **muscle atrophy and difficulty breathing** (due to constrictive effect of taut skin on chest)
  - Most likely form to have extracutaneous symptoms (fatigue, malaise, and myalgias/arthralgias)
  - Spontaneous resolution uncommon
  - Usually (+) ANA
  - Variant:
    - Pansclerotic morphea:
      - Children <14 yo
      - Type of generalized morphea involving deep structures → disability and contractures of extremities
- Bullous morphea
  - Rare, usually only seen in context of generalized morphea
  - Etiology: diffuse sclerosis of skin → impaired lymphatic flow → formation of lymphoceles/bullae
- Deep morphea (morphea profunda)
  - Morphea primarily involving subcutaneous tissue (fascia, muscle, and bone) w/ deep induration; overlying skin can appear normal, puckered (**"pseudocellulite"**), or hyperpigmented
  - Poor response to CS (vs. EF)
  - Can develop osteoma cutis in lesions
  - Complications: deformity, ulcers, SCC formation, joint restriction, and contractures
- Nodular morphea (keloidal morphea)
  - Hyperpigmented sclerotic nodules that mimic keloids; can be a/w classic plaque morphea
- Morphea-lichen sclerosis overlap
  - **Patients w/ combination of morphea and LS&A lesions**

Histopathology

- Early
  - **Lymphocytic infiltrate w/ plasma cells at dermal-SQ junction**
  - **Loss of CD34+ dendritic cells** (vs. ↑ in nephrogenic systemic fibrosis [NSF] and scleromyxedema)
- Later
  - Decreased inflammation
  - **"Square biopsy"** sign
  - Pale, edematous, and homogenized papillary dermis
  - Loss of pilosebaceous units/periadnexal fat
  - **"Trapped eccrine glands"** = eccrine glands/ducts compressed by surrounding sclerotic/keloidal collagen

Laboratory testing

- All forms of morphea **lack anti-Scl70 (Topo I) and anti-centromere** antibodies! (in contrast to SSc)
- All forms have **(+) anti-topoisomerase II** antibodies (75% overall, 85%–90% in generalized morphea)
- Plaque morphea:
  - Usually (−) ANA
  - Lacks anti-ssDNA and anti-histone antibodies
- Linear and generalized morphea:
  - More likely to be (+) ANA than other forms
  - Often (+) anti-ssDNA and (+) anti-histone antibodies → correlates w/ disease severity/activity
- ESR/CRP may be ↑, especially in linear or deep morphea

Treatment

- See treatment algorithm (Fig. 3.55)
- Treatment can halt disease progression
- Topical therapies used for superficial circumscribed lesions
  - Topical or intralesional CS can be used, but may cause atrophy
  - TCIs, vitamin D analogs, and imiquimod all have reported efficacy
- UVA1 phototherapy considered for more extensive disease, but can only penetrate the dermis so no benefit for deeper lesions
- **ToC for moderate to severe morphea is MTX**, often in combination with systemic CS for the first 2 to 3 months

Prognosis/clinical course

- **Superficial plaque morphea often self-limited**; softens over 3 to 5 years
- Generalized morphea has worse prognosis
- Important to **treat childhood linear morphea aggressively** → prevents limb shortening and joint contractures

Scleroderma (AKA systemic sclerosis, SSc)

Epidemiology

- F > M (3:1)
- Typical age of onset: 30 to 50 yo

Pathogenesis

- Key pathogenic features include vascular dysfunction, cellular and humoral immune dysregulation, and excess collagen/ECM protein deposition in skin and internal organs
- **Vascular dysfunction** (abnormal angiogenesis), primarily of microcirculation, is earliest feature and consists of endothelial injury (↑ VEGF) w/ vascular leakage, abnormal vasospasms, intimal proliferation, luminal obstruction, capillary destruction, and devascularization
- **Autoantibody production (anti-centromere, anti-Scl70, anti-RNA polymerase III)**, auto-antigen driven T-cell activation with a Th2-predominant profile, and ↑ **production of profibrotic cytokines**/growth factors (IL-2/-13/-17, **TGF-β**, PDGF, CTGF, IFN, endothelin-1) → accumulation of myofibroblasts in affected tissues → excess collagen production (types I and III) and other ECM proteins (e.g., proteoglycans, fibronectins, β1-integrins)

Clinical features

- Diagnostic criteria: score ≥ 9 classified as definite SSc (sensitivity 91%; specificity 92%)
  - Skin thickening of fingers of both hands extending proximal to MCP joints (9 points, sufficient criterion)
    - Early (edematous) phase: pitting edema of digits
      - Initial presenting sign in 50%

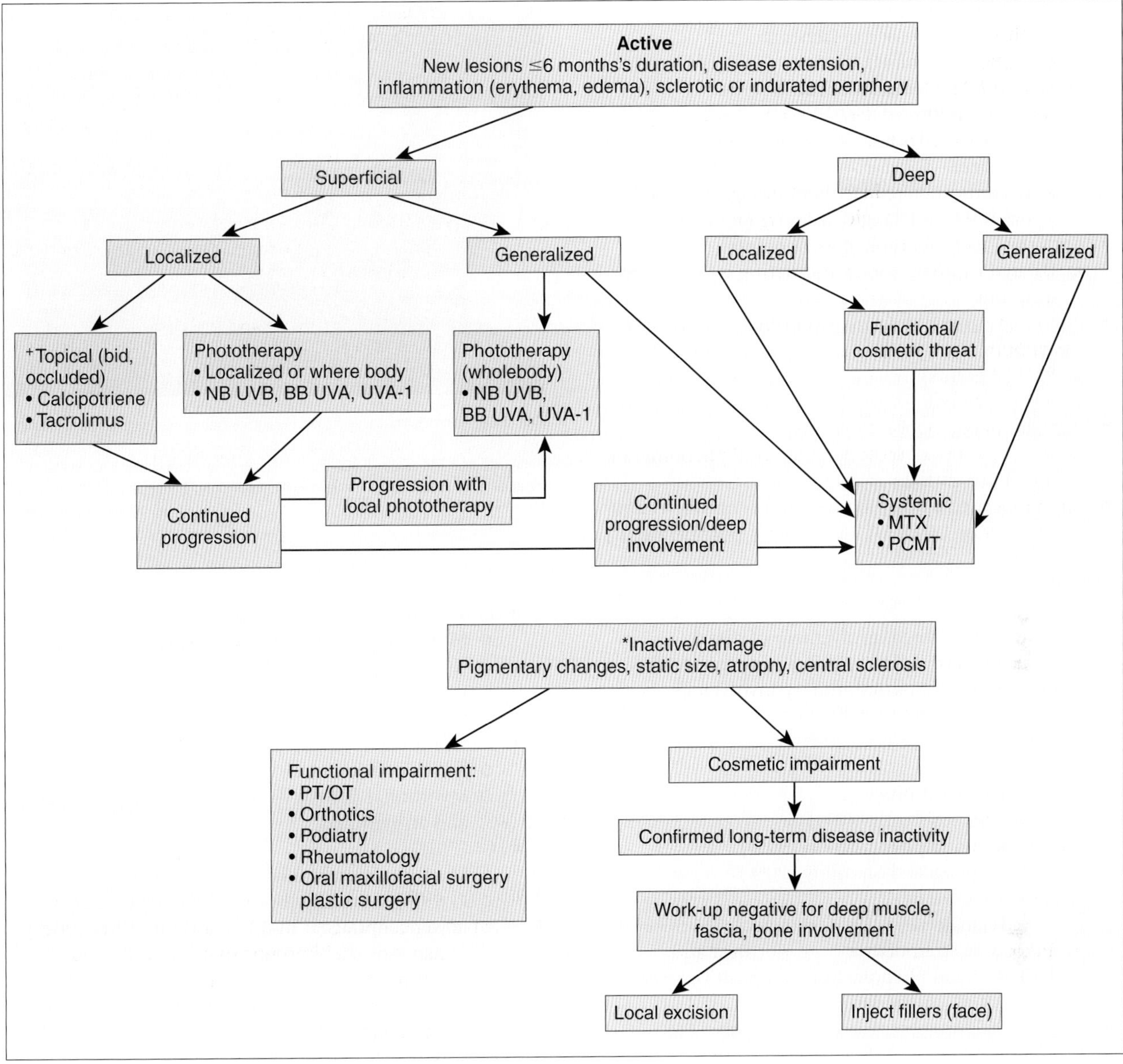

Fig. 3.55 Therapeutic algorithm for morphea based on existing evidence. Superficial involvement is defined by histologic evidence of papillary dermal involvement. Deep involvement is defined as sclerosis or inflammation of reticular dermis, subcutis, fascia, or muscle. Histologic examination and/or magnetic resonance imaging are encouraged to evaluate lesions for depth of involvement and, likewise, determine appropriate treatment and evaluation of therapeutic efficacy. *BB,* Broadband; *MTX,* methotrexate; *NB,* narrowband; *OT,* occupational therapy; *PCMT,* pulsed intravenous corticosteroids plus methotrexate; *PT,* physical therapy; *UV,* ultraviolet. *There is very little evidence for any therapy addressing disease damage in morphea. There is minimal evidence for efficacy of these measures. Risk of disease reactivation is also unknown, but surgical measures should only be undertaken in long-standing, inactive disease. +Topical therapies should not be used as monotherapy in the presence of active and progressively functional impairment (e.g., decreased range of motion, contracture, and limb length discrepancy). Systemic manifestations most commonly reported to occur in morphea include arthritis, seizures/headaches (en coupe de sabre), and ocular manifestations. All patients with morphea should be assessed for their presence and appropriate referrals made. (From Zwischenberger BA, Jacobe HT. A systematic review of morphea treatments and therapeutic algorithm. *J Am Acad Dermatol*. 2011;65[5]:925–941.)

- Indurated phase: edematous fingers harden and become tight and shiny
- Late (atrophic) phase: skin atrophy with flexion contractures

- Skin thickening of fingers (only count higher score)
  - Puffy fingers with diffuse, non-pitting increase in soft tissue (2 points)
  - **Sclerodactyly** of the fingers (distal to the four MCP joints, but proximal to the PIP joints) (4 points)
- Fingertip lesions with loss of substance from finger pad (only count higher score)
  - Digital tip ulcers (2 points)
    - Thought to be due to trauma

- Fingertip pitting scars (3 points)
  - Thought to be due to ischemia
- Telangiectasia (2 points)
  - **Matted telangiectasias** of face/lips/palms (more common in limited SSc/CREST):
    - Telangiectasias have smooth/"mat-like" squared-off edges
    - In contrast, hereditary hemorrhagic telangiectasia has irregular telangiectasias w/ radiating vessels
- Abnormal nail fold capillaries (2 points)
  - **Dilated capillary loops alternating w/ capillary drop out**
- Pulmonary arterial hypertension (PAH) and/or ILD **(maximum score is 2)**
  - PAH (2 points)
  - ILD (2 points)
- Raynaud phenomenon (3 points)
  - Leading cause of secondary Raynaud phenomenon
  - Initial presenting sign in 50% of SSc
- Any SSc-related autoantibodies: anti-centromere, anti-topoisomerase I (Scl-70), or anti-RNA polymerase III) (3 points)

- SSc subtypes:
  - Limited SSc
    - Definition: limited involvement of **distal extremities** (distal to MCP/MTP joints) and **face**
    - **Lacks severe renal/pulmonary involvement** → improved overall mortality
      - Commonly see isolated PAH
    - Variants:
      - **CREST syndrome**
        - Calcinosis cutis (40%)
        - Raynaud phenomenon (99%)
        - Esophageal dysmotility (90%)
        - Sclerodactyly
        - Telangiectasias (mat telangiectasias; 90%)
      - SSc sine scleroderma:
        - Raynaud phenomenon and positive serology, but no cutaneous involvement
  - Diffuse SSc ("progressive systemic fibrosis," PSS)
    - A/w **severe visceral disease** and worse prognosis
    - Sclerosis involving **distal and proximal extremities** as well as the face and **trunk**
- Other cutaneous findings
  - Raynaud phenomenon and hand edema are the two earliest and most common presenting features of SSc
  - **Beaked nose**, **microstomia**, and loss of wrinkles
  - Calcinosis cutis, usually over joints, may ulcerate
  - Xerotic itchy skin
  - Dyspigmentation: two types
    - Diffuse hyperpigmentation in sun-exposed or pressure-related areas
    - Hypopigmentation of the upper trunk/face with perifollicular sparing **("salt-and-pepper" sign)** (Fig. 3.56)
  - **Pterygium inversum unguis**: extension of hyponychium on undersurface of nail plate
- Extracutaneous findings ranging from asymptomatic to severe

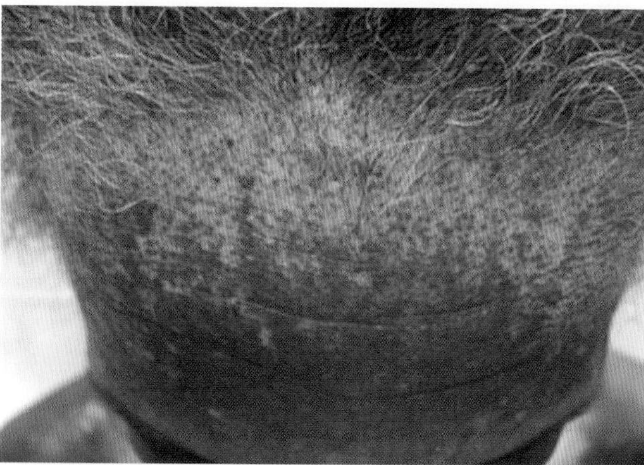

Fig. 3.56 Scleroderma-associated depigmentation with preserved perifollicular pigmentation. The salt-and-pepper appearance resembles repigmented vitiligo. (From Wigley FM, Boin F. Clinical features and treatment of scleroderma. In: Firestein GS, Budd RC, Gabriel SE, Koretzky GA, McInnes IB, O'Dell JR, eds. *Firestein & Kelly's Textbook of Rheumatology*. 11th ed. Philadelphia: Elsevier; 2021:1499–1538.)

  - Pulmonary (70%)
    - **Most common cause of mortality**
    - ILD (more common in diffuse SSc/PSS)
    - Pulmonary hypertension (more common in limited SSc/CREST)
  - Cardiovascular
    - ↑ Risk of atherosclerosis, MI, and stroke
    - Myocardial fibrosis → **restrictive cardiomyopathy** and arrhythmias
  - GI (90%)
    - **Most common site of visceral disease**
    - A/w **(↑) morbidity but no ↑ risk of mortality**
    - Lower **esophageal dysphagia/dysmotility (90%)** → aspiration and esophagitis
    - Gastroparesis
    - Gastric antral vascular ectasia (aka watermelon stomach) (1%–20%)
    - Small and large bowel dysmotility
    - Weak rectal tone → stool incontinence
  - Renal
    - Scleroderma renal crisis (SRC)
      - p/w rapid rise in creatinine
      - Affects 20% of **diffuse SSc** patients (PSS)
      - Almost never seen in limited SSc
      - **ACE-I will decrease risk**
  - Musculoskeletal
    - Arthralgias/arthritis
    - Palpable tendon friction rubs

Histopathology

- Same as morphea

Laboratory testing

- (+) ANA (>90%)
- Anti-centromere
  - a/w **Limited SSc** > diffuse SSc
  - ↑ Risk of PAH and digital ulcers

- Anti-topoisomerase I (anti-Scl-70)
  - a/w **Diffuse SSc** > limited SSc
  - ↑ Risk of ILD, digital ulcers, synovitis, joint contractures, and cardiac involvement
- Others: see Table 3.11
- CXCL4 is a biomarker for skin and lung fibrosis and PAH

Treatment

- **Most important goal = control internal organ involvement!**
  - Renal disease: **ACE inhibitors** for SRC and HTN
  - Pulmonary disease:
    - ILD: cyclophosphamide, rituximab, **MMF**, HSCT, and adjuvant N-acetylcysteine
    - PAH: endothelin receptor antagonists (e.g., bosentan), PDE-5 inhibitors, prostacyclin analogs (e.g., iloprost), lung transplant
  - GI involvement: PPIs for GERD symptoms, promotility agents
  - Cardiac involvement: ACE inhibitors
- Specific skin-directed treatments (often ineffective):
  - Raynaud phenomenon: tobacco cessation, cold temperature avoidance, and vasodilators (**CCBs [nifedipine]**, angiotensin II receptor blockers [losartan], PDE-5 inhibitors, endothelin receptor antagonists, prostaglandins, selective serotonin reuptake inhibitors [SSRIs])
  - Digital ulcers: same measures as Raynaud phenomenon; IV iloprost, ASA/clopidogrel
  - Cutaneous sclerosis: phototherapy **(PUVA, UVA1)**, ECP, glucocorticoids, immunosuppressives (MMF [w/ ILD], MTX [w/o ILD], rituximab), HSCT
  - Calcinosis cutis: **surgical excision** (can recur), **CCBs** (questionable efficacy), warfarin and extracorporeal shock-wave lithotripsy

Prognosis/clinical course

- Mortality (10-year survival):
  - Diffuse SSc (PSS): 50%
  - Limited SSc: 70%
- Due to the efficacy of ACE inhibitors for SRC, **ILD is now the #1 cause of death**
  - Screen for lung disease w/ **high-resolution CT and PFTs**
- Indicators of poor survival
  - Older age, male, African Americans, poor socioeconomic status
  - ↑ ESR and anemia
  - Major organ involvement: myositis, extensive cutaneous disease, heart involvement, ILD, and PAH
  - Presence of palpable tendon friction rubs

Additional boards factoids

Eosinophilic fasciitis (Shulman syndrome)

Epidemiology

- Female and Caucasian predominance
- Most present in fourth to sixth decades

Pathogenesis

- Pathogenesis unknown, but TGF-β levels markedly elevated
- A/w **recent history of strenuous activity** (30%)
  - Other potential triggers: trauma, borreliosis, and statin use

Clinical features

- Key feature = **rapid onset of symmetric edema/induration and pain** in extremities in a/w **peripheral eosinophilia**
  - Spares hands, feet, and face
  - Progresses to woody induration and fibrosis with a **peau d'orange** ("pseudocellulite" appearance)
  - **"Dry river bed" or "groove sign"** = linear depressions of veins within indurated skin
  - **Lacks Raynaud** phenomenon
- Disease associations (not very common): inflammatory arthritis, joint contractures, carpal tunnel syndrome, hemolytic anemia, myelodysplastic disorder, lymphoma/leukemia, MGUS, and multiple myeloma
- DDx:
  - SSc:
    - EF spares hands, feet, and face
    - EF lacks Raynaud phenomenon and visceral involvement
  - Eosinophilia-myalgia syndrome (L-tryptophan), Spanish toxic oil syndrome (rapeseed oil)
    - **EF lacks prominent systemic symptoms** (fever, myalgias, and pulmonary involvement)

Histopathology

- **Massive thickening and fibrosis of deep fascia** (10–50x the normal width); lymphoplasmacytic infiltrate +/− eosinophils
  - Must obtain deep biopsy (to fascia)
  - Eosinophils occasionally present in biopsy, but ***tissue* eosinophilia is NOT essential to diagnosis** → *peripheral* eosinophilia is more typical!

Laboratory testing

- **Peripheral eosinophilia (80%)**, ↑ ESR, hypergammaglobulinemia
- Metalloproteinase inhibitor-1 (TIMP-1) = serologic marker of disease activity
- MRI or CT scan demonstrates fascial thickening → may eliminate need for biopsy in some cases

Treatment

- **Excellent response to systemic steroids** (vs. deep morphea)
- Steroid-sparing agents: hydroxychloroquine, cyclosporine, dapsone, MTX, PUVA, UVA1 +/− acitretin, and TNF-α inhibitors
- **Physical therapy** to prevent joint contractures

Prognosis/clinical course

- Up to one third may resolve spontaneously, but some degree of induration usually persists
- Response to steroids can be appreciated after a few weeks

- Features a/w refractory disease:
  - Concomitant morphea-like skin lesions
  - Truncal involvement
  - Younger age of onset
  - Dermal fibrosis on histopathology

Nephrogenic systemic fibrosis (Nephrogenic fibrosing dermopathy NSF/NFD)

Epidemiology

- Typically presents in fifth decade
- No sex or race predilection

Pathogenesis

- Fibrosis of skin and internal organs occurs as a result of **gadolinium-containing contrast exposure** in the setting of **acute kidney injury or severe chronic kidney disease (CKD)**
  - Theory: gadolinium leaks into tissues → engulfed by macrophages → release profibrotic cytokines and growth factors → **"circulating fibrocytes" (CD34+, ProCollagen I+ cells)** recruited to skin → excess collagen and ECM production
- Onset: typically **2 to 4 weeks after gadolinium exposure**, but can occur after several years

Clinical features

- Cutaneous findings
  - Insidious onset of symmetrically distributed, painless, **hyperpigmented and indurated "patterned plaques"** (reticular or polygonal morphology) (Fig. 3.57 and Fig. 3.58)
    - **Extremities** > trunk
  - Deep induration of proximal extremities resulting in a "pseudocellulite" or cobblestone appearance
  - Marked **woody induration** with peau d'orange changes
  - Puckering or **linear banding** due to focal areas of bound-down skin on proximal extremities
  - **Dermal papules**: brawny to skin-colored papules or nodules with absent epidermal change
- **Scleral plaque** (exam favorite!): white-yellow plaques w/ dilated capillaries in patients < 45 yo (above this age, scleral plaques are less specific because of the clinical overlap w/ pinguecula) (Fig. 3.58)
- Extracutaneous involvement (very rare)
  - Fibrosis and calcification of rete testis, dura mater, diaphragm, renal tubules, heart, and lungs

Histopathology

- Very similar to scleromyxedema, but fibrosis usually extends more deeply (into fat and fascia)
  - Diagnostic findings are most prominent in subcutaneous fat septae → **must obtain deep biopsy (to fascia)**
  - ↑ **Collagen** (bundles only slightly thickened)
  - ↑ **Spindled fibrocytes** (positive staining for **CD34** and procollagen I) extending deeply into SQ fibrous septae
  - In contrast, morphea and scleroderma have loss/↓ CD34+ cells in dermis
- ↑ **Mucin (stains with Prussian blue)**

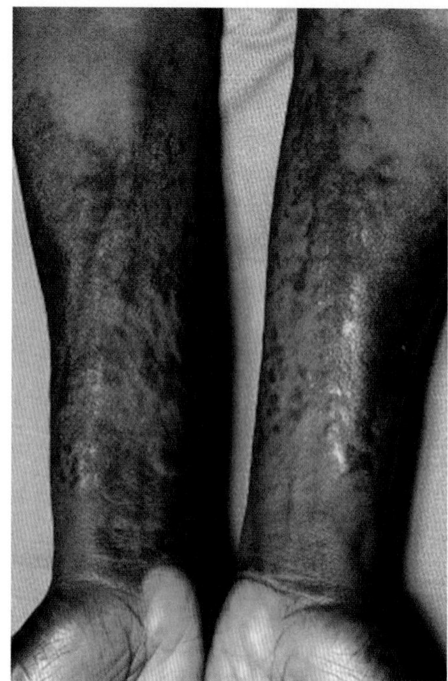

Fig. 3.57 Hyperpigmented sclerotic plaques of nephrogenic fibrosing dermopathy. (From James WD, Berger TG, Elston DM, Neuhaus IM. Connective tissue diseases. In: *Andrews' Diseases of the Skin*. 12th ed. Philadelphia: Elsevier; 2016:153–178.)

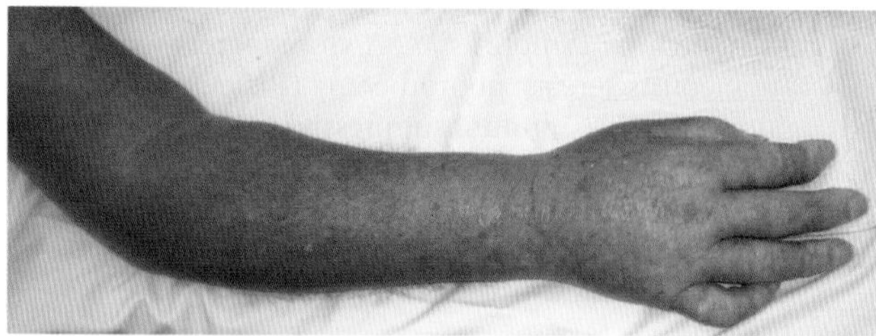

Fig. 3.58 Nephrogenic systemic fibrosis of the arm. (From Kribben A, Witzke O, Hillen U, Barkhausen J, Daul AE, Erbel R. Nephrogenic systemic fibrosis: pathogenesis, diagnosis, and therapy. *J Am Coll Cardiol*. 2009;53[18]:1621–1628.)

Laboratory testing

- ↑ Cr/BUN
- Calcium and/or phosphorus abnormalities

Treatment

- **Refractory to treatment** w/ CS and other immunosuppressives
- **Treatment of kidney disease is most important** → may slow or improve NSF
- **Physical therapy** for all patients to prevent joint contractures
- Anecdotal reports of improvement w/ imatinib, rapamycin, photodynamic therapy (PDT), UVA1, IVIG, plasmapheresis, extracorpeal photopheresis, and discontinuation of erythropoietin

Prognosis/clinical course

- Chronic, progressive course
- 2-year mortality rate ~50%

Additional boards factoids

- Know the differences between the major sclerosing/fibrosing dermopathies (Table 3.13)

Other sclerosing/fibrosing skin disorders (Table 3.14)

Abnormalities of dermal fibrous and elastic tissue

Perforating diseases (Elastosis perforans serpiginosa [EPS], reactive perforating collagenosis [RPC], acquired perforating dermatosis, and perforating calcific elastosis)

- Discussed in Table 3.15
- All are **characterized by transepidermal elimination** of dermal connective tissue
- All p/w papules and nodules with keratotic plugs
- Treatment
  - EPS/RPC generally mild; treat w/ local therapies, avoid trauma
  - Acquired perforating dermatosis: difficult to treat; BB- or NB-**UVB is most effective**

Abnormalities of connective tissue

- Discussed in Table 3.16

3.6 GRANULOMATOUS/HISTIOCYTIC DISORDERS

Non-infectious granulomas

Granuloma annulare (GA)

Epidemiology

- Children and young adults most commonly affected (2/3 arise before 30 yo)
- F > M (2:1)

Table 3.13 Major Clinical and Laboratory Manifestations of Systemic Sclerosis and Other Selected Conditions Characterized by Cutaneous Induration

	Systemic Sclerosis	Morphea	Eosinophilic Fasciitis	Scleredema	Scleromyxedema	NSF	Chronic GVHD
Major clinical variants	Limited Diffuse	Plaque-type morphea Linear morphea Generalized morphea		Post-infectious (type I) Monoclonal gammopathy-associated (type II) Diabetes mellitus-associated (type III)			Lichen sclerosis-like Morphea-like Scleroderma-like Fasciitis
Raynaud phenomenon	++	–	–	–	–	–	–
Symmetric induration	++[a]	– plaque-type and linear ± generalized	++[a]	++	++	+	+
Sclerodactyly	++	–		–	–	–	–
Facial involvement	+	– plaque-type and generalized + linear (en coup de sabre)		±types I and II – type III	+	–	±
Systemic involvement	++	– for plaque-type but ± for linear involving head (ocular, CNS)	+	–	++	+	+
Antinuclear antibodies	++	±generalized and linear – plaque-type	–	–	–	–	±
Anti-centromere antibodies	+ limited	–	–	–	–	–	–
Anti-topoisomerase I (Scl-70) antibodies	+ diffuse	–	–	–	–	–	–
Anti-RNA polymerase III	+ diffuse	–	–	–	–	–	–
Monoclonal gammopathy	–	–	±	+ type II	++	–	–
Spontaneous remission	–	++plaque-type + generalized ± linear	++	++type I ± types II and III	–	±[b]	–

[a]*May be preceded by edematous phase.*
[b]*With improved renal function.*
GVHD, *Graft-versus-host disease;* NSF, *nephrogenic systemic fibrosis;* ++, *almost always;* +, *common;* ±, *sometimes;* –, *rare or unusual.*
Courtesy of Vincent Falanga, MD. From Connolly MK. Systemic sclerosis (scleroderma) and related disorders. In: Bolognia JL, Schaffer JV, Cerroni L. Dermatology. *4th ed. Philadelphia: Elsevier; 2018:693–706.*

Table 3.14 Other Sclerosing/Fibrosing Skin Disorders

Disease	Clinical	Other
Mucinoses		
Scleredema	Erythema and woody induration of skin with a **peau d'orange** appearance; visceral involvement rare **Type 1** (55%): usually preceded by URI, especially ***Strep*** pharyngitis; typically affects middle-aged women, involving the face (expressionless face w/open mouth), neck, trunk, proximal upper extremities; usually resolves after 6–24 months **Type 2** (25%): same clinical presentation as type 1, but with associated **IgGκ** monoclonal gammopathy **Type 3** (20%, aka scleredema diabeticorum): a/w **IDDM**; typically in obese middle-aged men, involving posterior neck and upper back	Histologically shows wide spaces between collagen bundles filled with mucin
Scleromyxedema	Progressive condition, characterized by widespread, symmetric, linearly distributed **waxy papules**, typically involving **face/neck**, dorsal hands, extensor forearms, elbows, and upper trunk; diffuse infiltration can mimic scleroderma and result in leonine facies; **histologically similar to NSF**, but fibrosis does not extend as deeply into subcutis and fascia; **extracutaneous involvement common** (GI: dysphagia; MSK: arthritis, proximal muscle weakness, carpal tunnel; neuro: peripheral neuropathy)	a/w **IgGλ** paraproteinemia and HIV
Pretibial myxedema	Waxy indurated nodules or plaques with a peau d'orange appearance on the **shins**	Due to deposition of hyaluronic acid, most commonly in **Graves' disease**, but may also be seen with hypothyroidism and rarely euthyroid patients
Immunologic		
Chronic GVHD	Morpheaform plaques on trunk, which may become generalized	Usually still see some degree of interface dermatitis histologically
Paraneoplastic/neoplastic		
POEMS syndromes (polyneuropathy, organomegaly, endocrinopathy, M-protein, and skin changes)	Sclerotic skin changes favoring extremities, **hyperpigmentation**, hypertrichosis, hyperhidrosis, digital clubbing, leukonychia	**Glomeruloid hemangiomas** are strongly associated (only present in a minority of patients)
Amyloidosis (primary systemic form)	Diffuse induration of face, distal extremities, and trunk	N/A
Carcinoid syndrome	Sclerotic skin on legs	N/A
Carcinoma en cuirasse	Sclerodermoid induration of chest wall due to infiltration by cancerous cells	**Breast cancer** most commonly
Metabolic		
Diabetic cheiroarthropathy	Symmetric, painless loss of joint mobility, and stiffness of the small joints of the hand with scleroderma-like skin thickening of the dorsal aspects of the hands and feet; **"prayer sign"**	30%–50% of chronic DM2 patients; correlates w/ microvascular disease
Porphyria cutanea tarda	Morpheaform plaques in sun-exposed areas, hyperpigmentation, and hypertrichosis	Pseudoporphyria lacks sclerodermoid changes, hyperpigmentation, and hypertrichosis
Diffuse sclerodermoid conditions due to exogenous substances		
Toxic oil syndrome	p/w morbilliform eruption, **flu-like symptoms**, peripheral eosinophilia, and pulmonary edema; swelling and thickening of the skin occurs initially → followed by skin atrophy/fibrosis, dermal sclerosis, joint contractures, sicca symptoms, and Raynaud phenomenon	Due to ingestion of aniline-degraded **rapeseed cooking oil**; seen in **Spain** in 1981
Eosinophilia-myalgia syndrome	Presents initially with **fever**, **fatigue**, **weakness**, **severe myalgias**, peripheral **eosinophilia**, and a non-specific erythematous macular eruption; half develop sclerodermatous skin changes including eosinophilic fasciitis (30%), morphea, and diffuse/localized scleroderma	Due to ingestion of contaminated **L-tryptophan**, seen in 1989
Polyvinyl chloride	Workers exposed can develop skin findings that mimic scleroderma including diffuse sclerosis of the skin, sclerodactyly, Raynaud phenomenon, and hepatic/pulmonary fibrosis	Absent autoantibodies
Bleomycin	**Pulmonary fibrosis**, **Raynaud** phenomenon, and cutaneous changes indistinguishable from progressive systemic sclerosis	Absent autoantibodies
Taxanes (docetaxel, paclitaxel)	Diffuse edema (legs #1 site) → slowly becomes sclerotic; may result in flexion contractures	Absent autoantibodies; can occur after one or several courses of chemotherapy
Nephrogenic systemic fibrosis	Discussed in NSF section	a/w **Gadolinium-based contrast** agents in setting of kidney disease
Localized sclerodermoid conditions due to exogenous substances		
Radiation-induced morphea	Morphea-like plaques in radiation field (sometimes extend beyond irradiated area); chest wall most common site	Most common in breast CA pts with history of XRT
Sclerosis at injection sites	**Vitamin K (Texier's disease)**, silicone or paraffin implants/injections, **intralesional bleomycin**, **opioids** (**methadone**, pentazocine)	Bleomycin may cause SSc-like diffuse eruption if used systemically

Table 3.15 Major Perforating Diseases

	Clinical	Histopathology	High-Yield Facts/Associations
Familial reactive perforating collagenosis (RPC)	Rare, **childhood** onset; M = F; upper extremities; keratotic papules develop at sites of trauma (3–4 week latency); spontaneous resolution (6–10 weeks)	Hyper-/parakeratotic crusted plug; **COLLAGEN** fibers extend through epidermis into plug	Sites of minor trauma Collagen perforates Upper extremities
Acquired perforating dermatosis (includes acquired RPC, Kyrle disease)	Common; **adult** onset; M = F; diabetes/**renal failure**; intense pruritus; **legs** or generalized; koebnerize; central keratotic plug	Resembles RPC most commonly (may also resemble perforating folliculitis or less commonly EPS)	Almost always a/w **diabetes** or **renal failure** (10% of dialysis patients) **Lower extremities** (extensor)
Elastosis perforans serpiginosa (EPS)	Rare; **childhood or early adulthood**; **M** > F (4:1); annular/serpiginous plaques w/ **keratotic papules along rim**; most commonly on **lateral neck** > face, arms, flexural areas	Keratotic crusted plug surrounding epithelial hyperplasia **("crab-claw")** grabbing pink elastic fibers in superficial dermis (VVG stain: elastic fibers stain black vs. collagen pink)	**MAD**: **M**arfan's, **A**crogeria, **D**own's **PORES**: **P**enicillamine, **PXE**; **O**steogenesis imperfecta; **R**othmund-Thomson; **E**hlers-Danlos; **S**cleroderma May occur in Wilson's dz and cystinuria patients on **D-penicillamine**
Perforating calcific elastosis	Very rare; adulthood; mostly **black women**; plaques on abdomen **(periumbilical)** with peripheral keratotic papules	Transepidermal elimination of calcified elastic fibers **(PXE-like)**	Obese hypertensive **multiparous black women** Abdomen (especially periumbilical)

Data from Rapini RP. Perforating diseases. In: Bolognia JL, Schaffer JV, Cerroni L. Dermatology. *4th ed. Philadelphia: Elsevier; 2018:1690–1696.*

Table 3.16 Abnormalities of Connective Tissue

	Clinical Features	Histopathology	High-Yield Facts/Associations
Mid-dermal elastolysis	Uncommon; circumscribed areas of **fine wrinkling**; symmetric on **trunk**, lateral neck, extremities; Caucasian **middle-aged females**	Normal H&E, elastic tissue stains demonstrate selective loss of elastic fibers in the **mid dermis only**	**UV light** may have role in pathogenesis
Anetoderma	1–2 cm areas of flaccid/wrinkled skin, usually **elevated** (>depressed or flat); neck, trunk, upper extremities; primary form F > M, 15–25 yo	Normal H&E, elastic tissue stain shows near complete loss of elastic fibers in **papillary and reticular** dermis; **fragmented** elastic fiber remnants visible	Primary (idiopathic) Jadassohn-Pellizzari (inflammatory) Schweninger-Buzzi (non-inflammatory) Secondary Infection, penicillamine, inflammatory dermatosis, autoimmune (**lupus**, Sjögren's, Graves' dz), cutaneous tumors
Follicular atrophoderma	Dimple-like follicular-based **"ice-pick"** depressions; **dorsal hands/feet and cheeks**; onset birth to early childhood	Dilated follicles w/plugging, inflammation and dermal collagen sclerosis	Associated with: **Bazex-Dupre-Christol syndrome** (follicular atrophoderma, BCCs of face, milia, localized hypohidrosis above neck, hypotrichosis)
Atrophoderma vermiculatum	Variant of follicular atrophoderma that is on **face/cheeks exclusively**; may be (1) sporadic, (2) inherited as a sole finding (autosomal dominant), (3) part of a syndrome, or (4) presenting feature of KP atrophicans	Same as above	Associated with: **Rombo syndrome** (atrophoderma vermiculatum, milia, acral erythema, peripheral vasodilation with cyanosis, multiple BCCs) **Nicolau-Balus syndrome** (generalized eruptive syringomas, atrophoderma vermiculata and milia) **Others:** Tuzun (scrotal tongue), and Braun-Falco-Marghescu (PPK and KP)
Striae	Atrophic linear lesions along cleavage lines violaceous in color, Caucasians; F > M	Clinical diagnosis	Puberty, pregnancy; ↑ **in Marfan's syndrome**
Hypertrophic scar/keloids	Darker skin, often familial tendency; 10–30 yo; Hypertrophic scar **confined** to wound borders and raised; keloids delayed in onset, **extend beyond** wound borders	Hypertrophic scar: ↑ fibroblasts/collagen (type I >III) oriented both parallel to skin surface like normal scar and in **whorled nodules**; vertically oriented vessels Keloids: haphazardly-arrayed thick bundles of hyalinized collagen	Hypertrophic scars spontaneously resolve Keloids persist in absence of treatment; Rx: IL-steroids (first line), excision, XRT, topical imiquimod, lasers, IL 5-FU

Pathogenesis

- Unknown etiology; most likely Th1-type delayed hypersensitivity reaction to a variety of triggers (trauma/isomorphic Koebner response, insect bites, tuberculin skin test, mycobacterial/viral infection, drugs, or UV radiation)
  - Trigger → Th1 reaction → monocyte accumulation in dermis → release of lysosomal enzymes → degradation of elastic fibers
- Majority of affected patients are healthy (especially localized GA)
  - Generalized GA more commonly a/w **hyperlipidemia** (up to 45%), **type I diabetes**, HIV, thyroid disease, malignancy (clinical pattern atypical—e.g., palms and soles)

Clinical features

- Benign, self-resolving condition that p/w asymptomatic **annular**/arciform plaques comprising multiple small, **non-scaly**, flesh-colored to pink or violaceous papules
  - Solitary **umbilicated papules** are common presentation on **fingers**/hands
  - Previously involved skin in center of the **annulus** often has red-brown color
- Distribution: **isolated hands/arms most common** (60%; particularly dorsal hands/fingers and elbows) > isolated legs/feet (20%; particularly dorsal feet and ankles) > combined upper and lower extremities (7%)
  - Less commonly: isolated truncal lesions (7%) or trunk + other sites (5%)
- Variants:
  - <u>Patch GA</u>: symmetric erythematous patches commonly on bilateral dorsal feet (or trunk and extremities); often lacks annular configuration; **histology shows interstitial GA** most commonly
  - <u>Subcutaneous or deep dermal GA ("pseudorheumatoid nodule")</u>: most common in **children** < 6 yo; large, asymptomatic rheumatoid-like nodules on **dorsal foot (#1 site)**, palms, shins, buttocks, and scalp; often a/w **trauma**; 50% also have classic GA lesions
  - <u>Generalized (disseminated) GA</u>: occurs in minority of patients; later age of onset (40–50s); composed of innumerable small red-violaceous papules coalescing into **small annular plaques** especially on **upper trunk/proximal upper extremities** (Fig. 3.59); poor response to treatment; usually self-resolves over 3 to 4 years; **lipid abnormalities** in 45%; **diabetes** in 21% (vs. only 10% in localized GA); ↑ prevalence of HLA-Bw35
  - <u>Perforating GA</u>: 5% of GA cases; most commonly on **dorsal hands and fingers**; small papules with central keratotic plug, umbilication, or ulceration; transepidermal elimination of degenerated collagen seen histologically
  - <u>GA-like eruptions</u>: may be seen in association with solid organ tumors, B- and T-cell **lymphomas**, **HIV** (p/w generalized GA > localized), at sites of **prior herpes zoster scars**, or drug-induced (**TNF-α inhibitors** > amlodipine, allopurinol, diclofenac, gold)

Histopathology

- All forms are characterized by granulomatous dermal inflammation with foci of collagen/elastic fiber degeneration, ↑ mucin, and scattered eosinophils
- If LCV, granulomatous vasculitis, or thrombosis is present, there is ↑ risk of systemic disease (probably represents PNGD variant)
- Three common histologic patterns:
  - <u>Interstitial (most common; 70% of cases)</u>: most subtle pattern; singly-arrayed histiocytes between collagen fibers; minimal collagen/elastic fiber degradation; **key to diagnosis is ↑ dermal mucin between collagen fibers** (best appreciated w/ colloidal iron or Alcian blue) and perivascular eosinophils
  - <u>Palisaded granulomas (25%)</u>: best visualized at low power; consist of one or more palisaded granulomas w/ central degeneration of collagen/elastic fibers and ↑ **dermal mucin**
  - <u>Sarcoidal pattern (5%)</u>: rare histologic presentation comprising well-formed epithelioid histiocytic nodules

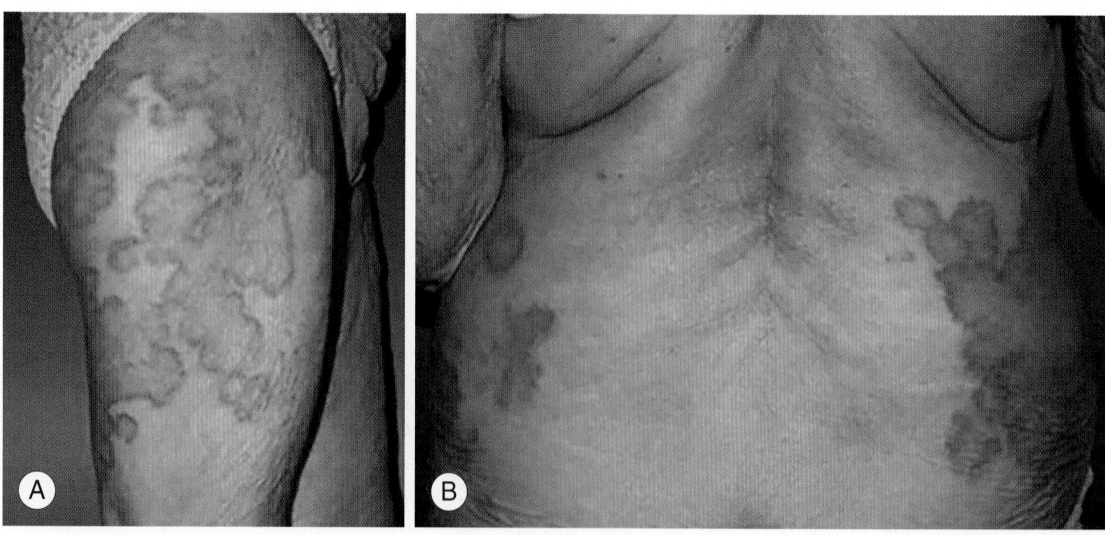

Fig. 3.59 (A) and (B) Disseminated granuloma annulare consisting of erythematous annular plaques. (From Solano-López G, Concha-Garzón MJ, de Argila D, Daudén E. Successful treatment of disseminated granuloma annulare with narrowband UV-B phototherapy. *Actas Dermosifiliogr*. 2015;106[3]:240–241.)

- Deep GA: palisaded granulomas w/ central blue-colored mucin (**vs. pink fibrin in RA**) in deep dermis/SQ
- Perforating GA: typical GA findings, plus transepidermal elimination of degenerated collagen and granulomatous debris

Treatment

- Localized/asymptomatic: reassurance, **high-potency topical or intralesional steroids**, TCIs, lasers, and light cryotherapy
  - In some cases, biopsy of lesion → resolution
- Severe disease: phototherapy, antimalarials, nicotinamide, isotretinoin, dapsone, pentoxiphylline, PDT, **triple antibiotic regimens** (minocycline, ofloxacin, and rifampin), and **TNF-α inhibitors**

Prognosis/clinical course

- Spontaneous resolution in 2 years for half of patients
- 40% recurrence rate, but recurrent episodes clear faster

Annular elastolytic giant cell granuloma (actinic granuloma of O'Brien)

- GA variant affecting **chronically sun-exposed skin** (face, neck, upper trunk, and arms)
- Possibly caused by inflammatory response to UV; most commonly middle-aged women
- Start as flesh-colored to pink papules → coalesce into **annular plaques** 1 to 10 cm in diameter; normally < 10 total lesions
- Histopathology: interstitial (> well-formed palisaded) granulomatous infiltrate w/ more **multinucleated foreign body GCs** than are typically seen in GA; **phagocytosed elastic fibers within histiocytes and GCs** ("**elastophagocytosis**"); no collagen alteration or lipid deposition, **lacks mucin**; Verhoeff-Van Gieson (**VVG**) **stain shows absence of elastic fibers** and loss of solar elastosis in affected areas
- Rx: typically persistent (vs. GA); poor response to standard GA treatments

Interstitial granulomatous dermatitis and arthritis (IGDA) and palisaded neutrophilic granulomatous dermatitis (PNGD)

- F > M
- These two granulomatous dermatitides exist on a spectrum (Table 3.17)
- Both are a/w systemic diseases:
  - **SLE** and ANCA vasculitides (PNGD > IGDA)
  - **RA** (both)
  - Other autoimmune diseases (both)
- Pathogenesis: autoimmune condition → immune complex deposition in/around dermal vessel walls → chronic, low-intensity vasculitis (more brisk and neutrophil-rich in PNGD) → gradual impairment of blood flow to dermal collagen → collagen degeneration → palisaded granulomatous inflammation in reaction to degenerated collagen

Table 3.17 Interstitial Granulomatous Dermatitis and Arthritis (IGDA)/ Palisaded Neutrophilic Granulomatous Dermatitis (PNGD)

IGDA	PNGD
Annular plaques or **linear red to skin-colored cords** (aka **"rope sign;"** usually in axilla)	**Red to violaceous tender papules/plaques** +/− **umbilication** +/− perforation/ ulceration
Trunk, buttocks, and intertriginous areas (symmetric)	Symmetric involvement of **extensor digits** (including palms), **elbows**, and other extensors
Histology: small **rosettes** of palisading histiocytes (w/ giant cells) in mid/deep reticular dermis ("bottom heavy") around small foci (smaller than GA) of degenerated collagen; interstitial lymphocytes; no mucin; +/−neutrophils; **no obvious vasculitis**	*Histology*: small vessel **LCV** w/**basophilic collagen degeneration** and neutrophilic infiltrates (early) → palisaded granulomas with basophilic collagen degeneration +/− perforating collagen (late)
Most common associations: **RA**, seronegative arthritis, autoimmune thyroiditis, SLE, IBD Arthralgias or arthritis (50%)	Most common associations: **RA, SLE, ANCA (+) vasculitides** (Wegener's/Churg-Strauss > others), malignancy (lymphoproliferative)

- ANA(+) in 50%
- No specific treatment exists other than treating underlying disease, +/− topical or IL-steroids
- 66% of patients achieve complete remission (months to years); 33% have persistent, chronic, relapsing course

Interstitial granulomatous drug eruption

- Clinically may resemble interstitial GA, IGDA, or PNGD
  - Annular, red, non-scaly papules and plaques w/ indurated border; favors creases and often photodistributed; spares mucous membranes
- Most commonly caused by **CCBs, statins, TNF-α inhibitors** (months to years after drug initiation)
  - Others: ACE inhibitors, furosemide, β-blockers, antihistamines, HCTZ, anakinra, thalidomide
- Histology: may resemble interstitial GA, IGDA, or PNGD but frequently has deeper dermal involvement (bottom two thirds of dermis), **interface dermatitis**, atypical lymphocytes, and lacks mucin
- Typically resolves months after drug discontinuation

Necrobiosis lipoidica (Necrobiosis lipoidica diabeticorum, NLD)

Epidemiology

- F > M (3:1)
- Only 0.03% of diabetics have NLD, but **22%** of patients with NLD have or will develop **diabetes/glucose intolerance**
  - Diabetics w/ NLD have ↑ risk of peripheral neuropathy, retinopathy, and joint immobility
- May be a/w smoking

Pathogenesis

- Vascular compromise from immunodeposition in vessel walls or diabetes-related microangiopathic changes → subacute **dermal ischemia** → dermal collagen degeneration → secondary granulomatous inflammatory response

Clinical features

- Early lesions manifest as firm, reddish papules → expand into atrophic plaques (usually multiple) on bilateral **shins** w/ a peripheral violaceous to **erythematous rim** and **atrophic central yellow-brown discoloration w/ telangiectasias** (Fig. 3.60)
  - Dermoscopy: comma-shaped vessels (early lesions), and irregular arborizing vessels (older lesions)
  - Minor trauma results in **ulceration** (30%)
- Adnexae and neural elements frequently lost within NLD plaques → ↓ pinprick/fine touch sensation, hypohidrosis, and localized alopecia

Histopathology

- "Square biopsy" sign
- **Horizontally arranged ("layered") palisaded granulomatous inflammation** w/ horizontal tiers of degenerated collagen fibers (irregular size and shape) and dermal sclerosis
- Process **diffusely involves** <u>**entire**</u> **dermis** and subcutaneous fat septae (vs. GA, which tends to have patchy dermal involvement with areas of normal intervening dermis)
- Lacks mucin
- **Plasma cells** and multinucleated GCs are abundant (both uncommon in GA)
- +/− epidermal atrophy; +/− vascular hyalinization (Fig. 3.61)

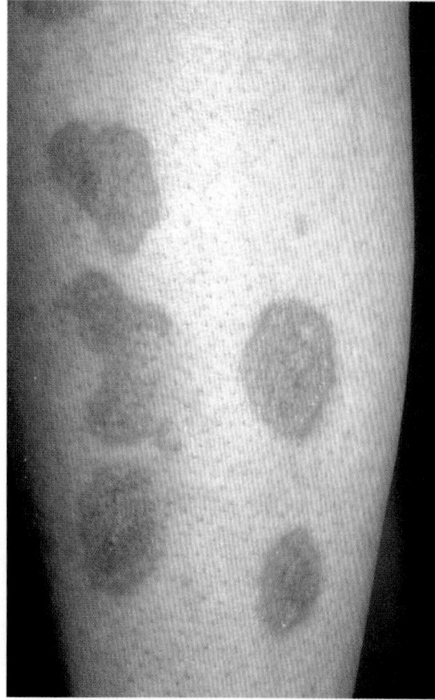

Fig. 3.60 Necrobiosis lipoidica with red-yellow atrophic plaques on anterior shin. (From James WD, Elston DM, McMahon PJ. Errors in metabolism. In: *Andrews' Diseases of the Skin: Clinical Atlas*. Philadelphia: Elsevier; 2018:361–378.)

Treatment

- First line: **potent topical and/or intralesional steroids** (injected into inflammatory rim); TCIs (early lesions)
- Systemic steroids, colchicine, cyclosporine, TNF-α inhibitors, CO_2 laser, stanozolol, pentoxyfylline in chronic/recalcitrant cases
- Surgical excision to fascia w/ skin grafting may be necessary in severe ulcerative cases

Prognosis/clinical course

- Rarely undergoes spontaneous remission (17% at 8–12 years)
- Control of blood glucose levels does **not** affect disease course
- No treatment has demonstrated efficacy in large double-blind studies
- SCC may arise in chronic ulcerative lesions

Necrobiotic xanthogranuloma (NXG)

- Peak in sixth decade; M = F
- Multisystem histiocytic disease that p/w firm **yellow xanthomatous** plaques and nodules, most commonly in **periorbital** region (Fig. 3.62) (> trunk, proximal extremities)
  - Often **ulcerates** and leads to scarring
- 50% have ophthalmic manifestations (ectropion, keratitis, uveitis, and proptosis); majority also have endocardial involvement; hepatosplenomegaly common
- Strongly a/w **IgGκ monoclonal gammopathy** (due to plasma cell dyscrasia or multiple myeloma)
  - Skin findings precede diagnosis of malignancy by 2–20 years
- Histopathology: diffuse (pandermal and into subcutis), palisading **xanthogranulomas** w/ necrobiotic collagen, foamy histiocytes, **"dirty dermis"** (scattered inflammatory cell debris), **abundant cholesterol clefts**, and multiple Touton and **bizarre foreign body GCs** (HUGE multinucleated cells w/ "horse-shoe" arrangement of 25 to 50 nuclei → these cells are not seen in NLD or GA)
- Rx: none effective; **treat underlying malignancy** or paraproteinemia

Cutaneous Crohn's disease

Epidemiology

- 20%–45% of Crohn's patients have skin or mucosal findings
- <u>Crohn's specific (uncommon)</u>: contiguous perianal/genital/oral Crohn's, distant ("metastatic") Crohn's
- <u>Non-specific/reactive (more common)</u>: **EN**, **PG (ulcerative colitis [UC] > Crohn's)**, pyostomatitis vegetans (UC > Crohn's), pathergy (pustular response to trauma), **EB acquisita** (IBD is the most common cause of EBA), and acrodermatitis enteropathica-like syndrome due to zinc deficiency
- F > M; average age = 35 yo
- Cutaneous Crohn's is more frequently a/w colorectal rather than small intestinal disease
- Skin findings may precede GI diagnosis of Crohn's (20% of cases)

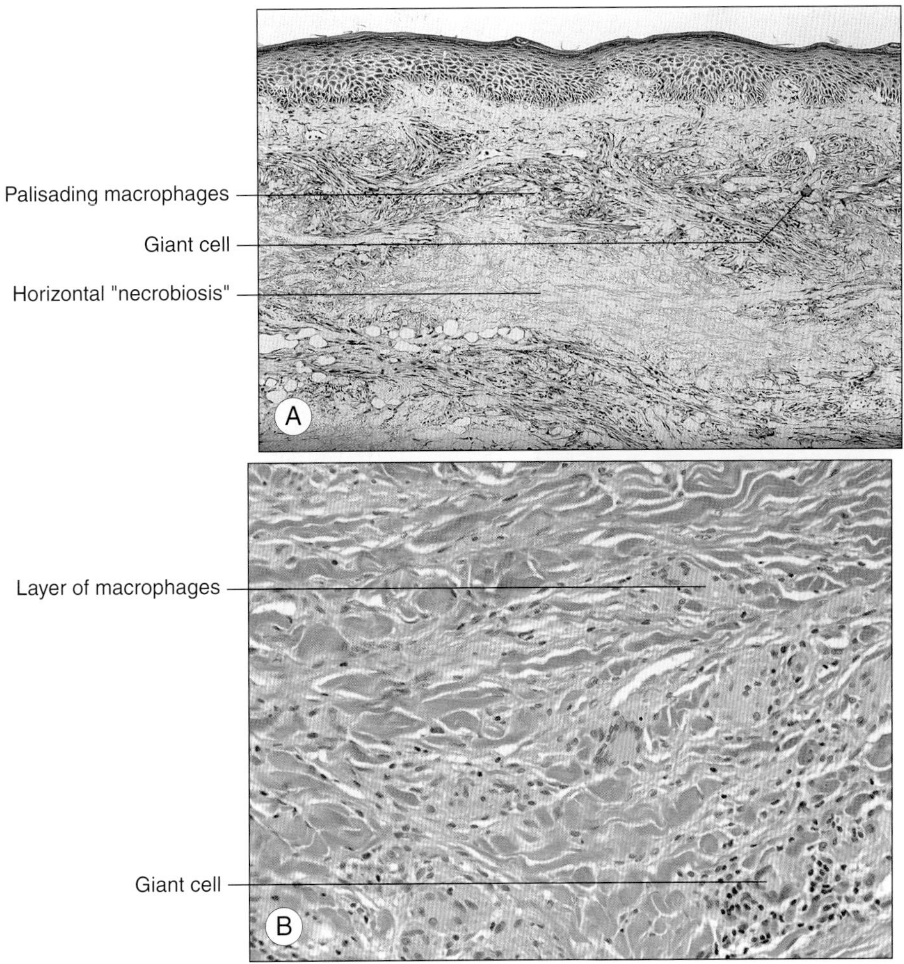

Fig. 3.61 Necrobiosis lipoidica. (A) Low magnification. (B) The layered cake appearance of granulomas is often subtle. (From Rapini RP: Noninfectious granulomas. In: Rapini RP, ed. *Practical Dermatopathology.* 3rd ed. Philadelphia: Elsevier; 2021:101–118.)

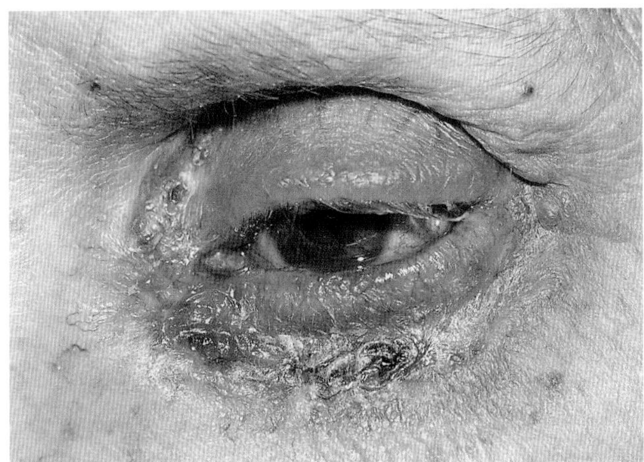

Fig. 3.62 Necrobiotic xanthogranuloma in a patient with a paraproteinemia. (From Piette WW. Dysproteinemias, plasma cell disorders, and amyloidosis. In: Callen JP, Jorizzo JL, Zone JJ, et al. *Dermatological Signs of Systemic Disease.* 5th ed. Philadelphia: Elsevier; 2017:171–182.)

Pathogenesis

- Genetic predisposition (e.g., NOD2) + defective microbial clearance, mucosal compromise or altered gut flora balance (dysbiosis) → exaggerated Th1 and Th17 response to gut flora → granulomatous lesions in gut and skin

Clinical features

- Genital Crohn's: **labial or scrotal edema** + erythema/ulceration/fissures (Fig. 3.63)
- Perianal Crohn's: ulcers, **sinus tracts**, **fissures**, or eroded vegetating plaques; lesions frequently extend to perineum, buttocks, abdomen, and abdominal surgical or ostomy sites
  - Peristomal Crohn's: fissures and fistulae around ostomy
- Oral Crohn's: "**cobblestoning**" of buccal mucosa, pyostomatitis vegetans, **cheilitis granulomatosa**, gingival hyperplasia, diffuse oral swelling, fissures, aphthous-like ulcers, linear ulcers, and small gingival nodules
- Extragenital ("metastatic") Crohn's: dusky red papules/plaques → ulcerations with undermined edges, fistulas, draining sinuses and scarring; most common sites = **lower extremities/soles** (38%) > abdomen/trunk (24%) > upper extremities (15%), face/lips (11%), flexures (8%), generalized (4%)

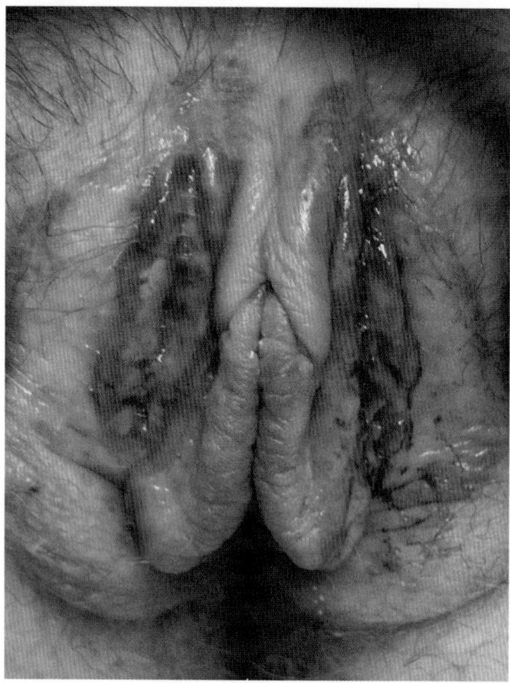

Fig. 3.63 Cutaneous Crohn's disease. Note the swelling and violaceous discoloration of the labia majora. (From Hagen JW, Swoger JM, Grandinetti LM. Cutaneous manifestations of Crohn disease. *Dermatol Clin*. 2015;33[3]:417–431.)

Histopathology

- Non-caseating tuberculoid granulomas w/ inflammatory rim of lymphocytes in superficial and deep dermis; frequent Langhans GCs

Treatment/prognosis

- First line: oral metronidazole, topical/intralesional steroids, and TCIs
- Severe cases: oral steroids, sulfasalazine, MTX, MMF, cyclosporine, thalidomide, AZA, 6-MP, and TNF-α inhibitors
- Disease tends to be chronic; severity of cutaneous and GI disease often not correlated

Sarcoidosis

Epidemiology

- Bimodal incidence peaks: 25–35 yo and 45–65 yo
- F > M
- **African Americans** have highest incidence and disease tends to be more severe/progressive
- ↑ Incidence of cases in spring/winter → environmental/infectious trigger hypothesis

Pathogenesis

- Multisystem granulomatous disease caused by upregulation of CD4+ **Th1** cells
- Genetic predisposition + **unknown antigen** presented by monocytes with MHC class II molecules → activation of CD4+ Th1 cells → ↑ IL-2, IFN-γ, TNF-α, and monocyte chemotactic factor → **monocytes** leave circulation and enter peripheral tissues, including skin, where they form granulomas → granulomas have potential to result in end-organ dysfunction
- Drug-induced sarcoid:
  - **Hepatitis C patients on treatment (IFN-α, ribavirin)**
  - HIV patients on HAART
  - Other meds: TNF-α inhibitors, vemurafenib, ipilimumab, and alemtuzumab

Clinical features

- **Cutaneous findings:**
  - 35% of patients with sarcoidosis develop skin lesions
  - Skin may be the only site of involvement
    - All patients w/ cutaneous sarcoid require CXR, PFTs, and regular eye exams
  - Lesions present as red-brown or erythematous papules and plaques w/ characteristic "**apple jelly**" color with diascopy (better appreciated on light-skinned patients)
    - Lesions typically lack secondary changes
    - Predilection for **face** (Fig. 3.64) (especially **lips and nose**), neck, and upper half of the body
    - Lesions often arise within **preexisting scars, piercings, or tattoos**
    - Less common presentations: hypopigmented, ichthyosiform, angiolupoid (prominent telangiectasias), psoriasiform, annular, verrucous, cicatricial alopecia, and erythrodermic
- **EN**: most important non-specific manifestation of sarcoidosis since it predicts **a benign, self-limited course**
- **Other areas of involvement:**
  - Lung disease (90%): alveolitis, bronchiolitis, and pleuritis; may culminate in "**honeycombing**" of lung, w/ fibrosis and bronchiectasis
  - Lymphadenopathy (90%): **hilar and/or paratracheal**; typically asymptomatic
  - Ocular involvement (20%–50%): **anterior uveitis** (most common), retinitis, lacrimal inflammation, and conjunctivitis → may result in blindness
  - Hypercalcemia (10%): due to **calcitriol synthesis by sarcoidal granulomas** (convert 25-hyroxyvitamin D into more active 1,25-dihyroxyvitamin D) → hypercalcemia, hypercalciuria, and **nephrocalcinosis** → renal failure
  - Other: nail changes (clubbing, onycholysis, and subungual hyperkeratosis), oral involvement (salivary

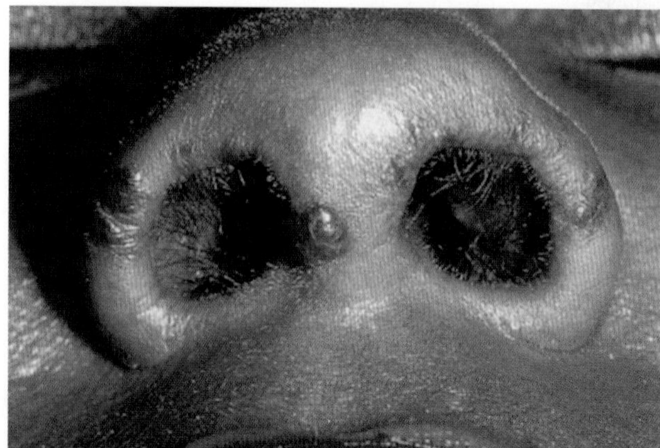

Fig. 3.64 Sarcoidosis characteristic papules on the nares. (From James WD, Berger TG, Elston DM, Neuhaus IM. Macrophage/Monocyte disorders. In: *Andrews' Diseases of the Skin*. 12th ed. Philadelphia: Elsevier; 2016:699–725.)

Table 3.18 Sarcoid Variants

Lupus pernio	**Violaceous** (rather than red-brown) papules coalescing into infiltrative plaques; **nose/earlobes/cheeks** = most common sites; **"beaded" appearance** along the nasal rim (Fig. 3.65); resolves with scarring (unlike most cutaneous sarcoid); **strongly a/w chronic sarcoid lung (75%) and upper respiratory tract (50%) disease**, cystic degeneration of bones of distal phalanges, ocular involvement, and reticuloendothelial involvement; rarely involutes and has **poor prognosis**
Darier-Roussy	**Subcutaneous sarcoid**; painless, firm, deep-seated mobile nodules; 90% have hilar adenopathy and multiple lesions; a/w **good prognosis**
Löfgren syndrome	**Acute** form of sarcoidosis; p/w **erythema nodosum** + **hilar adenopathy** + fever + migrating polyarthritis + acute iritis; most common in **Scandinavians**, rare in Blacks; a/w **good prognosis**
Heerfordt syndrome ("uveoparotid fever")	**Uveitis** + **parotid gland enlargement** + **fever** + **cranial nerve palsy** (facial nerve most commonly)
Mikulicz syndrome	Outdated, non-specific term (may be seen in TB, sarcoid, Sjögren's syndrome, lymphoma), referring to **enlargement of salivary, lacrimal, and parotid glands**
Blau syndrome	**Early-onset** (age < 5 yo) sarcoid-like disease; caused by **NOD2 mutation**; triad of skin, eye, and joint disease
Drug-induced cutaneous sarcoid	**IFN-α (hepatitis C patients)**, HIV patients on HAART, TNF-α inhibitors

gland, gingiva, hard/soft palate, and tongue), liver, and heart involvement
- Sarcoid variants (Table 3.18)

Histopathology

- Superficial and deep dermis packed w/ nodules of **well-formed, non-caseating, "naked epithelioid granulomas"** (epithelioid granulomas lacking a significant inflammatory rim of lymphocytes or plasma cells)
  - **Asteroid bodies** (star-shaped eosinophilic inclusions of collagen) and Schaumann bodies (basophilic calcium and protein inclusions) are commonly seen within histiocytic GCs

Laboratory testing

- **Kveim-Siltzbach test** (not routinely performed): injecting suspension of sarcoidal spleen into the skin of a patient w/ sarcoidosis → sarcoidal granuloma at injection site
- CXR or CT scan (most sensitive): hilar/paratracheal lymphadenopathy +/− pulmonary infiltrates

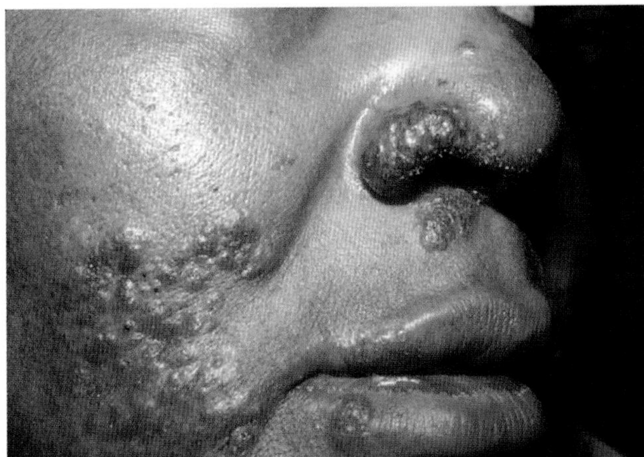

Fig. 3.65 Sarcoidosis, lupus pernio type, with coalescing violaceous papules on the nose. (From Marchell RM, Judson MA. Chronic cutaneous lesions of sarcoidosis. *Clin Dermatol*. 2007;25[3]:295–302.)

- PFTs: restrictive lung disease pattern → ↓ total lung capacity, ↓ diffusing capacity, and ↓ vital capacity
- ↑ **ACE level** (60%; more useful in **monitoring** response to treatment than for diagnosis)
- ↑ ESR; hypercalcemia, lymphopenia

Treatment

- First line: **oral prednisone** for systemic involvement +/− topical or IL-steroids for skin involvement; the degree of lung, eye, and other internal involvement determines how quickly you can taper prednisone
- Other treatments for chronic skin-predominant disease: **hydroxychloroquine**, chloroquine, **TNF-α inhibitors** (treat systemic symptoms), MMF, AZA, minocycline, leflunomide

Additional boards factoids

- **Granulomatous dermatitis summary** (Fig. 3.66, Tables 3.19 and 3.20)

Foreign body reactions
(Tables 3.21 and 3.22)

- Non-organic and high molecular weight organic materials that are deposited into the dermis/subcutis and are resistant to biologic degradation by inflammatory cells may → foreign body reaction
- p/w indurated red or red-brown papules coalescing into plaques +/− ulceration
- Histopathology: foreign body granulomas +/− recognizable foreign material
- Less common reaction patterns: pseudolymphomatous, lichenoid, and eczematous

Histiocytoses

- Group of proliferative disorders that share a common CD34+ progenitor cell in bone marrow
- This common ancestor later differentiates into a variety of so-called "histiocytes":
  - <u>Langerhans cell</u>: potent APC that migrates to and from **epidermis**, stains positively with **CD1a**, **S100**, and

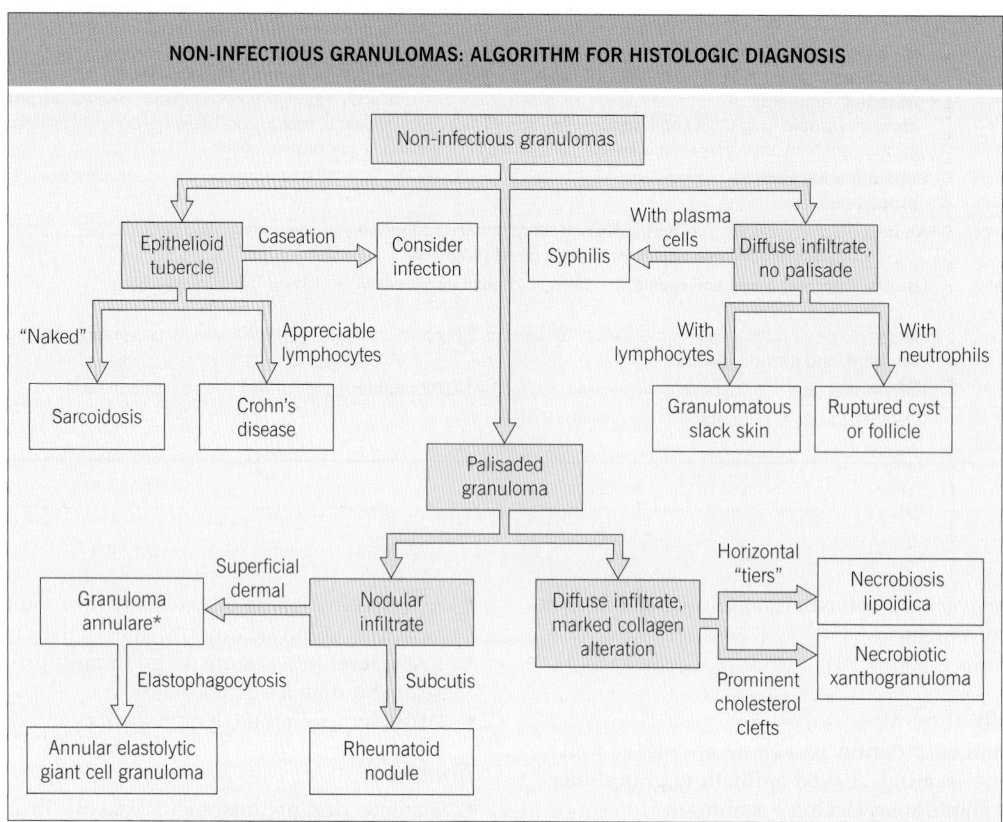

Fig. 3.66 Non-infectious granulomas: algorithm for histologic diagnosis. Interstitial granulomatous dermatitis and palisaded neutrophilic and granulomatous dermatitis may represent an additional diagnostic consideration. *May also have a patchy dermal interstitial pattern without palisades, or subcutaneous palisades with more mucin than rheumatoid nodules. (From Rosenbach MA, Wanat KA, Reisenauer A, White KP, Korcheva V, White CR Jr. Non-infectious granulomas. In: Bolognia JL, Schaffer JV, Cerroni L. *Dermatology*. 4th ed. Philadelphia: Elsevier; 2018:1644–1663.)

Table 3.19 Clinical Features of the Major Granulomatous Dermatitides

	Sarcoidosis[a]	Classic Granuloma Annulare[b]	Necrobiosis Lipoidica	AEGCG	Cutaneous Crohn's Disease	Rheumatoid Nodule
Average age (years)	25–35, 45–65	<30	30	50–70	35	40–50
Sex predilection	Female	Female	Female	None	Female	Male[c]
Racial/ethnic predilection in the United States	African American	None	None	Caucasian	Ashkenazi Jews	None
Sites	Symmetric on face, neck, upper trunk, extremities	Hands, feet, extensor aspects of extremities	Anterior and lateral aspects of distal lower extremities	Face, neck, forearms (sites of chronic sun exposure)	Genital areas, lower > upper extremities	Juxta-articular areas, especially elbows, hands, ankles, feet
Appearance	Red to red-brown papules and plaques; occasionally violaceous or annular	Papules coalescing into annular plaques	Plaques with elevated borders, telangiectasias centrally	Annular plaques	Dusky erythema and swelling, ulceration	Skin-colored, firm, mobile subcutaneous nodules
Size of lesions	0.2 to >5 cm	1–3 mm papules, annular plaques usually < 6 cm	3 to >10 cm	1–6 cm	Variable	1–3 cm
No. of lesions	Variable	1–10	1–10	1–10	1–5	1–10
Associations	Systemic manifestations of sarcoidosis; INF-α therapy for hepatitis C viral infection » melanoma	Rare diabetes mellitus, HIV infection, malignancy	Diabetes mellitus	Actinic damage	Intestinal Crohn's disease	Rheumatoid arthritis

Table 3.19 Clinical Features of the Major Granulomatous Dermatitides—cont'd

	Sarcoidosis[a]	Classic Granuloma Annulare[b]	Necrobiosis Lipoidica	AEGCG	Cutaneous Crohn's Disease	Rheumatoid Nodule
Special clinical characteristics	Occasional central atrophy and hypopigmentation; development within scars	Central hyperpigmentation	Yellow-brown atrophic centers, ulceration	Central atrophy and hypopigmentation	Draining sinuses and fistulas	Occasional ulceration, especially at sites of trauma

[a]*Clinical variants include lupus pernio and subcutaneous (Darier–Roussy), psoriasiform, ichthyosiform, angiolupoid, and ulcerative sarcoidosis.*
[b]*Clinical variants include generalized, micropapular, nodular, perforating, subcutaneous, and patch granuloma annulare.*
[c]*Although rheumatoid arthritis has a female:male ratio of 2–3:1.*
AEGCG, *Annular elastolytic giant cell granuloma;* HIV, *human immunodeficiency virus;* IFN, *interferon.*
Modified from Rosenbach MA, Wanat KA, Reisenauer A, White KP, Korcheva V, White CR Jr. Non-infectious granulomas. In: Bolognia JL, Schaffer JV, Cerroni L. Dermatology. *4th ed. Philadelphia: Elsevier; 2018:1644–1663.*

Table 3.20 Histologic Features of the Major Granulomatous Dermatitides

	Sarcoidosis	Granuloma Annulare	Necrobiosis Lipoidica	AEGCG	Cutaneous Crohn's Disease	Rheumatoid Nodule	Interstitial Granulomatous Dermatitis[a]	Palisading Neutrophilic and Granulomatous Dermatitis[a]
Typical location	Superficial and deep dermis	Superficial and mid dermis	Entire dermis, subcutis	Superficial and mid dermis	Superficial and deep dermis	Deep dermis, subcutis	Mid and deep dermis	Entire dermis
Granuloma pattern	Tubercle with few peripheral lymphocytes ("naked")	Palisading or interstitial	Diffuse palisading and interstitial; **horizontal "tiers"**	Palisading, irregular	Tubercle with surrounding lymphocytes	Palisading	Palisading in **small "rosettes"**	Palisading; prominent **neutrophils and leukocytoclasia**
Necrobiosis (altered collagen)	No	**Yes ("blue")**	Yes ("red")	No	No	**Yes ("red")**	Yes ("blue")	Yes ("blue")
Giant cells	Yes	Variable	Yes	Yes	Yes	Yes	Variable	Variable
Elastolysis	No	Variable	Variable	**Yes**	No	No	Variable	Variable
Elastophagocytosis	No	No	No	**Yes**	No	No	No	No
Asteroid bodies	**Yes**	Variable	Variable	Yes	No	No	Variable	Variable
Mucin	No	**Yes**	Minimal	No	No	Variable	Minimal	Variable
Extracellular lipid	No	Variable	Yes	No	No	Variable	No	No
Vascular changes	No	Variable	Yes	No	No	**Yes**	No	**Yes**

[a]*Interstitial granulomatous dermatitis and palisading neutrophilic and granulomatous dermatitis are often considered two ends of a spectrum.*
AEGCG, *Annular elastolytic giant cell granuloma.*
Modified from Rosenbach MA, Wanat KA, Reisenauer A, White KP, Korcheva V, White CR Jr. Non-infectious granulomas. In: Bolognia JL, Schaffer JV, Cerroni L. Dermatology. *4th ed. Philadelphia: Elsevier; 2018:1644–1663.*

Table 3.21 Foreign Body Reactions

Foreign Body	Clinical Presentation	Histopathology	Other Key Points
Tattoo inks	Red tattoos (**mercuric sulfide**, aka **cinnabar**) are most common cause of delayed reactions, usually lichenoid or pseudolymphomatous papules and nodules Eczematous dermatitis **Photoallergic reactions**, usually to **yellow** ink (**cadmium sulfide**), red ink (cadmium selenide) or yellow-red (azo dyes)	**Lichenoid** dermatitis or **pseudolymphoma** (red tattoo) Spongiotic dermatitis (many others) Granulomatous (**aluminum**, and others)	Tattoo pigment granules in dermis are smaller and darker than endogenous pigments (hemosiderin and melanin) Various Q-switched lasers are ToC for tattoos: QS-ruby (694 nm), QS-alexandrite (755 nm), QS-Nd:YAG (1064 or 532 nm) Ruby, alexandrite, and Nd:YAG (1064 nm) all treat **black, blue, dark brown** Ruby or alexandrite is ToC for **green** Only frequency-doubled Nd:YAG (532 nm) is effective for **red, yellow, light brown, violet, and white** If tattoo is inflamed, excise (instead of laser) to ↓ risk of systemic allergic rxn
Silica (silicon dioxide)	Penetrating injuries involving **sand**, **soil**, **rocks**, **glass**; prolonged incubation period (up to 25 years); p/w nodules, indurated plaques within scar Disseminated papules (blast injuries)	Sarcoidal granulomas containing **colorless, birefringent crystals**	Rx: excision

Continued

Table 3.21 Foreign Body Reactions—cont'd

Foreign Body	Clinical Presentation	Histopathology	Other Key Points
Talc (hydrous magnesium silicate)	Common component of **dusting powders** (umbilical stump, intertriginous areas of obese pts), surgical glove lubricants, and as filler for med tablets (IV drug abusers who mash up meds and inject) p/w sarcoid-like papules; may appear pyogenic granuloma-like	Sarcoidal or foreign body granulomas with needle-shaped or round crystals that are white and **birefringent on polarized light**	On H&E, the color of the needle-shaped or round talc crystals is highly variable (clear, blue-green or yellow-brown) Rx: excision
Zirconium	Zirconium in **antiperspirants** → persistent, soft brown **papules in axilla**	Sarcoidal granulomas; **no polarizable particles** seen	Zirconium particles are too small to be seen by polarized light microscopy → need advanced X-ray/electron imaging techniques Rx: excision
Beryllium	Used in manufacturing of **fluorescent lights** in the past; could result in systemic or local reactions: Systemic berylliosis: industrial exposure via inhalation → granulomatous lung disease with rare skin involvement (<1%) by scattered sarcoidal papules Localized cutaneous Berylliosis: puncture wound by fluorescent bulb → slowly healing nodules/ulcers	Caseating granulomas (localized cutaneous form); **no polarizable particles** seen	**Bronchioalveolar lavage recommended for Dx of systemic berylliosis** Beryllium particles are too small to be seen by polarized light microscopy → need advanced X-ray/electron imaging techniques Rx: excision
Aluminum	Persistent subcutaneous nodules at **vaccine injection sites**; arise several months after vaccination	Granulomas with central granular debris and palisade of surrounding histiocytes; **no polarizable particles** seen	Topical aluminum chloride for hemostasis can give similar stippled appearance to histiocytes in healing wound Aluminum particles are too small to be seen by polarized light microscopy → need advanced X-ray/electron imaging techniques Rx: excision
Zinc	Rare injection-reaction due to zinc-containing insulin shots; p/w furuncles at injection sites → heals with atrophic scars	Dense neutrophilic infiltrate with **birefringent rhomboidal crystals** → granulomas and fibrosis (end-stage)	Rx: excision
Starch	Due to contamination of wounds from **surgical gloves** with starch lubricant; p/w papules, nodules	Foreign body granulomas with **ovoid basophilic starch granules** that stain **PAS+**	
Cactus (*Opuntia* is most common genus)	Clusters of dome-shaped, skin-colored papules with a central black dot; occurs in those who peel/sell **prickly pear fruit**	Sarcoidal or foreign body granulomas w/ **PAS+ spines** (extra- and intracellular)	
Jellyfish, corals, sea urchin spines	Pruritic lichenoid papules and plaques (onset 2–3 weeks after exposure) **Linear, zig-zag, and whip-like (flagellate)** patterns of erythema/edema (early), hyperpigmentation or lichenoid papules (late)	Lichenoid dermatitis	May see birefringent calcite crystals (sea urchin spines) Rx: IL steroids for delayed-type reactions
Keratin	Ruptured epidermoid cysts Pseudofolliculitis/acne keloidalis Pyogenic granuloma-like lesions, ingrown nails Pilonidal sinus	Foreign body granulomas w/ birefringent keratin debris	
Intralesional corticosteroids	Due to failure of dispersion of injected material → weeks to months later develop FB rxn Skin-colored to yellow-white papules at site of prior IL-steroid injection	Foreign body granulomas with central **pale bluish material** (resembles mucin) on H&E	
Suture	Inflamed papule in wound that opens to form a fistula	Foreign body granulomas with **birefringent suture material**	

Modified from Abdallah MAR, Abdallah MMA, Abdallah M. Foreign body reactions. In: Bolognia JL, Schaffer JV, Cerroni L. Dermatology. 4th ed. Philadelphia: Elsevier; 2018:1664–1674.

Table 3.22 Distinguishing Staining Characteristics of Foreign Body Granulomas

Birefringent		Non-Birefringent
PAS (+)	*PAS (–)*	
Starch, cactus spines, wood splinters	Silica, talc, zinc, keratin, sea urchin spines, sutures, arthropod parts	Aluminum, beryllium, zirconium

PAS, *Periodic acid–Schiff.*

Langerin (**CD207** is most specific, stains Birbeck granules); has pathognomonic intracytoplasmic **Birbeck granules on electron microscopy**

- Mononuclear cell/macrophage: migrates to and from **dermis**, has phagocytic and APC abilities, and stains positively w/ **CD68 and HAM56**
- Dermal dendrocyte/dendritic cell (two types exist):
  - Type 1 dermal dendrocyte: versatile **factor XIIIa**$^{+}$ cell; resides in papillary dermis; involved in antigen presentation, phagocytosis, collagen production, and wound healing

- Type 2 dermal dendrocyte: less known about this **CD34+** cell; resides in reticular dermis
- Abnormal proliferation of any of these histiocyte cell types leads to the various forms of histiocytosis
- There is a high degree of clinical and histopathologic overlap between entities within a group (i.e., the various non-Langerhans cell histiocytoses are very similar to each other, but all are different than LCH)

Langerhans cell histiocytosis (LCH)

Epidemiology and pathogenesis

- Malignancy of immature hematopoietic myeloid precursors (not true Langerhans cells) affecting primarily young **(1–3 yo)** children **(White > Black)**
  - ***BRAF V600E* activating mutation (50%–60%)** → ↑ fibrosarcoma kinase activity → activation of RAS-RAF-MEK-ERK-**MAP kinase** pathway

Histology

- Dense proliferation of Langerhans cells (with **reniform nuclei**), regulatory T cells (FoxP3+, CD4+), and eosinophils in papillary dermis, with single and nested **LCH cells in the epidermis**
  - **S100+, CD1a+, Langerin (CD207)+, CD68+**
    - Negative for Factor XIIIA and HAM56

Clinical features and prognosis

- **Prognosis is primarily determined by <u>extent</u>** of systemic involvement
  - New classification systems classify LCH according to degree of systemic involvement (single vs. multisystem, **risk organ involvement [liver, spleen, bone marrow]**)
    - Bone marrow biopsy in all patients suspected of having multisystem disease
    - Testing: CBC, LFTs, electrolyte assessment, **skeletal survey**, CXR, U/S liver/spleen
  - Most commonly affected organs: bone (**80%; skull #1**) > skin (usually if skin is involved, other organs [liver #1] are too) > pituitary > liver/spleen/hematopoietic system/lungs (usually in adults, major cause of mortality) > lymph nodes > CNS (non-pituitary)
    - Skin presentation varies widely:
      - **Infants w/ petechial seborrheic dermatitis-like eruption (crusted papules) on scalp + groin involvement** (Fig. 3.67)
      - Tiny red flesh-colored papules/pustules w/ dermatitis/seborrheic dermatitis-like eruption, petechial/purpuric eruption, vitiligo-like lesions, xanthoma-like lesions
      - **Trunk, head, and face** most common sites
      - Ulcers in the genital and oral mucosa can occur
- Progression of skin-limited disease to systemic involvement is uncommon, but skin-limited disease only occurs in 2% of patients
- Most frequent sequelae: diabetes insipidus > orthopedic problems (facial asymmetry, vertebral collapse) > hearing loss > other neurologic issues (neurodegeneration)
- 5-year survival in patients with risk organ involvement ≈ 70%–80%; single system LCH and multisystem disease w/ NO risk organ involvement ≈ 100% survival rate

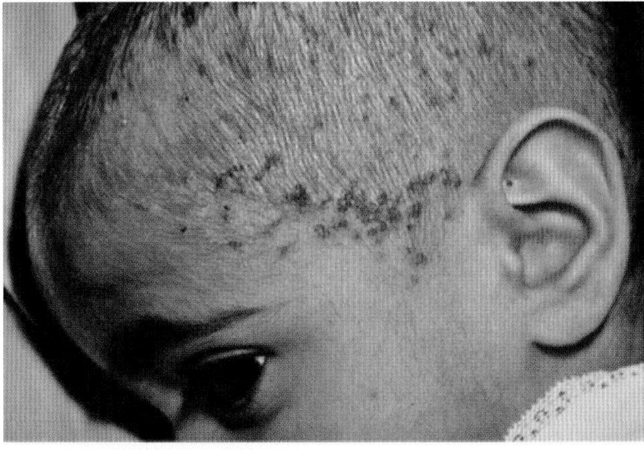

Fig. 3.67 Langerhans cell histiocytosis, seborrheic dermatitis–like eruption with hemorrhage. (From James WD, Elston DM, Treat JR, Rosenbach MA, Neuhaus IM. Macrophage/Monocyte disorders. In: *Andrews' Diseases of the Skin.* 13th ed. Philadelphia: Elsevier; 2020:704–730.)

- Features predictive of poor prognosis: **BRAF V600E mutation** (i.e., ↑ chance neurologic and pituitary issues), multisystem disease w/ risk organ involvement, craniofacial abnormalities, and failure to respond to treatment by 6 weeks

Treatment

- Mild cutaneous disease: potent topical steroids, spontaneous resolution; diffuse disease: **steroids + vinblastine**
  - Other treatment options: nitrogen mustard, imiquimod, PUVA/NB-UVB, MTX, AZA, 6-MP, retinoids
- Multisystem LCH: **vinblastine/prednisone** × 1 year; other options: cladribine, cytarabine, clofarabine; emerging options: BRAF inhibitors, MEK inhibitors, sorafenib

Non-langerhans cell histiocytoses (discussed in Table 3.23)

- All are CD68+, +/−Factor XIIIa+
- All are negative for Langerin
- S100 is negative in all (except ICH and Rosai-Dorfman)
- CD1a is negative in all (except ICH)

Malignant histiocytic disorders

- *Langerhans cell sarcoma* (high mortality, skin, Langerin/S100/CD1a (+)), *follicular dendritic cell sarcoma* (<20% mortality, cervical lymph node, CD21/CD35 (+)), *histiocytic sarcoma* (high mortality, skin, CD68/CD163 (+)), *indeterminate cell sarcoma, interdigitating dendritic cell sarcoma* (high mortality, single lymph node)

3.7 MONOCLONAL GAMMOPATHIES OF DERMATOLOGIC INTEREST

- Monoclonal gammopathies often arise in setting of plasma cell dyscrasia or multiple myeloma
- Their **associations w/ various dermatoses is important to know** (Table 3.24)
- IgG4-related disease: not a monoclonal gammopathy; seen in middle-aged men primarily

Table 3.23 Non-Langerhans Cell Histiocytoses

Histiocytosis	Age (Years)	Clinical Presentation	Other High-Yield Facts
Primarily cutaneous, self-resolving			
JXG	0–2 (15% at birth, 75% in first year of life)	**One** to few lesions » numerous/widespread; pink to red/yellow; **head/neck** > upper trunk, extremities (Fig. 3.68); mucosal JXG is rare; unilateral eye involvement in 0.5% (**iris** most common) → hyphema, glaucoma → blindness Can occur in adults (20–30s) and usually solitary papule/nodule	Spontaneous resolution in 3–6 years; rare visceral lesions; 40% of patients with ocular involvement also have skin involvement **Risk factors for ocular involvement**: multiple cutaneous JXGs and children < 2 yo **"Triple association" of JXG, NF-1, and >20x ↑ risk of juvenile myelomonocytic leukemia (JMML)** Histology: Well-circumscribed, dense dermal infiltrate of foamy lipidized histiocytes, **Touton giant cells** and **eosinophils**; loss of rete ridges +/– ulceration
Benign cephalic histiocytosis (likely a JXG variant)	Infants (<1 yo usually)	Numerous (more lesions than typical JXG) red-brown macules & papules of **face**/neck (Fig. 3.69) that may progress to upper torso	**Self-limited** **No internal or mucosal involvement** Historically known for intracytoplasmic "**comma-shaped/worm-like**" bodies on electron microscopy (not specific); histology: very similar to JXG but **no Touton giant cells,** minimal-to-no lipidized histiocytes
Generalized eruptive histiocytosis (likely a JXG variant)	**Adults** (20–50 yo) > kids	Recurrent eruption of hundreds of small (<1 cm) red-brown papules in **axial** distribution (trunk, proximal extremities > face); heal with hyperpigmentation	**Self-limited; no internal or mucosal involvement** Histology: Same as BCH → clinical distinction required
Indeterminate cell histiocytosis (ICH)	Any	Solitary and generalized variants exist; trunk, extremities; eruption clinically and histologically indistinguishable from BCH and GEH → need immunostains to distinguish	Rare visceral and bone lesions with occasional fatal cases **S100(+) and CD1a(+)** like LCH **Langerin(–)** since no Birbeck granules → differentiates from LCH
Primarily cutaneous, progressive			
Progressive nodular histiocytosis	Any	Generalized yellow papules/nodules, with predilection for face	Mucous membrane involvement may occur
Cutaneous + frequent systemic involvement			
NXG	50s	Destructive multisystem disease; yellow xanthomatous plaques +/– ulceration; **periorbital** » other face, trunk, extremities; **50% have ophthalmic complications**; hepatosplenomegaly, leukopenia and ↑ ESR	**IgGκ monoclonal gammopathy** (>80%), a/w plasma cell dyscrasia or multiple myeloma Histology: See NXG section
Reticulohistiocytosis (multicentric reticulohistiocytosis and solitary reticulohistiocytoma)	30–40s (very rare in kids)	**Multicentric form:** F > M; red-brown or yellow nodules; Acral sites favored (**head**, **dorsal hands** > elbows) (Fig. 3.70); 50% have **oral or nasopharyngeal** lesions; severe **destructive arthritis** → arthritis mutilans (45%); no effective treatment **Solitary form:** Solitary, asymptomatic < 1 cm yellow-red nodule; head (#1 site); young adults (M = F); no systemic involvement; self-resolving but may excise	Multicentric form: ↑ ESR, fever, anemia; **Solid organ malignancy in 30%** **"Coral bead"** appearance = papules along periungual region Histology: Dermal infiltrate of mono- and multi-nucleated histiocytes with granular, pink-purple (aka amphophilic, "**ground glass**") cytoplasm, often surrounded by empty white spaces (**lacunae**)
Rosai-Dorfman	10–30	Multisystem disease of children or young adults; massive but asymptomatic **bilateral cervical lymphadenopathy**; fever/night sweats/weight loss; ↑ ESR, polyclonal hypergammaglobulinemia; **any internal organ may be involved**; 10% have skin lesions (#1 sites = **eyelids** and **malar** cheek); p/w multiple red-brown or xanthomatous papules/plaques; disease **usually self-resolves**	↑ Incidence in West Indians Histology: pan-dermal infiltrate of very large, very foamy **$S100^+$/$CD68^+$ histiocytes with emperipolesis** (engulfment of intact lymphocytes and plasma cells), abundant **plasma cells** Skin-limited form: benign; usually pts are older and female (systemic involvement more often seen in males and younger pts)
Xanthoma disseminatum	<25 (60%), but any age	**Triad**: Cutaneous xanthomas, mucosal xanthomas (oral and upper airway most commonly), diabetes insipidus p/w 100s of red-brown or yellow papules → coalesce into **oddly patterned xanthoma-like plaques** (Fig. 3.71); symmetric **flexural/intertriginous** involvement	Normolipemic; a/w **monoclonal gammopathy**, **plasma cell dyscrasia**; histology: Dense dermal infiltrate of many foam cells and occasional Touton giant cells; chronic course; no effective treatment
Systemic, usually without skin involvement			
Erdheim-Chester	Any	Fever, **bone lesions**, diabetes insipidus, exophthalmos, CNS, multiple internal organs; skin involvement in minority (25%); eyelids and upper half of body; red-brown to yellow indurated nodules/plaques	**High mortality rate**

ICH, *indeterminate cell histiocytosis;* JXG, *juvenile xanthogranuloma;* NF-1, *type 1 neurofibromatosis;* JMML, *juvenile myelomonocytic leukemia;* BCH, *benign cephalic histiocytosis;* NXG, *necrobiotic xanthogranuloma;* LCH, *Langerhans cell histiocytosis;* GEH, *generalized eruptive histiocytosis;* ESR, *estimated sedimentation rate.*

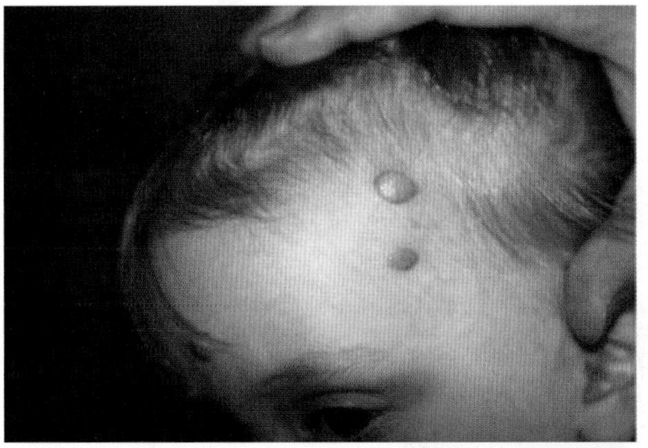

Fig. 3.68 Juvenile xanthogranuloma, multiple nodules. (From James WD, Berger TG, Elston DM, Neuhaus IM. Macrophage/Monocyte disorders. In: *Andrews' Diseases of the Skin*. 12th ed. Philadelphia: Elsevier; 2016:699–725.)

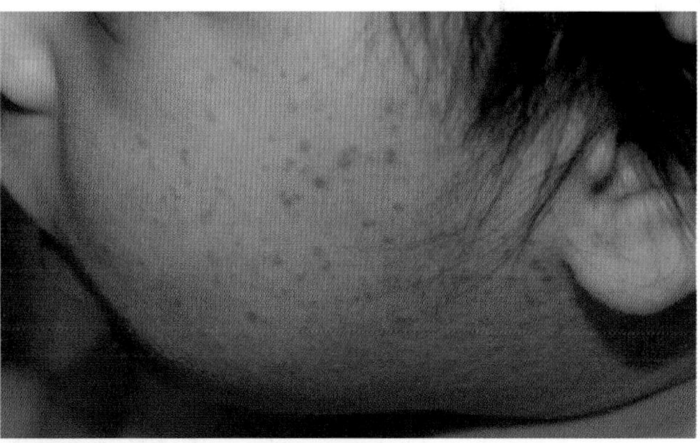

Fig. 3.69 Infant with benign cephalic histiocytosis. (From Prendiville JS. Lumps, bumps, and hamartomas. In: Eichenfield LF, Frieden IJ, Mathes EF, Zaenglein AL, eds. *Neonatal and Infant Dermatology*. 3rd ed. Philadelphia: Elsevier; 2015:422–442.)

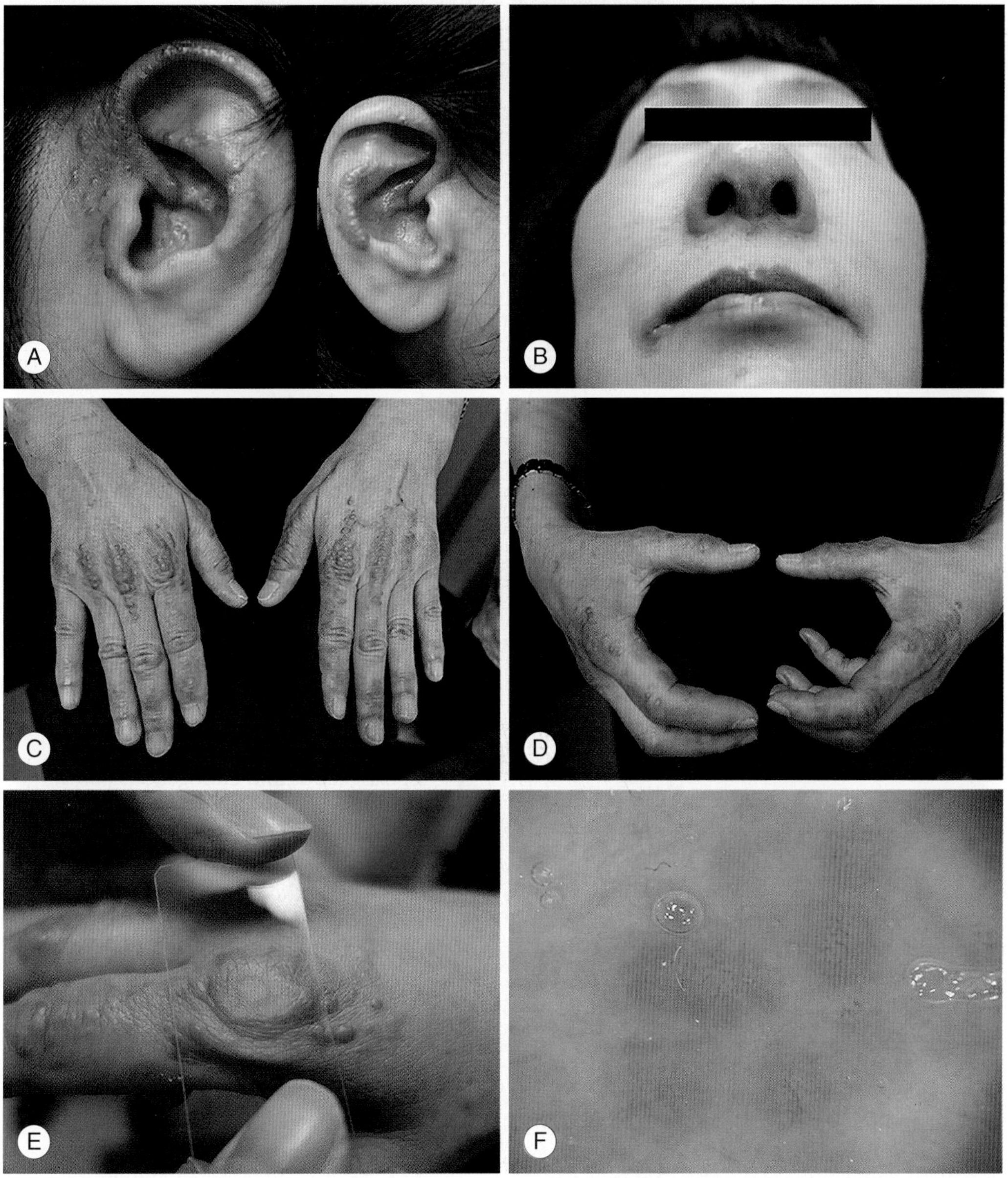

Fig. 3.70 Clinical manifestations and dermoscopic findings of the patient with multicentric reticulohistiocytosis. (A) Closely arranged reddish-brown papules ("coral beads") were located over the helices and antihelices of the ear. (B) Similar lesions were observed over the perinostril area. (C) and (D) Note the confluent papules and nodules forming erythematous plaques with a cobblestone surface over the knuckles, mainly involving the metacarpal joints, as well as the presence of periungual erythema and swelling of the distal phalangeal joints. (E) Diascopy revealed a negative "apple jelly" sign. (F) Delicate thin arborizing vessels within the papules were observed via gel immersion (contact) dermoscopy. (From Cheng LH, Chiang YY. Multicentric reticulohistiocytosis in Taiwanese woman with Sjögren syndrome. *Dermatol Sinica*. 2016;34[1]:42–45.)

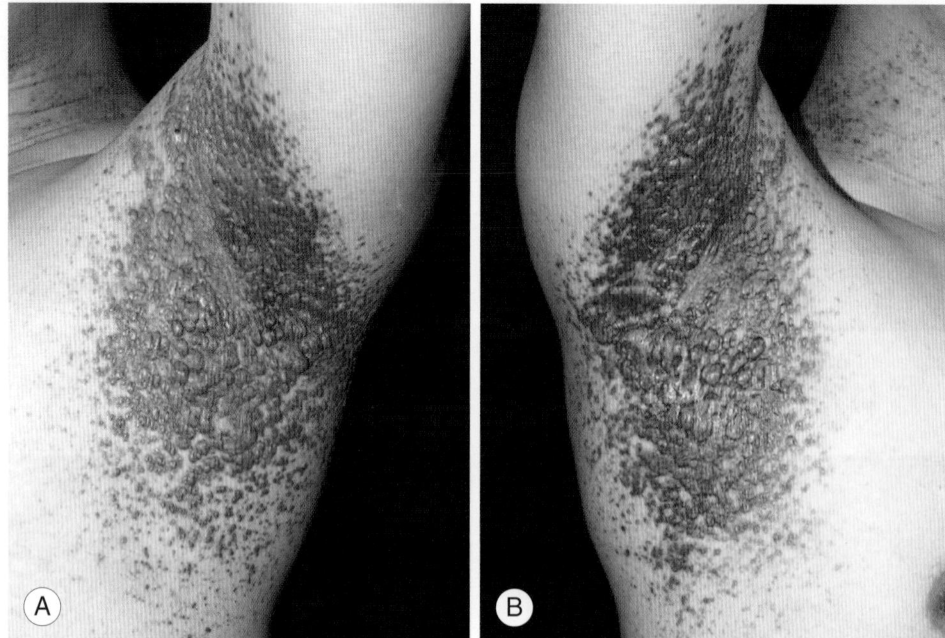

Fig. 3.71 (A) and (B) Cutaneous xanthoma disseminatum with many red-brown papules in the axillae. (From Gong HZ, Zheng HY, Li J. Xanthoma disseminatum. *Lancet*. 2018;391(10117):251. [Fig 1ab] Reprinted with permission from Elsevier).

Table 3.24 Monoclonal Gammopathies in Dermatology

Disorder	Immunoglobulin Type
Plane xanthoma	IgG
Sweet's syndrome	IgA
Primary (AL) amyloidosis	IgG
Necrobiotic xanthogranuloma	IgGκ
Scleredema	IgGκ
Scleromyxedema	IgG-λ
IgA pemphigus and subcorneal pustular dermatosis	IgA
Pyoderma gangrenosum	IgA
Erythema elevatum diutinum	IgA
POEMS syndrome	IgA and IgG
Schnitzler's syndrome	IgM
Cryoglobulinemia	Monoclonal IgM and IgG (type I) Monoclonal IgM + polyclonal IgG (type II) Polyclonal IgM and/or IgG (type III)
Waldenström macroglobulinemia	IgM

- Lymphoplasmacytic infiltration (with IgG4+ plasma cells) of various organs (e.g., **Mikulicz disease of lacrimal glands**, sclerosing cholangitis, retroperitoneal fibrosis, sclerosis sialoadenitis, inflammatory pseudotumor of the orbit, autoimmune pancreatitis) → sclerosis and organomegaly/pseudotumors
- Allergy symptoms, asthenia, weight loss, fever, ↑ IgG4 and IgE in plasma, lymphadenopathy
- Skin findings: papulonodules (plasmacytosis) on head/neck and proximal extremities (histology: fibrosis w/ storiform pattern and lymphoplasmacytic infiltrates w/ IgG4+ plasma cells), pseudolymphoma, psoriasis-like eruption, hypergammaglobulinemic purpura, and urticarial vasculitis
- Treatment: prednisone or steroid-sparing agent; rituximab

3.8 XANTHOMAS

- Intracellular and dermal lipid deposition → yellow appearance of lesions
- Prefer skin, tendons, and eyes
- Due to **abnormalities in lipid metabolism** (primary or secondary; may be a/w atherosclerosis) or **monoclonal gammopathy** (e.g., MGUS, multiple myeloma, CLL, Waldenström disease; usually IgG, but can be IgA or IgM)
  - Lipoproteins: transport plasma lipids to peripheral cells
    - Basic structure = inner core (triglycerides + cholesterol esters) + outer shell (phospholipids, free cholesterol, and apoproteins [bind receptors and activating enzymes])
    - Exogenous and endogenous pathways of lipoprotein synthesis exist
    - Types of lipoproteins:
      - Chylomicrons: mainly exogenous production
        - ➔ Central core of mainly triglycerides; outer shell contains various apoproteins (B-48, E, A-I, A-II, and C-II)
        - ➔ Becomes chylomicron remnant after most of the triglyceride content is hydrolyzed
      - Very-low-density lipoprotein (VLDL): mainly endogenous production in liver
        - ➔ Central core of mainly triglycerides; outer shell contains B-100, E and C-II
        - ➔ C-II needed for lipoprotein lipase activation
      - Intermediate-density lipoprotein (IDL): remnant of VLDL after hydrolysis of most of triglycerides by lipoprotein lipase
      - Low-density lipoprotein (LDL): product of further triglyceride hydrolysis of IDL (now

mainly cholesterol ester core and B-100 on surface)
➔ Uptake into hepatocytes by apo B-100/E
- High-density lipoprotein (HDL): removes cholesterol from tissues
  ➔ Free cholesterol esterified by lecithin: cholesterol acyltransferase
  ➔ Requires apoprotein A-I on HDL
- Hyperlipidemias have a variety of clinical findings (Table 3.25)

Cutaneous xanthoma types

- Eruptive xanthomas: numerous red-yellow papules on **extensor surfaces, buttocks**, intertriginous areas, and orally (Fig. 3.72)
  - Triglycerides usually **> 3000 mg/dL**
  - Pathogenesis: may be primary or secondary
    - Primary: type **I, IV, and V** hyperlipidemias
    - Secondary: obesity, diabetes, alcohol abuse, medication-induced (**oral retinoids**, protease inhibitors, olanzapine, and estrogen replacement)
- Tuberous xanthomas: yellow-pink indurated nodules mainly on **elbows and knees**
  - Most strongly a/w **type II and III**
- Tendinous xanthomas: firm nodules on **Achilles tendon** and extensor tendons of fingers/hands that develop in third decade
  - Usually seen in **type II** hyperlipidemia (>type III)
- Plane xanthomas: may be localized or diffuse
  - Occurrence on **palmar/finger creases** (xanthoma striatum palmare) nearly pathognomonic for **dysbetalipoproteinemia** (Fig. 3.73)
  - Occurrence in **intertriginous areas and web spaces of fingers** usually diagnostic of **homozygous familial hypercholesterolemia (type II hyperlipidemia)** (Fig. 3.74)
  - May occur in monoclonal gammopathy (plasma cell dyscrasia usually) with no lipid abnormalities; favors neck, upper trunk, intertriginous and periocular areas

Table 3.25 Important Hyperlipoproteinemias

			Clinical Findings	
Type	**Pathogenesis**	**Laboratory Findings**	**Skin (Types of Xanthoma)**	**Systemic**
Type I (familial LPL deficiency, familial hyperchylomicronemia)	Deficient or abnormal LPL Apo C-II deficiency Deficient glycosyl-phosphatidylinositol-anchored HDL-binding protein	Slow chylomicron clearance Reduced LDL and HDL levels Hypertriglyceridemia	**Eruptive**	No increased risk of coronary artery disease
Type II (familial hypercholesterolemia or familial defective apo B-100)	**LDL receptor defect** Reduced affinity of LDL for LDL receptor due to dysfunction of apo B-100 (ligand) Accelerated degradation of LDL receptor due to missense *PCSK9* mutations[a] Defective LDL receptor adaptor protein 1 (required for receptor internalization)	Reduced LDL clearance **Hypercholesterolemia**	**Tendinous, tuberoeruptive, tuberous, plane** (xanthelasma, intertriginous areas, interdigital web spaces[b])	**Atherosclerosis** of peripheral and coronary arteries
Type III (familial dysbetalipoproteinemia, remnant removal disease, broad beta disease, apo E deficiency)	Hepatic remnant clearance impaired due to apo E abnormality; patients only express the apo E_2 isoform that interacts poorly with the apo E receptor	Elevated levels of chylomicron remnants and IDLs **Hypercholesterolemia** Hypertriglyceridemia	**Tuberoeruptive, tuberous, plane (palmar creases** = strongly a/w dysbetalipoproteinemia) **Tendinous**	**Atherosclerosis** of peripheral and coronary arteries
Type IV (endogenous familial hypertriglyceridemia)	Elevated production of VLDL associated with glucose intolerance and hyperinsulinemia	Increased VLDLs Hypertriglyceridemia	**Eruptive**	Frequently associated with type 2 non-insulin-dependent diabetes mellitus, obesity, alcoholism
Type V	Elevated chylomicrons and VLDLs; subset related to apo A-V defect	Decreased LDLs and HDLs Hypertriglyceridemia	**Eruptive**	Diabetes mellitus

[a]*Gain-of-function mutations cause autosomal dominant hypercholesterolemia, whereas loss-of-function mutations (most prevalent in African Americans) result in low LDL levels.*
[b]*Said to be pathognomonic for homozygous state.*
Apo, *Apolipoprotein;* HDL, *high-density lipoprotein;* IDL, *intermediate-density lipoprotein;* LDL, *low-density lipoprotein;* LPL, *lipoprotein lipase;* PCSK9, *proprotein convertase subtilisin/kexin type 9;* VLDL, *very-low-density lipoprotein.*
Modified from Massengale WT. Xanthomas. In: Bolognia JL, Schaffer JV, Cerroni L. Dermatology. *4th ed. Philadelphia: Elsevier; 2018:1634–1643.*

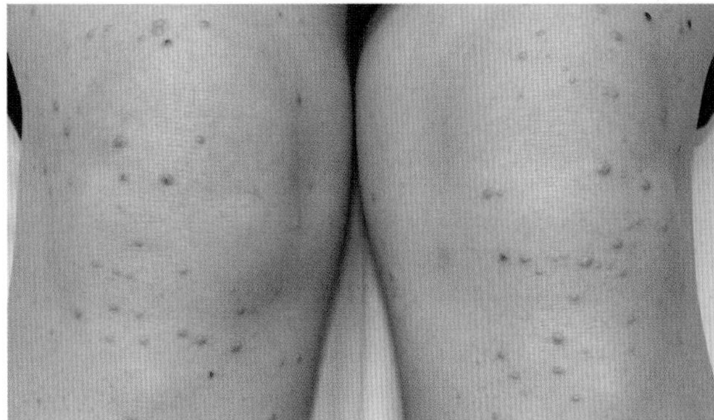

Fig. 3.72 Eruptive xanthomas (due to hypertriglyceridemia) typically occur on the extensor surface of the lower extremities, particularly the knees. (From Ko CJ, Cowper SE. Dermatologic conditions in kidney disease. In: Yu ASL, Chertwo GM, Luyckx VA, Marsden PA, Skorecki K, Taal MW, eds. *Brenner & Rector's the Kidney*. 11th ed. Philadelphia: Elsevier; 2020:1932–1944. Courtesy Yale Residents' Collection.)

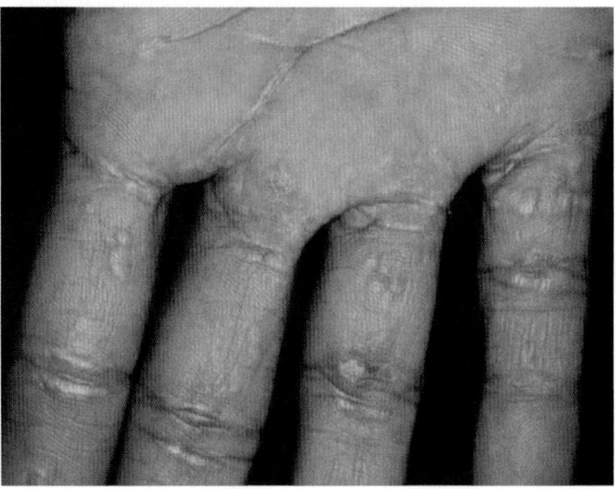

Fig. 3.73 Xanthomas of palmar striae. (From James WD, Elston DM, Treat JR, Rosenbach MA, Neuhaus IM. Pruritis and neurocutaneous dermatoses. In: *Andrews' Diseases of the Skin*. 13th ed. Philadelphia: Elsevier; 2020:46–62.)

- Xanthelasma = plane xanthoma on eyelids
  - Only 50% have hyperlipidemia
  - Surgical treatment is best option
- Verruciform xanthoma:
  - Benign verrucous plaque(s) typically occurring in **mouth** or **genital area**
  - Often confused for warts clinically and histologically
  - Not a/w hyperlipidemia
  - May be a/w CHILD (congenital hemidysplasia with ichthyosiform erythroderma and limb defects) syndrome and any disorder that causes epidermal damage (epidermolysis bullosa, GVHD, LS&A, and pemphigus)
  - Unique histology: papillomatous epidermal hyperplasia w/ **foam cells in dermal papillae**

Pathology

- **Foam cells** (macrophages w/ lipidized cytoplasm) in dermis
  - Foam cells located more superficially in plane xanthomas, and deeper in dermis/subcutaneous tissue in tuberous and tendinous xanthomas

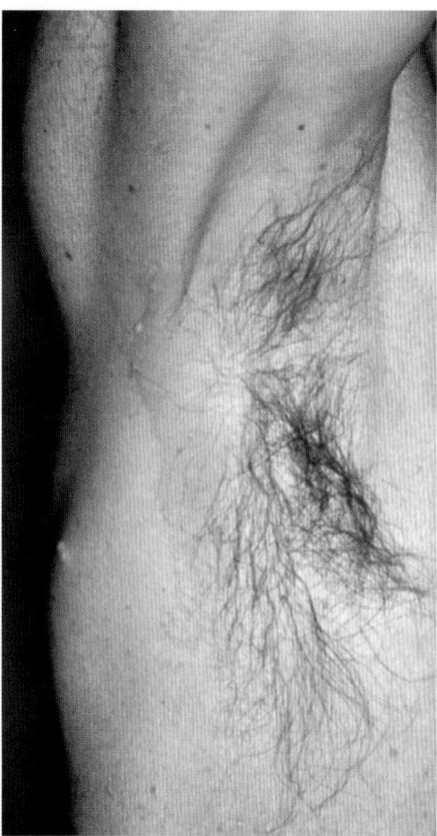

Fig. 3.74 Plane xanthoma. (From James WD, Berger TG, Elston DM, Neuhaus IM. Errors in metabolism. In: *Andrews' Diseases of the Skin*. 12th ed. Philadelphia: Elsevier; 2016:509–541.)

Treatment

- Determine underlying lipoprotein disorder and contributing factors, correct via various interventions (dietary modifications, lipid-lowering medications, surgical excision, and chemotherapy in certain monoclonal gammopathies)

3.9 URTICARIA AND ANGIOEDEMA

Urticaria

Epidemiology

- Up to 20% of population will have **acute urticaria (duration < 6 weeks)**
  - 1% may develop into chronic urticaria (duration ≥ 6 weeks)
- **F > M** overall, and for chronic urticaria, dermatographism, and cold urticaria
  - M > F for delayed pressure urticaria

Pathogenesis

- Many cases of urticaria are idiopathic and causes vary (e.g., allergy, autoimmune, infections, and drugs)
- In **children, the most common cause is viral or idiopathic**, but other causes include:
  - Infectious (assess for symptoms of UTI, URI, or GI infection)

- Allergic: foods, meds, and other environmental allergens
- Physical stimuli: pressure, solar, cholinergic, cold
- Arthropod bite reactions ("papular urticaria")
- Malignancy (most commonly lymphoma)

- Mast cell is the primary cell responsible for urticaria (though basophils and eosinophils play role)
  - Contains proinflammatory mediators:
    - Preformed: **histamine**, proteases, and heparin
    - Newly-formed: **prostaglandin D2, leukotrienes** C4/D4/E4, platelet-activating factor, and cytokines (TNF-α, IL-1, IL-4, IL-5, IL-6, and IL-8)
  - Degranulating stimuli → release of mediators by mast cells
    - **Immunologic mechanisms**: autoantibodies against FcεRI (seen in up to 30% of chronic urticaria patients; occurs via autoimmune cross-linking of receptors) or IgE; IgE-dependent allergic response (e.g., to food, med, latex, or infection); ↑ frequency of HLA-DR4 and -DQ8
      - Drug-induced immunologic urticaria: PCN and cephalosporins (>TMP-SMX, and minocycline), latex gloves, or medical devices
    - **Non-immunologic mechanisms**: opiate-mediated release of mast cell contents, C5a anaphylatoxin, stem cell factor, neuropeptides (e.g., substance P and vasoactive intestinal peptide)
- Other causes of urticaria include immune complex deposition (i.e., urticarial vasculitis), vasoactive stimuli like **nettle**, ASA/**NSAIDs**, **radiocontrast media**, **polymyxin B**, **ACE inhibitors (due to ↑ bradykinin)**, and dietary pseudoallergens
  - **ASA** → exacerbation of chronic urticaria in 30%

Clinical features

- Characterized by **wheals**: swelling and erythema of skin from plasma leakage in superficial dermis
  - May have **"flare" of erythema** surrounding them
  - Intensely itchy
  - Individual lesions **last < 24 hours**
- "Acute" versus "chronic" urticaria:
  - Acute:
    - Most common causes: **idiopathic (#1) > URIs (#2)** > drugs (**β-lactams** most common) and foods
    - Typically fast-onset (exception: drug-induced acute urticaria may start days after triggering agent)
  - Chronic:
    - Most common causes: "**ordinary**" (60%; consists of idiopathic and autoimmune autoantibodies against FcεRI or Fc portion of IgE, infection-related, and pseudoallergic) > **physical (35%) > vasculitic (5%)**
    - Autoimmune etiology in up to 50%
    - **a/w Autoimmune thyroid disease**, vitiligo, IDDM, RA, *Helicobacter pylori* gastritis, and parasitic infections
    - Mean duration: 3 to 5 years
- Physical urticaria: induced by physical stimuli
  - **Dermatographism**: urticaria develops at sites of friction/scratching/stroking
    - **Most common physical urticaria**
    - Reproducible by scratching back—occurs seconds to minutes after provocation
    - Worse in evening
  - **Delayed pressure urticaria**: deep red swelling (angioedema) at anatomic areas of high friction/pressure (e.g., waistline after wearing tight-fitting clothes)
    - May be quite delayed, up to 12 hours after stimulus
    - Painful, itchy, and possibly long lasting (72 hours) → ↓ QoL
    - May be a/w arthralgias, malaise, and flu-like symptoms
  - **Heat-induced:** very rare; urticaria after just a few minutes of heat contact
  - **Cold urticaria:** rapid itch, erythema, and swelling after exposure; triggers include cold weather, air conditioners, **aquatic activity**, and holding cold objects; "**ice cube" test** can aid in diagnosis (positive in primary cold contact urticaria [PCCU], negative in reflex cold and familial cold urticaria); patients should **never swim alone** as massive mediator release can → hypotension
    - PCCU: usually idiopathic; young adults; acute or chronic; can have systemic symptoms like syncope; **positive ice cube test**
    - Secondary cold CU: may be due to cryoglobulinemia, cryofibrinogenemia, hepatitis B/C, lymphoproliferative disease, or mononucleosis
    - Reflex cold urticaria: widespread urticaria after generalized cooling of body
    - Familial cold urticaria: cryopyrin-associated periodic syndromes (CAPS), PLAID (see Chapter 4)
  - **Cholinergic urticaria:** distinct lesions (multiple 2–3 mm slightly papular wheals with pronounced large flare) occurring after sweating/↑ **body temperature** in young adults (e.g., after exercise, hot bath, spicy foods, and strong emotions)
    - May be due to hypersensitivity to sweat components
    - May have systemic symptoms (e.g., faintness and wheezing) and be chronic
  - **Adrenergic urticaria:** blanched vasoconstricted halos around pink wheal
    - Responds better to **propranolol** than to antihistamines
    - Can reproduce lesions by intradermal norepinephrine injections
  - **Solar urticaria:** discussed in Section 3.15
  - **Aquagenic urticaria:** lesions similar to cholinergic, response to water exposure (independent of temperature)
    - Can be seen in cystic fibrosis
- Urticarial vasculitis: lesions that resemble urticaria but **last > 24 hours, burn/hurt** rather than itch and often **bruise**; histology shows mild **LCV** (+/– eosinophils)
  - Typically middle-aged women
  - Pain/burning > itch
  - Usually chronic
  - Angioedema in one third of patients
  - **Arthralgias (50%)**, GI involvement (20%), obstructive pulmonary disease (20%), and others (renal, ocular, cardiac, livedo, and intracranial HTN)
  - May be a/w **autoimmune CTDs** and infections
  - Can have ↑ ESR, ↓ complement, and (+)ANA
  - NSAIDs first line, but may need other agents (e.g., colchicine, dapsone, MTX, or steroids)

- Schnitzler's syndrome: chronic **urticaria** (burn > itch), **fevers**, **bone pain**, arthralgia/arthritis, ↑ ESR, and **IgM gammopathy**
  - Neutrophilic infiltrate on histopathology; **anakinra is a good treatment**

Histopathology

- Superficial dermal edema, vasodilation, scant perivascular and **interstitial infiltrate predominantly composed of neutrophils** (> eosinophils, lymphocytes)
  - Also see marginated neutrophils in vessel lumens
- Dermal neutrophilia seen 1 hour into process

Testing

- RAST and skin prick (intradermal) testing can help identify environmental allergens in acute urticaria
  - Most helpful to determine etiology of acute urticaria to foods, venom, and medications
  - RAST has 20% false-negative rate
- For recalcitrant chronic urticaria, consider CBC w/ differential, ESR/CRP, **thyroid antibodies**, thyroid function tests, anti-FcεRI and anti-IgE antibodies, immunoassays, functional assays (e.g., histamine release assay), and autoreactivity (e.g., autologous serum skin test)

Treatment/clinical course

- Soothing lotions (e.g., containing pramoxine and/or menthol); avoidance of triggers (e.g., overheating, cold exposure, and vibratory stimuli)
- May need to **avoid ASA**, NSAIDs, and opiates
- Exclusion diets/low-pseudoallergen diets may be helpful in some cases
- **First-line treatment = H1 antihistamines** (sedating and non-sedating; up to 4× dosing of non-sedating antihistamines is acceptable); can consider adding H2 antihistamine
- For more recalcitrant cases, consider doxepin, short courses of systemic steroids, montelukast (mixed results, second line), phototherapy, sulfasalazine, cyclosporine, colchicine, dapsone, antimalarials, MTX, MMF, and **omalizumab** (FDA approved for chronic idiopathic urticaria in patients 12 yo and older - monthly dosing)

Angioedema

Epidemiology

- Causes: idiopathic (#1 cause), physical stimuli (temperature, vibration), type I hypersensitivity reactions (drugs other than ACE inhibitors, arthropod bites, food allergies), "pseudoallergic" (NSAIDs, ASA, IV contrast), C1 inhibitor deficiency syndromes (hereditary angioedema [HAE], acquired angioedema [AAE]), and ACE inhibitor-induced angioedema
- HAE in 1:10,000–1:50,000; starts in first to second decade and more severe in adolescence
  - Type I HAE most common (80%–85% of HAE cases)
  - Sex predilections: types I and II (M = F); type III (F > M)
- AAE starts in middle age

Pathogenesis

- Similar to urticaria for majority of cases with urticaria + angioedema; **for cases of angioedema LACKING urticaria (HAE, AAE) and ACE inhibitor-induced angioedema, excess bradykinin is the cause**
- Must rule out C1 esterase inhibitor (C1 inh) deficiency in cases of angioedema without urticaria
- HAE:
  - Types I and II due to **mutations in C1 inh** (type I has ↓ C1 inh levels; type II has ↓ C1 inh function)
  - Type III due to an activating mutation in Hageman factor (FXII)
  - All forms of HAE are **autosomal dominant**
- AAE:
  - May be type I (consumption of C1 inh) or type II (inhibitory autoantibodies against C1 inh)
  - May be due to **B-cell lymphoproliferative** disorders, plasma cell dyscrasias, or **autoimmune CTDs**
- Acquired and hereditary forms result in ↑ **bradykinin** levels and ↓ **C4 levels (screening test of choice)**
  - ↓ **C1q levels** → seen in **AAE only!**
  - **C1 inh levels** → helps distinguish between types I and II HAE
    - ↓ **C1 inh** in type I HAE
    - **Normal/↑** C1 inh levels in type II (but decreased C1 inh function)
- Drug-induced angioedema
  - Most commonly **ACE inhibitors** (lisinopril, enalapril > captopril): occurs in 0.2% of all new users; **5× ↑ risk in Blacks**; 77% occur within first 3 weeks, and almost all within first year; ACE inhibitors block kinase II → ↑ **bradykinin**
  - Others causes (NOT bradykinin-induced): **PCN**, cephalosporins, NSAIDs, radiocontrast media, and monoclonal antibodies (biologics)

Clinical features

- Characterized by **deep swellings of skin/mucosa** (in deeper dermis and subcutaneous/submucosa)
  - Painful, non-erythematous
  - Non-pitting, non-pruritic (but may burn or cause pain)
  - **Commonly lasts 2–5 days** (worst in first 36 hours)
  - Face most commonly affected (**lips**, **eyelids**, throat, ears, and nose)
  - **May → anaphylaxis if throat involved** (laryngeal or epiglottic edema → stridor)
  - Associated symptoms: GI pain, N/V/diarrhea (edema of bowel wall), and urinary retention
  - Up to 50% of patients w/ chronic urticaria will also have angioedema at some point; however, if see angioedema in absence of urticaria, must consider HAE and AAE!
- Vibratory angioedema: vibration → localized swelling/itching lasting about half an hour
  - Causes include running, motorcycling, biking and operating machinery (e.g., lawnmower)
  - Familial form (activating mutation in ADGRE2) has systemic symptoms
- HAE:
  - Type I and II: estrogens and trauma can → attacks
    - Episodes last 2 to 3 days
    - Avoid ACE inhibitors (can trigger attacks)
  - Type III: later age of onset (in teens), ↑ **facial edema**

Table 3.26 Complement Alterations in Angioedema Due to C1INH Deficiency

	Antigenic C1INH	Functional C1INH	C4	C1q
HAE type I	↓	↓	↓	N
HAE type II	↑/N	↓	↓/N	↓
AAE type I	↓	↓	↓	↓
AAE type II	↓/N[a]	↓	↓	↓

[a]*In AAE, normal values of antigenic C1INH are due to elevated levels of its cleaved form of 96 kDa.*
AAE, acquired angioedema; *C1INH,* C1 inhibitor; *HAE,* hereditary angioedema; *N,* normal.
From Guilarte M, Luengo O, Nogueiras C, Labrador-Horrillo M, Muñoz E, López A, et al. Acquired angioedema associated with hereditary angioedema due to C1 inhibitor deficiency. J Investig Allergol Clin Immunol. *2008;18(2):126-130. Data from Bowen T, Cicardi M, Farkas H, Bork K, Kreuz W, Zingale L, et al. Canadian 2003 international consensus algorithm for the diagnosis, therapy, and management of hereditary angioedema.* J Allergy Clin Immunol. *2004;114(3):629-637.*

Diagnosis

- If HAE or AAE are suspected, check C4, C1 inh (quantification and function), and C1q Table 3.26

Treatment/clinical course

- Similar to treatments for urticaria
- Intensive support (e.g., intubation and tracheostomy) may be needed
- Should carry epi-pen in case of angioedema in oropharynx
- For **C1 inh deficiency**, oral **danazol** is ToC for prophylaxis, and **C1 inh concentrate is ToC for acute attacks**
  - Danazol and C1 inh concentrate can be used prophylactically prior to surgical procedures
  - Another option is icatibant, a synthetic **bradykinin B2 receptor antagonist**
- **Anaphylaxis**: life-threatening reaction to drugs that p/w both skin (urticaria/angioedema) and systemic (hypotension and tachycardia) findings; occurs **within minutes** of **parenteral** (> oral) administration of drugs; most common drugs: **PCN** (1/5000 patients), **latex** (especially mucosal contact), topical antibiotic use (**bacitracin**, Neosporin, and rifamycin); and radiocontrast media (anaphylactoid); Rx: hospitalization for serious cases + systemic steroids + subcutaneous epinephrine

3.10 NEUTROPHILIC DERMATOSES

Sweet's syndrome (Acute febrile neutrophilic dermatosis)

Epidemiology

- Usually middle-aged
- F > M (**3:1 for classic Sweet's**)
  - M = F for cancer-associated Sweet's
- Five major subtypes: classic (60%–70%), cancer-associated (10%–20%), inflammatory disease-related (10%–15%), drug-induced (5%), and pregnancy (2%)

Pathogenesis

- Unknown; may have (+) pathergy

Clinical features

- **Tender/burning**, red, well-demarcated, expanding, **edematous/"juicy"** papules/plaques (Fig. 3.75)

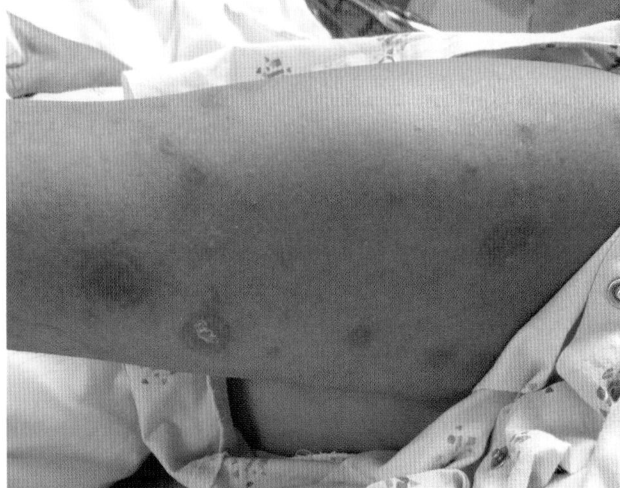

Fig. 3.75 Sweet's syndrome. Markedly edematous lesions on the upper arm. (Courtesy of Christopher Sayed, MD.)

  - Favors **head/neck and upper extremities**
  - Rapid onset
  - May become vesiculobullous or pustular, and may have a targetoid appearance
  - In drug-induced Sweet's, lesions occur 1–2 weeks after drug administration
  - **Ulcerative, bullous and oral lesions** → stronger a/w hematologic disorders/**malignancy**
- Extracutaneous features: **fever** (50%–80%), malaise, preceding URI or flu-like symptoms, **leukocytosis** (70%), **arthralgias**/arthritis, **ocular involvement** (conjunctivitis, episcleritis, scleritis, retinal vasculitis, and iridioyclitis), cardiac involvement (aortitis, cardiomegaly, coronary artery occlusion)
- Lab abnormalities:
  - ↑ ESR/CRP (90%)
  - Leukocytosis: neutrophilia w/ ↑ band forms ("left shift")
- Various triggers:
  - Infections: mainly **streptococcus** and yersiniosis; HIV, hepatitis C
  - Cancer: especially **acute myeloid leukemia (AML**; M2 and M4 subtypes), but also other hematologic malignancies and myeloproliferative disorders (e.g., **MDS**)

- Consider screening all patients without obvious causes with peripheral blood smear and bone marrow biopsy if the smear is abnormal
- **IBD**
- Drugs: **G-CSF, GM-CSF, ATRA, TMP-SMX, minocycline, OCPs**, furosemide, and hydralazine
- Other: autoimmune CTDs, **pregnancy**, vaccines (e.g., BCG, smallpox)

Histopathology

- **Diffuse dermal neutrophilic infiltrate** w/ karyorrhexis + massive **papillary dermal edema**
  - Generally **lacks LCV** (although some "bystander" damage is done to vessels within inflammatory soup)
  - Massive papillary dermal edema is responsible for "pseudovesicular" clinical morphology
- Variants:
  - Subcutaneous Sweet's: neutrophils involve subcutis in a lobular pattern; p/w deep-seated red nodules on extremities
  - Cryptococcoid Sweet's: presence of degenerated lymphocytes w/ vacuolization/acellular basophilic bodies mimicking *Cryptococcus* on H&E
  - Histiocytoid Sweet's (variant): deep dermal infiltrate of CD163+ macrophages (myeloid lineage), often associated with myeloproliferative disease **(myelodysplasia > AML)** or NSAIDs

Treatment/clinical course

- Resolves within 2–3 months without scarring (vs. PG)
- Recurs in up to one third of classical patients, but up to 69% of malignancy-associated cases
- **ToC = systemic steroids** (prednisone 0.5–1.0 mg/kg daily for 4–6 weeks; WORKS FAST!)
  - Others: saturated solution of potassium iodide (SSKI), dapsone (100–200 mg/day), and colchicine (1.5 mg/day)
- **Increased malignancy risk**: histiocytoid/lymphocytic subcutaneous histology, age, bullous morphology, leukopenia/anemia/thrombocytopenia, ↑ ESR, NO arthralgias

Mimickers of Sweet's syndrome

- CANDLE syndrome (Chronic Atypical Neutrophilic Dermatosis with Lipoatrophy and Elevated temperature): autoinflammatory disorder of children with mutations in PSMB8 gene that can mimic Sweet's
- Marshall syndrome: rare childhood disease that has Sweet's-like lesions that resolve w/ acquired cutis laxa at affected sites

Neutrophilic dermatosis of the dorsal hands

- Features of PG + Sweet's
- Ulcerative red-violaceous plaques on dorsal hands
- a/w Hematological disorders, infection, solid organ tumors, and IBD
- Rx: prednisone, dapsone, colchicine

Pyoderma gangrenosum

Epidemiology

- Adults (20–60 yo); F > M
- Half have an associated systemic inflammatory disorder (**IBD** most common, up to 30%), hematologic disorder (e.g., **IgA monoclonal gammopathy**, AML, **chronic myeloid leukemia** [CML], hairy cell leukemia, polycythemia vera), or inflammatory arthritis

Pathogenesis

- Likely immunologic disorder
- Genetic: some cases are caused by a mutation in CD2-binding protein 1 (**PAPA syndrome**)
- **Pathergy** (30%): minor trauma (e.g., incisions, needle sticks) may initiate and/or aggravate disease; may recur with surgical procedures in 15% of patients

Clinical features

- Major types include classic (ulcerative), bullous (less destructive than ulcerative type; strongly a/w myeloproliferative disorders), pustular, peristomal, and superficial granulomatous (aka vegetative; cribriform superficial ulcers on trunk)
- Classic (ulcerative) PG
  - Starts as inflamed papulopustule/bulla → **painful** undermining ulcer w/ **overhanging**, **irregular**, **violaceous border** and purulent/vegetative base; **satellite lesions** arise at the periphery of ulcer → break down and fuse with central ulcer (Fig 3.76)
    - a/w IBD, RA, and IgA gammopathies
    - Heals with atrophic **cribriform scar**
    - Most commonly on lower extremities (pretibial)
  - Related variants:
    - Pyostomatitis vegetans: chronic vegetative pyoderma of oral mucosa associated w/ IBD
    - Peristomal PG: painful, undermined lesions around ostomy; a/w IBD
    - **Classic PG in kids (rare)**: most common on head and anogenital region; usually a/w IBD or leukemia

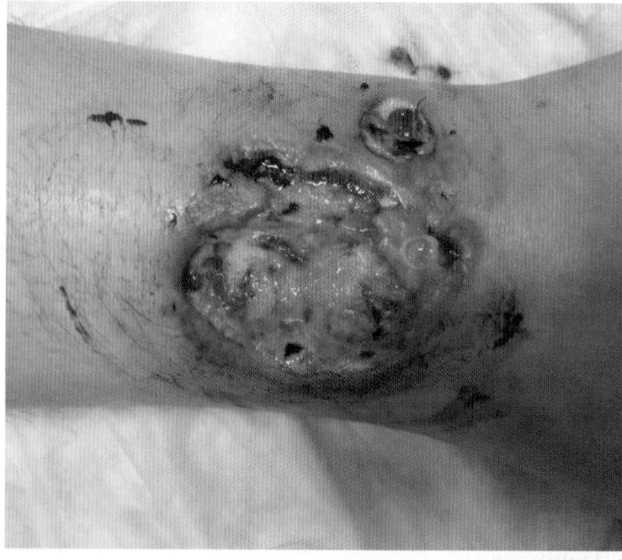

Fig. 3.76 Pyoderma gangrenosum. Ulcer with purulent exudate and violaceous, undermined border on the lower leg in a patient with ulcerative colitis. (Courtesy of Christopher Sayed, MD.)

- Pustular PG
  - **Multiple small pustules** that do not progress to ulcers
  - **a/w IBD in most cases**
- Bullous PG
  - More superficial, less destructive than classic PG
  - More widespread distribution (face, dorsal hands) → overlaps w/ bullous Sweet's disease
  - More strongly a/w **hematologic malignancy** (AML, CML, MDS, polycythemia vera)
- Vegetative PG
  - Least aggressive form
  - p/w superficial, **painless cribriform ulcers** w/ verrucous growths on trunk; responds well to conservative treatment
  - Usually arises as result of trauma (e.g., surgery)
  - **NOT** a/w underlying systemic diseases

Histopathology

- Epidermal ulceration w/ dense underlying **superficial and deep dermal neutrophilic infiltrate** (inflammation deeper than Sweet's), leukocytoclasis, epidermal pustules, and dermal edema
  - Neutrophilic infiltrate extends laterally beyond overlying ulcer ("undermining infiltrate")
- PG is a diagnosis of exclusion!!!
  - Histologic features are not entirely specific
  - **Must rule out infection, vasculitis, vasculopathy, and malignancy**

Treatment/clinical course

- Course varies depending on type of PG
- Good wound care is essential for all patients
- Must search for underlying diseases
  - GI: colonoscopy, stool studies, particularly in patients < 65 yo
  - Heme: CBC, peripheral smear, serum protein electrophoresis (SPEP), +/– bone marrow biopsy especially in patients > 65 yo
- Treatment:
  - Wound care is important (**DO NOT** surgically debride due to pathergy)
  - Initial: topical/intralesional steroids (mild disease); TCIs
  - Recalcitrant/severe disease: systemic steroids (1 mg/kg/day avg; first line); **cyclosporine** (first line); TNF-α inhibitors (**infliximab** has best data); other options (e.g., MMF, MTX, dapsone, minocycline, clindamycin/rifampin)

Behçet's disease

Epidemiology

- Japanese, **Middle Eastern, and Mediterranean** (highest prevalence in Turkey)
- Usually 20–35 years
- F > M in the United States and Japan; M > F in Middle East and Mediterranean
- May be familial in subset of cases

Pathogenesis

- Multifactorial (infectious trigger?); circulating immune complexes and neutrophil dysregulation → vascular injury
- Strongly a/w **HLA-B51 allele**

Clinical features

- Recurrent oral ulcerations (**aphthous stomatitis = first and most common symptom**) (Fig 3.77) at least three times in a year + two of the following:
  - **Recurrent genital ulceration:** large, irregular aphthae on scrotum (#1), penis, and vulva (labia majora #1) that heal with scarring
  - **Ocular lesions:** panuveitis is most common, and posterior > anterior when isolated also may have conjunctivitis, iridocyclitis, and retinal vasculitis (may → blindness)
  - Cutaneous lesions: pseudofolliculitis **papulopustules or acneiform** nodules, purpura, EN-like lesions on legs/buttocks, positive pathergy test
    - **Pathergy test:** needle stick or intradermal injection of saline → papulopustule at site of trauma within 24 to 48 hours
- Oral ulcerations can occur anywhere in oral cavity/lips, be single or multiple, painful, large in diameter, recurrent, and have a gray base w/ surrounding erythema
- Can affect all organs w/ unpredictable course:
  - Ocular (90%)
    - **#1 cause of morbidity**, including blindness
  - Vascular: superficial migratory thrombophlebitis (30%) and less frequently superior vena cava **thrombosis**
  - Other: joints (50% develop arthritis), neurologic (meningoencephalitis, multiple sclerosis-like symptoms), cardiopulmonary (cardiomyopathy, myocarditis, MVP), renal (glomerulonephritis), and GI (ileocecal inflammation/ulceration)

Histopathology

- Classically neutrophilic infiltrate around vessels w/ LCV
  - Lymphocytic vasculitis may be seen in older lesions

Treatment/clinical course

- Important to treat because of systemic involvement, but difficult to control (no ToC exists)
  - Options: mild (topical steroids, TCIs); moderate-severe (colchicine [first line for EN-like lesions and first line

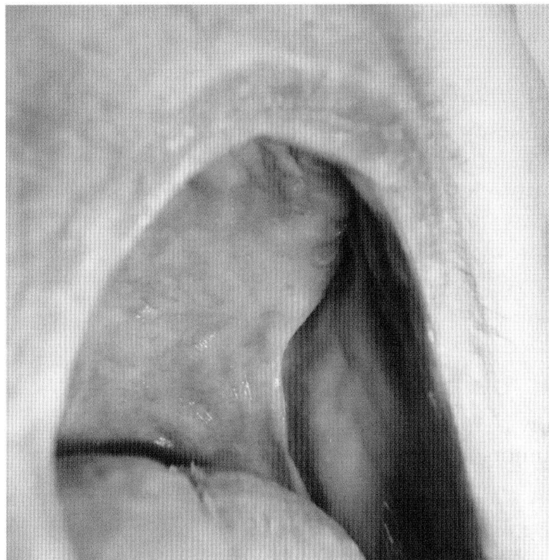

Fig. 3.77 Behçet's disease: oral aphthae on the gingiva and palate. (Courtesy of Christopher Sayed, MD.)

for mucocutaneous disease], dapsone [first line for mucocutaneous disease], minocycline, thalidomide, prednisone, IFN-γ, MTX, TNF-α inhibitors, anakinra/canakinumab, alemtuzumab, apremilast, AZA)
- Symptomatic relief (e.g., mild mouthwashes and sucralfate suspension, lidocaine gel, chlorhexidine) important

Additional information

- MAGIC syndrome = features of Behçet's and relapsing polychondritis

Bowel-associated dermatosis arthritis syndrome (Bowel bypass syndrome)

Epidemiology/pathogenesis

- Classically patients with **jejunoileal bypass surgery** and **blind loops of bowel**
  - Occurs 1–6 years after bowel surgery
  - Other causes: biliopancreatic diversion, gastric resection, IBD, peptic ulcer disease, and diverticulitis
- **Bacteria in blind loop** of bowel → immune complexes w/ bacterial antigens are deposited in skin/synovium

Clinical features

- Constitutional and serum-sickness like symptoms (e.g., malaise, fever, chills, arthralgias/myalgias) usually precede rash
- Classic rash = red to purpuric papulopustules over proximal extremities and trunk
  - May also have **tender subcutaneous nodules** (trunk, extremities; due to lobular panniculitis; heals w/ depressed scars) or **EN-like lesions** (lower legs; non-scarring)
- Diarrhea/malabsorption, hepatic failure, kidney stones, and gallstones

Histopathology

- Classic papulopustules: nodular or perivascular dermal neutrophilic inflammation
- Tender, scarring subcutaneous nodules: lobular neutrophilic panniculitis (→ loss of fat lobules and scar)
- EN-like lesions: resembles EN

Treatment/clinical course

- Skin lesions may last up to 1 month and **recur frequently**
- **Antibiotics** (e.g., tetracyclines) and immunosuppressive agents (prednisone, dapsone) → temporary improvement
- **Surgical correction** of blind bowel loop or revision of bypass is curative

Amicrobial pustulosis of the folds

- Chronic, relapsing disorder of grouped aseptic pustular lesions involving intertriginous sites
- May be due to immune-complex complement activation → neutrophil activation
- Commonly associated with autoimmune conditions (e.g., undifferentiated CTD, lupus, SjS, Hashimoto thyroiditis, APLS, IBD)

3.11 EOSINOPHILIC DISORDERS

- Various disorders can have significant numbers of eosinophils histologically, including: arthropod bites, urticaria, allergic contact and AD, drug reactions, and autoimmune blistering disorders (e.g., BP, PV, inflammatory EBA)

Granuloma faciale

- Discussed in Section 3.22

Eosinophilic folliculitis

- Discussed in Section 3.13

Papuloerythroderma of Ofuji

- **Elderly Japanese men** most commonly
- Generalized pruritic red-brown papules → erythroderma sparing skin folds ("**deck chair sign**"); lesions can become superinfected → cellulitis, erysipelas
- Eosinophilia, lymphopenia, ↑ IgE, lymphadenopathy common; can be a/w gastric carcinoma, hepatocellular carcinoma, CLL, B-cell lymphoma, T-cell lymphoma, hepatitis C, HIV
- Chronic, indolent course (remitting over several years) but responsive to **systemic steroids (ToC)**, PUVA, cyclosporine, retinoids; treat underlying cause if possible

Wells' syndrome (Eosinophilic cellulitis)

- Unknown etiology, but can be triggered by myeloproliferative diseases, infections, drugs, arthropod bites, and Churg-Strauss syndrome
- Exaggerated lymphocyte response to mosquito salivary gland extract may be present
- Recurrent tender/itchy erythematous indurated **cellulitis-like plaques** (occasionally arcuate)
  - Extremities > trunk
  - Malaise and **eosinophilia** typically present
  - Lesions resolve over 1 to 2 months
- Histology: striking eosinophilic infiltrate in interstitial dermis w/ classic **"flame figures"**
  - Flame figures = collagen fibers coated with eosinophil granule proteins (most importantly, **major basic protein**)
- **Systemic steroids are ToC** → quick improvement; alternatives include dapsone, colchicine, cyclosporine, minocycline

Hypereosinophilic syndrome (HES)

- Criteria:
  - Peripheral blood eosinophilia (eosinophils **>1500/mm^3** and/or tissue hypereosinophilia (e.g., eosinophils > 20% of cells in bone marrow)
  - No evidence of infectious, allergic, or other underlying causes
  - Symptoms/signs of end-organ involvement (due to eosinophil products)
- HES divided into **primary (neoplastic**; 75% cases) versus **secondary (reactive**; 25% cases)

- Primary HES (neoplastic):
  - Due to malignancy of stem cells/myeloid cells/ eosinophils (usually chronic eosinophilic leukemia)
  - Patients typically have ***FIP1L1-PDGFRA* fusion gene** → constitutively activated tyrosine kinase (rarely PDGFRB or FGFR1 fusion genes)
  - ~ 100% of cases are **men**
  - Systemic symptoms: fever, cough, malaise, and myalgias
  - May have ↑ serum tryptase and vitamin B12, **endomyocardial fibrosis, cardiomyopathy,** hepatosplenomegaly, CD25+ atypical mast cells on bone marrow biopsies, and constitutional symptoms (on presentation)
- Secondary HES (reactive):
  - Due to inflammatory, neoplastic, or other disorder
  - **Clonal T-cell proliferation** → ↑ Th2 cytokines (especially **IL-5**) → eosinophil activation/ hypereosinophilia)
  - Lymphocytic subtype of secondary (reactive) HES: itch, erythroderma, angioedema w/ ↑ **IgE** (due to ↑ IL-4/-13), eosinophilia, and **lymphadenopathy**
  - **Generally benign course (when compared with primary HES):**
    - Rarely develop cardiac complications
    - However, there is ↑ risk of T-cell lymphoma

- Mucocutaneous lesions in > 50% HES
  - Most commonly p/w **itchy red papules/nodules**, urticaria, angioedema
  - **Mucosal ulcers (a/w primary HES + more aggressive course**; responsive to imatinib)
- Treatment: successful treatment correlates w/ decreasing eosinophil count
  - Primary HES (neoplastic)
    - **Imatinib** (if fusion gene present) + prednisone (for possible cardiac issues), nilotinib/dasatinib/ sorafenib (other tyrosine kinase inhibitors), hydroxyurea, IFN-α, and mepolizumab/reslizumab (anti-IL-5 antibodies)
  - Secondary HES (reactive)
    - Treat underlying disorder
    - **Prednisone (first line—1 mg/kg/day)**, IFN-α, hyroxyurea, mepolizumab/reslizumab; imatinib can be considered as some patients may have occult PDGFRA/-B mutations
  - **#1 cause of death 5 congestive heart failure** (5-year survival = 80%)—patients need regular echocardiograms!

3.12 FIGURATE ERYTHEMAS

Erythema annulare centrifugum (EAC)

Epidemiology

- Peaks in fifth decade

Pathogenesis

- Unknown, but may be immune reaction to antigen (e.g., **tinea pedis**, other dermatophyte infections, other fungi, viruses, parasites), drug, pregnancy, malignancies (usually lymphoproliferative)

Clinical features

- Start as firm pink papule → erythematous annular lesions that **migrate centrifugally** (outward; up to 6 cm diameter in 2 weeks)
- **Trailing scale** (inner margin desquamation) is common in superficial lesions, but not deep lesions
- Most commonly on thighs/hips, but can become more generalized

Histopathology

- Superficial EAC: mild spongiosis, focal parakeratosis, and perivascular lymphohistiocytic infiltration, which is tight and dense (**"coat sleeve"**)
- Deep EAC: deep and tight perivascular lymphohistiocytic inflammation

Treatment

- Treat underlying disorder if present; otherwise topical steroids

Prognosis/clinical course

- Lesions last days to months

Erythema marginatum

Epidemiology

- Primarily seen in children 5 to 15 years old who are NOT treated for **group A β-hemolytic *Streptococcus* infections** of pharynx (≈3% of untreated patients)
- More prevalent in underdeveloped countries

Pathogenesis

- Seen in setting of **rheumatic fever** (aberrant humoral/ cellular immune response to group A β-hemolytic strep infection; may be related to cross-reacting epitopes)
  - Rheumatic fever: starts 2–5 weeks after infection; two major or one major + two minor criteria, in addition to evidence of group A strep infection (culture, anti-Dnase B titer, and antistreptolysin O [ASO])
    - Jones major criteria: carditis, migratory polyarthritis, **erythema marginatum**, subcutaneous nodules, or Sydenham's chorea
    - Jones minor criteria: fever, arthralgias, or abnormal laboratory findings (↑ ESR, ↑ CRP, and ↑ PR interval)

Clinical features

- Migratory expanding annular/polycyclic patches/plaques starting as macules
  - Can migrate 2 to 12 mm in half day
  - Usually trunk, axillae, and proximal extremities
- Typically resolves in a few weeks and is seen in active phase of rheumatic fever (in conjunction w/ carditis)

Histopathology

- Perivascular infiltrate of neutrophils and sometimes eosinophils without vasculitis

Treatment/clinical course

- No treatment shown to alter natural disease course

Erythema migrans

Epidemiology

- Most commonly seen in the United States (southern New England, SE NY, NJ, Eastern PA, Eastern MD, Delaware, and certain parts of MN/WI/MI) and Europe (particularly central Europe)
- White-footed mice and **white-tailed deer** are natural hosts for *Borrelia*

Pathogenesis

- Due to ***Borrelia burgdorferi*** (a spirochete) that is inoculated by ***Ixodes*** tick bites
  - Note: these ticks can also transmit babesiosis and human granulocytic anaplasmosis
  - ***Borrelia mayonii*** recently identified in Midwestern United States with higher spirochete burden and more severe disease
- Tick **MUST be attached for > 1 day** (and usually > 48 hours) to transmit disease

Clinical features

- **Large annular red expanding patch (≥5 cm)** at the site of *Borrelia*-infected tick bite 7–15 days after tick detachment lasting up to 6 weeks without treatment
  - Trunk and intertriginous areas
- Initial manifestation of Lyme disease (up to **90% of infected patients have erythema migrans**)
  - Smaller secondary lesions possibly due to lymphatic/hematologic spread or multiple tick bites
  - History of tick bite is not required for diagnosis
- Lyme disease has different symptoms in various phases
  - Early localized disease: flu-like symptoms and lymphadenopathy
  - Early disseminated disease: **Bell's palsy**, arthralgias, **AV block**, iritis
  - Chronic disease: chronic arthritis (usually monoarticular of large joints), encephalopathy, acrodermatitis chronica atrophicans (chronic sclerosing dermatitis)

Laboratory testing

- Confirmed diagnosis requires erythema migrans + either known exposure or laboratory evidence of exposure (positive tissue/fluid culture, tissue/fluid PCR, and anti-*Borrelia* antibodies via ELISA and Western blot—**peak IgM response occurs 3 to 6 weeks into infection**); agar for *Borrelia* = Barbour-Stoenner-Kelly medium
- <50% will have positive antibodies in the acute phase or in the convalescent phase after receiving treatment
- Histology: plasma cell-rich perivascular and interstitial pattern, though a significant minority may have GA-like or lichenoid features

Treatment

- Depends on stage of disease, age, and pregnancy status
- Typically **doxycycline** in early localized disease and mild early disseminated or chronic disease for non-pregnant adults and children ≥ 8 years
  - **Amoxicillin** in children < 8 years or pregnant women
- Ceftriaxone is best IV treatment (usually for Lyme meningitis)
- Jarisch-Herxheimer reaction with increased inflammation of erythema migrans may occur in up to 15% with start of treatment

Prognosis/clinical course

- If left untreated:
  - *Erythema migrans* lesions self-resolve in 6 weeks
  - 60% develop arthritis (usually knee)
  - 10% develop neurologic issues (usually Bell's palsy)
  - 5% develop cardiac issues (usually AV block)

Erythema gyratum repens

- **Paraneoplastic disorder** likely due to immune reaction against tumor-associated antigens, and subsequently cutaneous antigens (due to similarities/cross-reaction between tumor-associated antigen and cutaneous antigens)
  - Most common malignancies: **lung (most common)** > **breast and GI** (especially esophagus/stomach)
- Multiple lesions w/ **"wood grain"** (polycyclic and serpiginous) appearance of erythema in concentric rings (Fig. 3.78); **rapid expansion (1 cm/d)** with itch and trailing scale; hands and feet are spared
- M > F
- Lesions develop 1 year pre-cancer to 1 year post-cancer diagnosis, and resolve once cancer treated

Flushing

- Not a figurate erythema, but still an erythema (change in skin color due to dilation of blood vessels in dermis)
- Wide differential (Box 3.7), which includes common and serious medical issues, as well as medications and alcohol use; Table 3.27 discusses clinical findings and laboratory markers in malignancy-associated flushing

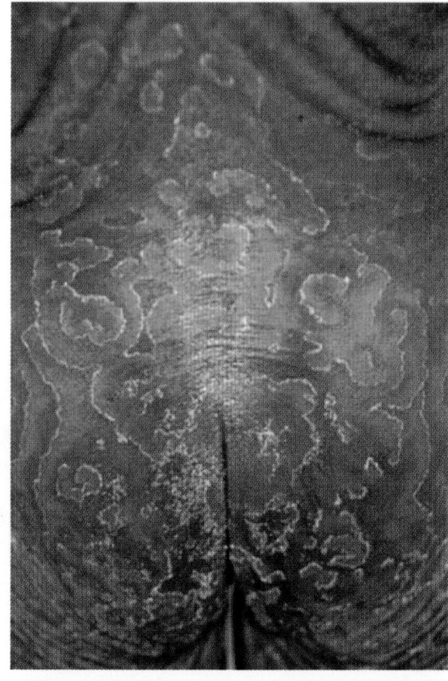

Fig. 3.78 Erythematous gyratum repens. (From James WD, Elston DM, Treat JR, Rosenbach MA, Neuhaus IM. Dermal and subcutaneous tumors. In: *Andrews' Diseases of the Skin*. 13th ed. Philadelphia: Elsevier; 2020:587–635.)

Box 3.7 Differential Diagnosis of Flushing

Common causes

- Benign cutaneous flushing
  - Emotion
  - Exercise
  - Temperature
  - Food or beverage
- Rosacea
- Climacteric flushing
- Fever
- Alcohol

Uncommon, serious causes

- Carcinoid tumors/syndrome, gastroenteropancreatic neuroendocrine tumors
- Pheochromocytoma
- Mastocytosis
- Medullary thyroid carcinoma
- Pancreatic cell tumor (VIP tumor)
- Renal cell carcinoma
- Anaphylaxis/hypersensitivity

Other causes

- Fish ingestion
  - Histamine (scombroid): poor refrigeration → bacterial overgrowth and conversion of histidine to histamine
  - Ciguatera fish poisoning from ciguatoxin (made by algae *Gambierdiscus toxicus*)
- Psychiatric or anxiety disorders
- Hyperthyroidism
- Idiopathic flushing
- Neurologic
  - Parkinson's
  - Migraines
  - Multiple sclerosis
  - Harlequin syndrome
  - Trigeminal nerve damage
  - Horner syndrome
  - Riley-Day syndrome
  - Frey syndrome
  - Autonomic epilepsy
  - Autonomic hyperreflexia
  - Paroxysmal extreme pain disorder
  - Orthostatic hypotension
  - Erythromelalgia
  - Streeten syndrome
- Medications (e.g., CCBs, vancomycin, metronidazole, cisplatin, cyclosporine, tamoxifen, disulfiram, glucocorticoids, morphine, opiates, NSAIDs, pilocarpine, serotonin agonists, niacin, nitroglycerine, sildenafil, prostaglandins)
  - Infusion reactions (e.g., vancomycin, ciprofloxacin, amphotericin B, blood)

Very rare causes

Sarcoid, mitral stenosis, dumping syndrome, male androgen deficiency, arsenic intoxication, POEMS syndrome, basophilic granulocytic leukemia, bronchogenic carcinoma, malignant histiocytoma, malignant neuroblastoma, malignant ganglioneuroma, peri-aortic surgery, Leigh syndrome, homocystinuria, superior vena cava obstruction, Rovsing syndrome, postherpetic gustatory flushing and sweating

VIP, vasoactive intestinal peptide; *CCBs*, calcium channel blockers; *NSAIDs*, nonsteroidal anti-inflammatory drugs; *POEMS*, polyneuropathy, organomegaly, endocrinopathy, monoclonal protein, skin changes

Modified from Izikson L, English JC 3rd, Zirwas MJ. The flushing patient: differential diagnosis, workup, and treatment. J Am Acad Dermatol. *2006;55(2):193–208; Data from Sadeghian A, Rouhana H, Oswald-Stumf B, Boh E. Etiologies and management of cutaneous flushing: malignant causes.* J Am Acad Dermatol. *2017;77(3):405–414.*

Table 3.27 Common Malignancies Associated with Flushing: Clinical Findings and Laboratory Markers

	Mastocytosis	Carcinoid Syndrome	Pheochromocytoma	Central Nervous System	Other
Clinical findings					
Flushing	X	X	X	X	
Blood pressure	May be low		Hypertension	May be low or high	VIPoma is associated with hypotension
Oropharyngeal edema/congestion			X		Medullary thyroid carcinoma
Dysphagia	Rare	Esophageal carcinoid			
Cardiac disease		X		X	
Pulmonary	X	X			Bronchogenic carcinoma
Gastrointestinal	X	X	X	X	VIPoma
Laboratory markers					
Serotonin/5-hydroxyindoleacetic acid		X (24-hour urine for 2 consecutive days)			
Total tryptase	X				Hypersensitivity/ anaphylaxis
Histamine	X				
Metanephrines			X		
Vanillylmandelic acid			X		
Norepinephrine			X		
Vasoactive intestinal peptide				VIPoma	
Creatinine		X (obtained to ensure adequate urine collection)			

VIPoma, *Vasointestinal polypeptide-secreting tumor.*

From Sadeghian A, Rouhana H, Oswald-Stumpf B, Boh E. Etiologies and management of cutaneous flushing: malignant causes. J Am Acad Dermatol. *2017;77(3):405–414.*

3.13 FOLLICULAR AND ECCRINE/ APOCRINE DISORDERS

Acne vulgaris

Epidemiology

- Peaks in adolescence; affects 85% between 11 and 30 yo
- >35% of women and 20% of men report acne in their 30s

Pathogenesis

- Disease of pilosebaceous unit with multifactorial pathogenesis: *Cutibacterium acnes*, sebum overproduction, abnormal keratinization, and/or inflammation
- **Abnormal follicular keratinization** (IL-1α trigger?) and microcomedone formation → comedo rupture → release of keratin and sebum → inflammatory papule/pustule → nodule/cyst
- Hormones
  - Androgens (especially dihydrotestosterone [**DHT**] and testosterone) → ↑ **growth of sebaceous glands/↑ sebum production**
    - Androgen receptors are found on the basal layer of sebaceous glands and outer root sheath of hair follicle
    - ↑ Androgen levels present during first 6 months (↑ luteinizing hormone [LH]) and at adrenarche (↑ DHEAS)
- *Cutibacterium acnes*
  - Gram-positive anaerobic rod; ribotypes 4 and 5 more prominent in acne
  - Produces lipases that break down triglycerides in sebum into FFAs, which are comedogenic and proinflammatory
  - Activates **TLR-2** on macrophages, which induces proinflammatory cytokines (**IL-1**α, IL-8, IL-12, MMPs, TNF-α) and attracts neutrophils
  - Activates **NLRP3** (part of inflammasome) of neutrophils/monocytes → ↑ IL-1β
  - Stronger peripheral macrophage response to *P. acnes* noted in patients with acne (i.e., tretinoin → CD209+ macrophages which are good good at killing *P. acnes*)
  - Produces **coproporphyrin III**, which fluoresces under Wood's lamp
- Inflammation: neutrophil predominant → pustule; lymphocytes + foreign body-type GCs + neutrophils → nodules/papules/cysts; scars more common in inflammation that is delayed and specific
- Dietary
  - Unclear, but skim milk, whey protein, vitamin B12, and **high glycemic load** may contribute to acne

Clinical features

- Most common sites (sebaceous areas): face, neck, behind ears, upper trunk, and upper arms
- Frequently start as open and closed comedones
- May develop more inflammatory lesions including papules, pustules, nodules, and cysts; nodulocystic lesions can coalesce into plaques and sinus tracts
- As lesions resolve may leave postinflammatory hyperpigmentation/erythema or scars (icepick, rolling, boxcar, anetoderma-like, hypertrophic, and keloidal)
- Women may **flare week prior to menstruation**

Histopathology

- Follicle filled with laminated keratin and debris, ± suppurative inflammation

Treatment/clinical course

- See Table 3.28 for treatment approach to acne
- Topicals/devices: retinoids (**downregulate TLR-2 expression**), benzoyl peroxide, azelaic acid, clindamycin, dapsone, erythromycin, sodium sulfacetamide/sulfur, clascosterone, salicylic acid, chemical peels, light/laser therapy (blue light safe in pregnancy)
- Orals: oral antibiotics (**tetracyclines**, penicillins/ cephalosporins, sulfonamides, and azithromycin/ erythromycin), hormonal agents (**spironolactone**, **OCPs** [5 are FDA-approved for acne]), **isotretinoin**, metformin

Table 3.28 Treatment Approach for Acne

	Mild	Moderate	Severe
1st Line Treatment	Benzoyl peroxide (BP) or topical retinoid -or- Topical combination therapy** BP + antibiotic or retinoid + BP or retinoid + BP + antibiotic	Topical combination therapy** BP + antibiotic or retinoid + BP or retinoid + BP + antibiotic -or- Oral antibiotic + topical retinoid + BP -or- Oral antibiotic + topical retinoid + BP + topical antibiotic	Oral antibiotic + Topical combination therapy** BP + antibiotic or retinoid + BP or retinoid + BP + antibiotic -or- Oral isotretinoin
Alternative Treatment	Add topical retinoid or BP (if not on already) -or- Consider alternate retinoid -or- Consider topical dapsone	Consider alternate combination therapy -or- Consider change in oral antibiotic -or- Add combined oral contraceptive or oral spironolactone (females) -or- Consider oral isotretinoin	Consider change in oral antibiotic -or- Add combined oral contraceptive or oral spironolactone (females) -or- Consider oral isotretinoin

The double asterisks (**) indicate that the drug may be prescribed as a fixed combination product or as separate component.
From Zaenglein AL, Pathy AL, Schlosser BJ, Alikhan A, Baldwin HE, Berson DS, et al. Guidelines of care for the management of acne vulgaris. J Am Acad Dermatol. *2016;74(5):945-973.e33.*

(especially polycystic ovarian syndrome [PCOS] patients), prednisone
- Complementary and alternative therapies: pantothenic acid, zinc, L-carnitine, probiotics, omega 3, borage seed oil, pumpkin seed oil; myoinositol and diindolmethane for women
- Intralesional CS for inflamed papulonodules
- Multiple modalities for scarring, including laser resurfacing, chemical peels, subcision, dermabrasion, fillers

Acne variants

Acne fulminans

- Males 13–16 years
- May occur after isotretinoin initiation or dose increase
- Most severe cystic acne, w/ **systemic manifestations**
  - Acute suppurative nodules and plaques
  - Lesions are friable w/ **hemorrhagic crust**; can ulcerate and form black eschar
  - Often scars
  - Chest, shoulders, and back; rarely on face
  - Fever, ↑ WBC, and ↑ ESR
  - **Sterile osteolytic bone lesions** (**sternum**, **clavicle**, and long bones), arthralgias, myalgias, and hepatosplenomegaly can also be seen
- Treat with **oral CS, followed by oral isotretinoin** when acute inflammation has subsided
  - If a patient on isotretinoin develops acne fulminans → ↓ isotretinoin dose immediately
- Polymorphisms in TLR-4 may be protective against acne fulminans

Acne conglobata

- M > F
- Severe eruptive nodulocystic acne, **without systemic manifestations** (vs. acne fulminans)
  - Cysts, nodules, and large abscesses with sinus formation
  - **Suppuration is characteristic** (lesions contain thick, yellow, blood-tinged fluid)
  - **Secondary comedones** can be white, firm, cyst-like or polyporous (clusters of blackheads)
  - Often scars
  - Usually on trunk (especially the back); less severe on face
- Treat with isotretinoin; may need to pretreat with prednisone to avoid acne fulminans

Solid facial edema in acne

- Swelling in midline face and cheeks
- Woody non-pitting, non-scaling induration (*peau d'orange* appearance)
- Acne predates edema by 2–5 years
- ToC = isotretinoin +/– ketotifen (antihistamine) or prednisone

Acne mechanica

- Repeated pressure/friction → obstruction of pilosebaceous unit (helmets, backpacks, collars, fiddler's neck)
- Unusual distribution pattern based on external provoking factor

Acne excoriée (de jeunes filles)

- Young women; may be **a/w underlying depression or anxiety disorder, obsessive compulsive disorder (OCD)**, body dysmorphic disorder, eating disorder, trichotillomania, or borderline personality disorder
- **Self-mutilation** of imagined acneiform lesions or mild acne lesions → excoriated crusted erosions
- Treatment: antidepressants, behavioral modification, and psychotherapy

Neonatal acne (Neonatal cephalic pustulosis)

Epidemiology

- Appears within first few weeks, resolves by 3 months
- 20% of healthy newborns
- M > F

Pathogenesis

- KOH may demonstrate *Malassezia*
- Other cases likely related to stimulation of sebaceous glands by **maternal androgens or transient androgen production**

Clinical features

- Cheeks and **nasal bridge** are common sites, but lesions may occur anywhere on the face/head/neck
- Inflammatory papules and pustules more common than comedones

Treatment/clinical course

- Usually regresses over few months
- If mild, cleanse with gentle soap and water
- Topical imidazole, topical retinoid, topical antibiotic or benzoyl peroxide
- Oral antibiotics (erythromycin) or isotretinoin if severe

Differential diagnosis

- Some neonates with trisomy 21 may develop a leukemoid reaction, which manifests as severe pustular eruption on the face, mimicking neonatal acne

Infantile acne

Epidemiology

- Appears around 3–6 months; usually resolves by 2–3 years
- M > F

Pathogenesis

- Hormonal imbalance (hyperandrogenism)

Clinical features

- More severe and persistent compared with neonatal acne
- Comedones (primarily) and inflammatory lesions including occasionally deep cysts
- Can result in **scarring**
- Usually limited to face

Treatment/clinical course

- Therapy is often necessary due to risk of scarring
- Topical retinoids, topical antibiotics, or in moderate-severe cases azithromycin or isotretinoin
- If acne arises between ages 1 and 7 (mid-childhood acne) and signs of pubertal development are noted (pubarche, thelarche, etc), an endocrinology evaluation should be considered along with the following laboratory analysis: DHEAS, androstenedione, 17-OH-progesterone, and bone age
- May predict propensity toward future acne

Transverse nasal crease

- Arise during early childhood
- Horizontal anatomical demarcation line at border of middle and lower third of the nose at junction of triangular and alar cartilage (Fig. 3.79)
- May contain milia/cysts/comedones

Acne in setting of endocrinologic abnormality

Epidemiology/pathogenesis

- Hyperandrogenism due to:
  - PCOS: **suspect in females with hirsutism or irregular menses**; most common endocrinopathy a/w acne
  - HAIR-AN syndrome (discussed below)
  - Congenital adrenal hyperplasia (CAH; children with acne)
  - Androgen-secreting tumors and Cushing's syndrome

Clinical features

- Signs: irregular menstrual cycles, androgenetic alopecia (AGA), hirsutism, deep voice, clitoromegaly
  - Distribution depends on underlying cause of androgen excess
- **Adult women** may have acne along **jawline or lower face** (adult female acne; hormonal pathogenesis)

Workup

- Initial workup: total/free testosterone, DHEAS, LH, and follicle-stimulating hormone (FSH); can also consider sex hormone-binding globulin [SHBG], 17-hydroxyprogesterone, prolactin, morning cortisol, and adrenocorticotropic hormone [ACTH] stimulation test
  - ↑ **Total testosterone** = **ovary** producing androgen
    - Testosterone 100 to 200 ng/dL +/– LH/FSH ratio > 2 to 3: PCOS
    - Testosterone > 200 ng/dL: ovarian tumors
  - ↑ **DHEAS or** ↑ **17-hydroxyprogesterone** = **adrenal gland** producing androgen
    - DHEAS 4000 to 8000 ng/mL or 17-hydroxyprogesterone > 3 ng/mL = CAH (**defects in 21-hydroxylase or 11-hydroxylase**)
    - DHEAS > 8000 ng/mL: adrenal tumors

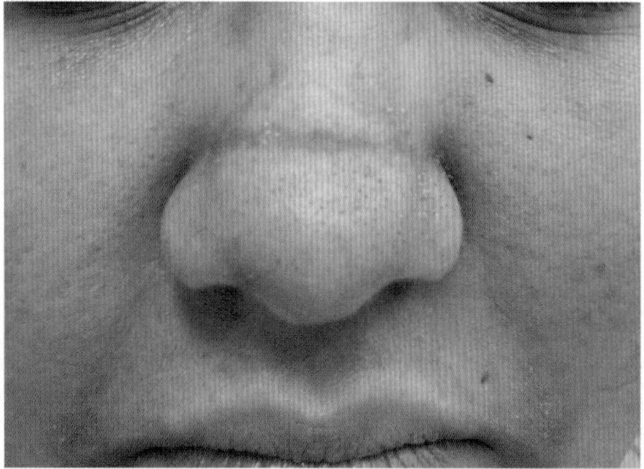

Fig. 3.79 Transverse nasal crease. (Courtesy of Christopher Sayed, MD.)

Treatment/clinical course

- Treat underlying abnormality
- OCPs or spironolactone

Additional information

- XYY genotype may have more severe acne

Acne cosmetica

- Frequent/heavy use of cosmetics containing lanolin, petrolatum, vegetable oils, butyl stearate, isopropyl myristate, sodium lauryl sulfate, lauryl alcohol, or oleic acid → small closed comedones, small papules and pustules

Pomade acne

- More common in **African Americans** using greasy/oily grooming substances on the scalp
- Closely set, monomorphic, small closed comedones on forehead and temples

Chloracne

- Type of occupational acne caused by exposure to **chlorinated aromatic hydrocarbons** (found in electrical conductors, insulators, and insecticides/fungicides/herbicides)
  - **Agent orange** was contaminated with 2,3,7,8-tetrachlorodibenzo-p-dioxin (**dioxin**), a chlorinated hydrocarbon
- Acne develops after several weeks of exposure
- May have recurrent outbreaks for many years after exposure
- Preferred sites are face, neck (including **retroauricular**), **axilla**, **scrotum**, and penis
- Treatment difficult; **ToC is isotretinoin** (high dose followed by low-dose maintenance), topical retinoids, surgical intervention for large lesions

Radiation acne

- Ionizing rays induce epithelial metaplasia in follicles → hyperkeratotic plugs
- Comedo-like papules in areas of previous radiation exposure
- Appears as the acute phase of radiation dermatitis resolves

Acneiform eruptions

Drug-induced acne

Epidemiology/pathogenesis

- A/w multiple meds:
  - **Anabolic steroids**
  - Androgens (testosterone)
  - **CS**
  - **Halogens** (iodides and bromides)
  - INH
  - OCPs (containing androgen-like progestins)
  - **Lithium**
  - **Phenytoin**
  - Upadacitinib
  - Vitamins B2, B6, and B12
  - **Epidermal growth factor receptor (EGFR) inhibitors** (monoclonal antibodies: cetuximab and panitumumab; tyrosine kinase inhibitors: gefitinib, erlotinib, and lapatinib)
  - Other chemotherapy a/w acneiform eruptions:
    - mTOR inhibitors (sirolimus and tacrolimus)
    - Multikinase inhibitors (sunitinib and sorafenib)
    - MEK inhibitors (trametinib)
- **Mnemonic:** "**SHIELD** yourself from acne with **vitamin** T:" **S**teroids (anabolic, CS), **H**alogens, **I**soniazid, **E**GFR inhibitors, **L**ithium, **D**ilantin (phenytoin), **Vitamin** B2, B6, B12, **T**estosterone

Clinical features

- Abrupt-onset monomorphous inflammatory papules or pustules (classic in CS-induced acne)
- Usually **lacks comedones**
- Trunk > face
- In setting of **EGFR inhibitors**, occurs in usual acne-prone areas and sun-exposed areas; starts 1 to 3 weeks after beginning treatment; severity of reaction positively correlates with clinical response to medication; occurs in > 80% of patients

Treatment/clinical course

- Discontinue offending medication if possible
- For EGFR inhibitors: prophylaxis with doxycycline or minocycline started on same day as EGFR inhibitor therapy; **DO NOT** use irritating agents like topical retinoids or benzoyl peroxide

Acne-associated syndromes

SAPHO (Chronic recurrent multifocal osteomyelitis)

- **S**ynovitis, **A**cne, **P**ustulosis, **H**yperostosis, **O**steitis
- Affects children and young adults (usually appears in third decade); more common in Japan
  - Inflammatory disorder of unclear etiology
  - Characterized by RF(–) osteoarthropathy with various skin manifestations
    - Bone disease precedes skin disease in the majority
    - **Sternoclavicular area** is the most common site of inflammation
    - Chest wall and mandible are most common areas of musculoskeletal pain
    - Of note, **"bull's head"** sign may be seen on X-ray
- Acne varies from mild to acne congolobata/fulminans; hidradenitis suppurativa and dissecting cellulitis can also be seen
- Pustulosis includes palmoplantar pustulosis and pustular psoriasis (psoriasis can also be seen)
- Associated with IBD
- Treatment: bisphosphonates, TNF-α inhibitors, MTX, NSAIDs, CS, colchicine, anakinra

PAPA

- **P**yogenic **A**rthritis (sterile), **P**yoderma gangrenosum, **A**cne conglobata
- Autosomal dominant mutation in CD2-binding protein 1 (**CD2BP1**; aka **PSTPIP1**)
  - Part of autoinflammatory disease group as CD2BP1 interacts with pyrin (mutation → unopposed inflammation)
- Treatment: systemic or local CS, dapsone, infliximab, anakinra
- Also know **PASH** (**P**yoderma gangrenosum, **A**cne, **S**uppurative **H**idradenitis) and **PAPASH** (**P**yogenic **A**rthritis, **P**yoderma gangrenosum, **A**cne, **S**uppurative **H**idradenitis)

HAIR-AN

- **H**yper **A**ndrogenism, **I**nsulin **R**esistance, **A**canthosis **N**igricans
- Can be considered a unique subtype of PCOS in women with high risk of diabetes and cardiovascular disease
- Treatment: anti-androgens (e.g., spironolactone), OCPs, and insulin-sensitizing medications (e.g. metformin)

Apert syndrome (Acrocephalosyndactyly)

- Autosomal dominant mutation in **fibroblast growth factor receptor 2 (FGFR2)**; ↑ FGFR2 signaling → follicular hyperkeratosis and sebaceous gland hypertrophy; FGFR2 mutations also found in some nevus comedonicus cases
- **Synostoses** of bones of hands/feet, vertebral bodies, and cranium
- Diffuse distribution of **moderate to severe acne**, especially on extensor arms, buttocks, and thighs
- Nail dystrophy and cutaneous/ocular hypopigmentation
- Treatment: isotretinoin

Rosacea

Epidemiology

- Peaks at 30–40 yo; F > M; usually skin types I and II

Pathogenesisv

- Chronic vascular inflammatory disorder
- Multifactorial: **vascular hyperreactivity**, dysregulated innate immunity, chronic solar damage, sensitivity to heat, hyperirritable skin, and possible association with *Demodex*
- Kallikrein 5, TPRV, cathelicidin LL-37, and TLR2 are upregulated

Clinical features

- Usually limited to central face
- Depends on subtypes (see Rosacea subtypes section)

Histopathology

- Perivascular and perifollicular lymphohistiocytic infiltrate, vascular ectasia, mild edema, and sebaceous hyperplasia

Treatment/clinical course

- **Avoid triggers** (sunlight, heat/cold, stress, strong emotions, alcohol, hot beverages, spicy foods, chemical irritation) and use sunscreen
- Topicals: **metronidazole**, sodium sulfacetamide/sulfur, azelaic acid, benzoyl peroxide, clindamycin, ivermectin, and green-tinted makeup
- Topical brimonidine (α2-adrenergic agonist) and oxymetazoline (α1 > α2-adrenergic agonist) reduce background erythema and flushing
- Systemic: **tetracyclines** (consider subantimicrobial modified release dosage doxycycline—fewer AEs), amoxicillin, and isotretinoin if severe
- Others: intense pulsed light (IPL) and pulsed dye laser (PDL); rhinophyma: CO_2 laser and electrosurgery

Additional information

- Haber's syndrome: genodermatosis w/ rosacea-like eruption and verrucous lesions

Rosacea subtypes

Erythematotelangiectatic (Vascular)

- Central face with recurrent blush that eventually becomes permanent flushing
- Burning, stinging sensation; easily irritated with roughness and scaling
- Can have associated edema
- +/– Telangiectasias

Papulopustular (Inflammatory)

- Similar to acne vulgaris, but lesions may have deeper red color and **no comedones**
- Persistent central facial erythema with transient papules/pustules

Phymatous

- Thickening of skin due to **overgrowth of sebaceous glands**
- Most common on nose (**rhinophyma**); can also involve chin (gnathophyma), forehead (metophyma), earlobes (otophyma), and eyelids (blepharophyma)

Ocular

- **~ 50% of rosacea patients affected**
- Many complaints including **dryness**, **foreign body sensation**, photosensitivity, burning/stinging, blepharitis, recurrent chalazion, conjunctivitis, keratitis, iritis, and scleritis
- Treatment: **doxycycline/minocycline**

Rosacea variants

Solid facial edema in rosacea (Morbihan disease and rosacea lymphedema)

- Unknown etiology; possibly due to chronic inflammation → obstruction of lymph vessels or fibrosis
  - There is a similar condition in acne
- **Hard non-pitting swelling** of forehead, glabella, nose, and cheeks
- May be more pronounced during **early morning hours**
- ↓ Vision if eyelids involved
- Spontaneous resolution DOES NOT occur
- ToC = **isotretinoin ± ketotifen** (antihistamine)
  - Other options: systemic steroids, antibiotics, and lymphatic drainage/compression therapy

Pyoderma faciale (Rosacea fulminans)

- **Females** in their 20s to 30s
- Rapid onset of intensely inflamed coalescent fluctuant nodules and cysts on background of dark red to cyanotic erythema; can have draining sinuses with purulent drainage
- Centrofacial region, no involvement elsewhere and no comedones (vs. acne fulminans)
- Most develop **scarring**
- Can have low-grade fever, myalgias, ↑ WBC, and ↑ ESR
- Treatment (same as acne fulminans): **prednisone** (with slow taper) and **isotretinoin**

Granulomatous rosacea

- Middle-aged women
- Discrete **yellow/brown-red firm papules** or nodules on background of diffusely reddened thickened skin on butterfly region; can be distributed around periphery of face and perioral areas
- Histology: non-caseating epithelioid granulomas (resembles sarcoidosis)
- Treatments: tetracyclines and isotretinoin

Lupus miliaris disseminatus faciei

- Young adults; more common in **Asians** (especially Japanese)
- Smooth, firm, **yellow-brown to red** 1 to 3 mm monomorphous papules with apple jelly color on diascopy
- Present in typical butterfly distribution, but also seen laterally (below mandible), periorificially, and involving the **eyelid skin** (characteristic site)
- Heals with **scarring**
- Histology often shows **caseating granulomas**
- Treatment is difficult—can try isotretinoin and tetracyclines

Perioral/periorificial dermatitis

Epidemiology

- Young women in their 20s to 30s
- Children can also be affected (of note, perialar intertrigo may be an overlap of seborrheic dermatitis and perioral dermatitis in kids)

Pathogenesis

- Inflammatory condition of unknown cause, perhaps related to rosacea
- Most commonly attributed to use of **topical fluorinated CS** or facial cosmetics

Clinical features

- Clusters of small, pink discrete scaly papules/pustules in perioral region with **clear zone around the vermilion border**
  - Can also involve opening of nares, nasolabial folds, and cheeks
- **Burning sensation**, minimal itching

Treatment/clinical course

- Self-limited, but resolution can take months to years
- Avoid cosmetics, topical steroids, and other irritating topicals
- **Tetracyclines** (or azithromycin/erythromycin in pediatrics) × 6 to 8 weeks with gradual tapering to avoid rapid rebounding, oral/topical ivermectin, TCIs, topical antibacterials, topical metronidazole

Variants

- Periorbital/periocular dermatitis
- **Periorificial dermatitis** is a combination of perioral and periorbital/periocular dermatitis

Folliculitis

Superficial folliculitis

- Culture of pustule usually = normal flora
  - When culture is positive, ***S. aureus* is most common** infectious etiology
- Perifollicular pustules often with erythematous base in areas with terminal hairs (scalp, beard, trunk, buttocks, and thighs)
- Treatment depends on culture results; if culture-negative: topical benzoyl peroxide, topical antibiotics, tetracyclines

Gram-negative folliculitis

- Occurs in acne **patients receiving prolonged antibiotic treatment** (esp. tetracyclines) More common in adult men
- Anterior nares become colonized with gram-negative organisms (*Proteus, Enterobacter, Escherichia coli,* or *Klebsiella*)
- Numerous **pruritic** pustules on an erythematous base; short-lived, but new lesions continue to appear
- Central region of face, **lesions fan out from nose**/mouth to involve perinasal/beard region
- **ToC = isotretinoin**; topical gentamicin or oral ciprofloxacin can be considered

Hot tub folliculitis

- A gram-negative folliculitis due to ***Pseudomonas aeruginosa***
- Use of hot tub 12 to 48 hours prior to onset
- Edematous pink to red perifollicular papules and pustules on the **trunk**
- **Self-resolves**

Eosinophilic folliculitis

- Three forms:
  - Eosinophilic pustular folliculitis (Ofuji's disease)
    - 30 yo; M > F; more common in **Japanese**
    - Recurrent explosive crops of intensely pruritic grouped follicular papules and pustules
      - Can also have erythematous patches and plaques with superimposed coalescent pustules
      - Central clearing and centrifugal extension leads to figurate/serpiginous lesions
      - Most common on face, back, and extensor arms
      - Peripheral eosinophilia
    - Spontaneous resolution followed by relapses every 3–4 weeks
    - Symptomatic treatment of pruritus and **oral indomethacin** may help
  - Immunosuppression-associated esosinophilic folliculitis (AIDS-associated eosinophilic folliculitis)
    - See Chapter 5, Infectious Dermatology
  - Neonatal eosinophilic pustular folliculitis
    - Early in infancy
    - Pruritic perifollicular pustules and vesicles on erythematous base usually on **scalp**
      - Secondary crusting is common
    - Self-limited, cyclical course for few months to years

Disseminate and recurrent infundibulofolliculitis

- Adults with **darkly pigmented** skin
- Hundreds of monotonous 1 to 2 mm pruritic flesh-colored follicular papules (similar to goose bumps in appearance) on **trunk** > neck and upper extremities lasting months-years
- Histology: edema and sparse lymphocytes and neutrophils infiltrating the follicular infundibulum
- Treatments: topical CS, lactic acid creams, urea creams

Viral-associated trichodysplasia

- Occurs in the context of immunosuppression
- Trichodysplasia spinulosa-associated polyomavirus → pink spiny papules on central face
- Histology: proliferation of inner root sheath cells with increased trichohyalin granules
- Treatment: topical cidofivir, tazarotene gel, oral valganciclovir

Pseudofolliculitis barbae

- Most common in **African American** curly-haired men who shave their **beard**
  - Keratin H6hf (Keratin 75) mutations have been implicated
- Tightly curled hairs curve back into skin after being shaved → inflammatory reaction with papules/pustules
- Hyperpigmentation, hypertrophic scars, and keloids are possible
- Treatment: **stop shaving**; laser hair removal, chemical depilatories, oral antibiotics and topical CS for anti-inflammatory effects, tretinoin can be used to "toughen" the skin
  - If patient must shave, instruct to gently dislodge ingrown hairs and shave in direction of hair growth

Acne keloidalis nuchae

- Males; **African American > Latinos** > Asians > Caucasians
- Dome-shaped, pruritic, follicular papules on **posterior neck and occipital scalp**
- Develop into **keloidal papules** which coalesce into large plaques in band-like distribution near posterior hairline; cicatricial alopecia in areas of involvement (Fig. 3.80)
- Keloidal collagen only present in severe disease; early disease has scar-like collagen
- Treatment: ↓ mechanical irritation to affected areas; tretinoin gel plus potent topical CS; intralesional CS; oral/topical antibiotics if inflamed; surgical excision; CO_2 laser

Follicular occlusion tetrad (acne conglobata, hidradenitis suppurativa, dissecting cellulitis of the scalp, and pilonidal cyst)

Hidradenitis suppurativa (acne inversa)

Epidemiology

- 0.3%–1% prevalence
- Starts after puberty
- F > M, but on average more severe in males
- More common in African Americans and those of lower socioeconomic status
- ~35% of patients have first-degree relative affected

Pathogenesis

- Immune dysregulation (both innate and adaptive immunity), follicular occlusion
- 1%–2% of patients have familial mutations seen in **gamma-secretase complex** (nicastrin, presenilin 1, presenilin enhancer 2) leading to atypical disease with diffuse involvement and many cysts
- Associations: obesity, **smoking, diabetes, metabolic syndrome, cardiovascular disease**, PCOS, lymphoma, anxiety, and depression

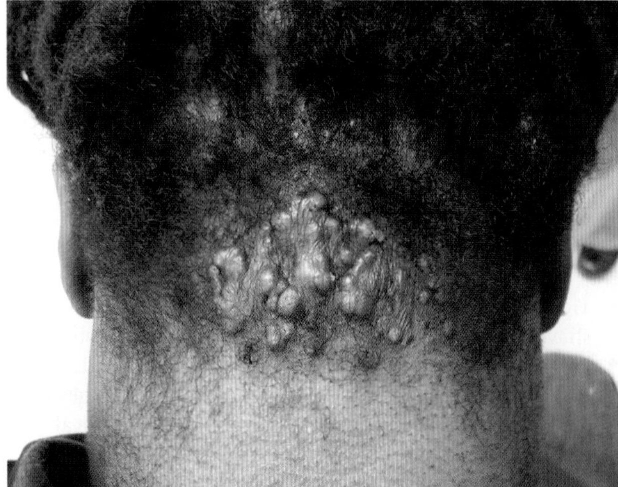

Fig. 3.80 Acne keloidalis nuchae. Crusted papules and pustules and keloidal plaques studded with papules on the occipital scalp. (Courtesy of Christopher Sayed, MD.)

Clinical features

- Criteria of (1) nodules and abscesses with (2) predilection for **intertriginous locations (axilla, inguinal, anogenital, and inframammary)** (3) with recurrence
- Hurley stage I: recurrent nodules and abscesses without sinuses or significant scarring
- Hurley stage II: stage I with the addition of limited sinuses and scarring
- Hurley stage III: widespread or interconnected sinuses and/or scarring
- **Sinus tracts** and **double or multi-headed comedones** are classic features
- Chronic thick viscous suppurative drainage; frequently malodorous; +/– secondary infection
- Anemia, secondary amyloidosis, lymphedema, fistula formation, and SCC due to chronic scarring
- Cultures most commonly grow skin flora (i.e., *Staphylococcus epidermidis*)

Histopathology

- Suppurative folliculitis with abscess formation, follicular plugging, granulation tissue, and inflammation that can involve apocrine glands; late stages can have fibrosis

Treatment/clinical course

- In early stage disease: ↓ weight, ↓ friction/moisture, oral antibiotics (clindamycin and rifampin, tetracyclines, R-O-M therapy), topical clindamycin, laser-based follicular ablation (i.e., Nd:YAG), PDT, and intralesional CS
- In severe disease: high-quality data for adalimumab (FDA approved for weekly 40 mg dosing or 80 mg every other week) and infliximab; lower-quality studies of anakinra, ustekinumab, apremilast, IL-17 inhibitors (though secukinumab has phase 3 data) and IL-23 inhibitors; ertapenem in extreme flares
- In female patients, spironolactone and OCPs can be considered
- **For sinuses, surgical excision, marsupialization**, deroofing, and CO_2 laser with secondary intention healing, may also be required
- Variable success: isotretinoin/acitretin, finasteride, MTX, metformin, colchicine

Pilonidal cyst

- M > F, 20–40 yo
- Associated with curly hair, obesity, poor hygiene, and prolonged sitting
- **Painful draining sinus in sacrococcygeal region**
  - Can be filled with nests of hair
- Treatment: surgical excision; if inflamed, oral antibiotics; moderate success with laser-based follicular ablation

Dissecting cellulitis of the scalp and acne conglobata (discussed in alopecia and acne sections)

- Discussed in Alopecia and Acne sections of Chapter 3

Other diseases of eccrine and apocrine sweat glands

Hyperhidrosis

Pathogenesis

- Sweating is a reflex controlled through the sympathetic nervous system; nerves are anatomically sympathetic but functionally cholinergic
- **Primary localized hyperhidrosis is most common type**
- 60%–80% have family history with possible autosomal dominant inheritance pattern for some
- **Secondary hyperhidrosis** is due to an **underlying condition**. There are many causes that can be classified based on the source of neural impulse:
  - Cortical (emotional)
    - ↑ Neural impulses from the cerebral cortex due to emotion or sensory stimuli
  - Hypothalamic (thermoregulatory)
    - Due to ↑ body temperature or direct hypothalamic stimuli
  - Medullary (gustatory)
    - Physiologic medullary hyperhidrosis: afferent impulses from taste receptors stimulate sweating (spicy foods, alcohol, and citrus fruits)
    - Pathologic medullary hyperhidrosis: auriculotemporal or **Frey's syndrome**
  - Spinal (cord transection)
    - Spinal disorders may result in lack of thermal sweating below the injury, hyperhidrosis at the injured level, or other unusual patterns of sweating
  - Axon reflex (local inflammatory)
    - Direct stimulation of a sympathetic axon can cause sweating (electrical, physical, or drug-induced)
    - Mediators from inflammatory skin disease (psoriasis and dermatitis) can elicit localized hyperhidrosis

Clinical features

- Shiny wet skin surfaces or excessive sweat stains on clothing
- Primary localized hyperhidrosis: **palmoplantar > axillary** > forehead
- Secondary hyperhidrosis: can be localized or generalized
- **Starch-iodine technique** can aid in determining the most active areas (highlighted by reaction changing to blue/black color)

Treatment/clinical course

- Topical antiperspirants **(aluminum chloride)**, iontophoresis, botulinum toxin, systemic anticholinergics (**glycopyrrolate, propantheline,** and **oxybutynin**), topical glycopyrrolate/glycopyrronium, α-adrenergic blockers (clonidine), thoracic sympathectomy (**risk of compensatory hyperhidrosis**), microwave ablation (miraDry®), liposuction, and behavioral modification/psychotherapy

Hypohidrosis and anhidrosis

Epidemiology/pathogenesis

- Central or neuropathic diseases (e.g., brain tumors and spinal cord injuries) or medications (e.g., **anticholinergics and α-adrenergic blockers**) that disrupt neural impulses
- Congenital alterations of sweat glands (e.g., ectodermal dysplasias)
- Acquired destruction/atrophy of sweat glands (e.g., burns, scleroderma, morphea, GVHD)
- Sweat gland obstruction (e.g., miliaria, ichthyoses, psoriasis, and eczematous dermatoses)

Clinical features

- Skin may appear unremarkable, but there is ↓ or absence of sweating and resulting **hyperthermia**
- Attempt to induce sweating (exercising in hot room or using electric blanket) followed by starch-iodide technique to demonstrate ↓ or absent sweating

Treatment/clinical course

- Discontinue offending medication(s)
- Avoid hyperpyrexia and maintain a cool environment
- Gentle exfoliation if obstructed sweat ducts

Miliaria

Epidemiology

- Most common in **neonates** who have not fully developed eccrine ducts
- **Adults in hot humid climates**

Pathogenesis

- Excessive sweating causes maceration of the stratum corneum → eccrine duct obstruction → sweat retention within the duct

Clinical features

- Table 3.29

Bromhidrosis

- **Apocrine bromhidrosis**: bacterial degradation of apocrine sweat yields ammonia and short chain fatty acids; exaggeration of typical axillary body odor

Table 3.29 Three Types of Miliaria

Type	Location of Obstruction	Cutaneous Lesions	Patient Population	Most Common Location
Crystallina	Stratum corneum	**Non-pruritic, clear**, fragile, 1 mm vesicles	Neonates < 2 weeks of age Children and adults in hot climates	Face and trunk
Rubra	Mid-epidermis	**Pruritic, erythematous**, 1–3 mm papules; may have pustules	Neonates 1–3 weeks of age Children and adults in hot climates	Neck and upper trunk
Profunda	Dermal–epidermal junction	Non-pruritic, white, 1–3 mm papules	**Adults in hot climates**; often with multiple bouts of miliaria rubra	Trunk and proximal extremities

- Eccrine bromhidrosis: three types
  - Keratogenic: bacterial degradation of stratum corneum macerated by excess eccrine sweat
  - Metabolic: abnormal secretion of amino acids or breakdown products as seen in heritable metabolic disorders (e.g., phenylketonuria has mousy odor and maple syrup urine disease has sweet odor)
  - Exogenous: odorogenic compounds such as garlic, asparagus, curry, DMSO, penicillins

Chromhidrosis

Pathogenesis

- Apocrine chromhidrosis: adrenergic stimuli causes myoepithelial contractions
- Eccrine chromhidrosis: contamination of colorless eccrine sweat by a chromogen

Clinical features

- **Colored sweat**
- Apocrine chromhidrosis:
  - Usually on face and axilla
  - Yellow = **lipofuscin** (if lipofuscin is more oxidized or concentrated, color can be blue, green, black)
- Eccrine chromhidrosis:
  - Blue or blue/green = copper
  - Brown = dihydroxyacetone-containing self-tanning products
  - Red = **clofazimine and rifampin**
  - Brown = ochronosis
- Pseudochromhidrosis: **sweat stained after excretion on the skin**
  - *Corynebacterium* (brown), *Serratia marcescens* (pink), copper salts (blue)

Fox-fordyce disease (Apocrine miliaria)

- Plugging of apocrine sweat glands in adolescent/**young adult females**
- **Extremely pruritic**, skin-colored or yellow dome-shaped follicular papules in apocrine areas (**axilla** > periareolar and anogenital) → ↓ hair density
- Treatment is difficult—options: tretinoin, topical CS, TCIs, topical antibiotics, microwave ablation, and surgical excision; pregnancy can lead to improvement

3.14 DRUG REACTIONS

See Pharmacology Section

3.15 PHOTODERMATOSES AND OTHER PHYSICAL DERMATOSES

Temperature-related dermatoses

Thermal burns

- Arise due to excess heat on skin
- First degree: erythema + epidermal peeling (e.g., ordinary sunburn)
- Second degree: two forms
  - Superficial: **painful** vesicles due to edema of superficial dermis and epidermis; **non-scarring**; may take 3 weeks to heal
  - Deep: pale, **anesthetic** skin; **results in scarring** (due to reticular dermis/appendageal injury)
- Third and fourth degree: third (full-thickness skin destroyed → ulcer → scar) and fourth (loss of skin and subcutaneous fat +/– underlying structures)
  - Grafting usually needed to help with function/contractures
  - May need to excise non-healing tissue
  - Silver-impregnated dressings may help to ↓ infection risk
    - Silver sulfadiazine absorption can → **leukopenia and argyria** (mafenide acetate is alternative)
  - Diligent wound care and monitoring for infection are key
  - More than two thirds of BSA = poor prognosis/↑ mortality (women, infants, toddlers)
  - For larger surface areas, will need IV fluid resuscitation

Erythema ab igne

- Thick **reticulated erythema** and/or pigmentation from chronic, non-burning, heat/infrared radiation exposure to a particular anatomic site (Fig. 3.81)
- F > M
- Classic sites and causes: shins (**space heaters**), lower back (**heating pad**), and anterior thighs (**laptop**)
- Possible ↑ SCC risk

Cold injuries

- Acrocyanosis
  - **Blue discoloration** of hands and/or feet +/– hyperhidrosis; ↑ with colder temperatures
    - **Young women** mainly

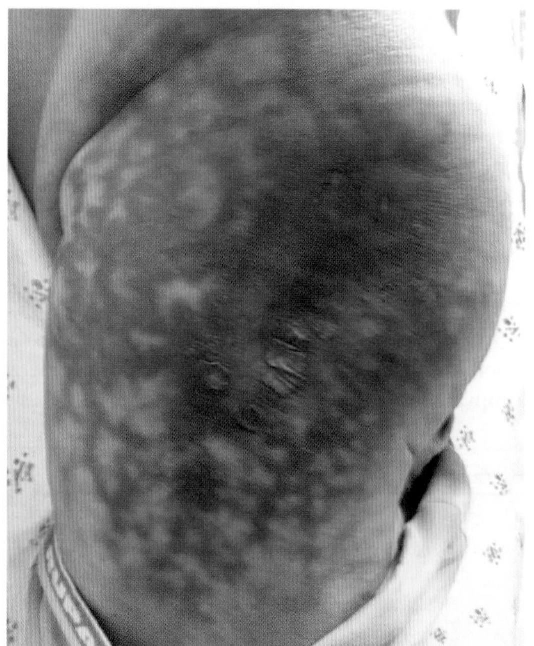

Fig. 3.81 Erythemat ab igne. Site of chronic heating pad use for hip pain demonstrating reticulated hyperpigmentation and erythema as well as scar at areas of previous ulceration. (Courtesy of Christopher Sayed, MD.)

- May be a/w butyl nitrite, IFN-α 2a, malignancy, anorexia nervosa
- Main DDx is **Raynaud syndrome** (episodic; **red/white/blue** phases a/w cold; can → ulceration and distal fingertip resorption)

- Pernio
  - **Symmetric red-blue/purple macules/papules of acral skin** (toes/fingers most commonly) + burning/itching after cold or wet exposure
    - Ulceration may be seen
    - Histology: dense superficial and **deep PV and peri-eccrine** lymphocytic infiltrate + **dermal edema**
  - DDx includes chilblain lupus (exclude via serologic testing and/or biopsy) and blood dyscrasias (exclude via CBC w/ diff, cryoglobulins, cryofibrinogens, cold agglutinin, SPEP/IF)
  - Treatment: warming measures (resolves in few weeks); **nifedipine** or topical CS may be used
- Frostbite
  - Erythema, edema, bullae w/ clear fluid, and pain indicate superficial injury w/ good prognosis
  - Cool, blanched, anesthetic, and woody/hard skin → red/purple color (from hyperemia) + hemorrhagic blisters (raise concern for deep tissue injury, scarring, and amputation when involving muscle and/or bone)
  - Pathogenesis: skin temperature drops below −2 °C → vasoconstriction and occlusion → skin damage
  - Most common locations = **ears and nose**
  - Treat with warm (37 °C–39 °C) water bath **rapidly**

Photodermatoses

Sunburns and pigment darkening

- ↑ UV exposure (UVB most commonly) → intense inflammation (↑ neutrophils, CD3+ lymphocytes, **prostaglandins**, eicosanoids)/erythema +/− blistering/edema **(peaks at 12–24 hours with UVB)** → desquamation
- Wavelengths **~300 nm are most erythemogenic**
  - Redness may take several days to fade; lasts longer with UVA exposure
- Severe cases may require hospitalization
  - Symptom relief with NSAIDs, CS, creams/lotions, water intake; early high-dose (200,000 IU) vitamin D may be effective
- Various forms of pigment darkening/tanning:
  - Immediate pigment darkening: within 10–20 minutes of **UVA light** or **visible blue light** exposure; secondary to photooxidation of melanin + melanin redistribution within melanocytes
  - Persistent pigment darkening: brown coloration present > 2 hours after **UVA light** exposure, lasting 24 hours; due to **oxidation of melanin**
  - Delayed pigmentation/tanning: develops over many days and lasts weeks-months; due to **UVB light** (mainly), resulting in ↑ **melanin synthesis**

Photoaging

- **Solar elastosis**: thickened, wrinkled, yellowish skin on chronically sun-damaged skin
  - **Cutis rhomboidalis nuchae**—solar elastosis variant affecting posterior neck with geometrically patterned leather-like wrinkled skin
- **Poikiloderma of Civatte**: reticular reddish-brown telangiectatic patches on lateral neck (central submental region spared)
- **Favre-Racouchot syndrome**: clusters of large open comedones on lateral/inferior periorbital area/temple + solar elastosis
- **Colloid milium**: 1–2 mm white-yellow subcutaneous papules, often grouped in sun-exposed regions of face
- **Erosive pustular dermatosis**: pustules + crusts + erosions on significantly photodamaged scalp of older, bald men, sometimes triggered by trauma (e.g., surgical excision)
  - No consistently effective treatment; topical steroids or calcineurin inhibitors may be tried

Polymorphous light eruption

- **Most common photosensitive dermatosis**; affects 5%–20% of Caucasians
- Erythematous, itchy papules, vesicles, or plaques (hence "polymorphous") on **sun-exposed areas** (V of neck, outer arms, and dorsal hands); face can be involved, but often spared due to consistent sun-exposure in most months; **arises within hours and lasts 1–4 days after UVA** (> UVB > visible light) exposure
  - In ethnic skin, may see clusters of pinpoint papules resembling lichen nitidus
  - **Juvenile spring eruption** is a variant seen in young males aged 5 to 12 yo **(see** Chapter 4**)**
- Young F > M (3:1)
- Occurs in **spring/early summer**, particularly in northern latitudes
- Lesions last days to weeks
- Improves as summer proceeds ("**hardening**" effect)
- Likely related to decreased suppression of delayed-type hypersensitivity reaction from UVR in some individuals → ↑ response to photo-induced antigens
  - Patients with PMLE may have less nonmelanoma skin cancer risk since UVR induces less cutaneous immunosuppression
- MED phototesting may be normal or may be decreased to UVA and/or UVB
- Histology: **marked papillary dermal edema** + dense perivascular dermal lymphocytic inflammation
- Treatment:
  - **Photoprotection (first line)**: broad-spectrum sunscreens that **block UVA (avobenzone, titanium dioxide, and zinc oxide**), DermaGard film for windows
  - Others: phototherapy (prophylactic, in early spring), antimalarial prophylaxis, AZA and CS for flares (may use systemic steroids if severe)

Hydroa vacciniforme (see Chapter 4)

Actinic folliculitis

- Photodistributed follicular eruption in young women developing up to 36 h after sun exposure (UVA specifically)
- Treatment: topical/oral retinoids, prophylactic NB UVB phototherapy

Chronic actinic dermatitis

- Chronic, pruritic, eczematous eruption in **photodistributed areas**
  - Spares skin furrows, upper eyelids, nasolabial folds, postauricular, and finger webs
  - Over time may spread to non-sun-exposed areas
  - Over time, eruption becomes **lichenified/thickened**
- Seen in **men > 50 years old**, primarily in temperate climates; worsens in the summer
- **Phototesting positive to UVA, UVB, and/or visible light (UVA + UVB most common)**
- Likely contact allergy-like response with delayed-type hypersensitivity reaction to UV-induced cutaneous antigens such as nucleic acids (history of contact or photocontact dermatitis are common)
- **Patch testing and photopatch testing may also be positive** (especially ***Compositae* or sunscreens)**
- Treatment: photoprotection, avoid possible sensitizers, PUVA, topical/systemic immunosuppressants; **severe UVB photosensitivity and ≥ two contact allergens are poor prognostic predictors**; up to 10% resolve in 5 years and 50% in 15 years

Actinic prurigo (see Chapter 4)

Solar urticaria

- Urticarial, itchy/burning, lesions appearing **within 5 to 10 minutes** especially on upper chest and outer arms (face and dorsal hands usually resistant) after exposure to **visible light (#1 cause)** or UVA (#2)
  - Type I (abnormal chromophore) versus type II (abnormal circulating IgE antibodies to a normal chromophore)
  - Lesions resolve within 24 hours
  - F > M; middle aged
  - **May occur with erythropoietic protoporphyria or PMLE**
  - Severe attacks rarely: bronchospasm, syncope, and nausea
- Etiology unknown, but felt to be **type I hypersensitivity** reaction (i.e., skin chromophore absorbs a photon → transforms into an endogenous photoallergen → recognized by IgE)
- Treatment: **photoprotection, antihistamines** (high dose, non-sedating), phototherapy, and immunomodulators (IVIG and omalizumab)

Porphyrias with cutaneous findings

- Cornerstone is diligent photoprotection with physical sunblock, avoidance of skin trauma, and good skin care
- Porphyria cutanea tarda
  - **Most common porphyria**
  - Due to ↓ hepatic **uroporphyrinogen decarboxylase (UROD)** activity
    - Three types—I: sporadic (no mutation; defective enzyme only in liver); II: familial (single allele mutation, defect present in all tissue); III: normal UROD gene, but multiple affected family members)
      - Type I **(sporadic/acquired) form most common (80%)**
  - Skin findings include: skin fragility, vesicles, bullae, **erosions, milia, scarring, hyperpigmentation**, and **hypertrichosis** in photodistributed areas (especially dorsal hands/forearms)
    - **Classic photo is hemorrhagic blisters on dorsal hands**
  - Hepatomegaly and cirrhosis may be seen
  - Laboratory: plasma fluorescence emission **peak at 620 nm**; ↑ uroporphyrin/↑ heptaporphyrin/↑ other porphyrins (including pentacarboxyporphyrin and coproporphyrin) in urine; ↑ isocoproporphyrin/↑ heptacarboxylporphyrin III in stool; ↑ ferritin
  - Multifactorial disease with various associations/triggers (**alcohol abuse, estrogen**, iron and **hemochromatosis**, hepatitis C, drugs [barbiturates, griseofulvin, rifampin, sulfonamides], and HIV)
  - Histology: **cell-poor subepidermal bulla** w/ **"festooning" of dermal papillae, "caterpillar bodies"** (pink BMZ material in blister cavity and epidermis)
  - DIF: IgG, IgM, fibrinogen, and C3 **linearly along BMZ and in superficial dermal vessels (see thickened deposits around vessels)**
  - Treatment: **avoid precipitating factors** (alcohol and estrogen), **photoprotection**/sun avoidance, treat underlying conditions (if any), **phlebotomy, low-dose (twice weekly) hydroxychloroquine** (equivalent efficacy to phlebotomy), and deferasirox
- X-linked dominant protoporphyria: presents similarly to erythropoietic protoporphyria (with more frequent liver disease) and is due to a gain of function mutation in the *ALAS2* gene that encodes 5-ALA synthase; ↑↑ plasma protoporphyrin
- Hepatoerythropoietic porphyria
  - **Homozygous** (or compound heterozygous) mutation of **UROD**
  - Laboratory: ↑ zinc protoporphyrin in RBCs and plasma fluorescence emission peak at 620 nm; ↑ uroporphyrin/↑ coproporphyrin in urine and stool
  - Starts in **childhood/infancy (dark urine in diapers often presenting sign)** → scarring, sclerodermoid changes, photosensitivity to point of **mutilation**, hypertrichosis, milia, and vesicles/bullae/erosions/ulcers
  - Treatment: photoprotection, sun, and trauma avoidance
- Variegate porphyria
  - AD mutation in **protoporphyrinogen oxidase** (located in mitochondria)
  - Rare—more common in **South Africa (1:300)** and Chile due to founder effects
  - Skin findings similar to **PCT +/− neurovisceral attacks**
  - Laboratory: plasma fluorescence emission peak = 626 nm only during acute attacks; ↑ ALA/↑ PBG/↑ coproporphyrin in urine **during acute attacks (can be normal at other times so stool testing mandatory)**; ↑ protoporphyrin IX/↑ coproporphyrin III : I ratio (protoporphyrin > coproporphyrin) in stool
  - Treatment: avoid triggers (e.g., porphyrinogenic drugs, alcohol, and hormones); for acute porphyric attacks, supportive care in ICU with sufficient caloric supplementation, IV hemin or heme arginate infusion, and supportive medical treatments (β-blockers, narcotics, phenothiazines, gabapentin, and laxatives);

luteinizing hormone-releasing hormone or growth hormone-releasing hormone agonists, prophylactic hemin and cimetidine may help prevent future attacks

- Hereditary coproporphyria
  - AD mutation in **coproporphyrinogen III oxidase** (located in mitochondria)
  - Acute attacks more common in women than men
  - **Neurovisceral attacks** + skin findings similar to **PCT**
  - Laboratory: ↑ ALA/↑ PBG in urine; ↑ coproporphyrin III:I ratio (coproporphyrin III > protoporphyrin)
  - Treatment is similar to variegate porphyria
- Congenital erythropoietic porphyria (Gunther's disease)
  - AR deficiency of **uroporphyrinogen III synthase (UROS)** → overproduction of uroporphyrin I and coporphyrin I in **erythrocytes, plasma, urine, and feces**
    - Also XLR mutation in *GATA1* (transcription factor that regulates expression of UROS)
  - Cutaneous features: photosensitivity with blistering, scarring, **mutilating cutaneous deformity**, sclerodermatous changes, hypertrichosis, dyschromia, and alopecia (Fig. 3.82)
  - **Red urine noted during** infancy due to ↑ porphyrins (pink/violet stained diapers), which are excited by visible light at **400** to **410 nm (Soret band)** and emit a red fluorescence
  - Splenomegaly, cholelithiasis, and hemolytic anemia
  - Pathologic fractures, osteopenia, vertebral compression, and contractures of fingers
  - Conjunctivitis and corneal scarring
  - **Erythrodontia (red discoloration of teeth)**—fluoresce under Wood's lamp
  - Laboratory: ↑ urinary/erythrocyte uroporphyrin I; ↑ urinary and fecal coproporphyrinogen I and uroporphyrinogen I
  - Treatment: strict photoprotection, hypertransfusions, and iron chelation such as with deferoxamine; splenectomy may be considered, use of **ascorbic acid** and **α-tocopherol** has been advocated; ocular lubricants, and allogeneic bone marrow transplantation
  - Poor prognosis for those with severe hematologic disease, or who present early unless treated with hematopoietic cell transplantation
- Erythropoietic protoporphyria
  - **Most common form of porphyria seen in children**
  - Caused by **ferrochelatase** mutations (resulting in ↑protoporphyrin IX in RBCs and plasma)
    - Autosomal dominant and AR forms
  - Usually becomes symptomatic between 1 and 6 years of age
    - **Adult onset may be linked to myeloproliferative disorders**
  - Manifests as burning/stinging/itching 5–30 minutes post-sunlight exposure (more so blue light than UV light)
  - Pruritic erythematous/edematous plaques that last 1–2 days post-sunlight exposure
  - Hypo-/hyperpigmentation, photoonycholysis
  - Shallow linear pits may develop on the face, along with a papular eruption over the knuckles
  - Hemolytic anemia and mild hypertriglyceridemia may be seen
  - **Cholelithiasis**; protoporphyrin accumulation in the liver may → hepatotoxicity and progressive hepatic dysfunction
  - Laboratory: ↑ free protoporphyrin in plasma, RBCs, and feces, but **NOT** in urine
  - Treatment: strict photoprotection, **oral β-carotene, afamelanotide** may be helpful in some patients, and hypertransfusion/plasmapheresis/exchange transfusion may be helpful in some patients; liver transplantation may be necessary with hepatic failure

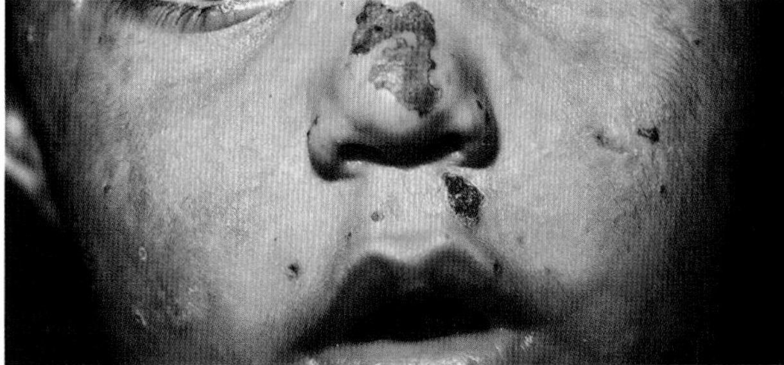

Fig. 3.82 Congenital erythropoietic porphyria. Vesicles, bullae, and crusts on sun-exposed areas. (From Paller AS, Mancini AJ. Photosensitivity and photoreactions. In: *Hurwitz Clinical Pediatric Dermatology: A Textbook of Skin Disorders of Childhood*:448–466.)

Mechanical injuries

- Callus: keratotic broad-based areas secondary to habitual trauma/friction on feet (e.g., poorly fitting footwear, anatomic bone structure of foot, and physical activity)
- Corn (clavus): smaller and more sharply defined than a callus, with two types (hard corn: firm w/ translucent central cores; soft corn: painful papules between toes)
  - DDx: warts do not have translucent central core, have thrombosed capillaries/pinpoint bleeding with paring, and disrupt dermatoglyphics (unlike callus which has normal dermatoglyphics)
  - Paring "core" of corn away provides symptomatic relief
- Chondrodermatitis nodularis helicis chronica
  - Tender pink crusted papules on cartilaginous portions of ear helix and antihelix (upper helix #1 site in men, mid antihelix #1 in women)
  - Seen in middle-aged and elderly patients
  - Histology: acanthosis and parakeratosis with **epidermal disruption/ulceration**; underlying dermis with reparative changes/fibrosis, **necrotic cartilage** (appears pale or pink instead of normal blue-purple color)
  - Treatments: specially designed pillows, surgical methods, nitroglycerin gel/patch, and IL steroid
- Piezogenic papules: herniation of fat through fascia of lateral heels—best seen when patient is standing with weight placed on heel (Fig. 3.83)
- Traumatic auricular hematoma: trauma to external ear → subperichondrial hematoma → **cauliflower ear** over time if not treated (hematoma organizes and develops fibroneocartilage +/− calcification)
  - Usually seen in **wrestlers** as tender induration on upper anterior ear
  - Treatment = hematoma evacuation + recurrence prevention (e.g., via splint)
- Black heel **(talon noir)**: cluster of black pinpoint macules on posterior heel(s)

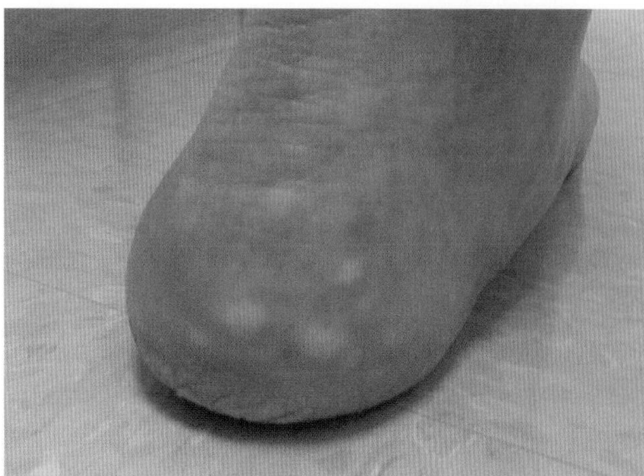

Fig. 3.83 Peizogenic pedal papules. Rubbery white papules that disappear when ankle is lifted. (Courtesy of Christopher Sayed, MD.)

- Athletic trauma → rupture of superficial dermal vessels → hemoglobin in stratum corneum
- Acanthoma fissuratum: firm skin-colored/red plaque on upper postauricular sulcus/upper lateral nose with groove running vertically through center of lesion; **due to poorly fitting eyeglass frames**

3.16 AMYLOIDOSES

- Group of disorders with extracellular amyloid deposition
  - Amyloid = fibril protein (various types including AL and AA) in a **cross-β-pleated sheet**
    - Histology = homogenous, eosinophilic, fissured masses that stain with **Congo red** and have **green birefringence with polarized light**
    - Amyloid also stains positively with **crystal violet, periodic acid–Schiff (PAS), and thioflavin T**
      - AA amyloid (secondary systemic amyloid) loses Congo red affinity after exposure to potassium permanganate
- Divided into systemic primary, secondary, genetic (e.g., autoinflammatory syndromes and MEN2A; see Chapter 4), hemodialysis-associated (β_2-macroglobulin) types, and localized (cutaneous, endocrine, and cerebral) types
  - Localized cutaneous amyloidosis
    - Three forms: **macular** (Fig. 3.84), **lichen, and nodular** (Table 3.30)
    - No great treatments—depending on depth, range from topicals to phototherapy/laser to surgery
    - More common in **Asians, Hispanics, and Middle Easterners**
  - Primary systemic (AL—Ig light chain, usually λ subtype) amyloidosis
    - Can involve several organ systems (worst prognosis if cardiac involvement)
    - Mucocutaneous lesions in one third of patients
    - Due to **underlying plasma cell dyscrasia** (15% with myeloma)
    - Papules/nodules/plaques (waxy, translucent, and/or purpuric), ecchymosis/**pinch purpura** (eyelids, neck, anogenital, and axillae), **macroglossia** (see teeth indentations on sides of tongue), **carpal tunnel syndrome**, and bullous amyloidosis (rare)
      - May have sclerodermoid presentation w/ alopecia and cutis verticis gyrata-like scalp changes
    - Histology: **amyloid throughout dermis and subcutis, in sweat glands, and blood vessel walls**
    - Check urine protein electrophoresis, **SPEP** and immunofixation serum test
    - Poor prognosis, though anti-CD38 antibody (daratumumab) and anti-amyloid antibodies are promising

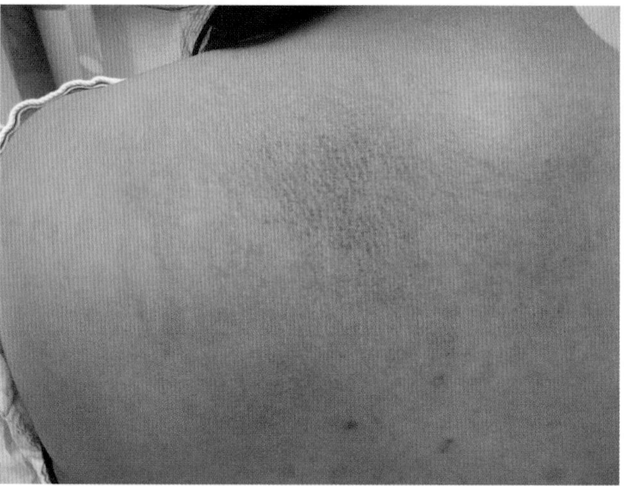

Fig. 3.84 Macular amyloidosis. Rippled hyperpigmented patches. (Courtesy of Christopher Sayed, MD.)

Table 3.30 Cutaneous Amyloidoses

Type	Description	Derivation	Protein	Other Facts	Histology
Macular amyloidosis	Confluent or rippled ("salt-and-pepper"), pruritic, hyperpigmented patches (**interscapular back** most commonly)	Keratinocyte tonofilaments (usually keratin 5)	Aker	Different but overlaps with notalgia paresthetica	Amyloid in papillary dermis
Lichen amyloidosis	Rippled, hyperpigmented, pruritic papules/plaques on extensor surfaces (esp. **shins**)	Keratinocyte tonofilaments (usually keratin 5)	Aker	Seen in **MEN 2A**	Amyloid in papillary dermis
Nodular amyloidosis	Pink to **yellow waxy nodules** and/or plaques	**Ig light chains**	AL	May be a/w **Sjögren's** (25% of nodular amyloidosis cases), scleroderma and rheumatoid arthritis **Progression to systemic amyloidosis in 7%**	Amyloid in reticular dermis, subcutis, **vessel walls**

- Secondary systemic amyloidosis (AA amyloidosis)
  - Sequela of severe **chronic inflammatory diseases** (e.g., ankylosing spondylitis, tuberculosis, JIA, dystrophic EB, scleroderma, and autoinflammatory syndromes like Muckle-Wells)
  - **SAA (serum amyloid A)** protein is processed to AA amyloid in tissues
  - **Rare skin deposition**; usually involves kidneys, liver, spleen, adrenals, and heart
    - Of note, **amyloidosis in hemodialysis** patients has **Aβ_2M amyloid (β_2-microglobulin)**—usually no skin involvement, but may see subcutaneous nodules on lower back

3.17 NEURODERMATOLOGY AND PSYCHODERMATOLOGY

Pruritus

- Divided into three groups: (1) itch of inflamed skin, (2) non-inflamed skin, and (3) with scratch-induced lesions (e.g., lichen simplex chronicus or prurigo nodules)
- Mediators of pruritus
  - C and **A-δ** nerve fibers in superficial skin produce **itch** sensation
    - Histaminergic C fibers respond to **histamine**, non-histaminergic to **cowhage**, via a protease called mucunain; relevance of non-histaminergic fibers in disease is unclear, but may explain lack of response to antihistamines in some forms of pruritus
  - **Histamine** produces pruritus via H1 receptor, though H4 receptor is likely also important in eosinophil chemotaxis and itch signaling
  - Other pruritogens: trypsin, serotonin, papain, bradykinin, substance P, VIP, kallikrein
  - Prostaglandins can exaggerate pruritus
  - **Opiates** can produce pruritus via central and peripheral μ-opioid receptor agonism

Internal causes of pruritus

- CKD to Chronic kidney disease
  - Localized or generalized **intractable, severe**, paroxysmal pruritus in 20%–80% of patients w/ chronic renal insufficiency; **worst at night and 2 days post-hemodialysis**
  - Treatments: **NB-UVB**, μ-opioid antagonists (e.g. naltrexone), κ-opioid agonists, emollients, gabapentin, pregabalin; renal transplant is curative
- Biliary pruritus
  - Patients w/ **obstructive hepatitides, including carcinoma**
  - Lipophosphatidic acid and autotaxin are potential mediators correlating to itch intensity
  - Generalized migratory pruritus not relieved by scratching; worse on hands, feet, and body areas covered by clothes and at night
  - Treat underlying hepatic disorder; possible improvement w/ **cholestyramine**, **ursodiol**, rifampin, naltrexone, naloxone, and sertraline
- Polycythemia vera
  - 30%–50% of PCV patients have pruritus, **usually aquagenic** (severe pruritus in absence of skin changes, within minutes of water contact)
  - Pathogenesis: platelet aggregation causing serotonin and histamine release; mutation in JAK2 → constitutive activation and agonist hypersensitivity in basophils
  - Treatment: **ASA**, NB-UVB, PUVA, **JAK-inhibition (e.g., ruxolitinib)** and oral antihistamines for pruritus; treatment of PCV
- Malignancy
  - Persistent, unexplained, intractable pruritus without primary skin lesion
  - a/w Hematologic (Hodgkin > non-Hodgkin; PCV > essential thrombocythemia; CLL) or biliary malignancies
  - In Hodgkin disease, **intense pruritus linked to worse prognosis** and may be sign of recurrence
  - Treatment: treat underlying malignancy; SSRIs, TCS, mirtazapine, thalidomide
- Endocrine
  - Severe generalized pruritus **(hyperthyroidism)**, generalized pruritus, or localized genital/perianal pruritus in **diabetes mellitus**
    - Localized pruritus of genitals is a/w poor glycemic control in women
  - Treatment: correct hyperthyroid state, improve glycemic control

Pruritus ani

- Pruritus of anus and perianal skin (1%–5% population); **male > female**
- Skin appearance: normal to severely irritated (erythema/crusting/lichenification, erosions/ulcerations)
- Pathogenesis:
  - **Primary** pruritus ani: pruritus in absence of cutaneous, anorectal, or colonic disorder; may be due to dietary factors, poor personal hygiene, or psychologic disorders
  - **Secondary** pruritus ani: due to irritation from stool or hemorrhoids, primary cutaneous disorders, infectious or infestations, previous radiation therapy, neoplasms, or contact allergy
- Treatment: reduce irritation w/ sitz baths, cool compresses, meticulous hygiene, mild topical steroids or TCIs, and treatment of underlying disorder

Pruritus scroti/vulvae

- Acute or chronic pruritus of scrotum or vulva; worse at night; **lichenification** secondary to repeated rubbing/scratching
- Pathogenesis—acute: infections, ACD or ICD; chronic: secondary to dermatoses, malignancy, atrophic vulvovaginitis, lumbosacral radiculopathy, irritation, or psychogenic (1%–7% patients)
- Treatment: specific to underlying etiology

Scalp pruritus

- May be **primary** (lacks skin lesions; a/w anxiety and depression) or **secondary** to dermatoses (psoriasis, seborrheic dermatitis, and folliculitis)
- Treatment: emollients and topical steroids; tar or salicylic acid shampoos, and low-dose doxepin

Aquagenic pruritus and aquadynia

- Severe **pruritus** or **burning pain after water contact**, irrespective of water temperature; within 30 minutes of contact with **no visible skin changes**; lasts up to 2 hours; spares head, palms/soles, and mucosae
- Pathogenesis: usually secondary to systemic disease (e.g., **polycythemia vera**) or other skin disorder
- Treatment: alkalization of bath water to pH 8 with baking soda, oral antihistamines, phototherapy, and capsaicin; clonidine and propranolol for aquadynia

Drug-induced pruritus

- Chronic pruritus with or without skin eruption
- Common culprits: **opioids** (secondary to action on various opioid receptors in skin and centrally), cocaine (formication), chloroquine, **CTLA-4 or PD-1 inhibitors, BRAF inhibitors, EGFR inhibitors**, hydroxyethyl starch (volume expander injected into skin → direct stimulation of cutaneous nerves)
- Rx: discontinue inciting medication

Lichen simplex chronicus

- Well-defined plaques w/ **lichenification**, hyperpigmentation, and varying erythema that are solitary or multiple and usually on **posterior neck**, occipital scalp, anogenital skin, **shins/ankles**, dorsal hands and feet, and forearms of older adults with xerosis, atopy, stasis, psychologic conditions, or pruritus secondary to systemic disease
  - Broader, thinner lesions than prurigo nodularis but w/ same **itch-scratch cycle** perpetuating the condition
- Rx: treat underlying systemic or psychiatric illness if present; **avoidance of scratching/rubbing**; topical/intralesional agents (CS and calcineurin inhibitors); topical antipruritics (menthol and pramoxine), antihistamines, and behavioral therapy

Prurigo nodularis

- Multiple pruritic, **dome-shaped**, firm, hyperpigmented papulonodules that may have central scale/crust/erosion/ulceration distributed symmetrically on **extensor extremities** with sparing of mid-back **("butterfly sign")**
- Caused by chronic repetitive scratching/picking secondary to pruritic systemic (diabetes, HIV, hepatitis B/C, malignancy, liver/renal/thyroid dysfunction) or dermatologic disease or psychologic condition
- Most commonly in **middle-aged adults** with underlying dermatologic/psychiatric disorder and occasionally in children with atopy
- Rx: topical capsaicin, topical lidocaine/ketamine/amitriptyline, TCIs, intralesional/topical steroids, calcipotriene, cryotherapy, **phototherapy**, **gabapentin**/pregabalin, **SSRIs/tricyclic antidepressants (TCAs)**, **doxepin**, aprepitant, MTX, thalidomide/lenalidomide, naltrexone, **dupilumab** (FDA approved), AZA, cyclosporine

Cutaneous manifestations of psychiatric illness or self-induction

Delusions of parasitosis

- Somatic delusional disorder; average onset 50 to 60 years; close contacts may share delusion
- Must be: (1) present > 1 month; (2) in absence of other delusions or bizarre behavior; (3) not in context of substance abuse or other psychiatric disorder
- Younger patients: low socioeconomic status w/ history of substance abuse
- Older patients: higher socioeconomic status
- **Fixed false belief** that they are infested w/ parasites in absence of clinical findings; may describe sensations of biting, crawling, or stinging; **"matchbox sign"** (patient brings in bits of skin and other materials he/she believes are parasites)
- Rx: **first step is building trust and rapport with patient**; **pimozide** is the classic treatment of choice (**QT prolongation** on EKG, extrapyramidal side effects, and drug-drug interactions); newer atypical antipsychotics (e.g., risperidone, aripiprazole, olanzapine) are effective w/ ↓ side effects

Excoriation disorder (Neurotic excoriations)

- Excoriations in different stages of evolution with **geographic/angulated shapes**; favors extensor arms, scalp, face, upper back, and buttocks
- Caused by conscious, repetitive, and uncontrollable picking/scratching; 3:1 female:male
  - Patients **admit to picking**, but cannot control behaviors; strong association with body dysmorphic disorder
- Rx: **doxepin (ToC)**, **N-acetylcysteine**, SSRIs, habit-reversal training, cognitive behavioral therapy, topical antipruritics, and wound care

Factitial dermatitis/dermatitis artefacta

- Patients self-inflict cutaneous lesions and **deny personal involvement**
- Geographic excoriations/erosions/ulcers within reach of hands
- Occurs in **adolescents/young adult females** who may work in healthcare fields or have personality disorders
- Rx: supportive wound and psychiatric care (psychotherapy); antidepressant, antianxiety, or antipsychotic medications may be necessary

Gardner-Diamond syndrome

- Patients traumatically induce lesions by various methods, causing sudden onset of **painful**, **swollen ecchymosis at sites of trauma**; affects any anatomic site, variable size, resolves within 2 weeks, and recurs
- Most often in women with underlying psychologic conditions
- Rx: very difficult, but antidepressants and psychotherapy can be beneficial

Trichotillomania (discussed in Alopecia section)

Body dysmorphic disorder

- Patients are **preoccupied by appearance** of their bodies and start obsessively checking in mirrors for perceived imperfections and may have **repeated cosmetic procedures**
- Typical areas of concern include face, hair, breasts, and genitalia
- Rx: **cognitive behavioral therapy (first line)** with high-dose SSRIs for increased benefit

Cupping/coining

- **Cupping**: method of traditional Chinese medicine used to stimulate acupuncture points by placing burning cotton in a jar that is then placed on skin → creates a vacuum → results in **circular areas** of erythema and/or ecchymosis after removal
- **Coining (cao gio)**: technique used in Southeast Asia to improve circulation; involves rubbing oiled skin with a coin or spoon in symmetric, linear patterns that creates **patterned/linear ecchymosis**

Other neurocutaneous dermatoses

Scalp dysesthesia/burning scalp syndrome

- Diffuse burning pain/pruritus/numbness/tingling of scalp without primary skin lesions, usually found in **depressed/ anxious middle-aged to elderly women**; can be associated with underlying neurologic and psychiatric disorders
  - Secondary causes: seborrheic dermatitis, LPP, contact dermatitis, folliculitis, dermatomyositis, and DLE
- Scalp is most frequent body region affected in correlation w/ stressful life events
- Rx: gabapentin, TCSs, and topical capsaicin

Burning mouth syndrome

- **Burning mucosal pain** of the **anterior two-thirds** of tongue, palate, and lower lip bilaterally (sparing buccal mucosa and floor of mouth) without primary lesions
- Type I is better in morning and worsens through day; type 2 is constant; type 3 has sporadic periods of activity and remission
- Middle-aged to elderly adult females primarily
- **Secondary causes must be excluded**: oral malignancy, xerostomia, contact dermatitis, medications, nutritional deficiencies, endocrinopathies, and psychiatric conditions
- Rx: antidepressants, benzodiazepines, doxepin, gabapentin, topical capsaicin/clonazepam, and "magic mouthwash" combinations

Brachioradial pruritus

- Chronic intermittent pruritus or burning pain on **dorsolateral forearms/elbows** (overlying the location of bradioradialis muscle; distribution of radial dorsal antebrachial cutaneous nerve)
- May be secondary to **photosensitivity** or **cervical nerve root impingement** (many patients have prior back injuries)
- Rx: **treat cervical spinal impingement** if present, sun protection, topical capsaicin/pramoxine/amitriptyline/ ketamine, gabapentin, physical therapy, and acupuncture

Notalgia paresthetica

- Adults w/ focal, intense **pruritus**, pain, paresthesias, hyperesthesias of upper back (most commonly near **medial scapular borders at T2–T6) +/– hyperpigmented patches** secondary to chronic rubbing
- Etiology likely sensory neuropathy; up to 60% have **spinal impingement**
- In children, consider MEN2A syndrome
- Rx: topical capsaicin, topical CS or anesthetics, gabapentin, acupuncture, paravertebral block, and local botulinum toxin injection

Meralgia paresthetica

- Localized numbness, burning, tingling, allodynia, or pruritus of **anterolateral thigh** secondary to **pressure on lateral femoral cutaneous nerve** as it passes under the inguinal ligament, often seen in middle-aged obese males
- A/w **Obesity**, pregnancy, prolonged sitting, **tight clothing**, heavy wallets in pant pockets
- Rx: manage eliciting factors, focal nerve block, surgical decompression, topical capsaicin/CS/anesthetics, gabapentin, and acupuncture

Complex regional pain syndrome/reflex sympathetic dystrophy

- Clinical presentation dependent on stage of disease
- Most common symptom is burning pain of upper limbs that is aggravated by movement or friction; affected **skin may become shiny**, **cold**, **atrophic**
- Five major components: pain, edema, autonomic dysregulation (LR, hypertrichosis, cyanosis, hyperhidrosis), alterations in motor function, and **dystrophic changes (can also affect nails)**
- Damage to regional peripheral pain receptors → complicated signal cascade that eventually amplifies the pain response of CNS → clinical manifestations
- Rx: directed toward interrupting autonomic nervous system; often ineffective

Trigeminal trophic syndrome

- Self-induced lesions of **central face** triggered by paresthesias/dysesthesias secondary to impingement or **damage of sensory portion of trigeminal nerve**
- May present as crusts or **ulcers of nasal ala** that can extend to cheek or upper lip w/ characteristic **sparing of nasal tip**
- Frequently occurs after treatment for trigeminal neuralgia w/ ablation of **Gasserian ganglion**; can also arise secondary to infection, stroke, and CNS tumors
- Rx: most successful is surgical repair with innervated skin flaps +/– various psychiatric medications, patient education, and protective barriers worn at night

Familial dysautonomia/Riley-Day syndrome

- Neurodegenerative disease → various cutaneous and systemic findings: **defective lacrimation**, **absence of tongue papillae** with taste disturbance and ↑ **salivation**, impaired regulation of temperature and blood pressure, ↓ pain sensation, **absent tendon reflexes**, **hyperhidrosis**, **transient erythema** of trunk, vomiting crises, and **acrocyanosis of hands**
- Pathogenesis: AR inheritance of ***IKBKAP*** (locus 9q31)
- Absence of PGP 9.5 staining indicates lack of sweat gland, blood vessel, and arrector pili nerves
- Rx: supportive; 50% mortality by 30 yo due to respiratory issues

Auriculotemporal nerve syndrome (Frey syndrome)

- Most common **complication of parotidectomy**
  - Nerve damage may also be caused by parotitis, parotid abscess, cerebellopontine tumors, or surgery
- Due to aberrant regeneration of parasympathetic fibers of auriculotemporal nerve after injury
- Most common cause in **children** is nerve damage from **forceps delivery** (presents after starting solid foods)
- P/w unilateral (> bilateral) flushing and/or sweating in the distribution of the auriculotemporal nerve
- Usually **stimulated by ingestion of certain foods**, especially sour or spicy foods; less commonly triggered by olfactory or tactile stimuli
- Changes are typically transient; botulinum toxin has been employed

3.18 PALMOPLANTAR KERATODERMAS

- Hyperkeratosis of palmar and/or plantar skin
- **Inherited PPKs** (see Chapter 4)
- **Acquired PPKs**
  - Keratoderma climactericum
    - Hyperkeratosis of pressure points on **heels in women > 45 yo** (or younger women after oophorectomy)
    - Can be tender
  - Aquagenic PPK
    - Thick clear-white pebble-like palmar eruption **after water immersion** (quick onset)
    - Swelling and pain
    - F > M; usually starts during teenage years; **50% of cystic fibrosis patients and 10%–25% of heterozygous carriers**
    - Aluminum chloride, botulinum toxin can help
  - Keratolysis exfoliativa
    - Spots of exfoliation on palms and soles that spread centrifugally
    - Annular collarette of scale around exfoliation with no erythema
    - Likely represents a **mild form of eczema**
  - Punctate keratosis of the palmar creases
    - 1 to 5 mm small plugs in creases of palms/fingers primarily in **African American patients**
  - Punctate PPK (spiny keratoderma)
    - Typically < 1 mm and usually multiple lesions
    - More common in Blacks and men; may be autosomal dominant
  - Circumscribed palmar/plantar hypokeratosis
    - Well-defined pink, **circular depression** on palm (especially thenar and hypothenar) or sole (especially medial)
    - F > M; middle-aged and older; loss of keratin 9 expression reported
    - Histology: **focally decreased** stratum corneum/granulosum, underlying angioplasia
- PPK associations:
  - Malignancy:
    - PPK can occur in various carcinomas (e.g., lung and breast)
    - PPK can also occur in genetic cancer-causing disorders (e.g., Huriez syndrome [acral SCC], **Howel-Evans syndrome [esophageal carcinoma]**)
    - **Arsenical keratoses** = focal keratotic papules on **palms/soles** → enlarge, ↑ number, spread → ulceration and **SCC**
      - Arise > 10 years after arsenic ingestion
  - Hypothyroidism: typically with myxedema of hypothyroidism; resolves with therapy
- Treatment: various keratolytic agents (e.g., ammonium lactate, urea); CO_2 laser

3.19 NUTRITIONAL DISORDERS IN DERMATOLOGY

- Can occur for a variety of reasons (inadequate intake, concurrent illnesses, problems with metabolism)
- Protein-energy malnutrition
  - Kwashiorkor: ↓ **protein intake** for at least several weeks (e.g., primarily rice diet)
    - Cutaneous findings:
      - **Dyschromia**
      - Hypopigmentation following trauma
      - Desquamation/erosion of skin (**"peeling/flaky paint"** appearance; most common finding on exam)
      - Bands of light and dark hair discoloration (**"flag sign"**) and sparse/dry/brittle hair with red tinge
      - Compromised wound healing with ulceration and erosion
      - **Edema/anasarca**
      - Secondary infections
  - Marasmus: ↓ **energy/calorie intake** for months to years
    - Cutaneous findings:
      - **Thin, dry, lax, pale, and wrinkled/loose skin**
      - Lanugo-like hair
      - Purpura
      - Follicular hyperkeratosis
      - Impaired hair and nail growth
      - Emaciated (**"monkey facies"—↓ buccal fat pads**)
- Essential fatty acid deficiency:
  - Secondary to malnutrition; other issues → fat malabsorption, parenteral nutrition w/o lipids, and **nephrotic syndrome**
  - Cutaneous findings: dry, rough, and scaly skin; erosions in flexures and rash similar to biotin and zinc

Table 3.31 Vitamin Deficiencies and Excesses

Vitamin	Cutaneous Findings: Deficiency	Cutaneous Findings: Excess	Interesting Facts
Vitamin A	**Phrynoderma (keratotic follicular papules resembling toadskin)**, night blindness, xerophthalmia	Desquamation, xerosis, cheilitis, epistaxis, dermatitis, alopecia **(think of SEs with systemic retinoids)**	
Beta-carotene		**Carotenemia** and carotenoderma (yellow discoloration best seen on **palms/soles, central face, sebaceous areas**)	Can see in **diabetes**, **nephrotic syndrome**, **and hypothyroidism** **From carrots, squash**
Biotin	Alopecia, **rash similar to zinc deficiency** (e.g., periorificial dermatitis)		Infantile type due to biotinidase defect; neonatal type due to holocarboxylase synthetase defects Acquired biotin deficiency: (1) diet rich in raw egg whites, which contain **avidin** (glycoprotein that complexes with and inactivates biotin), (2) parenteral nutrition lacking biotin, and (3) certain anticonvulsants (e.g., phenytoin, carbamazepine)
Selenium	**Hypopigmentation** of skin/hair, leukonychia, xerosis	Dermatitis, alopecia, abnormal nails	
Vitamin B1 (thiamine)	Glossitis, edema. "Wet" beriberi associated with edema and skin breakdown		
Vitamin B2 (riboflavin)	**Oral-ocular-genital syndrome** (cheilitis, angular stomatitis, seborrheic dermatitis-like rash, tongue atrophy/glossitis, genital and perinasal dermatitis)		Can be seen in breastfed infants of mothers who are deficient in riboflavin
Vitamin B3 (niacin)	**Pellagra** "**D**ermatosis" = **Casal's necklace** (upper chest/neck), **cheilitis/glossitis**, **photosensitivity** (esp. dorsal hands), perineal rash Plus other three Ds: **d**iarrhea, **d**ementia, and **d**eath	**Flushing**, pruritus, acanthosis nigricans	Causes of deficiency: **Hartnup** dz, alcoholism, **carcinoid** syndrome, **isoniazid**, 5-FU, **azathioprine**, anorexia, malabsorption syndromes
Vitamin B6 (pyridoxine)	**Periorificial seborrheic dermatitis-like** rash, angular **cheilitis**, intertrigo, atrophic **glossitis**	Photosensitivity	Highest risk of deficiency in **alcoholics**
Vitamin B9 (folic acid)	Hyperpigmentation (esp. sun-exposed sites) glossitis, angular cheilitis, hair depigmentation (cannities)		Goat milk diet can predispose
Vitamin B12 (cobalamin)	Hyperpigmentation (esp. hands, nails, face, palmar creases, intertriginous regions; oral sites can be involved), glossitis		Vitamin B12 deficiency may → **neurologic sequelae**, (not typically seen in folic acid deficiency) Malabsorptive states are a common cause
Vitamin C (ascorbic acid)	**Scurvy** (Fig. 3.85): corkscrew hairs, perifollicular hemorrhage/ hyperkeratosis (first cutaneous sign), hemorrhagic gingivitis, splinter hemorrhage of nails		Most manifestations due to impaired collagen synthesis
Vitamin D	**Alopecia**	Hypervitaminosis D	
Vitamin E		**Petechiae, ecchymoses**	
Vitamin K	**Purpura, ecchymoses, hemorrhage**		Antibiotics decrease **gut bacteria responsible for vitamin K production** → caution in pts on warfarin, as INR may become dangerously high
Zinc	**Perioral**, **perianal**, **and acral erosions**; erythema and crust **Alopecia**, paronychia, onychodystrophy, stomatitis, secondary infections **Classic triad** (dermatitis, diarrhea, depression) **seen in only 20%**		Deficiency can be inherited in AR pattern (**acrodermatitis enteropathica**, mutation in ***SLC39A4*** gene) Risk factors for acquired deficiency = **alcoholism**, vegan diets, anorexia, **cystic fibrosis**, HIV, certain drugs (e.g., penicillamine) See **low alkaline phosphatase** serum levels in zinc deficiency

deficiencies; alopecia w/ light-colored hair; secondary infections
- ↓ **Linoleic, linolenic, and arachidonic acids**
- ↑ Palmitoleic, oleic, and 5,8,11-eicosatrienoic acids

• Vitamin excesses and deficiencies
- See Table 3.31 for specific vitamin abnormalities
- Pathology (pellagra, acrodermatitis enteropathica, acquired zinc deficiency, and glucagonoma): **pallor of top one third of epidermis** +/− psoriasiform epidermal changes

• Anorexia nervosa: may see **lanugo-like hair**, carotenoderma, follicular hyperkeratosis, alopecia

• Bulimia nervosa: may see **calluses/scars on knuckles/** dorsal hands (**Russell's sign**), enlarged salivary glands, and **erosion of tooth enamel**

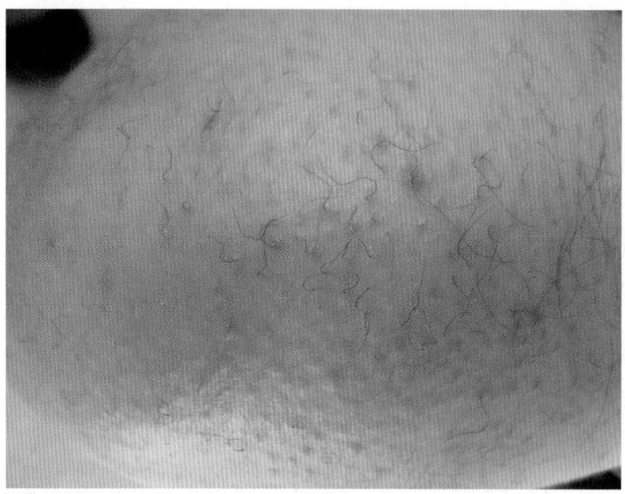

Fig. 3.85 Scurvy. Corkscrew hairs and perifollicular peteichiae on the knee. (Courtesy of Christopher Sayed, MD.)

3.20 DEPOSITIONAL AND CALCIFICATION DISORDERS NOT DISCUSSED ELSEWHERE (TABLE 3.32)

3.21 ULCERS (TABLE 3.33)

- Wound with loss of epidermis + dermis
- Various causes and types—important to look for clinical clues and order appropriate laboratory workup

3.22 VASCULITIDES, VASCULOPATHIES, AND OTHER VASCULAR DISORDERS

- Vasculitides are divided primarily according to vessel size that is targeted (Table 3.34)

Table 3.32 Depositional and Calcification Disorders Not Previously Discussed

Disorder	Histopathology	Clinical Findings	Pearls
Gout	Amorphous material with **needle-like clefts** in dermis Giant cells around material Negative birefringence	**Monosodium urate** crystals in tissue → gouty arthritis **(first MTP joint most common)**, nephrolithiasis/renal impairment, and gouty tophi (firm white/yellow subcutaneous nodules) M > F, middle-aged Risk factors: **obesity**, **alcohol**, renal issues, diuretic meds **Gouty tophi most common on ear helix** and skin overlying small joints **(fingers, toes)**; <10% pts get them, usually >10 years of disease	**Ethanol** based is best preservative (Carnoy's fluid) Diagnosis classically made by aspirating inflamed joint in acute arthritis → urate crystals in joint fluid Crystals stain black with 20% silver nitrate Treatment options: NSAIDs, **cochicine**, **allopurinol**, **febuxostat** DDx is pseudogout (deposition of **calcium pyrophosphate** crystals in joint and soft tissue) which can → tophaceous pseudogout
Pseudogout	**Calcium pyrophosphate** dehydrate crystals are positively birefringent, rhomboidal	Pseudogouty tophi over joints, esp. knee. Clinically indistinguishable from gout	Typically related to osteoarthritis, sometimes hemochromatosis or hyper-PTH
Colloid milium	Amorphous **homogenous pink nodular material** in superficial dermis +/– clefts Grenz zone **Solar elastosis** seen deep to nodules in adult form	<u>Adult type</u> (most common): pts usually middle-aged or older and **severely photodamaged**, M > F; multiple translucent yellowish papules in photo-exposed areas <u>Other types</u>: **juvenile**, pigmented (in setting of hydroquinone), nodular colloid degeneration	**Stains like amyloid** (congo red, thioflavin T, and crystal violet positive) PAS+
Dystrophic calcification	See appropriate sections	<u>AICTD</u>: most commonly seen in **CREST** and **childhood DM**; in DM, can → calcinosis universalis (severe form) <u>Panniculitis</u>: lobular, particularly **pancreatic panniculitis**, subcutaneous fat necrosis of the newborn, lupus profundus <u>Genodermatoses</u>: **PXE** (calcification of dermal elastic fibers), Ehlers-Danlos syndrome, PCT (longstanding) <u>Infections</u>: *Onchocera volvulus* and *Taenia solium* <u>Neoplasms</u>: **pilomatricomas (75%)**, BCCs, epidermal/pilar cysts	
Metastatic calcification	**Calciphylaxis**: perivascular and intravascular calcium in vessels of SQ fat → **thrombotic vasculopathy**	<u>Clinical</u>: violaceous reticulated patches (livedo) + subcutaneous nodules → **painful** necrotic, purpuric ulcers/bullae; F > M; RFs: obesity, DM2, poor nutrition; **high mortality**; **check protein C activity/function** <u>Histology</u>: **thrombotic vasculopathy** + **vascular calcification** + necrosis of skin/soft tissue <u>Treatment</u>: low calcium **dialysis**, phosphate binders, bisphosphonates, cinacalcet, **STS**, TPA, anticoagulation (i.e., heparin, tinzaparin; **DO NOT give warfarin**), vitamin K, parathyroidectomy, surgical debridement, management of tissue infections	**Chronic renal failure**: #1 cause of metastatic calcification; due to ↓ PO4-clearance, ↓ 1-α hydroxylation D3, ↓ Ca++ absorption, 2° hyperparathyroidism Other causes of metastatic calcification: chronic steroid use, liver disease, diabetes, **milk-alkali syndrome** and **hypervitaminosis D**

Table 3.32 Depositional and Calcification Disorders Not Previously Discussed—cont'd

Disorder	Histopathology	Clinical Findings	Pearls
Idiopathic calcification	Idiopathic calcified nodules of the **scrotum**: may see calcification in the setting of an epidermal cyst within scrotal skin	**Idiopathic calcified nodules of the scrotum**: multiple white small nodules of scrotum **Tumor calcinosis**: large painful calcium-phosphate subcutaneous nodules around joints → ulceration	Other causes include milia-like calcinosis (typically on dorsal hands/face in Down syndrome) and subepidermal calcified nodule
Osteoma cutis	Bone formation within dermis/SQ	Genetic causes: fibrodysplasia ossificans progressiva (process is endochondral; autosomal dominant; mutation in ACVR1 gene which encodes activin A receptor; may have malformed great toes), progressive osseous heteroplasia, plate-like osteoma cutis, **Albright hereditary osteodystrophy** **Miliary osteomas of the face**: white-skin colored tiny papules on faces of adults, common; **a/w prior acne and tetracyclines**	

MTP, *metatarsophalangeal joint;* PTH, *parathyroid hormone;* PAS, *periodic acid-Schiff;* AICTD, *autoimmune connective tissue disease;* DM, *dermatomyositis;* PXE, *psuedoxanthoma elasticum;* PCT, *porphyria cutanea tarda;* RFs, *risk factors;* DM2, *type 2 diabetes; STS, sodium thiosulfate;* TPA, *tissue plasminogen activator.*

Table 3.33 Key Features of Cutaneous Ulcers

Ulcer Types	Clinical Presentation	Useful Pearls
Venous	Irregular borders with shallow yellow fibrinous base Classically above **medial malleolus** (2° to Cockett's perforating veins) Usually in background of **venous stasis** changes (brown hemosiderin deposits + pinpoint purpura, LDS, edema) and varicosities	RFs: ↑ age, F > M, obesity, pregnancy, prolonged standing, ↑ height Due to venous HTN and insufficiency Duplex ultrasound +/– venography may help characterize dz Treatment: moisture/occlusion, debridement, dressings (create moist environment but absorb excess exudate), treatment of infection, compression (do NOT use in arterial insufficiency pts), negative pressure therapy, manual lymphatic drainage, pentoxifylline, ASA, G-CSF
Lymphedema	Classically starts as pitting edema of dorsal foot → moves to leg Skin changes: induration, ulceration, 2° infection **Elephantiasis nostras verrucosa**: chronic lymphedema of feet/legs → fibrosis of dermis and subcutis → verrucous, hyperkeratotic, cobblestone-like, papillomatous appearance	Due to ↑ interstitial lymph fluid due to poor drainage 1° (e.g., Nonne-Milroy dz, Meige dz, lymphedema tarda) vs. 2° (malignancy, radiation, LN dissection, CVI, recurrent cellulitis, obesity, filiriasis)
Arterial (peripheral arterial dz)	Painful ulcer w/ well-defined borders with round, **"punched out"** dry, necrotic base Classically at pressure points (e.g., **lateral malleolus**, first and fifth metatarsal heads) Usually in background of **atrophic skin w/ ↓ hair** Claudication	↓ **Pedal pulses** w/ ↑ capillary refill time and pallor w/ elevation **Diagnosis via ABIs**; may need CTA, MRA, invasive digital subtraction angiography Due to lack of blood perfusion (peripheral arterial dz) RFs: tobacco, DM2, HTN, hyperhomocysteinemia, HLD Do NOT use VAC treatment or sharp debridement May need surgical reconstruction and/or **angioplasty**
Diabetic/neuropathic ("mal perforans")	"Punched out," smelly, **moist base with callused borders** Classically at **pressure points** (e.g., metatarsal heads, great toes, heels) Usually in setting of **peripheral neuropathy** +/– foot deformity (e.g., hammer toes)	May have underlying **osteomyelitis** (MRI best for dx) which may require bone bx/cx 15% of DM2 pts with foot ulcer → lower extremity amputation Treatments: **off-loading measures** (e.g., total contact casting, therapeutic shoes), wound healing measures (e.g., debridement), treatment of infection, hyperbaric oxygen, negative pressure therapy, exogenous growth factors (e.g., becaplermin gel), skin substitutes, dressings, G-CSF
Decubitus/pressure	Ulcer due to prolonged pressure from ↓ ambulation/mobility → pressure to soft tissue from bony prominence and external surface Common sites: **sacrum**, heel, ischial tuberosities, greater trochanters, malleoli (lateral > medial) **Four stages**: I) non-blanchable erythema; II) skin loss of epidermis +/– dermis = erosion/shallow ulcer; III) skin loss + subcutis damage, but not fascia; and IV) tissue necrosis to muscle, bone or supporting structures	RFs: immobility, sensory deficit, poor nutrition, circulation issues Treatment: relief of pressure (e.g., position changes, support surfaces like foam wedges), good wound care Stage IV ulcers will likely need surgical treatment
Diffuse dermal angiomatosis	Violaceous/erythematous patches/plaques with ulceration on legs, **breasts**, forearms	Strongly a/w **vascular atherosclerosis** and **smoking** May need surgical intervention Isotretinoin recently described as treatment option
Arteriosclerotic ulcer of Martorell	**Painful** red blister → blue purpuric lesion → ulceration; ulceration is preceded by pigmented pretibial patches Anterior or medial **lower leg** Usually superficial ulcer w/ necrotic base and violaceous-erythematous edges, but may be deep and enlarging	Women 50–70 yo Poor healing and slow wound healing Typically a/w **HTN** Histology: impressive thickening of arteriole media and intima, +/– hyalinosis/**calcinosis of media**, +/– periarteritis, +/– endarterial proliferation Treatment involves multiple modalities (e.g., VAC, HTN control, compression stockings)

Continued

Table 3.33 Key Features of Cutaneous Ulcers—cont'd

Ulcer Types	Clinical Presentation	Useful Pearls
Hematologic causes		Anemia, particularly hemoglobinopathies Hematologic malignancy associations: pyoderma gangrenosum, vasculitis, type I cryoglobulinemia Clotting abnormalities: factor V Leiden deficiency, protein C/S deficiency, antithrombin III deficiency, prothrombin G20210A mutation, APLS, hyperhomocysteinemia, plasminogen activator inhibitor deficiency/increase
Inflammatory		Consider vasculitis, PAN, RA/Felty's syndrome, pyoderma gangrenosum and necrobiosis lipoidica, Behçet's—lower extremity common site in aforementioned Ulcerative LP, ulcerative sarcoid, livedoid vasculopathy Consider panniculitides (pancreatic, α_1-antitrypsin, erythema induratum)
Infectious		When suspected, culture broadly to r/o bacterial (e.g., anthrax), mycobacterial, viral (esp. **HSV**), fungal, parasitic (acanthamoeba, amebiasis)
Neoplastic		Almost all cutaneous malignancies can → ulcer (**SCC** most common, but also BCC, lymphomas, Kaposi's, angiosarcoma) **SCC can develop in chronic ulcers, scars, sites of chronic inflammation** (e.g., in hidradenitis suppurative or LS&A)
Metabolic		Ulcers can occur in depositional disorders (e.g., calcinosis cutis, gout) adjacent to joints, and higher fat areas in disorders like calciphylaxis
Genetic		Ulcers can be seen in **Adams-Oliver syndrome** (from aplasia cutis on scalp), **prolidase deficiency** (leg ulcers), familial tumor calcinosis, Werner syndrome (leg ulcers), Flynn-Aird syndrome, **Klinefelter syndrome** (leg ulcers)
Drugs		**Hydroxyurea** is a common culprit (malleolus, tibial crest; painful) Other culprits are **interferon** (injection sites), **MTX in psoriasis pts**, anticoagulants (warfarin [2° to acquired protein C deficiency] and heparin necrosis [2° to HIT])
Other		Dermatitis artefacta, **illegal drug use**, burns, frostbite, radiation-induced, chemical etching

RFs, *risk factors;* HTN, *hypertension;* ASA, *aspirin;* LDS, *lipodermatosclerosus;* LN, *lymph node;* CVI, *chronic venous insufficiency;* ABIs, *ankle-brachial index;* CTA, *computed tomography angiogram;* MRA, *magnetic resinance angiogram;* DM2, *type 2 diabetes;* HLD, *hyperlipidemia;* VAC, *vacuum-assisted closure;* MRI, *magnetic resonance imaging;* IV, *intravenous;* APLS, *antiphospholipid syndrome;* PAN, *polyarteritis nodosa;* RA, *rheumatoid arthritis;* LP, *lichen planus;* SCC, *squamous cell carcinoma;* HSV, *herpes simplex virus;* LS&A, *lichen sclerosus et atrophica;* MTX, *methotrexate;* HIT, *heparin-induced thrombocytopenia.*

Cutaneous small vessel vasculitis

Epidemiology

- Adults > children

Pathophysiology

- **Immune complex deposition** in **post-capillary venules** → activates complement → neutrophilic inflammatory response → vessel damage, hemorrhage, and tissue ischemia
  - Fibrinoid necrosis of blood vessels arises via lysosomal enzymes (collagenases and elastases) and reactive oxidative species
- Various triggers exist (Table 3.35)

Clinical presentation

- Crops of partially blanchable, **symmetric, palpable purpura** on the **lower extremities**, dependent areas, and under tight clothing or areas with pressure
  - Other manifestations: erythematous papules, urticaria, vesicles, pustules, and livedo reticularis
  - Rarely occurs on the face, palms, soles, or mucous membranes
- Timing: appears 7–10 days after exposure and resolves within 3–4 weeks with transient hyperpigmentation and/or atrophy
- Cutaneous symptoms: asymptomatic, pruritus, burning, or pain
- Systemic symptoms: 30% may have fever, malaise, arthralgias, myalgias, and GI/GU symptoms

Table 3.34 Categories of Vasculitis by Vessel Size

	Clinical Features	Examples
Small vessel vasculitis	**Palpable purpura** Petechiae Vesicles Pustules	Henoch-Schonlein purpura Acute hemorrhagic edema of infancy Urticarial vasculitis Erythema elevatum diutinum Granuloma faciale Secondary vasculitis Drug Infection Malignancy Autoimmune
Mixed small and medium vessel vasculitis	Mixture of features from small and medium vessel vasculitis	Mixed cryoglobulinemia (II and III) ANCA-associated: Microscopic polyangiitis Wegener's granulomatosis Churg-Strauss syndrome
Medium vessel vasculitis	**Livedo reticularis** Retiform purpura Ulcers **Subcutaneous nodules**	Polyarteritis nodosa Kawasaki disease
Large vessel vasculitis	Specific per disease Temporal arteritis: erythematous tender nodules or ulceration on the frontotemporal scalp Takayasu's arteritis: erythematous subcutaneous nodules, PG-like lesions on LE > UE	Temporal arteritis Takayasu's arteritis

LE, *lower extremity;* UE, *upper extremity.*

Table 3.35 Triggers of Cutaneous Small Vessel Vasculitis

Triggers	Examples
Primary cutaneous small vessel vasculitis	
Idiopathic (50%)	
Secondary cutaneous small vessel vasculitis	
Infection (15%–20%)	Bacterial: **group A β-hemolytic Streptococci**, *Staphylococcus aureus*, *Chlamydia*, *Neisseria*, *Mycobacterium* Viral: **hepatitis C** > B » A, HIV Fungal/yeast: *Candida*
Inflammatory disorders (15%–20%): can present as a small and/ or medium vessel vasculitis	Autoimmune CTD including: SLE, Sjögren's, RA > dermatomyositis, scleroderma, polychondritis IBD Behçet's disease
Drug (10%–15%): onset is 1–3 weeks after drug initiation, third most common cutaneous drug eruption (2%)	Most common: Antibiotics: **β-lactams** (penicillin, cephalosporins), **sulfonamides**, minocycline, quinolones Anti-inflammatory: **NSAIDs**, COX-2 inhibitors Other culprits: Leukotriene inhibitors Anti-thyroid: propylthiouracil Anti-hypertensives: thiazides, hydralazine Biologics: **TNF-α inhibitors**, MTX, Rituximab Hormonal: OCPs G-CSF Retinoid: isotretinoin **Levamisole-tainted cocaine** Allopurinol Radiocontrast media
Neoplasm (<5%)	Most common: Hematologic malignancy (Multiple myeloma Monoclonal gammopathies T-cell leukemia, MF, AML, CML Diffuse large cell leukemia Hairy cell leukemia) Less common: Solid organ (GU: prostate cancer, renal cancer GI: colon cancer)
Other	Thrombotic Embolic Cyroglobulinemia

Table 3.36 Evaluating for Systemic Vasculitis

General Workup	**If There Is No Concern for Systemic Involvement:**
	CBC [eosinophilia in EGPA], BMP [↑ Cr], ↑ ESR (>40 mm/hr), ↑ LFTs, UA [hematuria/proteinuria]
Extensive Workup	**If There Is Concern for Systemic Involvement Consider General Workup Plus:**
GI	Stool guaiac [+/– melena in HSP]
Renal	Serial UAs [hematuria, proteinuria]
Infectious	Hepatitis B and C HIV ASO titer (if (+), consider streptococcal infection) Abnormal CXR (infiltrates, opacities) Consider TTE and blood cultures in a patient with high fever or heart murmurs Consider other cultures based on history
Inflammatory	↑ ESR ↑ CRP (↑ in infection and autoimmune disease) ANA RF (if (+) consider Sjögren's, rheumatoid arthritis, cryoglobulinemia) C3, C4, CH50, C1q (WNL in NUV; ↓ C3/C4/C1q in HUV, SLE, other autoimmune vasculitides, atheroembolization) ANCA ((+)c-ANCA in GPA; (+)p-ANCA in MPA, EGPA, PAN) Antiphospholipid antibodies ((+) in APLS)
Neoplastic	SPEP/UPEP (if (+) consider hematologic malignancy) CXR (nodules or masses suggestive of malignancy) Abnormal peripheral blood smear
Other	Cryoglobulins (if (+), consider cryoglobulinemia) Immunoglobulins (IgA(+) in HSP, IgE(+) in EGPA)

CBC, *complete blood count;* BMP, *basic metabolic panel;* LFTs, *liver function tests;* UA, *urinalysis;* HSP, *Henoch-Schonlein purpura;* ASO, *anti-streptolysin;* HIV, *human immunodeficiency virus;* CXR, *chest xray;* TTE, *transthoracic echocardiogram;* ESR, *estimated sedimentation rate;* CRP, *C-reactive protein;* ANA, *anti-neutrophil antibody;* RF, *rheumatoid factor;* WNL, *within normal limits;* HUV, *hypocomplementemic urticarial vasculitis;* SLE, *systemic lupus erythematosus;* ANCA, *anti-neutrophil cytoplasmic antibody;* GPA, *granulomatous polyangitis;* PAN, *polyarteritis nodosa;* EGPA, *eosinophilic granulomatous polyangitis;* APLS, *antiphospholipid antibody syndrome;* SPEP, *serum protein electrophoresis;* UPEP, *urine protein electrophoresis.*

  - **If any are present → consider systemic vasculitis!**
  - Paresthesia and lack of painful lesions associated with systemic involvement
- Prognosis: 10% will have chronic and relapsing course with mean duration ≈ 2 years

Pathology

- H&E biopsy best **within 18 to 48 hours**; DIF best even earlier (within 8–24 hours)
  - After 48 hours, pathology is non-specific and may show mononuclear cells rather than neutrophils
- Perivascular **neutrophilic infiltrate (w/ leukocytoclasis)** centered around post-capillary venules w/ **fibrinoid necrosis of vessel walls** and endothelial swelling, and **RBC extravasation**
  - Concomitant involvement of the deeper larger vessels → suggests systemic vasculitis
- DIF: 80% w/ **perivascular C3 and IgM in first 48 hours; after 72 hours, only C3 in minority**

Laboratory testing

- ↑ ESR suggestive of systemic disease
- Significant complement consumption is suggestive of more extensive or systemic disease
- If systemic disease is suspected, evaluate as per Table 3.36

Treatment

- Depends on severity of disease (Table 3.37)

Subtypes of cutaneous small vessel vasculitis

Henoch-Schonlein purpura (HSP)

Epidemiology

- **Most common pediatric vasculitis**
- **90% of cases occur in children** < 10 yo with male predominance
- Seasonal variation, with winter predominance

Table 3.37 Treatment Approach for Cutaneous Small Vessel Vasculitis

Severity of disease	
Mild	Supportive measures: **90% will have spontaneous resolution**, 10% will have a chronic course Remove suspected meds Leg elevation and compression stockings NSAIDs for arthralgias is controversial H1 blockers, H2 blockers Topical steroids
Chronic or severe	Colchicine (0.6 mg, 2–3×/day) Dapsone (100–200 mg/day) Combination of **colchicine + dapsone** or colchicine + pentoxifylline is more efficacious than monotherapy
Severe ulcerating	Oral **prednisone** (0.5–1 mg/kg with a 4–6 week taper) Can add immunosuppressive agents including: Azathioprine (1–2 mg/kg/day) Mycophenylate mofetil (up to 2 g daily) Cyclophosphamide (1–2 mg/kg/day) Cyclosporine (2.5–5 mg/kg/day) IVIG (in an immunodeficient patient) Plasmapheresis (in refractory cases)

Pathophysiology

- **IgA vascular deposition** in small blood vessels results in:
  - Activation of several cytokines
  - Neutrophil activation of nitric oxide and ROS
- Triggers:
  - Occurs 1 to 2 weeks after a **URI**; **ASO titers elevated in 20%–50%**, but causal role of *Streptococcus* unclear
  - Other infections: *Bartonella henselae*, parvovirus B19, *S. aureus*, *H. pylori*, and coxsackievirus
  - Drug exposure reported in a minority of patients

Clinical presentation

- Tetrad:
  - Skin: palpable purpura on the **buttocks** and lower extremities (100%)
  - Musculoskeletal: **arthralgias** (75%); arthritis of the knees and ankles
  - GI: **colicky abdominal pain** (65%), diarrhea, +/− melena; hematochezia (20%)
  - **Renal (40%–50%)**: hematuria w/ risk of nephritis, end-stage renal disease **(1%–3%)**

Key features of adult HSP

- More likely to have aggressive course with diarrhea and **chronic renal insufficiency (30%)**
- Risk factors for chronic renal sequelae: preexisting renal disease, DM2, HTN, abnormalities in renal testing at time of vasculitis diagnosis (even very small anomalies)
- Adults who p/w fever, ↑ ESR, and **purpura above the waist are more likely to have IgA glomerulonephritis**
- A/w solid organ neoplasms (especially lung cancer) > hematologic neoplasms
- More frequent vesiculobullous lesions and cutaneous necrosis (60%)
- Prognosis: recurs in up to 40%

Key features of childhood HSP

- **Severe renal disease in 5%–7%; more common over 8 yo**
- Abdominal pain is a significant predictor of nephritis
- Orchitis and pulmonary hemorrhage are rare manifestations

Treatment

- First line: supportive measures (self-limited disease and resolves in weeks to months)
  - Add prednisone +/− AZA or cyclosporine if abdominal pain, arthritis, or severe nephritis
    - Controversial if prednisone is preventative of renal disease (Cochrane review did **not** show benefit)
  - Dapsone shortens duration and helps with skin findings
  - Ranitidine decreases duration and severity of abdominal pain
  - IVIG considered if rapidly progressive glomerulonephritis

Laboratory testing: see CSVV section

- DIF shows **IgA in blood vessel walls**
- Renal f/u (serial blood pressure, urinalysis [UA; hematuria, proteinuria], BUN, CRE, GFR) for at least 5 years in adults and 6 months in children!
- Guaiac if abdominal pain or suspect GI bleed

Pathology

- LCV
- DIF with IgA deposits, C3, and fibrin in dermal small blood vessels
- Rate of renal disease is greater if there are no eosinophils on skin biopsy

Acute hemorrhagic edema of infancy (Fig 3.86)

Epidemiology

- Occurs in **children < 3 years**
- 70% are boys

Pathophysiology

- Immune complex deposition in small blood vessels
- Triggers: (Table 3.37)

Clinical presentation

- Large **annular or targetoid/cockade**, edematous, hemorrhagic plaques on the **head (cheeks and ears)** and upper extremities

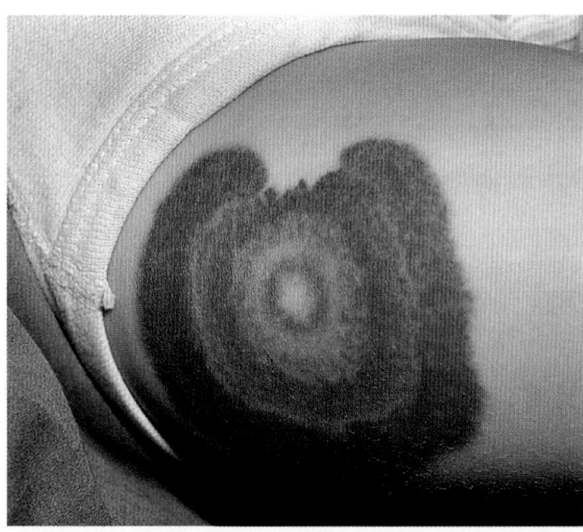

Fig. 3.86 Acute hemorrhagic edema; typical large annular hemorrhagic plaques. (From James WD, Elston DM, Treat JR, Rosenbach MA, Neuhaus IM. Cutaneous vascular diseases. In: *Andrews' Diseases of the Skin*, 13th Ed. Philadelphia: Elsevier; 2020, pp 813-861.e5.)

Table 3.38 Triggers for Acute Hemorrhagic Edema of Infancy

Triggers	
Infection: viral or bacterial	URI: adenovirus, coxsackievirus, EBV Diarrheal illness: hepatitis A, campylobacter, rotavirus UTI: *Escherichia coli* Other: HSV, VZV
Drug	Antibiotics: β-lactams, TMP-SMX Analgesic: NSAIDs, acetaminophen Vaccination

- Tender non-pitting acrofacial edema
- **Not ill-appearing**, but may be febrile
- Prognosis: resolves in 1–3 weeks

Pathology

- LCV
- DIF can have IgA deposits

Treatment

- Supportive with anti-histamines; resolves spontaneously in 1 to 3 weeks

Urticarial vasculitis

- NUV (70%–80%): normocomplemententemic urticarial vasculitis
  - Skin-limited and **idiopathic**
- HUV (20%–30%): hypocomplemententemic vasculitis
  - Highly **a/w systemic disease**

Epidemiology

- **Females > 50 years** most commonly affected, especially in HUV (same demographics as AICTDs)

Pathophysiology

- Complement and immune complex deposition in blood vessel wall and activation of the complement cascade
  - Hypocomplemententemic form: **IgG antibodies bind C1q → reduced serum levels of C1q**
- Causative agents: often idiopathic, but multiple triggers may play role (Table 3.39)

Clinical presentation

- **Painful/burning** urticarial lesions **lasting > 24 hours** (vs. <24 hours for normal urticaria) on trunk and LE; resolves w/ **hyperpigmentation or purpura**; may have concomitant angioedema

Table 3.39 Causes of Urticarial Vasculitis

Idiopathic	
Autoimmune disease	**SLE (associated w/ HUV)** **Sjögren's**
Infection—viral	Hepatitis B/C, EBV
Medications	NSAIDs MTX, TNF-α inhibitors Cimetidine Fluoxetine Potassium iodide
Malignancy	Leukemia/lymphoma Gammopathies (IgM, IgG)
Other	Serum sickness

Table 3.40 Systemic Involvement in Urticarial Vasculitis

System	Associated Symptoms or Disease
Musculoskeletal (50%)	Arthralgias, myalgias
Gastrointestinal (15%–30%)	Recurrent abdominal pain, diarrhea, nausea/vomiting
Pulmonary (20%)	SOB, severe COPD, laryngeal edema
Renal (20%–30%)	Glomerulonephritis or interstitial nephritis
Ocular (50%)	Uveitis, conjunctivitis, episcleritis
Constitutional symptoms	Fever, malaise, arthralgias, myalgias

- Recurrent episodes lasting months to years
- Systemic findings (more common in HUV) are highlighted in Table 3.40

Pathology

- LCV (**often subtle** in degree)
- Diffuse interstitial neutrophils seen more commonly in HUV and may be a/w SLE
- DIF: 70% have perivascular Igs and C3, but a lupus band (granular Ig or C3 along the BMZ) increases the risk for SLE and renal disease in HUV patients

Laboratory testing

- NUV: same as CSVV
- HUV: ↓ **CH50**, C3 and C4; **anti-C1q Ab** (~100% of HUV patients) and ↑ ESR
  - Check ANA given strong association of HUV with SLE (up to 50%)
- **Schnitzler's syndrome**: **urticarial vasculitis + IgM gammopathy** + two of the following: fever, arthralgia, **bone pain**, ↑ ESR, or ↑ WBC

Treatment (Table 3.41)

Erythema elevatum diutinum

Epidemiology

- Rare and chronic condition of middle-aged and older patients
- **A/w HIV**

Pathophysiology

- Immune complex deposition with repeat inflammation and partial healing → perivascular fibrosis
- May be a/w multiple systemic diseases (Table 3.42)

Clinical presentation

- Early lesions: **red-brown violaceous papulonodules** and plaques on **extensor** surfaces and near joints

Table 3.41 Treatment Approach for Urticarial Vasculitis

Primary	Antihistamines Oral steroids **Indomethacin**
Alternatives	**Dapsone** **Colchicine** Hydroxychloroquine
Severe	Prednisone+ mycophenolate mofetil Rituximab Intravenous immunoglobulin azathioprine

Table 3.42 Triggers of Erythema Elevatum Diutinum (EED)

Infection	β-Hemolytic Streptococci **HIV** HBV TB Syphilis
Autoimmune disease	IBD, celiac disease, SLE, RA
Hematologic malignancy	**IgA paraproteinemia/monoclonal gammopathy** Myelodysplasia

- Later lesions: **firm nodules** and masses at previously inflamed sites
- Systemic associations: ocular (scleritis/uveitis) and arthralgias

Pathology

- Early: LCV with interstitial neutrophils resembling neutrophilic dermatoses
- Late: perivascular storiform **fibrosis** (**"onion skin fibrosis"** around dermal vessels) with neutrophils

Treatment

- **Dapsone is the ToC**
- Other treatments: NSAIDs, tetracyclines, and colchicine
- Most resolve spontaneously in 5–10 years

Mixed cryoglobulinemia (see Cryoglobulinemia section)

Granuloma faciale

Epidemiology

- Adults (Caucasian > African American) and M > F

Clinical features

- Single or multiple discrete **red-brown papules**, **plaques**, and nodules on the **face**, especially the nose, malar prominence, forehead, and ear
  - Some consider granuloma faciale and erythema elevatum diutinum to be the same entity with different anatomic predilections
- May have **follicular prominence**, telangiectasias, or a **"peau d'orange"** appearance

Pathology

- LCV (findings may be difficult to identify)
- **Grenz zone**
- Dense **mixed dermal infiltrate** consisting of **eosinophils**, **neutrophils**, lymphocytes and plasma cells (Fig. 3.87)

Treatment

- **Intralesional triamcinolone** (2.5–5 mg/mL)
- Cryotherapy + intralesional triamcinolone
- Topical steroids
- Topical tacrolimus
- If unresponsive, consider dapsone (50–100 mg/day), colchicine, or plaquenil
- PDL

Small to medium vessel vasculitis

- General features:
  - Mixture of signs of CSVV and medium vessel disease
    - Livedo, retiform purpura, ulcers, and subcutaneous nodules
    - Consider especially if there is pulmonary and/or renal involvement
- Types:
  - **ANCA (+)**: granulomatosis with polyangiitis (GPA, formerly Wegener granulomatosis), microscopic polyangiitis (MPA), eosinophilic granulomatosis with polyangiitis (EGPA, formerly Churg-Strauss syndrome)
  - CTD (SLE and RA)
  - Mixed cryoglobulinemia (type II and III)

ANCA-positive vasculitis (Tables 3.42 and 3.43)

- General pathophysiology:
  - ANCA-mediated vascular injury is caused by neutrophils and monocytes that produce toxic oxygen metabolites
    - **Important ANCA associations** (boards tip: if you cannot remember the specific ANCA associations during the exam, just guess p-ANCA because it is the less specific autoantibody and is therefore associated w/ most of the diseases):
  - GPA (Wegener): **c-ANCA**
  - Levamisole-induced vasculitis: **p-ANCA**

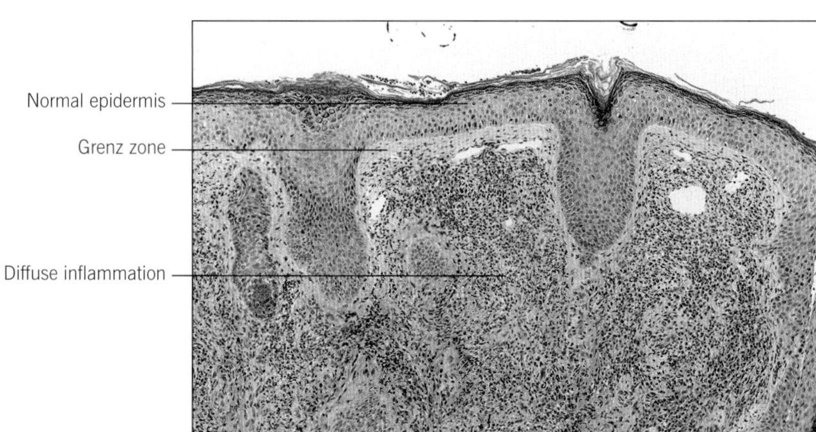

Fig. 3.87 Granuloma faciale (low magnification). (From Rapini RP. Vasculitis and other purpuric diseases. In: *Practical Dermatopathology*. 2nd ed. Philadelphia: Elsevier; 2012:73–86.)

Table 3.43 Features of ANCA Autoantibodies

p-ANCA (less specific)	Myeloperoxidase	Perinuclear staining	**EGPA, MPA** > PAN Other autoimmune disease Chronic infection
c-ANCA (highly specific)	Serine protease 3	Granular cytoplasmic staining	**GPA (Wegener's)** > MPA

ANCA, *Anti-neutrophil cytoplasmic antibody;* EGPA, *eosinophilic granulomatosis with polyangiitis;* MPA, *microscopic polyangiitis;* PAN, *polyarteritis nodosa.*

Table 3.44 ANCA(+) Vasculitides

Disorder	ANCA Type	Systemic Findings and Symptoms	Cutaneous Findings	Other Defining Features
Granulomatosis with polyangiitis (Wegener's)	c-ANCA	**Nasal/sinus**: sinusitis rhinorrhea **Pulmonary**: Cough Hemoptysis **Renal**: Glomerulonephritis with hematuria **CNS**: peripheral neuropathy, CVA	Palpable purpura **PG-like nodules** **Strawberry gums**	Granulomatous
Microscopic polyangiitis	p-ANCA > c-ANCA	**Nasal/sinus**: None **Pulmonary**: Alveolar hemorrhage **Renal**: Glomerulonephritis with hematuria **CNS**: Neuropathy, mononeuritis multiplex	Palpable purpura Livedo reticularis Retiform purpura Ulcers	**Non-granulomatous**
Eosinophilic granulomatosis with polyangiitis (Churg-Strauss)	p-ANCA	**Nasal/sinus**: Nasal polyps Allergic rhinitis **Pulmonary**: Asthma (adult-onset) **Renal**: less common **CNS**: mononeuritis multiplex, symmetric polyneuropathy **Cardiac**: cardiomyopathy, pericarditis, valvular disease **GI**: N/V, abdominal pain	Palpable purpura Painful subcutaneous nodules	Granulomatous eosinophilia

- EGPA: **p-ANCA** > c-ANCA
- MPA: **p-ANCA** > c-ANCA
- Minocycline-induced lupus erythematosus: **p-ANCA**

Granulomatosis with polyangiitis (Wegener)

Epidemiology

- Middle-aged adults + children

Pathophysiology

- **c-ANCA**-mediated (**anti-PR3**) Th1 immune response → granuloma formation
- PR3 expression on apoptotic neutrophils stimulates APCs → Th1-induced granulomas—this process is "neutrophil priming"
- Genetic predisposition; **nasal *S. aureus* carriage** may trigger flare that improves with antibiotics

Clinical presentation

- Triad of:
  - Necrotizing granulomas of the upper and lower respiratory tract
    - Respiratory: cough, hemoptysis, and shortness of breath
    - **Nasal/sinus inflammation**: rhinorrhea, sinusitis, and purulent or bloody nasal discharge
  - Systemic vasculitis
    - Musculoskeletal: arthralgias
    - Ocular: conjunctivitis, proptosis, and keratitis
    - CNS: peripheral neuropathy and cerebrovascular accident
  - Glomerulonephritis
    - **Death from renal disease** if left untreated (>80% 1-year mortality)
- Cutaneous findings: 10%–21% at initial presentation, 15%–46% throughout course of the disease
  - Palpable purpura in dependent areas
  - Oral ulcers are common—gingival hyperplasia with **"strawberry gums"** (Fig. 3.88) is rare, but pathognomonic
  - Painful PG-like nodules or necrotic ulcers
  - Cutaneous disease a/w earlier onset and more widespread vasculitis
- Limited form: cutaneous or pulmonary subtype
- Constitutional symptoms: fever, weight loss, anorexia, and malaise

Pathology

- LCV + extravascular necrotizing palisading **granulomas** with basophilic debris (**"blue granulomas"**)

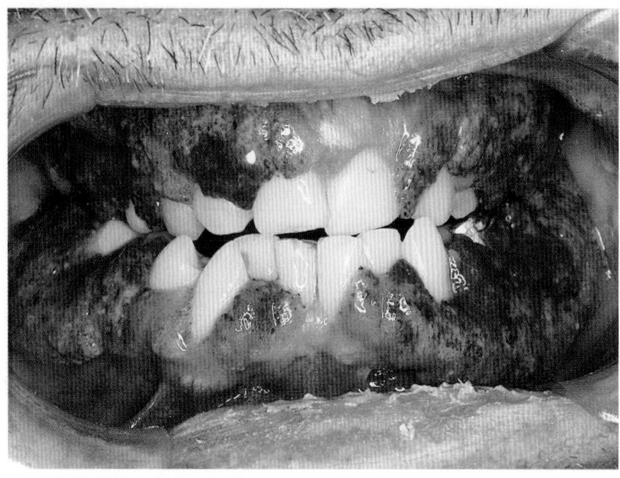

Fig. 3.88 Wegener granulomatosis; strawberry gingiva. (From James WD, Elston DM, Treat JR, Rosenbach MA, Neuhaus IM. Cutaneous vascular disorders. In: *Andrews' Diseases of the Skin*. 13th ed. Philadelphia: Elsevier; 2020:813–861.)

Laboratory testing

- ↑ ESR and ↑ WBC
- **(+) c-ANCA**
  - Sensitivity (up to 90%) and specificity (80%–100%)
  - May be absent in patients with localized GPA
  - May have a role in disease monitoring
- Abnormal UA: microscopic hematuria or RBC casts
- Abnormal CXR: nodules, infiltrates, and cavities often found
- Sinus involvement: abnormal sinus X-ray, CT sinus, or nasal biopsy

Treatment

- Induction: **cyclophosphamide (2 mg/kg/day) + steroids** (Prednisone 1 mg/kg/day); other options include MTX + steroids, rituximab (4 infusions of 375 mg/m^2 weekly) + steroids, plasma exchange (with cyclophosphamide + steroids)
- Maintenance:
  - MTX (20–25 mg/wk) + oral steroids
  - AZA (2 mg/kg/day) + oral steroids
  - Other options include: rituximab, MMF 2 g daily, IVIG, infliximab
  - **Rituximab > AZA > MMF for preventing relapses**
  - Consider adding TMP-SMX to treat nasal *Staphylococcus* carriage
- Prognosis:
  - Relapse rate: 50% within 5 years

Microscopic polyangiitis (MPA)

Epidemiology

- M > F; peaks at 65 to 75 years

Pathophysiology

- Unclear, may be ANCA-mediated
- a/w Infective endocarditis, meds, and malignancy

Clinical presentation

- 20%–70% have skin findings: cutaneous palpable purpura, petechiae > livedo racemosa, retiform purpura, ulcers, and splinter hemorrhages, acral erythematous macules

Table 3.45 Comparison of Microscopic Polyangiitis (MPA) and Polyarteritis Nodosa (PAN)

	PAN	MPA
Renal: glomerulonephritis	–	+
Hypertension and microaneurysms	+	–
Pulmonary symptoms	–	+
ANCA(+)	– (less likely)	+ (more likely)
Hepatitis B or C association	+	–

Table 3.46 Systemic Involvement in Microscopic Polyangiitis (MPA)

Renal (79%–90%)	**Focal segmental necrotizing glomerulonephritis**
Pulmonary (25%–50%)	Pulmonary capillaritis, pulmonary hemorrhage
Neurological (up to 33%)	Mononeuritis multiplex, peripheral neuropathy

- Constitutional symptoms may be present for months to years
- Systemic symptoms (Table 3.45):
  - Most common cause of **pulmonary-renal syndrome** (Table 3.46)

Pathology

- LCV with segmental small > medium vessel vasculitis
- **No granuloma formation, unlike GPA or EGPA**

Laboratory testing: see CSVV, especially:

- **p-ANCA (anti-MPO, 60%)** > c-ANCA (anti-PR3, 30%)
- Abnormal UA (proteinuria or hematuria)
- Abnormal CXR or CT (chest)
- Other: abnormal EMG or lung/nerve/kidney biopsy

Treatment

- Induction:
  - Cyclophosphamide (2 mg/kg/day) + oral steroids (1 mg/kg/day)
  - Other options: **rituximab** + steroids, MTX + steroids, plasma exchange (with cyclophosphamide + steroids)
- Remission:
  - MTX/AZA + steroids (similar to GPA); other options: MMF, rituximab, IVIG, infliximab
  - **Rituximab > AZA > MMF for preventing relapses**
- Localized
  - TMP-SMX + oral steroids

Eosinophilic granulomatosis with polyangiitis (Churg-Strauss syndrome)

Epidemiology

- Peaks in middle age

Pathophysiology

- Mixed inflammatory and ANCA-mediated tissue damage with granuloma formation and neutrophilic vasculitis with eosinophils
- Possible triggers: rapid steroid taper, vaccination, **leukotriene inhibitors**, and **anti-IgE antibody (omalizumab)**

Clinical presentation: three classic stages (Table 3.47)

- Cutaneous: presenting sign in 14%, but vast majority will develop at some point in disease course:
  - Palpable purpura on the lower extremities

Table 3.47 Stages of Churg-Strauss Syndrome

Stage	Presentation
1 (prodromal atopic phase)	**Adult-onset asthma (nearly 100% patients)** **Nasal polyps** **Allergic rhinitis**
2 (eosinophilic phase)	Eosinophilia Pneumonia GI: N/V, abdominal pain
3 (vasculitis phase)	Systemic necrotizing vasculitis Pulmonary: asthma, sinusitis, allergic rhinitis Neurologic: mononeuritis multiplex, symmetric polyneuropathy, sensorineural hearing loss, episcleritis, facial nerve palsy Cardiac: pericarditis, valvular disease, endocardiomyopathy (leading cause of death)

  - Painful symmetric subcutaneous nodules of the extremities and scalp; urticaria and erythema can occur also
- Systemic findings: see Table 3.47
  - **Limited renal involvement** unlike GPA and MPA

Pathology

- LCV w/ mixed infiltrate of **eosinophils**, neutrophils, lymphocytes, and macrophages
- Palisading neutrophilic and **eosinophilic extravascular granulomas** with degenerated collagen fibers **("red granulomas")**

Laboratory testing

- (+) ANCA: patients more likely to have neurologic and renal disease
- (−) ANCA linked to cardiac disease
- **p-ANCA** > c-ANCA in leukotriene-associated Churg-Strauss
- **Eosinophilia** (eosinophils > 1500/mm^3)
- Leukocytosis
- ↑ IgE
- CXR: patchy infiltrates, interstitial disease, and nodular masses; CT: bronchial wall thickening and ground glass opacities peripherally

Treatment

- TOC: Oral steroids (1 mg/kg/day)
- Severe multiorgan involvement:
  - Cyclophosphamide (2 mg/kg/day) + oral steroids
- AZA, MTX or MMF can be used for maintenance
  - Meplizumab (IL-5 MAB) approved for adults with EGPA w/ severe asthma

Medium vessel vasculitis

Subtypes: PAN and Kawasaki's disease

Polyarteritis nodosa

Epidemiology

- M > F; peaks 40 to 60 years
- 10% of cases overall are cutaneous form, but it is the most common form in children

Pathophysiology

- Possible triggers: medications, infections, inflammatory disease (IBD, SLE), **hairy cell leukemia**; may be immune complex-mediated
- a/w **Hepatitis B** (5%–7%) and hepatitis C
- Cutaneous form:
  - A/w Streptococcal infection in children
  - Has been a/w minocycline

Clinical presentation

- Two forms:
  - Classic subtype with multi-system vasculitis
    - Rare pulmonary involvement, unlike ANCA-associated vasculitides
  - Cutaneous (Fig. 3.89) subtype with limited systemic involvement (Table 3.48)

Pathology

- LCV
- **Necrotizing arteritis of medium-sized arteries**
  - In skin, these vessels are **located in subcutis** and at the dermopannicular junction
- **Microaneurysms** → thrombosis, ischemia, and necrosis
  - Microaneurysms seen on angiography of medium-sized vessels (coronary, **renal**, celiac, and mesenteric arteries)
- Later course defined by fibrosis
- DIF: IgM and/or C3 in the walls of cutaneous blood vessels

Laboratory testing: see CSVV

- CBC: anemia and leukocytosis
- UA for hematuria and RBC casts
- Hepatitis B and C
- ANCA (p-ANCA < 20% positive)
- **Consider angiography if suspect microaneurysm** or stenosis
- In children, consider ASO

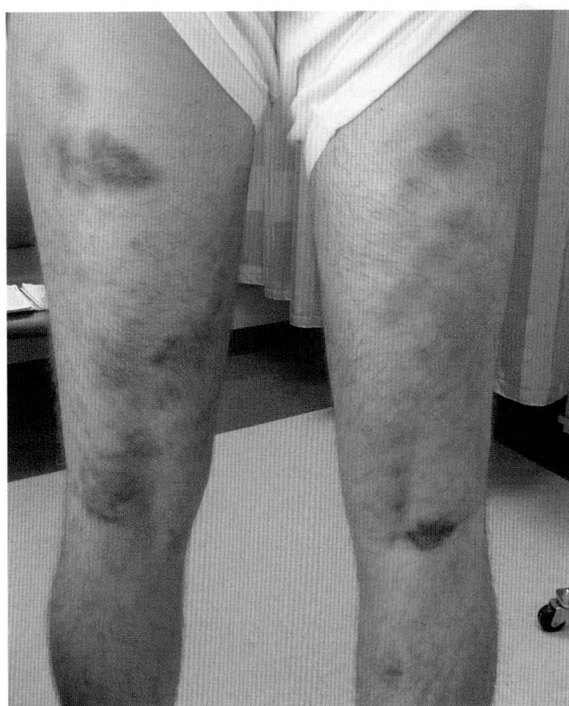

Fig. 3.89 Polyarteritis nodosa. Subcutaneous, tender, purpuric plaques and reticulated purpura on the legs. (Courtesy of Christopher Sayed, MD.)

Table 3.48 Features of Classic and Cutaneous Polyarteritis Nodosa (PAN)

	Key Cutaneous Features	Systemic Features
Classic subtype (PAN)	Palpable purpura on lower extremities Painful single/multiple **subcutaneous nodule(s)** on lower extremities that may ulcerate Nodules may follow course of superficial blood vessels, especially in the lower extremities **Livedo reticularis** Rare digital or penile infarction	Constitutional symptoms: fever, weight loss, arthralgias, malaise Multi-organ involvement: Renal: **HTN and renal failure** (most common cause of death) Cardiac: cardiomyopathy, MI, arrhythmias Nervous system: **paresthesias, motor or polyneuropathies (foot drop)** GI: N/V, bowel infarction, hemorrhage, mesenteric ischemia GU: orchitis Multi-organ infarcts from aneurysms
Cutaneous subtype (C-PAN)	Pink to purple-red nodules on lower extremities near the malleoli and may extend proximally Atrophie blanche: atrophic, ivory, stellate scars Livedo reticularis Digital gangrene	Constitutional symptoms: fever, myalgias Minimal organ involvement: Nervous: peripheral neuropathy Musculoskeletal: arthralgias, myalgias

Treatment

- Cutaneous subtype:
  - Oral steroids for 3–6 months or longer; may need to add colchicine, azathioprine, methotrexate or dapsone if ineffective
  - Children: consider penicillin or tonsillectomy, given the association with streptococcal infection
- Severe systemic disease:
  - Cyclophosphamide (2 mg/kg/day) + oral steroids for 12 months
  - Infliximab or rituximab
  - IVIG
- Hepatitis B (+):
  - IFN-α +/− vidarabine/lamivudine +/− plasma exchange

Kawasaki disease (acute febrile mucocutaneous lymph node syndrome)

Epidemiology

- 80% of cases in **kids < 5 years**; M > F
- ↑ Incidence in **Japanese**

Pathophysiology

- Unclear etiology, but likely due to infection by unknown agent
- Genetic and ethnic factors → ↑ susceptibility
- Inflammation, scarring, stenosis, and aneurysm formation in the small, medium, and large musculoelastic arteries including the **coronary artery**

Clinical presentation (Fig. 3.90)

- Fever for **at least 5 days** followed by:
  - **Conjunctival injection** (usually non-exudative)
  - Mucous membrane: lip/oral mucosa erythema, **fissured lips**, **strawberry tongue**, and injected oral and pharyngeal mucosa
  - **Cutaneous**: polymorphous eruption including psoriasiform, morbilliform, scarlatiniform (particularly **perineal** with **desquamation**), and EM-like lesions on hands/feet
  - **Cervical lymphadenopathy**
  - Extremity changes: **peripheral edema/erythema of hands/feet**, or periungual desquamation
- For diagnosis, need fever ≥ 5 days + four out of five of the above
- May get orange-brown or white transverse nail discoloration
- Systemic complications:
  - Cardiac: **coronary artery aneurysms/ectasia** (secondary to vasculitis) and myocarditis
  - Musculoskeletal: arthritis/arthralgias
  - Pulmonary: pneumonitis
  - CNS: aseptic meningitis and facial nerve palsies
  - Ophthalmology: anterior uveitis
  - GI: gastroenteritis, hepatomegaly, bile duct inflammation/hepatitis, jaundice, and pancreatitis

Laboratory testing

- **↑ CRP and ESR**
- CBC (**anemia, leukocytosis**, ↑ neutrophil/eosinophils, and thrombocytosis)
- ↓ Albumin, sodium, potassium, and HDL

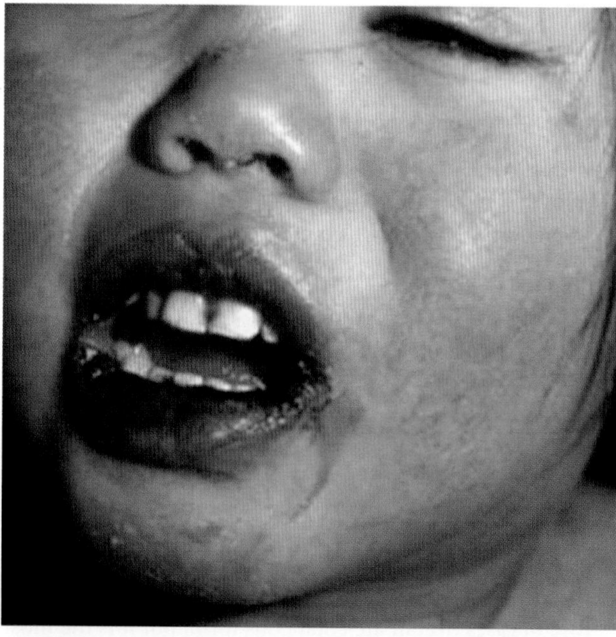

Fig. 3.90 Lip erythema, fissuring, and bleeding in a patient with Kawasaki disease. Oropharyngeal findings occur in 80% to 90% of patients, including redness of the lips, tongue, and throat. Lip fissuring and dryness are also common. (From Bayers S, Shulman ST, Paller AS. Kawasaki disease: part I. Diagnosis, clinical features, and pathogenesis. *J Am Acad Dermatol.* 2013;69[4];501.e1–e11, quiz 511–512.)

- LFTs ↑, GGT ↑
- Check **echocardiogram** at diagnosis, 2, 6, and 8 weeks

Treatment

- **High-dose ASA** (80–100 mg/kg/d) + **IVIG** (2 g/kg)
  - **If given within first 10 days → ↓ coronary artery issues**
- Resistant cases: IVIG + steroids, cyclophosphamide, cyclosporine/CIs, plasma exchange, TNF-α inhibitors, MTX, rituximab, anakinra
- **Maintenance: ASA**

Key testing facts

- A/w Myocardial infarction (**#1 cause of acquired pediatric heart disease in the United States**)
- Patients < 12 months do not respond as well to treatment

Large vessel vasculitis

Subtypes: temporal arteritis and Takayasu's arteritis

Temporal arteritis (giant cell arteritis)

Epidemiology

- More common in Caucasians, females
- >50 years

Pathophysiology

- Vessel involved: any medium to large vessel (especially temporal artery)
- **Granulomatous vasculitis** → ischemia, occlusion, infarction, and aneurysm

Clinical presentation

- Early: **tenderness and erythema along the scalp and temples** with possible cord-like nodule along temporal scalp
  - Other cutaneous symptoms: erythema, purpura, alopecia of overlying skin, and scalp necrosis
  - Unilateral **temporal headache**
  - **Loss of temporal pulse**
  - **Jaw claudication**
  - Glossitis, necrosis of anterior tongue (lingual artery)
- Late: ulceration or gangrene of **frontotemporal scalp or tongue**
- Systemic findings:
  - **Polymyalgia rheumatica** (40%–60%) with limb and girdle muscle pain, stiffness, and weakness
  - Fever and weight loss
  - Neurologic: **vision loss (14%)**, stroke, subarachnoid hemorrhage, and altered mental status

Pathology

- Segmental **granulomatous large vessel arteritis** with GCs
- Disruption of media with fragmentation of the internal elastic lamina

Laboratory workup

- ↑ **ESR** and ↑ CRP
- Anticardiolipin antibody (may be ↑)
- MRA
- **Temporal artery biopsy**

Treatment

- ASA 81 mg/day + oral steroids (40–60 mg/day)
- Consider methylprednisolone (1 g/day for 3–5 days) if acute visual loss
- Tocilizimab (anti-IL-6 Ab) approved for large vessel vasculitis—IL-6 levels may track with disease activity

Takayasu's arteritis

Epidemiology

- F > M; <40 years

Pathophysiology

- Vessel involved: **aorta** and its main branches
- Granulomatous vasculitis → stenosis, occlusion, and aneurysms

Clinical presentation

- Cutaneous symptoms seen in 50% of individuals, including:
  - Purpura
  - Erythematous subcutaneous nodules, EN-like lesions, **PG-like lesions**
  - Raynaud phenomenon and digital gangrene
- Systemic symptoms:
  - Constitutional symptoms: fever, fatigue, malaise, night sweats, and weight loss
  - HTN
  - Loss of carotid or radial pulse

Pathology

- Granulomatous inflammation of the aorta and its major branches

Laboratory workup

- ↑ ESR
- MRA with visualization of all branches of the aortic arch

Treatment

- Oral prednisone (1 mg/kg) for 1 to 3 months with a 6 to 12 month taper
- MTX 15 to 25 mg/wk + prednisone
- Cyclophosphamide
- Infliximab or etanercept
- Surgical intervention for cerebral hypoperfusion, valvular insufficiency, and aneurysms

Summary of organ system involvement in various vasculitides (Table 3.49)

Cryoglobulinemias

Epidemiology

- Varies geographically likely **related to HCV** prevalence
- F > M; average age = 50 yo

Pathophysiology

- Cryoglobulins are immunoglobulins that precipitate at colder temperatures; various triggers (Table 3.50)

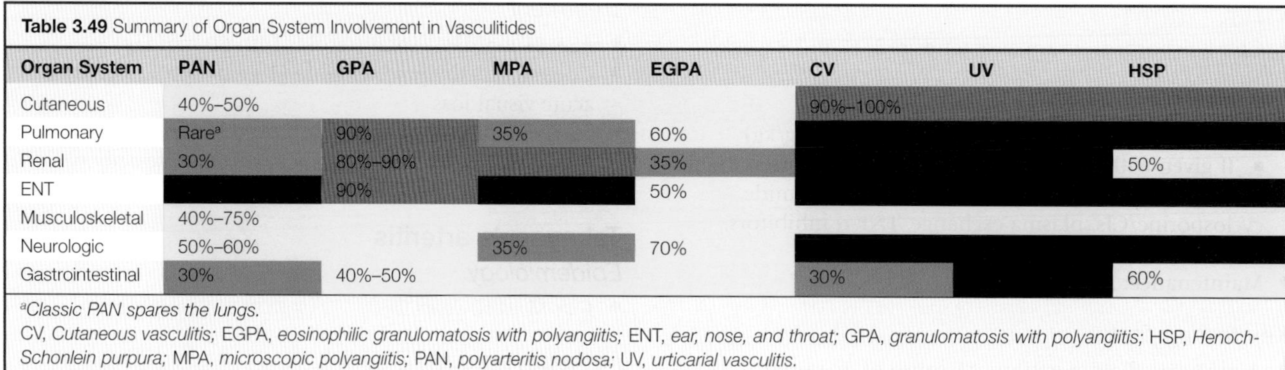

Table 3.49 Summary of Organ System Involvement in Vasculitides

Organ System	PAN	GPA	MPA	EGPA	CV	UV	HSP
Cutaneous	40%–50%				90%–100%		
Pulmonary	Rare[a]	90%	35%	60%			
Renal	30%	80%–90%		35%			50%
ENT		90%		50%			
Musculoskeletal	40%–75%						
Neurologic	50%–60%		35%	70%			
Gastrointestinal	30%	40%–50%			30%		60%

[a]*Classic PAN spares the lungs.*
CV, *Cutaneous vasculitis;* EGPA, *eosinophilic granulomatosis with polyangiitis;* ENT, *ear, nose, and throat;* GPA, *granulomatosis with polyangiitis;* HSP, *Henoch-Schonlein purpura;* MPA, *microscopic polyangiitis;* PAN, *polyarteritis nodosa;* UV, *urticarial vasculitis.*

Table 3.50 Comparison of Cryoglobulinemias

Type	Cause	Associations
Type 1 (20%–25%)	**Monoclonal** immunoglobulin (**IgM** » IgG, IgA, light chains)	**Lymphoproliferative disorders** Plasma cell dyscrasia MGUS CLL Multiple myeloma Waldenström macroglobulinemia B-cell non-Hodgkin's lymphoma
Mixed cryoglobulinemias		
Types 2 and 3 (75%–80%)	**Monoclonal (Type 2)** or **polyclonal (Type 3) IgM** complexes with **polyclonal IgG**	HIV Hepatitis B **Hepatitis C** (cutaneous symptoms more common) Other infections Autoimmune disease SLE (nephritis risk with cryo-globulins) Sjögren's RA

- Type I: ↑ **monoclonal cryoglobulins (IgM** > IgG, IgA, light chains) → complete occlusion of vessel lumens w/ **hyaline material**
  - **Lacks LCV**
- Type II and III (mixed type): complexed immunoglobulins will precipitate at cooler temperature and occlude vessels → triggers complement → **LCV**

Clinical presentation

- Cutaneous findings:
  - Type I findings:
    - Raynaud phenomenon
    - Purpura, **livedo reticularis/racemosa**, ulceration
    - Cold-induced **acrocyanosis** of helices
  - Type II and III findings:
    - **Palpable purpura** and urticarial lesions
    - Systemic findings common

Pathology

- Type I: **occlusive vasculopathy** with vessels completely filled by **homogenous hyaline material; lacks LCV**
- Types II and III: characteristic features of **LCV**

Laboratory testing

- ↑ Cryoglobulins
- Complement (**hypocomplementemia in 90%**; C4 ↓)
- **RF (+) (types 2 and 3)**
- **Hepatitis B/C**
- LFTs

Treatment: treat underlying disease

- Type I: treatment of lymphoproliferative disorder (e.g., rituximab, bortezomib, lenalidomide); plasmapheresis (for hyperviscosity symptoms)
- Type II
  - HCV-related: **IFN-α +/– ribavirin**; if symptoms severe, may need rituximab + high-dose steroids
  - Other infection: treat underlying infection; steroids if severe symptoms
  - AICTD: immunosuppression (e.g., rituximab, steroids, MMF, AXA, cyclophosphamide)

Thrombosis and thrombotic syndromes

- Consider occlusive vasculopathy if **livedo reticularis** and/or **retiform purpura** is present (signs of vascular occlusion); anatomic distribution can help (Fig. 3.91); *Journal of the American Academy of Dermatology* Continuing Medical Education article on retiform purpura from 2020 is very helpful for workup
- Two broad categories of thrombotic syndromes:
  - Acutely sick patient: disseminated intravascular coagulation (DIC), purpura fulminans, Coumadin necrosis, heparin-induced skin necrosis, TTP, paroxysmal nocturnal hemoglobinuria, HUS, cholesterol emboli, and septic vasculitis
    - **Purpura fulminans**: acute syndrome of progressive hemorrhagic skin necrosis and DIC; children > adults; may be idiopathic, triggered by an infection (most commonly meningococcal, **streptococcal**, staphylococcal, or varicella), or due to congenital deficiency in protein C or S; sudden onset of tender purpura and ecchymosis that often expand rapidly with a rim of erythema and central hemorrhagic bulla and/or necrosis; favor acral distribution and buttocks
  - Non-sick patient: APLS, livedoid vasculopathy, inherited coagulopathies (protein C, S, anti-thrombin III, Factor V Leiden), and type I cryoglobulinemia

Important subtypes

Calciphylaxis

- Discussed in Section 3.20 and Chapter 10

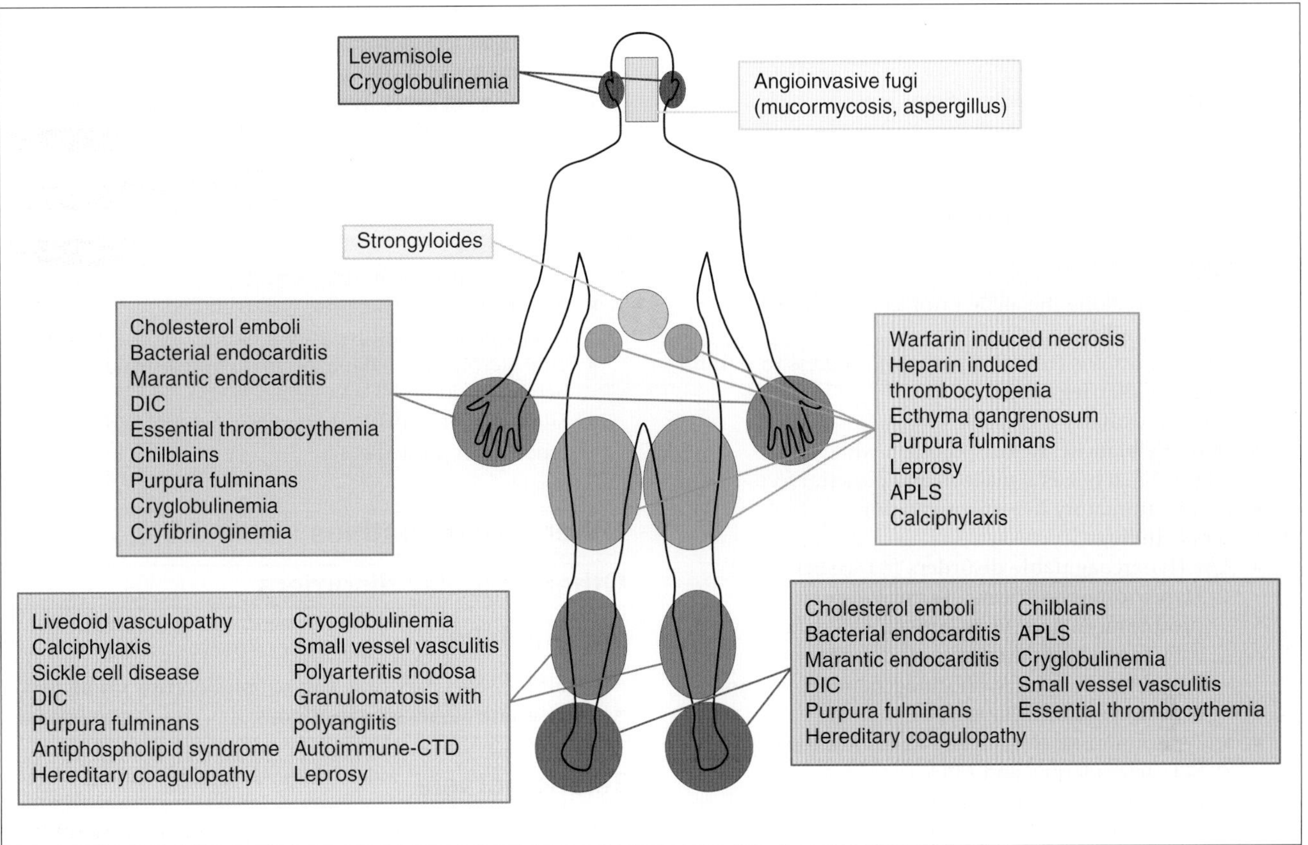

Fig. 3.91 Anatomic distribution of common causes of retiform purpura. *APLS*, Antiphospholipid antibody syndrome; *CTD*, connective tissue disease; *DIC*, disseminated intravascular coagulation. (From Georgesen C, Fox LP, Harp J. Retiform purpura: a diagnostic approach. *J Am Acad Dermatol.* 2020;82[4]:783–796.)

Antiphospholipid syndrome

Epidemiology

- Mainly young women

Pathophysiology

- Unclear etiology—50% primary, 50% with AICTD (SLE most commonly, up to 23% develop disease over 9 years)
- Associated with immunoglobulins that are reactive with phospholipids
- Predisposition to thrombosis

Clinical presentation

- History of vascular thrombosis (32%), **premature birth**, **miscarriage (8%)**, thrombocytopenia, and labile blood pressure
- Cutaneous features:
  - livedo reticularis (most common finding)
  - Leg ulcers, pseudovasculitis, digital gangrene, cutaneous necrosis, splinter hemorrhages, **anetoderma**, **retiform purpura (suggestive of occlusion)**
  - Atrophie blanche
- Systemic features:
  - DVT, PE, stroke, renal infarct, myocardial infarction, arthritis, and epilepsy
  - **a/w SLE (most common)** and other autoimmune conditions including RA and UC
  - Catastrophic antiphospholipid syndrome (CAPS) occurs when antiphospholipid syndrome progresses and results in multiple thrombotic events (e.g. multiorgan failure, diffuse microthrombosis of dermal/hypodermal vessels); mortality rate = 4%
- Precipitants: surgery, meds (HCTZ, OCPs, ACE inhibitors), malignancies, anticoagulation withdrawal/low INR, and infection

Pathology

- Occlusion of arteries and arterioles w/ **firbin thrombi**; minimal inflammation; **lacks LCV**

Laboratory findings

- (+) Antiphospholipid antibodies: **anti-cardiolipin antibodies (most sensitive**, most commonly positive), **lupus anticoagulant**, and **anti-β2-glycoprotein I** antibody (**most specific**)—one or multiple may be positive
- **False-positive syphilis serology**

Treatment

- Empiric anticoagulation, anti-platelet agents, and antimalarial agents in those with concurrent lupus

Livedoid vasculopathy (atrophie blanche)

Epidemiology

- F > M; mean age of onset = 45 yo
- Worse in summer

Pathogenesis

- Unknown, but linked to coagulation disorder

Clinical presentation

- Burning pain along the ankle prior to ulceration
- Cutaneous findings:
  - Purpuric lesions (retiform purpura) progress to **painful and irregular leg ulcers**
  - livedo reticularis
  - **Atrophie blanche**: stellate porcelain-white scar (Fig. 3.92) at bilateral malleoli and posterior feet
  - Postinflammatory hyperpigmentation
- Systemic findings
  - **A/w Hypercoagulable disorders (#1 association)**
    - Hyperhomocysteinemia, Factor V Leiden, prothrombin mutations, protein C/S deficiency, ↑ Factor VIII, antithrombin III deficiency, cryoglobulinemia, cryofibrinogenemia, plasminogen activator/inhibitor mutation
  - a/w Autoimmune conditions (#2 association)
    - SLE, scleroderma, and APLS
  - a/w Infections (e.g., hepatitis B/C) and paraproteinemia less frequently

Pathology

- Segmental **hyalinization and thrombosis of small vessels** in the upper and mid dermis
- Late stage with epidermal atrophy and **hyalinized vessels**

Laboratory findings

- Perform **coagulopathy workup and CTD serologies** (cryoglobulins, cryofibrinogen, homocysteine, protein C/S, antithrombin III, lupus anticoagulant, antiphosphatidylserine, anti-β2 glycoprotein I, ANA, anti-cardiolipin AB, Factor V mutation, Factor VIII, plasminogen activator/inhibitor, and prothrombin mutation); can also consider infectious and paraproteinemia workup (e.g., Ig levels, immunofixation, SPEP)

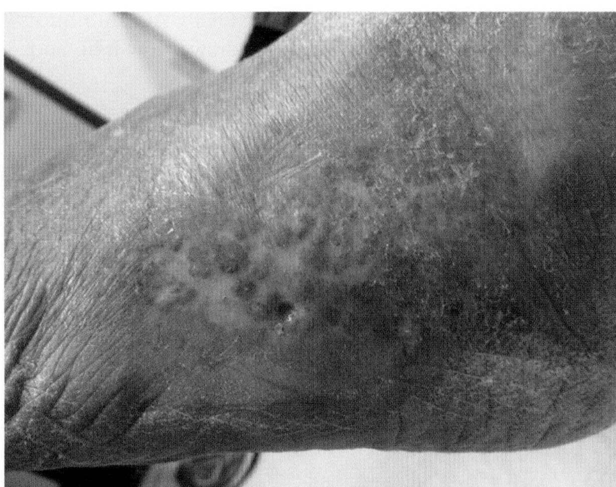

Fig. 3.92 Atrophie blanche with punched-out ulcer from livedoid vasculopathy. (Courtesy of Christopher Sayed, MD.)

Treatment

- **ASA**
- Dipyridamole
- **Pentoxyfilline**
- In recurrent or recalcitrant cases:
  - Anticoagulation (heparin, warfarin, and **rivaroxaban**)—best treatment data
  - Oral steroids (e.g., danazol, methylprednisolone, betamethasone)
  - Sildenafil, TPA, PUVA, hyperbaric oxygen, IVIG reported in limited cases

Other vasculopathies (Table 3.51)

Other vascular disorders

Venous lake

- Small (<1 cm) dark blue soft papules on **lips** primarily
- Large ectatic vessel seen in dermis

Telangiectasia

- Permanently dilated dermal vessels that appear red
  - Primary:
    - Spider telangiectasia (can also occur secondary to **↑ estrogen**)
    - Hereditary benign telangiectasia
    - Angioma serpiginosum
      - Females < 20 yo
      - Pinpoint punctate blanching red-purple petechiae in clusters/patches in serpiginous pattern typically on one **extremity**
    - Unilateral nevoid telangiectasia
      - Telangiectasias in trigeminal/upper cervical dermatomes +/− Blaschko's lines
      - Some cases are acquired, secondary to localized ↑ estrogen receptors on vessels
    - Generalized essential telangiectasia
      - Typically **adult women**
      - **Starts on lower extremities and spreads**, involving large areas
    - Cutaneous collagenous vasculopathy
      - Large anatomic areas—does not have female predominance or centripetal spread
      - Ectatic dermal vessels with **thick hyalinized BMZ surrounding vessels (stain (+) with collagen IV/PAS-positive)**
      - Not responsive to laser
  - Secondary:
    - Photodamage, post-radiation (including repeated fluoroscopy), telangiectatic rosacea, involuted hemangioma, estrogen-related (e.g., **liver disease**, **pregnancy**, hormone replacement therapy, or **OCPs**), CS use, AICTDs (e.g., **CREST syndrome**), HIV infection (chest), mastocytosis (telangiectasia

Table 3.51 Vascular Disorders Not Otherwise Discussed

Cause	Key Features	Laboratory Testing and Treatment
Emboli: cholesterol, bacterial or fungal endocarditis, oxalate		
Cholesterol emboli	**p/w livedo reticularis** > retiform purpura or gangrene of the distal extremities and digits. Clinical setting: **post-catheterization (hours–days), thrombolytics (hours–days), anticoagulation (1–2 months)**; may be febrile, hypertensive, and/or with altered mental status Pathogenesis: fragmentation of an atherosclerotic plaque that embolizes Histology: **cholesterol clefts in small vessels**	Laboratory findings: **Eosinophilia** common ↑ ESR ↑ **BUN/Cr** Treatment: supportive, aspirin, anti-platelet, statins
Inflammation: pigmented purpura, hypergammaglobulinemic purpura of Waldenström		
Pigmented purpura (capillaritis, PPD)	Group of disorders with clustered petechial hemorrhage Pathophysiology: inflammation of the capillaries with resultant hemorrhage **PPD Types:** **Schamberg's**: cayenne-pepper purpura on the lower extremities (esp. shin, ankles) that can extend; middle-aged to older adults **Purpura annularis telangiectodes of Majocchi**: annular patches with punctate petechiae on trunk and lower extremity in adolescent/young-adult women **Lichenoid dermatitis of Guogerot and Blum**: rust-colored lichenoid papules and Schamberg-like purpuric lesions in middle-aged to older men **Eczematid-like purpura of Doucas and Kapetanakis**: scaly and eczematous petechiae and purpura in middle-aged to older men **Lichen aureus**: solitary golden or rust-colored patch on the lower extremities **Linear pigmented purpura**: unilateral, linear eruption of yellow-brown macules, patches, and red-brown purpura; adolescents and children mainly Histology: hemosiderin containing macrophages with RBC extravasation, endothelial swelling, and a perivascular lymphocytic infiltrate. Guogerot: lichenoid infiltrate; Doucas and Kapetanakis: spongiosis and parakeratosis	Treatment: topical steroids for pruritus,TCIs, PUVA, NB-UVB, compression stockings, vitamin C + rutin
Hypergammaglobulinemic purpura of Waldenström	Crops of burning/stinging petechiae and/or purpura on the lower extremities, often seen in women. **a/w polyclonal gammopathy** (IgG and IgA RF), and CTD (Sjögren's) Pathophysiology: unknown cause, likely immune complex-mediated (IgG and IgA) Histology: hemorrhage, mild perivascular lymphocytic infiltrate, or LCV	Treatment: aspirin and compression stockings controversial; avoid triggers, including alcohol
Hemorrhage: trauma, thrombocytopenia, platelet dysfunction, medication (aspirin, steroids)		
Other: levamisole-induced vasculitis, Degos disease, Sneddon syndrome, Schnitzler's syndrome		
Levamisole-induced vasculitis	**Cocaine may contain levamisole**, an antihelminthic agent, which ↑ its stimulant effects and bulk It has recently been shown to cause **vasculitis/vasculopathy** Presentation: purpura and necrosis of the **earlobes** (but also nose, cheek, extremities), LCV-like lesions, ecchymoses, and systemic vasculitis, especially of the kidney/lung/testes Histology: thrombotic vasculitis/LCV +/– vascular occlusion	Laboratory findings: ↑ ABs to **p-ANCA (>80%)**, c-ANCA (50%), and human neutrophil elastase Agranulocytosis Leukopenia Treatment: Resolution once tainted cocaine stopped, occasionally immunosuppressants
Degos disease (malignant atrophic papulosis)	Crops of small **erythematous papules that develop a central depression/ ivory scar**, peripheral erythema and surrounding telangiectasias (~atrophie blanche) Systemic symptoms include: **GI (bowel perforation)** Seen in **young and middle-aged men** Pathophysiology: unknown, possible vasculopathy Histology: wedge-shaped area w/ dermal edema, mucin, sclerosis; vascular thrombosis	Treatment: No proven treatment Aspirin +/– pentoxifylline
Sneddon syndrome	**Livedo racemosa** and livedoid vasculopathy with labile blood pressure and **CNS disease (TIA, stroke, dementia)**, and extracerebral thrombosis. Seen in **young women** aged 20–30 Pathophysiology: a/w **APLS**, vasculopathy or vasculocoagulopathy Histology: endothelial inflammation; subendothelial intimal smooth muscle proliferation; partial or complete occlusion of arterioles	↑ Antiphospholipid antibodies Treatment: warfarin (INR 2–3)

macularis eruptiva perstan), carcinoid, and drugs **(CCBs → telangiectasias in sun-exposed areas)**
    - **Genodermatoses**: Cutis marmorata telangiectasia congenita, hereditary hemorrhagic telangiectasia, ataxia-telangiectasia, Klippel-Trenaunay syndrome, Rombo, Bloom, Rothmund-Thomson, dyskeratosis congenita, XP, Goltz (within Blaschko's lines), prolidase deficiency, and hypotrichosis-lymphedema-telangiectasia syndrome

Erythromelalgia

- **Red, painful/burning, edematous, hot distal extremities** (especially **lower extremities**—feet/lower legs)
- Episodes usually late day/night
- Many cases **a/w small fiber neuropathy**
- Worse with heat/activity; relieved with cooling, **classically "plunging feet into ice cold water"**
- Type 1: occurs with **thrombocythemia**
  - May → ischemic necrosis
  - Histologically see occlusive thrombi
  - ASA and hydroxyurea may be helpful
- Type 2: primary idiopathic
  - May occur in childhood and be familial
    - *SCN9A* mutations (Na+ channel subunit mutation ↓ sympathetic neuron activity, and ↑ pain receptor sensitivity)
  - May treat with sodium channel blockers (e.g., mexiletine and flecainide)
- Type 3: occurs with underlying condition (NOT thrombocythemia)
- Treatment: supportive treatments, capsaicin cream, amitriptyline-ketamine gel, lidocaine patches or IV, mexiletine, antidepressants, anticonvulsants (e.g., carbamazepine), CCBs, misoprostol, nitroprusside, prostaglandin E1, rizatriptan, and anesthetic epidural infusions/lumbar blocks and sympathectomies
- **Pediatric red ear syndrome** has similar features and may represent a subtype of erythromelalgia; **red scrotum** in older White men may represent a localized type of erythromelalgia (doxycycline and gabapentin may be helpful)

Livedo reticularis (LR)

- Reticulated vascular pattern that is usually benign (physiologic), but may be a/w an underlying disorder (e.g., AICTD or APLS)
  - **Physiologic**: secondary to vasospastic response to cold and improves with heat; processes that → ↓ blood flow to and within skin or ↓ blood draining out of skin → deoxygenated blood in venous plexus → livedo appearance
    - Physiologic type usually with fine complete network
  - **Idiopathic/primary LR**: persistent arteriole vasospasm → persistent LR of lower extremities
  - **LR secondary to vasospasm**: may be seen with AICTDs and Raynaud phenomenon
  - **LR secondary to vessel wall issues**: usually medium vessel vasculitis (especially cutaneous PAN; also systemic PAN, cryoglobulinemic vasculitis, vasculitis secondary to AICTDs); can also be seen in calciphylaxis
  - **Livedo racemosa** = larger branching and incomplete rings (vs. smaller complete rings of LR)
    - Seen in Sneddon syndrome, embolic phenomenon, APLS or other causes of occlusion
  - **LR secondary to intraluminal issues: slow blood flow within vessels** (cryoglobulinemia, cryofibrinogenemia, PCV, thrombocytosis, APLS, and protein C/protein S/anti-thrombin III deficiencies) versus **obstruction of vessels** (cholesterol emboli, APLS, heparin/warfarin necrosis, hyperoxaluria, and livedoid vasculopathy)
  - **Other LR causes: amantadine** pheochromocytoma, and reflex sympathetic dystrophy
- Biopsy technique: elliptical excisional biopsy from **normal appearing skin in center of net pattern**

Angiospastic macules (Bier spots)

- Benign physiologic vasoconstriction → blanched macules on lower > upper extremities that appear white
- Induced by tourniquet, resolve with tourniquet release and leg elevation
- Have been reported in pregnancy and cryoglobulinemia

3.23 PANNICULITIDES AND LIPODYSTROPHIES

Erythema nodosum

Epidemiology

- **Most common panniculitis,** especially women in second to fourth decades

Pathogenesis

- Delayed hypersensitivity response (Th1 cytokine pattern) to various antigens
- Idiopathic most common cause, followed by **streptococcal infections (#1 identifiable cause)**, other infections (bacterial GI infections [*Yersinia, Salmonella, Campylobacter*], viral URIs, coccidioidomycosis, TB, and histoplasmosis), drugs (estrogens/**OCPs, sulfonamides, and NSAIDs**), sarcoidosis, and **IBD (Crohn's > UC)**
  - Lofgren's syndrome: type of sarcoidosis w/ EN, hilar lymphadenopathy, fever, polyarthritis, and uveitis; a/w good prognosis

Clinical features

- Acute, **tender subcutaneous nodules** on **pretibial areas** (most commonly) bilaterally with overlying erythema to **bruise-like patches**
  - Develop over 1 to 2 weeks, then resolve spontaneously
  - New lesions may develop over 1 to 2 months
  - Can be a/w fever, arthralgias, malaise (may precede cutaneous findings)
- Chronic forms (**subacute nodular migratory panniculitis/EN migrans**) can occur
  - Women mainly; unilateral; migrating centrifugally expanding nodules (less tender than EN)
  - Usually idiopathic, but may be a/w *Streptococcus* infection; treat with SSKI

Histopathology

- **Septal panniculitis** with **thickening/fibrosis of septae**
- **Neutrophils** seen particularly in early lesions
- **Miescher's microganulomas**: small histiocytic aggregates surrounding a central stellate cleft; located in SQ fat septa
- +/– Thrombophlebitis (more common in EN-like lesions seen in Behçet's disease)

Treatment/clinical course

- Lesions last a few days to weeks, then **resolve w/o scarring**; recurrences may occur
- Treat underlying medical issue (if identified)
- Options for treatment of EN: bed rest/elevation, **NSAIDs, SSKI**, colchicine (especially for Behçet's-associated EN), dapsone, TNF-α inhibitors **(especially for IBD-associated EN)**, and systemic immunosuppressants
- **EN a/w improved prognosis of coccidioidomycosis and sarcoidosis**

Alpha$_1$-antitrypsin deficiency panniculitis

Pathogenesis

- Alpha$_1$-antitrypsin (serine protease inhibitor made in liver) deficiency → dysregulation of immune system and ↑ neutrophils → release of proteolytic enzymes → fat necrosis
- Various alleles:
  - M = medium (normal quantities of enzyme)
  - S = slow (moderately ↓ quantities of enzyme)
  - Z = very slow (severely ↓ quantities of enzyme)
- Heterozygotes with one copy of Z or S have mild/moderate deficiency (PiMS, PiMZ); **most severe dz = homozygous for Z allele (PiZZ)**

Clinical features

- Red/bruised tender plaques—lower trunk and proximal extremities → ulceration/necrosis → **oily discharge**
- Preceding trauma in one third
- Lesions quite resistant to treatment → permanent **scarring/atrophy**
- A/w **chronic liver dz (cirrhosis)**, **emphysema**, pancreatitis, membranoproliferative glomerulonephritis, c-ANCA vasculitis, and angioedema

Histopathology

- Lobular or mixed panniculitis w/ neutrophils
- **Liquefactive necrosis of SQ fat** (lobules and septa) and dermis

Treatment

- ToC = **alpha1-antitrypsin replacement** → rapid improvement
- Other treatments: doxycycline, colchicine, cyclophosphamide, dapsone, ↓ alcohol consumption, plasma exchange, and liver transplant

Erythema induratum/nodular vasculitis

Epidemiology

- Women primarily; 30 to 40 years old

Pathogenesis

- May be a/w **TB (erythema induratum of Bazin)** or idiopathic (nodular vasculitis)
  - Tissue culture for mycobacteria usually negative → PCR tests for *Mycobacterium tuberculosis* more sensitive
- Likely type IV cell-mediated response to antigen

Clinical features

- Tender, recurrent red-purple nodules and plaques on **calves** most commonly
- May ulcerate, drain, and scar

Histopathology

- **Lobular and septal panniculitis** (Fig. 3.93) w/ neutrophils, lymphocytes, macrophages, GCs + **medium vessel vasculitis** (found in connective tissue septa/fat lobules)
  - **Main DDx = PAN** (both affect medium-sized vessels, but **PAN does not have any significant involvement of the fat lobules** themselves)
- May have caseous or coagulative necrosis +/– palisading granulomas

Treatment

- Treat TB if present; otherwise supportive care + various systemic treatments (CS, NSAIDs, tetracyclines, and SSKI)

Pancreatic panniculitis

Pathogenesis

- A/w pancreatic disorders (e.g., **pancreatitis, carcinoma, and pseudocysts**)
- Due to hydrolysis of fat by **lipase, amylase, and trypsin**
  - ↑ Serum levels of any (or all) of these three enzymes are detectable

Clinical features

- **Subcutaneous nodules of legs** (most common site)
  - May occur prior to knowledge of pancreatic issues
  - Lesions are red/brown, firm, and tender → may ulcerate and release oily discharge

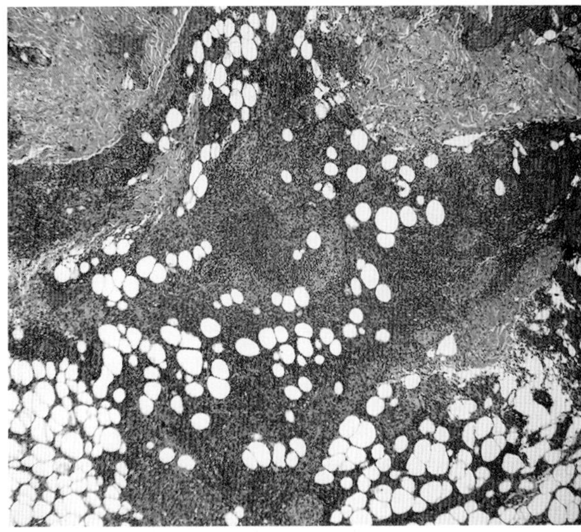

Fig. 3.93 Nodular vasculitis: vascular involvement as seen in this field is a characteristic feature. (Courtesy of Olayemi Sokumbi, MD.)

- May have concurrent systemic symptoms:
  - **Schmid's triad** (nodular lesions + polyarthritis + eosinophilia) → a/w **poor prognosis**

Histopathology

- Mixed panniculitis w/ **"ghost cell"** (anucleate necrotic adipocytes) formation and fat necrosis w/ **saponification** by calcium salts → basophilic color of damaged fat lobules

Treatment

- Treat underlying pancreatic disorder

Lipodermatosclerosis

Epidemiology

- Middle-aged/elderly
- F > M

Pathogenesis

- Due to combination of **venous insufficiency** and **fibrinolytic abnormalities** → ↑ capillary permeability → fibrinogen leakage → fibrin cuffs form around vessels → ↓ O_2 exchange/tissue anoxia → cystic fat necrosis +/– dermal stasis changes

Clinical features

- Acute (rubor, dolor, and calor) → chronic (well-defined induration, hyperpigmentation, **"inverted wine bottle"** appearance from sclerosis)
- **Medial lower leg**, superior to malleolus

Histopathology

- **Septal thickening** (Fig. 3.94) and fibrosis, **cystic fat necrosis** w/ surrounding lipophages (histiocytes that have engulfed lipid from necrotic lipocytes), mild non-specific inflammation, **lipomembranous change**, +/– signs of stasis changes (angioplasia, inflammation, and fibrosis)

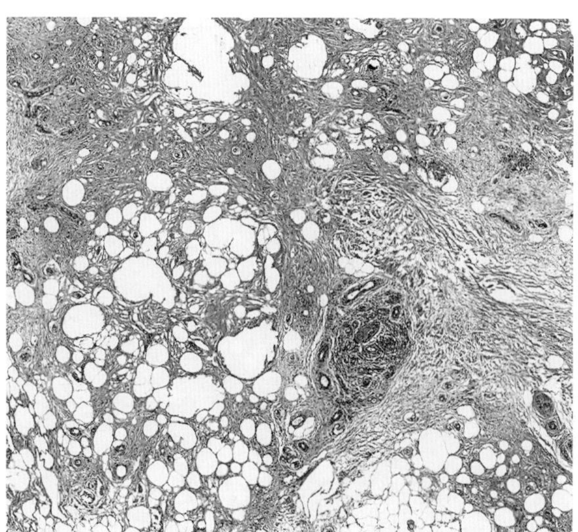

Fig. 3.94 Lipodermatosclerosis (sclerosing panniculitis) close-up view of micro-cysts. (Courtesy of Olayemi Sokumbi, MD.)

Treatment

- Leg compression and elevation +/– IL steroids
- Systemic options: **danazol**, oxandrolone, **pentoxifylline**, horse chestnut extract, tetracylines, HCQ

Panniculitis secondary to external factors

- Cold panniculitis: acute, firm, painful, cool (in temperature), and erythematous plaques/nodules that develop 1 to 3 days post cold exposure; **most commonly affects areas of prominent fat distribution (central cheek, thighs**, and back)
  - Named variants:
    - **Popsicle panniculitis**: seen in **infants** mainly on **cheeks** (due to higher saturated:unsaturated fatty acid ratio)
    - **Equestrian panniculitis: young women equestrians** on thighs
  - In neonates, risk factors include head or whole body hypothermia for hypoxic-ischemic encephalopathy and use of ice therapy for supraventricular tachycardia
  - Histology: **lobular panniculitis** + typical **pernio changes** (superficial and deep PV/peri-eccrine lymphohistiocytic infiltrate w/ papillary dermal edema)
  - Resolves over several weeks; lipoatrophy may develop in affected areas
- Physical trauma/foreign material:
  - **Sclerosing lipogranuloma**: male genitalia (penis mainly) due to injection of oil-based materials for augmentation
  - Other injectable agents (e.g., factitial, cosmetic)
  - Blunt trauma
  - Histologic clues: vacuolated spaces, foreign material (e.g., **"Swiss cheese" appearance in sclerosing lipogranuloma**), and evidence of needle stick injury

Lipodystrophies

- Disorders with selective loss of fat +/– fat accumulation in other areas (Table 3.52)

3.24 DERMATOSES OF PREGNANCY

Physiologic changes during pregnancy

- Vary widely, but most notable are **linea nigra, melasma, telogen effluvium (TE)**, striae gravidarum, and palmar erythema

Dermatoses of pregnancy (Table 3.53)

3.25 HAIR, NAIL, AND MUCOSAL DISORDERS

Non-scarring alopecia

Androgenetic alopecia

Epidemiology

- 80% men and 50% women by age 70

Table 3.52 Lipodystrophies

Disorder	Pathogenesis	Clinical Features	Other Facts
Congenital generalized lipodystrophy (Berardinelli-Seip syndrome)	Autosomal recessive AGPAT2 (type 1), BSCL2/ seipin (type 2), CAV1 (type 3) Highest frequency in Brazil	**Loss of fat in face** (e.g., preauricular), trunk, extremities, viscera +/– palmoplantar/retro-orbital/tongue/breasts/vulva/periarticular ((–) in type 1 and 3, (+) in type 2) Acanthosis nigricans, hypertrichosis, xanthomas Muscular hypertrophy appearance Osteosclerotic and lytic skeletal changes Masculinization in women/enlarged genitalia in kids only Starts at birth	Diabetes/insulin resistance more common, including metabolic syndrome ↑ Triglycerides ↓ HDL Vitamin D resistance in type 3 PCOS, infertility (women) **Hypertrophic cardiomyopathy** (usually fatal—mean lifespan = 32 yo; ↑ in type 2), atherosclerosis, liver failure, fatty liver/cirrhosis, organomegaly, acute pancreatitis, proteinuric nephropathy, developmental delay (↑ in type 2)
Familial partial lipodystrophy (Köbberling-Dunnigan syndrome)	Autosomal dominant LMNA, PPARγ (milder clinical features but worse metabolic features), AKT2, PLIN1	**Loss of fat on extremities/buttocks** +/– trunk (anterior > posterior) ↑ **Fat on face**/neck, labia majora **Muscular hypertrophy appearance** w/ prominent veins Starts at puberty Tuberous xanthomas, acanthosis nigricans, hirsutism	Diabetes/insulin resistance more common ↑ Triglycerides ↓ HDL (worse w/ PPARG type) Acute pancreatitis, fatty liver/cirrhosis, menstrual issues, PCOS, atherosclerosis, HCM Worse in women subtype with mandibuloacral dysplasia (LMNA or ZMPSTE24 mutation)
Acquired generalized lipodystrophy (Lawrence syndrome)	Unknown	Loss of fat on face, trunk, extremities **(including palms/soles)** Loss of visceral fat but bone marrow fat preserved (**unlike** congenital generalized lipodystrophy) Muscular appearance due to loss of fat Acanthosis nigricans, hyperpigmentation, eruptive xanthomas, hirsutism Starts in childhood/adolescence (7 yo in panniculitic variant, 15 yo in autoimmune variant, 20 yo in idiopathic variant)	Diabetes/insulin resistance more common ↑ Triglycerides ↓ HDL 30% have preceding AICTD (type 2 variant; e.g., juvenile DM) or infection, and one fourth have preceding **panniculitis** (type 1 variant) Clitoromegaly, PCOS, menstrual issues Coronary artery dz, PVD Organomegaly Fatty liver/cirrhosis (can be fatal, more so than in congenital generalized lipodystrophy) Cirrhosis, proteinuric nephropathy
Acquired partial lipodystrophy (Barraquer-Simons syndrome)	Sporadic vs. autosomal dominant LMNB2 Linked to infections and autoimmune diseases	**F » M** Loss of fat on face **(cadaveric facies)**, upper extremities, trunk (spreads in **cephalocaudal** direction, sparing lower extremities ↑ Fat in hips, legs, gluteal region Acanthosis nigricans, hirsutism starts in childhood/adolescence	↑ Triglycerides and DM2/ insulin resistance may occur but metabolic syndrome less common than other disorders may be preceded by infection and/or a/w AICTD (SLE, DM) Menstrual issues **Membranoproliferative glomerulonephritis** (several years after lipodystrophy, present in 20% of pts) ↓ **C3 and** ↑ **C3 nephritic factor** (polyclonal IgG; binds C3) → activates alternative complement pathway → adipocyte death and ↑ *Neisseria meningitides* infections

Table 3.53 Dermatoses of Pregnancy

Disorder	Onset	Appearance	Treatment/Course	Risk to Fetus	Interesting Facts
Pemphigoid gestationis (herpes gestationis)	Typically **second or third trimester** or immediately postpartum	Pruritic papules/plaques that → blisters/bullae mainly on trunk (**does NOT spare umbilicus**)	Topical or systemic corticosteroids depending on severity (taper once blisters resolve) Spontaneously resolves but may flare/recur around delivery, with menstruation, or OCPs May take weeks to months after delivery to entirely resolve Typically **recurs in future pregnancies** (more severe/earlier)	↑ **Risk prematurity and SGA** Baby may have mild transient pemphigoid lesions Risks to fetus correlate with dz severity	May occur with **choriocarcinoma** ↑ Risk of Graves' disease Due to IgG1 autoantibodies against **BP180** NC-16A segment (**DIF with linear C3 along perilesional BMZ**) Strongly a/w **HLA-DR3 and DR4**
Polymorphic eruption of pregnancy	**Third trimester** or immediately postpartum	Urticarial, pruritic papules/ plaques which prefer striae distensae (**spares umbilicus**) Usually spares face/extremities	Resolves over 4 weeks Topical steroids and antihistamines may help Typically does not recur	None	Mainly seen in **primiparous women** ↑ Risk in **multiple-gestation pregnancies**

Continued

Table 3.53 Dermatoses of Pregnancy—cont'd

Disorder	Onset	Appearance	Treatment/Course	Risk to Fetus	Interesting Facts
Intrahepatic cholestasis of pregnancy	Third trimester	**Extreme generalized pruritus without primary rash** Worse at night Bad on palm/sole Excoriations/ prurigo typically seen on extensor surfaces Jaundice in 10%	MUST ↓ serum bile acid levels—oral **ursodeoxycholic acid** May recur in future pregnancies and can flare with OCPs May have steatorrhea and vitamin K deficiency → postpartum hemorrhage Pruritus resolves shortly after delivery	↑ **Risk of premature birth, intrapartum fetal distress, stillbirth** Risks correlate with bile acid levels (i.e., >40 μmol/L)	↑ Total serum bile acid levels (>11 μmol/L) due to ↓ excretion
Atopic eruption of pregnancy (prurigo of pregnancy)	Usually first or second trimester	Eczematous or papular eruption usually in typical sites (e.g., flexural surfaces) typically in patients with **atopic history** May be flare of pre-existing dermatitis or first time they have had dermatitis (80%)	Treatments: topical steroids, emollients, antihistamines, UVB for symptom control Usually recurs with future pregnancies	None	Most have ↑ IgE May be Th2-mediated Most common pruritic disorder of pregnancy
Pustular psoriasis of pregnancy (impetigo herpetiformis)	Usually third trimester	Generalized **pustular psoriasis** starting in flexures (groin mainly)	Supportive, prednisone Resolves with delivery typically Recurs with future pregnancies and OCPs	**Placental insufficiency, stillbirth, neonatal death** in bad disease	**A/w Hypocalcemia** and ↓ vitamin D Mom may have cardiac/ renal failure

SGA, *small-for-gestational age*

Pathogenesis

- Strong genetic predisposition (polygenic)
- In men, ↑ **DHT** expression plays a role
  - **5α-reductase** enzymes catalyze **conversion of testosterone to DHT**:
    - Type I 5 α-reductase—**skin, hair follicles, and** sebaceous glands
    - Type II 5 α-reductase—**prostate mainly, but also hair (inner root sheath)**
      - Absence prevents male AGA

Clinical features

- Norwood-Hamilton classification system in men
  - Progressive **frontotemporal hairline recession** and thinning over frontal crown and vertex scalp
- Ludwig scale in women
  - **Preservation of frontal hairline** with progressive **thinning from vertex** to frontal scalp
  - Increased central part width creates "**Christmas tree pattern**"

Histology

- ↑ **Vellus hairs** and **miniaturized hairs** (both types are fine, short, non- or lightly pigmented)
  - Vellus hairs: have always existed as small hairs (never were terminal hairs)
  - Miniaturized hairs: hairs that were previously large terminal hairs but have shrunk over time to become small hairs roughly the size of vellus hairs
- ↓ **Terminal hairs** (thick, long, and deeply pigmented)
  - Due to progressive miniaturization process
- Anisotrichosis: ↑ variability in hair shaft size
  - Due to progressive process of terminal hairs becoming "miniaturized" to resemble native vellus hairs
  - This finding is a very helpful clue on horizontal sections
- **Shortened anagen phase** → slightly ↑ **telogen:anagen ratio** ("catagen/telogen shift")
  - Degree of catagen/telogen shift is mild in androgenetic → not nearly as dramatic of a catagen/telogen shift as in AA or trichotillomania/traction alopecia
- ↑ **Fibrous streamers**: fibromucinous tract remnants underneath miniaturized or telogen hairs
  - ↑ Streamers are a helpful clue that suggests one of two processes:
    - Hairs are undergoing **miniaturization process** (transforming from a robust terminal hair → wispy vellus-like hair)
    - Hairs are cycling more rapidly from anagen phase → telogen phase **("catagen/telogen shift")**
    - Both processes contribute to the ↑ in fibrous streamers seen in AGA
  - Note: ↑↑ fibrous streamers are also seen in **AA** and **trichotillomania/traction** alopecia
    - In these diseases, the massive catagen/telogen shift is primarily responsible for the dramatic increase in streamers

Treatment

- Only minoxidil and finasteride are FDA approved for AGA
  - **Topical minoxidil** 2% or 5% (5% is more effective)
    - Lengthens anagen phase and ↑ blood flow
    - Regrowth most effective on **vertex scalp (> frontal scalp)**; takes at least 4 months and must be continued indefinitely for hair retention
  - **Finasteride** 1 mg/day **(type II and III 5α-reductase** inhibitor)
    - Only approved for use in males but higher doses (2.5–5 mg/day) may help women

    - In pregnant females → risk of abnormal male genitalia in fetuses
    - Dutasteride 0.5 mg PO daily (**type I, II and III 5 α-reductase** inhibitor) appears to be more effective than finasteride, but not FDA approved
    - Mnemonic: "**DUtasteride = DUal action**" (inhibits both types I and II)
  - Antiandrogens: spironolactone (>100 mg per day), cyproterone acetate (women only)
  - Oral minoxidil (low dose) 0.25 to 5 mg/day demonstrates good efficacy and safety, but is not yet FDA approved
  - Low level light/laser therapy (infrared and red light)
  - Hair transplantation and scalp reduction (discussed further in Chapter 9, Cosmetic Dermatology)
  - Platelet-rich plasma
    - Stimulates hair regrowth by activating the stem cells in the hair bulge and dermal papillar cells located in the dermis; intradermal injections once monthly × three sessions followed by q3–6 monthly sessions for maintenance

Telogen effluvium

Clinical features

- ↑ Shedding due to telogen shift in response to stressor
- Normally lose about 100 to 150 hairs/day, but in TE may lose > 150 hairs/day
- Usually **occurs 3–4 months after inciting cause** (Box 3.8)
- Usually **temporary**; should subside in 6 to 12 months after the inciting factor corrected
  - Occasionally chronic, without inciting factor in some women
- Overall thinning and ↓ density of scalp hair
- **Positive hair pull test** (>4–6 telogen hairs released out of 40 pulled)—will see telogen hairs on hair mount

Histology

- **Mild ↑ percentage of total hairs in catagen/telogen** phase ("catagen/telogen shift"):
  - >20%, but less than 50% → indicative of TE (vs. <15% in normal scalp)
  - >50% → indicative of AA, trichotillomania/traction alopecia
- Normal total number of hairs

Anagen effluvium

- See Chapter 2, Section 2.10 Drug Reactions

Box 3.8 Common Causes of Telogen Effluvium

- Thyroid abnormality
- Iron deficiency
- Postpartum/pregnancy
- Drugs—oral contraceptive pills, retinoids, anticoagulants, anti-thyroid, anticonvulsants, interferon-α, heavy metals, beta-blockers
- Severe stress
- Hospitalization or surgery
- High fever
- Severe illness
- Malnutrition (e.g., ↓ protein, ↓ iron)

Trichotillomania

- Hair-pulling impulse control or OCD
- **Large, irregular/geometric areas of alopecia (scalp > eyebrows > eyelashes > genital hair)** with coexistent areas of completely normal, uninvolved scalp
  - Affected areas contain hair of **varying lengths**
- **a/w Trichophagy** (chewing and swallowing of hair) → may cause intestinal obstruction and **trichobezoars**
- **Female** > male (5:1)
- Average age of onset: 8 yo (boys), 12 yo (girls)
  - Histopathology: **massive "catagen/telogen shift"** (↑↑↑ catagen/telogen hairs; often > 50% of hairs in catagen or telogen phase), **pigmented hair casts**, empty anagen follicles (due to hair shafts being pulled out), **trichomalacia** (distorted hair shafts), and hemorrhage
- Trichoscopy: multiple broken hairs of different lengths and shapes without perifollicular changes
- Confirmatory test: **hair growth window**
  - During repeated shaving of a specific area, hair of normal density regrows (since hairs are too short to manipulate)
- Rx: behavior modification therapy, **clomipramine (ToC)**, SSRIs, N-acetylcysteine; **prognosis better in younger children** than in older children/adolescents

Alopecia areata

Pathogenesis

- Loss of immune privilege
- Autoreactive cytotoxic **CD8+ T cells** target hair follicle antigens
- Type 1 cytokines (IL-2, IFN-γ, and TNF-α)
- One fourth patients with **family history**

Clinical features

- Round patches of non-scarring hair loss (follicular ostia visible)
  - **Alopecia totalis**: complete scalp hair loss
  - **Alopecia universalis**: complete scalp and body hair loss
  - **Ophiasis pattern**: band-like loss across occipital and temporal scalp; **poor prognostic factor**
  - **Sisapho pattern** is opposite where there is hair growth in these areas, but loss of hair in other areas
- **Regrowth hair may be gray or white**
- Can have longitudinal lines of **regular nail pitting** and **trachyonychia**
  - Poor prognostic factor
- Dermoscopy: short "**exclamation point" hairs** and perifollicular yellow dots (small in size vs. larger in DLE)
- Can be chronic/relapsing and can occur at any age (>5-year duration = poor prognostic factor)
  - **Worse prognosis: childhood or diffuse patterns**
- Associated with:
  - Atopy (**atopic dermatitis = poor prognostic factor**)
  - **Autoimmune thyroid disease**
  - **Vitiligo**
  - Lupus erythematosus
  - IBD

Histology

- Classic findings: peribulbar lymphocytic cell infiltrate **("swarm of bees")**, marked **"catagen/telogen" shift** (↑ catagen and telogen hairs), ↑ miniaturized hairs (including super small **nanogen** hairs), occasionally trichomalacia +/− pigment casts
  - Note: trichomalacia and pigment casts may be seen in AA → can be confused for trichotillomania
- **Other helpful clues** in cases lacking classic "swarm of bees": lymphocytes (94%), melanin (84%), and eosinophils (44%) in fibrous tracts

Treatment

- Topical or **intralesional** CS, topical minoxidil 2%/5%, topical allergens (squaric acid, dinitrochlorobenzene, and diphenylcyclopropenone), calcipotriene, phototherapy (UV light), systemic CS, **JAK inhibitors** (baricitinib is FDA approved)

Temporal triangular alopecia

- Presents at birth or within the first decade
- Temporal scalp with **areas lacking terminal hairs** (only fine vellus hairs present)
- Normal total number of hairs within affected area
- Persists throughout life

Congenital atrichia with papules

- Inherited defect in **hairless gene** or vitamin D receptor
- P/w **failure to regrow almost all their hair** after shedding of their initial hairs after birth
- Also see **follicular cysts and milia** later in life

Cicatricial (scarring) alopecia

General points

- **Absence of follicular ostia + hair loss**
- It is important to either obtain two biopsies (one for horizontal and one for vertical sections), or to specify to your dermatopathologist whether you are suspecting scarring versus non-scarring alopecia
  - Vertical sections: **best for scarring alopecias**; does not show many follicles though, so it is a poor method for non-scarring alopecias (except may be AA)
  - Transverse/horizontal sections: show all follicular units in specimen → **best method for non-scarring alopecias**; can also be used for scarring alopecias but most dermatopathologists prefer vertical sections for this purpose since the epidermis is also visible (helpful particularly for DLE vs. LPP)

Primary cicatricial alopecia

- Hair follicle is the inflammatory target
- Classified by type of inflammation (Table 3.54)

Secondary cicatricial alopecia

- Hair follicle is "innocent bystander" (e.g., burns, radiation dermatitis, skin cancer, sarcoidosis, amyloidosis, and necrobiosis lipoidica)

Central centrifugal cicatricial alopecia

Epidemiology

- F > M; **African descent**

Pathogenesis

- *PADI3* mutation in some patients
- A/w use of **chemical relaxers, hot combs**, traumatic hairstyles, pomades

Clinical features

- Destructive, chronic, and progressive scarring hair loss
- Scarring starts on **vertex** scalp, then **spreads centrifugally**, with doll hairs present
  - Mildly tender

Histology

- **Premature desquamation of inner root sheath**
- **Concentric lamellar fibroplasia**
- **Eccentric thinning** of ORS
- Variable lymphocytic perifollicular inflammation (usually not as dense or lichenoid as LPP)
- Polytrichia (fusion of follicular infundibulae) = histologic correlate to "doll hairs"

Treatment

- STOP traumatic hair care practices
- Long-term tetracycline agent therapy, spironolactone, topical minoxidil, topical and/or intralesional CS
- Hair transplantation for severe cases

Lichen planopilaris

Epidemiology and pathogenesis

- Most common in middle-aged **Caucasian females**
- May be due to loss of **immune privilege** at hair follicle bulge → follicle stem cell loss and cicatrical hair loss

Clinical findings

- Inflammatory; scarring hair loss, with itching and burning
- Scattered patches of **perifollicular erythema, scaling, and scarring**
- 50% can have skin and nail LP findings
- <u>Frontal fibrosing alopecia</u>
  - Distinct clinical variant w/ similar histopathologic findings
  - Most common in postmenopausal Caucasian women; may be a/w sunscreen and moisturizer use
  - Progressive **frontal hairline recession** w/ atrophic scarring and perifollicular papules
  - **Eyebrow loss** (helpful clue)
- <u>Graham-Little syndrome</u>
  - Associated with LPP
  - Scarring hair loss on scalp
  - Non-scarring hair loss of axilla and pubic areas
  - Keratosis pilaris-like spinous follicular papules on trunk

Histology

- Dense **lichenoid interface dermatitis** of follicular epithelium at the level of the **infundibulum** w/ cytoid bodies, pigment incontinence, and dermal/**perifollicular fibrosis** (scar)

Table 3.54 Cicatricial Alopecias

Lymphocytic	Neutrophilic	Mixed
DLE	Folliculitis decalvans	Acne keloidalis
LPP	Dissecting cellulitis	Erosive pustular dermatosis
Frontal fibrosing alopecia		Acne necrotica
Pseudopelade of Brocq		
CCCA		
Alopecia mucinosa		
Keratosis follicularis spinulosa decalvans		

- **No interface dermatitis seen at DEJ (vs. present in DLE)**
- Lacks superficial and deep PV/PA inflammation (vs. DLE)

- DIF may show cytoid bodies + shaggy fibrin deposition at DEJ

Treatment

- Topical, oral, and/or intralesional CS
  - **Potent topical steroids are first line; TCIs** and minoxidil can be added
  - Oral steroids (i.e., prednisone 40–80 mg/d) if disease is aggressive or rapid
- Hydroxychloroquine most commonly used systemic treatment
- Doxycycline (second-line oral treatment); third-line options: naltrexone, acitretin, MTX, dapsone, MMF, PPAR-γ agonists (e.g., pioglitazone)
- For frontal fibrosing alopecia, finasteride/dutasteride are good options

Acne keloidalis nuchae

Clinical findings

- Firm, perifollicular papules on **occipital scalp and posterior neck** that can become keloidal and coalesce into plaques
- Most common in **Blacks**
- Eventual scarring alopecia

Histology

- Mixed (lymphoplasmacytic and neutrophilic) perifollicular inflammation at the isthmus and lower infundibulum
- Lamellar fibroplasia
- Loss of sebaceous glands

Treatment

- Topical or intralesional CS
- Systemic and topical antibiotics
- Surgical removal

Dissecting cellulitis of the scalp (Perifolliculitis capitis abscedens et suffodiens)

Epidemiology

- Most commonly young adult **Black men**

Clinical features

- Numerous inflammatory nodules forming **boggy, intercommunicating, purulent sinuses** with drainage → overlying scarring and alopecia (Fig. 3.95)
- Favors **vertex and occipital scalp**
- **Follicular occlusion tetrad**: acne conglobata, hidradenitis suppurativa, dissecting cellulitis, and pilonidal cysts

Histology

- Dense, pandermal neutrophilic inflammation with abscess formation, scarring, and sinus tracts
- Later inflammation may be lymphoplasmacytic or mixed, rather than purely neutrophilic

Treatment

- Very difficult to treat!
  - Options: **oral isotretinoin**, intralesional CS, **oral antibiotics** (e.g., tetracyclines, clindamycin/rifampin [if positive for *S. aureus*]), incision and drainage, excision, TNF-α inhibitors, intralesional injection of sinus tracts w/ sclerosing agents

Folliculitis decalvans

Epidemiology

- Most commonly in **Black men**

Clinical features

- Discrete, **crusted inflammatory papulopustules** arising **in crops** on vertex scalp → cicatricial alopecia
- Often colonized with ***S. aureus***

Histology

- Dense **neutrophilic** perifollicular inflammation at upper portion of follicles (same level as in LPP)
- Later inflammation often mixed (neutrophilic + lymphoplasmacytic)

Treatment

- Topical clindamycin, topical CS, selenium sulfide shampoo
- Oral tetracyclines, rifampin + clindamycin

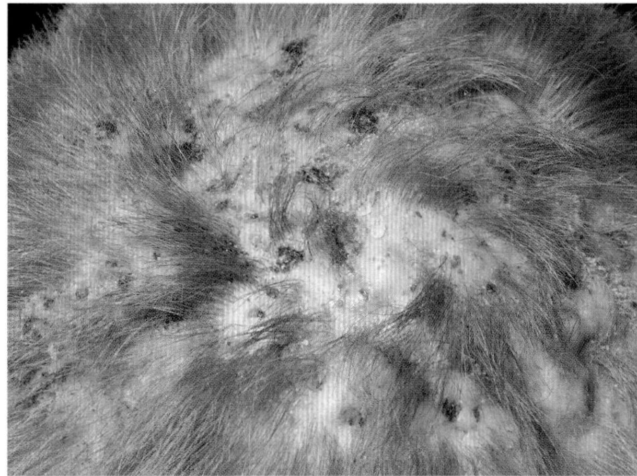

Fig. 3.95 Dissecting cellulitis of the scalp. (From McDonagh AJG. Dissecting cellulitis of the scalp. In: Lebwohl MG, Heymann WR, Berth-Jones J, Coulson I. *Treatment of Skin Disease: Comprehensive Therapeutic Strategies*. 4th ed. Philadelphia: Elsevier; 2014:195–196.)

Traction alopecia

Epidemiology

- Most commonly in **Black females**

Pathogenesis

- Tension from repeated **traumatic hairstyles** (e.g., tight ponytails, braids, weaves, extensions, and rollers)

Clinical features

- Hair loss/thinning along the frontotemporal hairline
- Biphasic in nature—initially temporary, but can become permanent
- "Fringe sign" = preservation of frontal rim of hair

Histology

- Non-scarring phase (early): histology same as trichotillomania
- Scarring phase (late): columns of connective tissue replace hair follicles; markedly decreased number of terminal hairs

Treatment

- Can try topical/IL steroids, minoxidil, PRP but may need hair transplantation

Hair shaft abnormalities

- Many of these disorders have been discussed elsewhere but are briefly reviewed here
- Hair shaft abnormalities are divided into those that are associated with **increased hair fragility** and those that are **not associated with increased hair fragility**
- See Table 3.55

Hypertrichosis and hirsutism

Hypertrichosis

- Definition: excessive hair growth
  - Versus hirsutism: female with ↑ terminal hair growth in a "male distribution" (upper lip, cheeks, central chest)
- Vellus hairs more so than terminal hairs
- May be generalized versus localized, congenital (see Chapter 4) versus acquired
- Most testable forms:
  - Acquired hypertrichosis lanuginosa
    - Paraneoplastic disease a/w **lung, colon, and breast cancer**
    - Lanugo hair quickly forms over entire body, especially **face → "simian" appearance**
  - Acquired generalized hypertrichosis
    - Slow growth of terminal hairs of medium thickness
    - Most prominent on forehead, temples, trunk, and flexor extremities
    - Reversible
    - **Medication-induced (most common): minoxidil, phenytoin, and cyclosporine**

Table 3.55 Structural Hair Abnormalities

Disease	Affected Gene/Pathogenesis	Findings
Structural hair abnormalities with increased hair fragility		
Bubble Hair	**Traumatic heat styling**	Young women with a localized area of uneven, fragile hairs Light microcopy: **hair shafts w/ large, irregularly spaced "bubbles"** that expand and thin the hair cortex → hair fractures at the site of larger bubbles
Monilethrix	Autosomal dominant inheritance: hair cortex-specific keratin genes ***KRT86*** (most often; previously referred to as *hHb6*) and ***KRT81*** (*hHb1*) AR inheritance: ***Dsg4***	p/w Normal-appearing hair at birth Within first few months of life, hairs are replaced by **short**, **fragile**, **brittle hair** w/ **perifollicular erythema** and **follicular hyperkeratosis** Scalp usually only site affected (occasionally eyebrows, eyelashes) Hairs have **uniform elliptical nodes** of normal thickness and **intermittent abnormal constrictions**
Pili torti	**Menkes kinky hair disease**: XLR, ***ATP7A*** (→ defective copper transport) **Bjornstad/Crandall syndrome**: autosomal recessive, *BCS1L* gene Netherton's: *SPINK5* gene (encodes serine protease inhibitor LEKTI) Urea cycle defects (**citrullinemia, argininosuccinic aciduria)** Acquired pili torti: **anorexia nervosa** and **oral retinoids**	Flattened shaft and twisting of hair fiber on its own axis Inherited forms: hair abnormal from birth, or normal at birth and then during infancy becomes replaced by brittle and fragile hair; body hair also sparse to absent; no treatment exists but improves at puberty Menkes: **pili torti** (sparse, lusterless hair on scalp/brows/lashes) and **trichorrhexis nodosa**; growth failure, wormian bones/fractures; neurologic abnormalities (seizures, lethargy, intellectual and psychomotor impariment, hypertonia), "**Cupid's bow**" upper lip; **doughy skin; diffuse hypopigmentation** (tyrosinase requires copper!) Bjornstad: pili torti + **hearing loss** **Crandall** syndrome = Bjornstad syndrome + **hypogonadism** (mnemonic "Crandall's = Cranberry balls") Bazex-Dupre-Christol: pili torti, **basal cell carcinomas, milia, follicular atrophoderma** (dorsal hands/feet, face, elbows, knees), **hypohidrosis, hypotrichosis** (+/– pili torti)
Trichorrhexis invaginata ("bamboo hair")	Netherton syndrome: ***SPINK5*** gene (encodes serine protease inhibitor LEKTI)	Netherton's: ichthyosis linearis circumflexa, atopy and hair abnormality (trichorrhexis invaginata, trichorrhexis nodosa) Hair abnormality arises in infancy, p/w **short**, **sparse and very fragile hair** Hair breakage points arise at intussusceptions of distal shaft ("ball") into proximal shaft ("socket") May also see proximal shafts with a **golf tee-shaped appearance**

Table 3.55 Structural Hair Abnormalities—cont'd

Disease	Affected Gene/Pathogenesis	Findings
Trichorrhexis nodosa	Congenital: **argininosuccinic aciduria (autosomal recessive**, arginosuccinate lyase) or **citrullinemia** (autosomal recessive, arginosuccinate synthetase) most commonly; also may see in Menkes, trichothiodystrophy, Netherton's Acquired (three variants): 1. *proximal* trichorrhexis nodosa: arises in patients after years of hair straightening 2. *distal* trichorrhexis nodosa: due to acquired, cumulative, cuticular damage 3. *circumscribed* trichorrhexis nodosa: affects scalp, moustache, or beard	**Most common** of all the structural hair abnormalities Characterized on light microscopic examination by a hair shaft fracture w/ adjacent fragments splaying out, resembling the **ends of two brushes pushed against each other** Citrullinemia: pili torti, trichorrhexis nodosa, hyperammonemia, lethargy, vomiting, seizures, CNS symptoms Argininosuccinic aciduria: pili torti, trichorrhexis nodosa, hyperammonemia, vomiting, seizures Neonatal form more severe—failure to thrive, hepatomegaly, lethargy Adult-onset form less severe but still have intellectual impairment and ataxia Treat with restricted protein diet + arginine supplementation; liver transplant may be curative
Trichothiodystrophy	AR disorder characterized by **sulfur-deficient hair**; due to several related genetic defects involving **TFIIH/XPD-XPB complex**	Microscopy: transverse fractures (**trichoschisis**), and **alternating light and dark bands under polarizing light** Clinical: may be isolated finding or **a/w PIBIDS**
Structural hair abnormalities without increased hair fragility		
Acquired progressive kinking of the hair	**Can be early sign of AGA**	Young men develop progressively curly, frizzy, lusterless hair in androgenetic areas → progresses to AGA
Loose anagen hair syndrome	Faulty cornification of inner root sheath → interference with normal interdigitation of the IRS cuticle and the hair cuticle → poorly-anchored anagen hairs	**Classic presentation**: **young girl w/ short blond hair that seldom needs to be cut**; see diffuse or patchy alopecia No ↑ hair fragility Anagen **hairs can be easily and painlessly pulled** from the scalp Hair microscopy: ruffled proximal cuticle, absence of root sheath, and a bent matrix
Pili annulati ("ringed hair")	Sporadic or autosomal dominant	Ringed hair with **light and dark bands** due to air-filled spaces **Do NOT need polarized light to see (vs. trichothiodystrophy)**
Pili bifurcate	–	Multiple bifurcations of the hair shaft; each ramus has its own cuticle
Pili multigemini	–	Multiple hair shafts arise from one papilla Each hair fiber has its own IRS but all the fibers are surrounded by a common ORS Most commonly occurs on **beard area**
Pili trianguli et canaliculi (aka "spun glass hair," "uncombable hair")	Uncombable hair syndrome: *PADI3* is most commonly mutated gene, but *TGM3* or *TCHH* can be mutated as well	Hair w/ **"spun glass" appearance** and **difficulty with combing** Due to light reflection off of flattened hair surfaces; **hairs have triangular shape** on cross-section w/ **longitudinal grooves** best seen by scanning electron microscopy
Wooly hair syndromes	Naxos disease (diffuse non-epidermolytic PPK, **RVH** and wooly hair): **plakoglobin** mutations Carvajal syndrome (striate epidermolytic PPK, **LVH**, wooly hair): **desmoplakin** mutations	Microscopy: elliptical cross-sections, axial twisting, +/– trichorrhexis nodosa Mnemonic: "Carvaja**L** has **L**VH" (vs. RVH in Naxos)
Wooly hair nevus	–	Well-defined, circumscribed patch of wooly hair

XLR, *x-linked recessive;* CNS, *central nervous system;* PIBIDS, *photosensitivity, ichthyosis, brittle hair, intellectual impairment, decreased fertility and short stature;* PPK, *palmoplantar keratoderma;* RVH, *right ventricular hypertrophy;* LVH, *left ventricular hypertrophy.*
Data from Sperling LC, Sinclair RD, El Shabrawi-Caelen L. Alopecias. In: Bolognia JL, Schaffer JV, Cerroni L. Dermatology. *4th ed. Philadelphia: Elsevier; 2018: 1162–1187.*

- Other causes: hypothyroidism, POEMS, porphyria, advanced HIV, dermatomyositis and SLE, and **anorexia nervosa**

▪ Acquired trichomegaly (primarily of eyelashes)
  - May be a/w **HIV**
  - May be a/w meds (most common cause of acquired): cyclosporine, phenytoin, minoxidil, EGFR inhibitors, topiramate, tacrolimus, IFN-α, danazol, **prostaglandin F-2α, and topical latanoprost/ bimatoprost**

▪ Localized hypertrichosis
  - Causes: **Becker's nevus**, melanocytic nevi, **spinal dysraphism** w/ **"hair collar sign," aplasia cutis** w/ **"hair collar sign,"** trauma (areas of chronic rubbing, or fractured limbs w/ plaster casts), or medication-induced (**prostaglandin analogs**, PUVA sites)

Hirsutism

- Definition: ↑ terminal hair growth in a **female**, with a **"male pattern"** (e.g., upper lip, cheeks, central chest, suprapubic area, back)
- Common; affects 5%–10% of women of reproductive age
- Related to ↑ **androgens** (from ovary or adrenal glands) or end-organ sensitivity to androgens from adrenal glands and ovaries
  - **DHEA-S** = marker for **adrenal** androgens
  - Δ-4-androstenedione = marker for ovarian androgens

- Useful rules of thumb:
  - **Rapid-onset** hirsutism w/ fast evolution → **tumor** (adrenal, ovarian, or pituitary)
  - Hirsutism limited to **areola**, **lateral face/neck** → **ovarian** source most likely
  - **Central hirsutism** (pubic triangle to upper abdominal area and sternal area up to chin) → **adrenal** most likely
  - Lateral face and back → iatrogenic hirsutism
- Labs: recommendations vary, but experts recommend checking total **testosterone**, **DHEA-S**, **24-hour urine cortisol**, Δ-4-androstenedione, SHBG, prolactin, and 3-α-androstanediol glucuronide (metabolite of DHT)
  - May add on 17-OH-progesterone (elevated in setting of CAH due to 21-hydroxylase deficiency) and other additional labs depending on results of these initial studies (Fig. 3.96)
- Four major causes:
  - PCOS (accounts for majority)
    - Characterized by infertility, large polycystic ovaries, secondary amenorrhea, and/or **menstrual cycle irregularities**
    - a/w **Hirsutism** (**90%**), **acne** (**70%**), obesity (50%), AGA, acanthosis nigricans, and insulin resistance
    - Labs: ↓ **FSH**, ↑ **LH**, **LH:FSH ratio > 3**, ↑ **testosterone**, ↑ estrone, ↓ SHBG, and **normal DHEA-S**
  - Congenital adrenal hyperplasia (CAH)
    - May be due to a variety of enzyme deficiencies but 95% of CAH is due to **21-hydroxylase** deficiency
      - Classic "salt-wasting form:" presents w/ **salt-wasting** in first 2 weeks of life w/ dehydration and electrolyte abnormalities (due to absence of cortisol); **female infants have ambiguous genitalia and virilization**; both sexes have premature growth of axillary and pubic hair during early childhood; ↑ **17-OH-progesterone** (build-up due to lack of 21-hydroxylase function), ↑ **DHEA-S**, ↑↑ ACTH, and normal or mildly elevated testosterone
    - Check 17-hydroxyprogesterone and ACTH stimulation test to r/o late-onset CAH (partial deficiency of 21-hydroxylase or other enzymes)
  - Neoplastic
    - If virilization also present or **very high testosterone** (**>200 ng/dL**) → **neoplastic etiology** most likely (e.g., arrhenoblastomas, Leydig cell tumors)
    - ↑↑↑ **Testosterone but normal DHEA-S** → **ovarian** tumor
    - ↑↑ **Testosterone and** ↑↑↑ **DHEA-S** → **adrenal tumor**
  - Constitutional hirsutism
    - No hormonal abnormalities present
    - More common in certain ethnicities (e.g., Southern/Eastern European, SW Asian)
- Treatment
  - **Antiandrogens** (e.g., spironolactone, leuprolide, flutamide, finasteride), **OCPs**, topical eflornithine, metformin, depilatory methods/agents, laser hair removal

Nail disorders

- Anatomy of the nail (Fig. 3.97)
- Disturbances of nail sites can → various clinical manifestations (Fig. 3.98; Table 3.56)

Mucosal disorders

- See Tables 3.57 and 3.58

3.26 PIGMENTARY DISORDERS

Disorders of hypopigmentation and depigmentation

Vitiligo

Epidemiology

- Average age of onset = 20 yo; females acquire disease earlier

Pathogenesis

- Multifactorial disease with genetic and non-genetic causes
- Absence of functional melanocytes secondary to **melanocyte destruction**
- Various hypotheses exist for the pathogenesis of vitiligo:
  - An **autoimmune theory** suggests that alterations in cellular or humoral immunity → melanocyte destruction
    - IFN-γ, CXCL10, IL-22 are important
    - Possibly secondary to cytotoxic activity of autoreactive T cells against melanocytes
  - Other theories: intrinsic defect in the structure/function of melanocytes, dysregulation of the nervous system → melanocyte damage, cytotoxic metabolites (extrinsic or intrinsic), biochemical anomalies (e.g., biopterin pathways), and oxidative stress (e.g., ↓ catalase levels, ↓WNT signaling); ↑PGF2α
- Genetics include incomplete penetrance, genetic heterogeneity, and multiple susceptibility loci (e.g., NLRP1, CTLA4, MC1R, FOXP3)
- Radiotherapy (e.g. external beam radiation) may cause vitiligo

Clinical features

- **Well-circumscribed, depigmented**, and asymptomatic macules/patches
  - Sites of predilection: fingers, wrists, axillae, groin, genital, and facial (around mouth/eyes)
  - Areas can enlarge over time, slowly, or rapidly
  - Köebner phenomenon: associated w/ more progressive course
- Can occur anywhere and is often classified as:
  - Acrofacial: face + distal extremities
  - Segmental: primarily in children; face most commonly; **stops at midline**; progresses quickly then stabilizes; **leukotrichia** seen frequently; less responsive to treatment
  - Focal: ≥1 macule(s) in an area, but not segmental
  - Mucosal: Wood lamp can be helpful
  - **Generalized/vulgaris (most common type)**: generalized patches
  - Mixed: segmental + generalized types
  - Universal (>80% of skin)

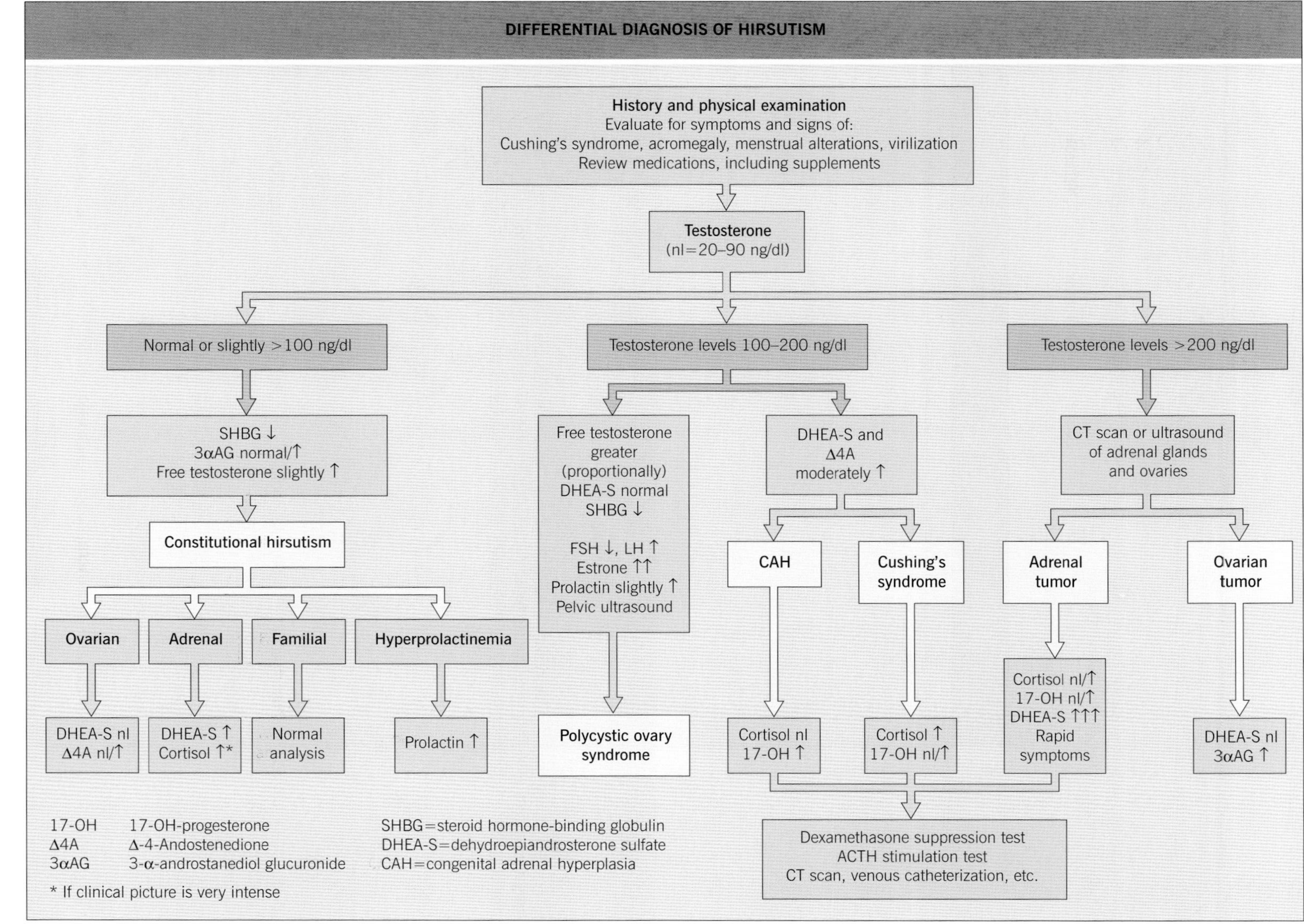

Fig. 3.96 Differential diagnosis of hirsutism. The optimum time to assess circulating follicle-stimulating hormone *(FSH)* and luteinizing hormone *(LH)* levels is 3–5 days after cessation of menses. (From Camacho FM. Hypertrichosis and hirsutism. In: Bolognia JL, Schaffer JV, Cerroni L. *Dermatology*. 4th ed. Philadelphia: Elsevier; 2018:1188–1202.)

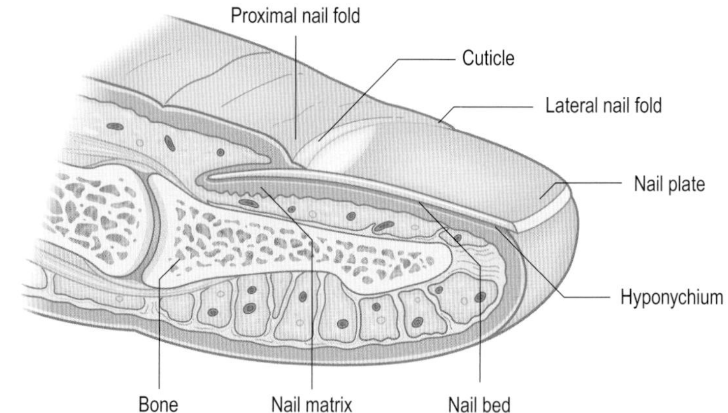

Fig. 3.97 Longitudinal drawing of the nail apparatus. (From Billingsley EM. Nail surgery. In: Vidimos AT, Ammirati CT, Poblete-Lopez C, Eds. *Requisites in Dermatology: Dermatologic Surgery*. Philadelphia: Elsevier; 2009:189–197.)

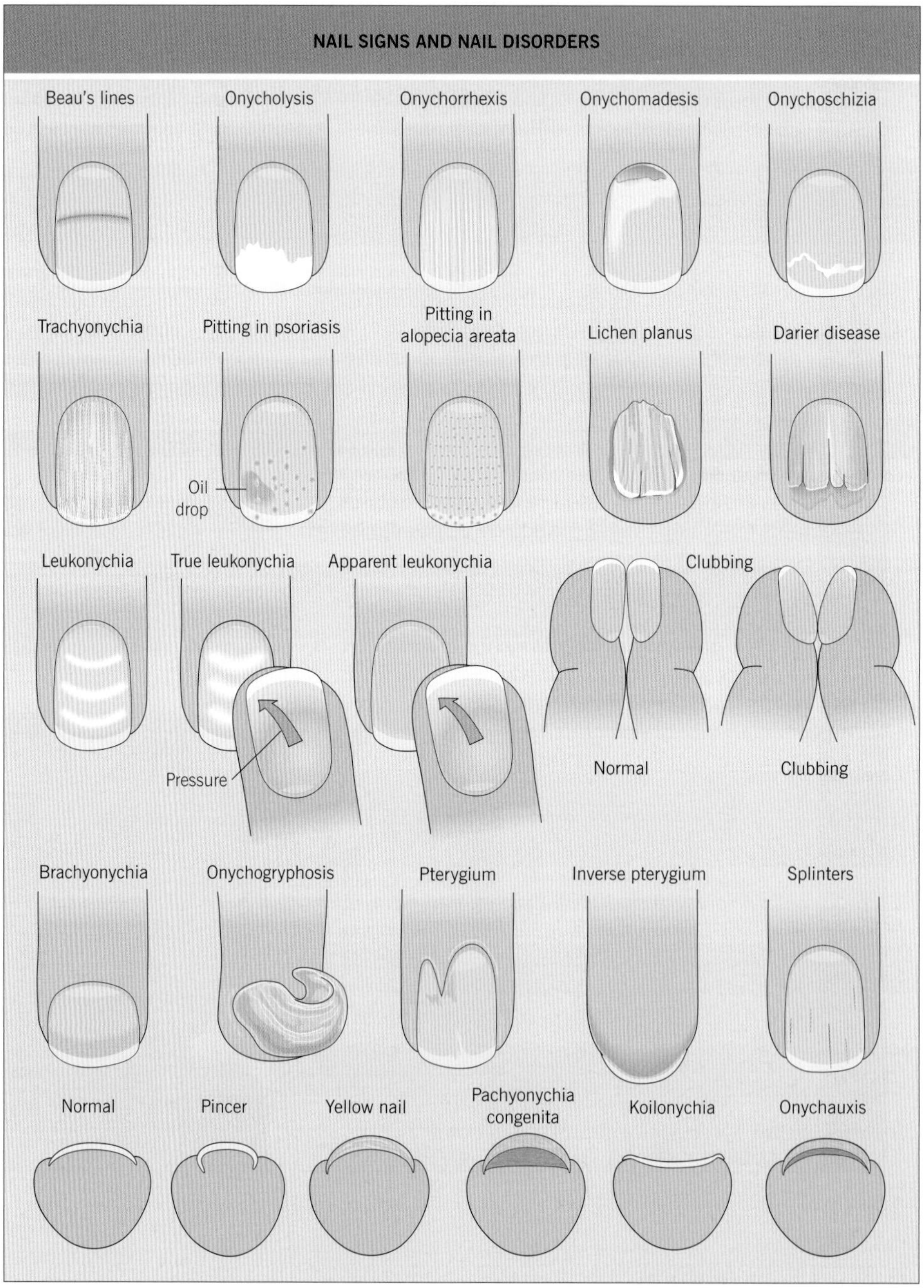

Fig. 3.98 Nail signs and disorders. (From Tosti A, Piraccini BM. Nail disorders. In: Bolognia JL, Jorizzo JL, Schaffer JV. *Dermatology*. 3rd ed. Philadelphia: Elsevier; 2012:1129–1147.)

Table 3.56 High-Yield Nail Disorders

Nail Sign/Disorder	Cause/Site of Injury	Associations
Beau's lines	Matrix (proximal)—**temporary stoppage of growth**	Usually due to mechanical trauma or skin diseases of proximal fold; also **chemotherapy**, stress on body (e.g., childbirth), **systemic illness**, major injury
Onychomadesis	Matrix (proximal)—temporary stoppage of growth	Same as above; also seen with ***coxsackievirus*** infection (hand-foot-mouth disease)
Pitting	Matrix (proximal)	**Psoriasis** **Alopecia areata** (**geometric, regularly distributed** grid-like small superficial pits)
Onychorrhexis (brittle nails)	Matrix	Lichen planus Chronic wet work, frequent nail polish use, eating disorders
Trachyonychia (sandpaper nails)	Matrix	**Alopecia areata** (children > adults) Lichen planus, psoriasis, and other autoimmune processes
True leukonychia	Matrix	Punctate: usually from trauma in kids Striate: fingernails in women from **manicures**; great toenails from shoe trauma; **Mee's lines** from arsenic and thallium Diffuse: rare—may be congenital
Koilonychia	Matrix	Normal in kids; in adults may be associated w/ **iron deficiency** (e.g., **Plummer-Vinson syndrome**)
Onycholysis	Nail plate detachment (distal)	**Psoriasis** **Onychomycosis** Trauma (e.g., great toenails with shoes), drugs (e.g., **photo-onycholysis w/ tetracyclines/ fluoroquinolones/chloramphenicol/psoralens + UV**) Systemic causes (e.g., thyroid issues)
Onychauxis	Subungual hyperkeratosis → thickened nail	Causes include psoriasis, onychomycosis, eczema
Onychocryptosis (ingrown nail)	Excess lateral nail growth into nailfold → pseudo-foreign body reaction/ inflammation	None, but may be mimicked by periungal pyogenic granuloma (which may be due to various meds like isotretinoin, protease inhibitors, and EGFR inhibitors)
Apparent leukonychia	Nail bed edema (white color that **fades w/ pressure**)	Chemotherapy Chronic hypoalbuminemia (**Muehrcke's nails** = transverse white bands parallel to lunula) Liver cirrhosis (**Terry's nails** = leukonychia of most of nail plate) Chronic renal disease w/ hemodialysis (**half and half nails** – leukonychia of half nail plate)
Longitudinal erythronychia	Erythema from matrix to distal onychodermal band	Seen in inflammatory conditions (e.g., lichen planus, **Darier disease**)
Splinter hemorrhages	Damage to nail bed capillaries	Distal (usually from **trauma**, psoriasis, onychomycosis) Proximal (**endocarditis**, vasculitis, trichinosis, APLS)—rarer
Longitudinal melanonychia	Melanin within nail plate (e.g., melanocyte activation or hyperplasia)	Matrix melanoma/nevus Non-melanocytic tumors Melanocyte activation (2/2 racial; e.g., **African Americans**), HIV, drugs (e.g., **AZT**, antimalarials, minocycline, gold), Addison's disease, Peutz-Jegher/**Laugier-Hunziker** syndrome, onychomycosis (*Trichophtyon rubrum,* ***Scytalidium*** **spp.**)
Hutchinson's sign	Pigmentation in proximal nail fold w/ longitudinal melanonychia	May be **sign of nail melanoma**, particularly in adults
Green nail syndrome	Green staining of nail plate due to **pyocanin** from *Pseudomonas*	Factors → infection or wet work (e.g., barbers, dishwashers), nail trauma, harsh exposures of note, **black nails may be caused by** ***Proteus mirabilis*** or *T. rubrum*
Red lunulae	Erythema of lunulae	**SLE, alopecia areata, rheumatoid arthritis, dermatomyositis, cardiac failure**, cirrhosis, lymphogranuloma venereum, psoriasis, vitiligo, chronic urticaria, LS&A, **carbon monoxide** poisoning, COPD
Brachyonychia	Shortening of distal phalynx → racquet thumb	Congenital finding—may be seen in **Rubinstein-Taybi** syndrome
Nail-Patella syndrome	**Mutation of** ***LMX1B*** (autosomal dominant)	Manifestations include: nail abnormalities (radial side of thumbs most commonly—**triangle-shaped lunula** may occur), bone findings (e.g., **absent/ underdeveloped patellae, iliac horns**), **nephropathy**/renal insufficiency, **Lester iris** (pigmentation of pupillary margin of iris)
Clubbing	Soft tissue growth in distal digit → curved, enlarged nail plate	Various causes, but **pulmonary** most common in acquired type; HIV is another reported cause
Yellow nail syndrome	Arrest in nail growth → yellow color, absent cuticle, thickening/curved (transversely and longitudinally)	A/w **lymphedema, pleural effusions, bronchiectasis**, chronic pulmonary infection/sinusitis
Acute paronychia	***Staphylococcus aureus*** or *Streptococcus pyogenes* infection → inflamed tender digit	Usually due to trauma Treat with drainage of abscess and treatment of infection

Continued

Table 3.56 High-Yield Nail Disorders—cont'd

Nail Sign/Disorder	Cause/Site of Injury	Associations
Chronic paronychia	Inflammation of proximal nail fold → fingernail issues and cuticle loss	Usually due to continuous contact exposure/**wet work** (e.g., food handlers) **Secondary infection with *Candida* common**
Habit-tic deformity	Due to manipulation of mid-cuticle of thumb → central longitudinal depression	**Median canaliform dystrophy may be subtype with "inverted fir tree" appearance**
Pincer nails	Overcurvature of nail plate	Can → pain due to pinching of distal nail bed Hereditary vs. acquired (trauma from shoes) **Lateral matricectomy is ToC**; r/o subungual exostosis
Onychomatricoma	Tumor → thickening of nail plate w/ multiple longitudinal hollow spaces (contain tumor)	Middle-aged patients on fingernails typically Frontal view of nail: **holes in thick free margin** Yellow-white thick longitudinal nail portion w/ splinter hemorrhages
Subungual exostosis	Subungual bony growth → nodule → nail plate elevation	Usually due to trauma in young patients; most commonly on hallux **X-ray** confirms diagnosis
Myxoid cysts (digital mucous cyst)	Outpouching of DIP joint space via a tract	**Most common nail tumor** Classic appearance is small **translucent nodule close to proximal nail fold** with nail plate groove distally
Pterygium unguis	Scarring between eponychium and matrix	Classically seen in **lichen planus**
Pterygium inversum unguis	Attachment of distal nailbed to ventral nail plate	a/w CTDs, esp. **scleroderma**

Table 3.57 High-Yield Mucosal Disorders

Disorder/Finding	Clinical Findings	Interesting Facts/Treatment
Fordyce granules (spots)	Pinpoint white-yellow papules on **vermillion and buccal mucosa**	Ectopic sebaceous glands like meibomian (eyelids), **Montgomery (areolae), Tyson (labia minora, prepuce)**
Geographic tongue	Well-demarcated patches of atrophy with surrounding erythema surrounded by white/yellow scalloped border on dorsal tongue	**A/w psoriasis** and atopy; histologically looks like psoriasis
Fissured tongue	Grooves on dorsum of tongue which can appear deep	A/w **Melkersson-Rosenthal syndrome** (along w/ recurrent or permanent facial nerve paralysis and swelling of face/lips), Down syndrome, Cowden syndrome
Torus palatinus	Bony prominence in middle of hard palate (normal variant)	
Hairy tongue	Dorsum of tongue with dark hairy-like appearance due to keratin retention → hypertrophic papillae from ↓ sloughing Color may be due to **bacteria** (porphyrin production), tobacco, food	Risk factors: **bad hygiene, smoking**, hot drinks Can treat with tongue scraper +/– dilute H_2O_2
Smooth tongue (atrophic glossitis)	**Atrophy of papillae** → smooth appearance Can be tender, sensitive, burning May assume a beefy red appearance	May be due to **vitamin deficiency** (e.g., B1, B2, B6, B12, iron (e.g., Plummer-Vinson), folate), or other disorders (e.g., Sjögren's syndrome)
Median rhomboid glossitis	Well-circumscribed erythematous smooth area on central dorsum of tongue (in front of **circumvallate papillae**; possibly a developmental defect)	A/w **oral candidiasis** May be sign of HIV infection or DM2 if more extensive Differentiate from herpetic geometric glossitis (geometrically shaped fissured patch on dorsal tongue a/w HSV1)
Necrotizing ulcerative gingivitis	**Gingivae are necrotic**, painful, swollen, red, bloody, and have ulcerated "punched out" interdental papillae due to **mixed bacterial infection**	Risk factors: immunosuppression, **malnutrition**, stress, smoking, poor oral hygiene
Fibroma	Pink smooth papule usually on buccal mucosa Usually along **bite line**	**#1 tumor of oral cavity** Middle aged women mainly
Cutaneous sinus of dental origin	Sequela of dental caries in which infectious abscess extends to apex of tooth, then medullary bone, then finally oral mucosal surface/facial skin where it drains Red eroded papule adjacent to teeth **Mandibular > maxillary**	
White sponge nevus	White, spongy well-defined small plaques on **buccal mucosa** most commonly, but can be found in other oral areas	**Keratin 4 and 13 mutation**
Morsicatio buccarum	White ragged, shredded surface changes of anterior buccal mucosa bilaterally due to **habitual chewing** of mucosa	
Gingival enlargement (drug)	Gingival growth seen in first year of med use Worse if oral hygiene is poor	Culprits: **phenytoin, nifedipine, cyclosporine**, though other anticonvulsants and CCBs can also cause

Table 3.57 High-Yield Mucosal Disorders—cont'd

Disorder/Finding	Clinical Findings	Interesting Facts/Treatment
Contact stomatitis	Mostly due to **cinnamon flavoring** and **dental amalgam** may see erythematous and/or white eroded, ulcerated patches, which may be adjacent to amalgam sites	Histologically, lichenoid mucositis is seen
Peripheral ossifying fibroma	Painful nodule usually < 2 cm on gingival mucosa Can → bone loss, tooth damage so best to excise	Histologically, fibroblast bands, calcifications, collagen and ↑ endothelial cells w/in periodontal ligament
Peripheral giant cell granuloma	Soft bleeding red papule < 2 cm typically on incisor/canine mandibular gingiva More aggressive in kids and can → local destruction so best to excise	Histologically, multinucleated giant cells w/ spindle-shaped mesnenchymal cells
Labial melanotic macule	Small brown/black/gray/blue maucles on vermillion lips (female > male) On dermoscopy, structureless pattern most likely to be malignant	Histologically, ↑ melanin in basal epidermis w/ ↑ melanophages and no change in # melanocytes
Amalgam tattoo	Most common oral pigmentation—homogeneous blue color	Due to dental amalgam deposition (mercury, then silver) into oral mucosa
Oral melanoacanthoma	Dark macules/papules that can be up to few cm; due to keratinocyte and dendritic melanocyte (S100+) proliferation due to trauma/mastication	See starburst pattern with peripheral streaks on dermoscopy
Recurrent aphthous stomatitis	Painful small oval ulcers—**white/gray base with erythematous border**, on **non-keratinized mucosa** Types are **minor** (most common, ulcers < 5 mm), **major** (ulcers larger (>1 cm), deeper, and last longer) and **herpetiform** (multiple small grouped ulcers which look like HSV infection)	Multifactorial etiology with a wide differential (r/o vitamin deficiencies, systemic disorders) M > F, teenagers most commonly Topical CS and/or local anesthetics first line, with colchicine or dapsone if needed
Eosinophilic ulcer of the oral mucosa	Rare self-limited ulceration of posterior **tongue** > mucosa indurated border with overlying pseudomembrane enlarge quickly, up to 1–2 cm	Plentiful eosinophils on biopsy likely due to trauma; some a/w HIV spontaneous resolution
Orofacial granulomatosis	Chronic swelling of lips ("granulomatous cheilitis"—may be seen in **Melkersson-Rosenthal** syndrome; upper lips then lower lips), face, and oral region young adults primarily	Non-caseating granulomas on histology May be seen in sarcoidosis or Crohn's disease
Oral leukoplakia/erythroplakia	<u>Leukoplakia</u> = well-defined white patch/plaque; risk of malignant transformation higher in nonhomogeneous (e.g., proliferative verrucous leukoplakia) vs. homogeneous Premalignant (to SCC) <u>Erythroplakia</u> = well-defined red patch/plaque **Higher likelihood of malignancy** (SCCIS, SCC) Risk factors are tobacco, alcohol, **high risk HPV**	Leukoplakia = most common premalignant oral lesion, M > F, peaks at > 50 yo A/w tobacco, alcohol, nut chewing ("betel quid chewing") Can occur on any mucosal site Erythroplakia is rare Most commonly on buccal mucosa, palate, ventral tongue, floor of mouth For both findings, obtaining biopsy is the first step
Mucocele	Soft translucent to bluish papule on mucosa (lower labial mucosa most commonly) Due to rupture of minor salivary gland duct → mucus in the submucosal tissue/pseudocyst formation	
Cheilitis exfoliativa	Desquamative/exfoliative inflammatory condition of lips → red/denuded/tender appearance	1°: upper lip; scaly/crusty 2°: lower lip; may be due to seborrheic dermatitis, atopic dermatitis or other factors
Angular cheilitis (perleche)	Erythema and fissuring involving labial commisures – irritant in nature +/– 2° *Candida* or staphylococcal infection	RFs: elderly (esp. w/ **dentures**), **riboflavin deficiency**, thumb sucking, Down syndrome, AIDS
Cheilitis glandularis	Enlargement/eversion of **lower lip** with pinpoint erythema (inflammation of secretory ducts) + **sticky mucoid film**; feels nodular due to enlarged glands	**Adult men with h/o sun exposure** **↑ SCC risk**
Pyostomatitis vegetans	Several to numerous **pinpoint yellow pustules** (in "serpentine" pattern) with red background → erosion/ulceration ("snail-track" ulcers) Labial, gingival; buccal mucosa most common **Deep edematous folds of buccal mucosa**	A/w **IBD (UC > Crohn's)** Treat IBD → improvement of dz M > F, young adults to middle-aged
Zoon's balanitis	Bright red, speckled, well-defined, smooth patches on **glans penis** (may have "kissing" lesions—e.g., glans of penis and inner foreskin) » vulva	M > F, middle-aged lichenoid interface dermatitis with ↑↑ **plasma cells** **Circumcision** curative in men

Table 3.58 Genodermatoses With Oral Cavity Manifestations

Genodermatosis	Mode of Inheritance	Description of Oral Cavity Lesion
Follicular keratosis (Darier disease)	Autosomal dominant	White papules on oral mucosa
Tuberous sclerosis	Autosomal dominant	Hemangiomas and gingival fibrous papules
Hereditary hemorrhagic telangiectasia (Osler-Weber-Rendu)	Autosomal dominant	Telangiectasias of oral and vermillion mucosa; hemorrhagic ulcers on gingival and oral mucosa
Lipoid proteinosis (Urbach–Wiethe disease)	Autosomal recessive	Cobblestone-appearing lesions in the oral mucosa
Gardner syndrome (FAP variant)	Autosomal dominant	Mandibular osteomas; dentigerous cysts
Peutz–Jeghers syndrome	Autosomal dominant	Mucosal hyperpigmentation, commonly found on the lip or periorally
Cowden syndrome	Autosomal dominant	Oral papillomas with a cobblestone pattern of the gingival, lip, buccal, and labial mucosa
Multiple endocrine neoplasia type 2B (MEN IIB)	Autosomal dominant	Mucosal neuromas on tongue and lips, can manifest on palatal, gingival, and buccal mucosa
Dystrophic epidermolysis bullosa	Autosomal dominant and recessive	Vesiculobullous lesions of the oral mucosa
Pachyonychia congenita	Autosomal dominant	Oral leukoplakia on buccal mucosa and tongue
White sponge nevus (of Cannon, hereditary mucosal leukokeratosis)	Autosomal dominant	Thick, spongy, white plaques on the gingival, labial, and buccal mucosa
Hereditary benign intraepithelial dyskeratosis	Autosomal dominant	White plaques on oral mucosa

From Maymone MBC, Greer RO, Burdine LK, et al. Benign oral mucosal lesions: clinical and pathological findings. J Am Acad Dermatol. *2019;81(1):43–56; Data from Wilder EG, Frieder J, Sulhan S, et al. Spectrum of orocutaneous disease associations: genodermatoses and inflammatory conditions.* J Am Acad Dermatol. *2017;77(5):809–830.*

- Various clinical variants of vitiligo: vitiligo ponctüe (confetti-like macules), inflammatory vitiligo (erythema at the edge of vitiligo), blue vitiligo (vitiligo in areas of post-inflammatory hyperpigmentation), and trichrome vitiligo (hypopigmented area between normal and depigmented skin)
- Insidious onset with unpredictable course

Associations

- A/w autoimmune diseases **(thyroid dysfunction [most common association]**, DM1, Addison's disease, and pernicious anemia), **halo nevi**, alopecia areata, and uveitis
- **Vogt-Koyanagi-Harada syndrome**: bilateral granulomatous uveitis, aseptic meningitis, dysacousia/deafness, poliosis/alopecia, vitiligo
- **Alezzandrini syndrome**: unilateral facial vitiligo/poliois with visual/hearing impairment on the same side
- Kabuki syndrome: developmental delay, congenital heart defects, skeletal anomalies/short stature, in addition to autoimmune issues (e.g., vitiligo)

Treatment

- Potent topical steroids, topical tacrolimus 0.1% (face, intertriginous areas), topical vitamin D analogs, **NB-UVB phototherapy**/excimer laser, PUVA, systemic immunosuppressants, surgical therapies (e.g., minipunch grafts, blister grafts, cellular grafts [i.e., **melanocyte-keratinocyte transplant procedure** for segmental vitiligo]), and depigmentation (only FDA-approved drug for vitiligo is **monobenzylether of hydroquinone**—depigments skin to create even pigmentation in severe cases; mequinol and monomethyl ether of hydroquinone work similarly)
- Emerging treatments: topical and oral **JAK** inhibitors (topical ruxolitinib is FDA approved), α-melanocyte-stimulating hormone (MSH) analogs + NB-UVB, helium-neon laser

Prognosis/clinical course

- **Bad prognostic indicators**: mucosal involvement, leukotrichia, trichrome lesions, koebnerization, inflammatory lesions, confetti-like depigmentation
- **Good prognostic indicators**: recent onset, younger, and lesions of face/neck/trunk
- **Follicular repigmentation** (migration of melanocytes from hair follicles) is typical

Halo nevus

- Melanocytic nevus with surrounding, well-demarcated hypo-/depigmented skin
  - Usually upper back; circumscribed scalp poliosis can occur if on scalp (seen in vitiligo as well)
- Histology: dense band-like infiltrate of lymphocytes and macrophages surrounding nests of melanocytes
- Many halo nevi regress over several months
- Warrants full skin exam as it can be melanoma marker; much more common in vitiligo patients

Chemical and physical agent-induced hypopigmentation

- Chemical leukodermas consisting of hypo-/depigmentation of skin/hair can result from various chemical and pharmacologic agents (e.g., **phenols/catechols,** arsenic, PPD, merury, imiquimod, azelaic acid, methylphenidate patches, and **sulfhydryls**)
  - The phenol derivative, monobenzyl ether of hydroquinone → depigmentation
  - Topical steroids, hydroquinone, chloroquine, and imatinib can → hypopigmentation
- Physical injuries from burns, freezing, radiation, lasers, surgery, UV irradiation, and physical trauma can damage melanocytes → hypo-/depigmentation

Idiopathic guttate hypomelanosis

- ↑ Incidence with age; more common in skin of color
- Thought to be related to sun exposure, aging, and genetics
- Presents w/ well-demarcated asymptomatic hypo-/depigmented macules on extremities

Progressive macular hypomelanosis

- Usually in **darker women from tropical regions**
- Unknown etiology, but *P. acnes* may be involved
- Presents w/ ill-defined, hypopigmented macules/patches on trunk/upper extremities, with no scale which can become confluent
- Treatments: benzoyl peroxide, topical clindamycin, UVA irradiation

Nevus anemicus

- Pale, typically unilateral area of skin (5–10 cm) with irregular outline
- Present **from birth** and typically on the trunk
- Caused by ↓ **blood flow/vasoconstriction in the dermal papilla due to localized hypersensitivity of blood vessels to catecholamines**; most noticeable when heat or emotional stress causes surrounding vasodilation with diascopy; nevus is no longer visible

Pigmentary mosaicism

Hypomelanosis of Ito

- Hypopigmentation **along Blaschko's lines** d/t mosaicism
- aka Linear nevoid hypopigmentation
- Present at birth or early infancy/childhood
- Affects trunk and extremities more commonly; can be unilateral or bilateral
- 30% of patients also have **CNS, musculoskeletal, or ophthalmologic abnormalities**

Nevus depigmentosus

- Hypomelanotic patches that are well-demarcated with irregular borders
- Typically appears in infancy on the trunk with distinct midline demarcation and less distinct lateral borders
- Throughout life it remains stable in size and distribution
- Histopathology: normal number of melanocytes with ↓ melanosomes in the melanocytes and keratinocytes
- **Segmental pigmentation disorder** represents a variant that can have a checkerboard pattern of hypopigmentation or hyperpigmentation

Disorders of hyperpigmentation

Melasma

Epidemiology

- Young to middle-aged women of Asian, Hispanic, African, or Middle Eastern descent

Pathogenesis

- Exact pathogenesis unknown; however, **UV irradiation and visible light** may activate hyperfunctional melanocytes to produce more melanin
- Exacerbating factors: **sun exposure, estrogen** (pregnancy, OCPs, and HRT), genetic influences, thyroid dysfunction, and meds (phenytoin and phototoxic drugs)

Clinical features

- Common acquired disorder characterized by symmetric, light to dark brown/gray irregular patches on face
  - Three patterns: centrofacial, malar, and mandibular
  - Four types: epidermal, dermal, mixed, and indeterminate
    - Epidermal areas accentuated with **Wood's lamp**, dermal areas are not

Histopathology

- ↑ Melanin in all layers of the epidermis, ↑ melanophages, and normal/↑ epidermal melanocytes

Treatment

- **Broad-spectrum sun protection/avoidance**
- Cosmetic camouflage
- Topical: **hydroquinone** (alone or in combination w/ topical steroid + retinoid), kojic acid, azelaic acid
- Procedural: chemical peels (e.g., glycolic, salicylic acid), fractional laser, IPL
- Systemic: Tranexamic acid 325 mg BID (SEs: venous thromboembolism, cerebral infarction)

Erythema dyschromicum perstans (ashy dermatosis) discussed in Section 3.3

Lichen planus pigmentosus

- Variant of LP in young to middle-aged adults with **skin types III–V** (may be associated with mustard oil, amla oil, and henna in Indian patients)
- Irregular oval, brown to gray-brown macules and patches in sun-exposed or intertriginous areas (Fig. 3.99)
  - Typically symmetric; may have reticulated or follicular pattern
- On histology, mild perivascular or band-like infiltrate in upper dermis, dermal melanophages, and basal cell degeneration; treatment option: topical tacrolimus, TCS, oral steroids, isotretionoin, dapsone

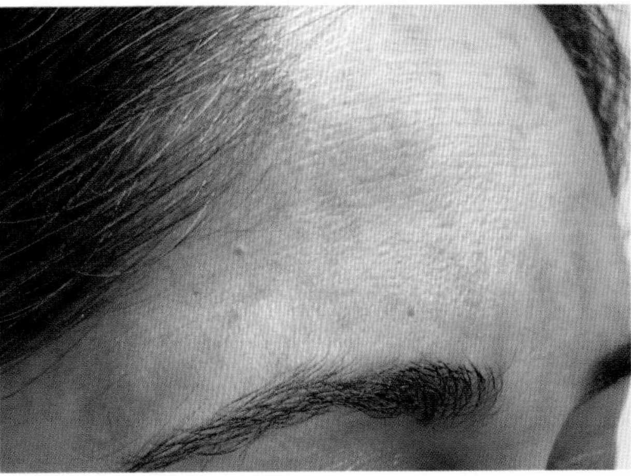

Fig. 3.99 Lichen planus pigmentosus of the face. (From Molinar VE, Taylor SC, Pandya AG. What's new in objective assessment and treatment of facial hyperpigmentation? *Dermatol Clin*. 2014;32[2]:123–135.)

Linear and whorled nevoid hypermelanosis

- Heterogeneous, sporadic mosaic skin condition in which a clone of skin cells leads to ↑ pigment production
- Hyperpigmented macular Blaschkoid whorls and streaks typically occurring before 1 year of age (Fig. 3.100)

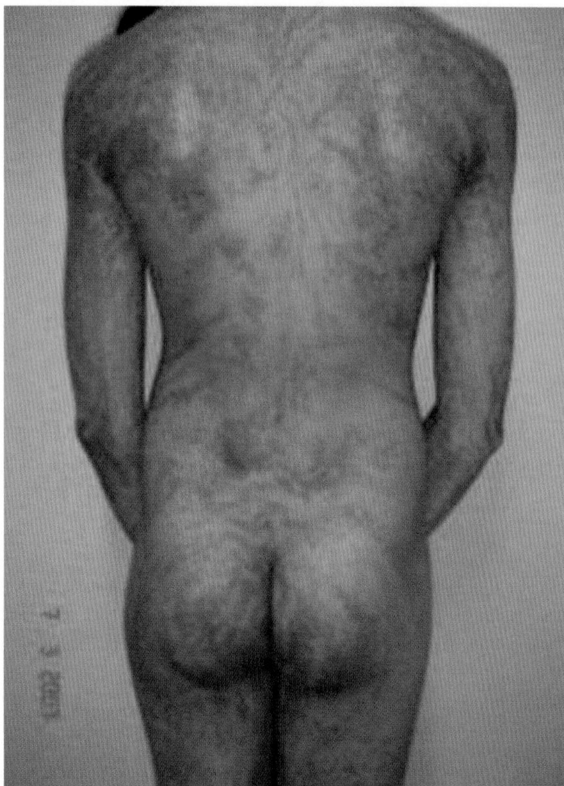

Fig. 3.100 Linear or circular arrangement of pigmented macules along the lines of Blaschko. (From Ertam I, Turk BG, Urkmez A, Kazandi A, Ozdemir F. Linear and whorled nevoid hypermelanosis: dermatoscopic features. *J Am Acad Dermatol*. 2009;60[2]:328–331.)

- +/− Associated systemic findings: neurologic, musculoskeletal, or cardiac
  - Persists indefinitely; no effective treatment

Prurigo pigmentosa

- Young adult F > M; Japanese especially
- Pruritic erythematous papules and papulovesicles on back/neck/chest, which develop rapidly and involute in < 1 week leaving residual reticulated macular hyperpigmentation
- Treatment: tetracyclines, dapsone

Familial progressive hyperpigmentation

- Autosomal dominant; mutation of KIT ligand gene (*KITLG*)
- Begins in infancy and hyperpigmentation increases in surface area with age
- Diffuse hyperpigmented patches involving palms, soles, lips, and conjunctiva

Endocrinopathies

- Addison's disease, Cushing's syndrome, acromegaly, and hyperthyroidism can all affect levels of ACTH and MSH, which can → generalized ↑ pigmentation.

Pigmentary demarcation lines (aka Futcher's lines, Voight lines, Ito's lines)

- Lines of demarcation between dorsal and ventral skin surfaces in which the dorsal side tends to be more hyperpigmented
- Often seen on anterolateral upper extremity and posteromedial thigh
- More apparent in darker-skinned individuals

4 Pediatric Dermatology

Brea Prindaville and Jennifer J. Schoch

CONTENTS LIST

4.1 NEONATAL DERMATOLOGY
4.2 VIRAL EXANTHEMS AND SELECT INFECTIOUS DISORDERS OF CHILDHOOD
4.3 INHERITED PIGMENTARY DISORDERS
4.4 EPIDERMOLYSIS BULLOSA
4.5 TUMOR SYNDROMES
4.6 VASCULAR TUMORS, MALFORMATIONS, AND RELATED VASCULAR DISORDERS
4.7 DISORDERS OF HAIR AND NAILS
4.8 INHERITED METABOLIC AND NUTRITIONAL DISORDERS
4.9 INHERITED CONNECTIVE TISSUE DISORDERS
4.10 AUTOINFLAMMATORY DISORDERS (PERIODIC FEVER SYNDROMES)
4.11 NEUROCUTANEOUS SYNDROMES
4.12 PREMATURE AGING SYNDROMES AND DNA REPAIR DISORDERS
4.13 PRIMARY IMMUNODEFICIENCY DISORDERS WITH CUTANEOUS MANIFESTATIONS
4.14 DISORDERS OF CORNIFICATION
4.15 MISCELLANEOUS PEDIATRIC DERMATOLOGIC DISORDERS

4.1 NEONATAL DERMATOLOGY

Newborn injuries may develop *in utero* or in the postpartum period, but most are sustained during birth (Table 4.1).

Transient skin lesions of the newborn are benign and generally do not require any active treatment as they are usually self-limited (Table 4.2).

Non-vascular birthmarks may be present at birth or during early childhood. Some are rarely associated with syndromes of systemic involvement, usually ocular, neurologic, and/or skeletal (Table 4.3).

Congenital malformations are present at birth, but may not become apparent until later in life. The majority of these are rare developmental abnormalities. Those on the face, scalp, or spine may herald abnormal neuroectodermal development, especially those in the midline. Common locations for congenital cysts and developmental remnants are detailed in Table 4.4. Congenital infections are discussed in Table 4.5.

4.2 VIRAL EXANTHEMS AND SELECT INFECTIOUS DISORDERS OF CHILDHOOD

Rubeola (measles, "first disease")

- **Outbreaks occur in areas where immunization rates are low**
- Caused by the measles virus (**RNA virus; paramyxovirus family**)
- Transmitted via **respiratory** droplets
- Infection begins in the nasopharynx or conjunctiva → subsequent spread to lymph nodes/blood (viremia)
- 1- to 2-week incubation period → fever and prodrome of cough/coryza/conjunctivitis (**3 Cs**)
  - Enanthem: **Koplik spots** (gray/white papules on buccal mucosa; resolve before exanthem)
  - Exanthem: morbilliform eruption (maculopapular) that **starts on frontal hairline and postauricular** areas, and subsequently spreads in a **cephalocaudal** fashion

Table 4.1 Newborn Injuries

Diagnosis	Epidemiology and Pathogenesis	Clinical Features	Histology and Laboratory Testing	Treatment	Prognosis/Clinical Course
Caput succedaneum	Occurs after prolonged labor Pressure during labor leads to extravasation of blood/serum **above the periosteum**	Diffuse swelling of the scalp; **crosses suture lines**; +/– ecchymoses		None	Presents at birth; resolves over several days Rarely leads to **halo scalp ring** (below)
Cephalohematoma	Occurs after prolonged labor Rupture of emissary/diploic veins during labor, resulting in **subperiosteal** hemorrhage	Unilateral swelling most commonly over parietal bones; **does not cross suture lines**; no bruising	CBC Bilirubin if severe	None	Presents hours to days after birth; resolves over weeks
Subgaleal hematoma	Occurs after traumatic/instrumented delivery Emissary veins rupture during traumatic delivery; bleeding into **subgaleal** space	Large area of dependent edema; +/– fluid waves; crosses suture lines and can extend from nape of neck to brow line; can lead to **anemia**, **DIC**, **and shock**	CBC; coagulation studies if severe	Close inpatient monitoring; fluids and blood products as indicated	Presents shortly after birth
Halo scalp ring	Occurs after prolonged labor Localized injury/soft tissue hypoxia during birth	Annular band of alopecia 1–4 cm wide over vertex, and scalp; associated caput; +/– necrosis and scarring		Wound care if necrotic; surgical excision for large areas; developmental monitoring	Presents shortly after birth; hair regrows in mild cases
Subcutaneous fat necrosis	Seen in **healthy** full-term and post-term neonates, and neonates receiving therapeutic hypothermia Hypoxic injury to fat; caused by trauma, perinatal complications	One to several indurated violaceous/red plaques/nodules; favors fat-rich anatomic sites, such as **back**, **cheeks**, buttocks, and thighs (Fig. 4.1)	Necrosis and crystallization of **fat with needle-shaped clefts**, granulomatous inflammatory infiltrate **Screen for hypercalcemia for 6 months**	Supportive care; avoid vitamin D supplementation; management of hypercalcemia as indicated	Presents in **first few weeks of life**; resolves over weeks to months; may leave scarring
Sclerema neonatorum	Occurs in **debilitated preterm** and term infants, now seen only in developing countries Impaired neonatal lipoenzymes and abundance of saturated fatty acids leads to fat solidification and sclerema	Sudden appearance of **diffuse hardening of skin** in first few weeks of life; spares palms, soles, and genitals	Lipid crystals form rosettes of fine needle-like clefts but **lacks granulomatous inflammation** (vs. SQ fat necrosis of newborn)	Intensive supportive care; systemic steroids controversial	**Most succumb to sepsis and shock**; process can reverse if underlying conditions are treated

Calcinosis cutis may be present on the heel from newborn blood draws (heel stick).
CBC, *Complete blood count;* DIC, *disseminated intravascular coagulation.*

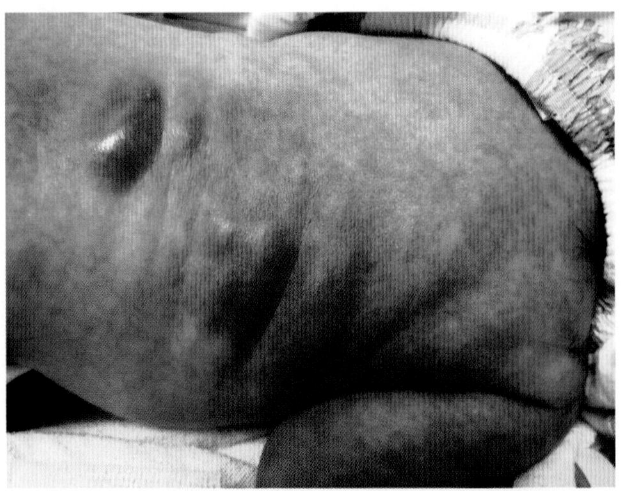

Fig. 4.1 Subcutaneous fat necrosis. (From Jensen CB, Galbraith SS. Iatrogenic and traumatic injuries. In: Eichenfield LF, Frieden IJ, eds. *Neonatal and Infant Dermatology*. 3rd ed. Philadelphia: Elsevier; 2015, pp 77–93.)

- Possible complications: upper or lower respiratory tract infection, otitis media, gastrointestinal (GI) symptoms, **encephalitis, myocarditis,** and **subacute sclerosing panencephalitis (occurs years after infection)**
- **Vitamin A** supplementation recommended for pediatric patients in communities with vitamin A deficiency, those aged 6 months to 2 years hospitalized with the disease, and those >6 months with risk factors
- Measles vaccine may be helpful if given within 3 days of exposure, and immunoglobulin may be given within 6 days of exposure
- Prevention of disease via a two-dose immunization series (**measles/mumps/rubella**); **first dose at age 12 to 15 months and second dose at age 4 to 6 years**

Rubella (German measles, "3-day measles," or "third disease")

- Caused by rubella virus (RNA virus; togaviridae family)
- Transmitted via respiratory droplets (like measles); nicknamed "3-day measles" because **resembles measles**

Table 4.2 Transient Skin Lesions of the Newborn

Diagnosis	Epidemiology and Pathogenesis	Clinical Features	Histology and Laboratory Testing	Prognosis/Clinical Course
Erythema toxicum neonatorm	**Full-term** infants, > 2500 g Common, may occur in up to one third of infants	Erythematous macules, papules, pustules, and wheals; may occur anywhere except palms and soles	Subcorneal and intrafollicular eosinophilic pustules Wright's stain of pustule fluid: **eosinophils**	Usually presents at **24–48 hours**, but can be seen from birth to 2 weeks Self-limited and resolves over several weeks
Transient neonatal pustular melanosis	Term infants; more common in **Blacks**	Three stages: **pustules** without underlying erythema; **collarettes of scale**; **hyperpigmented macules**. Lesions may be clustered together; may be seen anywhere, but most often forehead, ears, back, fingers, and toes (Fig. 4.2)	Subcorneal pustules with neutrophils, fibrin, and rarely eosinophils Wright's stain of pustule fluid: **neutrophils**	**Presents at birth, or shortly thereafter,** but collarettes or hyperpigmentation are occasionally noted at a few days to weeks of age; self-limited and resolves over several weeks
Congenital milia	16%–50% of newborns Tiny inclusion cysts in epidermis arising from infundibula of vellus hairs	Minute, white, and smooth papules typically seen on face; few to several dozen Of note, orofacial digital syndrome presents with numerous and persistent milia		Resolve over several months without treatment If numerous, consider oral-facial-digital syndrome, also w/ lobulated cleft tongue
Bohn's nodules/ Epstein pearls	Microkeratocysts of the mouth that form along embryonic lines of fusion	1–2 mm gray-white, smooth papules along the **palatal raphe** (**Epstein**) or the **alveolar ridge** (**Bohn**)		Most resolve spontaneously by 5 months
Neonatal cephalic pustulosis (neonatal acne)	*Malassezia* yeast is implicated; commonly seen in healthy infants	Onset typically first weeks to months with fine erythematous papules and superficial pustules on face > upper torso/scalp. NO comedones	No testing needed; follilcular neutrophilic pustules	Typically self-resolves over weeks; can use topical azole if needed
Eosinophilic pustulosis/ folliculitis	Mean age of onset 6 months; male > female Consider screening for **hyper-IgE syndrome**	Pustules and erythema Mainly involves **scalp** and face; occasionally trunk and extremities	Dense perifollicular mixed infiltrate with eosinophils CBC (eosinophilia)	Presents at birth or days to weeks of age May be pruritic Waxing and waning course over months with recurrent crops of pustules that eventually remit
Miliaria crystallina	Intracorneal obstruction of eccrine duct; typically a history of fever or overheating	Fragile, **clear-colored vesicles** without underlying erythema; forehead, upper trunk, and arms most commonly		May be seen in neonates and infants Self-limited
Miliaria rubra	Deeper intraepidermal obstruction of eccrine duct with inflammation; sometimes a history of overwarming, fever, or use of occlusive dressing or garment	**Erythematous papules** with superimposed pustules typically concentrated in one or two areas; favors **intertriginous/occluded sites** (neck, groin and axillae) most commonly affected areas	Dermal inflammation around occluded eccrine ducts	May be seen in neonates and infants Self-limited

in many ways, but has shorter and milder course; most important concern is to avoid infection during pregnancy (a/w **TORCH syndrome**)

- Infection begins in nasopharynx, then spreads to the lymph nodes; viremia subsequently develops
  - Prodrome: fever, headache, and upper respiratory infection (URI) symptoms
  - Exanthem: **morbilliform eruption** that **starts on the head/neck** (like measles) and spreads in a **cephalocaudal** fashion
  - Enanthem: **Forchheimer spots** (palatal petechiae)
  - Lymphadenopathy typically generalized/painful w/ involvement of **suboccipital/postauricular/anterior and posterior cervical lymph nodes**
- Complications (generally mild) include arthritis and arthralgias (~50% of females)
- Treatment is supportive; administration of immunoglobulin may be considered in exposed pregnant and unvaccinated women

Erythema infectiosum ("fifth disease," "slapped cheek disease")

- Caused by **parvovirus B19** (single-stranded DNA virus)
- Prodromal symptoms during viremia consisting of fever, myalgias, and headache
- Exanthem develops 1 to 1.5 weeks later, coinciding with IgG development

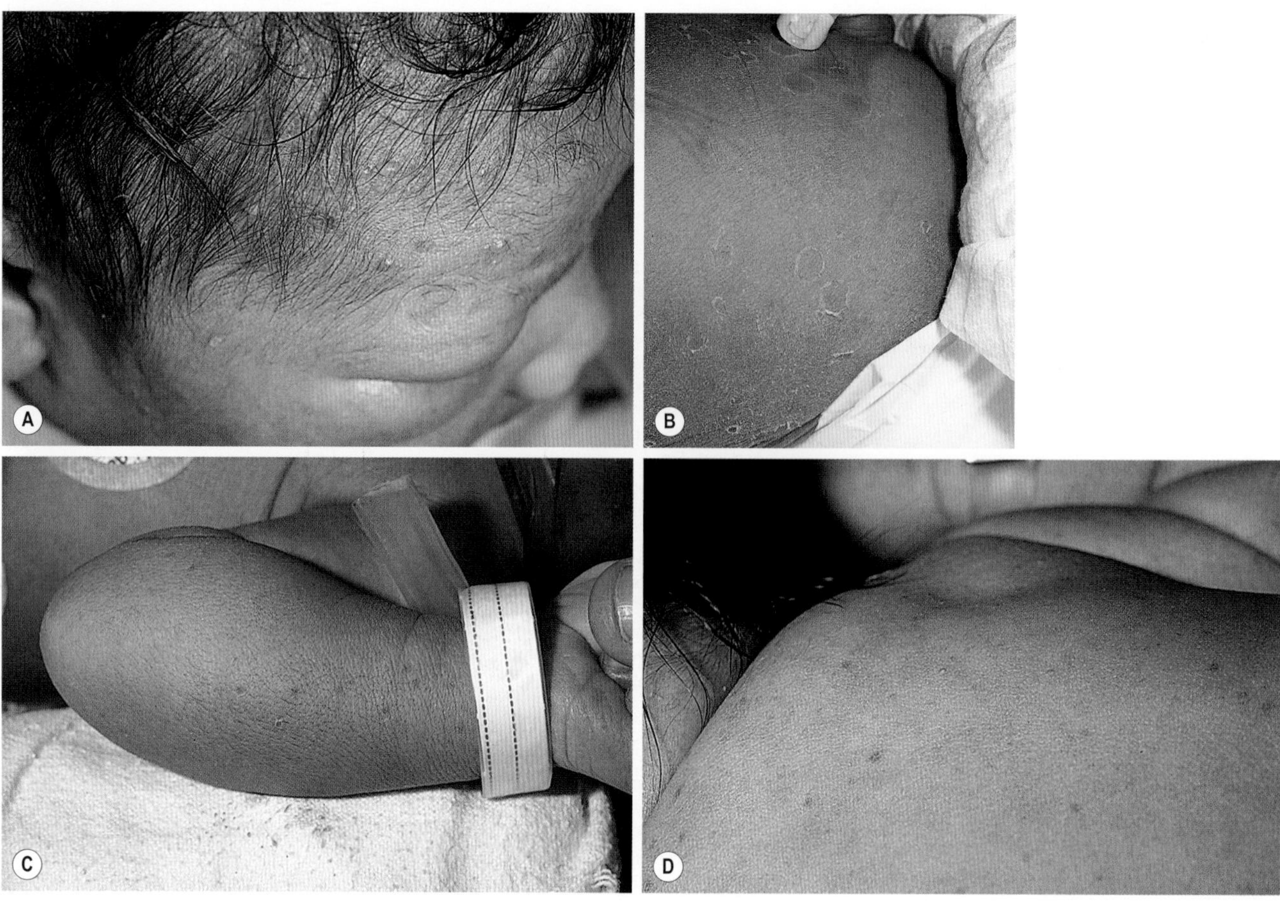

Fig. 4.2 (A) Transient neonatal pustular melanosis first appears as small, superficial pustules without inflammation. **(B)** Collarettes of scale, typical of the second stage, are occasionally seen at birth without evident pustules or **(C)** may develop after pustules have ruptured. **(D)** The final stage is that of small hyperpigmented macules resembling lentils, which gradually fade over weeks to months. (From Lucky AW. Transient benign cutaneous lesions in the newborn. In: Eichenfield LF, Frieden IJ, eds. *Neonatal and Infant Dermatology*. 3rd ed. Philadelphia: Elsevier; 2015:65–76.)

Table 4.3 Various Birthmarks[a]

Diagnosis	Epidemiology and Pathogenesis	Clinical Features	Histology	Treatment and Prognosis/Clinical Course	Additional Boards Fodder
Connective tissue nevus (CTN)	Hamartoma composed of excessive deposition of one or more components of dermal connective tissue (collagen, elastin, or glycosaminoglycans) Can occur sporadically or as a part of one of several AD familial genodermatoses	Asymptomatic, firm, and **skin-colored to yellowish nodules/plaques** on trunk/limbs; can be solitary or multiple; can have cobblestone, leather grain, or peau d'orange texture; present at birth or become evident in childhood/adolescence	Dermis shows excessive collagen or elastic tissue, or both Findings may be subtle, so need to take biopsy of adjacent normal uninvolved skin for comparison	No treatment needed; can be excised if cosmetically indicated Grows with somatic growth, stable over time; no malignant potential	Manifestations of CTN in genodermatoses: "Shagreen patch" or collagenoma (presents in later childhood) in **tuberous sclerosis** Multiple elastic tissue nevi with osteopoikilosis in **Buschke–Ollendorff** syndrome Familial cutaneous collagenoma: hypogonadism and cardiomyopathy Cerebriform collagenoma on sole of foot may be isolated or a component of **Proteus syndrome**

Table 4.3 Various Birthmarks—cont'd

Diagnosis	Epidemiology and Pathogenesis	Clinical Features	Histology	Treatment and Prognosis/Clinical Course	Additional Boards Fodder
Congenital smooth muscle hamartoma	Slight male predominance Hamartoma of reticular dermis composed of dense arrector pili muscle	Skin-colored to hyperpigmented plaque or patch with overlying hypertrichosis, sometimes perifollicular papules; most commonly on **lower back/lumbosacral area**, but also proximal extremities; typically single lesion, but (rarely) can be multiple; evident at birth or shortly thereafter	Many well-defined and variably oriented **bundles of smooth muscle** within reticular dermis	No treatment needed; can be excised if cosmetically indicated No malignant potential	**Becker's nevus** may have significant histological overlap with congenital smooth muscle hamartoma (both have increased bundles of smooth muscle in dermis and epidermal hyperpigmentation), but Becker's nevus tends to arise in peripubertal period, favors upper trunk and arms, and may be a/w hypoplasia of underlying structures (esp. breast hypoplasia)
Nevus simplex ("salmon patch")	**Very common** (up to 50% of all newborns), benign, transient vascular ectasia of capillary bed	**Ill-defined**, **pink** to light-red, blanchable macules and patches on glabella (**"angel's kiss"**), eyelids, and occiput (**"stork's bite"**); more rarely on nose, upper lip, and lumbosacral back	Superficial capillaries in upper dermis with normal overlying skin	Treatment not indicated unless lesions persist and cosmetically needed, in which use of pulsed dye laser may be considered Most **resolve over few months to years**, but lesions in occipital area often persist	More extensive lesions called "nevus simplex complex"; compared with port wine stains, nevus simplex lesions are far more common (50% vs. 1% of newborns), more poorly defined, lighter pink (vs. deep red or "wine-colored"), and transient
Dermal melanocytosis (DM)	African American (95%) > Asian (85%) > Latino (65%) > Caucasian (13%) neonates Defect in migration of pigmented neural crest cells that fail to migrate to dermoepidermal junction	**Slate blue**, **gray**, or black patches, often several cm in diameter, most commonly over **buttocks and sacrum**, but can occur anywhere (Fig. 4.3) Subtypes of dermal melanosis at specific sites: **nevus of Ota** (around eye/cheek and sclera; most common in Asians) and **nevus of Ito** (shoulder girdle; most common in Asians)	Collections of spindle-shaped melanocytes dispersed in normal, nonsclerotic dermal collagen (vs. sclerotic in blue nevus)	No treatment recommended for most dermal melanocytosis Use of **Q-switched lasers** (**ruby**, alexandrite or Nd:YAG) is ToC for nevus of Ota/Ito (90% effective!) **Sacral lesions tend to fade/disappear** over few years; other sites may persist	Blue color from the **Tyndall effect** (blue wavelengths reflected back from deep melanin in skin); extensive dermal melanocytosis described in infants with **mucopolysaccharidoses**, phakomatosis pigmentovascularis

[a]*Epidermal nevus, nevus sebaceus, nevus comedonicus, porokeratotic eccrine ostial, and dermal duct nevus are discussed in the Chapter 6, Neoplastic Dermatology.*

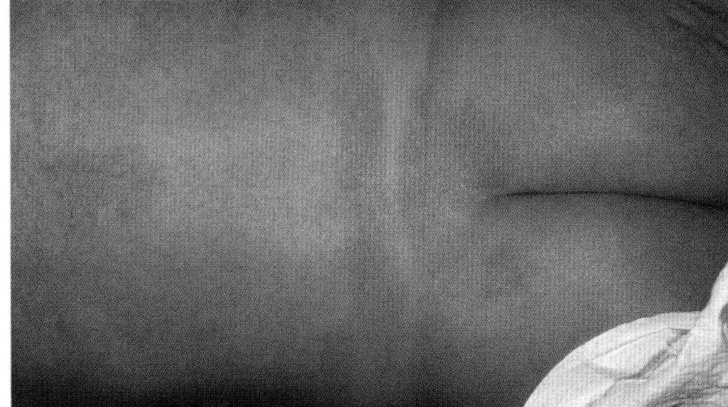

Fig. 4.3 Dermal melanosis (Mongolian spots) on the back and buttocks. (From Lucky AW. Transient benign cutaneous lesions in the newborn. In: Eichenfield LF, Frieden IJ, eds. *Neonatal and Infant Dermatology*. 3rd ed. Philadelphia: Elsevier; 2015. Courtesy of Dr. S. Friedlander.)

  - **Not contagious once eruption develops**
  - **Slapped cheeks**: erythema of cheeks, sparing central face
    - Facial rash may be absent in adults with infection
  - Subsequent maculopapular eruption with **"lacy, reticulated" pattern**, favoring **extremities** (Fig. 4.7)
- Fluctuates in intensity over several weeks
- **Arthritis with small joint predominance** may occur
  - More common in **adults** (females > males), rare in children (~10%)
  - May be present without skin findings
  - Those with arthritis are not infectious
  - Parvovirus B19 is tropic to bone marrow and replicates in erythroid precursors (binds to globoside—blood group P antigen); thus, during viremia, **transient decrease in hemoglobin**
- Relative anemia, which is asymptomatic in healthy individuals

Table 4.4 Developmental Abnormalities[a]

Diagnosis	Pathogenesis	Clinical Features	Histology and Laboratory Testing	Treatment and Prognosis/ Clinical Course	Additional Boards Fodder
Aplasia cutis congenita/hair collar sign	No single underlying cause; in midline cases, incomplete closure of neural tube; in lateral cases, incomplete closure of embryonic fusion lines	Solitary 0.5–10 cm (rarely multiple) well-demarcated round to stellate areas of **localized absence of epidermis, dermis, and sometimes subcutis and calvarium**; presents as an ulcer, erosion, or glistening membrane at birth that resolves leaving an **alopecic scar**; most (up to 90%) occur on scalp (near hair whorl), but may be seen on the face, trunk, and extremities; the **hair collar sign** is a congenital ring of dense, dark, and coarse terminal hair around an area of aplasia cutis or other congenital scalp lesion, suggesting **cranial dysraphism** (Fig. 4.4)	Epidermis is atrophic; superficial dermis replaced by loose connective tissue with absent adnexal structures; hair collar shows hypertrophic clustered hair follicles Radiologic imaging (MRI) if concern for underlying CNS extension/ calvarial defect	No intervention for small lesions Surgical excision if large (>4 cm^2) to minimize chance of complications (e.g., hemorrhage, meningitis, and thrombosis) Spontaneously resolves with scarring; if located in midline and associated with a palpable component, there is a higher risk of underlying calvarial/ CNS defect	Associated with teratogens (**methimazole**), **Adams-Oliver syndrome** (aplasia cutis w/cranial defect + congenital heart defects + CMTC + limb abnormalities), **Setleis syndrome** (bilateral temporal ACC, upslanting eyebrows, distichiasis, "leonine" facies, more common in Puerto Ricans, *TWIST2* mutation), **Bart syndrome** (aplasia cutis + DDEB), **fetus papyraceus** (multiple symmetric stellate areas due to death of twin/ triplet) omphalocele, gastroschisis, spinal dysaphism, meningomyelocele, **trisomy 13**, ectodermal dysplasias, focal dermal hypoplasia, amniotic band syndrome, and congenital infections (e.g., VZV, HSV)
Nasal glioma	Ectopic neuroectoderm	Firm, noncompressible, nontender usually skin-colored (can be blue-red) nodule at **root of nose**; can occur in extranasal (60%) or intranasal (30%) locations		Surgical excision Stable over time, no intracranial extension	May widen nasal bone, giving appearance of hypertelorism
Meningocele/ encephalocele	Herniation of cranial contents through skull defect; neuroectoderm did not properly separate from surface ectoderm in early gestation	Compressible subcutaneous nodule that **transilluminates**, typically at occiput; also can occur on dorsal nose, orbits, and forehead	Type of neural tissue present determines encephalocele (meningeal and glial tissue) versus meningocele (meningeal tissue only) **Radiologic imaging necessary** for surgical planning	Surgical excision Enlarge with increased intracranial pressure (e.g., crying, straining) as a result of connection to CNS	Can be associated with brain malformation, hypertelorism, and facial clefting; presence of hair collar sign, capillary stain, and mass highly suspicious for cranial dysraphism
Signs of spinal dysraphism	Neural tube developmental abnormality	**Highest risk: lipoma** Also midline lumbosacral IH > 2.5 cm, dimple > 2.5 cm from anal verge, tails/ pseudotails, sinuses, skin tags, aplasia cutis, multiple stigmata	MRI is gold standard		Low-risk lesions include simple dimple <2.5 cm from anal verge and <5 mm diameter, capillary malformations, melanocytic nevi
Accessory tragus	Congenital; faulty development of **first branchial arch**	Exophytic papule(s), with/ without cartilage, occur anywhere from **preauricular region to angle of mouth**; single to multiple; can be bilateral	Tiny hair follicles amidst connective tissue, sometimes with cartilaginous core	Careful surgical resection (cartilage can be contiguous with external ear canal)	Typically isolated, but can be associated with other branchial arch syndromes (e.g., oculoauriculovertebral or **Goldenhar syndrome**)
Congenital rests of the neck (wattles)	Remnants of branchial arches; occur along branchial arch fusion lines	Soft fleshy to firm cartilaginous nodules along the cervical neck (anterior border of sternocleidomastoid)	Mature cartilage lobules embedded in cartilage	Surgical excision (may contain cartilage)	
Midline cervical cleft	Congenital midline defect of ventral neck	Small skin tag above a vertically oriented linear atrophic patch; can be small sinus containing ectopic salivary tissue at bottom of atrophic patch		Surgical excision	Can be associated with cleft lip, palate, mandible, chin, tongue, or midline neck hypoplasia

Table 4.4 Developmental Abnormalities—cont'd

Diagnosis	Pathogenesis	Clinical Features	Histology and Laboratory Testing	Treatment and Prognosis/ Clinical Course	Additional Boards Fodder
Lip pits	Incomplete closure of furrows on mandibular process	Bilateral indentations on vermilion lower lip; can be unilateral Associated with cleft lip or palate (Van de Woude syndrome)	Fistulous lumen lined by stratified squamous epithelium with scattered mucinous acini Evaluate for cleft lip/palate, if indicated	Surgical repair May be associated with abnormal salivation	
Umbilical granuloma	Incomplete epithelialization after umbilical cord separation	**Bright red**, **friable**, broad-based papule; not present at birth	Inflamed vascular granulation tissue	**Silver nitrate** (caution in large lesions) Resolve over weeks to months	
Developmental anomalies of the umbilicus	Urachal remnant or omphalomesenteric duct fails to regress	Red to pink nodule within umbilicus, sometimes with mass underneath **Persistent drainage**	Abrupt transition from stratified squamous epithelium to glandular epithelium Consider abdominal ultrasound; referral to pediatric surgery	Surgical excision Can become infected and irritated	
Amniotic band syndrome	Premature rupture of the amniotic sac and formation of fibrous strands	Circumferential constriction band of the distal extremity; distal lymphedema, ischemia, and **amputation**; early rupture can lead to other extracutaneous malformations		Surgical correction Constriction can lead to ischemia and amputation	
Dermoid cyst	Faulty development along embryonic fusion lines	Firm, nontender, skin to blue-colored subcutaneous nodules most commonly seen on the **upper lateral forehead**, **near the eyebrow**, overlying the anterior fontanelle, or at the junctional of sagittal and coronal scalp sutures, but can be seen anywhere on the face, scalp, or spinal axis. May adhere to the underlying periosteum.	Imaging is recommended (MRI most often) for those present in the midline. Histology shows cysts lined by stratified squamous epithelium, and may contain hair follicles, sebaceous glands, and sweat glands.	Surgical excision is the treatment of choice. Lesions usually do not recur.	

[a]*Branchial cleft cysts, bronchogenic cysts, median raphe cysts, and thyroglossal duct cysts are discussed in the Chapter 6, Neoplastic Dermatology.*

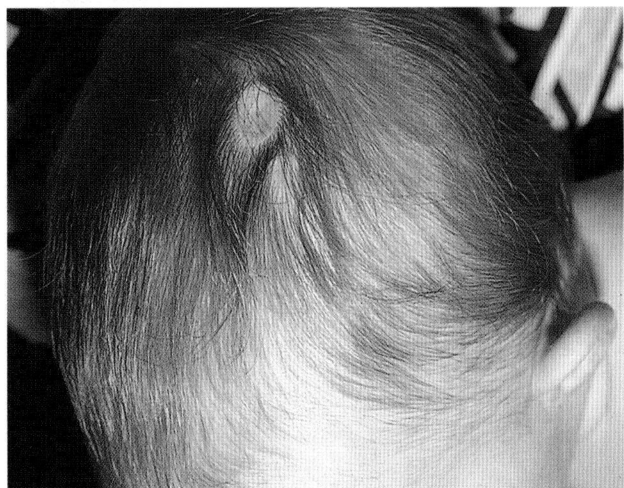

Fig. 4.4 Membranous aplasia cutis with a subtle hair collar sign. (From Drolet BA. Developmental abnormalities. In: Eichenfield LF, Frieden IJ, eds. *Neonatal and Infant Dermatology*. 3rd ed. Philadelphia: Elsevier; 2015, pp 94–110.)

  - **Aplastic crises and pancytopenia** may develop in those with predisposing conditions (e.g., **sickle cell anemia** and other hemoglobinopathies)
- Fetal infection
  - Highest risk if acquired before 20 weeks gestation
  - Fetal loss rate highest in second trimester
  - Possible fetal effects: anemia, high-output congestive heart failure (CHF), **hydrops fetalis**, and intrauterine fetal demise

Papular-purpuric gloves and socks syndrome

- **Young adult** predominance; due to **parvovirus B19 infection**; most common in spring
- Symmetric edema and erythema of palms/soles, may extend to dorsal surface
- Associated **petechiae and purpura with sharp demarcation at the wrists and ankles**
- Resolution over 1 to 2 weeks without treatment

Table 4.5 Congenital Infections

Diagnosis	Epidemiology/ Pathogenesis	Clinical Features	Histology and Laboratory Testing	Treatment Prognosis/ Clinical Course	Additional Boards Fodder
Congenital rubella	Maternal infection (in **first 12 weeks of gestation leads to most severe disease**), leads to infection of fetal cells and defective organogenesis	Skin: intradermal **extramedullary hematopoiesis** (EMH), which appears as soft spongy 2–20 mm erythematous to violaceous papules ("**blueberry muffin baby**"); hemorrhage, petechiae may be seen Other: small for gestational age, microcephaly, **deafness** (**most common symptom**), **cataracts**, chorioretinitis, retinopathy, **patent ductus arteriosus**, intracranial calcification, and hepatosplenomegaly	EMH: erythroid (nucleated RBCs) precursors, immature granulocytes, and megakaryocytes Viral culture of nasopharynx; serology less sensitive, but can do acute (cord blood) and convalescent (4–6 months) titers	No treatment Universal vaccination is designed to prevent congenital infection **Manifestations of congenital rubella are lifelong**, but can present later in childhood	
Congenital toxoplasmosis	Consumption of undercooked meats and exposure to **cat feces**	Congenital: chorioretinitis, hydrocephalus, **intracranial calcifications** +/– petechial rash, extrameddulary hematopoiesis (EMH; "blueberry muffin baby") Postnatal: majority are asymptomatic; very variable presentation	EMH Serology PCR of amniotic fluid Histology of lymph nodes	Pyrimethamine, sulfadiazine, folinic acid × 1 year Prognosis improves with therapy, but consequences can be severe	
Congenital CMV	**Most common congenital infection and most common cause of EMH** Three methods of infection: 1. Reactivation of latent maternal disease → no stigmata of disease 2. Primary maternal infection during pregnancy (earlier, more severe) 3. Postnatal exposure during delivery or while breastfeeding	**"Blueberry muffin"** spots (EMH), petechiae, intrauterine growth restriction, microcephaly, cerebral palsy, chorioretinitis, hepatosplenomegaly, and pneumonitis **Most common infectious cause of congenital deafness and developmental delay!**	EMH Culture: urine and saliva PCR: plasma Serology (rarely used in the neonate): rising IgG titer, IgM not sensitive in neonate	**IV gancyclovir** Oral valgancyclovir (limited data in newborns) Congenital CMV cannot be cured, only suppressed	
Congenital syphilis	Presents at birth or first few days of life; lack of prenatal care in ~30% of cases; mothers with primary or secondary syphilis; incidence increasing in some areas of the United States Invasion of placenta, bloodstream and organs by *Treponema pallidum;* adhere to endothelium and cause vasculitis	Early (<2 years of age): condyloma lata, bullae, or erosions favoring hands, feet, and perioificial areas; scaling, erythema, and **secondary syphilis-like papulosquamous lesions**, and mucous patches; hepatosplenomegaly, **snuffles**, jaundice, **Parrot pseudoparalysis** (due to painful epiphysitis), anemia, and edema Late (>2 years of age): interstitial keratitis, nerve deafness, **saber shins**, gummas of bone, frontal bossing, **Higoumenakis sign** (enlargement of medial third of clavicle), **mulberry molars**, **Hutchinson teeth**, **saddle nose**, perioral **rhagades/Parrot lines** and Clutton joints (painless, symmetric swelling of **knees**), tabes dorsalis	Swelling and proliferation of endothelial cells; perivascular infiltrate of plasma and lymphoid cells Dark-field exam of skin; DFA; syphilis serologies—VDRL, RPR titer in infant 4x mother's titer, but can have false negatives if disease acquired late in pregnancy; IgM FTA-ABS most specific; skin biopsy	**Penicillin** (route and course according to clinical features and per CDC and AAP guidelines) Depends on severity at presentation; prognosis for promptly treated syphilis is excellent	False positive nontreponemal tests (VDRL and RPR) in: infectious diseases, malignancies, and connective tissue diseases FTA-ABS, MHA-TP false positive with other spirochetes and Lyme disease

Table 4.5 Congenital Infections—cont'd

Diagnosis	Epidemiology/ Pathogenesis	Clinical Features	Histology and Laboratory Testing	Treatment Prognosis/ Clinical Course	Additional Boards Fodder
Congenital varicella	Fetal: infection in **first 20 weeks gestation** Neonatal: maternal primary varicella infection **7 days before to 2 days after delivery**	Fetal (presents at birth): stellate deep scars; limb paresis, hypoplasia, chorioretinitis, and low birth weight, developmental delay, microphthalmia, cataracts, nystagmus, and hydrocephalus Neonatal (presents at 0–14 days): vesicles on erythematous base; lesions usually in same stage of development; generalized distribution, often much more widespread than outside newborn period	Neonatal: intraepidermal blisters associated with intracellular edema and multinucleate epithelial cells with inclusion bodies Tzanck, FA, viral culture, and serology unreliable; prenatal imaging (ultrasound, MRI); virus usually not isolated from fetal varicella syndrome cases	**VZIG** Acyclovir Fetal: varies based on extracutaneous manifestations Neonatal: infection at <5 days has a **fatality rate of up to 30%**; infection after 5 days has a benign course	Zoster in first year of life without history of primary varicella infection is seen with exposure to varicella *in utero*; infants <1 year of age are more likely to develop secondary streptococcal infection
Congenital (intrauterine) herpes simplex	Birth, first few days of life Via ascending infection (secondary maternal infection) or viremia from primary maternal infection Congenital HSV is much less common than Neonatal HSV	Vesicles, pustules, widespread erosions, congenital scars, and areas of aplasia cutis Any site may be involved, but scalp often affected with aplasia cutis-like areas; signs of TORCH infections, e.g., low birth weight; microcephaly, and chorioretinitis; 50%–75% mortality if untreated	Tzanck; fluorescent antibody or immunoperoxidase slide test, PCR, and viral culture	IV acyclovir	
Neonatal herpes simplex	Presents at 5–14 days Infection during birth or perinatal period Risk is highest (~40%) for mothers with genital HSV acquired near delivery, risk is low (<~2%) for mothers with recurrence of genital HSV C-section decreases risk of transmission	Skin, eyes, and mouth (SEM); disseminated infection; **CNS infection** (**40% have neurologic sequelae**) Skin: vesicles, pustules, crusts, and erosions (predilection for scalp and torso); may involve mucosa (Fig. 4.5) Signs of sepsis; irritability and lethargy	Intraepidermal blisters associated with intracellular edema and multinucleate giant cells with inclusion bodies Tzanck; DFA or immunoperoxidase slide test, PCR, and viral culture	IV acyclovir Usually 5–14 days	
Congenital candidiasis/ neonatal candidiasis	Risk factors: prematurity, foreign body in cervix/ uterus, and maternal vaginal candida colonization Ascending intrauterine chorioamnionitis	Presents at birth or first few days to weeks of life with erythema, **small monomorphous papules, and pustules** (Fig. 4.6) In extremely premature infants presents as a **scald burn-like** dermatitis with scaling Favors upper torso, palms, and soles Systemic infection is rare in healthy term infants	Skin biopsy may be helpful if KOH negative and manifests subcorneal pustule with neutrophils; PAS will highlight yeast forms KOH: hyphae and budding yeast	If localized, can be treated with topical imidazole or nystatin; if extensive, or if the infant is ill, preterm, or very low birth weight, use of systemic antifungal is indicated Limited disease in healthy term infants resolves quickly with topical treatment Premature infants may have significant associated morbidity	

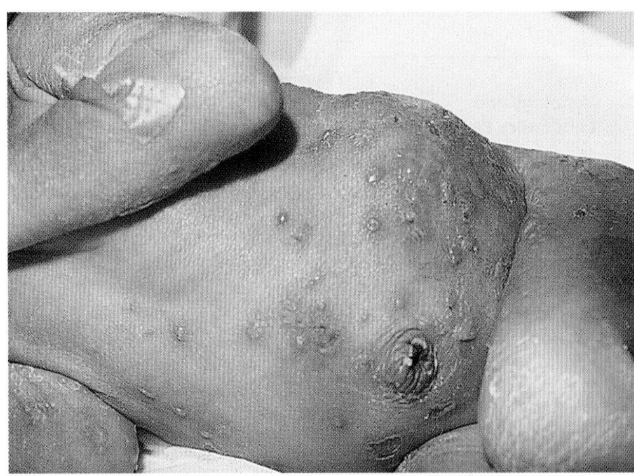

Fig. 4.5 Neonatal herpes simplex virus. Multiple vesicles and crusted papules on an erythematous base in the periumbilical area and left flank. (From Hunt RD, Friedlander SF. Viral infections. In: Eichenfield LF, Frieden IJ, eds. *Neonatal and Infant Dermatology*. 3rd ed. Philadelphia: Elsevier; 2015:176–197.)

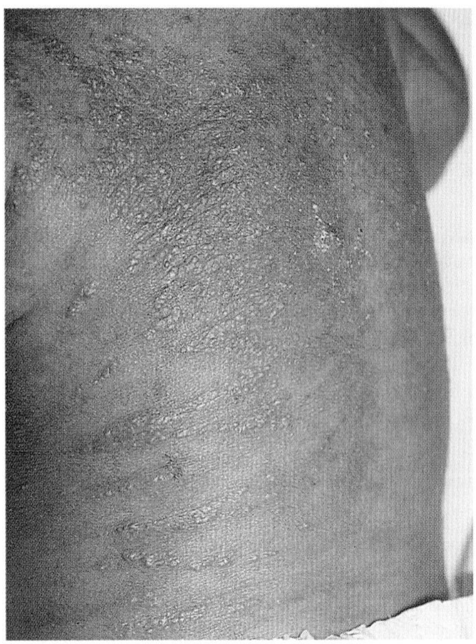

Fig. 4.6 Congenital candidiasis. Diffuse erythematous and pustular eruption. (From Morrell DS, Cathcart SD, Carder KR. Fungal infections, infestations, and parasitic infections in neonates and infants. In: Eichenfield LF, Frieden IJ, eds. *Neonatal and Infant Dermatology*. 3rd ed. Philadelphia: Elsevier; 2015:198–215.)

- Patients are viremic at the time of skin eruption; therefore, unlike erythema infectiosum, patients are considered infectious when rash is present
- Most infections resolve without sequelae

Exanthem subitum (roseola infantum, "sixth disease")

- 6 to 24 months of age; occurring most commonly in spring
- Infection with human herepesvirus (**HHV)-6** (HHV-7 less likely), a DNA virus
  - Two variants: HHV-6A (seen in HIV) and HHV-6B (cause of exanthema subitum)
  - Transmitted by oral secretions

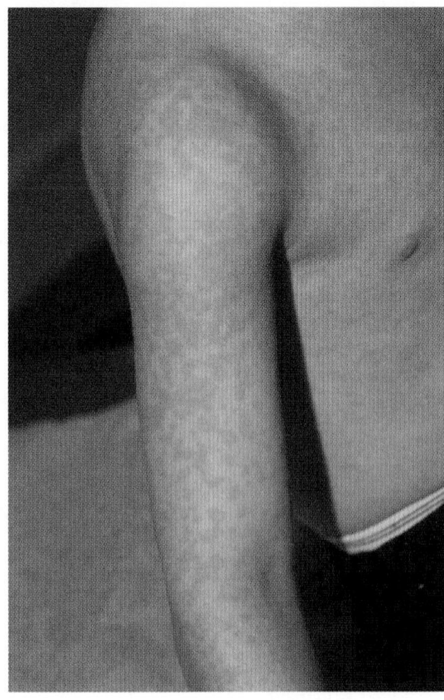

Fig. 4.7 Lacy eruption on extensor arm of child with parvovirus B19 infection. (From Weston WL, Lane AT, Morelli JG. Viral infections. In: *Color Textbook of Pediatric Dermatology*. 4th ed. Philadelphia: Elsevier; 2007:113–147.)

- Incubation period of 1 to 2 weeks → **high fever** (>40°C)
  - **Common cause of febrile seizures**
- **Fever resolves in 3 to 5 days as the exanthem begins (common clinical scenario: an infant has high fever resolving in 3 days at which point a rash develops)**
  - Exanthem: generalized but subtle maculopapular eruption, truncal predominance; typically resolves within 2 to 3 days
  - Enanthem: **Nagayama spots**, which are red macules on soft palate and uvula
- **Benign course**; resolves without complications, even in pregnant women; patients with febrile seizures are unlikely to suffer future seizures
- Remains latent in CD4+ T cells, which results in possibility of reactivation
  - **Implicated pathogenic factor in DRESS (Drug Reaction with Eosinphilia and Systemic Symptoms)**

Hand-foot-and-mouth disease (HFMD)

- Summer/fall predominance, most common in children up to 10 yo
- Infection caused by ***Coxsackie A16* virus** (> *Coxsackie A6* and *Enterovirus 71*)
- Transmitted by **fecal-oral and respiratory routes** → infection of pharyngeal or GI tract, followed by lymphoid involvement, subsequent viremia, and involvement of end organs, including skin
- Incubation period of 3 to 6 days → prodrome (fever and malaise) → onset of cutaneous eruption
  - **Vesicular eruption** most commonly involving palms/soles/buttocks/oral cavity
  - Erythematous macules and oval, deep-seated erythematous vesicles and bullae with **gray center**

- Erosive lesions can be found in the oral cavity "herpangina" (palate/uvula/tongue/buccal mucosa)
- **Onychomadesis/Beau's lines** often occur 1 to 2 months following a coxsackie infection (d/t nail matrix arrest at time of acute infection)
- Adult HFMD is more strongly associated with myocarditis
- Boards factoid: ***Coxsackie* A6** has recently been shown to cause more widespread and severe vesiculobullous eruptions and is a/w atypical HFMD presentations, including **eczema coxsackium** (in atopic patients, Fig. 4.8), that tend to be most predominant on the **perioral area** and extremities, and typically present with more superficial, polymorphic clustered vesicles and erosions (vs. eczema herpeticum which is more monomorphic and punched out). Coxsackie A6 can also present with **Gianotti-Crosti-like eruptions** and purpuric eruptions

Gianotti-Crosti syndrome (papular acrodermatitis of childhood)

- Peak age = 1 to 6 years of age (90% are younger than 4 yo)
- Exanthem arising in setting of viral trigger; may also be seen after vaccination
- #1 cause worldwide: **hepatitis B**
- **Symmetric monomorphic skin-colored to erythematous papular eruption** with predilection for **face (esp. cheeks), extremities, and buttocks** (Fig. 4.9); relative sparing of the chest, back, and abdomen
- Spontaneous resolution expected within 1 to 2 months

Parechovirus

- Infants with **erythema of the acral surfaces** combined with a **sepsis-like picture**
- Other symptoms include fevers, often with associated signs of sepsis/meningitis as well as an associated nonspecific morbilliform rash

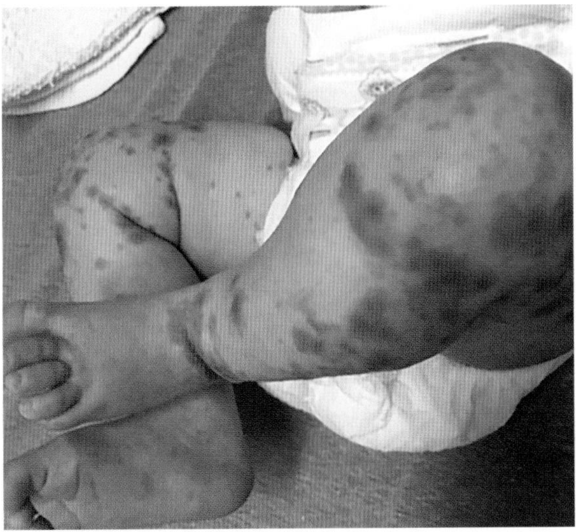

Fig. 4.8 Eczema coxsackium. (Personal collection, Dr. Brea Prindaville.)

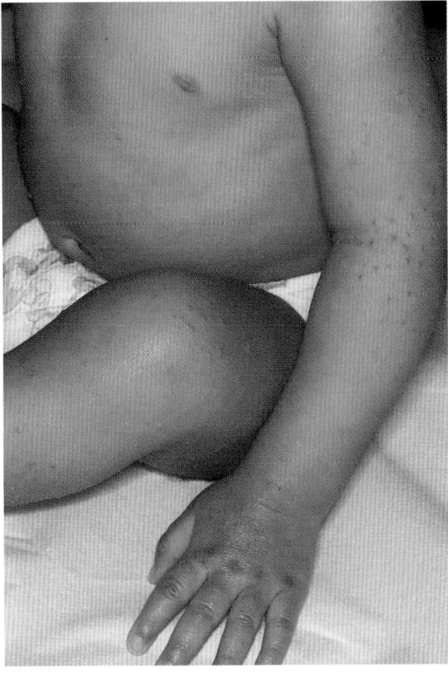

Fig. 4.9 Gianotti-Crosti syndrome. Grouped pink-red papules concentrated around the elbows and knees. (Personal collection, Dr. Jennifer Schoch.)

Unilateral laterothoracic exanthem (asymmetric periflexural exanthem of childhood)

- Average age = 1 to 5 years of age; female predominance; usually in spring
- Thought to be 2° to virus, but exact cause unknown
- May have preceding prodromal symptoms of URI or GI illness
- **Unilateral** erythematous macules and papules with flexural predominance, classically beginning in axilla and lateral trunk; "**Statue of Liberty sign**" (a boards clue) = picture of young child with one arm raised to the sky to show rash on axilla and lateral trunk
- Centrifugal spread to contralateral side may occur, but rash usually maintains unilateral predominance
- Resolves spontaneously after 3 to 6 weeks

Chronic mucocutaneous candidiasis (CMC)

- Most common skin manifestation of HIV in children
- If inherited, often autosomal recessive (AR)
- CMC is a heterogeneous group of disorders marked by chronic and recurrent infections of the skin/hair/nails/mucosa with *Candida albicans* (e.g., thrush, perlèche, chronic paronychia, diaper dermatitis/intertrigo, and dental enamel hypoplasia)
  - **APECED** (autoimmune polyendocrinopathy-candidiasis-ectodermal dystrophy syndrome): AR disease; CMC and other clinical features below
    - **AIRE** (*a*uto*i*mmune *re*gulator) mutation results in failure to delete autoreactive T cells with resultant autoimmunity—**affects regulatory T cells**

- Additional features seen in APECED
  - Endocrinopathies:
    - ➔ **Hypoparathyroidism (most common)**, hypoadrenocorticism (second most common), hypogonadism, thyroid disease, diabetes, and hypopituitarism
  - Cutaneous autoimmune conditions: **alopecia areata and vitiligo**
  - **Pernicious anemia**
- Additional CMC syndromes are seen in association with mutations in signal transducers and activators of transcription 1 (*STAT-1*), **interleukin-17F** (*IL-17F*) (important as candida infections are a side effect [SEs] of secukinumab), caspase recruitment domain-containing protein 9 (*CARD9*), and C-type lectin domain family 7 member A (*CLEC7a,* dectin)

4.3 INHERITED PIGMENTARY DISORDERS

Hypo-/depigmentation

Pigmentary mosaicism

- **Blaschkoid hypo- or hyperpigmentation**: faintly presents at birth and more apparent over first 1 to 2 years
- Most patients developmentally normal; if extensive, consider neurologic, skeletal, ocular anomalies

Oculocutaneous albinism (OCA)

- Group of AR disorders involving abnormal melanin and melanosome biosynthesis and transport within the melanocytes of skin, hair follicles, and eyes
  - There are four types (OCA 1–4), classified based on the affected gene (Table 4.6)
  - **OCA type 2 is the most common type**, followed by OCA type 1
- Variable pigmentary dilution of the skin, hair, and eyes
  - Many affected patients (**except classic OCA1a**) develop pigmented melanocytic nevi/lentigenes/ephelides
- **Photophobia**, **nystagmus**, and reduced **visual acuity** of variable severity
- On histology, ↓ melanin content w/ normal # of melanocytes
- ↑ Risk of basal cell carcinoma (BCC), squamous cell carcinoma (SCC; **most common type of skin cancer** in these patients), and melanoma (worse in OCA1)
- Boards factoid: OCA2-like hypopigmentation is seen in 1% of patients with **Prader-Willi** syndrome and **Angelman** syndrome, which are caused by deletions on chromosome 15q (which includes the *OCA2* gene), if a second mutation is present in the remaining *OCA2* gene

Silvery hair syndromes

- Includes Chédiak-Higashi syndrome (CHS), Griscelli syndrome (GS), and Elejalde syndrome (Table 4.7)
- All are **AR**
- Characterized by impaired synthesis, storage, and/or transport of melanosomes and in the case of CHS, other intercellular proteins
- All have **pigmentary dilution** of the skin and hair w/ variable **immunologic** and **neurologic** features
  - Under light microscopy, giant granules or melanosomes may be seen in the hair shaft and keratinocytes
- **CHS:** severe multisystem disease that presents in infancy with silvery hair, OCA, immunodeficiency, bleeding diathesis, and neurologic degeneration; **death typically occurs by age 10** as a result of the lymphoproliferative **accelerated phase**/hemophagocytic syndrome → pancytopenia and lymphocytic infiltration of liver/spleen/lymph nodes

Table 4.6 Oculocutaneous Albinism (OCA)

Type	Mutation (all are AR)	Phenotype	Comments
OCA1a	*TYR* (**absent**)	Tyrosinase negative	Generalized and **near-complete lack of pigmentation** at birth—white hair and skin (hair becomes light yellow over time) **Nevi are amelanotic/pink** Gray-blue irides **Markedly reduced visual acuity**, severe photosensitivity, markedly increased risk of **squamous cell carcinoma**
OCA1b	*TYR* (**decreased** to 5%–10% of normal level)	**"Yellow mutant** albinism"; minimal pigment	No pigmentation of skin/hair at birth → over time, develop some pigmentation Can have amelanotic or pigmented nevi Milder ocular complications compared to OCA1a **Temperature-sensitive variant (OCA1b TS):** tyrosinase functions at low temperatures, leading to hair pigmentation at cooler anatomic sites (mainly extremities) and white hairs in warmer sites (trunk, intertriginous zones)
OCA2	*OCA2* (previously called ***P gene***; pink-eyed dilution)	Tyrosinase positive	**Most common OCA**, usually seen in **Africans** Pigmentary dilution variable, but develop pigmented nevi/lentigines over time **Light brown hair** and gray/tan irides
OCA3	***TYRP1***	"Rufous"	Very rare; most commonly occurs in Africa and New Guinea Reddish-bronze skin and red hair color Blue-brown irides
OCA4	Solute carrier family 45 member 2 (*SLC45A2*, formerly *MATP*)	Resembles OCA2	Exceedingly rare except in **Japan** (where it accounts for 25% of OCA) Variable clinical presentation ranging from white skin/hair to mild pigmentation of skin/yellow-brown hair; distinguish from OCA2 via molecular studies

Table 4.7 Features of Chédiak-Higashi Syndrome (CHS) and Griscelli Syndrome (GS)

	CHS	GS1[a]	GS2	GS3
Gene defect	***LYST/CHS1***	***MYO5A***	***RAB27A***	***MLPH***
Major sites of gene expression	Melanocytes, platelets, granulocytes, and the CNS	Melanocytes, **CNS**	Melanocytes, **cytotoxic T cells**	Melanocytes
Cellular defect	Impaired biosynthesis and storage of melanosomes, platelet dense granules, and lysosomes within leukocytes	Aberrant translocation of melanosomes along microtubules within melanocytes	Aberrant translocation of melanosomes along microtubules within melanocytes	Aberrant translocation of melanosomes along microtubules within melanocytes
Pigmentary dilution of the skin[b]	+ Acral sun-exposed skin may be hyperpigmented	+	+	+
Silvery/metallic hair	+	+	+	+
Trichoscopy: clumps of melanin	**Small, regularly spaced**	**Larger, irregularly distributed**	+	+
Melanocytes	**Giant melanosomes**	Lacks giant melanosomes	Lacks giant melanosomes	Lacks giant melanosomes
Neutrophils	**Giant granules**	Normal-appearing granules	Normal-appearing granules	Normal-appearing granules
Ocular findings	+	–	–	–
Bleeding diathesis	+ **Prolonged bleeding time**, easy bruising	–	–	–
Recurrent infections	+ Especially skin, lungs, and upper respiratory May have EBV-induced lymphoproliferative syndrome	–	+	–
Other features/comments	**Severe gingivitis, periodontitis**, and oral mucosal ulceration	**Neurologic sequelae** are most severe complication	**Recurrent infections, immunodeficiency, and accelerated phase/HLH** are most prominent features	Generally mild disease; **skin-limited**
Accelerated phase	**+ 85%**	–	+ Development of HLH	–
Primary neurologic abnormalities	+ Progressive deterioration	+	–[c]	–

[a]**Elejalde syndrome likely represents a variant of GS1** *(MYO5A) and presents with the pigmentary features of GS with severe neurologic dysfunction but is not associated with immunodeficiency.*
[b]*Often accompanied by hyperpigmentation ± guttate hypopigmented macules in acral and sun-exposed sites.*
[c]*May develop neurologic symptoms secondary to the hemophagocytic syndrome of the accelerated phase.*
CNS, *Central nervous system;* EBV, *Epstein-Barr virus;* HLH, *hemophagocytic lymphohistiocytosis.*
Modified from Schaffer JV, Paller AS. Primary immunodeficiencies. In: Bolognia JL, Schaffer JV, Cerroni L, eds. Dermatology. *4th ed. Philadelphia: Elsevier; 2018:955–984.*

- Severe neurologic degeneration over time
- On peripheral blood smear, **characteristic giant granules** within cytoplasm of neutrophils, eosinophils, platelets, melanocytes, and granulocytes; on bone marrow smear, giant inclusion bodies within leukocyte precursors in CHS

Griscelli syndrome

- **GS1**: Myosin 5A, severe **neurologic impairment** developing during early childhood
- **GS2**: Rab27A, combined T- and B-cell **immunodeficiency** → numerous infections and hemophagocytic syndrome
- **GS3**: **least severe** GS subtype, **primarily cutaneous findings**
- **Elejalde syndrome**: pigmentary features of GS + **severe neurologic dysfunction** without immunodeficiency (may represent a variant of GS1, Myosin 5A)

Hermansky-Pudlak syndrome

- **AR** disorder with OCA, **bleeding diathesis** (due to platelet storage pool defect), and lysosomal accumulation of **ceroid lipofuscin**
  - Disorder of biogenesis of melanosomes and other lysosomal-related organelles, such as platelet-dense granules
- More common in **Puerto Ricans** (especially HPS1)
- Nine associated genes have been described: *HPS1, AP3B1/(HPS2), HPS3, HPS4, HPS5, HPS6, DTNBP1/(HPS7), BLOC1S3/(HPS8)*, and *BLOC1S6 (HPS9)*
- Variable pigmentary dilution of the skin, hair with a slight sheen, and pale irides
- Extensive **ecchymoses, nosebleeds, and menorrhagia**
  - Avoid aspirin and other anti-platelet medications
- Photophobia, strabismus, and nystagmus
- Other complications are **granulomatous colitis, progressive pulmonary fibrosis, cardiomyopathy, and**

renal failure as a result of lysosomal ceroid accumulation

- **Absence of dense bodies in platelets** noted on electron microscopy (EM)
- Most common cause of death is **pulmonary fibrosis**
- ↑ rates of skin cancer

Piebaldism

- **Autosomal dominant** (AD) disorder caused by mutations in the ***c-KIT* proto-oncogene** (c-KIT inhibitor imatinib can lead to leukoderma) or deletions in the snail family zinc finger 2 (*SNAI2, SLUG*)
- **Defective migration of melanoblasts** from neural crest to the ventral midline and failed differentiation of melanoblasts to melanocytes
- **White forelock (poliosis;** seen in 90%) + congenital patterned midline and ventral patches of leukoderma; in photos can often differentiate from vitiligo by the presence of hyperpigmented macules especially at the periphery (rare in vitiligo)
- Depigmentation is stable and permanent, but otherwise **benign**

Waardenburg syndrome

- Primarily AD disorder of neural crest development → absence of melanocytes in the skin/hair/eyes/striae vascularis of cochlea
- Features may include a depigmented patch on the forehead w/ **white forelock** (poliosis), congenital **deafness**, **heterochromia irides**, synophrys, broad nasal root, and **dystopia canthorum**
- Four clinical types have been described (WS 1–4) (Table 4.8)

Hyperpigmentation

McCune-Albright syndrome

- Caused by a **non-inherited postzygotic somatic activating mutation in the *GNAS1* gene**
- **Females >> males**
- **Triad: large café-au-lait macules (CALMs), polyostotic fibrous dysplasia, and endocrine dysfunction**
  - Typical CALMs are segmental and have jagged borders (**"coast of Maine"**) (Fig. 4.10)

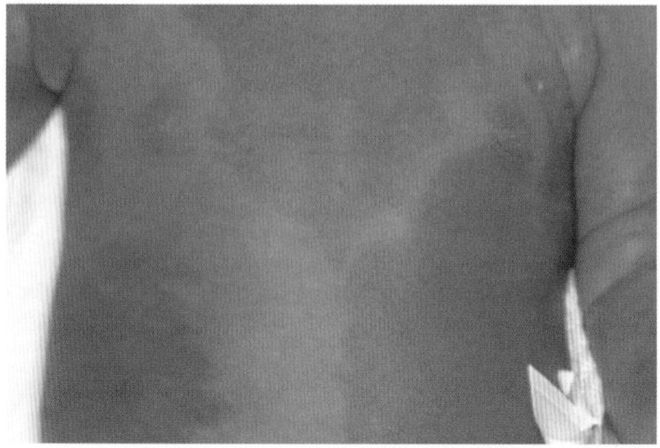

Fig. 4.10 Large, segmental café-au-lait macules with a "coast of Maine" border in an infant with McCune-Albright syndrome. (From Lucky AW, Powell J, Herbert AA. Cutaneous manifestations of endocrine, metabolic, and nutritional disorders. In: Schachner LA, Hansen RC, eds. *Pediatric Dermatology*. 4th ed. Philadelphia: Elsevier; 2011:1219–1268. Courtesy Philippe Backeljauw, Cincinnati Children's Hospital.)

Table 4.8 Disorders of Melanocyte Development

Human Disease	Inheritance	Gene	Protein	Clinical Features
Piebaldism	AD	***c-KIT***	KIT tyrosine kinase	Congenital patterned areas of **depigmentation**, **white forelock** (90%), and islands of normal **and hyperpigmented** skin within depigmented patches; **no internal sequelae**
	AD	*SNAI2*	Snail homolog 2 transcription factor	
WS1	AD	***PAX3***	Paired box 3 transcription factor	White forelock (20%–60%), synophrys, heterochromia irides, dystopia canthorum (eyes appear widely spaced due to lateral displacement of inner canthi; interpupillary distance is normal), and deafness (20%–40%)
WS2	AD	***MITF***	Microphthalmia-associated transcription factor	Similar to WS1, but **no dystopia canthorum**; +**deafness** is more common
	AR	*SNAI2*	Snail homolog 2 transcription factor	
WS3 (Klein-Waardenburg syndrome)	AD	***PAX3***[a]	Paired box 3 transcription factor	Similar to WS1, plus **upper limb abnormalities** (hypoplasia, contractures and syndactyly)
WS4	AD, AR	***EDNRB***	Endothelin B receptor	Similar to WS1, plus **Hirschsprung's disease**
	AD, AR	***EDN3***	Endothelin-3	
	AD	***SOX10***	SRY-box containing 10	

[a]*Homozygous PAX3 mutations have been described in individuals with WS3 whose parents were affected with WS1.*
AD, Autosomal dominant; AR, autosomal recessive.
Modified from Passeron T, Ortonne JP. Vitiligo and other disorders of hypopigmentation. In: Bolognia JL, Schaffer JV, Cerroni L, eds. Dermatology. *4th ed. Philadelphia: Elsevier; 2018:1087–1114.*

- Skeletal lesions (**polyostotic fibrous dysplasia**) usually occur under CALMs, and manifest as gait abnormalities, bone pain, visible skeletal deformity, and recurrent pathological fractures
- Endocrinologic abnormalities include **precocious puberty**, **hyperthyroidism**, acromegaly, **hypophosphatemic rickets**, and infantile **Cushing syndrome**

Reticulate acropigmentation of Kitamura

- Rare—majority of patients are **Japanese**
- AD—caused by mutations in *ADAM10* (encodes a disintegrin and metalloproteinase 10)
- Slightly depressed, lentigo-like hyperpigmented macules coalescing into a **reticulated pattern on the dorsal hands and feet**
- Hyperpigmented macules may darken, and distribution may expand over time
- Palmoplantar pits and abnormal dermatoglyphics may be noted

Dowling-degos disease (DDD)

- Rare—**AD** inheritance
- Mutations in **keratin 5 gene** (also a/w epidermolysis bullosa [EB] simplex with mottled pigmentation—K5 and 14 cause several genetic disorders with reticulate hyperpigmentation)
- **Onset usually during adulthood** w/ reticulated hyperpigmentation involving **axilla and groin**, may spread to gluteal and inframammary folds, neck, torso, inner thighs
- **Comedone-like lesions** on the back or neck and cystic lesions have also been reported
- **Galli-Galli disease**: variant of DDD in which suprabasilar **acantholysis** is noted on histology

Lentiginoses syndromes

See Table 4.9

Hereditary dyschromatoses

Dyschromatoses = both hypo- and hyperpigmentation

Dyschromatosis symmetrica hereditaria (acropigmentation of Dohi)

- Majority of patients are Japanese or Chinese
- AD—caused by heterozygous mutations in the ***ADAR (SRAD)* gene** (encodes an RNA-specific adenosine deaminase)
- Presents by 6 years of age with dyschromia and hyperpigmented/hypopigmented macules restricted to sun-exposed skin on the dorsal aspects of the extremities and face

Dyschromatosis universalis hereditaria

- Most cases are Japanese
- AD/AR—mutations in *ABCB6* (ATP-binding cassette subfamily B, member 6)
- Generalized or torso-predominant, well-demarcated brown macules interspersed with variously sized hypopigmented macules with a mottled appearance
- Nail dystrophy and pterygium

Dyskeratosis congenita (Zinsser-Engman-Cole syndrome)

- X-linked recessive (**XLR**) (**most common**), AD, and AR forms
- **Males** > females (females may have less severe clinical features)
- Occurs 2° to mutations in ***DKC1*** (**XLR inheritance**) > ***TERT, TERC*** (**AD inheritance**), or *TINF2* genes
  - Involved in **telomere maintenance**—affected patients manifest reduced **telomerase** activity and abnormally shortened telomeres → chromosomal instability
- Clinical features: **bone marrow failure** (up to 90%) + **triad of abnormal skin pigmentation, premalignant oral leukoplakia, and onychodystrophy**
  - Dyspigmentation: **reticulated, poikilodermatous patches** of the **face/neck**/upper torso
  - Nail abnormalities: anonychia, pterygium, and longitudinal ridging and splitting
  - Oral manifestations: **leukoplakia (premalignant)**
  - Other dermatologic features: palmoplantar hyperkeratosis and diffuse non-scarring alopecia
  - Other features: progressive periodontal disease, developmental delay, pulmonary fibrosis, and hepatic cirrhosis ↑ risk for malignancy (**SCC** [especially mucosal] and **hematopoietic malignancies)**
  - Causes of mortality include bone marrow failure (most common), pulmonary fibrosis, and malignancy (third to fourth decade)
    - Median age at death = 16 years

Naegeli-Franceschetti-Jadassohn syndrome (NFJS)/dermatopathia pigmentosa reticularis (DPR)

- Rare—AD inheritance
- Mutations in **keratin 14** (NFJS and DPR are allelic ectodermal dysplasia disorders that share many clinical features including **reticulate hyperpigmentation and absent dermatoglyphs**)
- NFJS: brown-gray reticulated hyperpigmentation typically localized to the abdomen, develops in early childhood (around age 2), and **improves after puberty**
  - Other findings: palmoplantar keratoderma (PPK), onychodystrophy, hypohidrosis, and **dental anomalies** (not seen in DPR) including early loss of teeth
- DPR: **diffuse non-scarring alopecia** (not seen in NFJS), onychodystrophy, and diffuse, **persistent reticulated hyperpigmentation** of the torso and proximal extremities
  - **Pigmentary changes fade in NFJS, but persist in DPR**; only DPR has alopecia; only NFJS has teeth abnormalities

Table 4.9 Lentiginoses Syndromes

Syndrome	Gene/Inheritance	Cutaneous Findings	Extracutaneous Findings
LEOPARD syndrome **L**entigines **E**CG defects **O**cular hypertelorism **P**ulmonic stenosis **A**bnormal genitalia **R**etardation of growth **D**eafness-sensorineural	Missense mutations in ***PTPN11/SHP2*** seen in 90% *RAF1* mutations in 3% **AD**	Lentigines involving the face, neck, and upper trunk are the most common presenting feature (86%) and develop at 4–5 years of age as pinpoint to 5-mm brown-black macules Café noir spots larger and more pigmented Numerous café-au-lait macules Abnormal dermatoglyphics	Hypertrophic cardiomyopathy in 71% Facial dysmorphism Genital abnormalities- gonadal hypoplasia, delayed puberty Skeletal–mandibular prognathism and short stature Granular cell myoblastomas
Carney complex **NAME:** nevi, atrial myxomas, ephelides **LAMB:** lentigines, atrial myxomas, blue nevi	50% with mutations in ***PRKAR1A*** gene, chromosome 17q22–24 Others with changes at chromosome 2p16 **AD**	Periorificial lentigines are seen in 77%; fade with time Blue nevi are seen in 43%; fade with time **Epithelioid blue nevi** (highly specific) Cutaneous myxomas Café-au-lait macules Skin myxomas involving the eyelids, ear, **nipple**, breast, and mucosa are seen in 33%	**Cardiac myxomas** (50%–80%; may embolize) Endocrine neoplasms, especially **primary pigmented adrenocortical disease** (26%–45%) **Sertoli cell tumor seen in 33%** Thyroid nodules/carcinoma **Psammomatous melanotic schwannoma** Breast ductal carcinoma
Peutz-Jeghers syndrome	Serine/threonine kinase ***STK11/LBK1*** gene, chromosome 19p.13.3 in up to 70% **AD**	**Pigmented macules on lips**, buccal mucosa, digits, and other mucosa are seen in 50%–60% by age 20 (Fig. 4.11) May fade with time No relationship between severity of pigmentation and polyps	**GI polyps, most common in the jejunum and ileum → can cause intussusception (most common), GI bleeding, anemia, and vomiting** 93% develop **cancer** before age 65: **GI most common** (small intestine, stomach, esophagus, colon or pancreas), lung, and breast Adenocarcinoma seen in younger patients
Laugier-Hunziker syndrome		Pigmented macules on **lips**, buccal mucosa, **genitals**, and other mucosa **Melanonychia** in ~50%	No increased cancer risk
Cronkhite-Canada syndrome	Acquired, usually older men	**Lentigines** of hands, feet, and buccal mucosa **Nail dystrophy** **Alopecia**	Intestinal polyposis
Centrofacial lentiginosis (Touraine's syndrome)	AD	Lentigines in first year of life—especially on nose and cheeks Sacral hypertrichosis	Developmental delay Congenital mitral valve stenosis Seizures Absent middle incisors Skeletal abnormalities Dwarfism Endocrine dysfunction
Bannayan-Riley Ruvalcaba syndrome	*PTEN* (on a spectrum with Cowden syndrome)	Lipomas **Penile lentigines**	**Macrocephaly** Vascular anomalies–deep, high flow **Developmental delay** Intestinal polyps Macrodactyly Pseudopapilledema Hashimoto thyroiditis Increased risk of malignancy

AD, *Autosomal dominant.*

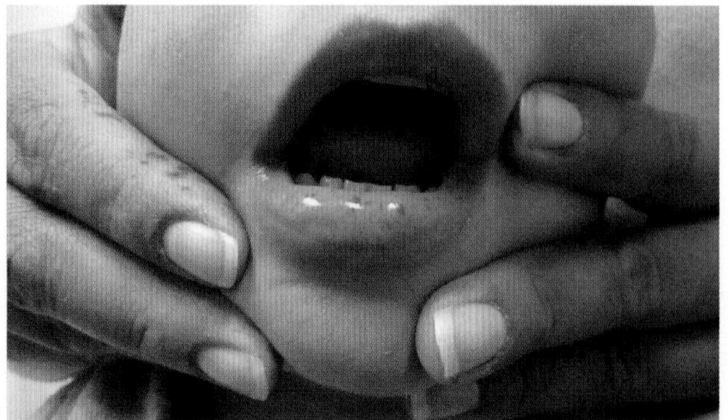

Fig. 4.11 Peutz-Jeghers syndrome. Note lentigines on mother's fingers also. (Personal collection, Dr. Megha Tollefson.)

4.4 EPIDERMOLYSIS BULLOSA

Epidermolysis bullosa (Table 4.10)

EB is a group of heterogeneously inherited mechanobullous disorders that are manifested as fragile skin leading to blisters. There are four major forms of EB, which are categorized by the level of blister cleavage. The fourth major form, Kindler syndrome, was added to the classification system of EB in 2008.

- EB simplex: **intraepidermal** blister with split at the **basal layer**
- Junctional EB: blister through the **lamina lucida** of the basement membrane zone (BMZ)
- Dystrophic EB: blister **below the lamina densa**
- Kindler: mixed levels

Congenital localized absence of skin may be associated with any of the subtypes of EB. Previously this was termed Bart

Table 4.10 Types of Epidermolysis Bullosa (EB)

EB Simplex (EBS)
- Level of split is intraepidermal
- Most common form of EB
- AD inheritance, except for EBS with muscular dystrophy (AR)
- Bullae generally heal without scarring

Subtype	Mode of Inheritance	Gene(s)	Protein(s)	Onset	Primary Cutaneous Features	Associated Clinical Features	Prognosis
EBS-localized (previously called Weber-Cockayne)	AD	*KRT5* *KRT14*	Keratin 5 Keratin 14	Birth through adolescence	Tense bullae predominantly on **hands and feet**, soles > palms (Fig. 4.12); non-scarring Worse with heat, ill-fitting shoes, and frictional trauma from walking	Rare oral blisters early in life Occasional palmoplantar hyperkeratosis Rare nail dystrophy	**Normal life span** May have worse blisters and severe pain during summer months
EBS-generalized intermediate (previously known as Koebner)	AD	*KRT5* *KRT14*	Keratin 5 Keratin 14	Birth or infancy	Tense bullae at **any site of friction**; non-scarring Bullae worse with heat	May have oral blisters Palmoplantar hyperkeratosis over time May have nail dystrophy	Normal life span
EBS-generalized severe (previously known as Dowling-Meara or EBS herpetiformis)	AD	*KRT5* *KRT14*	Keratin 5 Keratin 14	Birth, or within first few weeks of life	**Generalized blisters** After first few months of life, bullae take on characteristic **clustered herpetiformis appearance** May rarely heal with some scarring and milia	Oral blisters common Nail shedding, **nail dystrophy** and hyperkeratotic nails are common **Palmoplantar hyperkeratosis** Characteristic **clumped tonofilaments** on electron microscopy	**Most severe form of EBS** Usually normal life span Rare associated early death due to **sepsis**, anemia, or growth failure
EBS-mottled pigmentation	AD	*KRT5* *KRT14*	Keratin 5 Keratin 14	Childhood	Acral blisters Mottled hyperpigmentation on the trunk and limbs	Punctate palmoplantar keratoderma Common nail dystrophy	Very rare subtype, normal life span
EBS-muscular dystrophy	**AR**	*PLEC*	**Plectin**	Bulla develop at birth, but **muscle weakness is delayed** (may develop in infancy through adulthood)	Generalized blisters that lead to atrophic scars	Muscular dystrophy with onset in infancy or later in life Common nail hyperkeratosis Common dental abnormalities Associated cerebral and cerebellar atrophy, uretheral stricture, and scarring alopecia	Morbidity from muscular dystrophy

Continued

Table 4.10 Types of Epidermolysis Bullosa (EB)—cont'd

Junctional EB (JEB)

- Cleavage plane of blister is within the lamina lucida of the BMZ
- Rarest form of EB
- AR inheritance
- Enamel hypoplasia/pitting (and possible tooth loss due to caries) occurs in all forms of JEB

Subtype	Mode of Inheritance	Gene(s)	Protein(s)	Onset	Primary Cutaneous Features	Associated Clinical Features	Prognosis
JEB-generalized severe (previously known as JEB-Herlitz or EB Lethalis)	AR	*LAMA3* *LAMB3* *LAMC2*	**Laminin 332** (premature termination codon) **Absent Hemidesmosome** (or extremely rudimentary)	Birth	Generalized blisters; typically heals **without scarring** Common sites are **buttocks**, **perioral**, and pinnae of ears	Oral blisters common **Hoarse cry** as a result of **laryngeal involvement** Paronychial inflammation with nail dystrophy and nail loss Granulation tissue of nail beds **Perioral granulation** tissue may develop beyond 6 months of age	**Death** within first few years of life from **respiratory failure** or **septicemia** (90% die by age 1 year) Failure to thrive and anemia very common
JEB-generalized intermediate (previously known as non-Herlitz, generalized atrophic benign EB)	AR	*LAMA3* *LAMB3* *LAMC2* *COL17A1*	**Laminin 332** **Collagen XVII** (BPAG2/BP180)	Birth	Generalized blisters and oral involvement common in neonatal period, but improves as child ages; heals with **atrophic scars** Granulation tissue uncommon	**Scarring alopecia** Nail dystrophy common Dental enamel hypoplasia common Corneal erosions "EB nevi" seen in several forms including JEB—large, acquiried atypical nevi clinically resembling melanoma	Survival to adulthood
JEB-pyloric atresia	AR	*ITGA6* *ITGB4*	**α6β4 integrin**	Birth	Generalized blisters, often with large areas of congenital localized absence of skin	**Pyloric atresia** Scarring of urinary tract, leading to **ureteral stenosis** and hydronephrosis (requires urologic surgery) **Rudimentary and malformed ears**	Poor prognosis with mortality in infancy

Dystrophic EB (DEB)

- Level of split is below the lamina densa of the BMZ
- Two major subtypes are categorized by mode of inheritance: dominant dystrophic EB (DDEB) and recessive dystrophic EB (RDEB)
- In general, DDEB is more mild than RDEB, though there is considerable overlap between the milder forms of RDEB and DDEB
- DDEB may rarely manifest with only nail dystrophy

Subtype	Mode of Inheritance	Gene(s)	Protein(s)	Onset	Primary Cutaneous Features	Associated Clinical Features	Prognosis
DDEB	**AD**	*COL7A1* (missense mutation)	Collagen VII	Birth	Cockayne-Touraine Type: Generalized bullae, most prominent overlying extensor joints; tends to improve over time; heals with **atrophic scarring and milia** Pasini type: Similar to Cockayne-Touraine type but also has scar-like "**albopapuloid**" **papules** that favor trunk and arise spontaneously (without preceding blisters)	**Nail dystrophy common** Oral blisters may occur Rarely may have esophageal strictures Anemia uncommon	Disease activity tends to improve over time, typically milder overall disease similar to EBS
Transient bullous dermolysis of the newborn (TBDN)	Often AD	*COL7A1*	Collagen VII Likely a form fruste of DDEB	Birth	Blistering of the skin, can heal with milia and/or scarring		Often spontaneously resolves in the first several months of life
RDEB, generalized severe (previously known as Hallopeau-Siemens)	AR	*COL7A1* (premature termination codon leads to complete **lack of anchoring fibrils**)	Collagen VII	Birth	Generalized mucocutaneous blisters (Fig. 4.13) **Heals with atrophic scarring and milia**	**Pseudosyndactyly** ("**mitten deformities**" of hands/feet) common and pathognomonic **Contractures of digits and limbs** Scarring alopecia Corneal erosions Oral blisters common Microstomia Dental caries (severe) Esophageal strictures and other GI complications common Osteopenia Growth failure Anemia Dilated cardiomyopathy may (rarely) occur **Renal failure** **Aggressive SCC**	Many comorbidities of other organ systems **SCC is leading cause of death** (affects 50% of patients by age 35 years) Renal failure (12% mortality)
RDEB, generalized intermediate (previously known as non-Hallopeau-Siemens type)	AR	*COL7A1*	Collagen VII	Birth	Generalized blisters Heals with atrophic scars and milia May be difficult to distinguish from DDEB clinically	Fewer comorbidities than the severe form of RDEB	Like DDEB, disease activity may improve slightly over time
Kindler Syndrome (Acrokeratotic poikiloderma) • Rare disorder characterized by skin fragility, photosensitivity, and poikiloderma • In 2008, this disorder was grouped as a major form of EB, with mixed blister cleavage plane • Immunohistochemical analysis shows reduced or absent staining against fermitin family homolog 1 (***FERMT1*** gene, formerly known as kindlin-1; protein involved in keratinocyte adhesion and migration) • Electron microscopy shows **duplication of the lamina densa**; histology shows absence/fragmentation of elastic fibers							
Kindler syndrome	AR	*FERMT1*	Fermitin family homolog 1	Neonatal period	**Poikiloderma** **Acral blisters**, though may have more widespread involvement Cigarette paper-like atrophy of hands/feet	**Photosensitivity** Palmoplantar hyperkeratosis Hand/foot skin atrophy Nail dystrophy Gingivitis SCC of the lip and hard palate	Skin fragility, photo-sensitivity usually improves over time

AD, *Autosomal dominant* ; AR, *autosomal recessive* ; SCC, *squamous cell carcinoma.*

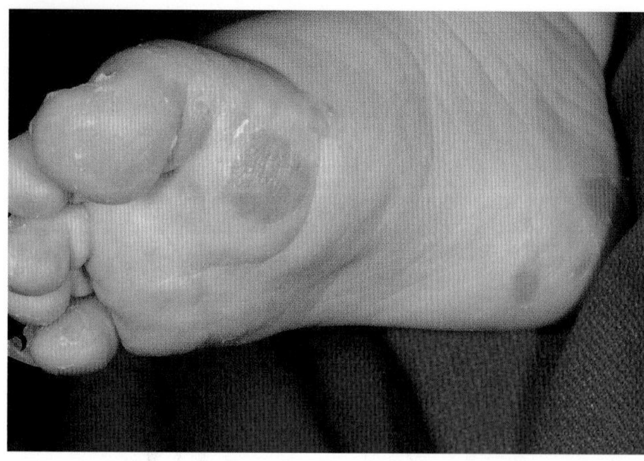

Fig. 4.12 Epidermolysis bullosa simplex, localized type. Note the superficial blistering with both intact bullae and denuded skin. This form tends to be limited to the palms and soles. (From Paller AS, Mancini AJ. Bullous disorders of childhood. In: *Hurwitz Clinical Pediatric Dermatology: A Textbook of Skin Disorders of Childhood and Adolescence*. 4th ed. Philadelphia: Elsevier; 2011:303–320.)

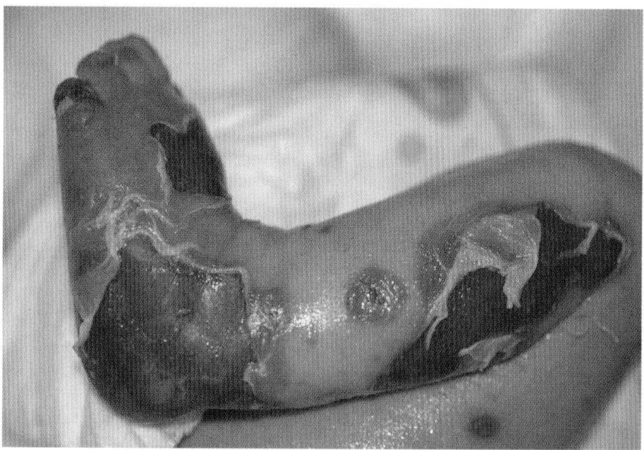

Fig. 4.13 Recessive dystrophic epidermolysis bullosa in a neonate. (Personal collection, Phuong Khuu.)

syndrome, but that eponym is no longer used in the current classification system.

The diagnosis of EB is made through ultrastructural evaluation of the cleavage plane of the blister and accompanying immunohistochemistry. **It is important that the biopsy specimen is obtained from an induced blister, rather than from a preexisting blister, in order to obtain an accurate result of the level of the split.** EM is the gold standard, but is not as readily available. Thus, immunofluorescence mapping is the more commonly used method for diagnosing EB. Once a subtype of EB is identified, genetic analysis may be pursued.

4.5 TUMOR SYNDROMES

- Note: Muir-Torre syndrome, dyskeratosis congenita, Peutz-Jeghers syndrome, and xeroderma pigmentosum (XP) are discussed elsewhere

Basal cell nevus syndrome (BCNS; gorlin syndrome)

- **AD mutations in the *PTCH* gene** (encodes the patched tumor suppressor protein of sonic hedgehog signaling pathway)
  - Patched normally inhibits smoothened (which, when uninhibited, signals intracellularly to activate GLI1/2 [transcription factors] to promote transcription of genes involved in cellular growth)
  - Mutations in *PTCH* → dysregulation of smoothened and ↑ transcription of *GLI* genes → neoplasia
- Diagnostic criteria include the presence of one major criterion + molecular confirmation, two major criteria, or one major and two minor criteria.
  - Major criteria:
    - BCCs (>5 BCCs or 1 before 30 years of age)
      - Multiple, early onset (typically around puberty)
      - May resemble melanocytic nevi, milia, acrochordons, or seborrheic keratoses
      - Favor sun-exposed areas (face, neck, and upper torso), but can occur in sun-protected sites
    - **Palmoplantar pits** (≥2), often present in childhood
    - **Odontogenic keratocysts of the jaw**, histologically proven
      - Generally asymptomatic
      - Typically present late in the first decade of life
    - **Calcification of the falx cerebri**
    - First-degree relative with BCNS
  - Minor criteria:
    - Rib anomalies (**bifid**, fused, or markedly splayed)
    - Cleft lip/palate
    - Other skeletal anomalies (pectus excavatum or pectus carinatum, polydactyly, syndactyly, kyphoscoliosis, Sprengel deformity, or other vertebral anomalies)
    - **Medulloblastoma**, which typically presents within the first 3 years of life
    - Macrocephaly
      - **Frontal bossing**, a broad nasal root, and hypertelorism may be seen
    - **Ovarian/cardiac fibroma**
    - Lymphomesenteric cysts
    - Ocular abnormalities (i.e., strabismus, hypertelorism, congenital cataracts, glaucoma, and colobomas)
  - Other features include: increased risk of fibrosarcoma and rhabdomyosarcoma, cryptorchidism, gynecomastia, agenesis of corpus callosum, **ovarian fibromas**, and cardiac fibromas
- Treatment: standard BCC treatment methods +/− targeted therapy with **vismodegib**, a smoothened inhibitor (essentially acts as "artificial PTCH")—of note, sonidegib is another option with similar mechanism of action to vismodegib
- **Syndromes a/w multiple BCCs (Boards favorite!)**: Gorlin, Bazex-Dupré-Christol, Rombo, Brooke-Spiegler, XP, and Schöpf-Schulz-Passarge

Birt-Hogg-Dubé syndrome

- AD disorder as a result of mutations in *BHD* gene (encodes **folliculin**)

- Manifestations begin in the third decade or later
- Cutaneous findings: **fibrofolliculomas, trichodiscomas, and acrochordons**
  - Fibrofolliculomas/trichodiscomas appear as multiple tiny skin-colored to white papules on the face
  - On histology, fibrofolliculomas/trichodiscomas have slender strands of basophilic cells radiating from a follicular unit, surrounded by a fibrous stroma
- Systemic findings: **renal cell carcinoma and spontaneous recurrent pneumothorax (w/ lung cysts and bullous emphysema)**

Brooke-Spiegler syndrome

- AD disorder as a result of mutations in cylindromatosis **(*CYLD*) gene** (a tumor suppressor); *CYLD* is a deubiquinating enzyme that normally interacts with NEMO to downregulate nuclear factor-κB (NF-κB) expression
- Skin findings (presenting in adolescence/early adulthood): **cylindromas** (papules/nodules on scalp), **trichoepitheliomas** (skin-colored to white small facial papules), **spiradenomas** (painful nodules on head/neck and elsewhere), and multiple **BCCs**; malignant degeneration into cylindrocarcinoma and spiradenocarcinoma may occur (increased risk compared with general population)
- Extracutaneous findings: **salivary and parotid gland tumors**

Multiple endocrine neoplasia (MEN) syndromes

- MEN I (Wermer)
  - AD disorder as a result of mutations in *MEN1* gene (menin)
  - Tumors in **p**ituitary (esp. prolactinoma), **p**arathyroid (usually hyperplasia or adenoma) and **p**ancreas (usually islet cell hyperplasia, adenoma, or carcinoma) **(three Ps = mnemonic)**
  - Cutaneous findings **may be similar to tuberous sclerosis**—facial angiofibromas, collagenomas, gingival papules, hypopigmented macules, and CALMs
- MEN IIA (Sipple)
  - AD disorder as a result of mutations in the ***RET*** proto-oncogene
  - **Parathyroid hyperplasia** (not seen in MEN IIB) + **medullary thyroid carcinoma** (~100%) + **pheochromocytoma**
  - Cutaneous findings: **lichen amyloidosis and macular amyloidosis** (+/– notalgia paresthetica)
- MEN IIB (multiple mucosal neuroma syndrome)
  - AD disorder as a result of mutations in ***RET***
  - Skin findings: **mucosal neuromas on tongue/lips**, thickened lips, and **marfanoid habitus**
  - Endocrine findings: **medullary thyroid carcinoma** (~100%; fatal if not caught early!) and **pheochromocytoma**
  - Ocular findings: conjunctival neuromas → thickened/everted upper eyelids
  - GI findings: ganglioneuromatosis → megacolon, diarrhea, and constipation

Cowden syndrome (multiple hamartoma syndrome)

- AD disorder as a result of mutations in the ***PTEN*** tumor suppressor gene → proliferation of cutaneous/GI/mucosal/thyroid/breast tissues; manifestations begin in second to third decade
- ***Other PTEN hamartoma syndrome* (Bannayan-Riley-Ruvalcaba)** has many features of Cowden syndrome + pigmented macules on glans penis, lipomas, macrocephaly, and developmental delay
- Cutaneous findings: **sclerotic fibromas**, **facial tricholemmomas** (skin-colored to light brown small papules), **punctate palmoplantar keratoses**, **keratotic papules (acral keratoses)** on dorsal hands/feet/forearms/legs, **lipomas**, skin tags, and inverted follicular keratoses
- Oral findings: small skin-colored grouped papillomas → "**cobblestone**" appearance on lips and gingival/buccal/labial mucosa
- Thyroid findings: goiter, adenomas, and carcinoma **(follicular carcinoma is the most common type)**
- Breast findings: fibrocystic disease, fibroadenomas, and **adenocarcinoma** (**most common malignancy** overall; in up to 50% of female patients)
- GI findings: **hamartomatous polyps** along the GI tract (most common in **colon**)—low risk of malignant transformation
- Other findings: ovarian cysts (benign), uterine leiomyomas, **endometrial carcinoma** (in up to 10% of female patients), menstrual irregularities, various GU carcinomas/cysts, **craniomegaly** (>80% of patients), adenoid facies, kyphoscoliosis, bone cysts, large hands/feet, myopia, angioid streaks, and intracranial venous anomalies
- **Lhermitte-Duclos disease** (dysplastic gangliocytoma of cerebellum): pathognomonic criterion for Cowden's; p/w overgrowth of cerebellar ganglion cells → ataxia, seizures, and ↑ intracranial pressure

Gardner syndrome

- AD mutations in adenomatous polyposis coli (***APC***) **gene** (tumor suppressor gene that regulates β-catenin)
- Cutaneous manifestations: **epidermoid cysts** (classically with **pilomatricoma changes**), fibromas (skin/subcutaneous/mesentery/ retroperitoneum), lipomas
- GI manifestations:
  - Premalignant polyposis throughout GI tract → ↑↑↑ risk **adenocarcinoma** (esp. colon/rectum; ~**100% affected**)
  - **Desmoid tumors:** locally aggressive, but do not metastasize; female > male; may arise post-surgically after colectomy; can → small bowel and/or ureter obstruction
- Ocular manifestations: congenital hypertrophy of retinal pigment epithelium (**CHRPE; 70%**)
- Other findings: **osteomas** (skull/mandible/maxilla; 80% patients; painless), odontomas of teeth, **supernumerary teeth**, papillary thyroid carcinoma (women), hepatoblastoma, adrenal adenomas, sarcomas, pancreatic carcinomas, and brain tumors (e.g., glioblastomas and

medulloblastomas; in subtype of Gardner syndrome called Turcot syndrome)
- **Treatment = prophylactic colectomy** when polyp formation is first evident (second to third decade)

4.6 VASCULAR TUMORS, MALFORMATIONS, AND RELATED VASCULAR DISORDERS

Vascular tumors

Vascular tumors are discussed more extensively in Chapter 6 (Neoplastic Dermatology).

PHACE syndrome

- **Female predominance; 9:1**
- Large segmental hemangioma on head/neck (**highest risk are S1, 3, and/or 4 distribution**)
- **Cerebrovascular anomalies most common extracutaneous finding**
  - Those with frontotemporal segment involvement may be at most risk of cerebrovascular abnormalities
  - Those with mandibular segment involvement may be at most risk of cardiac defects
- **P**osterior fossa malformations (e.g., Dandy-Walker and cerebellar hypoplasia)
- **H**emangioma, segmental
- **A**rterial anomalies (internal carotid arteries and cerebral arteries)
- **C**ardiac anomalies (**coarctation of aorta**, ventral and atrial septal defects, and patent ductus arteriosus)
- **E**ye anomalies (microphthalmos, optic atrophy, **cataracts**, strabismus, and exophthalmos)
- **S**ternal cleft or **s**upraumbilical raphe
- MRI/MRA of the head and neck to evaluate for cerebrovascular anomalies, echocardiogram, and ophthalmology evaluation
- **Oral propranolol is first-line therapy,** though coarctation of the aorta or other significant congenital heart disease should be ruled out before starting therapy

LUMBAR/SACRAL syndrome

- Segmental hemangioma of the **lower back** (lumbar or sacral spine) or buttocks and genitalia (Fig. 4.14)
- **L**ower body hemangioma
- **U**rogenital anomalies/**ul**cerations
- **M**yelopathy (myelomeningocele)
- **B**ony deformities
- **A**norectal malformation
- **R**enal anomalies
- **S**pinal dysraphism
- **A**nogenital anomalies
- **C**utaneous anomalies
- **R**enal and **a**nal anomalies
- Angioma with **L**umbosacral location
  - Evaluate with MRI of the pelvis and spine

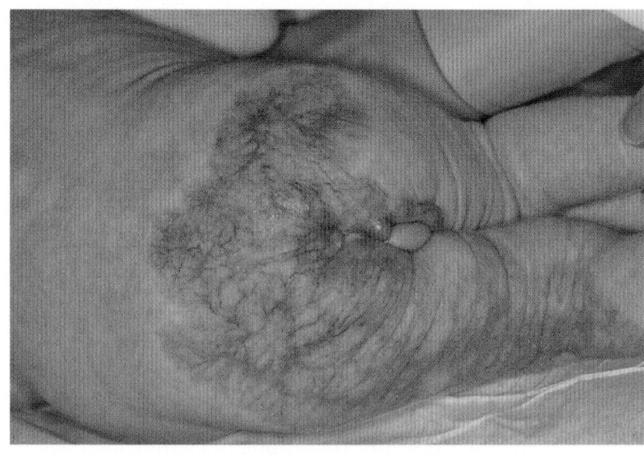

Fig. 4.14 LUMBAR (SACRAL) syndrome. (Personal collection, Dr. Jane Bellet.)

- If a segmental hemangioma crosses over the midline lower spine, imaging is required. Ultrasound can be considered in very young infants; however, MRI of the spine is the gold standard.
- **Propranolol** should be considered for large, ulcerated, or otherwise complicated segmental hemangiomas
  - Best to start in first 1 to 2 months of life
  - Goal dose 2 to 3 mg/kg/day, divided BID to TID
  - Documented normal cardiac exam and history before starting
  - SEs: hypotension, bradycardia, hypoglycemia

Multiple hemangiomas

- **If** five or more hemangiomas are present, especially small, miliary infantile hemangioma (IH), an ultrasound of the liver should be strongly considered to r/o hepatic hemangiomas (may also rarely occur in intestines, brain, eyes, spleen, kidney, and lungs)
- For cosmetic treatment of superficial IH, topical beta blockers (timolol) may be used judiciously
  - For patients with significant visceral involvement leading to **liver failure and/or high output CHF**, propranolol is first-line therapy
- When present, liver hemangiomas can produce the enzyme type 3 deiodinase, which can lead to **consumptive hypothyroidism**

Kasabach-Merritt phenomenon

- Usually occurs in the first few weeks to months of life
- Occurs in association with **tufted angioma** or **kaposiform hemangioendothelioma (KHE)**
- Pathogenesis: abnormal endothelium and convoluted architecture of KHE or tufted angioma promote platelet adhesion and trapping with subsequent **consumptive coagulopathy**
- Sudden growth of a vascular lesion with induration, edema, and advancing purpuric edge
  - Severe thrombocytopenia (from platelet trapping), consumptive coagulopathy, hypofibrinogenemia,

elevated D-dimer, hemolytic anemia, and **disseminated intravascular coagulation**
  - Hematuria, hematochezia, and epistaxis may occur
  - High-output cardiac failure and significant risk of internal hemorrhage → **10%–30% mortality**
- **Systemic corticosteroids and vincristine** are primary therapeutic interventions. Systemic sirolimus is an emerging treatment in this setting. Response to propranolol has been poor
- **Do not administer platelets as Kasabach-Merritt is due to platelet trapping and this may worsen the condition**

Vascular malformations

Capillary malformations (CM)

Capillary malformation ("Port Wine Stain," PWS, nevus flammeus)

- Sporadic, affecting 0.1%–2% of newborns
- Understanding of mutations is evolving; mutations in *GNAQ* reported in classic PWS; geographic CMs more commonly due to mutations in *PIK3CA*
- Red-purple vascular macule or patch **present at birth**
- Often located on the face, but may be found anywhere on the body
- Usually an isolated cutaneous finding, but may be seen in **many syndromes** (Sturge-Weber syndrome [SWS], Klippel-Trenaunay syndrome [KTS], Parkes-Weber syndrome, Proteus, PTEN hamartoma syndromes, Cobb syndrome, Beckwith-Wiedemann syndrome, phakomatosis pigmentovascularis, and capillary malformation-arteriovenous malformation [CM-AVM])
- On histology, dilated venules in dermis with normal number of vessels and no endothelial proliferation (is a malformation rather than true neoplasm)
  - In adults, fibrosis around the vessels and vascular dilation can be seen
- **Pulsed dye laser = first-line therapy; typical settings include 1.5-ms pulse duration;** areas over bony prominences on face (e.g., forehead) respond better than cheeks, distal extremities may respond less well
- Lesions do not resolve spontaneously; ↑ in size proportionately to the child's growth; may become gradually darker and hypertrophic over time, especially if located on the face

Sturge-Weber syndrome (encephalotrigeminal angiomatosis)

- 2° to somatic mosaic mutations in the *GNAQ* gene
- CM involving the frontonasal (forehead) placode (formerly **V1—ophthalmic branch of trigeminal nerve) distribution** (Fig. 4.15)
  - Only 5%–10% with a CM of the forehead will have SWS; more extensive often corresponds to increased risk
  - Soft tissue/skeletal hypertrophy often develop over time under the CM
- Ipsilateral leptomeningeal CM (angiomatosis) of the brain and eye

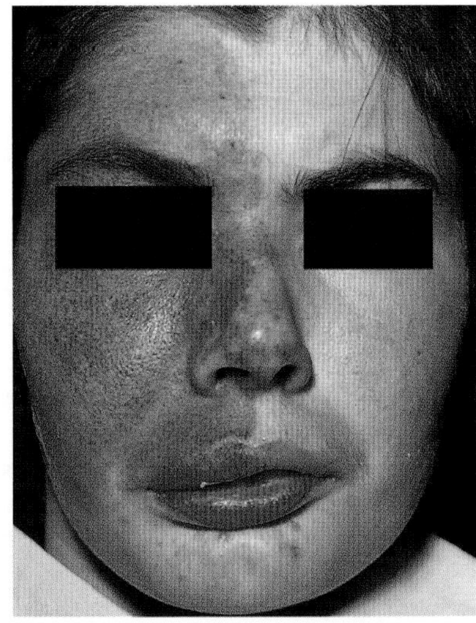

Fig. 4.15 Sturge-Weber syndrome. This patient has a classic capillary malformation in the distribution of the ophthalmic, nasociliary, and maxillary branches of the trigeminal nerve. The lesion extends backward over the anterior two thirds of the crown of the head. (From Forbes CD, Jackson WD. *Color Atlas and Text of Clinical Medicine*. 2nd ed. London: Mosby; 1996.)

- Neurologic complications include **seizures** (usually develop in first year of life), developmental delay, intellectual disability, and focal neurologic deficits
  - Head CT = cortical calcifications that resemble "**tram track** lines"
- Ophthalmologic complications affect 60% (#1 is **glaucoma**)
- Clinical course depends on extent of leptomeningeal involvement
- Bilateral facial CMs involving forehead distribution = worst prognosis (↑ risk of seizures and more profound developmental delay)

Phakomatosis pigmentovascularis

- Widespread CM in addition to other cutaneous findings
- Five defined types, a = no extracutaneous involvement; b = extracutaneous involvement
  - **I:** PWS + epidermal nevus
  - **II** (phakomatosis cesioflammea): **PWS** + **dermal melanocytosis** +/− nevus anemicus; **most common** form (85%); may have complications (SWS, overgrowth); identified mutation GNAQ in pluripotent progenitor cells
  - **III** (phakomatosis spilorosa): **PWS** + **nevus spilus** +/− nevus anemicus
  - **IV:** PWS + dermal melanocytosis + nevus spilus +/− nevus anemicus
  - **V** (phakomatosis cesiomarmorata): cutis marmorata telangiectatica congenital (CMTC) + dermal melanocytosis
- Extracutaneous features include neurologic, musculoskeletal, and ocular findings

Phakomatosis pigmentokeratotica

- 2° to post-zygotic mutation in *HRAS*

- **Speckled lentiginous nevus (nevus spilus) in conjunction with nevus sebaceus**
- Neoplasms (**trichoblastoma** > syringocystadenoma papilliferum > BCC) may develop within nevus sebaceus
- Neurologic abnormalities may be present and include seizures, hemiparesis, and intellectual impairment
- **Hypophosphatemic vitamin D–resistant rickets** can develop

PIK3CA-related overgrowth spectrum (PROS)

- Somatic mutations in the phosphatidylinositol/AKT/mTOR pathway cause segmental progressive overgrowth disorders often associated with enlarged, splayed digits, vascular malformations (esp. geographic CM), and lipomatous changes among other manifestations. This spectrum now encompasses a variety of conditions including Klippel-Trenaunay syndrome, CLOVES, and megalencephaly-capillary malformation (M-CM), all discussed below.

Klippel-Trenaunay syndrome

- Recently reported association with mutations in phosphatidylinositol-4,5-bisphosphate 3-kinase, catalytic subunit alpha (*PIK3CA*)
- CM, venous malformation (VM), and/or lymphatic malformation (LM) with soft tissue and/or bone **hypertrophy** of one limb
  - **Lower extremities** (95%) are affected much more commonly than upper extremities
  - Venous varicosities are common
- Complications include deep vein thrombosis and thrombophlebitis, pulmonary embolism (PE), GI bleeding, vascular blebs and pain, and **high-output cardiac failure**

Macrocephaly capillary malformation syndrome

- M-CM mutations in *AKT3*, ***PIK3CA***, or *PIK3R2*
- Macrocephaly and frontal bossing
- Widespread reticulated CM often prominently involving **mid-face (philtrum** and glabella)
- **Hemihypertrophy** involving contralateral side of the body from the CM
- **Progressive neurologic dysfunction** → developmental delay, seizures, and hypotonia
  - Polymicrogyria, cerebral asymmetry, white matter abnormalities, ventriculomegaly, cortical dysplasia, and/or cerebellar tonsillar herniation
- **Syndactyly** (esp. second–third toes), polydactyly, joint laxity, and hyperplastic skin
- ↑ Risk of Wilms' tumor

CLOVES syndrome

- Congenital lipomatous overgrowth (asymmetric, progressive)
- Vascular malformations (including geographic CM)
- Epidermal nevi
- Scoliosis/spinal and skeletal anomalies
- *PIK3CA* postzygotic activating mutation
- ↑ Risk of Wilms' tumor; screening protocol with ultrasound q3mo until age 8
- Risk for thromboembolic events, PE, cerebrovascular accident (CVA)

Proteus syndrome

- Sporadic, due to ***AKT1*** **somatic activating mutation** → asymmetric progressive overgrowth
- Skin:
  - **Cerebriform connective tissue nevi** (plantar collagenoma): pathognomonic if present
  - **CM/VM/LM**
  - Epidermal nevi
  - Lipomas
  - CALMs
  - Focal atrophy/dermal hypoplasia
  - Varicosities
  - Partial lipohypoplasia
- Central nervous system (CNS): hemimegalencephaly and **impaired intelligence**
- Ophthalmologic: nystagmus, strabismus, cataracts, and myopia
- Musculoskeletal
  - Typical facies: dolichocephaly, down-slanting palpebral fissures, depressed nasal bridge, anteverted nares, and open mouth position at rest
  - **Overgrowth** of one or more of the following (involves soft tissue and bone): **extremities, digits, cranium** (hemifacial macrosomia), vertebrae, and external auditory meatus
  - Hyperostoses
  - Scoliosis
- **Bilateral ovarian cystadenoma** and parotid monomorphic adenoma
- **Organomegaly**
- Cystic lung malformations
  - Restrictive lung disease
  - Pulmonary emphysema
  - Recurrent pneumonia
- Risk of venous thrombosis and PE

Beckwith-Wiedemann syndrome

- Associated with chromosome 11 abnormalities at p57(*KIP2*) gene
- 85% of cases are sporadic
- Clinical features:
  - **Macrosomia/gigantism** (height and weight > 97%)
  - **Facial CM** of glabella, mid-forehead, and upper eyelids
  - Hemihyperplasia (asymmetric overgrowth)
  - **Macroglossia**
  - **Omphalocele/exomphalos**
  - Anterior **linear earlobe creases** and posterior helical ear pits
  - **Visceromegaly** (kidney, liver, pancreas, spleen, and heart)
  - Neonatal hypoglycemia
- ↑ risk for embryonal tumors (**Wilms' tumor [#1]**, rhabdomyosarcoma, neuroblastoma, and hepatoblastoma)

Diffuse capillary malformation with overgrowth (DCMO)

- More extensive reticulate CMs, can be one extremity or truly diffuse
- Proportional nonprogressive overgrowth 2° to hypertrophy of the bones and soft tissues

- Overgrowth may affect only one extremity, ipsilateral or contralateral to the stain, or, less frequently, an entire side of the body
- Otherwise healthy

Venous malformations

- Sporadic, but 50% of sporadic VMs have *TIE2* (aka *TEK*) mutations
  - Familial cutaneous and mucosal venous malformation syndrome (VMCM): widespread VMs of skin, mucosa and visceral organs due to ***TIE2*** (aka *TEK*) mutations; has significant overlap w/ Blue rubber bleb syndrome!
- Present at birth, but may become more apparent in childhood
- Erythematous to violaceous, soft, compressible nodule or plaque without warmth, vascular thrill, or pulsations +/− radiating veins
- On histology, dilated vascular spaces with single-layer endothelial wall that is surrounded by fibrous tissue; involves deep dermis or subcutaneous fat
- Ultrasound shows **slow-flow lesion**; MRI is the best imaging modality to determine the extent; on plain films, calcification can be seen 2° to phleboliths; fibrinogen may be ↓ and D-dimer may be ↑

Maffucci syndrome (enchondromas with multiple angiomas)

- 80% cases caused by mutations in isocitrate dehydrogenase (***IDH1*** and ***IDH2***); characterized by mesodermal dysplasia of skin and skeletal systems
- First sign in early infancy = deep VMs (soft, compressible, and bluish nodules) on the **hands and feet**
- **Enchondromas** develop on the phalanges and long bones, and predispose to **short stature**, **fractures**, and limb length discrepancies; can occur in cranium/vertebrae → neurological problems
- LMs, hemangioendotheliomas, and spindle cell hemangiomas may be present
- Extracutaneous sites of vascular malformations: leptomeninges, eyes, oropharynx, and GI tract
- Clinical course: bone fractures 2° to non-ossification; **50% risk for chondrosarcoma (occurs within enchondromas)**; lymphangiosarcoma and hemangiosarcoma also reported

Blue rubber bleb nevus syndrome

- Usually sporadic
- Presents at birth to early childhood with VMs (**multiple blue-violaceous compressible papules and nodules** with hyperhidrosis overlying lesions; with compression, an empty wrinkled sac is noted that quickly fills with release of pressure)
  - VMs involve the **trunk/extremities, mucosa, GI tract** (esp. small intestine), liver, and CNS
  - ↑ Size/# with age
- **Small intestine blebs** → **hemorrhage** (which may → death if severe) or occult/chronic bleeding (melena and iron-deficiency anemia)

Glomulovenous malformations (GVMs; previously termed "glomangiomas")

- Variant of VM (is not a neoplasm → no longer referred to as "glomangioma") where ectatic vessels are lined by a small number of glomus cells
  - Glomus cells are modified smooth muscle cells of **Sucquet-Hoyer canal** origin
  - **AD** inheritance, due to loss-of-function mutations in **glomulin** (*GLMN*) gene
- Clinical presentation: presents in **infancy** or childhood with **multiple lesions** (soft, partially compressible blue nodules > confluent plaques); favors **lower extremities**; usually **asymptomatic** (pain is more common with glomus tumors)
- Histology: large, dilated vessels surrounded by a small number of glomus cells
- Treatment: sclerotherapy, CO_2 laser, and Nd:YAG laser may help
  - Surgical excision generally not feasible for GVM, since multiple lesions and high rate of recurrence
- Comparison with glomus tumor
  - Glomus tumor: **more common** (accounts for 80% of all glomus lesions); affects **young adults** (20–40 yo); **solitary** blue papule or nodule with triad of **tenderness, sensitivity to cold, and paroxysmal pain**; most common on palms and **subungual area** (may result in bony erosion); histology shows dense proliferation of **many glomus cells** surrounding small vascular spaces; easily treated with excision

Lymphatic malformations

Microcystic lymphatic malformations (superficial lymphatic malformation, "lymphangioma circumscriptum")

- More common than macrocystic LMs
- Present in first few months to years of life
- Always **confined to one anatomic region**; most common sites = **abdomen**, axillae, mouth (esp. **tongue**), and genital region
- Presents w/ **clusters of papulovesicles** with clear or **blood-tinged** fluid (red-purple in color), either discrete or coalescing into a plaque, resembling **"frog spawn"** (Fig. 4.16)
- On histology, collections of small dilated lymphatic channels in the dermis are lined by endothelial cells
  - **D2-40** (podoplanin) and **LYVE-1** positive
- Can perform surgical excision, sclerotherapy or destructive measures (CO_2 or pulsed dye lasers) for localized lesions

Macrocystic lymphatic malformations (cystic hygroma)

- Congenital lesions are thought to result from abnormal lymphatic development during embryogenesis
- Associated with fetal aneuploidy, including **Turner syndrome and Down syndrome**; also associated with Noonan syndrome and achondroplasia (note: congenital lymphedema of the hands and feet may also be a clue to these conditions)

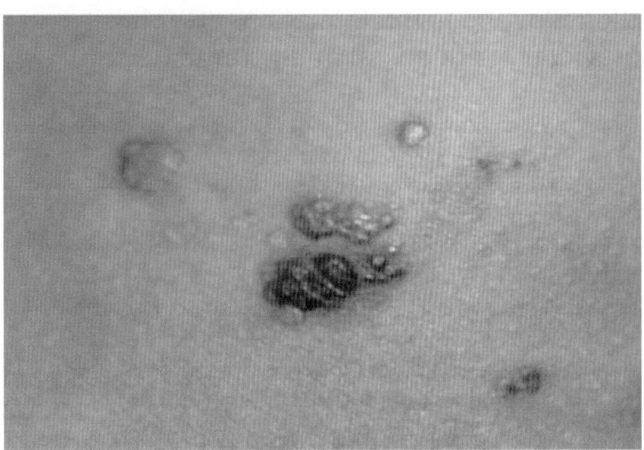

Fig. 4.16 Microcystic lymphatic malformation—irregularly grouped, translucent, and red papules. (From Marks JG Jr, Miller JJ. Dermal and subcutaneous growths. In: *Lookingbill and Marks' Principles of Dermatology*. 6th ed. Philadelphia: Elsevier; 2019:75–94.)

- Majority (~60%) are present at birth
- Presents as a large, soft, bluish, and sometimes translucent mass, with normal overlying skin
  - Transilluminates with light
  - Head, neck, and axilla/chest most common locations, favoring left side
- Sudden size ↑ may herald infection or intralesional hemorrhage
- On histology, large, multicystic, irregular lymphatic sinuses with a single layer endothelial lining, a fibrous adventitia, and both smooth and striated muscle component
  - **D2-40** (podoplanin) and **LYVE-1** positive
- Mortality (<6%), usually as a result of airway obstruction or pneumonia
- Complications include pleural/abdominal/pericardial effusions, lymphedema, cardiac failure, and respiratory failure

Gorham-Stout (disappearing bone) disease

- LM proliferates to involve the underlying bone and leads to osteolysis; may also be associated with chylothorax if upper trunk is involved

Congenital lymphedema (hereditary congenital lymphedema, Nonne-Milroy syndrome)

- **Female** > male
- Developmental aplasia, hypoplasia, and/or functional failure of lymphatic vessels
- **AD** inheritance; due to loss-of-function mutations in ***FLT4* gene** (encodes VEGFR3, which is required for lymphatic development)
- Presents at birth (or soon after) and persists for life
- Painless pitting edema of **bilateral lower extremities**
  - Over time, involved area becomes firm and fibrotic
  - Associated features: **hydrocele**, prominent veins, and upslanting toenails
- Treatment options: massage (manual lymphatic drainage), use of compression garments, and surgical interventions
- Contrast with **lymphedema-distichiasis syndrome**: also a form of hereditary lymphedema but has **peripubertal-onset** (10–30 yo); AD inheritance; *FOXC2* mutation; lower-limb lymphedema + distichiasis (extra eyelashes ranging from a single hair to a full set)

Arteriovenous malformations

AVMs

- Rarest but most dangerous type of vascular malformation
- Developmental anomaly arising early in embryogenesis → abnormal communication between an artery and vein causing high-flow (**fast-flow**) shunting of blood from the arterial circulation to the venous circulation (AV shunting)
- Erythematous to violaceous patches/nodules/tumors that are warm to touch and have **palpable thrill or pulsation**; most commonly **cephalic** (70%)
- Peripheral edema, pain, varicosities, ulceration, and limb hypertrophy may develop
- Small, hemodynamically stable AVMs are asymptomatic, but larger, hemodynamically unstable **AVMs may → tachycardia/CHFs**
- Puberty, **pregnancy**, and trauma are common exacerbating factors
- **MRI and ultrasound** studies confirm diagnosis and assess disease extent
- On histology, circumscribed, unencapsulated, and thick-walled **arterioles w/ direct connection to veins** (thin-walled), and abundant superficial capillaries
- **Embolization** + **excision** is the treatment of choice for symptomatic lesions; amputation may be required as a result of aggressive growth
- Consumptive coagulopathy may develop in larger AVM

Parkes-Weber syndrome

- Mutations in *RASA1* have been noted, can be isolated or noted in patients with CM-AVM (also caused by *RASA1*)
- Characterized by CMs, VMs, LMs, and **multiple fast-flow AVMs/shunts (differentiates it from KTS,** which only has slow-flow malformations)
- Typically affects the **lower extremities**
  - **Soft tissue and bony hypertrophy**
- Diagnose with **duplex ultrasound and MRI/MRA**
- **High-output cardiac failure** can occur in infancy or later in life
- The development of **lytic bone lesions** can be seen
- Poor prognosis after puberty with continued growth of the AV malformation

Cobb syndrome (cutaneomeningospinal angiomatosis)

- Spinal hemangioma or **AVM (most common)** + **cutaneous AVM or CM (depending on source cited) of the same metamere of the torso**
- Cutaneous manifestations: faint erythema (elicited with rubbing the affected area, often with Valsalva maneuver) to violaceous patches and plaques
  - Located on lumbar back
  - Painful throbbing (due to AVM) may develop
- **Neurologic abnormalities (due to enlarging AVM,** which causes a mass effect on spinal cord) typically develop in

childhood and include back pain or headache, muscle atrophy, weakness/numbness, and bowel/bladder dysfunction 2° to spinal compression

- MRI = **imaging modality of choice**

Bonnet–Dechaume–Blanc syndrome is the similar association of a facial metameric AVM extending to the brain/orbit.

Other vascular disorders

Cutis marmorata telangiectatica congenita

- Unknown etiology; may represent mosaicism
- Present **at birth** as reticulated erythematous-violaceous vascular network (Fig. 4.17)
  - Usually on **lower extremities and unilateral**
  - Cold exposure may accentuate cutaneous features
  - **Atrophy and ulceration** can occur within the lesion → scarring
  - Often fades somewhat over first 2 to 3 years of life
- Ipsilateral limb atrophy may occur (girth and length)
- Neurologic abnormalities in some: seizures, macrocephaly, developmental delay, and/or ophthalmologic anomalies (e.g., **glaucoma**)
- **Adams-Oliver syndrome:** CMTC with scalp aplasia cutis congenita and transverse limb defects

Angiokeratoma corporis diffusum (ACD)

- Finding seen in **Fabry disease**, **fucosidosis, sialidosis,** GM1 gangliosidosis, galactosialidosis, aspartyl-glycosaminuria, and Kanzaki disease
- Histology: numerous thin-walled ectatic blood-filled capillaries in the papillary dermis with a hyperkeratotic epidermis
- Fabry disease:
  - **XLR** lysosomal storage disease 2° to deficiency of alpha-galactosidase (***GLA* gene** mutation)
    - Glycosphingolipids accumulate in the vascular endothelium and in epithelial, perithelial, and smooth muscle cells of multiple organs (skin, eye, heart, brain, kidney, and peripheral nervous system) → endothelial swelling and proliferation
  - Pubertal males develop thousands of angiokeratomas in **"bathing trunk" distribution** between umbilicus and knees, as well as oral mucosa/conjunctiva; a/w hypohidrosis
  - **"Whorl-like" corneal opacities**, and **posterior capsular cataracts**
  - Episodic and/or chronic paresthesias, often triggered by stress/temperature/fatigue (**"Fabry crisis"**); often the **initial manifestation in early childhood**; can develop **peripheral neuropathy**
  - Cardiac rhythm/conduction abnormalities, cardiomegaly, CHF, **CVAs**, angina/myocardial infarction (MI), peripheral edema, and hypertension
  - Renal destruction → polyuria, hematuria, and **renal failure**
    - Urinalysis typically reveals birefringent lipid globules (**"Maltese crosses"**)
  - Female heterozygotes have much milder presentation (30% w/ ACD; 70% w/ corneal opacities)
  - **Recombinant enzyme therapy is the treatment of choice**, and can reverse/delay cardiac, renal, and neurologic complications
    - Progressive neuropathy, renal failure, and cardiac disease
    - Symptomatic strokes in fourth decade, w/ recurrence
    - In patients receiving enzyme replacement, cardiac complications and cerebrovascular disease are the main causes of mortality
  - Median age of death = 50 years of age
- Fucosidosis:
  - AR lysosomal storage disease as a result of a mutation/deficiency in **α-L fucosidase**
  - ACD occurs earlier in life (around 5 years old) and is more generalized
  - Hypo- or hyperhidrosis, coarse facies, progressive neuromotor and cognitive deterioration/seizures, growth failure, visceromegaly, recurrent infections, and dysostosis multiplex
  - Ultimately fatal

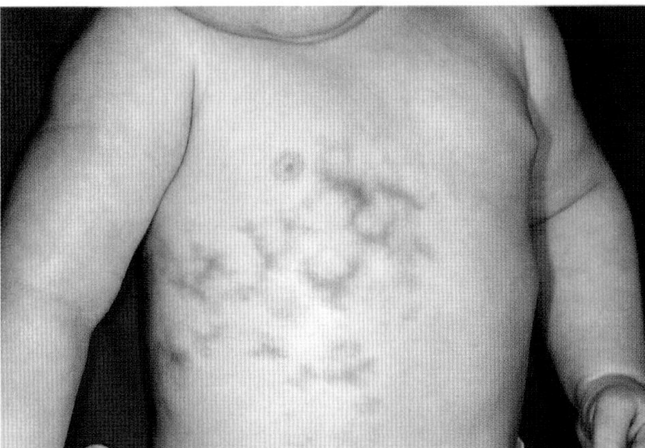

Fig. 4.17 Cutis marmorata telangiectatica congenita. The reticulate mottling was limited to the chest in this newborn male. (From Paller AS, Mancini AJ. Vascular disorders of infancy and childhood. In: *Hurwitz Clinical Pediatric Dermatology: A Textbook of Skin Disorders of Childhood and Adolescence*. 5th ed. Philadelphia: Elsevier; 2016:279–316.)

Vascular disorders characterized by telangiectasias

See Table 4.11

4.7 DISORDERS OF HAIR AND NAILS

Pachyonychia congenita

- **AD** mutations in *KRT6A*, *KRT6B*, *KRT16*, and *KRT17* genes
- Three characteristic features: **onychodystrophy, plantar keratoderma, and plantar pain**, which develop during childhood
  - Onychodystrophy: discoloration and progressive hyperkeratosis of the nail plate most pronounced at the free edge with a pincer-like appearance (does not have to affect all nails) (Fig. 4.18)

Table 4.11 Vascular Disorders Characterized by Telangiectasias

Diagnosis	Etiology	Key Characteristics of Telangiectasia(s)	Distribution of Telangiectasia(s)	Other Clinical Features
Spider angioma (nevus araneus)	Usually **idiopathic in children** and not indicative of underlying systemic disorder Associated with **liver disease, pregnancy, and estrogen therapy more in adults**	Central erythematous papule (arteriole) with radiating linear macules Blanches with diascopy	Most commonly on cheeks, nose, or dorsal hands	None when idiopathic, treat with PDL if desired
Unilateral nevoid telangiectasia	Rarely congenital When acquired may be idiopathic or associated with puberty, pregnancy, estrogen therapy, or liver disease	Usually macular, but may have papular center Pallor or vasoconstriction around telangiectasias represents "vascular steal"	Unilateral distribution on upper extremity, trunk, neck, or face May have dermatomal distribution	None when idiopathic
Angioma serpiginosum	Unclear if this represents a vascular malformation or proliferation	Pinpoint red to violaceous papules usually in a serpiginous pattern May be purpuric	Most commonly on **lower extremities**, but may be more extensive	More common in females (90%)
Generalized essential telangiectasia	Sporadic and idiopathic	Macular, retiform, or linear May coalesce to form large patches	Usually **begins on legs** and spreads proximally Eventually widespread, but usually spares face	More common in **females** Slowly progressive May be asymptomatic or associated with paresthesias (numbness, tingling, or burning)
Hereditary benign telangiectasia	AD mutations in *TELAB1* gene on 5q14	Variable morphology including macular, punctate, or plaque-like Surrounding pallor first appear between 2 and 12 years of age	Predominantly on face, arms, and upper trunk May be on lips and palate	Slowly progressive No associated systemic disease
Hereditary hemorrhagic telangiectasia (HHT, Osler-Weber-Rendu syndrome)	**AD** mutations in **endoglin** (**HHT1**), activin receptor-like kinase 1 (***ALK1***) (**HHT 2**) or growth/differentiation factor-2 (*GDF2*) gene; other genes may be involved Juvenile polyposis with HHT (JPHT) caused by mutations in *SMAD4* gene	Dark red and may be elevated May not appear until third or fourth decade of life	Predilection for **lips**, tongue, palate, nasal mucosa, ears, palms, soles, and nail beds	Most common **initial presentation is epistaxis** (night time) Can also get anemia from GI bleeding AVMs: pulmonary (HHT1 typically), cerebral, and hepatic (HHT2 typically)
Ataxia telangiectasia (Louis-Bar syndrome)	**AR** mutations in ataxia-telangiectasia mutated (***ATM***) **gene** (regulates cell cycle control and the cellular damage response to double-strand DNA breaks and confers radiosensitivity and chromosomal instability)—see ↑ chromosomal breakage *in vitro* w/ ionizing radiation **Of note, female carriers of the *ATM* gene have ↑ risk of breast cancer**	**Oculocutaneous telangiectasias** appear around 3–5 years of age Ocular lesions often striking Skin lesions may be subtle and pinpoint Not present in all patients	Typically **first appear on bulbar conjunctivae** at 3–5 years of age Skin telangiectasias tend to be symmetric and predilection for sun-exposed areas	**Truncal ataxia usually first manifestation**, followed by choreoathetosis, myoclonus, and oculomotor signs (progressive neurologic deterioration) Other dermatologic manifestations: **noninfectious granulomas**, progeroid/sclerodermoid changes of skin, hypo- or hyperpigmented patches, and canities Growth failure, thymus hypoplasia, developmental delay, and endocrine anomalies (hypogonadism and diabetes) **↑ alpha-fetoprotein** **Immunodeficiency (↓ IgA/↓ IgG/↓ IgE/↑ IgM)** Chronic **sinopulmonary infections** w/ *Streptococcus pneumoniae* **Bronchiectasis → respiratory failure = #1 cause of death** (average 20 years of age) **↑ Risk of malignancies (esp. leukemia and lymphoma in adolescence; also breast CA)**

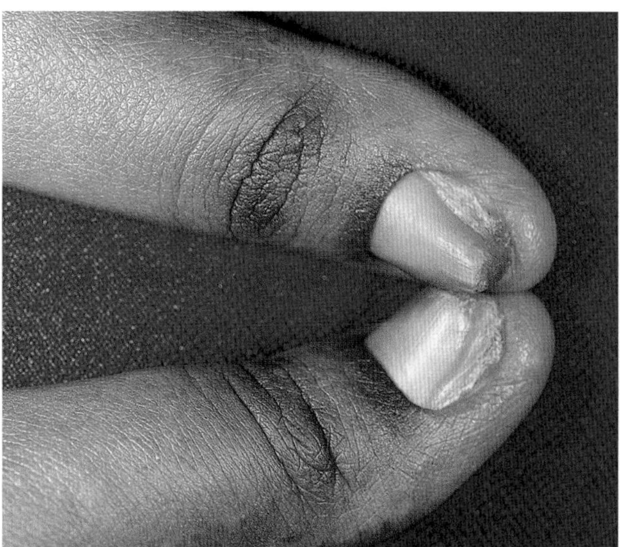

Fig. 4.18 Pachyonychia congenita. Nails show progressive discoloration, tenting, and thickening, particularly owing to accumulation of a horny, yellowish-brown material of the undersurface that causes the nail to project upward from the nail bed at the free margin. Although unusual, this adolescent's nail changes began during the teenage years. (From Paller AS, Mancini AJ. Disorders of hair and nails. In: *Hurwitz Clinical Pediatric Dermatology: A Textbook of Skin Disorders of Childhood and Adolescence*. 5th ed. Philadelphia: Elsevier; 2016:136–174.)

- Painful focal plantar keratoderma with hyperhidrosis and secondary bullae and fissures develop during childhood; palmar involvement is less severe
- Other manifestations may include pilosebaceous cysts, cheilitis, corneal dystrophy, and hoarseness
- Type I: Jadassohn-Lewandowski
  - *KRT6A* and *KRT16*
  - Full expression usually not until late childhood or adulthood
  - Recurrent paronychia
  - **Benign oral leukoplakia** of the tongue and buccal mucosa (vs. premalignant in dyskeratosis congenita)
  - **Follicular hyperkeratosis** of knees, elbows, back, and buttocks
- Type II: Jackson-Lawler
  - ***KRT6B*** and ***KRT17***
  - **Natal teeth**
  - Minimal oral leukokeratosis
  - **Steatocystomas**
  - Milder keratoderma
- EGFR inhibitors (e.g. erlotinib) may be useful for the painful plantar keratoderma

Ectodermal dysplasias

Heterogeneous group of genetic disorders w/ variable abnormalities of hair, teeth, nails, and eccrine glands

Hypohidrotic ectodermal dysplasia (Christ-Siemens-Touraine syndrome)

- **XLR mutations in ectodysplasin (*ED1*)** classically; AD/AR mutations in ectodysplasin receptor (*EDAR*) and ectodysplasin receptor-associated death domain (*EDARDD*)
  - Female carriers may demonstrate features as a result of random x-inactivation of *ED1* (e.g., alopecia, dental defects, and Blaschkoid linear patches of hypohidrosis)
- Clinical triad: ↓ **sweating, hypotrichosis, and abnormal dentition**
  - Facial features: **frontal bossing, flat nasal bridge (saddle nose),** large nostrils, wide/flat malar cheeks, **thick everted lips**, and prominent chin (Fig. 4.19)
  - Hair: **hypotrichosis** with thin, light hair; eyelashes absent
  - Skin: soft/smooth, thin wrinkled skin; periorbital hyperpigmentation; hypoplastic breast/areola, mild onychodystrophy
  - Teeth: dentition delayed; may have **peg-shaped, conical or missing teeth**
  - Eccrine glands: **risk for hyperthermia (may present as fever of unknown origin)** as a result of ↓ perspiration; ↓ lacrimation may be seen
  - Notably: nails are NORMAL (unlike hidrotic ED)
  - May develop chronic sinus disease, pulmonary infections, and asthma

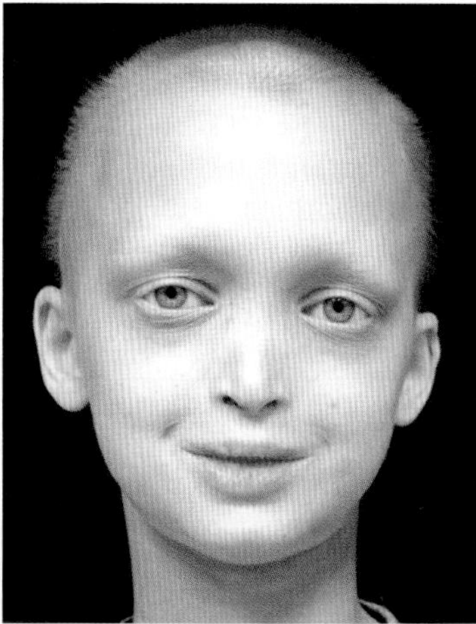

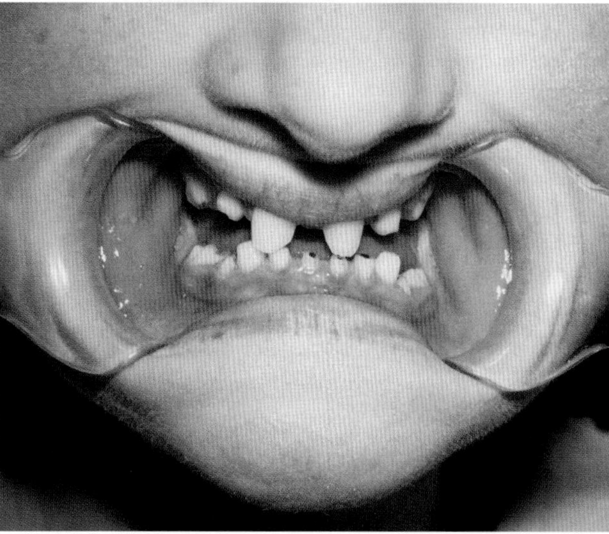

Fig. 4.19 (A) and **(B)** Hypohidrotic ectodermal dysplasia with flat nasal bridge, depressed nasal tip, sparse hair (scalp, eyebrows, and eyelashes), and peg-shaped teeth. (From James WD, Elston DM, McMahon PJ. Genodermatoses and congenital anomalies. In: *Andrews' Diseases of the Skin Clinical Atlas*. Philadelphia: Elsevier; 2018:379–404. *A*, Courtesy of Scott Bartlett, MD.)

- Boards factoid: **hypohidrotic ectodermal dysplasia with immunodeficiency** is a result of mutations in ***IKBKG/NEMO* (XLR)** or *NFKBIA* (AD); susceptible to recurrent pyogenic or atypical mycobacterial infections

Hidrotic ectodermal dysplasia (Clouston syndrome)

- AD mutation in ***GJB6* (connexin 30)**
- Clinical triad: **marked onychodystrophy**, **PPK (with stippling, a common feature in connexin PPKs)**, and **hair abnormalities**
  - Onychodystrophy with variably hyperkeratotic/thin/striated/discolored nails; **hypotrichosis with thin/brittle hair**
  - Normal sweating, facial features, and teeth
  - Possible ophthalmologic (e.g., conjunctivitis, strabismus, and cataracts) and musculoskeletal (**tufted distal phalanges**) anomalies

Ectodermal dysplasias due to *p63* mutation

- **AD** mutation in ***p63*** (critical transcription factor required for ectodermal, orofacial, and limb development)
- Overlapping features of clinical disease from *p63* mutations (thought to be a disease spectrum)
- Defined clinical syndromes include:
  - Rapp-Hodgkin syndrome: clefting of lip/palate/uvula, hypoplasia of maxilla, small narrow nails, and small conical teeth
  - Ankyloblepharon-ectodermal dysplasia-clefting syndrome (AEC; Hay-Wells syndrome): congenital fusion of eyelids (**ankyloblepharon**) a/w facial clefting or mid-face hypoplasia; diffuse collodion-like peeling/erythema seen at birth; **scalp w/ chronic erosive dermatitis → frequent *Staphylococcus* infections**
  - Ectrodactyly ectodermal dysplasia-cleft lip/palate syndrome (EEC): **ectrodactyly** (developmental anomaly of median ray of feet > hands → **"lobster claw"** deformity/missing digits), facial clefting, mild PPK, **conductive hearing loss**, and **genitourinary anomalies**
  - *p63* mutations also underlie acro-dermato-ungual-lacrimal-tooth (ADULT) syndrome, limb-mammary syndrome (LMS), and split hand/foot malformation (SHFM)
- All syndromes may have wiry/sparse hair, dystrophic nails, ↓ number of teeth/hypoplastic enamel, hypohidrosis, ↓ tearing, and short stature or poor weight gain

Schöpf-Schulz-Passarge syndrome

- AR, *WNT10A* mutation
- Ectodermal dysplasia with multiple eyelid apocrine hidrocystomas, increased risk of BCC, hypodontia, hypotrichosis, PPK, and nail dystsrophy

Other disorders

Rubinstein-Taybi syndrome

- **Sporadic** mutation in ***CREBBP***
- Broad thumbs/halluces w/ racquet nails (**brachyonychia**)
- CMs, short stature, severe **developmental delay**, cryptorchidism, **congenital heart defects**, and typical facies (beaked nose, downslanting palpebral fissures, low-set ears, epicanthal folds, and grimacing smile), **multiple pilomatricomas**

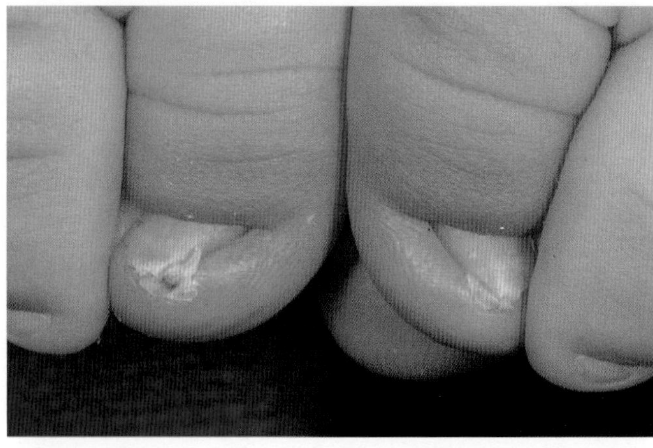

Fig. 4.20 Congenital malalignment of the great toe. (From Paller AS, Mancini AJ. Disorders of hair and nails. In: *Hurwitz Clinical Pediatric Dermatology: A Textbook of Skin Disorders of Childhood and Adolescence*. 5th ed. Philadelphia: Elsevier; 2016:136–174.)

Parakeratosis pustulosa

- **Subacute paronychia**, school-aged **girls**
- **Fingers** (thumb, first finger most common; toes rare), typically **single digit**
- **Associated with underlying inflammatory disease** (atopic dermatitis, psoriasis, contact dermatitis)

Congenital Malalignment of the great toenails

- **Likely AD,** with variable expression
- **Lateral deviation of nailplate** (due to lateral deviation of nail matrix), first toe, with nail ridging, thickening, darkening, and triangular shape (Fig. 4.20)
- **50% spontaneously improve**

Other nail changes are discussed in Chapter 3, General Dermatology. Menkes disease, Björnstad syndrome, Crandall syndrome, argininosuccinic aciduria, and citrullinemia are also discussed in Chapter 3, General Dermatology. See Table 4.12 and Figs. 4.21 and 4.22 for selected pediatric hair disorders.

4.8 INHERITED METABOLIC AND NUTRITIONAL DISORDERS

Acrodermatitis enteropathica (genetic form)

- **Primary form is AR—mutations in *SLC39A4*** (encodes intestinal zinc-specific transporter ZIP4)
  - Acquired/secondary zinc deficiency (acrodermatitis-like syndrome): similar clinical findings and histology, but due to low zinc intake (**alcoholics**, anorexia) or malabsorption (IBD); also may arise in **infants who are initially breastfed but switch to formula (lower**

Table 4.12 Selected Pediatric Hair Disorders

Disorder	Pathogenesis	Clinical Features of Alopecia	Additional Clinical Features	Microscopy/Trichoscopy
Temporal triangular alopecia	Unknown	May be present at birth Usually diagnosed between 2 and 9 years of age Localized triangular patch of alopecia involving the **frontotemporal scalp** Often unilateral (left > right)	If large areas of involvement, consider cerebellotrigeminal dermal dysplasia	Trichoscopy and microscopy: ↓ terminal hairs and ↑ vellus hairs
Atrichia with papules	Mutations in **hairless (*HR*) gene**	**Hair is normal at birth, then is quickly shed** after birth Follicular cysts and **milia-like papules** appear later	May be associated with vitamin D–resistant rickets (early-onset rickets, hypocalcemia, 2° hyperparathyroidism, and ↑ 1,25-OH vitamin D3)	Disintegration of the lower two third of the hair follicle Multiple small cystic structures
Wooly hair	Nonsyndromic forms may be AD or AR Syndromic forms are AR	Poor hair growth noted from birth Hair is fine, dry, and curly with a corrugated appearance	<u>Naxos syndrome:</u> PPK, wooly hair, and **right** ventricular dysplasia/ cardiomyopathy <u>Carvajal syndrome:</u> PPK, wooly hair, and **left**-sided cardiomyopathy	NA
Uncombable hair (pili trianguli et canaliculi)	Unknown	Presents during infancy or early childhood Hair is pale/blonde, dry, and unruly w/ **shiny/"spun glass"** appearance	Mild onychodystrophy Various ectodermal dysplasias	Light microscopy or scanning EM of hair: in cross section, hair shaft appears triangular or reniform with a canalicular longitudinal depression
Monilethrix	Mutations in hair keratins (e.g., ***KRT81, KRT83,*** and ***KRT86***) and desmoglein 4 (***DSG4***) Mutations in hair keratins are AD but mutation in **DSG4 is AR**	Hair typically appears normal at birth During infancy, hair becomes **short and brittle** with a **beaded appearance**	Koilonychia **Keratosis pilaris** (most common association)	Light microscopy/ trichoscopy of hair: **uniform elliptical nodes along hair shaft**
Pili torti	Depending on associated syndromes	Hair typically sparse or absent at birth Poor hair growth Hair appears spangled	**Menkes kinky hair syndrome** **Bazex-Dupre-Christol syndrome** **Rombo syndrome** **Björnstad syndrome** **Crandall syndrome**	Light microscopy/ trichoscopy of hair: flattened, twisted hair shafts occurring at irregular intervals
Trichorrhexis nodosa (Fig. 4.21)	Most commonly acquired as a result of trauma, such as from chemical and thermal treatments AD form also exists	**Most common hair shaft anomaly** Variably dry, lusterless, sparse hair Inherited form presents in infancy Acquired form presents in adolescence	Argininosuccinic aciduria Citrullinemia Oculo-dental-digital dysplasia Trichothiodystrophy Netherton syndrome	Light microscopy/trichoscopy of hair: intermittent **nodules with the appearance of broom bristles**
Trichorrhexis invaginata ("bamboo hair") (Fig. 4.22)	AR mutation in ***SPINK5*** (encodes LEKT1)	Dry, lusterless, sparse hair Poor hair growth	Marker for **Netherton syndrome**	Light microscopy/ trichoscopy of hair: hair shaft intussuscepts into itself, creating the appearance of a **"golf tee"** or "ball in cup" joint seen
Marie Unna hypotrichosis	AD mutations in *U2HR*	Absence of scalp hair, eyebrows, and eyelashes at birth Hair grows in coarse and twisted Beginning in adolescence, hair is progressively lost	Widely spaced central incisors	Histology: mild-moderate inflammation, w/ ↓ # of hair follicles, and without scarring or fibrosis Scanning EM: longitudinal grooves and peeling of the cuticle Light microscopy of hair: hair shafts have variable diameter and a twisted, bent appearance
Alopecia mucinosa (follicular mucinosis)	In children, usually an **idiopathic** inflammatory dermatosis **In children, rarely a presentation of cutaneous T-cell lymphoma**	Favors **head**, neck, and upper torso in children; may involve scalp or eyebrows **Usually solitary** Presentation may include grouped follicular papules, with or without erythema, and scaling, which may coalesce into a boggy plaque Alopecia is a prominent feature	NA	Follicular degeneration Accumulation of mucin within hair follicles Periappendageal, perivascular, and/or interstitial lymphocytic/mixed inflammatory cell infiltrate If histologic features suggest mycosis fungoides, check **T-cell receptor gene rearrangement assay** from a skin biopsy

Continued

Table 4.12 Selected Pediatric Hair Disorders—cont'd

Disorder	Pathogenesis	Clinical Features of Alopecia	Additional Clinical Features	Microscopy/Trichoscopy
Loose anagen syndrome	Typically sporadic AD inheritance may be seen Defective anchoring of the hair shaft (**defective inner root sheath keratinization**) to the follicle resulting in **easily and painlessly plucked hair**	**Common in young, fair-haired girls 2–6 years of age** Diffuse hair thinning Hair may appear fine, limp, and matted Girls typically grow out of this without any intervention	Noonan-like syndrome cause by *SHOC2* mutations	Trichoscopy: **multiple anagen hairs with ruffled cuticles** and misshapen bulbs ("hockey stick")
Short anagen syndrome	Shortened anagen growth phase	Fine, short hair present at birth Poor hair growth	NA	Histology and trichogram: ↑ telogen hairs
Nevoid hypertrichosis	Unknown	Localized patches of terminal hair of abnormal length, color, and/or diameter Common sites include lumbosacral area, anterior neck, and elbows (**hypertrichosis cubiti**)	Rare associations with neurodevelopmental abnormalities	NA
Congenital hypertrichosis, generalized	Unknown; XLD inheritance has been reported, with both syndromic and nonsyndromic presentations	Universal overgrowth of terminal hair	Ambras syndrome: excessive vellus-like hairs on the face, ears, and shoulders; associated with mutations in tricho-rhino-phalangeal syndrome gene *TRPS1* Hypertrichosis lanuginosa: persistence of generalized lanugo hairs Hypertrichosis and gingival hyperplasia: diffuse overgrowth of terminal hair, gingival hyperplasia **Cornelia de Lange syndrome**: AD mutation in *NIPBL* in some cases; hirsutism, **synophrys**, **trichomegaly**, low hairline, developmental delay/psychomotor retardation, **cutis marmorata,** hypertonicity, short stature, fifth finger clinodactyly, cryptorchidism, congenital heart defects, and recurrent lung infections/aspiration → death or hearing loss	NA
Keratosis pilaris	Abnormal keratinization of hair follicles	Affects 25%–60% of adolescents and adults Multiple small, scaling, and skin-colored to pink follicular papules Favor the **cheeks, upper arms, thighs, and buttocks** Treatments: keratolytics (e.g. salicyclic acid, TCA, glycolic acid, ammonium lactate), chlorine dioxide, lasers (e.g. diode, Nd:YAG)	Often associated w/ **atopy**, xerosis, or ichthyosis vulgaris Trisomy 21 Some ectodermal dysplasias	Histology: keratotic plugging of the pilosebaceous follicles; mild hypogranulosis and hyperkeratosis
Keratosis pilaris atrophicans, atrophoderma vermiculatum subtype	Usually sporadic; AD inheritance reported	Erythematous papules with follicular plugging, horn cysts, and **atrophic cribriform scarring** **Cheeks** and forehead; less commonly neck and extremities Typically presents between 5 and 12 yo	Trisomy 21 **Rombo syndrome** (atrophoderma vermiculatum, basal cell carcinoma, milia, telangiectasias, acral erythema)	Histology: epidermal atrophy; atrophic hair follicles with keratotic follicular plugs and dermal cysts; variable perifollicular inflammation

Table 4.12 Selected Pediatric Hair Disorders—cont'd

Disorder	Pathogenesis	Clinical Features of Alopecia	Additional Clinical Features	Microscopy/Trichoscopy
Keratosis pilaris atrophicans, ulerythema ophyrogenes subtype	Usually sporadic; AD inheritance reported	Erythematous papules with **follicular plugging and atrophic scarring** Scarring alopecia of **eyebrows** Eyebrows, cheeks, and scalp; less commonly extremities Boys > girls; presents during infancy	**Noonan syndrome** Cardio-facio-cutaneous syndrome Cornelia de Lange syndrome Rubenstein-Taybi syndrome Wooly hair	Histology: keratotic plugging of pilosebaceous follicles and mild perifollicular inflammation (early) Dermal fibrosis and atrophy of the hair follicles and sebaceous glands (late)
Keratosis pilaris atrophicans, keratosis follicularis spinulosa decalvans subtype	XLR mutations in spermidine/ spermine N(1)-acetyltransferase (SSAT) Mutations in membrane-bound transcription factor protease site 2 reported (similar to IFAP) AD inheritance also described	Pink hyperkeratotic papules with follicular plugging Progressive scarring alopecia Eyebrows, eyelashes, and scalp Extensive keratosis pilaris begins in early childhood Scarring alopecia begins in adolescence	Palmoplantar keratoderma Corneal dystrophy with photophobia Atopic disease	Histology: concentric perifollicular fibrosis w/ mixed perifollicular inflammation and follicular plugging
Eruptive vellus hair cysts	Unknown, but may represent developmental anomaly of vellus hair follicles Often sporadic AD reported	1- to 3-mm skin-colored to **hyperpigmented** follicular papules Seen in school-aged children and adolescents Favor the **mid chest**, but may also be seen on the face, neck, extremities, buttocks, back, and abdomen	Hidrotic ectodermal dysplasia Hypohidrotic ectodermal dysplasia Pachyonychia congenita	Histology: cystic dilation of the infundibulum; cysts contain vellus hairs and laminated keratinaceous debris

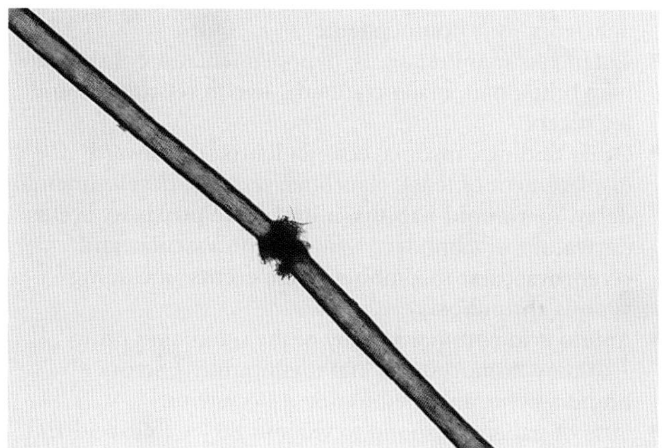

Fig. 4.21 Trichorrhexis nodosa. Light microscopic appearance. (From Lam JM, Wong LC. Hair disorders. In: Eichenfield LF, Frieden IJ, eds. *Neonatal and Infant Dermatology*. 3rd ed. Philadelphia: Elsevier; 2015.)

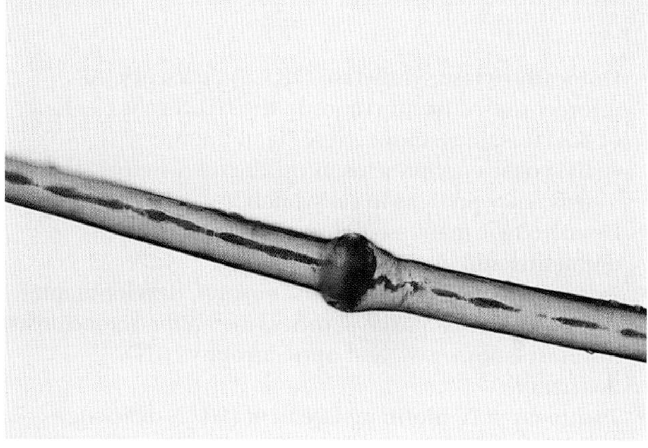

Fig. 4.22 Trichorrhexis invaginata in Netherton syndrome. Light microscopic appearance. (From Lam JM, Wong LC. Hair disorders. In: Eichenfield LF, Frieden IJ, eds. *Neonatal and Infant Dermatology*. 3rd ed. Philadelphia: Elsevier; 2015.)

bioavailability) or breastfeed from a mother who has a low serum/breastmilk zinc level or premature infants (have lower baseline zinc stores)

- Triad of **erosive vesiculopustular eczematous lesions involving the diaper area, face (periorificial), and acral areas,** along with **diarrhea** and **alopecia** (Fig. 4.23)
  - Severe irritability, failure to thrive, photophobia, stomatitis/ glossitis/perlèche, and nail dystrophy commonly seen
- On histology, **cytoplasmic pallor of keratinocytes in upper epidermis**, with ballooning and reticular degeneration; necrosis of keratinocytes in early lesions
- On laboratory, ↓ **serum zinc** (<70 μg/dL), ↓ **serum alkaline phosphatase** (zinc-dependent enzyme); if zinc is normal in a patient with suspected acrodermatitis enteropathica, consider screening for biotin deficiency and cystic fibrosis as these can present similarly
- Treatment: life-long zinc sulfate supplementation → fast resolution

Biotinidase (BTD) deficiency and multiple carboxylase deficiency

- Biotin is required for the function of four carboxylase enzymes (pyruvate carboxylase, propionyl-CoA-carboxylase, alpha-methylcrotonyl-CoA carboxylase, and acetyl-CoA carboxylase); in BTD deficiency and multiple carboxylase deficiency, loss of function of these enzymes results in disruption of fatty acid oxidation and accumulation of toxic metabolites
- **BTD deficiency:** AR disorder caused by mutations in *BTD* gene

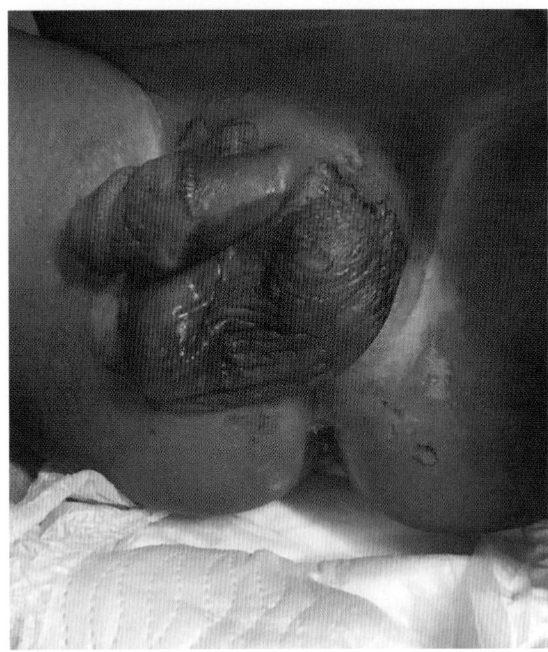

Fig. 4.23 Zinc deficiency. Erosions with a peripheral collarette of scale in the diaper area. (Personal collection, Dr. Jennifer Schoch.)

- **Holocarboxylase synthetase (HLCS)** deficiency: AR disorder caused by mutations in the *HLCS* gene (→ loss of BTD function), more severe (**fatal** if untreated)
  - BTD deficiency presents in childhood, whereas HLCS deficiency presents in early infancy
- Dermatologic manifestations: perioral/generalized **dermatitis and alopecia**
- Extracutaneous manifestations: seizures, developmental delay, hypotonia/ataxia, diarrhea, metabolic ketoacidosis, hepatosplenomegaly, and **optic atrophy** (BTD deficiency)
- Treatment = **IV biotin** replacement (HLCS deficiency requires ↑ doses)

Hartnup disease

- AR disorder caused by **mutations in *SLC6A19*** (encodes B(0)AT1, the intestinal and renal **neutral amino acid transporter**) resulting in low tryptophan
  - ↓ Tryptophan → ↓ nicotinic acid and **pellagra-like symptoms** (e.g., photosensitivity)
- Cutaneous eruption presents in **childhood as an acute photodermatitis with erythema, blistering, scaling, crusting, and scarring occurring after sun exposure in sun-exposed areas of the face, neck, arms, dorsal hands, wrists, and lower legs**
  - Atrophic glossitis, angular stomatitis, hair loss/fragility, and longitudinal nail streaks
- Untreated patients may develop cerebellar ataxia, seizures, intellectual disability, and emotional lability/psychosis
- Treatment: avoid sunlight; oral nicotinamide supplementation

Phenylketonuria

- AR disorder 2° to loss-of-function mutation in **phenylalanine hydroxylase** (*PAH* gene) → inability to convert phenylalanine to tyrosine
- Cutaneous features: **diffuse hypopigmentation** with blonde hair and blue eyes, **eczematous dermatitis, photosensitivity, and sclerodermatous changes** of the torso and thighs
  - **Hypopigmentation** of skin/hair 2° to inhibitory effect of ↑ phenylalanine on tyrosinase
  - **Mousy odor of urine**, short stature, and microcephaly
- **Developmental delay**, seizures, irritability, limb posturing and purposeless movements, psychosis, hyperactivity, and autistic features may develop if untreated
- Neonatal screening for phenylketonuria is included in the newborn screen in all states
- **Treatment with low-phenylalanine diet**/formula under the guidance of a nutritionist → good prognosis; **AVOID aspartame**

Homocystinuria

- AR disorder → deficiency of **cystathionine beta-synthetase** (*CBS* gene), which catalyzes the formation of cystathionine from homocysteine and serine; thus deficiency → ↑ **homocysteine**
- Cutaneous manifestations: hypopigmentation of skin and hair, brittle hair, malar erythema, **livedo reticularis, and leg ulcers**
- Other findings: myopia, **ectopia lentis** (**downward** displacement of lens), glaucoma, seizures, **developmental delay**, **marfanoid habitus**, **mitral valve prolapse**, pectus excavatum, arachnodactyly, and **cardiovascular and cerebrovascular thromboembolic events** (including **venous thrombosis**)
- Amino acid chromatography of the serum and urine: ↑ urinary homocysteine and methionine; ↑ serum homocysteine and methionine + ↓ cysteine
- 50% of patients respond to vitamin B6 (+ folic acid and vitamin B12)
  - Otherwise, methionine-restricted, cysteine-supplemented diet

Lesch-Nyhan syndrome

- **XLR disorder** 2° to hypoxanthine-guanine phosphoribosyl transferase mutation (*HGPRT* gene) → ↑ uric acid, ↓ dopamine
- **Orange uric acid crystals in the diaper** or hematuria may be seen in the first few months of life
- Neurodevelopmental delays, spastic cerebral palsy, choreoathetosis, and **intellectual impairment**
- **Significant self-mutilation** is characteristic
- Short stature/sstugrowth retardation, **uric acid nephropathy, gout,** and megaloblastic anemia
- Treatment of choice = allopurinol (100–300 mg/day) in divided doses; other hypouricemic agents may be considered
- Renal failure → morbidity and mortality

Prolidase deficiency

- AR disorder 2° to mutations in **peptidase D (*PEPD*)** (encodes prolidase, a ubiquitous metalloenzyme involved in the catabolism of proteins)
- Cutaneous manifestations: **severe, progressive ulceration of lower extremities**, diffuse telangiectasias, photosensitivity, and an eczematous dermatitis
  - **Recurrent infections** contribute to morbidity and mortality
- Other findings: intellectual impairment, and abnormal facies with **hypertelorism**/ptosis/beaked nose/frontal bossing

Alagille syndrome

- AD mutation in Jagged 1 (*JAG1*) (encodes ligand for Notch receptor; pathway plays role in determining cell fates in early development)
- Typical triangular facies
- **Tuberous xanthomas, hypercholesterolemia, and hypertriglyceridemia**
  - **High serum cholesterol (>200 mg/dL) and triglyceride (500–2000 mg/dL) levels**
- **Congenital intrahepatic biliary hypoplasia** (cholestasis, pruritus, and failure to thrive)
- Treatment: liver transplantation is treatment of choice; pharmacologic management of hyperlipidemia → resolution of cutaneous xanthomas
  - Without treatment, death before 5 years of age

Hunter syndrome

- **XLR** disorder 2° to mutation in ***IDS* gene** (encodes the lysosomal enzyme iduronate 2-sulfatase → accumulation of glycosaminoglycans in almost all organs and tissues)
- Cutaneous features: hypertrichosis, coarse facies (thick nose, thick lips, and tongue), **pebbled ivory-colored plaques between scapulae on upper back**, as well as the upper arms/thighs
- Cardiomyopathy, hepatosplenomegaly, skeletal deformities, progressive neurodegeneration
- ↑ Urinary heparin sulfate and dermatan sulfate (chondroitin sulfate B)
- Part of a family of disorders termed mucopolysaccharidoses—**Hurler syndrome** has dermal melanosis, developmental delay and "**gargoyle**" appearance; **all mucopolysaccharidoses have hypertrichosis and coarse facies and may be associated with extensive dermal melanosis (Mongolian spots)**

Alkaptonuria

- **AR** disorder 2° to mutation in **homogentisic 1,2-dioxygenase (*HGO*) gene**
- **Blue-gray pigmentation** (ochronosis) on face, nose, **ears** (seen well on cartilage), and sclera
- Dark sweat, cerumen, and urine (pH > 7.0; adding NaOH to urine → darkening)
- Mitral/aortic valvulitis w/ ↑ MI risk
- Intervertebral disc calcification; **severe arthritis**

4.9 INHERITED CONNECTIVE TISSUE DISORDERS

Cutis laxa/generalized elastolysis

- AD forms (less common): **elastin gene (*ELN*) or fibulin 5 (*FBLN5*)** mutations → dysregulation of elastic fiber network in the **skin** mainly (internal involvement uncommon); presents in early adulthood
- AR forms (**most common**): ***FBLN5***, *EFEMP2/FBLN4*, *LTBP4*, ATPase, *ATP6V0A2*, *PYCR1*, and *ALDH18A1*; presents at birth to early childhood; **skin + severe internal involvement**
- XLR form (**occipital horn syndrome**, previously Ehlers-Danlos syndrome **[EDS] type IX**): mutations in ATPase, Cu(2+)-transporting, alpha polypeptide **(*ATP7A*) (allelic to Menkes disease)**
- **"Aged" facial appearance (hound-dog facies)** with down-slanting palpebral fissures and a long philtrum (Fig. 4.24)
- **Loose, sagging skin** with reduced elasticity and resilience; deep voice 2° to vocal cord laxity
- Histology: sparse and/or fragmented elastic fibers
- AD cutis laxa
  - Primarily generalized cutaneous findings, cardiac valve abnormalities, aortic dilatation (variable), emphysema (uncommon), and hernias
- AR cutis laxa (ARCL)
  - ***ARCL type I***
    - ***FBLN5***, *EFEMP2*, or *LTBP4* mutations
    - Potentially fatal involvement of lungs (**hypoplastic lungs and emphysema**)
    - Cardiovascular abnormalities (aortic tortuosity and aneurysms)
    - Inguinal/diaphragmatic/umbilical hernias
    - **GI/GU diverticula**
    - Joint laxity, arachnodactyly, and fractures (variable)

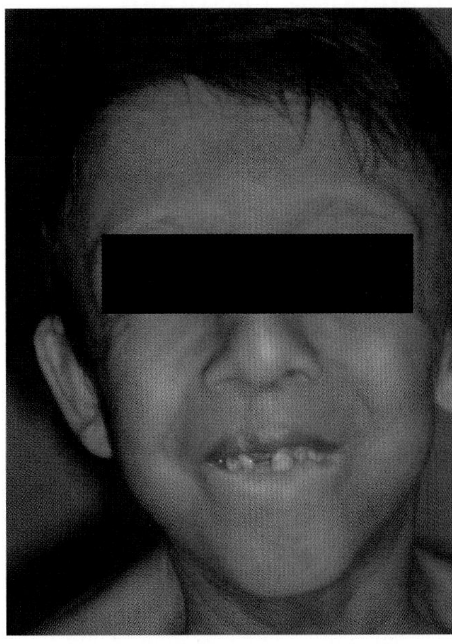

Fig. 4.24 Cutis laxa. (Personal collection, Dr. Helen Shin.)

- *ARCL type II*
  - *ATP6V0A2* (type IIA) or *PYRC1* (type IIB) mutations
  - Craniofacial anomalies
  - Cutaneous features may be primarily acral
  - Pachygyria (IIA) and absent corpus callosum (IIB)
  - Translucent skin (IIB)
- *ARCL type III (De Barsy syndrome)*
  - *ALDH18A1* (type IIIA) or *PYRC1* (type IIIB) mutations
  - Developmental delay/dystonia/neurologic deterioration
  - Progeroid appearance
  - Athetosis
  - **Corneal clouding/cataracts**
- XLR cutis laxa (now termed occipital horn syndrome)
  - Easy bruising and coarse hair (variable)
  - Tortuous arteries
  - GU diverticula
  - Inguinal, diaphragmatic, and umbilical hernias
  - Long face w/ high forehead and hooked nose
  - **Wedge-shaped occipital calcifications** (occipital horns)
  - Hip dislocations (joint laxity)
- Acquired cutis laxa
  - Primarily adults w/ sagging of skin and little associated internal involvement
  - Cutaneous involvement may be primarily acral; generalized involvement typically begins on the face/ neck
  - May occur in association with drugs (**penicillamine** and isoniazid), other cutaneous disorders (e.g., cutaneous lymphoma, **Sweet's syndrome-like eruption**, interstitial granulomatous dermatitis, and cutaneous mastocytosis) or **systemic disease** (rheumatoid arthritis, sarcoidosis, SLE, and infectious disorders)

Pseudoxanthoma elasticum

- AR disorder as a result of mutations in ***ABCC6*** (ATP-binding cassette, subfamily C, member 6) gene → 2° calcification of the elastic tissue of the eyes, skin, and arteries
- Presents during childhood or second/third decade of life
- Cutaneous manifestations
  - **Thin, yellowish papules in flexural areas** arise during the first or second decade of life (Fig. 4.25)
    - Typically first appear on the lateral aspects of the neck
    - Papules coalesce to form cobblestone-like plaques resembling **"plucked chicken skin"**
    - Antecubital and popliteal fossae, wrists, axillae, groin, and periumbilical area (in multiparous women) are involved; can also occur inside lips
    - **Perforating pseudoxanthoma elasticum**: in advanced disease, ↑ dermal calcium deposition and extrusion of this yellowish material through the epidermis may occur
    - Loss of recoil and sagging skin in axillae and groin
    - Yellow papules may develop in oral/anogenital mucosa

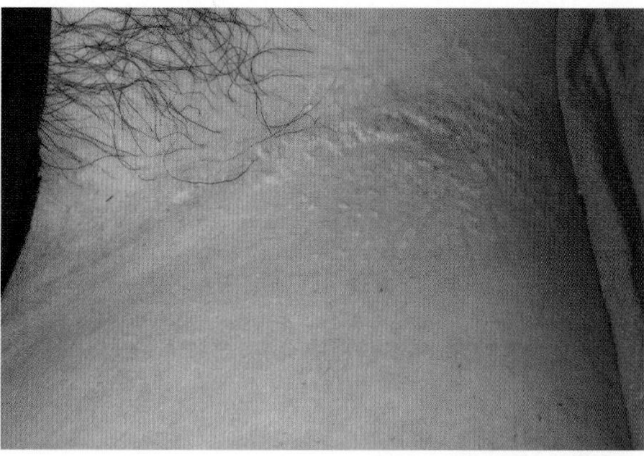

Fig. 4.25 Pseudoxanthoma elasticum. (From Neldner KH, Lebwohl MG. Pseudoxanthoma elasticum. In: Lebwohl MG, Heymann WR, Berth Jones J, Coulson I, eds. *Treatment of Skin Disease: Comprehensive Therapeutic Strategies*. 4th ed. Philadelphia: Elsevier; 2013:638–639.)

- Ocular manifestations
  - Asymptomatic **angioid streaks** (**Bruch's membrane rupture**) usually in first decade
    - "Owl's eyes": paired areas of hyperpigmented spots straddling an angioid streak
    - Agioid streaks also seen in **Paget's disease of bone**, **sickle cell anemia**, **thalassemia**, **EDS**, **lead poisoning**, and age-related degeneration
  - Macular degeneration, optic drusen, and retinal hemorrhage (→ blindness)
  - Mottling of retinal pigment epithelium
    - Most prevalent ophthalmologic finding; may precede development of angioid streaks
- Cardiovascular manifestations
  - Intermittent claudication, loss of peripheral pulses, renovascular **hypertension**, **mitral valve prolapse**, angina/**MI**, and **stroke**
  - Progressive calcification of elastic media and intima → atheromatous plaques involving predominantly medium-sized arteries (esp. in extremities)
- GI manifestations
  - **Gastric artery hemorrhage**, hematemesis, epistaxis
- Obstetric complications
  - ↑ Risk of **first trimester miscarriage** and maternal cardiovascular complications
- On histology, **distorted, basophilic, and fragmented calcified elastic fibers** in mid/deep reticular dermis (Figs. 4.26 and 4.27)
- Morbidity and mortality **2° to GI hemorrhage, cerebral hemorrhage, atherosclerotic disease, and MI**

Osteogenesis imperfecta (OI)

- Mutations in **type I collagen** → fragile bones (poor cortical modeling and less trabecular bone formation)
- There are at least eight well-defined types of OI, but types I to IV account for 90%
  - Types I (**most common form**, accounts for 50% of OI; generally **mild**; fractures in childhood and adolescence), II (**most severe** form, **fatal** in perinatal period), III (progressive and deforming—skull fractures [soft at birth] and respiratory infection), and IV (milder form)

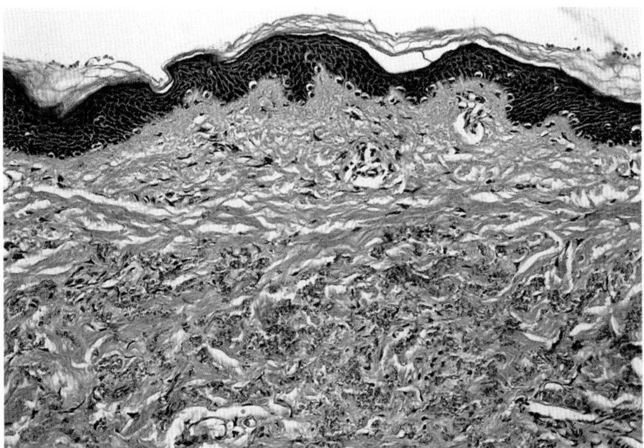

Fig. 4.26 Pseudoxanthoma elasticum. Note the short, curled elastic fibers in the reticular dermis. (From Patterson JW. Disorders of elastic tissue. In: *Weedon's Skin Pathology*. 5th ed. Philadelphia: Elsevier; 2021:413–436.)

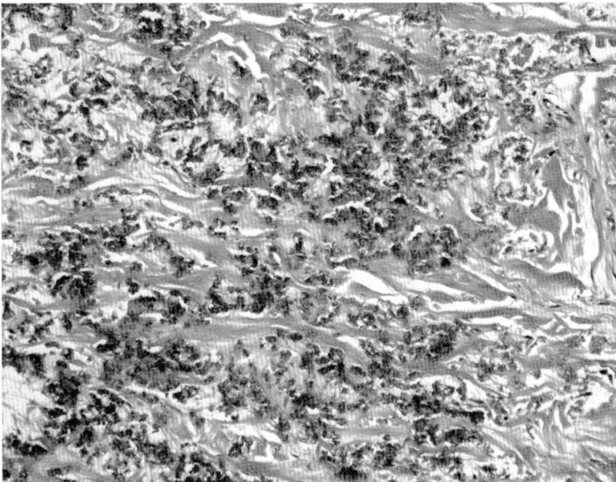

Fig. 4.27 Pseudoxanthoma elasticum. Note the short, curled elastic fibers in the reticular dermis. They are basophilic. (From Patterson JW. Disorders of elastic tissue. In: *Weedon's Skin Pathology*. 5th ed. Philadelphia: Elsevier; 2021:413–436.)

    - **AD** inheritance; due to mutations in type I collagen genes ***COL1A1* and *COL1A2***
  - Onset (birth to adulthood) and severity depend on type
- Cutaneous manifestations
  - Thin, atrophic, and **translucent skin**
  - **Easy bruisability**
  - Scars may be atrophic or hypertrophic
- Musculoskeletal manifestations
  - Hyperlaxity of ligaments and hypermobility of joints
  - **Brittle bones + fractures** (skull, long bones, and vertebrae; occurs *in utero* in severe forms)
  - **Beaded ribs**
- Other manifestations
  - **Blue sclerae are seen ~90% of patients (not seen in type IV)**
  - Otosclerosis with **hearing loss** may begin during adolescence
  - Fragile/discolored teeth
  - Dentinogenesis imperfecta (DI)
  - Mitral and aortic valve prolapse/dilatation and regurgitation
- Variable prognosis depending on disease type and severity:
  - Types I and IV: normal life span
  - Type II: **death in perinatal period**
  - Type III: increased mortality in third/fourth decade due to **respiratory failure** (2° to kyphoscoliosis) or head trauma

Ehlers-Danlos syndrome

- Heterogeneous group characterized by abnormal collagen structure and/or function within the skin, joints, and vasculature (Table 4.13)
- <u>Classical EDS (most common subtype)</u>
  - May deliver/be delivered preterm as a result of early rupture of fetal membranes; normal life span
  - Mucocutaneous manifestations
    - Velvety, soft, and doughy consistency of skin
    - **Marked hyperextensibility of skin**
    - **Poor wound healing ("cigarette paper" scars)**
    - Widened atrophic cutaneous scars **("fishmouth" wounds)**
    - Piezogenic pedal papules
    - Fragile blood vessels → hematomas and **easy bruising**
    - Subcutaneous spheroids (fat lobules that have **calcified** after losing their blood supply)
    - **Molluscoid pseudotumors** associated with scars over knees and elbows
    - **Blue sclerae**
    - **Gorlin's sign:** ability to touch tip of nose with tongue (50%)
  - Musculoskeletal manifestations
    - Generalized joint hypermobility
    - **Double-jointed fingers**
    - **Frequent subluxation of larger joints**
    - Chronic joint and limb pain
    - **Kyphoscoliosis**
    - **Pes planus**
  - GI manifestations
    - Hiatal/inguinal hernia, postoperative hernias, and anal prolapse
    - GI bleeding/rupture
  - Cardiac manifestations
    - **Mitral valve prolapse**
    - Aortic root dilation
- <u>Vascular EDS</u>
  - **Life-threatening risk of blood vessel and organ rupture** → sudden death in third/fourth decade (arterial or colonic rupture; **maternal death may occur as a result of uterine or arterial rupture**)
  - Cutaneous manifestations
    - Easy bruising
    - **Thin and translucent skin with visible underlying blood vessels**
    - Skin is not hyperextensible, but can be fragile
    - Lack of subcutaneous fat
  - Facial features: thin, pinched nose; prominent sunken eyes; thin upper lip; and lobeless ears

Table 4.13 Ehlers-Danlos Syndrome Classification

Type	Genes	Inheritance	Skin Findings	Joint Changes	Other
Classical (formerly **type I**, "gravis" and **type II**, "mitis")	***COL5A1***, *COL5A2*	AD	Hyperextensibility Easy bruising Fragile skin Widened atrophic ("**fish mouth**" or "**cigarette paper**") scars **Molluscoid pseudotumors** (overlying extensor joints and pressure points) Spheroids	Hypermobility and joint dislocations	**(+) Gorlin's sign** Absence of lingual frenulum
Hypermobility (formerly **type III**)	*TNXB*	AD/AR	Mild	**Hypermobility** Chronic joint pain + arthritis Recurrent **dislocations and subluxations**	Deficiency of **tenascin X**
Vascular (formerly **type IV**)	***COL3A1***	AD	Thin, translucent skin Extensive bruising Early varicosities (can **visualize veins under skin** easily) Acrogeria	Small joint hypermobility	Mnemonic: "IV = blood vessels" **Rupture of bowel, uterus, or arteries** Most life-threatening form
Kyphoscoliotic (formerly **type VI**)	Lysyl hydroxylase 1 (*PLOD1*)	AR	Mild	Hypermobility **Severe scoliosis**	Severe muscle hypotonia **Ruptured globe, blindness, retinal detachment, or keratoconus** Marfanoid Osteopenia Ascorbic acid supplementation may help
Arthrochalasic (formerly **types VIIa and VIIb**)	*COL1A1*, *COL1A2*	AD	Mild	**Most severe hypermobility** with recurrent subluxations/dislocations (much more severe than hypermobility type)	**Congenital hip dislocation** Short stature
Dermatosparaxis (formerly **type VIIc**)	Procollagen N-proteinase (***ADAMTS2***)	AR	Severe fragility **Sagging, redundant skin**, and bruising	Mild	Umbilical/inguinal hernias Premature rupture of fetal membranes
Periodontitis type (formerly **type VIII**)	Unclear	AD	Hyperextensible skin with scarring (esp. pretibial) and bruising	Mild	**Severe periodontitis → teeth loss**

AD, Autosomal dominant; AR, autosomal recessive
Modified from Paller AS, Mancini AJ. Hereditary disorders of the dermis. In: Hurwitz Clinical Pediatric Dermatology: A Textbook of Skin Disorders of Childhood and Adolescence. *5th ed. Elsevier. 2016:119–135.*

- **Blue sclera** (>90%)
- Acrogeria
- **Hypermobility limited to digits**
- Congenital talipes (club foot)
- Recurrent pneumothoraces
- Arterial (including aorta) dissection, rupture, and aneurysm of medium-sized vessels
  - **Spontaneous rupture of arteries** (medium-sized) may occur during childhood, and incidence peaks during third and fourth decade
  - **Intestinal rupture is common** (sigmoid colon #1 site)
- Intracranial aneurysms a/w CVAs
- Obstetric complications, including uterine and arterial rupture, massive postpartum hemorrhage, and severe laceration from tearing at vaginal delivery
- Short stature

- Hypermobile EDS
  - Not prone to life-threatening complications
  - **Severe joint laxity**, recurrent **dislocations/subluxations**, and chronic joint pain +/– arthritis
  - Mitral valve prolapse
  - Symptoms of autonomic dysfunction, including postural orthostatic tachycardia syndrome (POTS)

Marfan Syndrome

- **AD** mutations in the ***FBN1* gene** (encodes **fibrillin-1**)
- Manifestations may not present until adolescence or in 30 to 40s
- **Tall with long extremities** (marfanoid habitus)
  - Arm span is characteristically greater than height
  - After puberty, upper segment (vertex to pubis) to lower segment (pubis to sole) ratio is <0.86
- Lack of subcutaneous fat, presence of **striae** on upper chest, arms, thighs, and abdomen and increased risk of **elastosis perforans serpiginosa**
- Skeletal manifestations
  - **Arachnodactyly**
  - Kyphoscoliosis, pectus excavatum, and dolichocephaly
  - Pes planus
  - Joint laxity, patellar dislocation, and hip dislocation

- Ocular manifestations
  - **Ectopia lentis (upward lens displacement;** 60% of patients**)**
  - Ocular globe elongation leading to myopia (~40%)
  - Retinal detachment, cataracts, and glaucoma
- Cardiovascular manifestations (70%)
  - **Dilatation of ascending aorta → regurgitation, CHF, dissection/aneurysm, and rupture**
  - **Mitral valve prolapse**
  - Left ventricular dilation
  - Cardiac complications may → death
- Pulmonary manifestations
  - **Spontaneous pneumothorax**, apical blebs, and bullous emphysema

Buschke-Ollendorff syndrome

- **AD** disorder due to mutation in ***LEMD3/MAN1*** (LEM domain-containing-3/MAN antigen 1) gene → ↑ TGF-β signaling
- **Dermatofibrosis lenticularis disseminata** (typically elastomas) on buttocks, proximal trunk, and limbs
  - Symmetric, small, uniform, yellow to skin-colored dermal papules coalescing into plaques; onset in childhood (typically in the first year of life)
- **Osteopoikilosis ("spotted bones")**
  - **Asymptomatic circular densities** in carpal bones, tarsal bones, phalanges of hands and feet, pelvis, and **epiphyses and metaphyses of long bones**
  - Often noted incidentally on plain films (1- to 10-mm round opacities)
- Histology: abundant thickened elastic > collagen fibers (often fragmented and clustered into nets)

Infantile systemic hyalinosis (ISH) and juvenile hyaline fibromatosis (JHF)

- Allelic **AR** diseases caused by mutations in *ANTXR2*/***CMG2*** gene (capillary morphogenesis protein-2) → abundance of hyalinized fibrous tissue in skin and internal organs
  - ISH presents within first 6 months of life with cutaneous, mucosal, skeletal, and internal organ involvement and **death in early childhood**
  - JHF presents during early childhood with cutaneous, mucosal, and skeletal/joint (often debilitating) involvement only; **survival into adulthood**
- Cutaneous manifestations
  - Thickened skin and hyperpigmentation overlying bony prominences is characteristic of ISH
  - Perianal nodules
  - **Small pearly papules** on **ears** and face (perinasal and perioral)
  - Scalp nodules are characteristic of JHF
- Oral manifestations
  - Thickening of oral mucosa
  - **Gingival hypertrophy**
  - Marked curvature of dental roots
  - Replacement of periodontal ligament by hyaline fibrous material
  - Feeding difficulty
- Musculoskeletal manifestations
  - **Debilitating joint contractures** and tumors
  - Osteolytic bone lesions are characteristic of JHF
- Normal intelligence
- Visceral involvement (ISH only): hyaline deposits develop in multiple internal organs w/ recurrent infections, malabsorption, protein-losing enteropathy, and failure to thrive
- Histology: ↑ # of fibroblasts embedded in **hyalinized connective tissue stroma** that is homogeneous, amorphous, and acidophilic (PAS-positive)
- ISH has a poor prognosis with death by 2 years of age **from recurrent pulmonary infection and GI complications**
- In JHF, survival into adulthood (death often by fourth decade)

Lipoid proteinosis (hyalinosis cutis et mucosae, Urbach-Wiethe disease)

- **AR** disorder due to mutations in the **extracellular matrix protein 1 (*ECM1*) gene**; ↑ in South Africa
- Thickening of basement membrane and deposition of hyaline material in dermis → characteristic thickening of the skin, mucous membranes, and certain viscera
- **Hoarse cry** or weak cry from infiltrated vocal cords is the **first clinical sign** (occurs in infancy and persists for life)
- Cutaneous lesions develop during first few 2 years of life in two overlapping stages
  - First stage: vesicles and hemorrhagic crusts involving the face, extremities, and oral mucosa develop in association with trauma and resolve with **"ice-pick" scars**
  - Second stage: ↑ hyaline deposition within the dermis → yellow, waxy, and coalescing papules/nodules on the face/neck and extremities; **beaded eyelid papules resembling "string of pearls"** (50%); verrucous nodules on elbows/knees/hands
- Infiltration by yellow papules/plaques of the mucosa of pharynx, soft palate, tonsils, and lips
- **Thickened "woody" tongue; inability to protrude tongue** (due to shortened frenulum)
- **Respiratory difficulty** a/w upper respiratory tract infections and may require tracheostomy; occasionally fatal in infancy (major cause of early death)
- Neurologic manifestations include **seizures** and neuropsychiatric symptoms, a/w pathognomonic sickle or **"bean-shaped" calcifcations in temporal lobes or hippocampus**
- Histology: **deposition of amorphous or laminated basement membrane-like material containing collagen (types II and IV) and laminin** around blood vessels, dermal-epidermal junction, adnexal epithelia, and in connective tissues (appears as vertically oriented pink dermal deposits)
  - Deposits are PAS-positive and diastase-resistant

Cutis verticis gyrata

- Thick furrowing of skin on scalp (vertex) +/– neck, due to increased dermal collagen

- **Primary: associated with pachydermoperiostosis** (cutis verticis gyrata, clubbing, periostosis of long bones); also seen in Turner, Noonan syndromes
- **Secondary: manifestation of hyperpituitarism**

Focal dermal hypoplasia (Goltz syndrome, Goltz-Gorlin syndrome)

- X-linked dominant (**XLD**) disorder due to mutations in the ***PORCN*** (porcupine) gene (regulator of Wnt signaling proteins, which are critical for embryonic development of skin, bone, teeth, and other structures)
- Majority of patients are heterozygous females (90%); **lethal in males**
- Cutaneous manifestations:
  - Widely distributed linear/**Blaschkoid** areas of **hypoplasia**/atrophy of the skin, with **telangiectasias** (Fig. 4.28)
  - **Soft, yellow to reddish-yellow nodular outpouchings caused by herniation of subcutaneous fat through thinned dermis**
  - Dysmorphic facies (notched nasal ala and malformed ears)
  - Large cutaneous ulcers (from a congenital absence of skin) that heal w/ atrophic scarring
  - Streaky hyper- and/or hypopigmentation
  - **Red ("raspberry-like") papillomas**; favors **lips**, **anogenital** region, larynx and acral skin
  - Hair is thin or absent
  - Dystrophic or completely absent nails

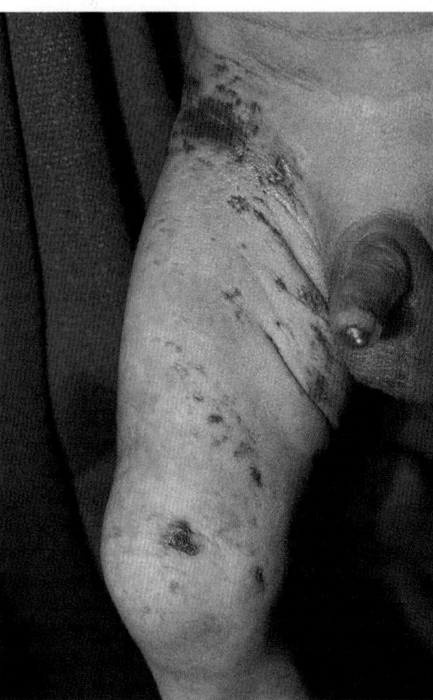

Fig. 4.28 Goltz syndrome (focal dermal hypoplasia). Linear streaks of dermal hypoplasia with visible telangiectasia in an affected boy. The condition is presumed to be lethal in males, suggesting that this boy's manifestation reflects post-zygotic mosaicism. (From Paller AS, Mancini AJ. Hereditary disorders of the dermis. In: *Hurwitz Clinical Pediatric Dermatology: A Textbook of Skin Disorders of Childhood and Adolescence*. 5th ed. Philadelphia: Elsevier; 2016:119–135.)

- Skeletal manifestations
  - Oligodactyly, syndactyly, **ectrodactyly (lobster claw deformity)**, and polydactyly
  - Microcrania, scoliosis
  - **Osteopathia striata**: vertical striations in long bone metaphyses on X-ray
- Ophthalmologic manifestations (40%)
  - **Colobomas** of iris/choroid/retina/optic disc
  - Strabismus
  - Anophthalmia, microphthalmia, and incomplete development of the retina and optic nerve
- Dental manifestations
  - **Underdeveloped, dysplastic, or absent teeth**
  - Delayed eruption of primary dentition
  - **Enamel hypoplasia**
- Intelligence usually normal, though severe developmental delay has been reported
- Histology: markedly **decreased/absent dermis** with herniated fat located abnormally close to epidermis
- **FOCAL** has been suggested as an acronym that incorporates the key clinical features of this disorder:
  - **F**emale, XLD
  - **O**steopathia striata
  - **C**olobomas
  - **A**plasia ectoderm elements
  - **L**obster claw deformity

Congenital contractual arachnodactyly (Beals syndrome and distal arthrogryposis type 9)

- AD mutation in **fibrillin 2** (*FBN2*) gene
- Crumpled ears, Marfanoid habitus, arachnodactyly, congenital contractures of small and large joints that usually improve over time, kyphoscoliosis, and pectus excavatum
- Characteristic facial features
  - High forehead
  - Down-slanting palpebral fissures
  - Hypertelorism
  - Anteverted nostrils
  - Low-set and abnormal auricles
  - Retromicrognathia
  - Short neck
- Cardiac manifestations: **mitral valve prolapse and aortic root dilation**

Restrictive dermopathy (tight skin contracture syndrome)

- AR disorder as a result of mutations in **lamin-A** (*LMNA*) or zinc metalloproteinase STE24 (*ZMPSTE24*) → ↑ prelamin A (accumulates in the nucleus → nuclear membrane toxicity)
- Prenatal manifestations
  - Intrauterine course characterized by **fetal akinesia or hypokinesia deformation sequence**
  - **Polyhydramnios** with reduced fetal movements noted beginning at about 31 weeks
  - Clavicular hypoplasia develops *in utero*

- Birth typically occurs before 35 weeks of gestation as a result of premature rupture of membranes (**PROM**)
- Cutaneous manifestations
  - **Taut translucent, thin skin with erosions and fissures**
  - Skin tears in response to stress of delivery, resuscitation, and neonatal movements
  - Complications include infection and dehydration after fluid loss
  - Increased transepidermal water loss leads to hypoalbuminemia and electrolyte imbalance
- **Dysmorphic facies**
  - Fixed round open mouth with micrognathia
  - Small pinched nose
  - Hypertelorism
  - Enlarged fontanelles
  - Widened cranial sutures
- **Flexion contractures**
- **Restrictive pulmonary disease as a result of thoracic stiffness and severely restricted movements**
- **Death 2° to respiratory insufficiency shortly after birth**

Stiff skin syndrome (congenital fascial dystrophy)

- AD disorder due to mutations in ***FBN1*** (**fibrillin-1**)
- Progressive development of **stony-hard skin** on thighs, buttocks, lower back, and shoulders
- **Joint contractures** (esp. large joints), scoliosis, tiptoe gait, narrow thorax in relation to arm girdle, restrictive pulmonary changes, growth retardation, and postural and thoracic wall irregularities
- On histology, **fascial sclerosis**; ↑ fibroblast cellularity; thickened, sclerotic, horizontally oriented collagen bundles in deep reticular dermis and/or subcutaneous septa

4.10 AUTOINFLAMMATORY DISORDERS (PERIODIC FEVER SYNDROMES)

Epidemiology

- Predominantly hereditary (rarely acquired) syndromes characterized by **recurrent**, **spontaneous**, **inflammatory episodes** w/ varying degrees of severity and duration; presenting w/ fever and variable cutaneous, serosal, mucosal, ocular, neurologic, and osteoarticular manifestations

Pathogenesis

- **Disorders of innate immunity** caused by ↑ production of proinflammatory cytokines (e.g., IFN-α, IFN-γ, IL-6, IL-1, and TNF-α) as a result of aberrant signaling of cell surface or intracellular innate immune receptors
- Cytokine receptors, receptor antagonists, and components of the **inflammasome** are involved and result in intracellular protein complexes that enable the **autocatalytic activation of inflammatory caspases, driving the release of proinflammatory cytokines**
- These innate immune cells are activated by endogenous or exogenous stimuli, so-called pathogen-associated molecular patterns (PAMPs) and damage-associated molecular patterns (DAMPs)
- Clinical features
  - Most patients present in infancy to early childhood; adult-onset reported for familial Mediterranean fever (FMF) and TNF-receptor-associated periodic syndrome (TRAPS)
  - **Fever** = key feature of most of the autoinflammatory syndromes and is periodic in nature
  - **Know the key clinical features for each syndrome** (Table 4.14)

Table 4.14 Features of Selected Autoinflammatory Syndromes

Diagnosis	Gene (Protein)	Inheritance	Clinical Features	Rx	Other Comments
Cryopyrin-associated periodic syndromes					
Familial cold autoinflammatory syndrome	***CIAS-1/NLRP3*** (cryopyrin) Mild on a spectrum with below MWS and NOMID	AD	Age of onset: Infancy Skin: Cold-induced urticaria, favors extremities (> face, trunk) Systemic: Arthralgia, conjunctivitis	IL-1 antagonists	Short attacks (minutes to 3 days)
Muckle-Wells syndrome	***CIAS-1/NLRP3*** (cryopyrin)	AD	Age of onset: Any Skin: Widespread urticaria Systemic: Abdominal pain, **"lancing" extremity pain**, conjunctivitis, optic disk edema, arthralgia/arthritis, and sensorineural **hearing loss**	**IL-1 antagonists**	Febrile attacks last 1–2 days High risk of **secondary AA amyloidosis** (25%)
Neonatal-onset multisystem inflammatory disease (NOMID)/chronic infantile neurologic cutaneous articular syndrome (CINCA)	***CIAS-1/NLRP3*** (cryopyrin)	AD	Age of onset: Neonatal Skin: Widespread urticaria +/– oral ulcers; **dysmorphic facies** (frontal bossing and protubierant eyes) Systemic: **Deforming arthropathy**, arthritis, epiphyseal overgrowth, significant ocular involvement (may → **blindness**), sensorineural hearing loss, lymphadenopathy, HSM, seizures, **aseptic meningitis**	IL-1 antagonists	**Febrile attacks occur continuously** Secondary AA amyloidosis Significant morbidity/mortality in childhood (if untreated)

Continued

Table 4.14 Features of Selected Autoinflammatory Syndromes—cont'd

Diagnosis	Gene (Protein)	Inheritance	Clinical Features	Rx	Other Comments
Monogenic periodic fever syndromes					
Hyper-IgD syndrome (Mevalonate kinase deficiency)	***MVK*** (mevalonate kinase)	AR	Age of onset: Infancy Skin: Widespread polymorphous eruption (morbilliform or urticarial most commonly) Systemic: Arthralgia, abdominal pain, vomiting, diarrhea, arthritis, cervical LAN, HSM	IL-1 antagonists, TNF-α antagonists	Febrile attacks last up to 7 days ↑ Incidence in Dutch and Northern Europeans ↑ **Serum IgD** and urinary mevalonate levels
TNF-receptor-associated periodic syndrome (TRAPS)	***TNFRSF1A*** (TNF receptor superfamily 1A/p55 TNF receptor)	AD	Age of onset: Any Skin: **Painful migratory/serpiginous plaques** (often edematous) on extremities; may become ecchymotic Systemic: Serositis, periorbital edema, scrotal pain, **migratory myalgias** (underlying rash)	Corticosteroids, TNF-α antagonists	Febrile attacks often long (1–6 weeks) **Secondary AA amyloidosis** (15%) Labs: ↓ serum soluble TNF receptor levels
Familial Mediterranean fever (FMF)	***MEFV*** (pyrin/marenostrin)	AR	Age of onset: Any Skin: **Erysipelas-like** rash, favors **legs/feet** Systemic: Serositis and arthritis	**Colchicine**, NSAIDs, IL-1 antagonists, and TNF-α antagonists	Febrile attacks last 1–3 days ↑ Incidence in Mediterranean populations **Secondary AA amyloidosis** (mainly in homozygotes; prevented by colchicine)
Autoinflammatory pyogenic disorders					
Pyogenic arthritis, pyoderma gangrenosum, acne syndrome (PAPA)	***PSTPIP1/ CD2BP1*** (Proline-serine-threonine phosphatase-interacting protein 1/CD2 antigen binding protein 1)	AD	Age of onset: Childhood Skin: Pyoderma gangrenosum and nodulocystic acne Systemic: **Sterile pyogenic oligoarthritis**, afebrile	TNF-α antagonists, IL-1 antagonists	
Deficiency of the IL-1 receptor antagonist (DIRA)	***IL1RN*** (IL-1 receptor antagonist)	AR	Age of onset: Neonatal Skin: Neutrophilic pustular dermatosis, ichthyosis Systemic: Sterile multifocal osteomyelitis, periostitis, afebrile	**IL-1 antagonists**	
Generalized pustular psoriasis/Deficiency of the IL-36 receptor antagonist (DITRA)	***IL36RN*** (IL-36 receptor antagonist)	AR	Age of onset: Infancy, childhood Skin: **Generalized pustular psoriasis** Systemic: Malaise, multiorgan failure	NSAIDs, Vitamin D analogs, systemic retinoids, TNF-α inhibitors, IL-1 inhibitors	Multiorgan failure
Autoinflammatory granulomatous disorders					
Blau syndrome/early-sarcoidosis	***NOD2/CARD15*** (nucleotide-binding oligomerization domain 2/caspase recruitment domain 15)	AD, sporadic	Age of onset: Childhood Skin: Sarcoidal granulomatous dermatitis, ichthyosiform dermatitis Systemic: Fever (30%), polyarticular arthritis (favors hands/feet), synovitis and tenosynovitis	Corticosteroids, IL-1 antagonists, TNF-α antagonists	
Newly described autoinflammatory disorders					
Chronic atypical neutrophilic dermatosis with lipodystrophy and elevated temperature (CANDLE) syndrome	*PSMB8* (encodes Proteasome subunit β type)	AR	Almost **daily fever** in early infancy Pernio like lesions of hands and feet **Recurrent annular plaques** worst on trunk that progress to purpura and hyperpigmentation Swollen, violaceous eyelids and lips Also **lipodystrophy,** lymphadenopathy, hepatosplenomegaly, **arthralgias**, other systemic inflammation	May respond to JAK inhibitor (tofacitinib)	

Table 4.14 Features of Selected Autoinflammatory Syndromes—cont'd

Diagnosis	Gene (Protein)	Inheritance	Clinical Features	Rx	Other Comments
STING-associated vasculopathy with onset in infancy (SAVI) syndrome	*TMEM173*	AD	**Acral vasculopathy** with violaceous plaques of cold exposed acral surfaces, ears, and nose Progresses to soft tissue loss, with ulceration, necrosis, and sometimes **auto-amputation** and nasal septum perforation Can also have **fevers,** nail dystrophy, adenopathy, **severe interstitial lung disease**	May respond to JAK inhibitor (tofacitinib)	
Aicardi-Goutières	Several reported including *TREX1, SAMHD1*	Mainly AR	**Chilblains-like lesions** and acrocyanosis especially of cold exposed areas of fingers, toes, ears Variable **neurodevelopmental** abnormalities including encephalopathy, abnormal tone, seizures, fever, hepatosplenomegaly, thrombocytopenia, glaucoma	Mainly symptomatic treatment	
Deficiency of ADA2 (DADA2)	*ADA2*	AR	**Vasculopathy** leads to livedo reticularis, necrosis, and Raynaud's phenomenon. **Recurrent strokes**, intermittent fevers, and hepatosplenomegaly may occur along with mild immunodeficiency including hypogammaglobulinemia	May respond to anti-TNF agents Replacement of ADA2 with fresh frozen plasma	
VEXAS (Vacuoles, E1 enzyme, X-linked, Autoinflammatory, Somatic) syndrome	UBA1 gene on X-chromosome	Somatic mutation in males 40–80 years old	Systemic features: MDS, MGUS, uveitis, fever, LAD, pulmonary infiltrates, vasculitis, VTE Cutaneous features: relapsing polychondritis, EN, livedo reticularis, Sweet syndrome-like erythematous nodules, periorbital edema, PAN Lab features: macrocytic anemia, thrombocytopenia, vacuolization of erythroidand myeloid precursors in bone marrow	May respond to systemic steroids (+/- colchicine)	Long-term prognosis is poor with high mortality rate

Histopathology

- Histology (all except PAPA and Blau): moderate-dense dermal perivascular and interstitial neutrophils (**"neutrophilic urticarial dermatitis"**) +/– dermal edema

Treatment

- The treatment of each autoinflammatory syndrome is disease-specific—agents such as **anakinra**, etanercept, and **canakinumab** are commonly used
- **Colchicine is crucial in preventing amyloidosis in patients with FMF**

Prognosis/clinical course

- Untreated, many of the autoinflammatory syndromes → significant morbidity and mortality
- **DITRA, DIRA, and NOMID may be fatal** during infancy or childhood
- **Secondary AA amyloidosis is a complication of FMF and the cryopyrin-associated periodic syndromes (CAPS)**

4.11 NEUROCUTANEOUS SYNDROMES

Neurofibromatosis (NF)

- Encompasses three distinct disorders (NF1, NF2, and schwannomatosis), characterized by ↑ propensity toward tumor development, particularly of the nerve sheath
  - 90% of cases are NF1
- NF1 (von Recklinghausen's disease)
  - AD disorder caused by mutations in **neurofibromin** (*NF1*), a tumor suppressor gene
    - Neurofibromin is a cytoplasmic protein that **negatively regulates Ras activation**
    - 50% are sporadic mutations and mosaic/segmental disease can occur
    - Diagnostic criteria for NF1 (Box 4.1)

Box 4.1 Diagnostic Criteria for NF1

Must have two or more of the following:

Six café-au-lait macules ≥0.5 cm prepubertal or ≥1.5 cm postpubertal
Intertriginous freckling
Plexiform neurofibroma or >2 dermal neurofibromas
>2 Lisch nodules
Optic nerve glioma
Pathogenomic skeletal dysplasia (tibial or sphenoid wing dysplasia)
Affected first-degree relative

- Manifestations by age of presentation listed in Table 4.15
- Cutaneous manifestations:
  - **Neurofibroma**: soft papule that invaginates upon finger pressure ("buttonholing")
  - Plexiform neurofibroma: overlying CALMs and/or hypertrichosis; "**bag of worms**" texture (seen in ~25% of patients)
  - **Malignant peripheral nerve sheath tumor** (MPNST): rapid enlargement or pain of plexiform neurofibroma (**10% risk**)
  - **CALMs** (typically ≥ 6, ↑ #/size in first 5 years)
  - Axillary and/or inguinal freckling (**Crowe's sign**)
- Ocular manifestations
  - **Lisch nodules** (>90% of patients by 10 years of age)
  - Optic glioma, choroid nevus, and glaucoma
- Skeletal manifestations
  - **Sphenoid wing dysplasia**: pulsating exophthalmos may be noted, though often asymptomatic
  - Macrocephaly
  - Scoliosis
  - **Congenital tibial pseudarthroses (tibial)**
  - Additional skeletal abnormalities: thoracic cage asymmetry, osteoporosis, and pathologic fractures
  - Short stature
- Neurologic manifestations:
  - Learning disability, **ADHD**, and autism
  - Seizures
  - Hydrocephalus
  - **Optic glioma** (can → blindness; seen w/ precocious puberty), astrocytomas, meningiomas, vestibular/acoustic schwannoma/neuroma, and ependymoma
- Other manifestations:
  - Other tumors: neurofibrosarcoma, rhabdomyosarcoma, **pheochromocytoma**, Wilms' tumor, and **chronic myelogenous leukemia**
  - **Hypertension** may develop as a result of a pheochromocytoma (rare) or **renal vascular stenosis** (most common cause in children) 2° to fibromuscular dysplasia; most common cause of HTN **in adults is essential**

Table 4.15 Manifestations of NF1 by Age of Presentation

Average Age of Onset	Cutaneous	Ocular	Neurologic	Skeletal
Infancy to early childhood	Café-au-lait macules Plexiform neurofibromas (first cutaneous sign—probably all congenital according to Bolognia)	Optic gliomas	Learning disabilities Attention deficit disorder Autism Macrocephaly	Tibial dysplasia Sphenoid wing dysplasia
Prepubertal	Intertriginous freckling (Fig. 4.29)		Brainstem gliomas Meningiomas	Scoliosis
Adolescence	Dermal or subcutaneous neurofibromas	Lisch nodules		
Adulthood	Malignant peripheral nerve sheath tumors			

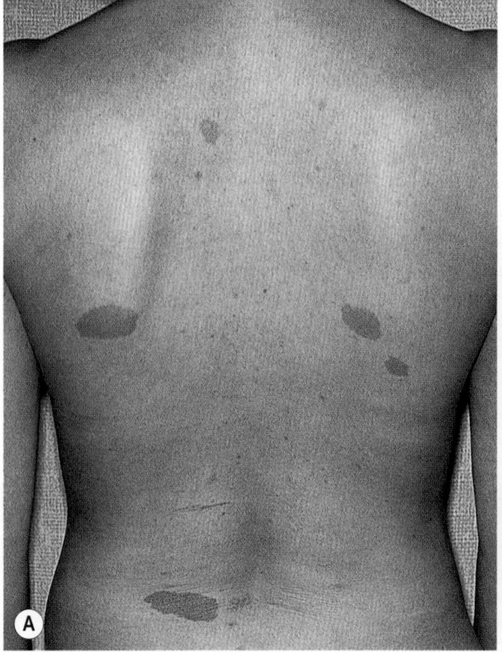

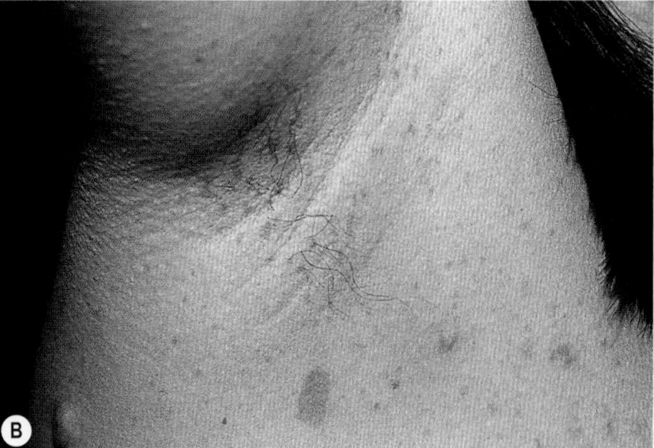

Fig. 4.29 von Recklinghausen's neurofibromatosis. **(A)** Café-au-lait spots vary in size and have a smooth border. **(B)** Axillary freckling (Crowe's sign) is a pathognomonic sign. (From Dinulos JGH. Cutaneous manifestations of internal disease. In: *Habif's Clinical Dermatology: A Color Guide to Diagnosis and Therapy*. 7th ed. Philadelphia: Elsevier; 2021:990–1012.)

  - Vascular anomalies of the CNS, including stenoses, moyamoya disease, and aneurysms
  - **Nevus anemicus** found in up to 50% of patients; also associated with **glomus tumor**
  - Malignant transformation of neurofibroma 2° to second mutation, most commonly in **p53**
  - **Possible triple association** between **NF1, juvenile xanthogranulomas,** and **juvenile chronic myelogenous leukemia** (questionable but still asked on exams)
  - Of note, Watson syndrome = NF1 features + **pulmonic stenosis** ↑
- NF2 (bilateral acoustic schwannomas)
  - AD disorder caused by mutations in *SCH* gene (encodes schwannomin/**merlin**; tumor suppressor gene)
  - Symptoms appear later than NF1 (usually in second to third decade)
  - Cutaneous findings: neurofibromas (in lower #s than NF1)—more commonly **subcutaneous** type w/ **overlying pigment/hair** rather than intradermal (seen mainly in NF1), **CALMs** (usually ≤ 2 lesions)
  - Neurologic findings: **bilateral vestibular schwannomas (acoustic neuromas)** is diagnostic; may → deafness, **tinnitus**, unsteadiness, headache; patients should NOT swim alone, meningiomas, astrocytomas, and ependymomas
  - Ocular findings: juvenile posterior subcapsular lenticular opacity/cataract
  - Poor prognosis with worsening hearing, vision, ambulation; CNS tumors are most common cause of death
  - Selumetinib — mitogen-activated protein kinase (MEK) inhibitor approved for patients aged >2 years, for inoperable symptomatic plexiform neurofibromas; SEs: ↑ creatine kinase, acneiform rash, paronychia, and GI symptoms (most common SE) like nausea, vomiting, and diarrhea

Tuberous sclerosis complex (TSC)

- AD disorder caused by mutations in **hamartin** (***TSC1***) or **tuberin** (***TSC2***) (tumor suppressor genes); TSC2 is most common and is contiguous with polycystic kidney disease (PKD)
  - Tuberin and hamartin form a complex that inhibits signal transduction of downstream effectors of **mTOR** (mammalian target of rapamycin) → abnormal regulation of cellular differentiation, proliferation, and migration of affected cell types with the formation of multiple hamartomas
- Mosaic/segmental disease can occur
  - Cutaneous findings: **adenoma sebaceum** (facial angiofibromas), hypopigmented **"ash-leaf"** macules (confetti pattern pretibially; first cutaneous finding), **Shagreen patch** (collagen connective tissue nevus), periungual fibromas ("**Koenen tumors**"), and **CALMs**
  - Histology of angiofibromas: dermal fibrosis with stellate fibroblasts, atrophic sebaceous glands, dilated capillaries, and loss of elastin
  - Histology of Shagreen patch: broad sclerotic collagen bundles and reduced elastin
  - Histology of hypomelanotic macules: normal # of melanocytes with ↓ pigmentation
- Treatment of facial angiofibromas: pulsed dye laser, ablative laser, excision, and **topical rapamycin**
- Neurologic findings: **cortical tubers**, subependymal nodules (may → hydrocephalus), subependymal giant cell astrocytomas, seizures/**infantile spasms**, hypsarrhythmia, intellectual impairment, and **paraventricular calcification**
  - Infantile spasms, large number of cortical tubers, and early age of onset of seizures or intractable seizures associated with **worse prognosis**
  - **#1 cause of mortality** = complications related to seizures
- Renal findings: renal cysts, **angiomyolipomas**, and renal cell carcinoma
  - Systemic mTOR inhibitors (i.e., sirolimus and everolimus) used for management of renal and hepatic angiomyolipomas and subependymal giant cell astrocytomas
  - Complications of renal disease (renal failure, catastrophic hemorrhage within a renal angiomyolipoma, and renal hypertension) = **#2 cause of premature death**
- Ocular findings: **retinal phakomas** (hamartomas)
- Cardiac findings: **cardiac rhabdomyomas** → Wolff-Parkinson-White arrhythmia; notably most rhabdomyomas spontaneously involute in early childhood
- GI findings: hepatic cysts, hepatic angiomyolipomas (usually asymptomatic), and GI polyps/hamartomas
- Dental findings: **pits in enamel** and **gingival fibromas**
- Lung findings: pulmonary **lymphangioleiomyomatosis** and pulmonary cysts
  - Pulmonary complications: pneumothorax, chylothorax, hemoptysis, and pulmonary insufficiency
- Definite diagnosis of TSC requires either the presence of a pathogenic mutation in *TSC1* or *TSC2* **OR** the presence of two major criteria or one major criteria and two minor criteria (Table 4.16)
- A possible diagnosis of TSC requires the presence of one major or two minor criteria (see Table 4.16)
- Cutaneous features are seen in 90% of affected patients, and may be the first presenting sign Table 4.17

Table 4.16 Diagnostic Criteria for Tuberous Sclerosis Complex

Major Features	Minor Features
≥3 Angiofibromas or fibrous cephalic plaque	≥3 Dental enamel pits
≥3 Hypomelanotic macules >5 mm in diameter	≥2 Intraoral fibromas
≥2 Ungual fibromas	"Confetti"-like skin lesions
Shagreen patch	Nonrenal hamartomas
Multiple retinal hamartomas	Multiple renal cysts
Cortical dysplasias	Retinal achromic patch
Subependymal nodules	
Subependymal giant cell astrocytoma	
Cardiac rhabdomyoma	
Lymphangioleiomyomatosis	
≥2 Angiomyolipomas	

Table 4.17 Cutaneous Manifestations of Tuberous Sclerosis Complex by Average Age of Presentation

Average Age of Onset	Cutaneous	Other
Infancy to early childhood	**Hypomelanotic macules** "Confetti"-like skin lesions	Cardiac rhabomyomas Subependymal nodules Seizures
Prepubertal	Angiofibromas (Fig. 4.30) Shagreen patch Fibrous cephalic plaque Dental pits	Renal hamartomas
Adolescence	**Ungual fibromas** (Fig. 4.31)	
Adulthood	Intraoral fibromas	Pulmonary lymphangioleiomyomatosis (females) Renal cysts

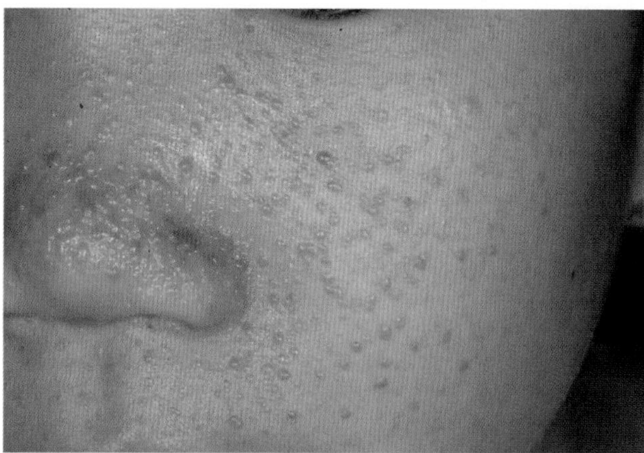

Fig. 4.30 Tuberous sclerosis. Facial angiofibromas ("adenoma sebaceum") are typically 1- to 4-mm, skin-colored to red, dome-shaped papules with a smooth surface. (From Paller AS, Mancini AJ. Disorders of pigmentation. In: *Hurwitz Clinical Pediatric Dermatology: A Textbook of Skin Disorders of Childhood and Adolescence*. 4th ed. Philadelphia: Elsevier; 2011:234–267.)

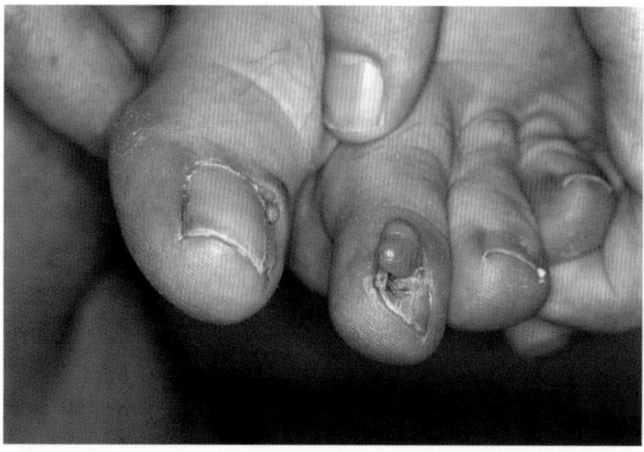

Fig. 4.31 Periungual fibrous nodules (Koenen's tumors) on the toes of an adolescent with tuberous sclerosis.(From Weston WL, Lane AT, Morelli JG. Disorders of pigmentation: the white lesions and the brown lesions. In: *Color Textbook of Pediatric Dermatology*. 4th ed. Philadelphia: Elsevier; 2007:309–333.)

Incontinentia pigmenti (IP)

- **XLD** loss-of-function mutation in NF-κB essential modulator (*NEMO*; *IKBKG*)
  - Mutation in ***NEMO*** **prevents activation of** NF-κB, a regulator of cell proliferation, inflammation, and **TNF-α–induced apoptosis**
  - Mutation is **lethal in males**; seen primarily in women and possible in XXY (Klinefelter's) males
  - Functional mosaicism from lyonization in affected females (random inactivation of affected X chromosome) results in **Blaschkoid pattern** of cutaneous involvement
- IP is a neuroectodermal disorder that affects the skin, teeth (hypodontia/anodontia), CNS, and eyes
  - Cutaneous lesions are typically arranged in streaks and whorls, following Blaschkoid pattern
  - **Four distinct morphologic stages** (Table 4.18)

Table 4.18 Findings in Incontinentia Pigmenti

Stage	Manifestation	Timing	Comments
Vesicular	Inflammatory vesicles or pustules (Fig. 4.32)	Birth to 1 month	Reactivation may occur with illness or trauma
Verrucous	Warty papules	Up to 2 years (usually resolved by 8 weeks)	
Hyperpigmented	Blue to brown streaks	Up to adolescence (may resolve by 1 year)	May not involve previously vesicular or verrucous areas
Hypopigmented	Atrophic hypopigmented streaks	May persist through adulthood	

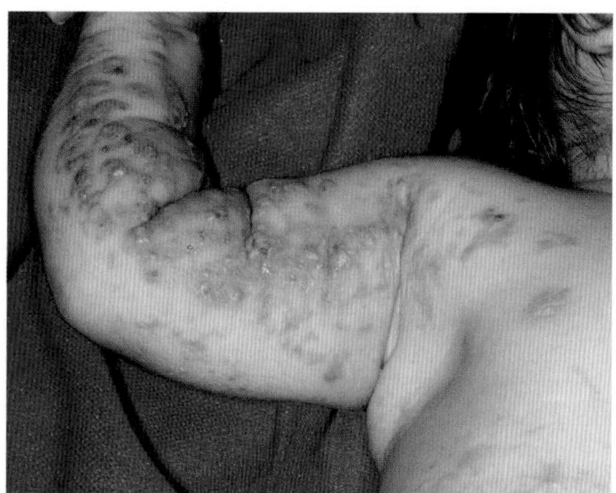

Fig. 4.32 Incontinentia pigmenti. The lesions of incontinentia pigmenti tend to follow a curvilinear pattern along lines of Blaschko, lines of the embryological development of ectoderm, as a manifestation of functional mosaicism (i.e., the X chromosome with the mutation in the NEMO gene is the activated X chromosome in the skin at these sites). The lesions of the vesicular phase may range from largely papular with a minor vesicular component to vesiculopustular as shown here and occasionally to bullous. (From Paller AS, Mancini AJ. Disorders of pigmentation. In: *Hurwitz Clinical Pediatric Dermatology: A Textbook of Skin Disorders of Childhood and Adolescence*. 4th ed. Philadelphia: Elsevier; 2011:234–267.)

- Patients may not develop all four cutaneous stages and there may be some overlap of stages
- Alopecia may affect the scalp and other parts of the body
- See Table 4.19.

- Histology varies by stage:
  - Vesicular stage: **eosinophilic spongiosis**; intraepidermal vesicles containing eosinophils; **apoptotic keratinocytes** in epidermis
  - Verrucous stage: papillomatosis, hyperkeratosis, and acanthosis of the epidermis; apoptotic cells in epidermis forming squamous eddies
  - Hyperpigmented stage: marked pigment incontinence with numerous melanophages in the dermis; apoptotic cells may be seen in epidermis
  - Hypopigmented stage: epidermal atrophy, loss of melanin in basal layer, complete absence of pilosebaceous units and eccrine glands; apoptotic cells may be seen in epidermis
- Severely affected patients may develop **seizures, developmental delay and intellectual impairment, and** ↓visual acuity/blindness (due to **retinal vascular changes** and optic atrophy)
- **Females with missense mutations in NEMO (milder phenotype of IP) can bear children (usually male) with hypohidrotic ectodermal dysplasia with immunodeficiency**
- Review neurocutaneous syndromes in Table 4.20.

Table 4.19 Other Clinical Manifestations of Incontinentia Pigmenti

Organ	Manifestation	Frequency
Other cutaneous	**Cicatricial alopecia**	10%–20%
	Nail dystrophy	10%
	Subungual tumors (resembles squamous cell carcinoma!)	Up to 10%
Teeth	**Pegged or conical teeth**	50%
	Anodontia (dental = most common extracutaneous feature)	
	Delayed dentition	
Central nervous system	**Seizures**	30%
	Developmental delay	
	Spastic paresis	
Eyes	**Retinal vascular anomalies** (e.g., vascular changes → blindness)	30%
	Nonretinal anomalies (strabismus, cataracts, and optic atrophy)	
Breast	Supernumerary nipples	11%–30%
	Nipple hypoplasia	
	Breast hypoplasia or aplasia	

4.12 PREMATURE AGING SYNDROMES AND DNA REPAIR DISORDERS

Hutchinson-Gilford progeria

- AD disorder caused by specific mutation (1824C>T) in the ***LMNA*** **gene** (encodes **lamin A**)
  - Mutation introduces a splice site that results in the protein being abnormally farnesylated
  - Lamin A protein **contributes to the structure/function of the nuclear envelope**
  - With abnormal farnesylation, lamin A cannot insert normally into the nuclear envelope
- Cutaneous manifestations begin around 6 to 18 months:
  - Localized sclerodermatous changes of lower trunk/thigh

Table 4.20 Neurocutaneous Syndromes: Genetic Basis and Clinical Findings

Disease	Gene/Inheritance	Gene Function	Cutaneous Features	Neurologic Features	Other Distinct Features
Neurofibromatosis type 1	Neurofibromin/AD Incidence ~1/3000	Cytoplasmic protein; negatively regulates Ras activation	Café-au-lait macules Intertriginous freckling Dermal neurofibromas Plexiform neurofibromas	Learning disabilities Attention-deficit disorder Autistic spectrum Pilocytic astrocytomas Meningiomas	Lisch nodules Optic gliomas Tibial dysplasia Sphenoid wing dysplasia Scoliosis
Legius syndrome	SPRED1/AD	Interacts with Ras	Café-au-lait macules Intertriginous freckling	Learning disabilities	
Neurofibromatosis type 2	Merlin/AD	Cytoskeletal protein; tumor suppressor	Schwannomas Neurofibromas Café-au-lait macules (33%)	Vestibular and cranial schwannomas Cranial meningiomas Spinal cord tumors	Juvenile posterior subcapsular cataract Hearing loss
Tuberous sclerosis	Hamartin or tuberin/AD	Inhibits signal transduction of downstream effectors of mTOR	Hypomelanotic macules Angiofibromas Fibrous cephalic plaque Shagreen patch Ungual fibromas Intraoral fibromas	Subependymal nodules Seizures Subependymal giant cell astrocytoma	Cardiac rhabdomyoma Renal angiolipomas and cysts Pulmonary lymphangioleiomyomatosis (females)
Incontinentia pigmenti	NEMO/XLD	Activates NF-κB, a regulator of cell proliferation, inflammation, and apoptosis	Four stages: vesicular, verrucous, hyperpigmented, and hypopigmented Alopecia Nail dystrophy Subungual tumors	Seizures Developmental delay Spastic paresis	Dental anomalies Ocular (retinal) defects Breast anomalies Male children with hypohidrotic ectodermal dysplasia with immunodeficiency

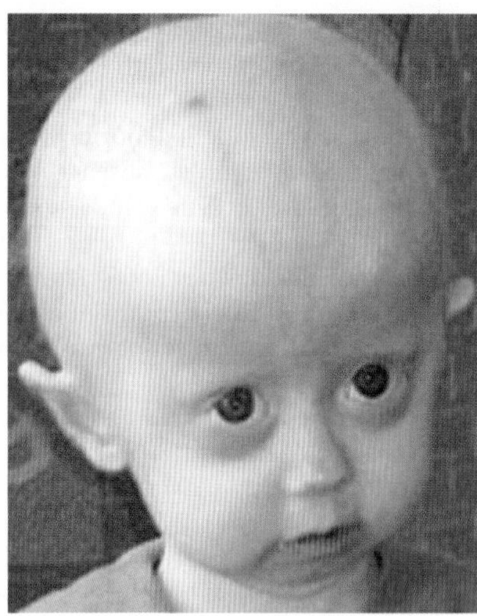

Fig. 4.33 Progeria syndrome. (From Scaffidi P, Gordon L, Misteli T. The cell nucleus and aging: tantalizing clues and hopeful promises. *PLoS Biol.* 2005;3[11]:e395.)

- Cyanosis around mouth or nasolabial folds
- Dyspigmentation
- Also see failure to thrive early on
- Over time, patients show **signs of premature aging**
  - Early skin wrinkling and xerosis
  - Hair loss (scalp, eyebrows, and eyelashes)
  - Skin atrophy with prominent veins
  - **Atherosclerosis and angina**
  - Bone density loss/osteoporosis (w/ susceptibility to fractures), coxa valga, and osteolysis of distal phalanges
- Other dermatologic manifestations: lipodystrophy, onychodystrophy, and breast hypoplasia
- Facial features: **enlarged head**, micrognathia with dental crowding, small ears, and beaked nose (Fig. 4.33)
- A **high-pitched voice** is characteristic
- **Rapid and progressive features of premature aging develop**—complications include cerebrovascular and cardiovascular events (CHF and MI), limited mobility and exercise tolerance, and poor growth; intelligence is typically normal
- **Complications of cardiovascular disease are the most common cause of mortality** (mean age of death = 13 years)

Werner syndrome

- AR disorder as a result of mutations in the ***RECQL2/WRN*** gene (encodes a **DNA helicase** that helps maintain genomic stability)
  - Mutations in *RECQL2/WRN* → ↑ expression of inhibitors of DNA synthesis and ↑ telomere-driven replicative senescence → **accelerated aging**
  - Symptoms/signs seen in third to fourth decade
- Cutaneous findings: premature canities, progressive alopecia, bird-like facial appearance, **sclerodermatous/atrophic change acrally/facially**, mottled pigmentation, telangiectasias, hyperkeratotic ulcers over pressure points, leg ulcers, calcinosis cutis, and loss of subcutaneous fat
- Extracutaneous findings: short stature, muscle wasting, atherosclerosis (can → CVA/MI), diabetes mellitus, hypogonadism, osteoporosis, arthritis, posterior subcapsular cataracts, DM2, and hypogonadism
- ↑ Risk of malignancy: **fibrosarcoma, osteogenic sarcoma**, carcinoma of breast or ovary, thyroid adenocarcinoma, skin cancers
- **Malignancy** and **cerebrovascular/cardiovascular events** are main causes of mortality (mid-50s typically)

Xeroderma pigmentosum

- **AR** disorder due to mutations in ***XPA*** to ***XPG* genes** (as well as variant ***XPV*** gene)—each gene encodes a protein important in the **nucleotide excision repair (NER) pathway**: *XPA* encodes DNA damage-binding protein 1 (DDB1), *XPB* encodes excision-repair cross-complementing 3 (ERCC3), *XPC* encodes endonuclease, *XPD* encodes ERCC2, *XPE* encodes DDB2, *XPF* encodes ERCC4, *XPG* encodes endonuclease, and XPV is unique in that it encodes a DNA polymerase
  - Subtypes (complementation groups) of XP (XPA to XPG) correspond to the affected genes
  - In the variant subtype XPV, the **post-replication repair pathway** is abnormal because of mutations in the gene that encodes **DNA polymerase-η**
  - Affected individuals have ↑ **sensitivity to UV-induced skin damage** caused by **abnormalities in DNA repair pathways** (i.e., recognition of damaged DNA, unwinding of DNA [helicases], and incision/removal of damaged DNA [endonucleases])
  - Most common subtypes in the United States are XPA and XPC; XPA is the most common subtype in Japan
  - Different mutations in the XP genes may lead to different phenotypes and overlap syndromes:
    - ***XPB, XPD, and XPG:*** a/w XP-Cockayne overlap syndrome; possess signs of both XP (skin cancers, lentigines) and **Cockayne** syndrome (retinal degeneration, basal ganglia calcification)
    - ***XPB, XPD:*** also a/w **trichothiodystrophy (TTD)**
- Typical cutaneous manifestations appear after 6 months, with development of persistent erythema, scaling, and ephelides on sun-exposed areas
- Eventually poikiloderma develops, followed by development of numerous cutaneous malignancies (Fig. 4.34)
  - **1000-fold increased risk of cutaneous malignancy** in patients <20 years of age, including BCC, SCC, melanoma, and fibrosarcoma; mean onset of cutaneous malignancy = 8 years of age
  - ↑ Risk of solid and CNS tumors, though rare
- Ophthalmologic complications: photophobia, conjunctivitis, ectropion, and symblepharon
- Neurodevelopmental complications, including developmental delay, intellectual impairment, sensorineural hearing loss, hyporeflexia, and/or ataxia occurs in **20%–30% of XP patients** (esp. XPA and XPD groups); **XPV patients have no neurologic complications**
  - **De Sanctis-Cacchione syndrome:** rare XP phenotype with severe neurologic deficits (severe developmental delay, deafness, ataxia, and paralysis)
- Severely affected individuals usually die as a result of complications from metastatic melanoma or invasive SCC by ~20 years of age

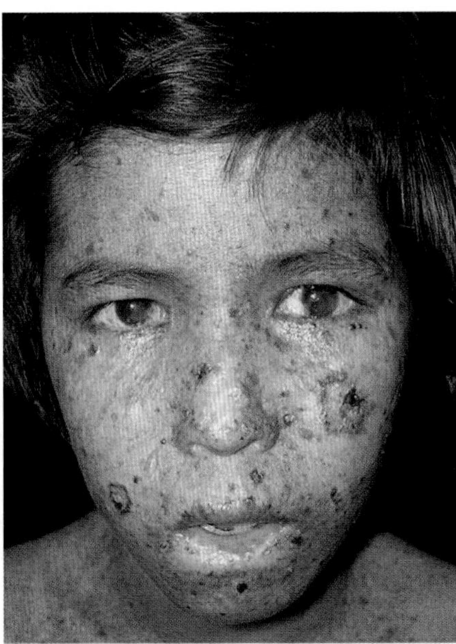

Fig. 4.34 Xeroderma pigmentosum. An 8-year-old girl presenting with dry and parchment-like skin with hyperpigmentation and multiple pigmented basal cell carcinomas on the face. Both eyes show corneal opacification. (From Chantorn R, Lim HW, Shwayder TA. Photosensitivity disorders in children: part II. *J Am Acad Dermatol*. 2012;67[6]:1113.e1–1113.e15. Photograph courtesy of Dr. Wisuthsarewong, Bangkok, Thailand.)

Bloom syndrome (congenital telangiectatic erythema)

- AR disorder due to mutations in *BLM/RECQL3* (DNA helicase) → ↑ **rates of sister chromatid exchange and chromosomal instability**
- Presents early in life w/ prenatal and postnatal growth impairment (**short stature**; do not exceed 5 feet in height)
- Cutaneous manifestations: **photosensitivity**, **telangiectatic erythema in a malar distribution**, cheilitis, CALM, and hypopigmentation
- Facies: narrow face w/ prominent ears, malar hypoplasia, and prominent/**bird-like nose**
- Other features: **primary hypogonadism** (men are sterile, women have decreased fertility), high-pitched voice, ↓ **IgA and IgM** → bronchiectasis/chronic lung disease/recurrent **respiratory and GI infections**, ↑ risk **lymphoma and leukemia** (150- to 300-fold ↑ risk), ↑ risk of some solid tissue tumors (SCCs and adenocarcinomas ([esp. GI])
- A characteristic pattern of **chromosomal breakage and rearrangement may be seen on chromosomal instability testing**, which can be performed at specialized centers
- Cutaneous and immunologic findings improve with age, but ↑ risk of mortality from **malignancy** (**#1 cause of death**, esp. leukemia) in the second to third decade; patients do not survive beyond 50 yo

Rothmund-Thomson syndrome (poikiloderma congenitale)

- **AR** disorder caused by mutations in *RECQL4* (**DNA helicase** that facilitates DNA replication and repair of UV damage)
- Cutaneous manifestations (present in first year of life): **erythema, edema, and blisters that begin on the cheeks** and subsequently progress to involve the extensor surfaces of the extremities and buttocks; **poikiloderma** (hypo- and hyperpigmentation + atrophy) is subsequently noted at these sites; acral verrucous keratoses (may → **SCC**), photosensitivity (in 30%), alopecia of scalp/lashes/brows, and dystrophic nails
- Short stature and skeletal dysplasia (e.g., **absence or hypoplasia of thumbs, radius, and ulna**); triangular-appearing face with frontal bossing/saddle nose/micrognathia; **juvenile cataracts**; dental anomalies; **hypogonadism**
- Malignancy may lead to premature death
  - **Osteosarcoma** (mean onset = 14 years of age) in ~30% patients
  - Non-melanoma skin cancer (esp. SCC)—mean age = 34 years of age

Cockayne syndrome (CS)

- **AR** disorder due to defective **transcription-coupled** NER = inability to resume RNA synthesis after UVR exposure (differs from XP, which has defective global genomic NER)
- Identical phenotype may occur due to mutations occur in either of two genes:
  - CS-A (20%): mutations in excision repair, cross-complementing group 8 (*ERCC8*)
  - CS-B (80%): mutations in *ERCC6*
- Classic CS (CS I) presents at the end of first decade
- CS II (severe CS) presents at birth; progresses more rapidly
- Cutaneous manifestations: **photosensitivity**, with telangiectatic erythema; unlike XP, has **NO ↑ risk of skin cancer** and **LACKS pigmentary changes**
- Typical facies: pinched, narrow "bird-like" face w/ beaked nose, large protuberant ears, and sunken eyes; growth failure and cachexia
- Neurologic manifestations: basal ganglia calcification, **progressive deterioration/demyelination of CNS**/PNS with ataxia and spasticity, intellectual impairment, microcephaly, and progressive sensorineural hearing loss
- Skeletal manifestations: short stature + cachectic/thin body ("**cachectic dwarfism**"), joint contractures, and kyphosis
- Ophthalmologic manifestations: **salt-and-pepper retinopathy**, optic atrophy, cataracts, and nystagmus
- Hypogonadism may be seen in affected males
- Most patients die by fourth decade from **progressive neurologic disease** complications

Trichothiodystrophy (Tay syndrome and PIBIDS syndrome)

- AR
  - A heterogeneous group of diseases w/ brittle hair and nails (↓ **content of cysteine-rich proteins**), ichthyosis, and neurodevelopmental disability; **classified as photosensitive or non-photosensitive**
    - <u>TTD with photosensitivity (TTD-P)</u>: caused by mutations in three genes (***ERCC2***, ***ERCC3***, and *GTF2H5*) encoding proteins (**XPD**, **XPB**, and TTDA),

respectively, that function in the transcription repair protein IIH complex, which is involved in DNA transcription and excision repair.
  - TTD, non-photosensitive (TTD-NP): results in about 10%–20% of cases from mutations in the *C7Orf11* gene, M-phase-specific PLK1-interacting protein (MPLKIP), which is thought to regulate transcription efficiency; **lacks ichthyosis**
- Photosensitivity (unlike XP, has **NO increased skin cancer risk**)
- Ichthyosis
- Brittle hair (short/sparse on scalp/brows/lashes w/ alternating light and dark bands on **polarizing light microscopy ("tiger-tail" abnormality)**
  - **Trichoschisis** and **trichorrhexis nodosa** may be seen
- Intellectual impairment and ataxia
- Decreased fertility/hypogonadism
- Short stature
- Other findings: **hypogammaglobinemia** with recurrent infections

4.13 PRIMARY IMMUNODEFICIENCY DISORDERS WITH CUTANEOUS MANIFESTATIONS

- Categorized by defects in the various components of the innate and adaptive immune system; overlap or combined defects often occur
  - Tables 4.21–4.23 summarize primary immunodeficiency disorders (PIDs) that are most commonly associated with cutaneous findings
  - Majority have AR inheritance, but some are X-linked (anhidrotic ectodermal dysplasia with immunodeficiency, chronic granulomatous disease, severe combined immunodeficiency syndrome (SCID) (IL2Rγ), Wiskott-Aldrich syndrome, Bruton's agammaglobulinemia, and IPEX syndrome)
- Signs that raise suspicion for PID
  - ↑ Frequency/severity/duration of bacterial, viral, and/or fungal infections
  - Opportunistic infections including atypical mycobacterial or deep fungal infections
  - Failure to thrive

Table 4.21 Cutaneous Infections Associated With Primary Immunodeficiency Disorders

Mucocutaneous Candidiasis	Chronic Mucocutaneous Candidiasis Syndromes
Recurrent bacterial pyodermas	AD hyper-IgE syndrome (STAT3) Chronic granulomatous disease Leukocyte adhesion deficiency Chédiak-Higashi Griscelli
Extensive viral infection (HPV, molluscum)	AR hyper-IgE syndrome (DOCK8) WHIM EDV Monomac

AD, *Autosomal dominant* ; AR, *autosomal recessive* ; EDV, *epidermodysplasia verruciformis*; WHIM, *warts, hypogammaglobinemia, infections, myelokathexis*.

Table 4.22 Cutaneous Findings Associated With Primary Immunodeficiency Disorders

Erythroderma	Omenn Syndrome > Other SCID[a]
Atopic phenotype (eczematous dermatitis and elevated eosinophils and IgE)	Hyper IgE syndrome (STAT3 > DOCK8) Wiskott-Aldrich syndrome IgA deficiency Omenn syndrome IPEX syndrome
Noninfectious cutaneous granulomas	Ataxia telangiectasia SCID (RAG1) Common variable immunodeficiency Chronic granulomatous disease
Pigmentary dilution (silvery hair and hypopigmentation)	Griscelli syndrome Chédiak-Higashi syndrome

[a]*Maternal graft-versus-host disease should be considered.*
IPEX, Immune dysregulation, polyendocrinopathy, enteropathy, X-linked; SCID, severe combined immunodeficiency syndrome.

- Cutaneous infections may include any or all of the following:
  - Recurrent staphylococcal or other bacterial pyodermas
  - Extensive viral infections (warts, molluscum, and HSV)
  - Widespread dermatophyte infections
  - Mucocutaneous candidiasis
- Hematopoietic stem cell transplantation may be indicated in those with severe PIDs including:
  - SCID
  - Chronic granulomatous disease
  - Wiskott-Aldrich syndrome
  - IPEX
  - Hemophagocytic lymphohistiocytosis (CHS and GS)
  - MonoMAC syndrome
- **Transplacental transfer of maternal T lymphocytes** may occur in neonates with **SCID**, and may → clinical and histologic signs of graft-versus-host disease (e.g., morbilliform, LP-like, seborrheic dermatitis-like, and sclerodermatous change)
- Cutaneous infections predominantly caused by one family of organisms may ↑ suspicion of specific PIDs (see Table 4.21)
- Distinct non-infectious cutaneous findings may lead to the diagnosis of a specific PID (see Table 4.22)

4.14 DISORDERS OF CORNIFICATION

- Inherited ichthyoses generally present at birth or in infancy/early childhood
  - Heterogeneous group of genetic disorders linked by a common finding of abnormal epidermal differentiation or metabolism → hyperkeratosis and/or epidermal hyperplasia
  - Dysfunction of cornified cell envelope disrupts skin barrier function → ↑ **transepidermal water loss** with possible resultant **hypernatremic dehydration**
  - Inherited ichthyoses characterized by localized or generalized hyperkeratosis, scaling, or both, along with variable additional cutaneous and/or systemic manifestations; +/– erythema

Table 4.23 Primary Immunodeficiencies Most Commonly Associated With Cutaneous Findings

Class	Mutation	Characteristic Infections	Distinct Cutaneous Features	Extracutaneous Features
Combined immunodeficiencies				
Omenn syndrome	***RAG1*** ***RAG2***	Any	Erythroderma Alopecia	Hepatosplenomegaly and lymphadenopathy
SCID	***IL2RG*** (IL-2Rγ chain)—most common; **XLR** inheritance ***ADA*** → ↑ adenosine → lymphocyte toxicity; **AR inheritance** *ZAP70* ***JAK3*; AR inheritance**	**Any** *Candida albicans* (esp. oral), *Staphylococcus. aureus*, and *Streptococcus pyogenes* Cutaneous infections caused by various organisms, including those listed above Sepsis of blood Viral diarrhea Otitis media Pneumonia (PCP and parainfluenza, in addition to bacteria)	Erythroderma (less common) See above re: GVHD-like presentation	**No palpable lymph nodes** No tonsillar buds/lymphoid tissue Failure to thrive
Leiner syndrome	Encompasses a variety of conditions, often **low C3 and/or C5**	Recurrent skin infections	Severe, generalized **seborrheic dermatitis-**like eruption	Failure to thrive, diarrhea
Combined immunodeficiencies with associated or syndromic features				
Wiskott-Aldrich	*WAS* (XLR)	**Recurrent encapsulated bacterial infections** (e.g., otitis media, pneumonia, and meningitis), HSV (as eczema herpeticum), HPV, and PCP Infection can → death in first decade	**Eczematous dermatitis** (scalp, face, and flexures) w/ 2° infections	Thrombocytopenia (→ **petechiae/purpura/epistaxis**), small platelets, and bloody diarrhea ↑**Food allergies/asthma/urticaria** ↑ **IgA**, **IgD**, **and IgE**; ↓ **IgM** Both cell-mediated and humoral immune response are compromised ↑ **Risk non-Hodgkin's lymphomas** (and other hematologic malignancies)
Ataxia telangiectasia	*ATM*		Telangiectasias of skin and conjunctivae Noninfectious granulomas	Truncal > peripheral ataxia Neurologic deterioration **Sensitivity to ionizing radiation** ↑ Risk of **hematologic malignancies** Female heterozygotes at increased risk for breast cancer
AD hyper IgE	*STAT3*	Pyodermas, cellulitis, furuncles, abscesses, and paronychia *S. aureus*, *Candida*, and *Streptococcus* **30% of abscesses are cold** Bronchitis, otitis media, empyemas, sinusitis, pneumatoceles, lung abscesses, and pneumonia (can → early death) *S. aureus*, *H. influenzae*, and fungal infections	**Coarse facial features** (broad nasal bridge and big nose) Diffuse dermatitis	**Retained 1° teeth w/ issues in 2° teeth** Osteopenia → fractures, scoliosis, and hyperextensibility ↑ IgE and eosinophilia
AR hyper IgE	*DOCK8*	Any	No dysmorphic features	
Antibody deficiencies				
IgA deficiency	*IGAD1*	**Sinopulmonary bacterial infections** and Giardia gastroenteritis	Eczematous dermatitis Autoimmune conditions	Must test for IgA deficiency (is the **most common immunoglobulin deficiency**) before giving ANY patient IVIG!

Continued

Table 4.23 Primary Immunodeficiencies Most Commonly Associated With Cutaneous Findings—cont'd

Class	Mutation	Characteristic Infections	Distinct Cutaneous Features	Extracutaneous Features
CVID (heterogeneous disorder currently classified into types CVID1-CVID11)	*ICOS* *CD19* *CD20* *CD21* *CD81* *LRBA1* *TACI* *BAFFR* *NFKB2* *IL21* *PRKCD*	Bacterial infections	Noninfectious granulomas Autoimmune conditions	Hypogammaglobinemia ↑ risk for hematologic malignancies
Bruton's hypogammaglobinemia	*BTK*	*Helicobacter bilis* associated pyoderma gangrenosum	Noninfectious granulomas	↑ risk for hematologic malignancies
Defects in phagocyte number or function				
Chronic granulomatous disease	***CYBB*** (p91- phagocyte oxidase (phox) beta subunit ***CYBA*** (p22-phox alpha subunit) *NCF1* (neutrophil cytosolic factor 1/p47-phox) *NCF2* (p67-phox) *NCF4* (p40-phox)	Pneumonia (*Nocardia*, Aspergillosis, and *Staphylococcus*), perianal abscesses, perioral dermatitis, and pyodermas due to **catalase-(+) organisms *(Staphylococcus aureus* #1**)	Noninfectious granulomas (cutaneous AND extracutaneous, esp. GI tract) Gingivitis/stomatitis	Hepatosplenomegaly, diarrhea, and lymphadenopathy (cervical #1; suppurative → abscess/fistula), granulomas of lung/liver/GU/GI **Female carriers of x-linked CGD may have higher risk of lupus** Can test diagnosis with nitroblue tetrazolium test
Leukocyte adhesion deficiency type 1	AR, ITGB2 ↓ β2 integrin (CD18)	Pyodermas Bacterial ulcerations can mimic pyoderma gangrenosum	**Delayed separation of umbilical cord** **Poor wound healing → ulcers**	Periodontitis → loss of teeth
Chédiak-Higashi	*LYST*	Pyodermas Bacterial ulcerations can mimic pyoderma gangrenosum	**Pigmentary dilution** (silvery hair and hypopigmentation of skin) Hyperpigmentation may develop in acral sun-exposed areas	**Accelerated lymphohistiocytic phase** Neurologic deterioration Giant granules or melanosomes in leukocytes and melanocytes
Griscelli (Fig. 4.35)	*Rab27A*	Pyodermas	**Pigmentary dilution** (silvery hair and hypopigmentation of skin)	**Accelerated lymphohistiocytic phase** Neurologic deterioration (primarily with MYO5A mutation)
Innate immunity				
Hypohidrotic ectodermal dysplasia with immunodeficiency	***NEMO***		Conical incisors Decrease or absence of sweat glands and hair follicles	Allelic to incontinentia pigmenti
Chronic mucocutaneous candidiasis/familial candidiasis	*CARD9* *IL-17RA* *IL-17F* *CLEC7A* *STAT1* *TRAF3IP2*	Mucocutaneous candidiasis and deep dermatophytosis		
WHIM	*CXCR4*	**HPV (extensive verrucae)**		**Myelokathexis** (peripheral neutropenia with retention of neutrophils in bone marrow)
EDV	*EVER1* *EVER2*	**HPV 5**, **8**, 10, 14, 20, 21, 25 and 47 (extensive verruca plana, along with thicker verrous warts)		Malignant transformation of warts to **SCC**
MonoMAC	*GATA2*	HPV, atypical mycobacteria, and deep fungal infections		Pulmonary alveolar proteinosis ↑ risk for hematologic malignancies
Immune dysregulation				
Immune dysregulation, polyendocrinopathy, enteropathy, and X-linked (IPEX)	***FOXP3***		Eczematous dermatitis	Severe diarrhea (enteropathy) Type 1 diabetes mellitus Hypothyroidism Autoimmune hemolytic anemia

CVID, *Common variable immunodeficiency;* EDV, *epidermodysplasia verruciformis;* SCID, *severe combined immunodeficiency;* WHIM, *warts, hypogammaglobinemia, infections, myelokathexis.*

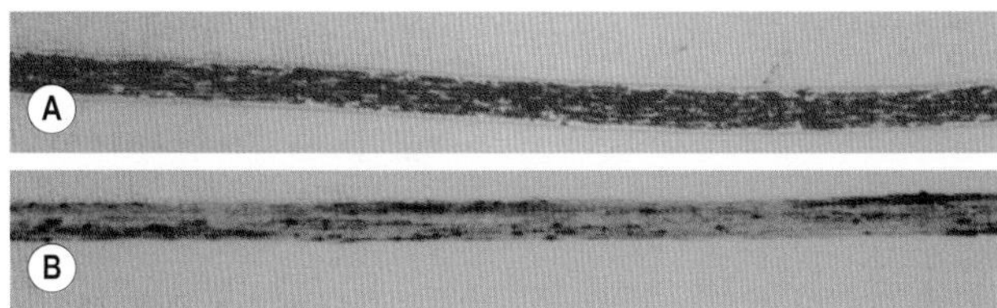

Fig. 4.35 Silvery hair syndromes. The giant melanosomes are easily seen in the hair shaft of individuals with Chédiak-Higashi syndrome **(A)** and Griscelli syndrome **(B)**. Note the more regular spacing of the melanosomes in the hair from a patient with Chédiak-Higashi syndrome. (From Paller AS, Mancini AJ. Disorders of pigmentation. In: *Hurwitz Clinical Pediatric Dermatology: A Textbook of Skin Disorders of Childhood and Adolescence*. 5th ed. Philadelphia: Elsevier; 2016:245–278.)

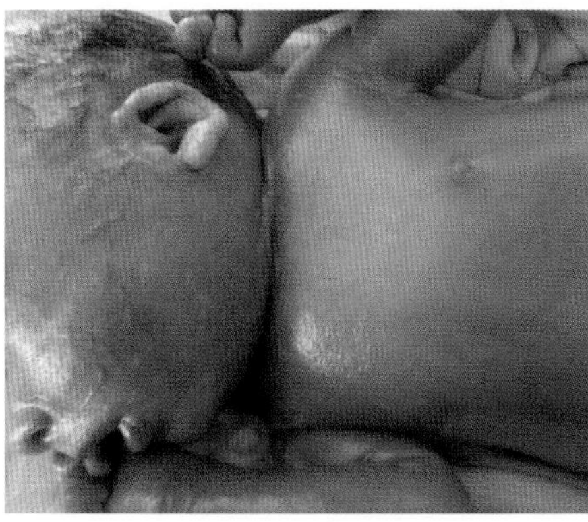

Fig. 4.36 Collodion baby: collodion membrane in a 1-day-old newborn. (From Prado R, Ellis LZ, Gamble R, Funk T, Arbuckle A, Bruckner AL. Collodion baby: an update with a focus on practical management. *J Am Acad Dermatol.* 2012;67[6]:1362–1374.)

- Collodion membrane at birth seen with AR congenital ichthyosis (**non-bullous congenital erythroderma most commonly; transglutaminase 1 is the most common mutation to result in collodion)** and lamellar ichthyosis; also Sjögren-Larsson syndrome, Gaucher disease type 2, Hay-Well syndrome, TTD, Netherton syndrome, ectodermal dysplasia, and neutral lipid storage disease); monitor for **hypernatremia**, approximately 5% are "self-healing" and shedding reveals normal skin; phenotype reveals itself once the collodion resolves, after several weeks (Fig. 4.36)
- Routine histology is generally non-diagnostic, but may demonstrate epidermal hyperplasia and variable orthohyperkeratosis; **ichthyosis vulgaris shows a diminished or absent granular layer** and epidermolytic ichthyosis shows epidermolytic hyperkeratosis
- Treatments for inherited ichthyosis: **emollients and keratolytics**; topical and systemic **retinoids** can help reduce hyperkeratosis and are useful for some disorders; neonatal care includes humidified incubators, emollients and close observation for infection, dehydration, and electrolyte abnormalities

- PPKs are a heterogeneous group of inherited and acquired disorders marked by hyperkeratosis of the palms and soles
  - Three types of PPK: focal (localized areas of hyperkeratosis, usually over pressure points), diffuse (hyperkeratosis involves entire palmoplantar surface), and punctate (1- to 2-mm keratotic papules)
  - PPK can be an isolated finding or a/w other abnormalities
  - Treatment: topical keratolytics (salicylic acid 2%–5%, lactic acid 5%–12%, and urea 10%–40%), topical retinoids, and topical corticosteroids when inflammation is present; use of oral retinoids may be helpful in some disorders; CO_2 laser ablation and surgical paring or excision helpful for more severe PPK
- See Tables 4.24 and 4.25

4.15 MISCELLANEOUS PEDIATRIC DERMATOLOGIC DISORDERS

Hydroa vacciniforme

- Mean age = 8 years; equal sex ratio
- UVA is most common trigger, but mechanism unclear
  - Probable role of chronic or latent Epstein-Barr virus **(EBV)** infection
    - a/w Atypical hydroa vacciniforme or hydroa vacciniforme-like lymphoproliferative disorder
    - EBV also detected in lesional skin and blood of patients with classical hydroa vacciniforme
- Outbreaks typically occur only in **summer**; eruption begins within a few hours of sun exposure
- Most common on **face and dorsal hands**, but can occur on any sun-exposed area
- Starts with burning or itching sensation that may be associated with mild constitutional symptoms
- Primary lesion is a pink macule or papule that progresses to vesicles and crusted erosions
- **Lesions resolve, leaving punched out varioliform scars**
- Ocular involvement: photophobia, keratoconjunctivitis, or uveitis
- Histology: dense perivascular infiltrate composed of lymphohistiocytes and neutrophils
  - The epidermis is **edematous** with reticular degeneration and necrotic keratinocytes
  - Dermal vessels may demonstrate thrombosis or hemorrhage
- Photoprovocation testing with **UVA** can be performed to help confirm diagnosis
- **Children with severe or atypical cutaneous involvement or constitutional symptoms of fever, lymphadenopathy, and hepatosplenomegaly should be evaluated for a concomitant EBV-associated lymphoproliferative disorder**
- Treatment: sun avoidance/photoprotection, narrowband UVB (NB-UVB) phototherapy in the spring to "harden" skin; hydroxychloroquine, beta-carotene, thalidomide, azathioprine, and cyclosporine may help
- **Usually resolves during adolescence or young adulthood**

Actinic prurigo

- Most common in **Native American** children; female > male; onset < 10 years of age
- Caused by UVR (**esp. UVA**)

Table 4.24 Features of Selected Ichthyoses and Erythrokeratodermas

Diagnosis	Gene	Inheritance	Onset	Primary Cutaneous Features	Associated Clinical Features	Histology and Ultrastructural Features	Ancillary Diagnostic Studies
Ichthyosis vulgaris	*FLG*	Autosomal semidominant	Infancy/ childhood	Fine, adherent scales on **extremities** and trunk with sparing of flexures; larger scale on lower legs; **hyperlinear palms/ soles**, and furrowed heels	**Keratosis pilaris; atopic diathesis**	Diminished/**absent stratum granulosum** w/ overlying **orthohyperkeratosis**; absent/reduced filaggrin immunostaining	Genetic testing
Steroid sulfatase deficiency (X-linked recessive ichthyosis)	*STS*	XLR Contiguous gene deletion may → Kallmann syndrome	Infancy	Fine to large, **dark/brown**, **adherent scales** on extremities, trunk, neck, and lateral face **spares flexures**, palms, soles, and face	**Corneal** (**comma-shaped**) **opacities**; **cryptorchidism**; ↑ Risk of **testicular cancer**, and hypogonadism *Female carriers:* corneal opacities; **prolonged labor** with affected child (placental sulfatase deficiency)	Retained corneodesmosomes within stratum corneum	Lipoprotein electrophoresis (increased mobility of β-fraction); plasma cholesterol sulfate increased; decreased steroid sulfatase activity in leukocytes; FISH, array CGH, genetic testing Maternal carriers may have abnormal triple/ quad screen during affected pregnancy with decreased serum estriol
Lamellar ichthyosis (Fig. 4.37)	***TGM1*** *ABCA12*[a] *CYP4F22*[a] *CERS3*	AR	Birth	Frequently collodion membrane at birth with ectropion and eclabium; after collodion resolves, presence of large, **thick**, **plate-like brown scales** in generalized distribution w/**significant flexural involvement**; absent or mild erythroderma; variable palm/sole involvement (PPK)	**Heat intolerance** (hypernatremic dehydration); frequent **scarring alopecia**; dystrophic nails Hypohidrosis	TGM1: thin cornified envelope and disorganized lamellar bilayers ABCA12: absence of lamellar body content NIPAL4: defective lamellar bodies and perinuclear membranes within stratum granulosum	*In situ* transglutaminase-1 expression and activity assay; genetic testing
Congenital ichthyosiform erythroderma (CIE)	*TGM1* ***ALOXE3***[b] ***ALOX12B***[b] *NIPAL4 (ICHTHYIN)*[b] *PNPLA1*[b]	AR	Birth	Frequently **collodion membrane** (#1 cause) at birth; after collodion resolves, fine, **white scale** in generalized distribution (**flexures involved**); erythroderma; variable palm/sole involvement	Heat intolerance/ hypohidrosis; variable scarring alopecia and ectropion	Same as for lamellar ichthyosis	Genetic testing
Congenital self-healing collodion baby	*TGM1ALOXE3, ALOX12B*	AR	Birth	**Collodion membrane** at birth; after resolution, skin appears normal without features of ichthyosis	None	Nondiagnostic	Genetic testing
Harlequin ichthyosis	*ABCA12*	AR	Birth	Very thick, yellow-brown plates of scale with large, deep and bright red fissures that tightly encase the neonate; **extreme ectropion**, **eclabium**, **and ear deformities**; survivors develop severe CIE-like phenotype; **early initiation of systemic retinoids** and specialized neonatal intensive care reduce mortality	Premature delivery; risk of neonatal hypothermia, and hypernatremic dehydration; **often neonatal death from sepsis or respiratory insufficiency**	Vesicular lamellar body ghosts, paucity of secreted lamellar structures in stratum corneum	Genetic testing

Epidermolytic ichthyosis (bullous CIE)	*KRT1* (has PPK) *KRT10* (no significant PPK)	AD May have somatic mosaicism → extensive epidermal nevi (ichthyosis hystrix); if it is gonadal mosaicism, then may have offspring with full blown disease	Birth	*At birth:* erythroderma, **blistering**, and erosions *Later:* **hyperkeratosis** with cobblestone pattern (most prominent over joints), ridging of the flexures; generalized or localized; variable degree of erythroderma, palmoplantar involvement, and blistering/bullae; **retinoids can exacerbate** skin fragility	Frequent skin infections; **malodor**; gait and posture abnormalities	Hyperkeratosis, keratinocyte vacuolization, and a prominent granular layer with **clumped keratin in suprabasal cells**; lamellar body accumulation	Genetic testing
Superficial epidermolytic ichthyosis (ichthyosis bullosa of Siemens)	*KRT2*	AD	Birth	Erythroderma and **superficial blistering** at birth; later, hyperkeratosis with accentuation over joints, flexures, and dorsal hands/feet; "**molting**" of the skin; palms and soles spared		Cytolysis of granular cells	Genetic testing
Ichthyosis prematurity syndrome	*SCL27A4*	AR	Birth	Thick caseous desquamating scale at birth Progresses to perifollicular hyperkeratosis	Patients are often born premature Often associated eosinophilia And respiratory distress		
Ichthyosis hystrix Curth-Macklin	*KRT1*	AD	Birth	Mild to severe, mutilating palmoplantar keratoderma; hyperkeratosis with verrucous, cobblestone, or hystrix-like pattern on extremities and trunk	Pseudoainhum; digital contractures	Binuclear cells; particular concentric perinuclear "shells" of aberrant putatively keratin material	Genetic testing
Ichthyosis en confetti	*KRT10*	AD		At birth, erythroderma and scaling; later, confetti-like areas of scaling (result from revertant mosaicism); palmoplantar keratoderma	Joint contractures	Affected skin: loss of epidermal differentiation above the basal layer with nucleolar vacuolization, loss of granular layer, and acanthosis, Revertant skin: normal	

Continued

Table 4.24 Features of Selected Ichthyoses and Erythrokeratodermas—cont'd

Diagnosis	Gene	Inheritance	Onset	Primary Cutaneous Features	Associated Clinical Features	Histology and Ultrastructural Features	Ancillary Diagnostic Studies
Netherton syndrome (Fig. 4.38)	*SPINK5* (encodes LEKT1, serine protease inhibitor)	AR	Birth/infancy	**Congenital erythroderma** and scaling; two principal phenotypes: **ichthyosis linearis circumflexa** (annular or serpiginous plaques w/ **double-edged scale**) and CIE-like; pruritus and eczematous plaques are common **Caution with tacrolimus ointment** (↑ absorption → toxic) or keratolytics (irritating)	**Trichorrhexis invaginata**, trichorrhexis nodosa, and pili torti (short/sparse hair and brows; ↑ **IgE**; neonatal temperature instability, electrolyte imbalance (hypernatremia), and failure to thrive; recurrent infections; **food and other allergies/ anaphylaxis**; nonspecific aminoaciduria	Psoriasiform histopathology; light microscopy of hair shafts may reveal trichorrhexis invaginata ("**bamboo hair**")	Genetic testing
Sjögren-Larsson syndrome	*ALDH3A2/**FALDH***	AR	Birth	At birth, erythema and hyperkeratosis; later, fine to plate-like/dark scaling or nonscaling hyperkeratosis; favors abdomen, neck, flexures; lichenification; palmoplantar keratoderma; pruritus can be severe	**Progressive spastic di- and tetraplegia**; developmental delay; intellectual disability; seizures; **perifoveal glistening white dots**; white matter disease of the brain; **photophobia**	Nonspecific; hyperkeratosis, acanthosis, and preservation of granular layer	Fatty aldehyde hydrogenase activity assay in cultured fibroblasts; genetic testing (preferred method)
Neutral lipid storage disease with ichthyosis/Chanarin-Dorfman syndrome	*ABHD5 (CGI-58)*	AR	Birth	Generalized, fine, white scales with variable erythema	**Developmental delay**; **hepatomegaly** with liver fibrosis, elevated liver enzymes, and creatine kinase; myopathy; hearing impairment; cataracts	**Globular electron-lucent inclusions in epidermis**	Peripheral blood smear to detect lipid vacuoles in granulocytes, eosinophils, and monocytes; oil stains of frozen tissue; genetic testing
Refsum disease	*PHYH* *PEX7*	AR	childhood to adulthood	Fine, white scales on extremities and trunk, resembling ichthyosis vulgaris (50%)	Peripheral motor and sensory neuropathy; cranial nerve dysfunction (deafness, anosmia); **cerebellar ataxia**; atypical retinitis pigmentosa ("**salt-and-pepper** pigment"); cardiomyopathy, arrhythmias w/ heart block; muscle wasting	Orthokeratotic hyperkeratosis and lipid-containing vacuoles in basal keratinocytes	**Increased plasma phytanic acid**; phytanoyl-CoA hydroxylase activity assay in cultured fibroblasts; genetic testing Diet is essential: ↓ green vegetables, dairy products, and ruminant fats

Keratitis-ichthyosis-deafness (KID) syndrome	*GJB2* (encodes connexin 26)	AD (nearly all reported cases are sporadic)	Birth/infancy	Transient neonatal erythroderma; erythematous, **hyperkeratotic plaques w/ well-demarcated, borders on face and extremities**; follicular keratoses; thickening of the skin with an appearance of "coarse-grained leather;" stippled palmoplantar keratoderma	Congenital **sensorineural hearing impairment**; progressive keratitis with corneal neovascularization that may lead to **blindness**, conjunctivitis; recurrent mucocutaneous infections, especially with *Candida albicans;* increased susceptibility to oral and cutaneous **squamous cell carcinoma**; nail, hair, and dental anomalies; cheilitis	Nonspecific; acanthosis, papillomatosis, and follicular plugging	
Erythrokeratodermia variabilis	*GJB3* *GJB4* (encode connexin 31 GJA1 and 30.3)	AD	Birth/infancy	**Transient**, **variable**, **erythematous patches**; more **stable**, **geographic**, **hyperkeratotic plaques** over knees, elbows, Achilles tendons, extremities, buttocks, and lateral trunk; face and scalp often spared; less common generalized hyperkeratosis; palmoplantar keratoderma in ~50% of patients	Burning or stinging sensation preceding or accompanying erythema	Nonspecific; may reveal reduced lamellar bodies in stratum granulosum and reduced keratinization	Genetic testing
Progressive symmetric erythrokeratoderma	*LOR* *GJB4* other unknown gene(s)	AD or AR	Infancy/ childhood	Fixed, slowly progressive, erythematous, hyperkeratotic plaques with sharp, figurate borders; on cheeks, over knees, elbows, extremities, and rarely trunk; palmoplantar keratoderma common		Nondiagnostic; acanthosis, hyperkeratosis, and prominent granular layer	
Acral peeling skin syndrome	*TGM5*	AR		Recurrent spontaneous painless superficial peeling on dorsal hands and feet, followed by the development of mild erythema; resolves without scarring; exacerbated by heat and humidity		Separation occurs between the junction of the stratum granulosum and the stratum corneum	

Table 4.24 Features of Selected Ichthyoses and Erythrokeratodermas—cont'd

Diagnosis	Gene	Inheritance	Onset	Primary Cutaneous Features	Associated Clinical Features	Histology and Ultrastructural Features	Ancillary Diagnostic Studies
Congenital hemidysplasia with ichthyosisiform erythroderma and limb defects (**CHILD**) **syndrome** (Fig. 4.39)	*NSDHL* *(3β-hydroxysteroid-dehydrogenase)*	**XLD**	Birth	At birth, unilateral (right > left-sided) erythema and waxy, yellowish adherent scale on **half of the body** (trunk/ extremities); later, verrucous hyperkeratosis of variable extent, with affinity for skin folds	**Ipsilateral skeletal hemidysplasia** (hypoplastic limbs); **ipsilateral organ hypoplasia**; ipsilateral alopecia; may also see stippled epiphyses/ chondrodysplasia punctata (similar to Conradi-Hunermann-Happle)	Nonspecific; acanthosis, papillomatosis, and superficial perivascular infiltrate	Genetic testing
Conradi-Hünermann-Happle syndrome (X-linked dominant chrondrodysplasia punctata) (Fig. 4.40)	*EBP* (emopamil-binding protein)	**XLD**	Birth	At birth, ichthyosiform erythroderma (**generalized**, vs. unilateral in CHILD syndrome) with feathery, adherent scale along Blaschko's lines; **erythema resolves** in first few months of life (unlike CHILD syndrome) and is replaced by follicular **atrophoderma** along Blaschko's lines, most prominently on the forearms and dorsal hands	Unilateral cataracts; **stippled epiphyses/ chondrodysplasia punctata** seen only during infancy; asymmetric skeletal abnormalities, including scoliosis and rhizomelic limb shortening, but less severe than CHILD syndrome; frontal bossing w/ macrocephaly; patchy scarring alopecia	Nonspecific; hyperkeratosis and focal parakeratosis; may see dystrophic calcification in keratotic plugs	**Epiphyseal stippling on X-ray** only visible during infancy; accumulation of plasma cholesterol; genetic testing
Ichthyosis follicularis-atrichia-photophobia (IFAP) syndrome	*MBTPS2*	XLR	Birth	Erythroderma, scaling, and follicular hyperkeratosis; generalized alopecia, including eyebrows and eyelashes	Growth retardation and microcephly; corneal opacities and ulcerations; photophobia; vascularizing keratitis; variable hearing loss; nail dystrophy; variable intellectual impairment, developmental delay, seizures, and structural CNS anomalies; genitourinary anomalies and skeletal anomalies	Follicular plugging and hypoplastic pilosebaceous structures	

[a]*Also occasionally associated with CIE or intermediate LI/CIE phenotypes; a CIE-like phenotype is also seen in harlequin ichthyosis survivors.*
[b]*Also occasionally associated with mild LI or intermediate LI/CIE phenotypes.*
CGH, Comparative genomic hybridization; FISH, *fluorescence* in situ *hybridization;* PPK, *palmoplantar keratoderma.*
Modified from Richard G, Ringpfeil F. Ichthyoses, erythrokeratodermas, and related disorders. In: Bolognia JL, Schaffer JV, Cerroni L, eds. Dermatology. *4th ed. Philadelphia: Elsevier; 2018:888–923.*

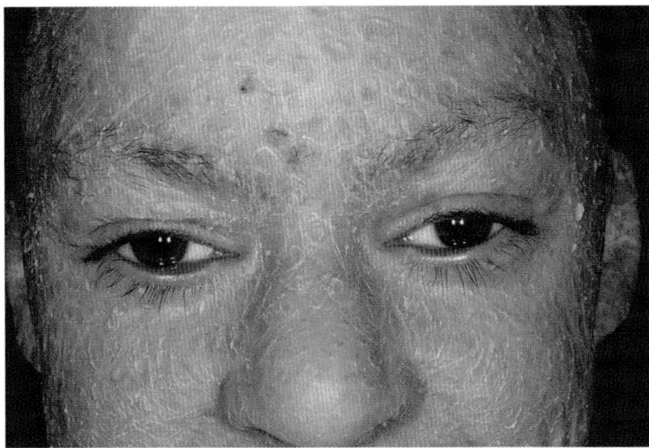

Fig. 4.37 Lamellar ichthyosis phenotype of autosomal recessive congenital ichthyosis. Large plate-like scaling on the forehead and cheeks. This patient shows moderate ectropion. (From Paller AS, Mancini AJ. Hereditary disorders of cornification. In: *Hurwitz Clinical Pediatric Dermatology: A Textbook of Skin Disorders of Childhood and Adolescence*. 5th ed. Philadelphia: Elsevier; 2016:95–118.)

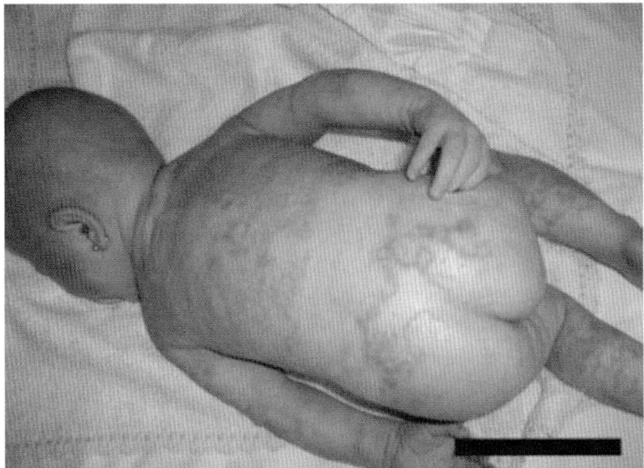

Fig. 4.38 Erythroderma, hypotrichosis, and areas with ichthyosis linearis circumflexa. (From Pastore S, Gorlato G, Berti I, Barbi E, Ventura A. Successful induction of oral tolerance in Netherton syndrome. *Allergol Immunopathol (Madr)*. 2012;40[5]:316–317.)

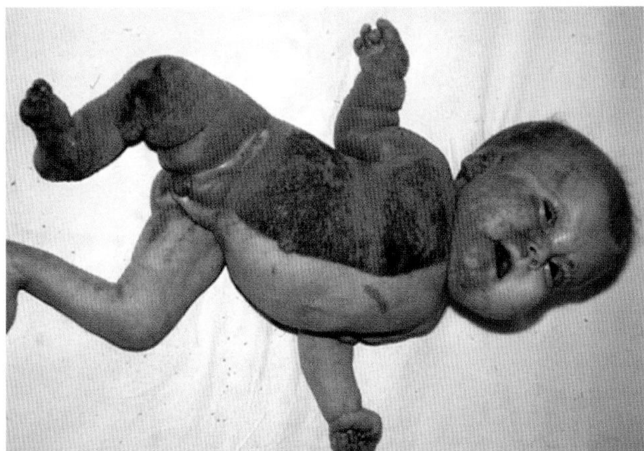

Fig. 4.39 CHILD syndrome. Unilateral erythema and scale with ipsilateral limb defects. (From Baden HP, DiGiovanna JJ. Ichthyosiform dermatoses. In: Rimoin DL, Pyeritz RE, Korf BR. *Emery and Rimoin's Principles and Practice of Medical Genetics*. 6th ed. Philadelphia: Elsevier; 2013.)

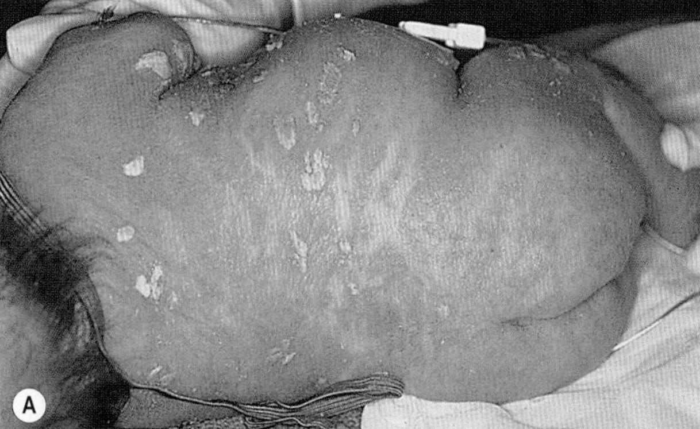

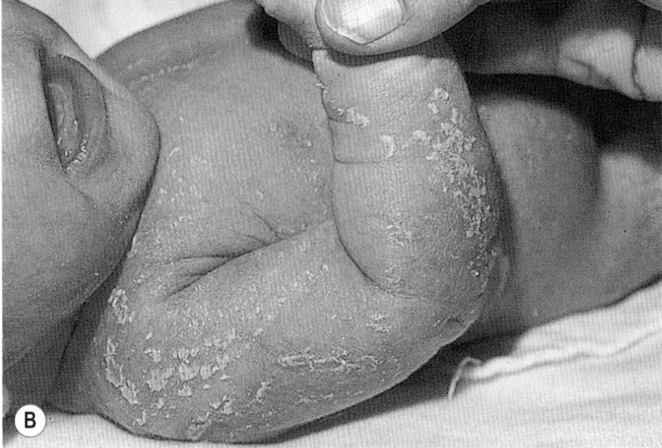

Fig. 4.40 Conradi-Hünermann syndrome. **(A)** Thick, psoriasiform scaling overlying erythema in a 1-month-old girl with the syndrome and chondrodysplasia punctata. As the scaling desquamated, the underlying erythema along Blaschko's lines became more apparent. **(B)** The pattern of scale along Blaschko's lines is more evident in this neonate with Conradi-Hünermann syndrome. (*A*, from Foley CC, Paller AS, Irvine AD. Disorders of cornification (ichthyosis). In: Eichenfield LF, Frieden IJ, eds. *Neonatal and Infant Dermatology*. 3rd ed. Philadelphia: Elsevier; 2015; *B*, from Paller AS. Ichthyosis in the neonate. In: Dyall-Smith D, Marks R, eds. *Dermatology at the Millennium*. London: Parthenon Publishing Group; 1998, with permission.)

- May be an AD inheritance pattern with incomplete penetrance
  - **HLA-DR4 DRB1*0407 polymorphism present in 60%–70% of patients**
- Seasonal variability in severity
  - **Flares in spring and persists through summer**
  - Improves in fall, but usually **does not completely remit in winter**
- Intensely pruritic eruption on sun-exposed areas, though covered skin may also be involved
  - Presents as papules and nodules that are frequently excoriated and crusted
  - Progresses to eczematous plaques with lichenification; secondary bacterial infection may occur
  - Dyspigmentation and scarring are common (vs. polymorphous light eruption [PMLE])
- **Actinic cheilitis is a characteristic feature**
  - 65%–85% of patients will have lip involvement with pruritus, edema, scale, and crusting
  - Actinic cheilitis without other features may be seen in 10%–25% of children

Table 4.25 Selected Hereditary Palmoplantar Keratodermas (PPKs) With Known Genetic Basis

Type	Gene	Gene Product	Synonyms	Inheritance	Onset	Transgrediens	Comments
Diffuse							
Unna-Thost (Fig. 4.41)	***KRT1*** *KRT6c*	**Keratin 1** Keratin 6c	Nonepidermolytic PPK (NEPPK)	AD	2–5 years, sometimes later	No	Second most common type of diffuse PPK (after EPPK) Diffuse, well-demarcated PPK w/ yellow hue; hyperhidrosis Histology w/ prominent orthokeratosis
Vörner	*KRT1* *KRT9*	Keratin 1 Keratin 9	Epidermolytic PPK (EPPK)	AD	0–3 years	No	Clinically identical to diffuse NEPPK, but histology shows epidermolytic hyperkeratosis
Mal de Meleda	*SLURP-1*	Secreted Ly6/Plaur domain-containing protein-1	Mal de Meleda	AR	0–3 years	Yes	Atopic dermatitis; **transgradiens** PPK erythematous w/ fissures/hyperhidrosis/maceration/ **horrible odor**/often infected; **dystrophic nails**
Greither	*KRT1* (in some families)	Keratin 1	Transgrediens and progrediens PPK	AD	Infancy	Yes	
Mutilating (Vohwinkel) (Fig. 4.42)	*LOR* (+ ichthyosis) *GJB2* (+ deafness)	Loricrin Connexin 26	Vohwinkel syndrome; keratoderma hereditaria mutilans	AD	Infancy	Yes	**Honeycombed palmar PPK**, **pseudoainhum** (esp. fifth finger – constriction bands → autoamputation), **starfish keratoses** on the knuckles/ feet/ elbows/knees, linear keratoses on elbows/knees, **sensorineural deafness** (**connexin 26**), and generalized **ichthyosis** (**loricrin**)
Papillon-Lefèvre syndrome	*CTSC*	Cathepsin C	PPK with periodontitis	AR	Birth to early infancy	Yes, diffuse	**Transgradiens** PPK w/ erythema/hyperhidrosis/ terrible odor (soles > palms); pyogenic infections; **periodontitis/gingivitis → premature loss of teeth**, psoriasiform lesions on elbows/knees, and pyogenic infections; **dural calcification**
Naxos disease	*JUP*	Plakoglobin	Diffuse NEPPK with woolly hair and cardiomyopathy	AR	Infancy	No	Woolly hair; arrhythmias and **right ventricular cardiomyopathy** develop during adolescence
Focal							
Striate type Areata type	*DSG1* *DSP* *KRT1* *KRT16* *KRT6c*	Desmoglein 1 Desmoplakin Keratin 1 Keratin 16 Keratin 6c	Wachters type, Brünauer-Fuhs-Siemens type	AD	4–10 years	No	Striate on palms and islands on feet; variable phenotype
Richner-Hanhart syndrome	*TAT*	**Tyrosine amino-transferase**	**Tyrosinemia type II**, oculocutaneous tyrosinemia	AR	Infancy (ocular) Early childhood to adolescence (skin)	No	**Focal painful PPK on weight-bearing areas**; **dendritic keratitis**, **corneal ulcers**, **and blindness** (ocular findings prior to skin findings); hyperkeratosis of elbows/knees; developmental delay
Pachyonychia congenita	*KRT16* *KRT6a* *KRT17* *KRT6b*	Keratin 16 Keratin 6α Keratin 17 Keratin 6b	PC1, Jadassohn-Lewandowsky type PC2, Jackson-Lawler type	AD	Infancy to early childhood	No	PC1: more severe NEPPK PC2: steatocystoma multiplex and eruptive vellus hair cysts more common; natal teeth
Carvajal syndrome	*DSP*	Desmoplakin	Striate PPK with woolly hair and cardiomyopathy	AR > AD	Infancy	No	Woolly hair; **dilated left ventricular cardiomyopathy** (variable onset); occasionally skin fragility, nail dystrophy, hypodontia
Howel-Evans syndrome	*RHBDF2/ IRHOM2*	Rhomboid 5, drosophila, homolog of 2/inactive rhomboid protein 2	**Tylosis with esophageal cancer**	AD	Childhood	No	**Thick yellow PPK on weight-bearing areas** (heels and balls of feet) starting in second decade Significant risk for development of esophageal cancer in third to fifth decade

AD, Autosomal dominant; AR, autosomal recessive; SCC, squamous cell carcinoma.
Modified from Krol AL, Siegel D. Keratodermas. In: Bolognia JL, Jorizzo JL, Schaffer JV. Dermatology. *3rd ed. Philadelphia: Elsevier; 2012:871–885.*

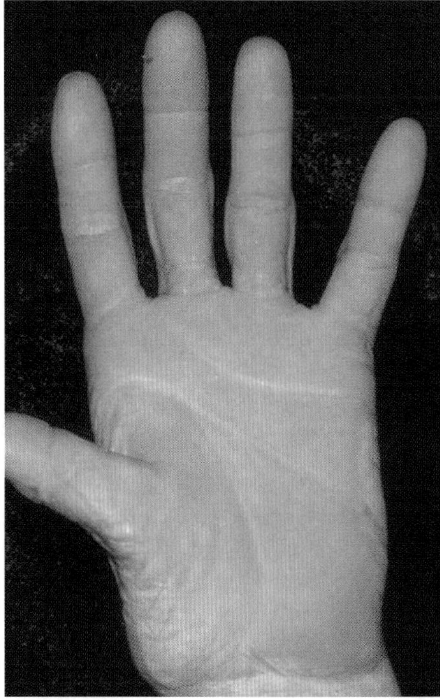

Fig. 4.41 Unna-Thost syndrome. (From Gehris RP, Ferris LK. Genodermatoses. In: Schwarzenberger K, Werchniak AE, Ko CJ, eds. *Requisites in Dermatology: General Dermatology*. Philadelphia: Elsevier; 2009:277–296.)

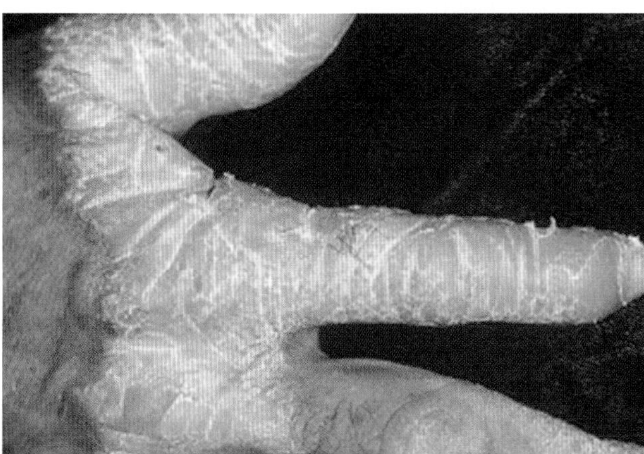

Fig. 4.42 Vohwinkel's syndrome. Mutilating keratoderma. (From Gehris RP, Ferris LK. Genodermatoses. In: Schwarzenberger K, Werchniak AE, Ko CJ, eds. *Requisites in Dermatology: General Dermatology*. Philadelphia: Elsevier; 2009:277–296.)

- **Actinic conjunctivitis** can manifest as epiphora and photophobia
- Biopsy of the lips commonly shows lymphoid follicle formation and is a distinguishing feature
- Phototesting shows ↓ minimal erythema dose in 60%
- Treatments: sun avoidance/photoprotection, NB-UVB phototherapy in the spring can minimize flares, topical corticosteroids, and short courses of oral prednisone may help with flares; mainstay of treatment is **thalidomide**
- Often has a **chronic course** that continues into adulthood

Juvenile spring eruption

- **Boys** > girls; 5–12 years of age
- Triggered by UVA, UVB, and rarely visible light
- Thought to be a **variant of PMLE**
- Occurs in **early spring** with improvement through the season
- Pruritic, skin-colored to pink edematous papules that can progress to vesicles and crusting
  - Most common on the **helical ears**, but can affect the hands or face
  - Lesions self-resolve in 1 week w/o scarring
- Treatment: sun avoidance and photoprotection; NB-UVB phototherapy for a 4- to 6-week course at the beginning of spring may prevent recurrence; topical and systemic corticosteroids; oral antihistamines
- Lesions self-resolve in several weeks, but may recur each spring; disease remits after puberty

Diaper dermatitis

- Peak incidence at 9 to 12 months
- Risk factors: contact with urine/feces, friction/maceration, and 2° infection with bacteria and/or yeast
- Irritant contact dermatitis: erythema of convex surfaces, but tends to spare the folds
- Seborrheic dermatitis: salmon-colored erythema in the folds
- Allergic contact dermatitis: most often due to blue dye or mercaptobenzothiazole in the elastic band
- Psoriasis: diaper area is often the presenting area in infancy; may be due to koebnerization from irritant contact; presents as well-demarcated erythema +/– scale
- **Candidiasis:** beefy red erythema and pustulovesicular "satellite" lesions
- **Granuloma gluteale infantum**: purple red nodules, often appearing after use of high-potency topical steroids and/ or prolonged use of cloth diapers (nonabsorbent)
- **Perianal pseudoverrucous papules and nodules:** flat topped, wart-like papules and nodules appear in incontinent patients as a form of severe irritant contact dermatitis
- **Jacquet's erosive dermatitis**: severe erosive dermatitis with ulcerated papules and nodules; presents more pinpoint than other erosive diaper dermatoses
- Acrodermatitis enteropathica: similar to "erosive psoriasis" of the diaper area; also affects perioral area
- Langerhans cell histiocytosis: severely erosive in the folds, petechial papules
- Treatment:
  - Meticulous diaper hygiene with frequent diaper changes and gentle cleansing, avoid packaged wipes when possible
  - Application of thick barrier ointments
  - Low-potency topical steroid ointments (**avoid in granuloma gluteale infantum**)

Juvenile plantar dermatosis

- **Boys** > girls
- May be worse in summer and cold weather
- Most likely represents a **frictional irritant dermatitis**

- Erythematous, symmetrical, **smooth** red plaques, affecting the **plantar surfaces** of the distal soles and toes, with sparing of the web spaces
  - 5% may have similar changes on fingertips
  - May be associated with hyperhidrosis ("**sweaty sock syndrome**")
- Treatments: cotton or super absorbent socks and avoidance of occlusive footwear, absorbent foot powder, emollients, and medium-/high-potency topical corticosteroids

Acropustulosis of infancy

- Onset is typically between birth and 2 years of age
  - Most common in **black infants**
- Etiology unknown; some cases **a/w preceding scabies** infection
- Recurrent crops of vesiculopustules over the **palms, soles, and distal extremities**
- Biopsy not necessary but demonstrates neutrophils
- Treatment: systemic antihistamines and high-potency topical corticosteroids
- Typically resolves spontaneously by 3 years of age

Trichorhinophalangeal syndrome

- Mainly AD, *TRPS1* gene
- Cone-shaped epiphyses of the phalanges
- Short stature
- **Pear-shaped nose** with a rounded tip, long philtrum; and thin upper lip
- Sparse hair, with possible total alopecia, mainly in males

Nail-patella syndrome (onycho-osteodysplasia; Fong disease)

- AD, *LMX1B* (encodes collagen synthesis transcription factor)
- Hypoplastic or absent nails, most often on the thumb, sometimes fingers (esp. medial), with dystrophy typically worse on the radial side
- **Triangular lunula**
- Bony abnormalities including hypoplastic or absent patellae, radial head dysplasia, and posterior iliac "horns" (exostoses)
- Nephropathy, especially glomerulonephritis, sometimes causing renal insufficiency
- Lester iris (darker pigmentation of central iris)

MIDAS syndrome (also MLS or microphthalmia with linear skin defects)

- XLD, *HCCS* gene
- <u>Mi</u>croopthalmia (among other ocular defects), <u>d</u>ermal <u>a</u>plasia, <u>s</u>clerocornea
- Linear skin defects → aplasia cutis congenita (ACC)—mostly red-brown Blaschkoid on the face and neck, limited to upper body
- Can also get agenesis of corpus callosum, seizures, intellectual disability, and cardiac arrythmias

H syndrome

- AR, *SCL29A3* (nucleoside transporter)
- **H**yperpigmentation, **H**ypertrichosis with induration and varicose veins characteristically of the thighs sparing knees, **H**allux valgus with flexion contracture of toes, **H**epatosplenomegaly, **H**eart abnormalities, **H**ypogonadism, decreased **H**eight, **H**yperglycemia/DM

Cutaneous findings in patients with chromosomal abnormalities

- Down syndrome (trisomy 21): transverse palmar crease, **syringomas**, **elastosis perforans serpiginosa**, **transient myeloproliferative disorder** (often presents as vesiculopustular eruption) autoimmune diseases including **alopecia areata**, epicanthic folds, predisoposition to yeast and fungal infections, hidradenitis suppurativa, and scrotal tongue
- Turner syndrome (XO): **cystic hygroma** → webbed neck, transient peripheral lymphedema, ↑ **numbers of nevi** (but no increased melanoma risk), **multiple pilomatricomas**, propensity towards keloid formation, nail dystrophy, and low posterior hairline, coarctation of the aorta
- Noonan syndrome (AD, *PTPN11*): lower extremity lymphedema, CALMs, multiple nevi, light/curly/rough hair, hypertelorism, **ulerythema ophryogenes**, webbed neck, lowered nuchal hairline, and low-set ears **(note: allelic with LEOPARD syndrome—both have pulmonic stenosis)**
- Cardio-facio-cutaneous (CFC) (AD, *BRAF* > *KRAS*): generalized ichthyosis-like scaling, keratosis pilaris including ulerythema ophryogenes, CALMs, many nevi, sparse curly hair, cardiac including pulmonary stenosis
- Costello syndrome (AD, HRAS > KRAS): lax skin especially of the hands and feet, periorofacial papillomas, acanthosis nigricans, curly hair, unusual body odor and heat intolerance, cardiac including pulmonary stenosis, increased risk of rhabdomyosarcoma
- Klinefelter syndrome (XXY): ↑ **varicosities**, **leg ulcers**, ↓ body hair, marfanoid habitis, and gynecomastia

Cutaneous mastocytosis

- Childhood and adulthood types; most cases present before 15 years of age
- Adults more likely than children to develop systemic symptoms/disease
- ***c-KIT* mutations** (activating mutations typically, as tyrosine kinase accounts for increased pigmentation of mastocyotmas)
  - D816V activating mutation found in 42% of children and adults
  - Of note, *c-KIT* encodes KIT (CD117) on mast cells; stem cell factor is the ligand for KIT and essential for survival of mast cells
- Childhood forms
  - <u>Solitary mastocytoma</u>
    - Usually occurs as single tan/yellow-tan plaque/nodule with an overlying peau d'orange appearance
    - Most commonly seen on distal extremities
    - Generally self-resolves over 1 to 3 years
  - <u>Urticaria pigmentosa</u> (Fig. 4.43)
    - **Most common presentation in children**

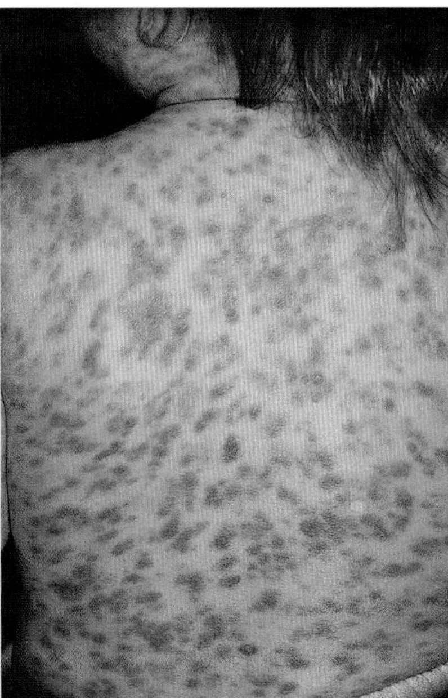

Fig. 4.43 Multiple tan to brown lesions of urticaria pigmentosa. (From Tharp MD. Mast cell disease. In: Callen JP, Jorizzo JL, Zone JJ, Piette WW, Rosenbach MA, Vleugels RA, eds. *Dermatological Signs of Systemic Disease*. 5th ed. Philadelphia: Elsevier; 2017:370–376.)

- Multiple light brown to red-brown macules and papules, which can occur anywhere; start on trunk; spare palms/soles/face
- Pruritus and flushing may be seen; blistering (bullous mastocytosis) in about one fourth patients
- Symptoms improve by early adolescence, and skin lesions often resolve
- Patients with more lesions are more likely to have systemic symptoms
- Diarrhea, abdominal pain are most common symptoms
- Anaphylaxis is rare, but possible

- Diffuse cutaneous mastocytosis
  - Infiltrated, red-brown, leathery plaques with **peau d'orange** appearance that can involve large areas of body
  - Skin lesions frequently blister → erosions
  - ↑ Incidence of systemic symptoms and progression to systemic mastocytosis
  - Can also occur in adults, although rarely
- **Adult Forms**
  - Reddish-brown macules/papules: occur on trunk/ proximal extremities; ↑ in # over time; hyperpigmented; **most common presentation in adults**
  - Telangiectasia macularis eruptiva perstans: telangiectatic macules and patches with no hyperpigmentation
- **Darier's sign** (local erythema or urticarial wheal after friction or rubbing) is present in all forms; more pronounced in childhood forms due to increased numbers of mast cells
- Systemic manifestations commonly occur in the systemic mastocytoses (e.g., indolent systemic mastocytosis, mast cell leukemia, and aggressive systemic mastocytosis)
  - Prognosis is poor for many of these disorders
  - Symptoms include skeletal lesions, bone marrow involvement, hepatosplenomegaly, lymphadenopathy, GI symptoms (diarrhea, abdominal pain, nausea/ vomiting, and GI hemorrhage), and mixed organic brain syndrome
- On histology, mast cell infiltrates are seen in the dermis of lesional skin
  - Eosinophils and hyperpigmentation of the basal layer may be present
  - Stains: **toluidine blue**, **Giemsa**, **Leder**, **tryptase**, **and CD117 (kit) antibodies**
  - Bone marrow biopsy should be performed when considering systemic disease, especially in adults
- **Serum tryptase may be elevated** but is often normal; urinary histamine and histamine metabolites (1,4-methylimidazole acetic acid and N-methylimidazoleacetic acid) may be detectable
- Treatment:
  - Avoid mast cell degranulators (e.g., alcohol, anticholinergics, nonsteroidal anti-inflammatory drugs [NSAIDs], aspirin, opiates including **morphine and dextromethorphan**, polymyxin, and systemic anesthetics)
  - Antihistamines (H1 and H2 antagonists), topical/ systemic steroids, topical calcineurin inhibitors, **oral cromolyn** (best treatment for associated **GI symptoms**), PUVA/UVA1, intramuscular epinephrine, and imatinib (**in some with systemic mastocytosis—e.g., those who have *FIP1L1-PDGFRA* gene rearrangement**)

Neutrophilic eccrine hidradenitis of childhood

- **Acute onset, painful palmoplantar** papules and nodules in children (6 months to 15 years)
- May be associated with chemotherapy or idiopathic
  - **Pseudomonas hot foot syndrome** is a variant due to *Pseudomonas* in swimming pools or hot tubs
- **Neutrophilic infiltration around eccrine glands** on histopathology

5

Infectious Diseases

Ali Alikhan and Thomas L.H. Hocker

CONTENTS LIST

5.1 VIRAL DISEASES
5.2 HIV/AIDS DERMATOLOGY
5.3 BACTERIAL INFECTIONS
5.4 FUNGAL DISEASES
5.5 PARASITES AND OTHER CREATURES

5.1 VIRAL DISEASES

I. Human papillomavirus (HPV)

- **Double-stranded DNA virus** that infects skin and mucosal epithelial cells → **warts** and malignancies (e.g., **cervical cancer** and squamous cell carcinoma [SCC])
  - Capsid
    - Contains DNA
    - Composed of L1 (major structural protein) and L2 (minor structural protein)—important for binding/entering epithelial cells
  - HPVs are species-specific and require fully differentiated squamous epithelia for their life cycle
    - Productive infection/hyperproliferation can only be accomplished if virus infects basal layer keratinocytes; early proteins (**E1–E7**) are responsible for **DNA replication** and keratinocyte immortalization; late proteins (**L1–L2**) are expressed in superficial epidermis and encode **structural proteins** required for virion formation
    - E1 and E2 genes are first to be expressed at strata basale and spinosum—control transcription of other genes + replication of viral DNA (using host cell machinery)
    - E4 protein disrupts cytokeratin network → koilocytosis
    - E5, E6, and E7 genes allow viral replication above stratum basale → **amplification**
      - E6 and E7 decrease host immune response (e.g., TLR-9 and IL-8)
      - **E6 and E7** in high-risk mucosal subtypes are **oncoproteins**
        - E6 → ubiquitin-mediated **p53** destruction → ↓ apoptosis/↑ replication/↑ mutations
        - E7 binds **RB** → loss of inhibition of **E2F** transcription factor → ↑ expression of genes important for DNA replication
    - More superficial epidermal layers have higher L1 and L2 levels; **complete virus observed in granular layer and above**
    - Host response is primarily cell-mediated in nature, along with help from the innate immune system (e.g., TLR-3 and TLR-9)
  - Genus **α (most of the mucosal and cutaneous HPV types)** and **β (epidermodysplasia verruciformis** [EV]-associated HPV types) account for most known types
- Typically spread via sexual contact or skin-to-skin/fomite contact; HPV DNA found in normal skin and perilesional skin
- Most warts resolve in 1 to 2 years without treatment
- <u>Cutaneous manifestations of HPV infection</u>
  - Common warts: hyperkeratotic papules with pinpoint black dots (thrombosed capillaries), most commonly on fingers, dorsal hands/elbows/knees; usually **HPV-1, -2**, -4, -27, and -57 (HPV-57 can cause 10 nail dystrophy)
  - Palmar/plantar warts: thick/deep endophytic papules with black dots on palms/soles
    - **Myrmecia** refers to anthill appearance of some plantar warts; **mosaic** refers to coalescence of several warts on plantar surfaces
    - **HPV-1**, **HPV-2**, -4, -27, and -57
    - Histology: "**church spire**" **papillomatosis** + hyperkeratosis, acanthosis (with elongated rete ridges), **hypergranulosis**, **koilocytosis** (granular layer); ↑ dermal vessels
  - Flat/plane warts: light pink/brown, **soft/smooth**, slightly raised, occasionally linear flat-topped papules on **dorsal hands/face**
    - More common in **children; adult women** >> adult men
    - **HPV-3**, **-10**, -28, and -29
    - Histology: alternating orthokeratosis/parakeratosis, mild papillomatosis, hypergranulosis, acanthosis, koilocytosis (granular/upper spinous layer; "bird's eyes")

- Butcher's warts: extensive lesions on hands in meat/fish-handlers; **HPV-7** and **HPV-2**
- Ridged warts retain normal dermatoglyphics—**HPV-60**; pigmented variant is more common in Japan
- EV: genetic disorder in which host has susceptibility to **genus β HPV types** (HPV-3, **-5**, **-8**, -9, -12, -14, -15, -17, -19–25, -36–38, -47, -49)
  - Autosomal recessive inheritance—mutations in TMC6 (**EVER1**) and TMC8 (**EVER2**) (encode transmembrane proteins in endoplasmic reticulum, which interact with Zn transporter 1 → ↓ Zn intracellularly → ↓ Zn-associated transcription factors)
  - **Acquired form may be seen in HIV**
  - HPV types 5 and 8 can → Actinic keratoses and **SCC** (generally patients ≥30 years old in sun-exposed areas; >30% of patients will develop SCC)
  - Generalized polymorphic papules (generally **flat wart-like appearance** (dorsal hands, neck, face, and extremities), but **also scaly, pink macules or hypopigmented, guttate macules/patches**, and seborrheic keratosis-like lesions on forehead/neck/trunk)
  - Some cases have extensive and confluent warts → generalized verrucosis
  - Histology: flat wart-like architecture + large cells w/ perinuclear halos and **blue-gray granular cytoplasm** (Fig. 5.1)
- WHIM syndrome: autosomal dominant, primary immunodeficiency caused by a CXCR4 mutation—**w**arts, **h**ypogammaglobinemia, **i**nfections (bacterial), and neutropenia (2° to **m**yelokathexis)
- WILD syndrome: **w**arts, **i**mmunodeficiency, **l**ymphedema, and **d**ysplasia (anogenital)
- Treatments: destructive (cryotherapy, electrodessication and curettage, scissors/shave removal, laser [pulsed dye laser or CO_2]/photodynamic therapy (PDT), cantharidin, and salicylic acid preparations), immunomodulatory/antiviral (diphenylcyclopropenone, cidofovir gel, and intralesional immunotherapy [e.g., *Candida*]), 5-FU (topically w/ salicylic acid usually or intralesional), intralesional bleomycin

- Mucosal/genital manifestations of HPV infection
  - Genital warts (condyloma acuminata)
    - **Most common sexually transmitted disease**
    - Occur on external genitals/perineum/perianal/groin/mons/vagina/urethra/anal canal
    - Smooth, sessile, raised, skin-colored to brown lobulated papules
    - **HPV-6, HPV-11, HPV-16, HPV-18,** HPV-31, HPV-33, and HPV-45
    - Condylomata plana (flat cervical warts) best seen w/ **acetic acid → whitening**
    - Most cases resolve spontaneously within 2 years
    - Risk factors: sexual intercourse at young age, # of sexual partners, and men who have sex with men (MSM)
    - Circumcision → ↓ risk HPV transmission
    - May → **cervical cancer**
      - Most common scenario = persistent cervical infection with high-risk HPV type (**HPV-16, HPV-18, HPV-31, HPV-33, and HPV-45**)
      - Immunosuppression (e.g., HIV+) can ↑ risk
    - Histology: epidermal hyperplasia, koilocytosis (should be seen in stratum spinosum too), papillomatosis (less severe and more rounded than in common warts), and parakeratosis
    - Treatments: destructive (cryotherapy, tricyclic antidepressants [higher concentrations], electrosurgery, scissors/shave removal, laser [CO_2]/PDT, and podophyllotoxin/podophyllin), immunomodulatory/antiviral (imiquimod, sinecatechins, intralesional immunotherapy, and cidofovir gel/intralesional)
    - **HPV vaccines:** contain L1 major capsid protein (self-assembles into virus-like particles → allow for development of immunity without any harm because they do not contain DNA)
      - Three types: **quadrivalent** (Gardasil; HPV-6, -11, -16, and -18), **bivalent** (Cervarix; HPV-16 and -18), and 9-valent (Gardasil 9; HPV-6, -11, -16, -18, -31, -33, -45, -52, and -58)
      - Best to use before sexually active—FDA-approved for females and males ≥9 years old
  - Bowenoid papulosis: multiple **brown papules**/smooth plaques on genitals/perineum/perianal that are high-grade

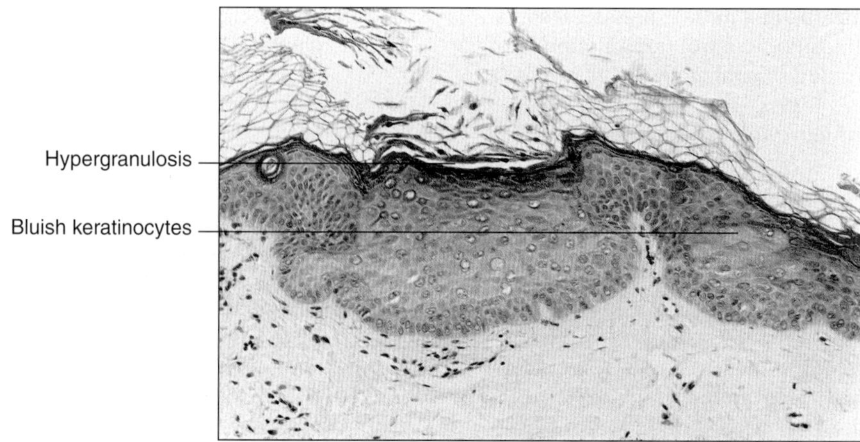

Fig. 5.1 Epidermodysplasia verruciformis histology—note the blue-gray cytoplasm of the keratinocytes. (From Rapini RP. Viral, rickettsial, and chlamydial diseases. In: Rapini RP, ed. *Practical Dermatopathology*. 3rd ed. Philadelphia: Elsevier; 2021:209–220.)

squamous intraepithelial lesions (HSIL) or squamous cell carcinoma *in situ* (SCCIS); **progression to invasive SCC is very rare**; a/w **high-risk HPV types**

- Erythroplasia of Queyrat: **red smooth plaque** on glabrous penis/vulva that is HSIL or SCCIS; increased risk of **progression to invasive SCC**; has **high-risk HPV types**
- Buschke-Lowenstein tumor (arises on genitals)
  - Part of a group of **verrucous carcinomas** (slow growing and locally destructive) that includes **oral florid papillomatosis** (HPV-6, -11; Risk factors: smoking, radiation, and inflammation), **epithelioma cuniculatum** of the sole (HPV-2, -11, and -16), and papillomatosis cutis carcinoides
  - **HPV-6 and HPV-11**
  - **Cauliflower-like tumors** that infiltrate deeply on external genitals and perianally
  - Histology: papillomatous acanthotic epidermis with bulbous ("**pushing**") **downward-extending** rete ridges; no cellular atypia/basement membrane penetration
  - Treatment: **excision** with clear margins
- Oral warts: soft pink-white papules on any oral surface; HPV-6 and -11; more common in HIV (HPV-7, -71, and -73)
  - Focal epithelial hyperplasia **(Heck's disease):** multiple flat wart-like papules on gingival/buccal/labial mucosa (South American children, South Africans, Greenlanders); **HPV-13 and HPV-32**
- Recurrent respiratory papillomatosis: papillomas of airways due to HPV-6 and HPV-11; #1 benign tumor of larynx; hoarseness + stridor + respiratory distress; childhood (2° to vertical transmission) and adulthood (2° to genital-to-oral contact) onsets; can → SCC, especially in smokers

II. Human herpesviruses

- A total of **eight distinct human herpesviruses (HHV-1 to HHV-8)** belong to the *Herpesviridae* family; all are characterized by an icosahedral capsid containing **linear double-stranded DNA**, surrounded by a glycoprotein-containing envelope; **replicate in host nucleus**
- Pathogenesis involves infection, latency, and reactivation

Herpes simplex virus (HHV-1/HSV-1 and HHV-2/HSV-2)

- Recurrent vesicular eruptions occurring in **orolabial (classically HSV-1)** and **genital (classically HSV-2)** regions
- Primary infection = first infection with virus (may → symptoms); latency = virus **lies dormant in sensory (dorsal root) ganglia**; reactivation/recurrence (may → symptoms)
- Genital herpes risk factors: 15 to 30 years old, ↑ sexual partners, lower income/education, **HIV(+)** (vice versa too—genital HSV-2 → ↑ HIV risk), and homosexuality
- **Pathogenesis**
  - Infection can occur without clinical lesions (and often does), and virus may still be shed
  - HSV-1 spread by saliva/secretions and HSV-2 spread by sexual contact → viral replication at skin/mucous membrane → retrograde axonal flow to dorsal root ganglia → latency and subsequent reactivation
  - HSV can evade host immune system (e.g., ↓ expression of CD1a by antigen-presenting cells [APCs], ↑ Langerhans cells apoptosis, ↓ TLR signaling, interferes w/ MHC class I/II); $CD8^+$ T cells and TLRs control infection
  - Reactivation triggers: **stress, UV** (UVB > UVA), fever, injury (e.g., **chemical peel or fractionated laser**), and immunosuppression
- **Clinical presentation**
  - Classic appearance: grouped/**clustered vesicles on a red base**
    - Can become pustules, erosions (with classic scalloped borders due to coalescence), and ulcers, ultimately crusting over and healing within 6 weeks
  - 1° infection: 3 to 7 days post infection → prodromal symptoms (tender lymphadenopathy [LAD], malaise, anorexia, and fever) → mucocutaneous lesions +/− pain/tenderness/burning/tingling just before lesions erupt
  - **Recurrent infections: generally milder than 1° infections,** have 24-hour prodrome of tingling/itch/burning
  - Orolabial infection
    - 1° HSV can be severe (gingivostomatitis in children; pharyngitis/mononucleosis-like in adults)
    - Mouth (esp. buccal mucosa and gingivae; favors anterior mouth unlike herpangina) and lips (recurrent lesions prefer **vermilion border**) affected
  - Genital herpes
    - 1° infection often asymptomatic, but can → **painful/tender** erosions on external genitalia, vagina, cervix, buttocks, and perineum (women) +/− LAD/dysuria (women mainly)
      - 1° worse in women—↑ % extragenital involvement, urinary retention, and aseptic meningitis (10%)
    - Recurrent—mildly symptomatic with few vesicles lasting ≈10 days; frequency of outbreaks usually decreases over time
  - Other HSV presentations
    - **Eczema herpeticum:** widespread, sometimes **severe** HSV infection in areas of **atopic dermatitis** (Fig. 5.2) +/− **systemic symptoms**, LAD, may be **life-threatening**; *Strep*/*Staph* superinfection can occur
      - ↑ With filaggrin mutations
      - **Usually HSV-1;** associated with Th2 shift in immune system
      - ↑ In patients with severe atopic dermatitis w/ **onset < 5 years old**, ↑ IgE levels, ↑ eosinophils, and food/environmental allergies
      - Have been a/w topical calcineurin inhibitors
    - Herpetic whitlow: infection of **digits (HSV-1 in children, HSV-2 in adults)** w/ vesiculation/pain/swelling; recurrence seen; bimodal peaks at <10 years old and 20 to 40 years old (digital-genital contact)

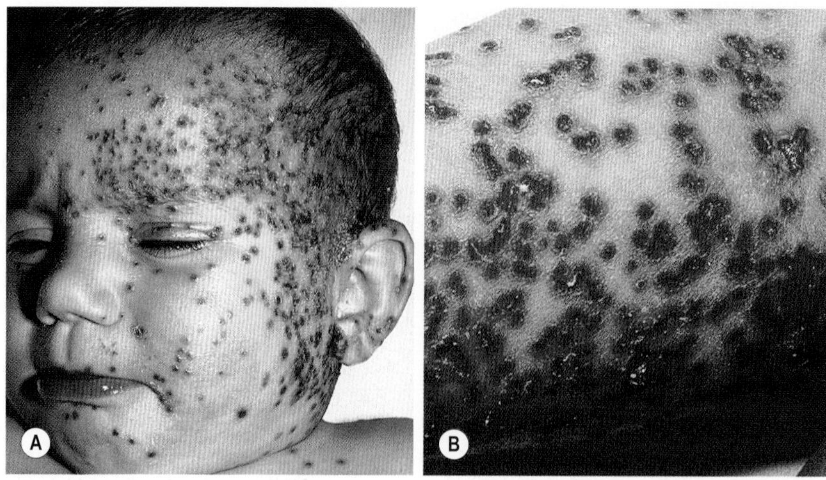

Fig. 5.2 Eczema herpeticum infection in a patient with atopic dermatitis. Numerous punched out vesicles and erosions involving the face **(A)** and extremities **(B)**. (From Cohen BA. Papulosquamous eruptions. In: *Pediatric Dermatology*. 4th ed. Philadelphia: Elsevier; 2013:68–103.)

- Herpes gladiatorum: HSV-1 infection 2° to athletic contact (classically **on lateral neck/side of face** and forearm)
- HSV folliculitis (herpetic sycosis): follicle-based vesicles/pustules in beard area (HSV-1) typically in HIV/immunocompromised
- Severe/chronic HSV: large, chronic ulcers may involve oral mucosa, respiratory/GI tract in immunocompromised
- Ocular HSV: keratoconjunctivitis w/ LAD and **branching dendritic corneal ulcer**; blindness may occur (HSV-2 in newborns; HSV-1 otherwise)
- **HSV encephalitis:** most common fatal viral encephalitis in the United States (>**70% die** without treatment); a/w TLR-3 or UNC-93B mutations; usually **HSV-1**; fever/altered mentation/strange behavior; **temporal lobe #1 site;** ↑ risk w/ **natalizumab**
- Neonatal HSV—see Chapter 4, Pediatric Dermatology

- **Diagnosis**
  - Viral culture (high specificity, low sensitivity), direct fluorescent antibody (DFA) assays, serology (Western blot = gold standard), **PCR (most sensitive/specific)**, and **Tzanck smear** (multinucleated epithelial giant cells; best when done on acute lesions)
  - Histology: intraepidermal vesicle + slate-gray enlarged keratinocytes (ballooning degeneration) which are **multinucleated with margination of chromatin**
    - +/– Cowdry A inclusions (eosinophilic inclusion bodies) within nucleus, epidermal necrosis, multicellular dermal infiltrate, and perivascular cuffing
- **Treatment**
  - Orolabial: oral penciclovir/valacyclovir, topical penciclovir/acyclovir ± hydrocortisone
  - Genital: oral acyclovir/famciclovir/valacyclovir
    - Use meds w/in first 48 hours → ↓ pain/healing time/viral shedding
    - Suppressive daily doses may be given in patients with >6 outbreaks of orolabial/genital HSV per year (also ↓ viral shedding)
  - May need **IV acyclovir in eczema herpeticum, neonatal HSV, or severe HSV in immunosuppressed**
  - **Foscarnet or cidofovir for acyclovir-resistant HSV** (more common in immunosuppressed); both are **nephrotoxic**
- Boards factoid: **HSV-1** is the most common cause of **erythema multiforme (EM) minor** (herpes-associated EM)

Varicella zoster virus (VZV; HHV-3)

- Causes varicella (chickenpox) and herpes zoster (shingles)
- Varicella is the 1° infection and herpes zoster is the reactivation of the latent infection (more common in **immunosuppressed and elderly** and can → death, e.g., via SIADH development in disseminated zoster patients)
- **Primary varicella incidence has decreased because of VZV vaccination**
- Herpes zoster occurs in 20% of adults, 50% of immunocompromised
  - Elderly at highest risk; Whites > non-Whites
  - Risk factors: physical/emotional stress, fever, trauma, immunosuppression, tofacitinib, proteasome inhibitors
- **Pathogenesis**
  - Transmitted via aerosolized droplets and direct contact with lesional fluid
    - Contagious from 1 to 2 days before lesion develops in varicella until all lesions crusted over
  - After primary varicella infection, **VZV travels to dorsal root ganglion and stays—dormant**—if reactivated later will replicate, travel down sensory nerve to the skin, and present as herpes zoster (zoster w/ 15% transmission rate vs. 80%–90% for varicella)
- **Clinical presentation**
  - <u>Primary varicella</u>
    - Primarily self-limited in healthy individuals
      - **More severe disease in adolescents and adults**
    - Prodromal symptoms: fever, fatigue, and myalgias
    - Cephalocaudal progression of classic lesions over 12 hours—"**dew drops on rose petal:**" vesicles on an erythematous base that become pustular, then crust over
      - Crops of lesions in **various stages** (Fig. 5.3)

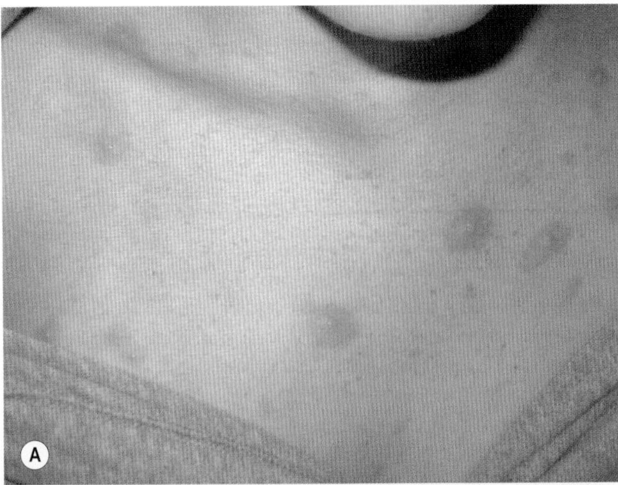

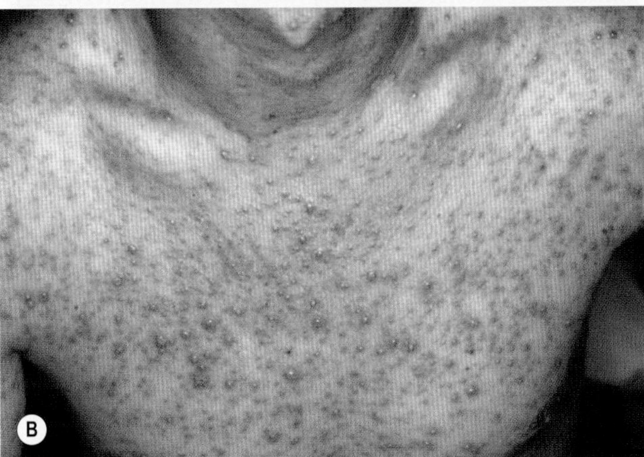

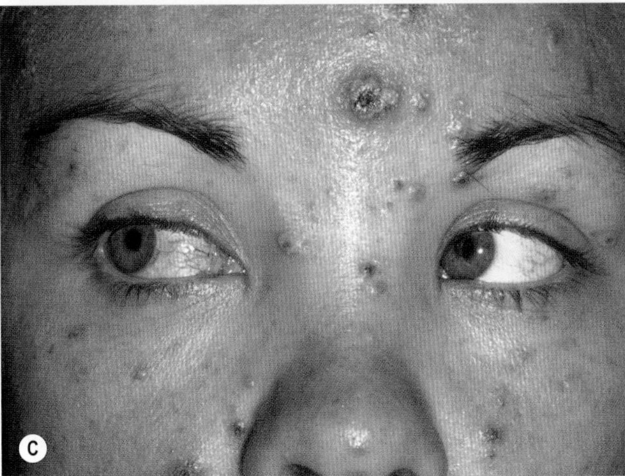

Fig. 5.3 (A) to **(C)** Varicella occurs in various stages including vesicles, pustules, and hemorrhagic crusts. (From James WD, Elston DM, McMahon PJ. Viral diseases. In: *Andrews' Diseases of the Skin Clinical Atlas*. Philadelphia: Elsevier; 2018:263–289.)

- Vaccine-associated varicella zoster may rarely develop after the vaccine is administered—represents mild case of chickenpox that may start at injection site
- Primary varicella in pregnancy
  - **Congenital varicella syndrome:** cutaneous scarring; **CNS (cortical atrophy, psychomotor retardation)/ocular/limb anomalies**; risk greatest if infected during **first 20 weeks of gestation**; exposed fetus may develop reactivation (herpes zoster) in childhood
  - **Neonatal varicella:** perinatal varicella transmission (within **5 days before delivery until 2 days post-delivery**); disease is severe (up to **30% mortality**) because of the lack of protective maternal antibodies

- Herpes zoster: **prodrome** (itch, tingling, hyperesthesia, and pain) → painful grouped vesicles on red base in a **dermatomal pattern**
  - **Trunk = most common location** (thoracic); face #2 (cranial; trigeminal nerve most common nerve involved); lumbar #3, and sacral #4
  - Postherpetic neuralgia (PHN): pain, potentially chronic, after lesions have cleared; **more common, severe, and chronic in elderly**
  - In HIV patients, lesions more persistent/thickened, postherpetic hyperhidrosis
  - Complications: granulomatous/pseudolymphomatous lesions, bacterial superinfection
  - Disseminated disease = dermatomal disease + **>20 lesions outside of dermatome** +/– visceral involvement; almost exclusively seen in **immunosuppressed** (AIDS; lymphoreticular malignancy, long-term immunosuppressive medication use, etc.); increased risk of **life-threatening pneumonitis, hepatitis, and encephalitis**
  - Vasculopathies (usually of CNS, but also peripheral arteries) are a worrisome delayed complication
  - **Dermatomal-specific herpes zoster findings:**
    - Ramsay Hunt syndrome: disease of **geniculate ganglion** of facial nerve (CN-VII) may → ear pain, vesicles on tympanic membrane/external auditory canal/anterior two thirds of the tongue; **ipsilateral facial nerve paralysis**, dry mouth/eyes, **anterior two thirds of the tongue taste loss**, and auditory (e.g., **deafness and tinnitus**) and equilibrium issues (vestibulocochlear nerve)
    - Aseptic meningitis and/or vasculopathy (encephalitis) if CN-V affected
    - Hearing impairment/deafness if CN-VIII affected
    - Eye involvement (**herpes zoster ophthalmicus**) if CN-II, CN-III, or CN-V affected
      - **Hutchinson's sign** (involvement of the side and **tip of nose**): indicates disease of the **external division of the V1 nasociliary branch**; may → to ocular involvement (e.g., keratitis, **uveitis**, acute retinal necrosis, and **visual loss**) half of the time
      - Uveitis is the most common form of ocular involvement; keratitis #2
    - **Bell's palsy if CN-VII affected**
    - Back dermatome complications
      - Cervical: motor neuropathy of arm (with possible atrophy) and diaphragm weakness
      - Thoracic: abdominal wall pseudohernia and weakness of muscles
      - Lumbar: motor neuropathy of leg (with possible atrophy)

- Possible urinary hesitancy/retention if sacral dermatomes involved
- Possible dilatation, constipation, pseudo-obstruction, reduced anal sphincter tone w/ thoracic/lumbar/sacral zoster

- **Diagnosis**: Tzanck smear, DFA, **PCR (sensitive, fast)**, viral culture (specific, not sensitive), serology (four-fold increase in IgG titer can retrospectively confirm prior infection), and skin biopsy (similar appearance to HSV, but immunohistochemistry can differentiate)
- **Treatment**
  - Primary varicella
    - Systemic acyclovir/valacyclovir **within 3 days of lesion onset** → ↓ severity/duration disease, though symptomatic treatment alone sufficient for healthy children
      - Oral acyclovir/valacyclovir approved for children, and acyclovir for adults (acyclovir)
      - IV acyclovir in immunocompromised patients
    - Postexposure prophylaxis
      - Varicella vaccine may be given within 72 to 120 hours of exposure in nonimmune, immunocompetent individuals >12 months
      - VZIg (Varicella zoster immunoglobulin) should be administered within 96 hours of exposure in immunocompromised, pregnant females, and neonates
        - ➔ Intravenous immunoglobulin (IVIG) may alternatively be administered
      - Oral acyclovir can be administered within 7 to 10 days of exposure
    - Primary prevention = varicella vaccination
      - Live attenuated virus recommended as a two-dose vaccination series; part of primary immunization series (≥99% effective)
      - Initial dose at 12 to 15 months, booster dose at 4 to 6 years
      - **Contraindicated in pregnancy and in immunocompromised patients**
    - Sequelae of primary varicella
      - **Reye's syndrome** (encephalitis + fatty liver) with concomitant **aspirin** use
      - **Pneumonia more common in older individuals;** high mortality if untreated
      - Encephalitis, cerebellar ataxia, glomerulonephritis, optic neuritis, keratitis, hepatitis
      - In immunocompromised, varicella can → death; extensive w/ hemorrhagic/purpuric lesions
  - Herpes zoster
    - **Antiviral treatment** with acyclovir (IV form in immunosuppressed), famciclovir, or valacyclovir is best given within 72 hours; prednisone helps with acute pain but has no effect on course or development of PHN
      - ↓ Duration of lesions/pain
      - ↓ Rate of PHN in patients >50 years old
      - Valacyclovir and famciclovir preferable to acyclovir
    - PHN: tricyclic antidepressants (e.g., nortriptyline), gabapentin, 8% capsaicin patch, pregabalin, opioid analgesics, EMLA cream, lidocaine patch
    - **Vaccines:** (1) **live attenuated vaccine → ≈50% ↓ in disease and 67% ↓ in PHN**, immunocompetent patients >60 years old; (2) **adjuvanted, non-live recombinant vaccine → >90% ↓ in disease and PHN**, patients >50 years old

Epstein-Barr virus (HHV-4)

- Causes **infectious mononucleosis** plus many other disorders (e.g., **oral hairy leukoplakia, hydroa vacciniforme, Gianotti-Crosti** syndrome, genital ulcers, and various hematologic disorders/malignancies (e.g., **Burkitt's lymphoma**, NK/T-cell lymphoma, post-transplant lymphoproliferative disorder, and **nasopharyngeal carcinoma**)
- Pathogenesis: transmission via saliva/blood → infects mucosal epithelial cells initially → **B cells via CR2/CD21 receptors** (where virus can lay dormant and evade immune system via production of EBNA-1 protein and latent membrane protein-2)
  - Incubation period of 1 to 2 months; symptoms develop with viral replication
  - **In patients with ↓ cell-mediated immunity, infected B cells may continue to replicate → lymphoproliferative disorders** (cell-mediated immunity appears to be more important than humoral, conferring immunity after first mononucleosis episode)
- Clinical features
  - Mononucleosis: typically **young adults** w/ **pharyngitis**, fever, and **cervical LAD**
    - **Splenomegaly** (and possible rupture) +/− hepatomegaly
    - ↑ LFTs in subset of patients
    - **Lymphocytosis** (up to 40% atypical lymphocytes)
    - May have indistinct polymorphous (e.g., urticarial, morbilliform) eruption in 10% occurring within first week of illness
      - Centrifugal spread
      - Petechial lesions on eyelid and hard/soft palate junction
      - +/− **Genital ulcers** (>1 cm, painful, esp. **adolescent females**)
    - **Ampicillin/amoxicillin → "hypersensitivity" skin reaction (itchy generalized morbilliform eruption → desquamation)**
  - Oral hairy leukoplakia: corrugated white plaque typically on lateral tongue, with strong **HIV association (CD4+ T cell <200/mm^3)**; more common in smokers
  - Gianotti-Crosti syndrome and papular-purpuric glove and socks syndrome (more common w/ parvovirus B19, though) may occur in setting of Epstein-Barr virus (EBV) infection
- Diagnosis:
  - Monospot test: nonspecific, confirms presence of **IgM heterophilic antibodies** which are often present in EBV infection and may persist for months after infection; 85% of older children/adults are positive during second week of infection, but Monospot is **often negative in younger children**
    - Positive heterophilic antibody (>1:40) and >10% atypical lymphocytes suggests acute infection

Table 5.1 Epstein-Barr Virus–Specific Serology Interpretation

	Viral Capsid Antigen (VCA)			
Status	**IgG**	**IgM**	**EA**	**EBNA**
No past infection	–	–	–	–
Acute IM	+	+	±	–
Convalescent IM	+	±	±	±
Past infection	+	–	Low + or –	+
Reactivated/chronic	++	±	++	±

From Paller AS, Mancini AJ. Exanthematous diseases of childhood. In: Hurwitz Clinical Pediatric Dermatology. *5th ed. Philadelphia: Elsevier; 2016:382–401.*

- EBV-specific antibodies: **higher sensitivity in younger children**; can be useful in determining current versus prior infection (Table 5.1)
  - Viral capsid antigen (VCA) IgM/IgG, EA (early antigen) IgG, and EBNA IgG
- CBC: lymphocytosis with atypical lymphocytes and thrombocytopenia
- Transaminitis may be present
- PCR to EBV DNA may be performed from tissue or blood; RT-PCR available from lymphoid cells; *in situ* hybridization for EBER can detect EBV in tissue, including skin

- Treatment:
  - Supportive care
  - Oral corticosteroids may be considered for severe cases of tonsillitis
  - **Avoid contact sports** until splenomegaly resolves (risk for **splenic rupture**)
  - Rare sequelae: **upper airway obstruction**, aseptic meningitis, meningoencephalopathy, myocarditis, pericarditis, and renal failure

Cytomegalovirus (HHV-5)

- Transmitted via body fluids, fomites, vertical transmission, **transplanted organs**, and hematopoietic stem cells
- Infects leukocytes → dissemination → various organs → latency
  - Most infections are **asymptomatic in healthy adults;** can cause **severe disease** *in utero* **(TORCH**; discussed in Chapter 4, Pediatric Dermatology) or in **immunosuppressed/transplant patients (CMV retinitis/blindness**, meningoencephalitis, pneumonitis, GI ulcers)
  - After the 1° infection, **very low risk of reactivation, except for immunocompromised** patients
- Cutaneous features in adults
  - **Mononucleosis-like presentation** (e.g., sore throat, fever, LAD, and hepatosplenomegaly) may be associated with nonspecific exanthem (e.g., morbilliform); Guillain-Barré syndrome = rare complication
    - If ampicillin given → eruption (as in infectious mononucleosis)
  - **Recalcitrant ulcers of perineum or leg in HIV** patients; these patients may also get verrucous plaques, vesicles, and/or nodules
- Diagnosis via human fibroblast culture (gold standard), but faster methods include shell vial assay, PCR, and serologic testing; **histology of ulcers may show enlargement** (cytomegaly) **of endothelial cells with pathognomonic "owl's eye"** (intranuclear) **inclusions**
- **Ganciclovir** (IV) and valganciclovir (oral) are first-line

HHV-6 (Roseola infantum, exanthem subitum, sixth disease)

- One of the most common viral exanthems of childhood (see Chapter 4, Pediatric Dermatology); up to 15% of infants may develop febrile seizures, but otherwise follows a self-limited course in healthy patients
  - 95% of patients are between 6 months and 3 years of age
- Virus remains latent in CD4+ T cells for life → reactivation has been a/w **pityriasis rosea** (along with HHV-7), Rosai-Dorfman, and **DRESS syndrome** (along with EBV, CMV, and HHV-7)

HHV-7

- Lymphotropic virus that shares significant homology with HHV-6 and may participate in coinfection w/ HHV-6
- Although not definitively causative of any disease, it has been a/w **pityriasis rosea** (along with HHV-6), and a subset of exanthem subitum cases (coinfection with HHV-6; lesions = later, lighter colored)

HHV-8

- Etiologic factor for **Kaposi sarcoma (KS)**—see Chapter 6, Neoplastic Dermatology
- Also associated with **multicentric Castleman disease**, **primary effusion lymphoma**, and paraneoplastic pemphigus

III. Other viruses not covered elsewhere

Poxviruses

- Smallpox (Variola virus; genus = Orthopox)
  - Infection **via respiratory tract** → 7 to 17 days incubation period → 1 to 4 days prodromal period (fever, headache, prostration, myalgias, and malaise) → **centrifugal (face/arms/legs > trunk)** vesiculopustular eruption and may involve hands/feet (lesions in any given anatomic region will be in **same stage**) w/ lethargic/"toxic" appearance
    - Rash: macule → papule → vesicle → **pustules; typically scarring; lesions spread over 1 to 2 weeks**
    - Lesions **first appear on palms/soles**
    - Patients infectious from eruption onset till 7 to 10 days post-eruption
    - Oral lesions (tongue, mouth, and oropharynx) often appear before cutaneous **lesions** by 1 day
  - Complications: blindness, **encephalitis**, toxemia, hypotension, pneumonitis, arthritis, and osteitis
  - Diagnosis: PCR, viral culture
  - Treatment: supportive; vaccine as prophylaxis
- Vaccinia (Vaccinia virus; genus = Orthopox): used for **live smallpox vaccine**
  - SEs: LAD, ocular vaccinia, generalized vaccinia, single crusted papule at vaccination site, vesiculopustular/

urticarial/morbilliform eruption, **eczema vaccinatum** (patients with **atopic dermatitis**, Darier, or Hailey-Hailey disease), EM/SJS, postvaccinial CNS disease, and progressive vaccinia (immunosuppressed patients; can → death)

- Monkeypox (Monkeypox virus; genus = Orthopox): Central/Western Africa, though US outbreak from **prairie dogs**
  - Can spread via cutaneous inoculation or inhalation (hosts = monkeys, rodents, humans)
  - Prodrome (fever/sweating/chills) → smallpox-like lesions, but usually milder/fewer
    - Lesions may present in **various stages** and favor face and extremities (esp. **palms/soles**), with **centrifugal spread**; may scar
    - May have systemic symptoms (respiratory, fever, and LAD in 67%)
  - Most recent worlwide outbreak primarily in MSM (98%) with over half of lesions on genitals/perianal region; fever, LAD and myalgia were most common systemic features; JYNNEOS and ACAM2000 vaccines can be used to prevent smallpox and monkeypox (both are live vaccines; ACAM2000 should not be given to those with exfoliative skin conditions/eczema, immunosuppression, or HIV infection, and may cause myocarditis and pericarditis)
- Cowpox (Cowpox virus; genus = Orthopox): Europe and Asia
  - Spread via cutaneous contact (hands and face) with infected animal (**usually cats**)
    - Incubates 7 days → painful red papule at contact site → vesicular → pustular → hemorrhagic → ulcer w/ eschar → large scars
    - Lesions usually solitary and occur on hands/fingers and face
    - Can have LAD and fever
- Orf (ecthyma contagiosum; Orf virus; genus = Parapox): as a result of contact with infected animals (**sheep, goats, or reindeer**; usually on udders/perioral areas of ewes)
  - Develop one to few lesions at contact site (usually **hands**)
  - Risk factors: certain jobs (**shepherds, butchers, and veterinarians**)
  - **Six lesion stages:** maculopapular (umbilicated) → targetoid → acute (weeping nodule) → regenerative (nodule w/ thin crust and black dots) → papillomatous → regressive (crust overlying resolving lesion); self-resolves
  - Diagnosis: histology (intracytoplasic eosinophilic inclusion bodies, keratinocyte vacuolization, epidermal necrosis, finger-like acanthosis) or PCR
- Milker's nodules ("Pseudocowpox;" Paravaccinia virus; genus = Parapox): papules at the site of contact (**usually muzzles of calves and teats of cows**)
  - Distal upper extremities usually with single lesion(s), which look like orf
  - Most common in farmers/ranchers, veterinarians, and butchers
  - Diagnosis: histology or PCR
- Molluscum contagiosum (Molluscum contagiosum virus [MCV]; genus = Molluscipox)
  - Common in **school-aged children**; may be sexually transmitted in adolescents/adults
  - Cause by molluscipox infection (**MCV-I and MCV-II**)
  - Infection spread by contact with infected skin or fomites, or possibly via water
  - Prototypical lesion is an **umbilicated, pink, and pearly papule**
    - Most common distribution: intertriginous areas, torso, lower extremities, and buttocks
    - Lesions can become widespread in patients with impaired skin barrier (atopic dermatitis [molluscum dermatitis] or ichthyosis) or immunodeficiency (chemotherapy-induced or HIV; may also see **giant molluscum** lesions)
  - Histology: **molluscum bodies** within dermis
  - Treatments: cryotherapy, cantharidin, extraction/curettage, cimetidine, candida antigen immunotherapy, topical retinoids, cidofovir, berdazimer gel, and imiquimod
  - **Self-limited** with resolution after weeks to years of infection

Chikungunya virus

- Single-stranded (+) sense RNA virus belonging to Togaviridae family
- Transmitted by *Aedes* (***Aedes aegypti*** > *Aedes albopictus*) mosquitoes; endemic to Africa/India/Southeast Asia
- Symptoms: **high fever, marked joint symptoms**, ("Chikungunya" is an African word for "crooked/bent joints") neuropathic acral findings, and headache/nausea/vomiting
- Cutaneous presentation: → **morbilliform eruption** (50%–75% of patients), mucosal aphthous-like **ulcers**, **postinflammatory pigmentation** of face/extremities, acral/facial edema, bullous eruptions in infants, and ecchymoses

Zika virus

- Icosahedral, single-stranded **RNA virus** within the **Flaviviridae** family
  - Most commonly transmitted via ***A. aegypti*** and *A. albopictus* mosquitos; also transmitted via blood transfusions, **sexual contact**, and **vertically (from mother to fetus)** → **microcephaly** and other fetal anomalies
- Clinical features:
  - Incubation period of 3 to 12 days → 20% develop mild symptoms lasting up to 1 to 2 weeks
    - Systemic symptoms: fever, myalgia, arthralgia, headache, and conjunctivitis; possibly a/w Guillain-Barré syndrome
    - Mucocutaneous symptoms:
      - **Nonspecific**, diffuse **morbilliform/scarlatiniform eruption** (begins 3–12 days after initial infection w/ **cephalocaudal** progression) → rash completely resolves within 1 week, sometimes with desquamation
      - Mild hemorrhagic manifestations (petechiae and bleeding gums)
- Diagnosis:
  - Confirmed with **RT-PCR** or **ELISA** during initial phase (first 7 days) of infection
    - Later in disease course, may check Zika-specific IgM antibodies and plaque reduction neutralization tests

- Treatment:
  - Currently no vaccine exists and no specific anti-viral therapies; avoid aspirin and non-steroidal anti-inflammatory drugs (NSAIDs; can worsen hemorrhagic sequelae)
  - **Prevention is critical; pregnant women should avoid travel to Zika-endemic areas!**

Dengue virus

- Arbovirus in the **Flaviviridae** family; transmitted by *A.* ***aegypti*** mosquitoes
- Wide range of clinical presentations:
  - Asymptomatic infection: **most common** presentation (75% of cases)
  - Classic Dengue fever: fever, diffuse **morbilliform/ scarlatiniform rash (50% of cases;** classically **white islands** of sparing **in sea of red** widespread erythema), **severe headache/myalgia/arthralgia**, retroorbital pain, +/− **petechial mucosal lesions**, epistaxis and gingival bleeding (thrombocytopenia due to non-neutralizing, fucosylated IgG1 antibodies that bind **activating Fc receptor FcγRIIIA**)
  - Dengue hemorrhagic fever: **more severe** than classic Dengue fever; most likely to develop when a patient **previously infected with one serotype is subsequently infected with a different viral serotype**
    - Most common in **children** <15 years
    - Symptoms: lethargy/weakness, vomiting, facial flushing, and circumoral cyanosis
- Diagnosis:
  - Confirmed with **RT-PCR** or **ELISA** during initial/acute phase of disease, NSI antigen detection, or IgM serologies later in disease course
- Treatment: supportive; avoid aspirin and NSAIDs (can worsen hemorrhagic sequelae)

Viral hepatitides (Table 5.2)

Viral-associated trichodysplasia of immunosuppression

- Occurs in **solid organ transplant patients** or leukemia/ lymphoma patients on chemotherapy
- **Polyomavirus** → collections of pink/flesh-colored spiny papules on face (esp. **mid face**), eyebrow/eyelash loss, thickening of facial skin

Table 5.2 Cutaneous Manifestations of Hepatitis B and/or C Infection

Small vessel vasculitis (B, C)	**Necrolytic acral erythema (C)**
Cryoglobulinemic vasculitis (C > B)	Porphyria cutanea tarda (B, C)
Urticarial vasculitis (B, C)	Pruritus (B, C)
Polyarteritis nodosa (B (classic) > C)	**Lichen planus**—particularly erosive oral disease (C)
Livedo reticularis (C)	
Serum sickness-like reaction (B, C)	**Sarcoidosis (with interferon and/or ribavirin therapy; C > B)**
Urticaria (B, C)	
Gianotti–Crosti syndrome (B > C)	
	Erythema multiforme (B, C)
	Erythema nodosum (B > C)

From Mancini AJ, Shani-Adir A, Sidbury R. Other viral diseases. In: Bolognia JL, Schaffer JV, Cerroni L, eds. Dermatology. *4th ed. Philadelphia: Elsevier; 2018:1425–1446.*

- Histology: **eosinophilic keratinocytes w/trichohyalin granules w/ in dilated anagen follicles**
- Decreasing immunosuppressive agents can help, as can topical cidofovir and oral ganciclovir

COVID-19

- Caused by severe acute respiratory syndrome coronavirus 2 (SARS-CoV-2)
- Characterized by fever/chills, shortness of breath/difficulty breathing, cough, anosmia, dysgeusia, fatigue/muscle aches, diarrhea/nausea/vomiting; can progress to severe morbidity and death through multiorgan failure, kidney failure, respiratory failure/acute respiratory distress syndrome, septic shock, brain swelling, clotting/ thrombosis/embolism
- Cutaneous manifestations typically occur after classic COVID-19 symptoms
- Various cutaneous manifestations (in decreasing order of incidence): morbilliform, pernio-like (**long duration**), urticarial, macular erythema, vesicular, papulosquamous, **retiform purpura**
- Pernio-like lesions seen in young/healthy patients w/ mild disease, while retiform purpura seen in severe disease (acral ischemia, livedo racemosa, EM-like lesions, and petechiae/purpura may also be seen in severe disease)

5.2 HIV/AIDS DERMATOLOGY

HIV

- Enveloped, single-stranded RNA lentiviruses in retroviridae family (HIV-1 > HIV-2 in causing AIDS)
  - AIDS = CD4+ T cells < 200/mm^3 + AIDS-defining condition
- Gp120 and gp41 on viral envelope interact with CD4 and CCR5/CXCR4 on CD4+ T cells (CXCR5 is a fusion cofactor) → fusion/internalization of virus (Fig. 5.4)
- First-line treatment: dual nucleoside reverse transcriptase inhibitors (NRTIs) + integrase inhibitor; second-line treatment: dual NRTIs + non-nucleoside reverse transcriptase inhibitor (NNRTI) or protease inhibitor (PI)

HIV-associated inflammatory dermatoses

- Acute exanthem of primary HIV infection
  - ≤50% of newly infected patients; presents in conjunction with classic **mononucleosis-like syndrome** of primary HIV infection, within 6 weeks of transmission
  - Rash usually generalized, asymptomatic, morbilliform, lasting ≈5 days
- Eosinophilic folliculitis
  - Characterized by eosinophil-rich inflammatory infiltrate in or around hair follicles
  - **Intensely pruritic**, erythematous, and follicular-based **papules** located on the upper trunk, face, neck, and scalp
- Aphthous stomatitis
  - Lesions most often occur on mobile, nonkeratinized oral mucosal surfaces, but esophageal and anogenital aphthae are not uncommon in HIV patients

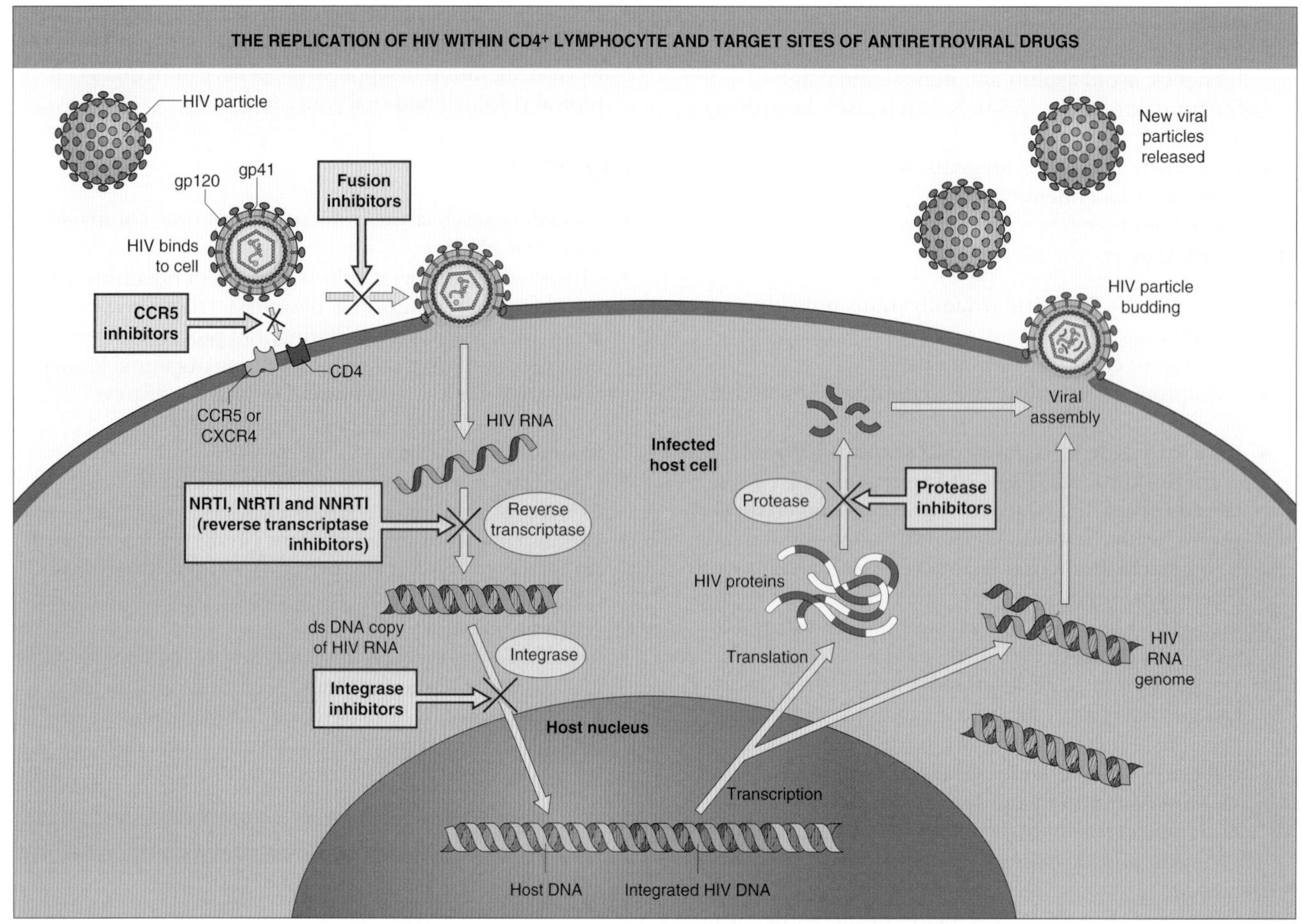

Fig. 5.4 Replication of HIV within CD4+ lymphocyte and target sites of antiretroviral drugs. *CCR5*, CC-chemokine receptor 5; *NNRTI*, non-nucleoside reverse transcriptase inhibitor; *NRTI*, nucleoside reverse transcriptase inhibitor; *NtRTI*, nucleotide reverse transcriptase inhibitor. Information on FDA-approved antiretroviral drugs is available at: https://aidsinfo.nih.gov/understanding-hiv-aids/fact-sheets/21/58/fda-approved-hiv-medicines. (From Chan RKW, Chio MTW, Koh HY. Cutaneous manifestations of HIV infection. In: Bolognia JL, Schaffer JV, Cerroni L, eds. *Dermatology*. 4th ed. Philadelphia: Elsevier; 2018:1364–1382.)

- Treatments: topical anesthetics, potent topical steroids, intralesional steroids, systemic corticosteroids, and thalidomide (severe or refractory disease)
- Erythema elevatum diutinum
  - In HIV, often associated with β-hemolytic strep infection
  - **Dapsone is treatment of choice**
  - Oral antibiotics indicated for streptococcus-associated cases
- Pruritic papular eruption
  - Intensely pruritic condition seen in advanced HIV in developing world
  - May represent aberrant immunologic response to insect bites or reactivation of prior bites
  - Patients present with extensive, non-follicular skin-colored to hyperpigmented, excoriated papules
- HIV photodermatitis
  - Group of photodistributed rashes with multiple clinical manifestations including **lichenoid** (most common), eczematous, hyperpigmented, and vitiliginous
  - Exposure to certain photosensitizing medications (e.g., **trimethoprim-sulfamethoxazole [TMP-SMX]** and NSAIDs) can increase risk
  - Treatment difficult; strict photoprotection and topical steroids; thalidomide in refractory cases
  - **Chronic actinic dermatitis** (CD4+ < 200/mm^3) and **porphyria cutanea tarda** more common in HIV
- Seborrheic dermatitis more common in HIV
- Type VI (HIV-associated) pityriasis rubra pilaris (see Chapter 3)

HIV-associated infectious dermatoses

- Oral hairy leukoplakia (see EBV section)
- HSV
  - Can present in the anogenital region as exophytic, **verrucous lesions**, termed herpes vegetans, or **hypertrophic HSV**
    - Herpes vegetans is **often acyclovir-resistant** and intralesional cidofovir can be used
  - Large, longstanding, chronic ulcerative lesions refractory to treatment can be seen with low CD4+ (typically perianal, genitals, tongue but weird sites like oropharynx/esophagus too)
- Herpes zoster
  - HIV testing indicated for patients <50 years presenting with herpes zoster
  - Atypical presentations, such as disseminated zoster, multidermatomal zoster, systemic complications

(e.g., pneumonitis), chronic lesions/verrucous plaques
  - Give VZV Ig ≤10 days postexposure
- HPV
  - Large, extensive, and/or treatment-resistant HPV-induced lesions, with higher rate of malignant transformation (anal/penile/cervical cancer, anal intraepithelial neoplasia, cervical intraepithelial neoplasia, SCCIS)
  - Unusual presentations of HPV infection can be observed (e.g., acquired EV-like lesions a/w HPV types 5 and 8)
- Bacillary angiomatosis (see Bartonella section in 5.3 Bacterial Infections)
- Molluscum contagiosum
  - Lesions commonly seen on face lack classic dome shape and central umbilication; may be >1 cm (**giant molluscum**)
  - Treatment: destructive therapies (e.g., curettage, cryotherapy, and trichloroacetic acid)
  - Topical/intravenous cidofovir useful in refractory cases
- CMV
  - Retinitis, esophagitis, colitis, ulcers of oral and GI mucosa if CD4+ <100/mm^3
  - Typically colonizes areas of HSV ulceration in patients with CD4+ <50 cells/mm^3 and treating HSV usually → clearance of CMV, but CMV can also cause ulceration in HIV patients
- Proximal white subungual onychomycosis and candidiasis (most common fungal disease in HIV; oropharyngeal may be first HIV manifestation)
- Disseminated mycoses
  - Disseminated infection caused by *Cryptococcus neoformans, Coccidioides immitus, Histoplasma capsulatum,* or *Penicillium marneffei* should be considered in AIDS patients presenting with **umbilicated, molluscum-like lesions**
- Crusted (Norwegian) scabies and exaggerated arthropod bite reactions

HIV and cutaneous malignancies

- Basal cell carcinoma (BCC), SCC, and melanoma
  - HIV patients at ↑ risk of developing NMSCs and melanoma (BCC > SCC > melanoma)
  - HIV infection → ↑ risk of post-treatment recurrence and metastasis in SCC
  - In addition to photo-induced SCCs, also ↑ risk of developing HPV-induced intraepithelial neoplasia and SCCs, most commonly of anogenital skin
- Kaposi sarcoma
  - Involvement of oral mucosa, face, and genitals more common in HIV-associated KS
  - May even be seen in patients with longstanding/ well-controlled HIV and can be aggressive without treatment
  - Treatment options for limited/localized disease: initiation or resumption of antiretrovirals, intralesional chemotherapy (e.g., vinblastine), radiation, cryotherapy, excision, and topical retinoids (e.g., alitretinoin)
  - Treatment for extensive cutaneous disease, or disease involving lymph nodes or viscera: initiation or resumption of antiretrovirals in addition to systemic chemotherapy (doxorubicin most common)
- Lymphomas
  - Typically **B-cell**, intermediate/high-grade, **non-Hodgkin lymphoma** (EBV frequently associated)
  - Pink/purple papules/nodules w/ possible CNS/GI involvement

HIV treatment-associated dermatoses

- Immune reconstitution inflammatory syndrome (IRIS)
  - Pathologic **inflammatory response** that develops 2 weeks to 3 months after initiation of antiretroviral therapy, particularly if CD4+ <50/mm^3, in the **setting of decreasing viral load** and immunologic improvement
  - Cutaneous manifestations of IRIS: development or worsening of infectious entities, neoplastic conditions, and inflammatory dermatoses (summarized in Tables 5.3 and 5.4)
  - Cutaneous IRIS events rarely require discontinuation of antiretroviral therapy
- Antiretroviral-associated lipodystrophy
  - Caused by PIs, NRTIs, and to lesser extent, NNRTIs

Table 5.3 Correlation of CD4+Cell Count With Specific HIV-Associated Disorders

System[a]	>500 CD4+ Cells/mm^3	<500 CD4+ Cells/mm^3	<250 CD4+ Cells/mm^3	<50 CD4+ Cells/mm^3
Dermatologic	• Acute retroviral syndrome • Oral hairy leukoplakia • Vaginal candidiasis • Seborrheic dermatitis	• Oropharyngeal candidiasis (thrush) • Herpes zoster • Psoriasis, severe or refractory • Eruptive atypical melanocytic nevi and melanoma • Kaposi sarcoma	• Eosinophilic folliculitis • Seborrheic dermatitis, refractory • Mollusca, extensive • Bacillary angiomatosis • Miliary/extrapulmonary tuberculosis • Herpes simplex virus infection, disseminated • Cryptococcosis, disseminated • Histoplasmosis, disseminated • Coccidioidomycosis, disseminated • Botryomycosis • Non-Hodgkin lymphoma	• Large, non-healing mucocutaneous herpes simplex virus infections (e.g., perianal) • Papular pruritic eruption • Giant mollusca • Perianal ulcers due to cytomegalovirus • Aspergillosis • Acquired ichthyosis • *Mycobacterium avium* complex infections • Major aphthae
Respiratory	Bacterial pneumonia and sinusitis	• Pneumococcal pneumonia • Pulmonary tuberculosis • Lymphocytic interstitial pneumonia (pediatric)	*Pneumocystis jiroveci* pneumonia (PCP)	*Pseudomonas* spp. pneumonia

Continued

Table 5.3 Correlation of CD4+Cell Count With Specific HIV-Associated Disorders—cont'd

System[a]	>500 CD4+ Cells/mm^3	<500 CD4+ Cells/mm^3	<250 CD4+ Cells/mm^3	<50 CD4+ Cells/mm^3
Nervous	• Aseptic meningitis • Guillain–Barré syndrome	Mononeuritis multiplex	• HIV-associated dementia • Cerebral toxoplasmosis • Peripheral neuropathy • Progressive multifocal leukoencephalopathy	Primary CNS lymphoma
Hematologic	Persistent generalized lymphadenopathy	• Anemia • Idiopathic thrombocytopenic purpura	Non-Hodgkin lymphoma	
Other	Myopathy	• Cryptosporidiosis • Cervical/anal intraepithelial neoplasia • Cervical cancer • Anal cancer	• Esophageal candidiasis • Wasting • Microsporidiosis • Vacuolar myelopathy • Cardiomyopathy	• Cryptosporidiosis, refractory • Cytomegalovirus retinitis, extraocular systemic cytomegalovirus infection

[a]*Diseases occur with increasing frequency and severity at lower CD4+ cell counts.*

From Chan RKW, Chio MTW, Koh HY. Cutaneous manifestations of HIV infection. In: Bolognia JL, Schaffer JV, Cerroni L, eds. Dermatology. *4th ed. Philadelphia: Elsevier; 2018:1364–1382.*

Table 5.4 Common Cutaneous IRIS Events

Infectious	Inflammatory	Neoplastic
HSV-1 and HSV-2	Eosinophilic folliculitis	Kaposi sarcoma
VZV (Herpes-zoster)	Acne vulgaris	
HPV	Acne rosacea	
CMV	Seborrheic dermatitis	
Molluscum contagiosum	Foreign-body reactions	
Mycobacteria (leprosy, tuberculosis, and atypical mycobacteria)		
Disseminated fungal (*Cryptococcus* and histoplasmosis)		
Leishmaniasis		

CMV, *Cytomegalovirus;* HPV, *human papillomavirus;* HSV, *herpes simplex virus;* IRIS, *immune reconstitution inflammatory syndrome;* VZV, *varicella zoster virus.*

- Can manifest as lipoatrophy (loss of fat in face, extremities, and buttocks) or lipohypertrophy (accumulation of fat in upper back, neck, or abdomen)
- Typically seen ≤2 years of starting therapy
- Associated with **metabolic abnormalities** (e.g., hyperlipidemia and insulin resistance)
- **Poly-L-lactic acid** and **calcium hydroxylapatite** approved for treatment of antiretroviral-associated facial lipoatrophy and tesamorelin approved for abdominal obesity

• Pigmentary alteration
- **Zidovudine** can cause nail and mucocutaneous hyperpigmentation (longitudinal streaks or diffuse hyperpigmentation of fingernails/toenails); of note, zidovudine can also cause **trichomegaly**

• Morbilliform eruptions
- **NRTIs** and TMP-SMX (#1) are common cause of morbilliform eruptions
- Typically mild and variably symptomatic—pruritus most common complaint
- In most cases, treatment with inciting agent can be continued—rash will resolve

• Drug-induced hypersensitivity syndrome (DIHS/DRESS)
- **Abacavir** is the most common antiretroviral to cause DIHS/DRESS (up to 8% patients; can be **fatal**)
- HLA-B*5701 linked with abacavir hypersensitivity syndrome—screen patients before initiating therapy
- Other common causes of DIHS/DRESS in HIV patients: efavirenz, nevirapine, **TMP-SMX,** and **dapsone**

• Retinoid-like effects
- Associated with PIs, particularly **indinavir**
- Clinical manifestations: chronic paronychia, **periungual pyogenic granulomas**, alopecia, cheilitis, and xerosis

• Injection-site reactions
- Reported in most patients treated with enfuvirtide
- SEs: erythema, ecchymosis, induration, nodules, cysts, and localized sclerosis

5.3 BACTERIAL INFECTIONS

I. Gram-positive skin infections

Staphylococcal skin infections

• Impetigo
- **Most common bacterial infection in children**
- 35% of population carry *Staphylococcus aureus* (**anterior nares** > perineum > axilla, toe webs) → ↑ risk impetigo
- Nonbullous impetigo (70%): ***S. aureus*** (>*Streptococcus pyogenes*); **children** > adults
  - Most commonly see erosion + **"honey-colored" crust**; affects **traumatized, abraded, or eczematous skin**; most commonly **face** (perioral/perinasal); self-resolves in 2 weeks
  - Histology: neutrophilic microvesiculopustules, spongiosis, and Gram-positive cocci
- Bullous impetigo (30%): **phage group II (types 55 and 71)** *S. aureus* → produce **exfoliatoxins A and B** (ETA and ETB) → cleaves **desmoglein 1 → subcorneal/intragranular acantholysis**
  - Children > adults; presents with (p/w) **flaccid bullae** + erosions w/ **collarette of scale**, minimal

surrounding erythema; **affects intact skin,** has more **generalized** distribution
  - Histology: **subcorneal/intragranular acantholysis, neutrophils** in blister cavity, Gram-positive cocci
- Treatment:
  - Localized: **topical** mupirocin, retapamulin, or fusidic acid
  - Widespread: **oral** β-lactamase–resistant PCN or first-generation cephalosporin (CSN; clindamycin or clarithromycin if PCN-allergic)
- **Decolonization**: used for patients w/ recurrent infections; topical mupirocin BID to nares for 7 to 10 days +/– skin decolonization w/ mupirocin ointment, bleach baths or chlorhexidine washes
- **Other high-yield facts**
  - Nonbullous impetigo caused by ***S. pyogenes*** serotypes 1, 4, 12, 25, and 49 → **poststreptococcal glomerulonephritis** in 5%; risk not altered by antibiotics
  - **No risk of rheumatic fever** from streptococcal impetigo (vs. streptococcal pharyngitis)
  - **Bullous impetigo + renal insufficiency** or immunodeficiency → exfoliatoxin may disseminate → **staphylococcal scalded skin syndrome (SSSS)**
  - ETA is chromosomally encoded; ETB is plasmid encoded
  - Bullous impetigo and pemphigus foliaceus have nearly identical histology → need DIF and culture (positive culture in bullous impetigo)

- Bacterial folliculitis
  - ***S. aureus* folliculitis**: most common form; most commonly on **face** (beard area typically)
    - Superficial form (Bockhart's impetigo): small papulopustules on erythematous background
    - Deep form ("**sycosis barbae**"): large red papulopustules +/– plaques with small pustules
  - **Gram-negative folliculitis**: seen in **acne** patients on **long-term antibiotics**
  - **Pseudomonal folliculitis**: a/w poorly chlorinated **hot tubs**/whirlpools
  - Treatment:
    - Superficial staph folliculitis: chlorhexidine washes, topical mupirocin/clindamycin
    - Widespread staph folliculitis: β-lactamase–resistant PCN or first-generation CSN, tetracyclines
    - Gram-negative folliculitis: **isotretinoin**
    - Pseudomonal folliculitis: **self-resolves**; ciprofloxacin if severe
    - Decolonization of nares/skin helpful if recurrent
- Abscesses, furuncles, and carbuncles
  - All are walled off collections of pus, most commonly from ***S. aureus*** (often methicillin-resistant *S. aureus* **[MRSA]**); may be complicated by surrounding **cellulitis/phlebitis**
  - Abscess: inflamed and fluctuant nodule; arises on **any site**
  - Furuncle: only occurs in a/w hair follicles/on **hair-bearing sites** ("FURuncle = FURry sites"); **head/neck (#1 site)** > intertriginous zones, thighs, other sites of friction
  - Carbuncle: collection of furuncles, often **deeper** w/ **multiple draining sinuses**; most often affects thick skin of **posterior neck, back, and thighs**; systemic symptoms typically present
  - Treatment:
    - Simple abscesses/furuncles: warm compresses
    - Larger/deeper lesions: incision and drainage (I&D)
    - Complicated (sensitive locations, extensive disease, a/w cellulitis/phlebitis, systemic symptoms, recalcitrant, and immunosuppressed): **doxycycline, TMP-SMX**, and **clindamycin** (depending on local resistance patterns)
    - **Culture necessary since frequently due to MRSA**
    - Decolonization of nares/skin helpful if recurrent
- MRSA
  - #1 cause of purulent infections in emergency department; usually p/w **furunculosis**; may be a/w cellulitis, and necrotic plaques
  - Resistance: specific ***mecA* genes** (from SCC*mec* types I–VI, mobile genetic elements) → encodes mutated penicillin-binding protein, **PBP2a** → ↓ affinity for β-lactams
  - Possible resistance to macrolides (active drug efflux pump [*msrA/msrB* gene], inactivating enzymes, cross-resistance to clindamycin by alteration of bacterial ribosome by erythromycin ribosomal methylase [*erm* genes])
  - Community-associated MRSA (CA-MRSA; majority) also has Panton-Valentine leukocidin (**PVL**) virulence factor; a/w **increased virulence**, leading to more severe necrosis of skin and other tissues
  - CA-MRSA susceptible to more antibiotics than hospital-associated MRSA
  - Treatment:
    - Minor infection: **TMP-SMX**, **minocycline/doxycycline**, or **clindamycin**
    - Severe infection: **vancomycin** (best choice); linezolid, daptomycin, ceftaroline, and telavancin as second line
- Staphylococcal scalded skin syndrome (SSSS)
  - Most commonly **infants/young children (low mortality, <5%)** who lack neutralizing antibodies and have ↓ renal clearance
  - Also seen in **adults w/ chronic renal failure (high mortality, >50%)**; M > F (2-4:1)
  - p/w **febrile prodrome**, widespread **skin tenderness**; skin eruption **begins on face (periorificial radial fissuring)** and **intertriginous** zones (Fig. 5.5) → generalizes within 48 hours as **wrinkled-appearing**

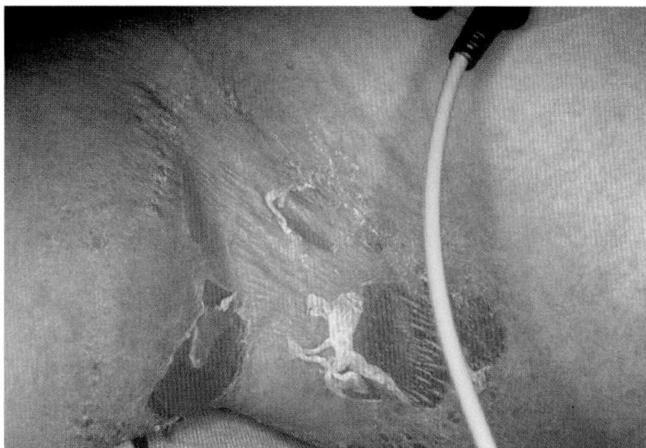

Fig. 5.5 Staphylococcal scalded skin syndrome with a wrinkled appearance of the erythematous skin in addition to peeling and denudation. (From James WD, Elston DM, McMahon PJ. Bacterial infections. In: *Andrews' Diseases of the Skin: Clinical Atlas*. Philadelphia: Elsevier; 2018:185–202.)

skin w/ **flaccid bullae** and positive Nikolsky sign → desquamation continues for up to 1 week, then **heals without scarring**

- Pathogenesis: infection by **phage group II (types 55 and 71)** *S. aureus* at a different/distant site → production of ETA and ETB) → exfoliatoxins disseminate via bloodstream → widespread cleavage of **Dsg1** → **subcorneal/intragranular acantholysis**
- Histology: resembles pemphigus foliaceus; **lacks inflammatory cells and bacteria** in blisters (vs. bullous impetigo)
- **Cultures from bullae are negative**; blood cultures almost always negative in children, but often positive in adults
- Treatment:
  - Mild disease: β-lactamase–resistant PCN (**dicloxacillin**) or first-generation CSN (**cephalexin**)
  - Severe disease: hospitalization (manage fever, pain, fluids, electrolytes, skin care) + IV antibiotics (nafcillin, methicillin)
- Other high-yield facts
  - Same exfoliatoxins as bullous impetigo (ETA/ETB), but hematogenously disseminated
  - Most common **primary sites of infection in children** = **nasopharynx or conjunctivae** (vs. pneumonia and bacteremia in adults)

- Staphylococcal toxic shock syndrome (TSS)
  - Severe multisystem disease with **cutaneous and internal involvement** (**renal** > GI, MSK, CNS, hepatic, hematologic, and mucosal)
    - Typically affects **young, healthy adults; occult primary site of infection**
    - Two forms: "**menstrual TSS**" (<50% of cases; young women w/ superabsorbent tampons; mortality rate less than 5%) or "**nonmenstrual TSS**" (>50%; **M = F; a/w nasal packing**, surgery, skin, or internal infections; mortality rate <20%)
      - Both forms p/w high fever (>102°F) + rash + systemic symptoms (e.g., myalgias, headache) + **hypotension (100%)**
      - Mucocutaneous eruption classically starts w/ **scarlatiniform eruption** (initially on trunk → becomes generalized), **redness and edema of palms/soles**, **"red strawberry tongue," conjunctival hyperemia → palmoplantar desquamation** (1–3 weeks later), Beau's lines, onychomadesis; usually **negative blood cultures** (<15% positive); **low mortality** (<5% for menstrual TSS and <20% for nonmenstrual TSS)
  - Pathogenesis: production of **toxic shock syndrome toxin-1 (TSST-1)** by certain strains of *S. aureus* → TSST-1 acts as **superantigen**, binding to **Vβ region** of TCR and class II MHC on APCs → **nonspecific activation of T cells** + cytokine storm (↑ TNF-α, IL-1, IL-6, TLR2, and TLR4)
  - Treatment:
    - β-lactamase–resistant antibiotics, **clindamycin (suppresses toxin** production) +/– IVIG; IV fluids for hypotension; hospitalization
  - Other high-yield facts
    - Compared with strep TSS, staph TSS has **lower mortality** (3%–20% vs. 30%–60%), **less florid primary site infection, more frequent rash, and less frequent blood culture positivity** (<15% vs. >50%)
- Pyomyositis
  - *S. aureus* **infection of skeletal muscle**; usually have predisposing factors (immunosuppression, diabetes, trauma, and intravenous drug abuse [IVDA]); p/w 1- to 2-week febrile prodrome, muscle pain, and a soft tissue mass w/ surrounding woody induration → muscle abscess +/– septicemia
  - Treatment: I&D + IV antibiotics, then long oral antibiotic course
  - **MRI** is best diagnostic tool
- Botryomycosis
  - **Deep** granulomatous and suppurative infection most frequently caused by *S. aureus*
  - May extend to skeletal muscle and bone; affects all ages; a/w ↓ **T-cell counts** and other defects in cellular immunity
  - 70% have **skin-limited** disease (rarely visceral in severely immunosuppressed patients; **lung** most common); p/w deep, **ulcerative plaques/nodules** with multiple **draining sinuses** that **drain yellow granules**
  - Histology: large **granules w/ basophilic center** (nonfilamentous bacteria) and **eosinophilic/hyaline periphery (Splendore-Hoeppli phenomenon;** composed of **IgG** and **C3** deposits), granules are surrounded by abscess and granulomatous inflammation (Fig. 5.6); granules are **PAS+**, Giemsa+, and **Gram(+)**
  - Treatment:
    - Surgical debridement/excision + antistaphylococcal antibiotics

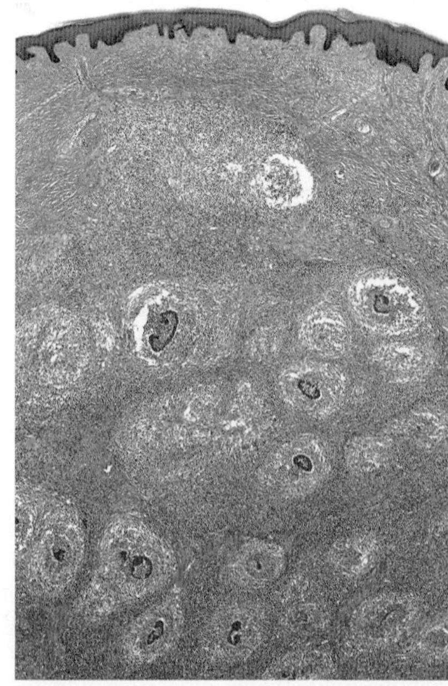

Fig. 5.6 Botryomycosis: there are multiple dermal abscesses surrounding discrete bacterial colonies. (From Grayson W, Calonje E. Infectious diseases of the skin. In: Calonje E, Brenn T, Lazar AJ, Billings SD, eds. *McKee's Pathology of the Skin*. 5th ed. Philadelphia: Elsevier; 2020:826–975.)

Streptococcal skin infections

- Ecthyma
  - Deep variant of impetigo; most common in **children**; caused by *S. pyogenes;* p/w few vesicopustules, most commonly on **legs** → develop into **"punched-out" ulcers** with purulent base and **hemorrhagic crust** → slowly self-resolves w/ **scarring**
    - Frequently as a result of scratching bug bites
  - Diagnosis: wound culture confirmatory, blood culture-negative, biopsy + Gram stain in difficult cases
  - Treatment: β-lactamase–resistant PCN (**dicloxacillin**) or first-generation CSN (**cephalexin**)
- Erysipelas ("St. Anthony's Fire")
  - **Superficial variant of cellulitis** (upper-mid dermis vs. deep dermis/SQ) with sharply defined ("**ridge-like**") **borders, fiery-red** color, and pain/**burning sensation**; prominent **lymphatic involvement**; most common sites = **lower extremity** (#1 site) > **face** (Fig. 5.7)
    - Lymphedema is a major risk factor
  - Usually caused by **group A β-hemolytic strep**
  - Labs: wound/blood **cultures usually negative**; best confirmatory tests = ↑ **DNase B and ASO titers**
  - Treatment: **PCN** (treatment of choice) for 2 weeks; erythromycin if PCN-allergic
- Perianal streptococcal skin infection
  - Classically **boys > 4 years old**; p/w **sharply defined** red plaques spreading up to 3 cm from anus (girls can get similar presentation on vagina/vulva); a/w pain upon defecation, blood in stool, **guttate psoriasis** outbreak
  - Labs: skin culture confirmatory
  - Treatment: oral **cefuroxime** (treatment of choice) or PCN (slightly less effective)
- Blistering distal dactylitis
  - Initially p/w darkening of skin of **distal finger** (>toe) **volar fat pad** → progresses to purulent vesicle/bulla on erythematous background within 1 week; affects **children**; results from picking nose or local skin trauma; ***S. pyogenes*** > *S. aureus*
  - Treatment: I&D + 10-day course oral β-lactam
- Scarlet fever
  - **Young children** (1–10 years old); caused by group A β-hemolytic streptococcus → produces **streptococcal pyrogenic toxins A, B, and C** (SPE-A, B, and C)
  - Most commonly in setting of streptococcal **pharyngitis/ tonsillitis**; p/w **sore throat**, high fevers, and systemic symptoms → 1 to 2 days later, macular erythema on upper trunk/neck → soon develop classic "**sandpaper-like**" papular eruption, **Pastia's lines** (linear petechiae; favors flexural sites), flushed cheeks with **circumoral pallor**, and "**white strawberry tongue**" (white background + red papillae) → later "**red strawberry tongue,**" **purulent exudate** from throat → 1 to 2 weeks later, **palmoplantar desquamation**
  - Labs: **positive throat/nasal culture** confirmatory; elevated DNase B and ASO titers
  - Treatment: **PCN** (treatment of choice), amoxicillin, or first-generation CSN/erythromycin/clindamycin (if PCN-allergic)
  - Other high-yield facts:
    - Notable complications: **acute glomerulonephritis and rheumatic fever**
    - **Purulent pharyngitis** almost always present (helpful clue)
    - 10% of all patients w/strep throat develop scarlet fever; mortality rate has dropped hugely since the advent of antibiotics (1% currently vs. 20% mortality in pre-antibiotic era)
- Streptococcal toxic shock syndrome
  - Similar clinical features as staph-TSS, but **affects young/healthy adults**, is **more severe** w/ **higher mortality** (30%–60%), usually a/w **florid skin/ soft tissue infections** (often necrotizing fasciitis [NF] vs. occult infections in staph-TSS), **much less frequent generalized macular erythematous rash**, and **far more frequent blood culture positivity** (>50%)
  - **Most common primary source = skin infection** from skin barrier breakdown (excoriation, bug bite, and infected surgical site)
  - Classically p/w **severe localized pain in extremity** w/ redness, swelling, or **NF**→ within 24 to 48 hours, systemic symptoms (**hypotension [100%]**)
  - Pathogenesis: group A β-hemolytic strep (**M types 1 and 3**) produce various toxins:
    - **SPE A, B, and C**
    - Streptococcal mitogenic toxin Z (SMEZ)
    - Streptolysin O
  - Toxins act as **superantigens**, binding to **Vβ region** of TCR and class II MHC on APCs → nonspecific activation of T cells + cytokine storm (↑ TNF-α, IL-1, IL-6, TLR2, and TLR4)
  - Treatment: most cases severe, requiring hospitalization + **surgical debridement** of soft tissue infection (possibly fasciotomy or amputation) + **clindamycin** (inhibits toxin production) + **PCN +/- IVIG**

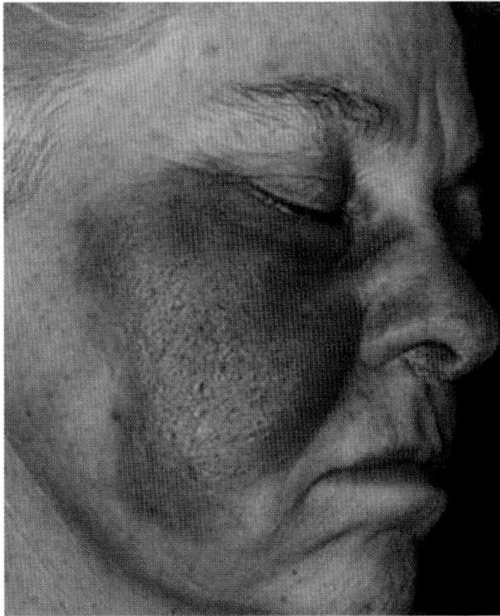

Fig. 5.7 Erysipelas on the malar cheek. (From Dinulos JGH. Bacterial infections. In: *Habif's Clinical dermatology: a color guide to diagnosis and therapy.* 7th ed. Philadelphia: Elsevier; 2021:331–375.)

Polymicrobial Gram-positive skin infections

- Cellulitis
  - Infection of **deep dermis/SQ** most commonly affecting **adults** w/ skin barrier disruption; p/w **tender/red/warm, ill-defined plaques** w/ fever/chills/**lymphangitis**
    - In severe cases, may see necrosis, bullae, vesicles
  - Most commonly caused by **group A β-hemolytic strep** > ***S. aureus*** (most common cause in children); most common sites: **head/neck** (children), **lower extremities** (adults), and IV injection sites on **arms** (IVDA)
  - Labs: blood cx ~**always negative** in immunocompetent patients
  - Notable variants:
    - *Haemophilus influenzae* (discussed in Gram-negative infection section)
    - Cellulitis a/w diabetic ulcers or chronic decubitus wounds: mixed infection w/ Gram-positive cocci and Gram-negative aerobes and anaerobes
  - Treatment:
    - Uncomplicated cases: oral **dicloxacillin, cephalexin, or clindamycin** for 10 days (must empirically cover for staph and strep)
    - Cellulitis a/w diabetic/decubitus ulcers: **piperacillin/tazobactam**, or ciprofloxacin + metronidazole
    - Severe cases: hospitalize and IV antibiotics
    - MRSA cellulitis: TMP-SMX, minocycline/doxycycline, and clindamycin
  - Other high-yield facts
    - Lymphatic damage (e.g., prior cellulitis, lymph node dissection, vein harvesting) → ↑ risk of recurrent cellulitis
    - Presence of **abscess** or necrotizing cellulitis are clues to **MRSA**
- Necrotizing fasciitis
  - **Rapidly progressive**, **life-threatening** (up to 50% mortality) **necrotizing infection** of skin, SQ, and fascia
  - Most common site = **extremities** (>trunk)
  - Caused by **group A β-hemolytic strep M types 1 and 3** (#1 cause in children) or **polymicrobial** (#1 cause in adults; mixture of *Streptococci, S. aureus, E. coli, Clostridium,* and *Bacteroides*)
  - Initially p/w severely painful indurated/"woody" plaque ("pain out of proportion to visible skin changes") → over 1 to 2 days and **rapidly progresses** → color changes from **erythematous** → **dusky purple/gray** +/− hemorrhagic bullae/ulceration, **crepitus**, **foul-smelling discharge**; patients **always severely toxic-appearing** (fever, tachycardia, and septic shock) → late in course and skin becomes **anesthetic** (nerves destroyed)
  - Imaging: **MRI may demonstrate gas**
  - Fournier's gangrene: NF of genitalia/perineum/lower abdominal wall
  - Meleney's gangrene: polymicrobial NF arising as a postoperative complication
  - Treatment: **fasciotomy** + **IV antibiotics** (piperacillin/tazobactam + clindamycin + ciprofloxacin)
  - Other high-yield facts
    - Risk factors: diabetes, immunosuppression, peripheral vasular disease (PVD), CRF, trauma, bevacizumab, IVDA, and recent surgery
    - **Prognostic factors a/w ↑ mortality**: older age, ↑ time to first debridement, ↑ extent of infection, females, ↑ lactic acid, and ↑ creatinine

Corynebacterial skin infections

- Erythrasma
  - Caused by ***Corynebacterium minutissimum*** **(Gram-positive filamentous rod)**
  - Affects stratum corneum of **moist, intertriginous zones (groin and toe webs [particularly fourth]** > axillae, inframammary, umbilicus, and intergluteal)
    - Fluoresces **"coral red" w/ Wood lamp** (bacterial **coproporphyrin III** production)
    - Groin: **light red-pink** (later brown) slightly scaly patches w/ thin scale
    - Toe webs: chronic, asymptomatic fissuring and maceration
    - Histology: filamentous Gram-positive rods within stratum corneum
  - Treatment:
    - Localized: **topical clindamycin/erythromycin/** mupirocin, Whitfield ointment
    - Widespread/recalcitrant: oral erythromycin, clarithromycin, tetracyclines
- Pitted keratolysis
  - Caused by ***Kytococcus sedentarius***, which digests keratin in stratum corneum
  - Non-inflammatory infection of **weight-bearing** areas of **plantar** (>palmar) skin
  - p/w **Small crateriform pits** and **foul odor** → may coalesce into arciform pits
    - Risk factors: hyperhidrosis and occlusion
  - Histology: deep pits in stratum corneum with **Gram-positive bacteria** at base
  - Treatment: topical **erythromycin** (or clindamycin, mupirocin, benzoyl peroxide) +/− 20% aluminum chloride, botulinum toxin
- Trichomycosis axillaris
  - Asymptomatic, **adherent yellow**-red concretions on **axillary hair shafts**; fluoresces with Wood lamp; caused by ***Corynebacterium tenuis***
  - Treatment: **shaving** of axillary hair (treatment of choice); may use topical erythromycin/clindamycin/benzoyl peroxide

Clostridium skin infections

- Clostridial anaerobic cellulitis and myonecrosis
  - Very rapid, potentially fatal **necrotizing soft tissue infections** with localized gas production (**"gas gangrene"**)
    - Caused by ***Clostridium perfringens*** **(Gram-positive, spore-forming rod)**
      - Obligate anaerobe (only reproduces in hypoxic tissues)
  - Due to **traumatic inoculation (surgery or crush/penetrating injuries)** of *C. perfringens* into oxygen-poor deep tissues; bacteria produces two pathogenic toxins: **α-toxin** (cleaves lipids) and **perfringolysin O** (induces vascular clots and worsens tissue hypoxia) → bacteria

proliferates freely in anaerobic environment, producing CO_2 and cleaving lipids → clinically p/w **crepitus, foul-smelling brown exudate ("dirty dishwater" color)**, w/ variable skin changes
  - Myonecrosis more likely to have **swelling, overlying skin changes, pain, toxemia, bacteremia**, but less likely to have **crepitus** than anaerobic cellulitis
  - Risk factors: diabetes, PVD
- Imaging: **X-ray reveals gas** in soft tissues
- Labs: blood culture usually negative
- Treatment: immediate **aggressive surgical debridement** (most important) + clindamycin and piperacillin-tazobactam +/− hyperbaric oxygen

Filamentous bacteria

- Actinomycosis
  - Agent: ***Actinomyces israelii***
  - Gram-positive, **non-acid fast**, and anaerobic/microaerophilic filamentous bacteria
  - Actinomycetes spp. are part of **normal flora** of mouth, GI/GU tracts → infection arises after **trauma (dental procedures** or surgical interventions)
  - Subacute-chronic granulomatous lesions with **suppurating abscesses 1 sinus tracts**
  - Forms:
    - **Cervicofacial (most common**, accounts for 70%): **"lumpy jaw disease,"** red-brown nodules with fistulous abscesses draining characteristic **yellow sulfur granules** (= clumps of bacteria); a/w **poor dental hygiene** and **dental procedures**
    - Pulmonary/thoracic: as a result of aspiration, p/w **pulmonary cavities** at base of lungs
    - Pelvic: due to intrauterine devices in women
    - GI: as a result of trauma or inflammatory disease, p/w granulomatous lesions in bowel wall
  - Histology: dense granulomatous and suppurative inflammation with **"granules"** with basophilic center (Gram-positive branching filaments of *Actinomyces*) and **eosinophilic rim (Splendore-Hoeppli** phenomenon)
  - Treatment: **penicillin G** or ampicillin
    - Chronic or deep-seated infections: 2 to 6 weeks of IV antibiotics followed by 3 to 12 months of oral PCN
    - Acute infections: 2 to 3 weeks of oral PCN + I&D of abscesses + surgical excision of sinus tracts
- Nocardiosis
  - Agent: ***Nocardia brasiliensis* (#1 cause of actinomycotic mycetoma)**, *Nocardia asteroides* (#1 cause of pulmonary/systemic nocardiosis), other *Nocardia* spp.
  - Gram-positive, **weakly acid-fast**, filamentous bacteria
  - **Ubiquitous in soil** (explains why **foot** is the most common site of actinomycotic mycetoma!)
  - Four major forms of disease (Table 5.5), but actinomycotic mycetoma is most testable
  - Histology: intense neutrophilic infiltrate + **sulfur granules** (only seen in actinomycotic mycetoma form); branching filaments are **Gram-positive**, acid-fast bacteria **(AFB)+ (Fite** > Ziehl-Neelsen), and GMS+
  - Treatment: **sulfonamides** (treatment of choice) +/− surgical drainage (Box 5.1)

Table 5.5 Four Major Clinical Forms of Cutaneous Nocardiosis

Primary	
Actinomycotic mycetoma	Half of all cases of actinomycotic mycetoma are caused by the *Nocardia* species[a] **Traumatic inoculation** causes a painless nodule that enlarges, suppurates, and drains via the sinus tracts Purulent discharge contains sulfur granules The **foot** is the usual site of involvement May involve underlying muscle and bone
Lymphocutaneous	Occurs days to weeks after trauma Appears as a crusted pustule or abscess resistant to antibiotics Ascending lymphatic streaks, a **sporotrichoid** pattern of papulonodules, and tender palpable lymph nodes may be seen
Superficial cutaneous	Traumatic implantation of foreign objects (including soil and gravel) into the skin The diagnosis is based on a high index of suspicion, lack of response to routine antibiotic treatment, and laboratory results
Secondary	
Pulmonary/systemic	Subcutaneous abscesses of the **chest wall** Pustules, nodules, and cutaneous fistulae Almost universally fatal if left untreated Most commonly caused by *Nocardia asteroids*

[a]*In Mexico and Central and South America,* ***Nocardia brasiliensis*** **is the etiologic agent of 90% of actinomycotic mycetomas**, *whereas in the United States, most mycetomas are caused by true fungi.*
From Sommer LL, Reboli AC, Heymann WR. Bacterial diseases. In: Bolognia JL, Shaffer JV, Cerroni L, eds. Dermatology. *4th ed. Philadelphia: Elsevier; 2018:1259–1295.*

Box 5.1 "SNAP" Mnemonic

Antibiotics of choice for *Nocardia* versus *Actinomyces* = "SNAP"

Sulfonamides = ***N****ocardia*, ***A****ctinomyces* = **P**enicillin

Other Gram-positive infections

- Anthrax
  - Agent: ***Bacillus anthracis***
  - **Gram-positive, spore-forming** rod
  - Three forms (**pulmonary, GI, and cutaneous** anthrax)
  - Cutaneous anthrax: **most common** (>95%) and **least fatal** form
    - Arises via **occupational exposure ("Woolsorter's disease")** from direct contact w/ infected animals/carcasses
    - Presents 1 week postexposure with purpuric papulovesicle (**"malignant pustule"**) that drains serosanguinous fluid → vesicle ulcerates to form **painless**/black/necrotic **eschar** w/ satellite vesicles and edema
    - 20% mortality if untreated
  - Treatment:
    - First line (cutaneous anthrax): **quinolone** or **doxycycline** × 2 weeks (treat for 60 days if suspect bioterrorism or possible inhalation exposure); vaccine and immune globulin are available for postexposure prophylaxis
  - Other high-yield facts:
    - **Early treatment critical!** (20% mortality if untreated vs. ~0% if treated)

- Virulence factors:
  - Poly-D-glutamic acid **capsule** (resists phagocytosis)
  - **Lethal toxin** = protective antigen + lethal factor (↑ TNF-α and IL-1β → septic shock, death)
  - **Edema toxin** = protective antigen + edema factor (↑ cAMP → edema)

- Erysipeloid
  - Acute, **self-limited** infection; **occupational** disease of **fisherman** or **poultry/fish handlers**; as a result of traumatic inoculation of ***Erysipelothrix rhusiopathiae*** (Gram-positive rod); most commonly p/w localized form: **red-violaceous** non-suppurative cellulitis +/− hemorrhagic vesicles; classically affects **finger web spaces** w/ **sparing of terminal phalanges**
  - Treatment: **PCN** (treatment of choice), ciprofloxacin (if PCN-allergic)
- Listeria
  - Most commonly affects **pregnant women**, elderly, and the immunosuppressed as **GI illness** caused by the ingestion of ***Listeria monocytogenes*** (motile Gram-positive rod) → fever, bacteremia, and meningitis
  - **Rarely see skin lesions**—mostly occurs in setting of neonatal septicemia (from vertical transmission), which p/w disseminated papules/pustules/vesicles/purpura
  - Treatment:
    - First line: **ampicillin**
    - Second line: TMP-SMX
- Cutaneous microbiome: Most bacteria on the skin are Actinobacteria (e.g., *Propionibacterium*, *Corynebacterium*), Firmicutes (e.g., *Staphylococcus*), Proteobacteria, and Bacteriodetes—help protect skin from pathogenic organisms

II. Gram-negative skin infections

Pseudomonas

- Green nail syndrome
  - **Green/blue-black** nail discoloration; a/w excessive water exposure, nail trauma; from ***Pseudomonas aeruginosa* pyocyanin** pigment production
  - Treatment: **topical quinolone**, topical sodium hypochlorite, or **aminoglycoside** solution
- Pseudomonal pyoderma
  - Superficial erosive infection w/ **blue-green purulent exudate**, "**moth-eaten**" appearance to skin surface, with "**mousy**" **or** "**grape-like**" **odor**; may arise at burn sites, in **mixed toe web infections** (Fig. 5.8), and other chronic wounds
  - Treatment: systemic antipseudomonal antibiotics, topical antiseptics, debridement, and drying agents
- Otitis externa ("swimmer's ear")
  - *P. aeruginosa* infection of external auditory canal; p/w edema, skin maceration, and purulent green exudate; tympanic membrane intact; classically **severe pain upon pinna manipulation**
  - Malignant otitis externa (severe variant): usually only in **diabetics** or **immunosuppressed**; persistent drainage w/ excessive granulation tissue extending to bony portion of ear → may result in osteomyelitis of skull base

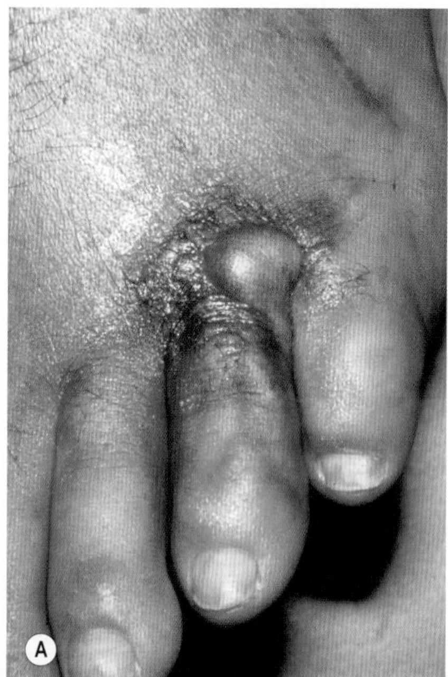

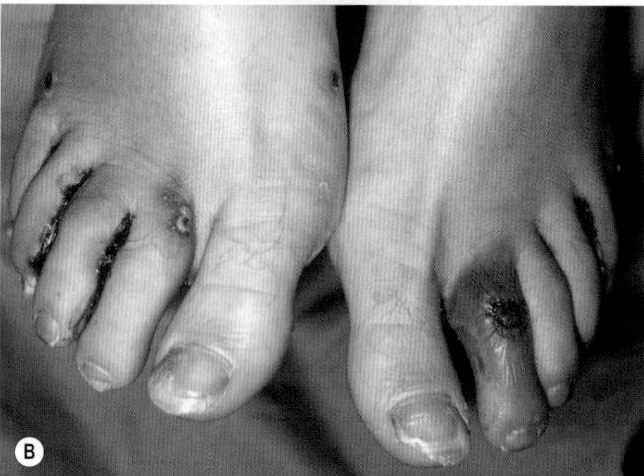

Fig. 5.8 (A) and **(B)** Pseudomonas skin infection of the feet. Note the erosions and blistering of the skin. (From James WD, Elston DM, McMahon PJ. Bacterial infections. In: *Andrews' Diseases of the Skin Clinical Atlas*. Philadelphia: Elsevier; 2018:185–202. B, Courtesy of Ken Greer, MD.)

  - Treatment: topical antipseudomonal agents, but systemic for malignant otitis externa
- Pseudomonal folliculitis ("hot tub folliculitis")
  - Self-resolving *P. aeruginosa* infection arising from poorly chlorinated **hot tubs/whirlpools**; p/w red, perifollicular papulopustules 1 to 2 days postexposure; commonly affects **areas covered by bathing suit**
  - Treatment:
    - Immunocompetent: spontaneous resolution in ≤ 2 weeks
    - Widespread, immunosuppressed: oral quinolone
- Pseudomonas hot-foot syndrome
  - Self-resolving *P. aeruginosa* infection arising from **wading in pools** w/ high concentrations of *Pseudomonas*; p/w **painful**, red-violaceous plaques/nodules on **weight-bearing areas** of plantar surface
  - Histology: perivascular/perieccrine neutrophils
  - Treatment: none required; self-resolves

- Ecthyma gangrenosum
  - Cutaneous lesion indicative of *P. aeruginosa* **septicemia**; most commonly occurs in immunosuppressed patients w/ **severe neutropenia** (often bone marrow transplantation patients); p/w a small number of **purpuric macules** → progresses to hemorrhagic bullae → bullae rupture → **ulcer w/ necrotic black eschar** and tender, red skin surrounding eschar; most common sites = **anogenital region and extremities**
  - Histology: sharply demarcated epidermal necrosis w/ hemorrhagic crust, and underlying dermal infarction w/ septic vasculitis (**Gram-negative rods in vessel walls**)
  - Labs: blood/wound cultures positive
  - Treatment: **IV aminoglycoside + antipseudomonal PCN**
  - Other high-yield facts
    - Prognostic factors a/w poor outcomes: ↑ # lesions, delay in diagnosis, and prolonged neutropenia

Bartonella

- Small, facultative **intracellular** Gram-negative bacilli
- Three species cause human disease (Table 5.6):
  - ***Bartonella henselae*** (cat scratch disease, bacillary angiomatosis, and peliosis hepatitis)
  - ***Bartonella quintana*** (trench fever and bacillary angiomatosis)
  - ***Bartonella bacilliformis*** (Carrion's disease/Oroya fever/verruga peruana)
- Both *B. henselae and B. quintana* may cause: bacillary angiomatosis, chronic afebrile bacteremia, and endocarditis
- **Bacillary angiomatosis** mostly occurs in **HIV-positive** patients w/ **CD4 count < 200**; only **20% recall cat bite/scratch** (vs. 90% w/ cat scratch disease); vascular proliferation caused by bacterial angiogenic factor
  - Can involve lymph nodes, bone, and viscera
  - Lesions are dome-shaped, vascular papulonodules
  - More developed lesions can have a friable eroded appearance, resembling pyogenic granulomas
- Death in Oroya fever usually secondary to ***Salmonella enterica*** superinfection; **chloramphenicol + β-lactam** is treatment of choice (alt. is quinolone)
- Histopathology (verruga peruana and bacillary angiomatosis): resembles pyogenic granuloma (lobular capillary proliferation), but has **dense neutrophilic infiltrate,** and extra- and intracellular **organisms (within endothelial cells—Rocha-Lima inclusions)** seen w/ **Warthin-Starry stain** (Fig. 5.9)
- Labs: *B. bacilliformis*—PCR, culture, immunologic testing; *B. henselae* and *B quintana*—**PCR assay** (rapid, sensitive), **serologies** (sensitive, specific; not for *B. quintana*), **chocolate agar** culture (slow!)

Rickettsia

- Small, obligate intracellular Gram-negative organisms
- **Transmitted** by **arthropod** host/vector (ticks, fleas, lice, and mites)
- Target = **endothelial cells**
- Transmitted from arthropod (tick, flea, mite, and louse) via saliva or feces → bacteria enter dermis via bite or scratching → bacteria **attach to endothelial cells** → spread hematogenously and destroy infected vessels via **reactive oxygen species** formation → ↑ **vascular permeability** → vascular skin findings (petechiae, purpura, and vasculitis = "**spotted fever**") and life-threatening end organ damage (**meningoencephalitis** and **pulmonary edema/pneumonitis** most important causes of mortality), **thrombocytopenia**, hypovolemia, and hypotension
- **Three groups** (Table 5.7):
  - Spotted fever group (rash in 85%–100%): *R. rickettsii, R. conorii, R. akari, R. africae, R. japonica,* and *R. australis*
  - Typhus group (rash in 50%–80%): *R. typhi* and *R. prowazekii*
  - Scrub typhus (rash in 50%): *R. tsutsugamushi*
- **Eschar at inoculation site** ≈1 week prior to illness is constant and important feature seen in majority of spotted fever group, and scrub typhus
  - **No eschar** in Rocky Mountain spotted fever (RMSF) and typhus group
- Variable prognosis:
  - Severe: **RMSF** (**most severe**, 25% mortality if untreated, and 4% if treated) > **epidemic typhus** (15% mortality if untreated and 3% if treated)
  - Intermediate: Mediterranean spotted fever (3%–5% mortality)
  - Benign: **endemic typhus** (≤1% mortality) and **Rickettsialpox** (0% mortality)

Other Gram-negative skin infections

- *Neisseria meningitidis*
  - **Gram-negative diplococcus** (strains A, B, C, Y, and W-135)
  - Most commonly affects children/**young adults** living in close quarters (**military recruits** and college students); M > F (4 : 1); humans are only reservoir; 10% to **15% population are asymptomatic carriers (in nasopharynx)**; disease transmitted via **respiratory secretions**
  - **Acute meningococcemia**: 1 to 10 days postexposure, p/w fever, chills, headache, **petechial rash** (30%–50%), **retiform purpura** w/ classic "**gunmetal gray**" color (Fig. 5.10), or **hemorrhagic bullae** on **legs and trunk**; may progress to **septic shock with DIC** (purpura fulminans)
    - Histology: **LCV w/ vascular thrombosis** and **Gram-negative rods** in 70% biopsies
    - Labs: PCR assay most sensitive/specific (>blood/tissue/CSF cultures or latex agglutination studies)
    - Prognosis: **10% to 15% mortality**; up to 15% who survive have **hearing loss** or CNS sequelae
  - **Chronic meningococcemia**: less common; p/w recurrent fevers, arthralgias, and macular/papular eruption; condition self-resolves, only to recur days to weeks later
  - Treatment: early treatment is critical!
    - First line: high-dose IV **PCN** (treatment of choice)
    - Second line: quinolones or chloramphenicol (if PCN-allergic); third-generation CSN (resistant disease)

Table 5.6 Major Human Diseases Caused by *Bartonella* Species and Their Treatment

Species	Disease	Vector	Reservoir/ Host	Epidemiology	Clinical Presentation	First Line	Second Line	Notes
Bartonella bacilliformis	**Bartonellosis** (Carrion's disease, Oroya fever, and verruga peruana)	Phlebotomine sand fly (***Lutzomyia verrucarum***)	Human	Andean mountain valley regions of Peru, Ecuador, and Southwestern Columbia (altitudes of 2500–8000 feet) More common in immunologically naive tourists and transient workers Milder in children	Oroya fever (acute phase)	**Chloramphenicol**[a] plus β-lactam antibiotic Quinolone (norfloxacin and ciprofloxacin) (>6 years of age and not pregnant)	Trimethoprim-sulfamethoxazole Macrolide Doxycycline	Successful treatment does not eliminate risk for developing verruga peruana Adjunctive treatment needed with chloramphenicol, as treatment failures have been seen with monotherapy Death occurs in ~40% of untreated individuals
					Verruga peruana (chronic phase)	Azithromycin	Ciprofloxacin Rifampin + streptomycin (traditional)	Only 5% of patients recall an acute febrile illness Disappearance of skin lesions within 1 month with treatment
Bartonella henselae	**Cat scratch disease**	Cat flea (***Ctenocephalides felis***)	Cat	Primarily seen in young people (<18 years) in the fall and winter Immunocompetent > immunocompromised	Mild to moderate, uncomplicated	Supportive care (analgesics) only Needle aspiration of suppurative lymph nodes	Azithromycin Doxycycline plus rifampin	Azithromycin shown to decrease lymph node volume, but not effective in preventing dissemination or complications
					Severe, complicated	Doxycycline plus rifampin		Severe disease includes retinitis, encephalopathy, and visceral spread
	Bacillary angiomatosis *Bacillary peliosis hepatis* Bacteremia (chronic afebrile) Endocarditis			**Immunocompromised** (e.g., common in HIV) Immunocompromised Immunocompetent or immunocompromised Late complication of chronic bacteremia	Mild, uncomplicated bacillary angiomatosis Severe, complicated bacillary angiomatosis	Erythromycin Erythromycin Doxycycline plus rifampin	Doxycycline Azithromycin Clarithromycin	Jarisch–Herxheimer-like reaction may occur Treatment failures seen with quinolones, trimethoprim-sulfamethoxazole, and narrow-spectrum cephalosporins Use of IV antibiotics recommended for GI intolerance or poor absorption states
Bartonella quintana	**Trench fever** "Five day fever" "Urban trench fever" "Quintan fever" **Bacillary angiomatosis** Bacteremia (chronic afebrile) Endocarditis	**Human body louse** (*Pediculosis humanus*)	Human	First reported in World War I troops, now associated with **homelessness and poor hygiene** ("urban trench fever") Immunocompromised (e.g., common in HIV) Immunocompetent or immunocompromised Late complication of chronic bacteremia		Doxycycline plus aminoglycoside		Doxycycline plus rifampin recommended for CNS disease, because of better CNS penetration

Fever and splenomegaly caused by bacteremia with Bartonella rochalimae *(a recently recognized species) has also been described.*
[a]*Gray baby syndrome can develop in premature neonates who receive chloramphenicol.*
From Sommer LL, Reboli AC, Heymann WR. Bacterial diseases. In: Bolognia JL, Shaffer JV, Cerroni L, eds. Dermatology. *4th ed. Philadelphia: Elsevier; 2018:1259–1295.*

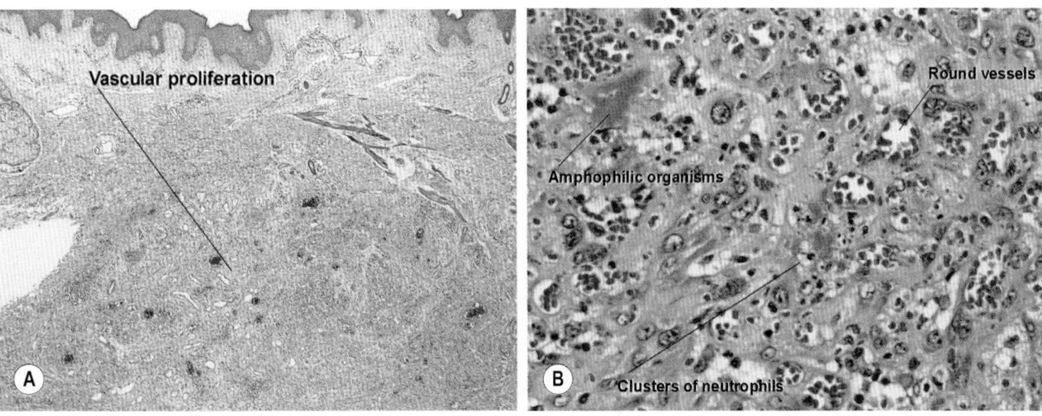

Fig. 5.9 (A) and **(B)** Bacillary angiomatosis histology. Note the vascular proliferation in the dermis with plump endothelial cells, as well as clusters of neutrophils and amphophilic collections of organisms. (From Elston DM: Vascular tumors. In: Elston DM, Ferringer T, eds. *Dermatopathology*. 3rd ed. Philadelphia: Elsevier, 2019:433–495.)

Table 5.7 Rickettsial Diseases

Disease (Bacterium)	Vector	Clinical Features	Rx	Other High-Yield Facts
Spotted fever group: "spotted fever" = high fevers (>102°F) + erythematous-petechial skin eruption (85%–100%) + constitutional symptoms				
Rocky Mountain Spotted Fever (RMSF) ***(Rickettsia rickettsii)***	***Dermacentor variabilis*** (#1 vector, Eastern 2/3rd and Pacific Coast of the United States) ***Dermacentor andersoni*** (#2 vector, Rocky Mountain states) *Rhipicephalus sanguineus* (Southwestern United States) Less commonly *A. cajennense, A. aureolatum, A. imitator, and A. sculptum*	7–14 days post-tick bite, develop fever, headache, myalgias, and GI symptoms → **90% develop rash** 3–5 days later with faint red **macules** on acral sites **(wrists and ankles** are most common initial sites) → subsequent **centripetal spread** to trunk; **spares face** → over time, lesions become papular and **petechial/purpuric** as a result of edema and RBC extravasation from vessel destruction; **mortality rate** = **25%** if untreated (vs. <4% if treated early)	**Doxycycline** is treatment of choice in ALL patients, **even children**! Only exception: **chloramphenicol** is treatment of choice for **pregnant** patients (→ risk of "**gray baby syndrome**")	RMSF is the **most severe** Rickettsial infection 40% of patients do not recall tick bite! Cutaneous necrosis in 4% **Lacks eschar!**
Mediterranean spotted fever/"Boutonneuse fever" (*Rickettsia conorii)*	***Rhipicephalus sanguineus*** (brown dog tick)	p/w Necrotic papule at site of tick bite ("**Tache noir**") → maculopapular eruption favoring **legs**	First line: **doxycycline** Mild disease in children: azithromycin, clarithromycin	
Rickettsialpox (***Rickettsia akari***)	**Liponyssoides sanguineus** (house mouse mite)	Within 48 hours of bite p/w **papulovesicle** at bite site → progresses to **eschar** (>90%) → fever and systemic symptoms w/ **widespread cutaneous eruption** (**face**, trunk, and extremities) of red macules and papulovesicles w/ **hemorrhagic crusts** +/– oropharyngeal enanthem	**None required; self-resolves** within 3 weeks May hasten resolution w/ doxycycline	The only spotted fever to be caused by a **mite** Most common in **urban areas** of Northeastern United States Weil-Felix test does **not** identify Rickettsialpox
Typhus group: similar to spotted fever group in most regards; p/w erythematous macules starting around **axillae**; **rash in only 50%–80%** (vs. 85%–100% in spotted fever group)				
Endemic/murine typhus ***(Rickettsia typhi)***	***Xenopsylla cheopis*** (Oriental rat flea)	p/w Fever + similar systemic symptoms as spotted fever group + erythematous macules and papules initially on **axillae**	**Doxycycline**	***X. cheopis*** is also the vector for bubonic plague
Cat flea typhus ***(Rickettsia felis)***	***Ctenocephalides felis*** (cat flea)	Clinically identical to endemic (murine) typhus	**Doxycycline**	
Epidemic typhus ***(Rickettsia prowazekii)***	***Pediculus humanus var. corporis*** (human body louse)	Epidemic typhus: a/w crowded living conditions Brill-Zinsser disease: recurrence of latent infection (occurs decades later) Flying squirrel typhus: caused by contact w/ **flying squirrels** and their fleas/lice	**Doxycycline**	

Continued

Table 5.7 Rickettsial Diseases—cont'd

Scrub typhus: solitary member comprising the third group of rickettsial infection; rash in only 50%				
Scrub typhus (***Orientia tsutsugamushi***)	**Larval trombiculid mites** ("chiggers")	**Eschar** forms at bite site (60%–90%) → fever, lymphadenopathy, and macular rash (50%) starting **initially in axilla → subsequent centrifugal spread**; variable prognosis	First line: **doxycycline** Pregnant women: azithromycin	Most common in **Asia**; particularly areas w/ dense **scrub** vegetation Interstitial pneumonia common
Rickettsia-like bacteria				
Human monocytic ehrlichiosis (HME) ***(Ehrlichia chaffeensis)***	***Amblyomma americanum*** (lone star tick)	Most common in Southern United States; p/w fever, myalgias, thrombocytopenia, **leukopenia**, and **maculopapular or petechial** rash (30%–40%) most commonly on **trunk, extremities**; mortality rate = 3%	**Doxycycline**	Obligate intracellular organism targets and kills **monocytes/ macrophages** Reservoir = **white-tailed deer** **No eschar** seen ↑ LFTs
Human granulocytic anaplasmosis (***Anaplasma phagocytophilum***)	***Ixodes scapularis and Ixodes pacificus*** (same as Lyme and Babesiosis)	Found in same geographic distribution as Lyme disease; similar clinical presentation as HME, but **↓ fatality rate, ↓ skin findings,** and **↑** peripheral neuropathy	**Doxycycline**	Obligate intracellular organism targets and kills **neutrophils** **Coinfection** w/ Lyme and Babesiosis is common
Q fever (***Coxiella burnetii)***	Usually transmitted via aerosols from infected **sheep and cattle**	**Rare skin findings** Fever, pneumonia, hepatitis	**Doxycycline**	Rare cause of erythema nodosum and mixed cryoglobulinemia vasculitis

GI, *Gastrointestinal;* LFTs, *liver function tests.*

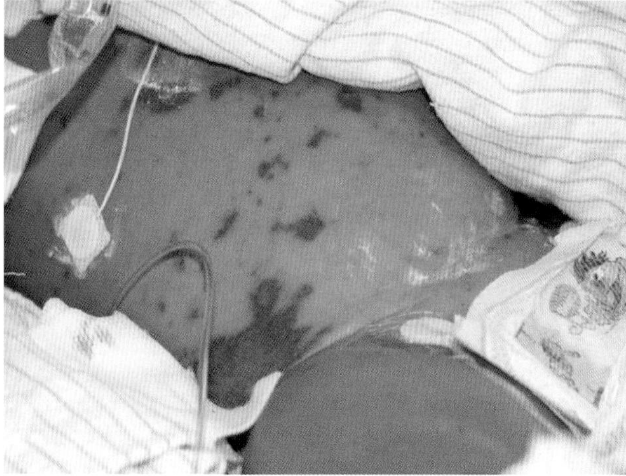

Fig. 5.10 Stellate purpura with a central gunmetal-gray hue suggestive of meningococcemia. (From Mishkin DR, Rosh AJ. Female infant with fever and rash. *Ann Emerg Med.* 2009; 54[2]:155–180.)

- **Prophylactically treat all close contacts** w/ ciprofloxacin, rifampin, azithromycin
- Other high-yield facts
  - Risk factors: **asplenic** patient or **terminal complement deficiency** (C5–C9)
  - **Main virulence factor = polysaccharide capsule**
  - **Endotoxin** → septic shock and **purpura fulminans**
  - In the United States, types B, C, and Y are most common causes of acute meningococcemia
  - Quadrivalent vaccine protects against types A/C/Y/W-135

- Brucellosis (Malta fever, "undulant fever")
  - Caused by Gram-negative coccobacillus, *Brucella* spp.
  - Endemic in Middle East (consuming **unpasteurized goat milk/cheese**)
  - In the United States, occupational disease (**farmers, butchers, and veterinarians**) from **direct contact or inhalation**
  - p/w **Undulating fevers**, arthralgias, LAD, hepatosplenomegaly, endocarditis, **foul-smelling sweat**, and **rare (<10%) skin findings** (disseminated violaceous papules, purpura, erythema nodosum-like)
- Glanders
  - Gram-negative bacillus, ***Burkholderia mallei***
  - Caused by contact w/ **infected horses**, mules, or donkeys
  - Four forms:
    - **Localized**—hemorrhagic, ulcerative papulopustule at inoculation site
    - Chronic—multiple soft tissue nodules ("**farcy buds**") on skin overlying lymphatics
    - **Septicemic form**—mortality rate >95% without treatment and 50% w/ treatment
    - Pulmonary form—mortality similar to septicemic form
  - Treatment:
    - Localized disease: 60- to 150-day course of amoxicillin/clavulanate, doxycycline, or TMP-SMX
    - Septicemic: IV carbapenems + ciprofloxacin or doxycycline
- Melioidosis
  - Gram-negative bacillus ***Burkholderia pseudomallei***
  - Caused by direct contact w/ contaminated **water or soil**
  - Risk factors: diabetes, chronic kidney disease, immunosuppression, and IVDA
  - Clinical presentation and mortality rates ~same as glanders
  - Treatment: IV ceftazidime or a carbapenem × 2 weeks → 3+ month TMP-SMX
- Malakoplakia (malacoplakia)
  - Chronic granulomatous infection as a result of the inability of macrophages to kill phagocytosed ***E. coli***

- Most commonly affects **immunosuppressed (esp. kidney transplant patients)**
- Most commonly affects **GU tract**; may affect **skin of perianal/genital** region (ulcerated abscesses and soft polypoid lesions)
- Histology: dense granulomatous infiltrate composed of **von Hansemann cells** (large macrophages w/ eosinophilic cytoplasm [**Michaelis-Gutmann bodies**]; stain w/ CD68, lysozyme, α-1 antitrypsin)
  - **Michaelis-Gutmann bodies**: round, laminated, calcified basophilic intracytoplasmic inclusions; comprised of incompletely killed bacteria within calcified phagolysosomes; stain w/ **von Kossa, PAS,** Perls, Giemsa)
- Treatment:
  - Localized: **surgical excision**
  - Nonsurgical candidates: difficult to treat; may try long courses of ciprofloxacin, TMP-SMX, or clofazimine

- Tularemia (rabbit fever and deer fly fever)
  - Gram-negative coccobacillus, ***Francisella tularensis***
  - Mode of transmission = contact w/ **rabbit carcasses (classic!)**, deer flies, and ticks; increased risk in **hunters** and animal handlers
  - Most common presentation is **ulceroglandular** = 80% (> pneumonic > glandular, typhoidal > oropharyngeal > oculoglandular), which p/w **necrotic, punched-out ulcer** at inoculation site w/ **suppurative LAD** (Box 5.2)
  - Treatment: **streptomycin** (treatment of choice)
- *H. influenzae* cellulitis
  - Gram-negative coccobacillus
  - Classically affects **infants**, p/w deep **red-violaceous/ blue facial cellulitis** (most commonly **periorbital** or **buccal**) following an upper respiratory infection-like illness
  - Usually **positive blood cultures**
  - Treatment: third-generation CSN
  - Incidence has decreased since development of **Hib vaccine**
- Rhinoscleroma
  - Chronic granulomatous infection of **nose** and upper respiratory tract
  - Affects adults, mainly in **tropical** locations
  - Transmitted by **inhalation** of ***Klebsiella rhinoscleromatis***
  - a/w Cellular immune defects: inability of macrophages to kill phagocytosed bacteria → **Mikulicz cells** (large, vacuolated histiocytes containing bacteria)
  - Three clinical phases:
    - **Catarrhal phase** (rhinitis, obstruction from soft tissue edema)
    - **Granulomatous/infiltrative phase** (granulomatous nodules in nose/upper respiratory tract, epistaxis, **dysphonia, anesthesia of soft palate**, and **Hebra nose**)

Box 5.2 Differential Diagnosis of Ulceroglandular Diseases Mnemonic

"My Aunt's Temperamental Tall Rats Plague Glands"

Melioidosis, Anthrax, Tularemia, TB chancre, Rat-bite fever, Plague, Glanders

    - **Sclerotic phase** (extensive scarring requires tracheotomy and nasal reconstruction)
  - Histology: dense pan-dermal infiltrate of **Mikulicz cells** containing bacteria (seen w/ **Warthin-Starry, Giemsa**) and **Russell bodies**
  - Treatment: **tetracycline** (treatment of choice) for 6 months along with surgical correction of airway; ciprofloxacin is second line
- Salmonellosis (typhoid fever)
  - Enteric infection caused by ***Salmonella typhi***
  - Spread by direct contact w/ infected individuals or carriers
  - p/w Fever, nausea/vomiting, diarrhea, headache, and characteristic **"rose spots"** of skin (2- to 8-mm pink, grouped papules on **trunk**); bacteria can be cultured from rose spots
  - Treatment: **quinolones** (treatment of choice); use third-generation CSN in children
- Rat-bite fever ("Haverhill fever")
  - ***Streptobacillus moniliformis***
  - As a result of a **rat bite** ("rat-bite fever"), or occasionally, ingestion of contaminated food ("Haverhill fever"); ↑ **incidence in urban areas** w/ high rat concentration
  - Classic triad (paroxysmal fever, migratory polyarthritis, and acral rash)
    - p/w Redness, edema, and ulceration at bite site (w/ LAD) → paroxysmal fever w/ systemic symptoms → 2 to 4 days later, migratory polyarthritis + acral eruption (**palms and soles** most common) of petechial red macules/papules, vesicles, or pustules
    - Up to **15% mortality**
  - Treatment: **PCN** (treatment of choice) for 1 week (6 weeks if septicemic)
- Plague
  - Caused by ***Yersinia pestis***, a Gram-negative **bipolar bacillus**
    - Characteristic "**safety pin**" **appearance** of bacteria on Gram or Giemsa stain
  - **Reservoir = rodents**; usually transmitted to humans by **flea bites** (>rodent contact, inhalation)
  - Forms:
    - **Bubonic (most common)**: pustule or ulcer at inoculation site (10%) + **painful, suppurative regional LAD = "buboes"** (groin, axillae most common); ≈50% mortality rate if untreated
    - Septicemic: vesiculopustular eruption w/ petechiae, purpura; hemorrhagic and necrotic lesions in nasopharyngeal and GI tracts; 100% mortality if untreated
    - Pneumonic: acute pneumonitis; 100% mortality if untreated
  - Treatment:
    - First line: **aminoglycosides** (streptomycin and gentamicin)
    - Plague meningoencephalitis: chloramphenicol
    - Postexposure prophylaxis: doxycycline or ciprofloxacin × 7 days
- *Vibrio vulnificus*
  - Most commonly affects **men > 40 years old** who have predisposing factors: **liver disease (hemochromatosis, cirrhosis**, or alcoholism), **diabetes** (peripheral

neuropathy/vasculopathy predisposes to wound infections), GI disease (peptic ulcer disease w/ antacids), immunosuppression, and end-stage renal disease
- Reservoir = **shellfish**
- Two modes of infection:
  - **Cutaneous exposure to contaminated seawater/ shellfish**: affects shellfish handlers; trauma → painful cellulitis → **hemorrhagic bullae** → may progress to **NF**, **myositis**, or septicemia
  - **Consumption of raw/undercooked shellfish**: most commonly from **raw oysters**; septicemia, abdominal cramps, and hypotension; 75% have skin findings—red-purple macules/vesicles → progress to **hemorrhagic bullae and necrotic plaques**
- Treatment: **doxycycline** + third-generation CSN

• Bite-induced infections
- **Dog bites are most common** (>cats >humans); human bites are most likely to get infected
  - Dog bite: ***Pasteurella multocida, Pasteurella canis, or Capnocytophaga canimorsus*** (potentially fatal in asplenic or immunosuppressed patients)
  - Cat bite: ***P. multocida*** > *Streptococcal* spp.
  - Human bite: ***Eikenella corrodens*** (a/w chronic infections), *S. aureus* (a/w severe infections), *Peptostreptococcus, Enterococcus,* and *Bacteroides*
- Treatment:
  - **Amoxicillin/clavulanate** (treatment of choice)
  - Also important to irrigate the wound and give tetanus vaccine

III. Nonvenereal spirochete infections

Borrelia

• Lyme disease
- Agent: ***Borrelia burgdorferi*** (#1 in the United States); ***Borrelia garinii*** and ***Borrelia afzelii*** (#1 in Europe)
- Reservoir: **white-tailed deer** and white-footed mouse
- Vector: ***Ixodes*** spp. (hard body) ticks; specific type varies by geographic region:
  - ***Ixodes scapularis (Ixodes dammini)*** → #1 cause in the United States (prevalent in Eastern United States and Great Lakes region)
  - ***Ixodes pacificus*** → the Western United States
  - ***Ixodes ricinus*** → Europe, ***Ixodes persulcatus*** →Asia
- Pathogenesis: *Ixodes* tick feeds on infected animal reservoir → spirochetes stored in tick's salivary glands → tick bites human and releases Borrelia spirochetes into dermis → erythema migrans develops at bite site 1 to 2 weeks later → if untreated, hematogenous dissemination + systemic symptoms
- Three clinical stages of Lyme disease:
  - Early localized:
    - **Erythema migrans (90%):** initial cutaneous manifestation; develops 7 to 14 days post-tick attachment; p/w **expanding annular plaque w/ central clearing** ("bull's eye" appearance) → **reaches > 5 cm** diameter; favors **trunk** (#1 site in children), **legs** (#1 site in adults), and intertriginous areas; lesion **self-resolves in 4 weeks** if untreated
    - **Disseminated erythema migrans lesions (25%–50%)**: multiple smaller annular lesions; arise days to weeks after primary erythema migrans lesion
    - **Other**: nonspecific flu-like symptoms and regional LAD
  - Early disseminated: as a result of hematogenous spread of spirochetes; arises if initial phase untreated
    - **Borrelial lymphocytoma** (1%, Europe only): strongly a/w ***B. afzelii*** and ***B. garinii***; p/w firm, plum-colored tender nodule/plaque on **earlobes (children)**, or **nipple/areola (adults)**
    - **Arthritis** (60%): mono/oligo-articular (**knee** = most common site); arises weeks to months after initial infection
    - Neurologic abnormalities (10%): most commonly **Bell's palsy**
    - Cardiac complications (5%): **AV block**, myopericarditis
  - Chronic:
    - **Acrodermatitis chronica atrophicans** (10%, **Europe only**): strongly a/w ***B. afzelii and B. garinii;*** occurs months to years after initial infection in middle-aged women; two clinical phases: erythematous plaques with "doughy"/ swollen skin on distal extremities (early phase; easily treated/reversible) → progresses to atrophic "**cigarette-paper**" skin w/ telangiectasias (chronic phase; recalcitrant to treatment) and subcutaneous fibrous nodules overlying joints
    - **Other:** encephalopathy, neuropathy, and chronic arthritis
- Diagnosis:
  - Recognition of **erythema migrans rash = most sensitive** way to confirm Lyme!
  - **Serologic evidence of Lyme infection is often lacking early** (only 41% positive at 1 to 2 weeks, and 88% positive when checked > 2 weeks into infection) → cannot rule out Lyme via negative serologies early in disease course!
  - Tissue PCR/culture: specific, but not sensitive
  - Treatment discussed in Table 5.8
- Other high-yield facts:
  - Peak incidence in **summer** (80% of cases in the United States arise between June and August)
  - **Tick must be attached for > 24 hours** to transmit Lyme → ↑↑↑ risk if > 48 hours of attachment
  - Frequent **coinfection** with Lyme + **Babesiosis** + human granulocytic anaplasmosis **(HGA)** → doxycycline covers all three agents
  - European Lyme disease has: **larger erythema migrans lesions** that persist longer, ↓ **arthritis**, and ↑↑ **neurologic sequelae**

• Other borrelial infections (see Table 5.8)

Nonvenereal (endemic) treponematoses

• Yaws, pinta, and endemic syphilis (bejel) are **all caused by *Treponema pallidum* subspecies** that are morphologically and antigenically identical to the organism responsible for venereal syphilis

Table 5.8 *Borrelia* Infections

Disease	Agent	Vector	Clinical Features	Prescription
Lyme disease	Borrelia *burgdorferi*	***Ixodes dammini*** (Northeast United States and Great Lakes area) ***Ixodes pacificus*** (Western United States) *Ixodes ricinus* (Europe)	As previously discussed in text	First line: **doxycycline** In pregnancy or children <8 years old → **amoxicillin** is treatment of choice
Borrelial lymphocytoma	***B. afzelli*** >*B. garinii*	***I. ricinus*** (Europe)	As previously discussed in text	Doxycycline
Acrodermatitis chronica atrophicans	***B. afzelli*** >*B. garinii*	***I. ricinus*** (Europe)	As previously discussed in text	Doxycycline
Louse-borne relapsing fever (Africa)	*B. recurrentis*	***Pediculus humanus*** var. *corporis* (human body louse)	**3–4 relapses of paroxysmal fevers** w/ nonspecific flu-like symptoms and nonspecific macular or petechial eruption; **more severe** than tick form	Doxycycline
Tick-borne relapsing fever (Western United States)	*B. duttonii* *B. hermsii*	***Ornithodoros*** (soft-bodied ticks)	Like Louse-borne relapsing fever, but only **1–2 relapses** and less severe	Doxycycline

Table 5.9 Nonvenereal Treponematoses

Disease (bacterium)	Most Common Age and Geographic Location	Clinicopathologic Features	Other High-Yield Facts
Yaws (*T. pallidum pertenue*)	Age: children < 15 years old Location: warm, humid, and tropical climates (Africa, Asia, Central and South America, and Pacific Islands)	1° stage: legs most commonly affected; p/w indurated, red, painless papule(s) that enlarges to 1–5 cm, then ulcerates ("Mother Yaw"); occurs at site of inoculation; lower extremities most common; histology shows spongiosis, acanthosis/papillomatosis w/ dermal plasma cell infiltrate 2° stage: multiple, smaller, symmetrical, widespread eruption w/ "daughter yaws" (smaller "mother yaws" vs. "miniature yaws" (firm pink papules); face and intertriginous most common; hyperkeratotic plaques on soles ("crab yaws"); osteoperiostitis, polydactylitis, periosteal thickening 3° stage: **necrotic and ulcerative abscesses** that heal with severe/deforming scars; palmoplantar keratoderma; bony damage (periostitis, osteitis, osteomyelitis)	3° stage only occurs in 10% Mnemonic: **"Yaws = Jaws"** (big, destructive "bites" are taken out of affected skin and bone)
Pinta (*T. pallidum carateum*)	Age: **all ages** equally affected Location: Western hemisphere only (Central and South America)	Skin-only disease 1° stage: legs most commonly affected; p/w papules surrounded by red halo; enlarges over months up to >10 cm plaques 2° stage: smaller scaly papules and psoriasiform plaques erupt ("pintids") and change in color from **red** → **blue** → **brown** → **gray/black** 3° stage: symmetric **vitiligo-like lesions** over bony prominences w/ atrophic epidermis; palmoplantar hyperkeratosis; histology shows lichenoid interface + complete loss of melanin + epidermal atrophy	Mnemonic: "Pinta **only paints the skin** different colors" Mnemonic: "Pinta is a Spanish word → limited to **Spanish America**"
Endemic syphilis/"bejel" (*T. pallidum endemicum*)	Age: children < 15 years old Location: dry, warm climates (North Africa and Southeast Asia)	1° stage: rarely noticed; p/w inconspicuous papule or ulcer in **mouth or on nipples of breastfeeding women**; may have hypomelanotic macules on extremities, genitalia, areolae, and trunk 2° stage: **mucous membrane lesions** (mucosal patches, condyloma lata, and angular stomatitis) + generalized lymphadenopathy + laryngitis +/– skin lesions 3° stage: Gumma formation of mucous membranes (nasopharynx), skin, cartilage and bones (exostosis, periostitis of tibia/fibula; palate/nasal septum affected)	Mnemonic: "similar to venereal syphilis, but **mucosal disease predominates** over skin" or "ENDemic syphilis attacks ENside surfaces"

- All three diseases have primary, secondary, and tertiary stages (Table 5.9)
- Route of transmission: skin, mucous membrane, or fomite contact
- **All except pinta most commonly affect children**
- **All except bejel most commonly begin on legs**
- Serologic assays used for venereal syphilis are also positive in these diseases, but cannot differentiate between them
  - Treponemal tests (FTA-ABS, MHA-TP, and TPHA): specific for treponemal infections, may remain positive for life
  - Non-treponemal tests (RPR and VDRL): less specific, but useful for identifying current or recent infections, or

monitoring response (**four-fold decrease** = successful treatment; **four-fold increase** = reinfection/relapse)
- Histology for all three resembles venereal syphilis
- Treatment: **benzathine PCN** (treatment of choice for all)

IV. Sexually transmitted bacterial infections

Syphilis

- Agent: *T. pallidum* (Gram-negative spirochete)
- Congenital syphilis
  - **Early congenital (<2 years old):** snuffles, perioral fissures, dactylitis, Parrot's pseudoparalysis, syphilitic pneumonitis, epiphysitis, marasmic syphilis, pemphigus syphiliticus, and hepatitis
  - **Late congenital (>2 years old):** keratitis, mulberry molars, Hutchinson's teeth (notched/peg-shaped incisors), rhagades (linear scars at angles of mouth), saddle nose, Higoumenakis syndrome, Clutton's joints, optic atrophy, corneal opacities, and eighth nerve deafness
- Primary (10- to 90-day incubation [avg. = 3 weeks] until chancre)
  - **Chancre (painless**, well-defined, and **indurated** ulcer) w/ enlarged lymph nodes
- Secondary (3–10 weeks postchancre; dissemination to other tissues; clears in 3–12 weeks, but relapses in 25%)
  - Prodromal signs (e.g., malaise, fever, lymph node enlargement, conjunctivitis, hepatosplenomegaly [HSM], arthralgia)
  - Papulosquamous/maculopapular generalized, non-itchy, rash **("copper-colored") w/ papules/plaques on palms/soles** (Fig. 5.11), annular plaques of face
  - **"Moth eaten" alopecia**
  - Split papules (syphilitic perlèche)
  - Mucous patches in oropharynx (condyloma lata-like lesions of the mouth)

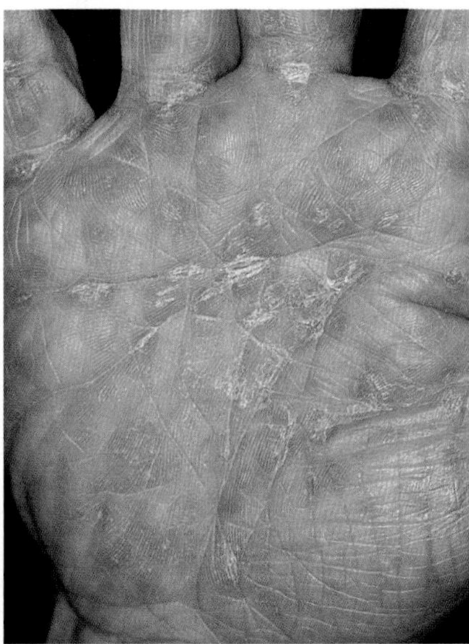

Fig. 5.11 Secondary syphilis. A classic presentation for secondary syphilis with copper-colored scaly plaques on the palms and soles. (From Dinulos JGH. Sexually transmitted bacterial infections. In: *Habif's Clinical Dermatology: A Color Guide to Diagnosis and Therapy.* 7th ed. Philadelphia: Elsevier; 2021:376–412.)

  - Hypopigmented macules on neck ("necklace of Venus")
  - Condyloma lata (analogous to "plaques muqueuses" in oropharynx)
  - HIV patients may have multiple chancres, palmoplantar keratoderma, **lues maligna** (fever/arthralgia/headache → papules/pustules/nodules w/ necrosis/crusting/ulceration)
- Tertiary (months to years after secondary in one third of untreated patients—the period in between is called **latency** and two third of untreated patients stay latent indefinitely)
  - **Gummas** (skin, bones, liver, and organs)
  - Cardiovascular syphilis (e.g., aortitis)—25%
  - Neurosyphilis (e.g., paresis, dementia, meningitis, ataxia, tabes dorsalis, optic atrophy, gummas, and Argyll Robertson pupil (accommodates to light, but does not react)—25%
- Treatment: **IM benzathine PCN** (2.4 M IU × 1 dose for primary/secondary/early latent disease; 7.2 M IU total for late latent disease and cardiovascular/gummatous), aqueous PCN G 18 to 24 M IU daily × 10 to 14 days—neurosyphilis/ocular
  - Doxycycline can be used in allergic patients
- Other high-yield facts:
  - M > F, **↑ in MSM**
  - ↑ Risk of coinfection w/ HIV (any disease that → genital ulcers will increase HIV risk)
  - HIV → ↑ risk of neurosyphilis
  - Serologic studies are divided into **treponemal** (FTA-ABS, MHA-TP, FTA-ABS-19S-IgM, SPHA) and **non-treponemal** (RPR, VDRL; IgG/IgM to **cardiolipin**); FTA-ABS and MHA-TP more sensitive/specific, used mainly to confirm positive non-treponemal tests
  - **RPR and VDRL:** first serologic test to become positive (within 1–2 weeks vs. after third week for treponemal tests); used to monitor response to therapy as titers decrease and then **become negative after successful treatment** (vs. treponemal tests, which remain positive throughout life); **higher false-positive rate** than treponemal tests (esp. pregnancy and systemic lupus erythematosus)
  - Warthin-Starry stain identifies spirochetes
  - Positive darkfield examination (overall most sensitive and specific test for diagnosis of **primary** syphilis, but operator-dependent)
  - Perform **lumbar puncture** for CSF examination in secondary patients with ocular/neurologic symptoms and all tertiary patients
  - Histology of secondary syphilis: **slender, elongated psoriasiform** epidermal hyperplasia + lichenoid interface changes + **"dirty"** dermal inflammatory infiltrate (neutrophils, cell debris, and **abundant plasma cells**)

Other bacterial venereal diseases (Table 5.10)

V. Mycobacterial infections

Cutaneous tuberculosis

- *Mycobacterium tuberculosis* = acid-fast, alcohol-fast, aerobic bacillus, and ↑ risk in HIV

Table 5.10 Venereal Diseases Other Than Syphilis

Disease	Organism	Dermatologic Signs	Treatment	Interesting Facts
Chancroid	***Hemophilus ducreyi*** (Gram-negative coccobacilli)	**Painful**, purulent ulcers with **ragged/ undermined** borders and fibrinous base (may get "kissing ulcers" from apposition of skin with initial ulcer) Prepuce/coronal sulcus/frenulum are common sites Painful, inguinal, typically unilateral, lymphadenitis (40%)	**Azithromycin** 1 g PO × 1 dose (ceftriaxone, ciprofloxacin are alternatives)	**"School of fish"** sign on Giemsa stain of exudate smear M > F; **prostitutes** are major reservoir More common in Africa and Asia
Gonorrhea	*Neisseria gonorrhoeae* (Gram-negative diplococci)	Most findings are not cutaneous, but can get **hemorrhagic acral pustules** w/**arthritis** (of larger joints), and fever (arthritis-dermatosis syndrome) if hematogenous dissemination occurs (more common in menstruation and C5–9 complement deficiencies)	**Dual therapy:** Ceftriaxone 250 mg IM × 1 dose + Azithromycin 1 g PO × 1 dose	F > M Culture is gold standard for diagnosis and susceptibility testing (**Thayer-Martin** media is used) Often see coinfection w/ chlamydia
Lymphogranuloma venereum	*Chlamydia trachomatis* (serotypes L1–3)	**Stage 1** (after 3–12 days of incubation period): painless ulcer which resolves (transient) +/– lymphangitis **Stage 2** (10–30 days, up to 6 months after stage 1): **buboes** (unilateral, painful, erythematous, and enlarged inguinal lymph nodes) w/ "**groove sign**" (enlarged nodes above and below Poupart ligament); buboes may rupture → pus drainage and sinus tracts **Stage 3** (months-years after stage 2; aka ano-genito-rectal syndrome): **proctocolitis** w/ perirectal abscesses, fistulas, strictures/stenoses, and "lymphorrhoids" (perirectal/intestinal lymphatic hyperplasia)	**Doxycycline** 100 mg PO BID × 21 days	**"Gamna-Favre bodies"** in macrophages on Giemsa stain More common in Asia, Africa, and South America M > F
Granuloma inguinale	***Klebsiella granulomatis*** (intracellular Gram-negative bacillus)	Enlarging chronic **painless ulcer** with "**beefy red**," friable, hypertrophic **granulation tissue** (avg. incubation = 17 days) Get "pseudobuboes" (nodules), genital swelling, and secondary infections (→ bad odor) Most common sites: prepuce/glans/ frenulum/coronal sulcus (men); vulvar area (women) May get extragenital lesions as a result of dissemination or autoinoculation (skin, bones, oral, and abdominal)	**Azithromycin** 1 g PO once weekly (or 500 mg daily) for at least 3 weeks AND until all lesions have resolved	**"Safety pin" Donovan bodies** on Wright or Giemsa stain of smears More common in Papua New Guinea, Australia, and South Africa

- Diagnosis made with tuberculin skin test versus interferon-γ release assays (QuantiFERON Gold)
  - Skin test better in children; interferon-γ test better for patients who have had BCG (live, attenuated *Mycobacterium bovis*) vaccination (false-positive with skin test)
- Inoculation-induced
  - Tuberculous chancre: in patients w/o previous infection (hence **no immunity** against TB); 2- to 4-week inoculation period; painless, red, and indurated papule that ulcerates—heals ≤ 12 months; may spread to lymph nodes
  - **TB verruca cutis**: reinfection via inoculation, in patients w/ previous infection w/ moderate to high immunity; #1 form of cutaneous TB; **warty/verrucous**, growing papule may heal over years
- Spread of endogenous infection
  - **Lupus vulgaris**: contiguous spread or hematogenous/ lymphatic; **red-brown**, sometimes annular, papules/plaques (with **"apple jelly"** color on diascopy) that → scarring centrally; head/neck #1 site; **moderate to high immunity** (Fig. 5.12)
  - **Scrofuloderma**: result of **contiguous spread** of infection to skin from underlying disease (usually **cervical lymph nodes** and bones); fluctuant nodules that develop sinus tracts, draining to skin, with tethered appearance; **low immunity**
  - Orificial TB: patients with advanced TB and poor cell-mediated immunity; **autoinoculation of mucosa/skin** close to anatomic orifice draining active systemic TB infection → ulceration/drainage
  - Acute miliary TB: hematogenous dissemination from lung, most often in **immunosuppressed patients**; **pinpoint blue-red crusty papules** → small scars
  - Tuberculous gumma: hematogenous dissemination → deep nodule that ulcerates/drains; immunosuppressed patients

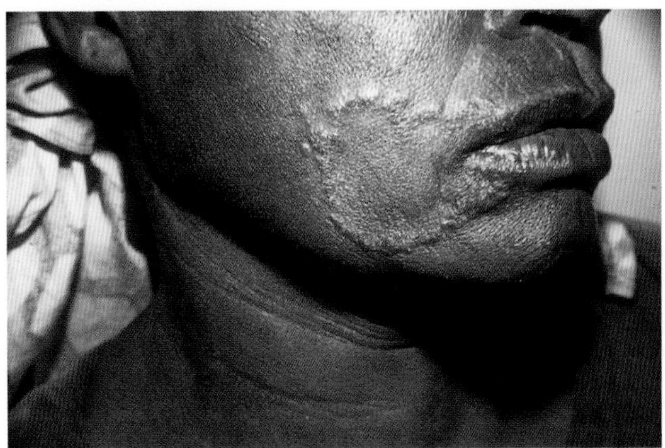

Fig. 5.12 Lupus vulgaris: a perioral annular plaque with a papulomatous border and signs of central clearing in a male patient with pulmonary tuberculosis. (From the collection of Jan and Titia Warndorff, Department of Dermatology, Amsterdam UMC, Amsterdam, The Netherlands.)

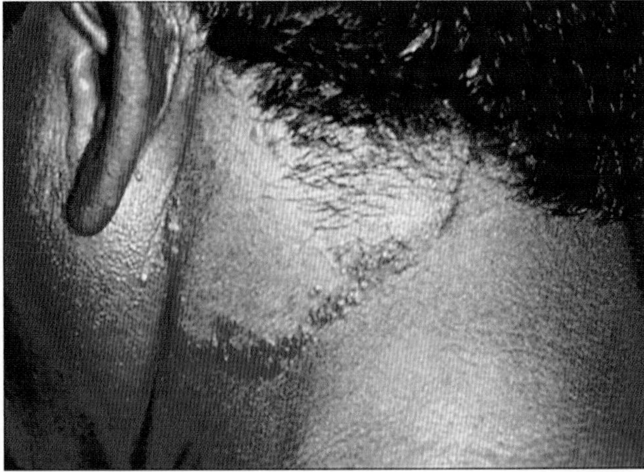

Fig. 5.13 Tuberculoid leprosy. Sharply defined plaque with a raised border and an absence of hair. (Courtesy, Dr. Omar Lupi. From Tyring SK, Lupi O, Hengge UR. Mycobacteria. In: *Tropical Dermatology*. 2nd ed. Philadelphia: Elsevier; 2017:252–279.)

- First-line combination therapy for TB: **rifampin, isoniazid, pyrazinamide, and ethambutol**; isoniazid and/or rifampin can be used in latent infection

Leprosy (Hansen's disease)

- Agent: *Mycobacterium leprae*
  - Obligate intracellular, **weakly acid-fast** bacillus that **parasitizes macrophages** and **Schwann cells**
  - Requires **cool temperatures** (30°C–35°C) for growth → predilection for cooler areas of skin (**nose, testes, and ear lobes**) and **peripheral nerves that lie close to skin surface**
  - Transmitted primarily by **nasal/oral droplets**; also **nine-banded armadillos** in SE United States
  - **Cannot be cultured *in vitro*** → must be cultivated in **mouse footpads** or in armadillos
- Chronic, deforming disease **characterized by skin and nerve involvement**
- **Prolonged incubation period** (avg. 4–10 years, but up to 30 years!); bimodal age range (10–15 years old and 30–60 years old); M > F
- Characterized by **granulomas** and **neurotropism**, both within skin and peripheral nerves
- Primary skin lesion = erythematous, or **hypopigmented**, annular anesthetic/hypoesthetic plaque w/ mild scaling (Fig. 5.13)
- **Peripheral nerves are enlarged in all forms** (except indeterminate)
  - Most commonly affects superficially located nerve trunks (CN-5, CN-7, median, radial, ulnar, greater auricular, posterior tibial, and common peroneal nerves)
  - Damage results in: "**claw hand**" and "papal hand" flexural deformities, **stocking-glove anesthesia**, **neuropathic ulcers** of plantar surfaces, foot drop, atrophy of interosseous muscles, and **ocular damage** (because of CN-7 dysfunction)
- *M. leprae*–specific **cell-mediated immunity** (assessed by lepromin skin test) plays a major role in the **Ridley-Jopling scale** → divides leprosy into **two polar forms** (Lepromatous/LL [Th2 response] and Tuberculoid/TT [Th1 response]), and **three borderline forms** (BL, BB, and BT) (Table 5.11)
  - **Polar forms are stable!** → patients in either polar form (LL or TT) remain in this form throughout their disease course
  - **Borderline forms are unstable** and have clinicopathologic features somewhere in between the polar forms
- **Indeterminate leprosy** (earliest stage of leprosy): p/w solitary, ill-defined hypopigmented macule, without enlargement of peripheral nerves
  - Disease will either self-resolve, or evolve into one of five leprosy forms (LL, BL, BB, BT, or TT)
- Reactional states: abrupt-onset skin lesions that arise in 50% of patients during or after initiation of therapy
  - Type 1 (reversal reaction): result of change in cell-mediated (Th1) immunity against *M. leprae*. May either be **downgrading** (borderline leprosy patient who "downgrades" toward lepromatous pole) or **upgrading** (increase in cell-mediated immunity). Both may p/w **ulceration of existing lesions** and preferential targeting of nerves, resulting in **dangerous neuritis** (= emergency!); generally lacks systemic symptoms (unlike type 2 reactions); highest risk with **borderline forms** (**BL** > BB, BT); treatment = **prednisone**
  - Type 2 (erythema nodosum leprosum): **Th2** (humoral)-mediated formation of **immune complexes**, resulting in multisystem **vasculitis and EN-like lesions** scattered at **previously unaffected** skin sites (medial thighs and extensor forearms are #1 sites); prominent systemic symptoms; **highest risk with LL and BL** patients receiving antimicrobial therapy; **treatment = thalidomide**
  - Lucio phenomenon: **severe necrotizing vasculitis** w/ thrombosis; occurs in patients from **Mexico and Central/South America** with diffuse lepromatous leprosy; p/w purpuric macules and ulcerative bullous lesions below the knees → superinfection/sepsis; **treatment = prednisone**

Table 5.11 Polar and Borderline Leprosy

Clinical Findings	Lepromatous (LL)	Borderline (BB)	Tuberculoid (TT)
Type of lesions	Small hypopigmented macules, papulonodules, and **diffuse infiltration** (→ **leonine facies**, elongated earlobes, and madarosis)	Plaques and dome-shaped lesions	**Dry, scaly, hypopigmented, and anesthetic plaques** with raised peripheral rim and central atrophy +/– alopecia and anhidrosis
Lesion number/size	**Innumerable, small**	Multiple (but countable); variable sizes	**One or few** (<5); large
Distribution	**Widespread and symmetric (face, buttocks, legs)**	Generalized but asymmetric	Localized, asymmetric
Circumscription	**Poorly defined** lesions and difficult to discern edges	Not as sharply defined as TT	**Well-defined**; sharply demarcated raised/indurated borders
Sensation within lesions	**Normal**	↓	Absent
Site of nerve enlargement	Symmetric and **not a/w skin lesions**	Variable	Asymmetric and localized around skin lesions
Lepromin test	Negative	+	+++
Cell-mediated immunity	None (**Th2** >> Th1) IL-4, -5, -10, -13	Unstable	**Strong** (**Th1** >> Th2) IL-2, IFN-γ
Humoral immunity	**Strong**	Unstable	None
Bacilli in skin lesions	**++++ (globi)** **Multibacillary**	++ Multibacillary	None Paucibacillary
AFB stain (Fite-Faraco stain is best)	++++	++	Negative
Histology	**Grenz zone**, diffuse infiltrate of **parasitized foamy histiocytes (Virchow cells)**, plasma cells, free-floating **clumps of bacilli (globi)** in dermis, and "onion-skin" pattern around nerves; lacks well-formed granulomas	Overlap of LL and TT findings, organisms easily seen	Well-formed sarcoidal **granulomas w/ linear arrangement (East-West) along nerves**, numerous Langhans giant cells, fragmented nerve fibers, lacks organisms (no globi or Virchow cells), and Grenz zone
Associated findings	Acquired ichthyosis, **saddle nose**, lagophthalmos, corneal anesthesia, blindness, and orchitis (→ sterility and gynecomastia)		One-sided neuropathic changes of extremities (e.g., bone resorption → short digits)
Other comments	**High risk for type 2 reaction** Lesions do not have anhidrosis or alopecia Histoid leprosy (subtype of LL)—dermatofibroma- and neurofibroma-like lesions **Ziehl-Neelsen, Fite, Gram stains** all (+) for bacilli False (+) VDRL, FTA-ABS	Borderline categories (BL, BB, and BT) are **highest risk for type 1 reactions** BL is high risk for type 2 reaction	Skin lesions favor face, extremities, and cool areas of trunk TT often self resolves in 3 years

- Treatment (WHO recommendations):
  - Multibacillary (duration = 12 months): **rifampicin** 600 mg Qmonth + **dapsone** 100 mg QD + **clofazimine** 300 mg once a month and 50 mg daily
  - Paucibacillary (duration = 6 months): **rifampicin**: 600 mg Qmonth + **dapsone** 100 mg QD
  - Single skin lesion paucibacillary leprosy (duration = single dose): **rifampicin** 600 mg + **ofloxacin** 400 mg + **minocycline** 100 mg

Atypical mycobacteria

- *Mycobacterium avium* complex: more commonly seen in **AIDS patients**; found in **environment** (water, soil, and animals); pulmonary infection is most common finding; skin findings w/ primary inoculation or via dissemination (pustules, ulcers on legs, and nodules); ↑ alkaline phosphatase; clarithromycin/azithromycin + ethambutol +/– rifampin
- *Mycobacterium marinum:* acquired via **cutaneous contact** (usually hands w/ abrasions) with aquatic environments (e.g., **fish tanks** and swimming pools) → erythematous/blue ulcerating nodules in a **sporotrichoid** pattern; diagnosis is confirmed with culture: *M. marinum* **grows best at 31°C** (~3 weeks required for growth), as opposed to the usual 37°C for most other mycobacteria; treatment: **clarithromycin** +/– rifampin/ethambutol, **minocycline**, and TMP-SMX
- *Mycobacterium ulcerans:* aka **Buruli ulcer**; usually in Africa, in areas close to water bodies; minor trauma → nodule → ulcer on **extremities; can become . 15 cm** and extend to bones; treatment: **excision (treatment of choice)**, local heating, rifampin + streptomycin + clarithromycin, and amputation
- *Mycobacterium fortuitum, chelonae, and abscessus:* **rapid growing mycobacteria** (Table 5.12); saprophytic organisms; can get infections post-trauma/surgery or **medical treatments (e.g., implant placement, liposuction, and botulinum toxin)**/tattoo/**nail salon footbaths**; skin presentations vary, but **most common** is **inflamed subcutaneous nodules in sporotrichoid pattern; clarithromycin is treatment of choice**, but surgical treatment may be needed

Table 5.12 Mycobacteria That Cause Cutaneous Disease

Group and Pigment	Rate of Growth	Pathogens
Slow growers		
Photochromogens[a]	2–3 weeks	*M. kansasii, M. marinum, M. simiae*
Scotochromogens[b]	2–3 weeks	*M. scrofulaceum, M. szulgai, M. gordonae, M. xenopi*
Nonchromogens[c]	2–3 weeks	*M. tuberculosis, M. avium, M. intracellulare, M. ulcerans, M. haemophilum, M. malmoense, M. terrae, M. genavense, M. bovis,*[d] *M. nonchromogenicum*
Rapid growers	3–5 days	*M. fortuitum, M. chelonae, M. smegmatis, M. abscessus, M. immunogenum, M. goodii, M. wolinskyi, M. cosmeticum, M. mucogenicum*
Non-cultured (to date)		M. leprae

[a]*Capable of yellow pigment formation upon exposure to light.*
[b]*Capable of yellow pigment production without light exposure.*
[c]*Incapable of pigment production.*
[d]*Including bacillus Calmette-Guérin.*
Modified classification of Runyon.

5.4 FUNGAL DISEASES

I. Superficial mycoses

Dermatophytes

- Species—three genera: *Microsporum, Epidermophyton,* and *Trichophyton*
  - Generally cause superficial skin infections and nail infections
  - The most common organism(s) that cause(s) various manifestations are as follows:
    - **Tinea capitis—*Trichophyton tonsurans*** (#1 cause in United States), ***Microsporum canis*** (#1 cause worldwide; more inflammatory), and *Tinea violaceum* (East Africa)
      - **Endothrix (black dot** appearance from breakage near scalp; **arthroconidia within hair shaft)**: *T. rubrum, T. tonsurans, T. schoenleinii, T. yaounde, T. violaceum, T. gourvilli,* and *T. soudanense* (mnemonic: "Ringo Gave Yoko Two Squeaky Violins")
      - **Ectothrix (**gray patch appearance = scaly patches of alopecia; **arthrospores around hair shaft)**
        - → Fluorescent (via Wood lamp—**pteridine**): *M. canis, M. audouinii* (formerly #1 cause in children), *M. gypseum, M. ferrugineum, M. distortum,* and *T. schoenleinii* (mnemonic: "Cats And Dogs Fight and Growl Sometimes")
        - → Nonfluorescent: *T. mentagrophytes, T. rubrum, M. nanum, T. megninii, T. gypseum,* and *T. verrucosum*
      - **Favus**—*T. schoenleinii* > *M. gypseum, T. violaceum*
      - **Kerion**—*M. canis, T. verrucosum, T. mentagrophytes,* and *T. tonsurans*
    - **Majocchi granuloma**—*T. rubrum* most common
    - **Tinea corporis**—*T. rubrum* most common
      - Zoophilic species (i.e., in farmers and pets)—*T. verrucosum* and *M. canis*
    - **Tinea imbricata**—*T. concentricum*
    - **Tinea barbae**—*T. verrucosum, T. mentagrophytes, T. tonsurans,* and *T. rubrum*
    - **Tinea faciei**—usually zoophilic species (*M. canis* and *T. metagrophytes*) > *T. rubrum*; most commonly in kids after visiting rural areas
    - **Tinea cruris**—*T. rubrum, E. floccosum,* and *T. interdigitale*
    - **Tinea pedis** (Tinea manuum has same causative organisms)
      - Moccasin, interdigital, and ulcerative—*T. rubrum* > *E. floccosum* (mocassin), *T. interdigitale* (interdigital)
      - Vesicular/bullous—***T. mentagrophytes***
    - **Onychomycosis**
      - Distal subungual: ***T. rubrum,*** *T. interdigitale,* and *E. floccosum*
      - Proximal white subungual—*T. rubrum*
      - **↑ Risk in HIV**
      - White superficial—*T. mentagrophytes* (adults) versus *T. rubrum* (children)
      - Less common causes: *Candida albicans* (most commonly in setting of mucocutaneous candidiasis), *Fusarium* spp. (white superficial onychomycosis), *Scytalidium* spp. (dark onychomycosis with chronic paronychia), and *Scopulariopsis brevicaulis* (white superficial onychomycosis)
  - Geography—ubiquitous; fungi are classified according to their normal habitat:
    - Anthropophilic: restricted to humans and cause a chronic, mild inflammatory response; includes **all *Trichophyton* spp.** (except *T. mentagrophytes* and *T. verrucosum*), ***E. floccosum, M. audouinii,*** and *M. ferrugineum*
    - Zoophilic: primarily affect animals; cause massive inflammatory response in humans; includes ***M. canis*** (cats and dogs), ***M. nanum*** (pigs), ***T. verrucosum*** (cattle), and ***T. mentagrophytes*** (rodents)
    - Geophilic: found in soil; cause severe inflammatory response and scarring in humans; ***M. gypseum*** (soil) is the only common species in this class
  - Histology—septate hyphae in stratum corneum or nail plate, **brisk dermal inflammation** (vs. minimal in tinea versicolor) +/− neutrophilic microabscesses in epidermis or corneum/nail plate
    - PAS (red) and GMS (black)
  - Diagnosis—KOH (helps break down keratin making fungi more visible) +/− culture
    - Chlorazol black E—**chitin stain**—hyphae will be green
    - Calcofluor white—chitin stain—blue or green with **fluorescence** microscopy
  - Pathogenesis: virulence factors (hydrolases and keratinases) allow penetration into stratum corneum

and the released enzymes induce inflammation (Th1 response)
- Clinical presentation:
  - Tinea corporis/cruris: annular/arcuate scaly patches/plaques with inflamed and possibly palpable borders +/− pustules; **tinea cruris spares scrotum** (unlike candidiasis)
  - Tinea pedis: erythema with scale, especially between toes (maceration) and sides of feet
- Tinea manuum: **non**-erythematous scaling (+/− collarettes of scale) of palm of one hand + moccasin-type tinea pedis; treat with systemic antifungals
  - Tinea capitis: circular scaling patches +/− pustules +/− **LAD**; may have black dots from broken hairs in endothrix infections; treat with systemic antifungals
    - Usually school age children; **↑ in blacks/males**
    - Kerion: boggy inflamed nodule/abscess with pustules and possible LAD which may → scarring
    - Favus: yellow cup-shaped crusts **(scutula)** that cluster together, resulting in a honeycomb appearance and can → scarring
    - Green fluorescence of infected hairs with Wood lamp may be seen with *Microsporum* infection
    - Dermatoscopy: comma and corkscrew hairs
  - Tinea imbricata: concentric and **polycyclic** rings of scale
  - Majocchi's granuloma: erythematous papules/nodules around hair follicles, particularly lower legs (may arise from tinea pedis); treat with systemic antifungals
  - Tinea faciei: erythematous follicular-based papules, often in an annular distribution most common in kids; treat with systemic antifungals
- Treatment: topical or systemic terbinafine or azole antifungals, topical naftifine
  - Terbinafine and griseofulvin have equivalent safety/efficacy in children in the treatment of tinea capitis; **terbinafine more effective for *T. tonsurans*** and **griseofulvin more effective for *Microsporum***
  - Onychomycosis: systemic terbinafine is most effective but itraconazole/fluconazole can be used particularly in non-dermatophyte onychomycosis; tavaborole, ciclopirox, and efinaconazole solutions are not as effective but safer

Tinea versicolor (pityriasis versicolor)

- Species: ***Malassezia globosa* and *M. furfur***; yeast form is normal skin flora; transforms to filamentous/hyphal form in disease states; culture requires **olive oil** for growth
- More common in darker skin/adolescents/summer
- Histology: hyphae and spores **("spaghetti and meatballs")** seen in stratum corneum (also on KOH)
- Pathogenesis: overgrowth of normal flora, which is ubiquitous (esp. with warmth and humidity in the right host); **hypopigmentation** due to **melanocyte inhibition by azelaic acid** (dicarboxylic acid byproduct of *Malassezia*)
- Clinical presentation: hyper- or hypopigmented finely scaling circular/oval macules/patches in sebaceous distribution (scalp, face, neck, upper chest, and upper back)
- Treatment: topical or systemic **azole-antifungals**, selenium sulfide shampoo, or topical ciclopirox

Piedra

- Species:
  - Black—***Piedra hortae***
  - White—***Trichosporon asahii*** (most strongly linked to white piedra; may cause **disseminated disease in immunocompromised** patients), ***T. ovoides, T. inkin,*** *and T. cutaneum*
- Geography: tropical
- Pathogenesis: found in water and soil in tropics
- Microscopy: black or white **concretions along hair** (encircle hairs, unlike the sac-like appearance of lice)
  - **White piedra with soft mobile nodules; black piedra with hard nonmobile nodules**
- Clinical presentation: asymptomatic hair breakage on scalp, axillary, and pubic region
- Treatment: **hair shaving/cutting** and antifungal shampoos; systemic antifungals if recalcitrant

Tinea nigra

- Species: ***Hortaea werneckii***
- Geography: tropical and subtropical, especially coastal
- Microscopy: dark brown septate hyphae with budding yeast in thickened stratum corneum
- Pathogenesis: overgrowth of fungus
- Clinical presentation: dark-brown/**black macule or small patch on palms/soles**, limited to stratum corneum
- Treatment: azole creams, Whitfield's ointment; oral terbinafine if recalcitrant

II. Subcutaneous mycoses

Sporotrichosis

- Species: *Sporothrix schenckii*
- Geography: **ubiquitous saprophyte**; endemic to Central/South America and Africa
- Microscopy: usually not well-visualized with stains; granulomatous inflammation with plasma cells and asteroid corpuscles (Splendore-Hoeppli phenomenon); organisms are **cigar-shaped budding yeast**
- Pathogenesis: traumatic inoculation from soil via plant thorns, **wood splinters, and sphagnum moss** >> cats/rodents/armadillo bites; inhalation of spores
- Clinical presentation: **multiple ascending ulcerated nodules** or subcutaneous abscesses, most frequently in gardeners, agriculture/farm workers, and veterinarians
  - May → erythema nodosum
- Treatment: obtain fungal culture (difficult to find in tissue samples), **itraconazole (treatment of choice)**, **SSKI**, and amphotericin B in disseminated disease (Box 5.3)

Box 5.3 "No SALT" Mnemonic

Sporotrichoid spread: **No**cardia, **S**porotrichosis, **A**typical mycobacteria, **L**eishmaniasis, **T**ularemia (**No SALT**)

Lobomycosis

- Species: *Lacazia (Loboa loboi)*
- Geography: infects **freshwater dolphins** in South American rivers
- Microscopy: thick-walled yeast with tubular connections between cells—**"pop bead" or "chain of coins" appearance**
- Pathogenesis: unable to be cultured *in vitro*
- Clinical presentation: **keloid-like** verrucous fibrotic nodules that can ulcerate; **ear helix** #1 site; men >> women; rural areas
- Treatment: **surgical excision**

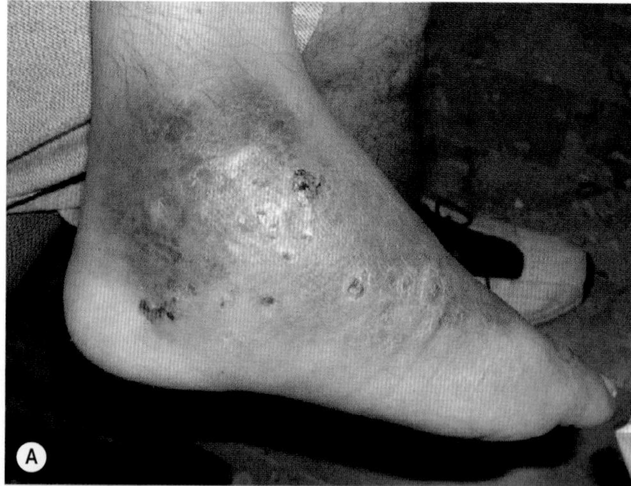

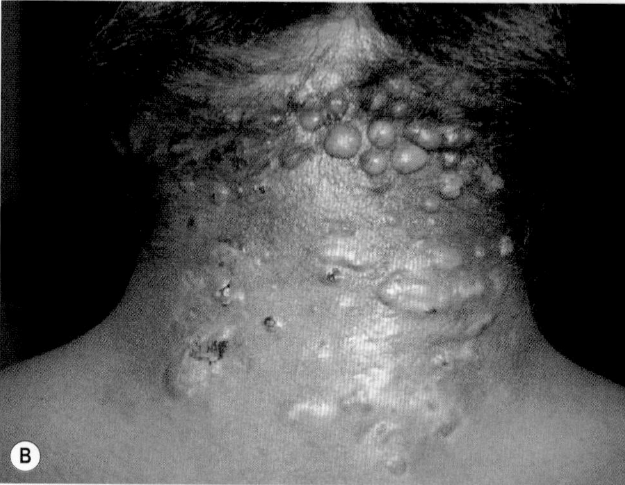

Fig. 5.14 Mycetoma cases produced by *Nocardia brasiliensis*. **(A)** Inflammation of the dorsum of the foot and ankle showing abscesses and sinuses. **(B)** Mycetoma of the back of the neck. (From Welsh O, Vera-Cabrera L, Salinas-Carmona MC. Mycetoma. *Clin Dermatol.* 2007;25[2]:195–202.)

Mycetoma (madura foot)

- Species:
  - **Eumycetoma (fungus)**—*Madurella* spp. *Pseudallescheria boydii* (most common), *Exophiala jeanselmei*, and *Acremonium* spp.
  - **Actinomycetoma (bacteria)**—*Nocardia* (*N. brasiliensis* [#1 bacterial cause] and *N. asteroides* both have **white grains**), *Actinomadura* spp. (***A. pelletieri* = red grains**; *A. madurae* = cream or pink grains), and *Streptomyces somaliensis* (**yellow grains**)
- Geography: southern tropics (Latin America, India, and Africa), a/w poverty and bare feet; young men
- Microscopy: granulomatous reaction with grains; serologic testing used because of culture difficulty
- Pathogenesis: traumatic inoculation
- Clinical presentation (Fig. 5.14): slow progression of tumors (tumefaction) with **sinus tracts draining grains**, which are fungal or bacterial aggregates; most common on **feet/lower legs**; long-standing lesions → bone and visceral involvement
  - **Black grains only seen in eumycetoma** and **red grains only seen in actinomycetoma** (specifically *A. pelletieri*)
- Treatment:
  - Actinomycetoma: streptomycin/amikacin + TMP-SMX
  - Eumycetoma: surgical debridement and several month courses of azole antifungals

Chromoblastomycosis

- Species: ***Fonsecaea pedrosoi*** (most common), *Fonsecaea compacta* and *Fonsecaea monophora, Rhinocladiella aquaspersa, Phialophora verrucosa,* and *Cladophialophora carrionii*
- Geography: tropical and subtropical climates; found in decaying vegetation and soil
- Microscopy (Fig. 5.15): pseudoepitheliomatous hyperplasia (PEH), granulomatous dermal inflammation with **medlar bodies** (pigmented muriform cells, **"copper pennies"**)
- Pathogenesis: traumatic inoculation by thorns or splinters
- Clinical presentation (Fig. 5.16): weeks to months after inoculation of lower extremity, pruritic papules/nodules expand → verrucous plaque with black dots; does not invade muscle or bone; chronic lesions can → SCC
- Treatment: itraconazole, 5-flucytosine + amphotericin B, voriconazole; surgical excision for small lesions

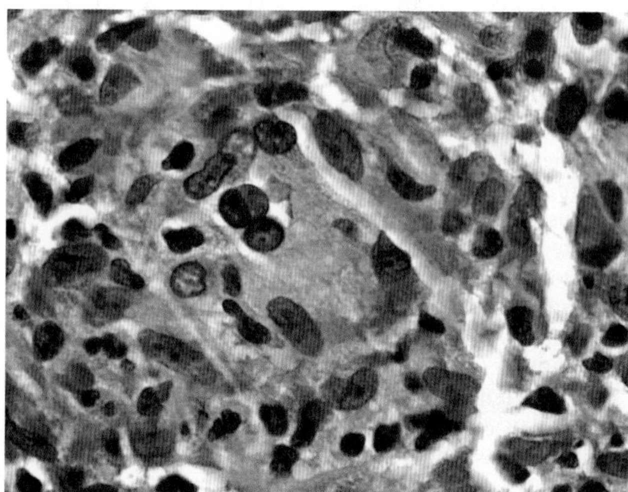

Fig. 5.15 Fumagoid cells, or sclerotic or Medlar bodies. (H&E, original magnification 40×) (Courtesy of Dr. Derek Marsee, Diagnostic Pathology Medical Group.)

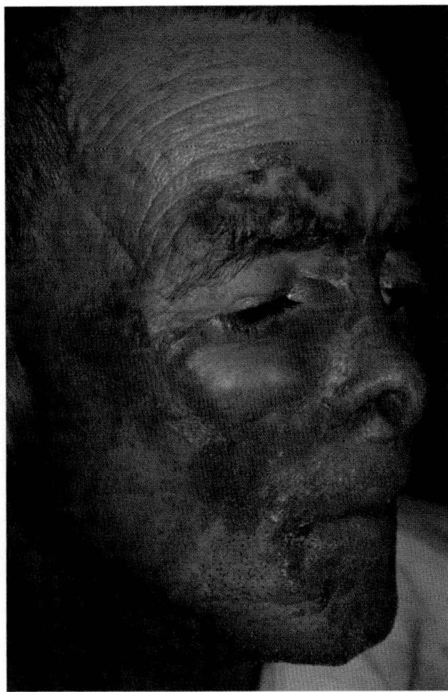

Fig. 5.16 Chromoblastomycosis, facial lesions. (From Torres-Guerrero E, Isa-Isa R, Isa R, Arenas R. Chromoblastomycosis. *Clin Dermatol*. 2012;30[4]:403–408.)

III. Systemic (dimorphic) mycoses

Histoplasmosis

- Species: *Histoplasma capsulatum* var. *capsulatum*
  - African: *Histoplasma capsulatum* var. *duboisii*
- Geography: **Ohio and Mississippi River valley**
- Microscopy (Fig. 5.17): tuberculoid **granuloma with intracellular 2 to 4 μm yeast** in histiocytes (looks like leishmaniasis, but see yeast have **surrounding halo** and are more evenly distributed throughout histiocyte cytoplasm; **lacks "marquee sign" and kinetoplast**) (Box 5.4)

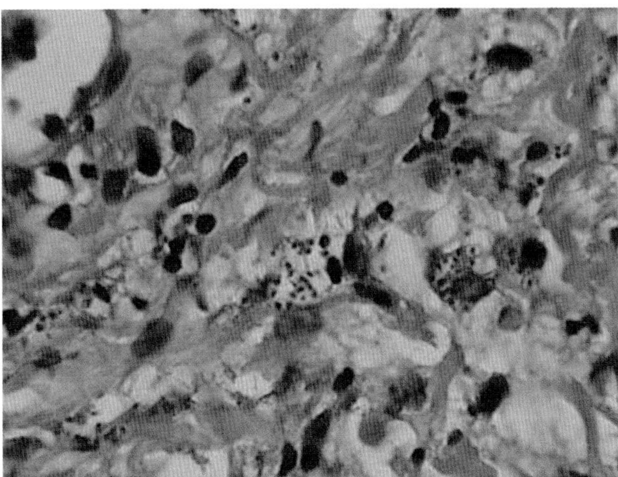

Fig. 5.17 Histoplasmosis. Biopsy specimen shows periodic acid Schiff-positive intracellular yeast. (From Chang P, Rodas C. Skin lesions in histoplasmosis. *Clin Dermatol.* 2012;30[6]:592–598.)

Box 5.4 Diseases With Parasitized Macrophages

Rhinoscleroma	Leishmaniasis
Granuloma inguinale	Penicilliosis
Histoplasmosis	Emmonsiosis

- Pathogenesis: inhalation (esp. **bird and bat feces**) with hematogenous spread (can go to liver, spleen, bone marrow, and brain; **skin involvement more common in HIV**, often p/w **umbilicated** or "molluscoid" papules)
- Clinical presentation: primary cutaneous chancre with lymphangitis and lymphadenitis (rare); more commonly, secondary cutaneous molluscoid nodules, cellulitis, **ulcers (particularly oral)**, and panniculitis
  - Pulmonary manifestations = most common presentation
- Treatment: itraconazole (mild-moderate disease), or amphotericin B (severe disease)

Blastomycosis ("North American blastomycosis")

- Species: *Blastomyces dermatitidis*
- Geography: **Eastern United States** (esp. SE), Great Lakes, Ohio, and **Mississippi River valleys**
- Microscopy: PEH, granulomatous dermal inflammation with unipolar budding yeast (8–18 μm) (**broad-based buds**)
- Pathogenesis: inhalation with subsequent hematogenous spread to skin (>75% of cases), bones, and genitourinary tract (e.g., prostate, spleen, liver, and brain)
- Clinical presentation: primary cutaneous form (rare) presents with lymphangitis and lymphadenitis at injury site; **secondary cutaneous form** (more common; due to hematogenous dissemination from lungs to skin), presents with verrucous plaques, papulopustules, and ulcers (can occur orally as well)
  - **Pulmonary manifestations** = most common presentation
- Treatment: polyene and azole antifungals (mainly **itraconazole**) and amphotericin B (severe disease)

Coccidioidomycosis

- Species: *Coccidioides immitis* and *Coccidioides posadasii*
- Geography: desert Southwest United States (esp. **Central Valley/San Joaquin Valley, California**), Mexico, and Central/South America
- Microscopy (Fig. 5.18): **large (up to 100 μm) spherules containing endospores**; also has PEH and granulomatous inflammation
- Pathogenesis: inhalation with hematogenous spread to skin (as well as **CNS** and bone); very rarely primary cutaneous infection
- Clinical presentation: face #1 site; verrucous nodules/papules (can be molluscum-like), pustules, abscesses, or ulcerative lesions
  - Pulmonary manifestations = most common presentation
- Treatment: limited and cutaneous: itraconazole; severe: amphotericin B; meningeal: amphotericin B and fluconazole; voriconazole also an option

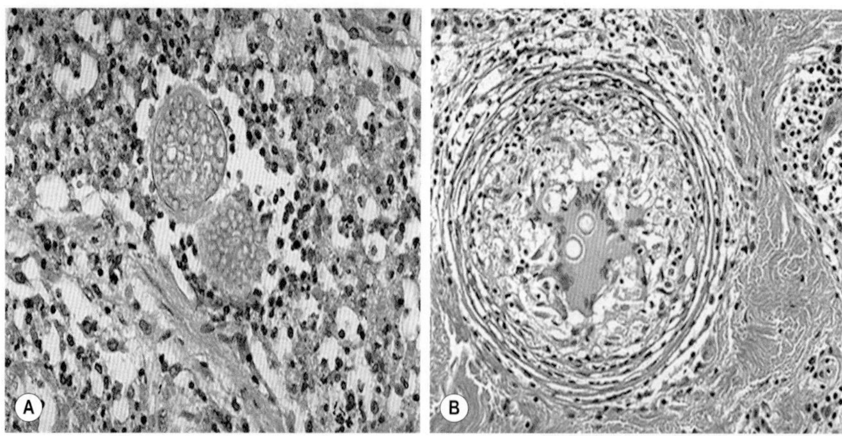

Fig. 5.18 Coccidioidomycosis. Granulomas show large spherules and a giant cell containing small spherules (H&E; original magnification 400×). (From Welsh O, Vera-Cabrera L, Rendon A, Gonzalez G, Bonifaz A. Coccidioidomycosis. *Clin Dermatol*. 2012;30[6]:573–591.)

Paracoccidioidomycosis ("South American blastomycosis")

- Species: *Paracoccidioides brasiliensis*
- Geography: southern United States, Mexico, and Central/**South America**
- Microscopy: PEH, granulomatous dermal inflammation with multipolar budding yeast (**mariner's wheel** or **Mickey Mouse**)
- Pathogenesis: inhalation of infected soil (can disseminate to skin, liver, adrenal glands, lymph nodes, gastrointestinal tract, and spleen); rarely may arise from direct inoculation in skin
- Clinical presentation: granulomatous ulcerative **oropharyngeal and perioral** involvement in 70% of adults; cutaneous lesions can be contiguous, hematogenous, or via inoculation; clinical appearance of ulcers with infiltrated borders (verrucous) and hemorrhagic dots, and associated LAD (can be massive)
  - **Men** >>> women
  - Pulmonary disease (granulomatous and chronic) most common presentation
- Treatment: mild: TMP-SMX; moderate: itraconazole; meningeal: fluconazole or voriconazole; severe: amphotericin B

IV. Opportunistic systemic mycoses

Candidiasis

- Species: ***C. albicans*** (most common in systemic and localized infections), ***C. tropicalis*** (also very common; in systemic infection, frequently disseminates to skin), *C. parapsilosis* (commonly seen in chronic paronychia), *C. glabrata* (fluconazole resistance), *C. krusei* (fluconazole resistance), and *C. dubliniensis* (oropharyngeal candidiasis in HIV patients)
- Geography: ubiquitous
- Microscopy: KOH = **yeast and pseudohyphae**
- Pathogenesis:
  - *Candida* species form biofilm on plastic medical devices
  - SAPs (secretory aspartyl proteinases) and phospholipases aid in fungal adhesion and tissue invasion
  - Chitin, mannoprotein, and glucan may function as adhesins, which allow *Candida* to adhere to mucosal surfaces
  - *C. albicans* exists in normal flora of skin and digestive/GU tracts with pathologic state with immunosuppression, and debilitation and imbalances in microbiome
- Clinical presentation:
  - Mucocutaneous candidiasis: vaginal candidiasis, **oral thrush** ("cottage cheese" like), **median rhomboid glossitis** (central smooth erythema of tongue), onychomycosis, **chronic paronychia** (not always involved but often), **candidal intertrigo** (typically see beefy red color + satellite pustules +/– erosions), **angular cheilitis** (perlèche; risk factors: edentulous, elderly, atopic dermatitis, and vitamin deficiencies), and **erosio interdigitalis blastomycetica (third web space of fingers**; also fourth web space of toes)
    - Risk factors: **DM2** and corticosteroids/immunosuppression (if chronic/severe may be sign of HIV)
  - Deep-seated candidiasis: usually starts in GI tract; 10% of bloodstream infections; 30% mortality in systemic candidiasis despite antifungal therapy
    - Usually in immunosuppressed patients who are neutropenic
    - See scattered papules/nodules, occ. hemorrhagic and ecthyma gangrenosum-like
    - Also infect muscles, retina, internal organs, and heart valves
  - Treatment:
    - Mucocutaneous: polyenes (e.g., nystatin) and azole preparations (e.g., clotrimazole and fluconazole)
      - ***C. glabrata* and *C . krusei* have lower sensitivity to azole antifungals; *C. albicans* is developing resistance to fluconazole**
    - Systemic: amphotericin B, azoles, and echinocandins (first-line in disseminated candidiasis)

Cryptococcosis

- Species: ***C. neoformans*** and *C. gattii*
- Geography: in bird droppings (particularly **pigeons**) and bark/fruit of tropical trees; *C. neoformans*—ubiquitous, *C. gattii*—tropical, subtropical

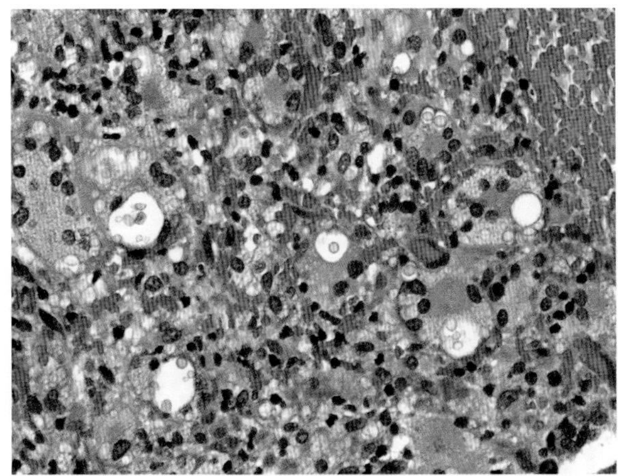

Fig. 5.19 Cryptococcosis. Soap bubble appearance of organisms (H&E, 40x). (Courtesy of Dr. Derek Marsee, Diagnostic Pathology Medical Group.)

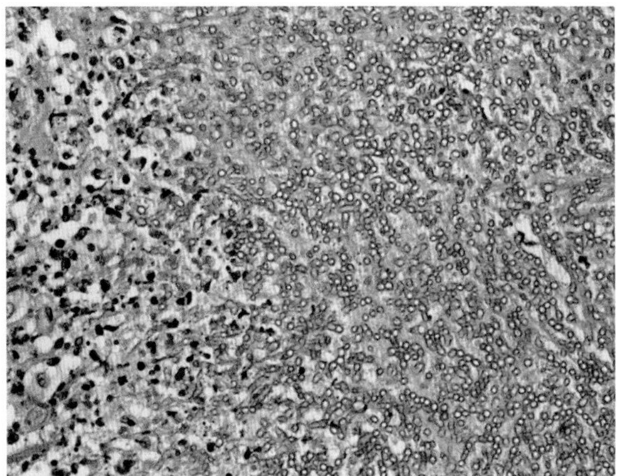

Fig. 5.20 Septated hyphae of Aspergillus spp. in the dermis. (Courtesy of Dr. Derek Marsee, Diagnostic Pathology Medical Group.)

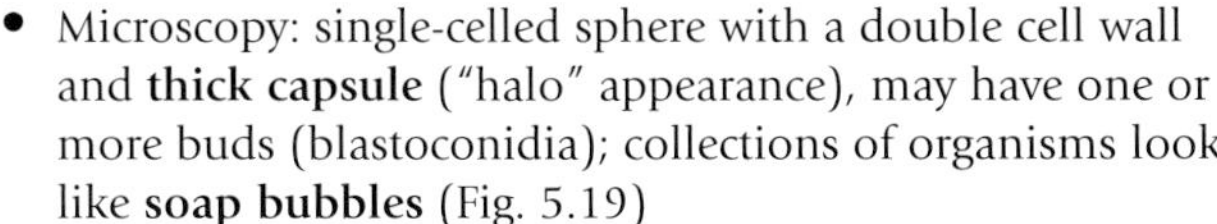

- Microscopy: single-celled sphere with a double cell wall and **thick capsule** ("halo" appearance), may have one or more buds (blastoconidia); collections of organisms look like **soap bubbles** (Fig. 5.19)
  - Stains: **India ink, PAS, mucicarmine, GMS,** and Fontana-Masson
- Pathogenesis: inhalation → lungs (1° pulmonary infection, usually mild) → hematogenous spread (CNS, bones, and skin); can also arise from primary inoculation of skin (rare)
  - More common in immunosuppressed individuals (esp. in **HIV/AIDS**, but also associated with sarcoidosis and pregnancy)
  - Glucuronoxylomannan polysaccharide capsule is a virulence factor
- Disease manifestation
  - **Papules/nodules (often molluscum-like)** that can be **umbilicated** and/or ulcerated, and prefer **head/neck, mouth, and nose**
    - Patients with 2° cutaneous lesions have high mortality rate
  - Nodular lymphangitic syndrome—nodule at inoculation site, nodular lymphangitis, and adenopathy
  - **Meningoencephalitis** is a serious and common manifestation
- Treatment—mild: **oral fluconazole**; CNS: amphotericin B and flucytosine

Aspergillosis

- Species: ***Aspergillus fumigatus* most common**, *A. flavus* (second most common), and *A. niger* (can → otomycosis)
- Geography: ubiquitous in soil
- Microscopy (Fig. 5.20): **septate hyphae with 45° angle branching**
- Pathogenesis:
  - Can be **1° cutaneous** disease (most commonly ***A. flavus***) via direct inoculation (e.g., **IV catheter**, trauma sites, **burn sites**, and disturbed skin under dressings) versus **2° cutaneous** disease (most commonly ***A. fumigatus***; more common, typically in immunosuppressed, esp. neutropenic) via inhalation → pulmonary aspergillosis → disseminated disease
    - Both can → hematogenous spread with a tendency for **vascular invasion causing thrombus and necrosis**
- Clinical presentation: six clinical forms including erythematous edematous plaques, nodules with necrotic centers, subcutaneous nodules (2° cutaneous) hemorrhagic bullae, and necrotic ulcers
  - Can involve CNS, heart, kidneys, bone, and GI tract
- Treatment: azoles (e.g., **voriconazole—first line**), echinocandins, and amphotericin B

Fusarium

- Species: *Fusarium solani* most common
- Geography: ubiquitous in soil
- Microscopy: **45° angle branching**, similar to *Aspergillus*
- Pathogenesis: more common in immunosuppressed; severe burns (**most common fungus cultured in burn patients**); cutaneous disease via direct inoculation and hematogenous spread with a tendency for vascular invasion causing thrombus/necrosis
- Clinical presentation: erythematous; edematous plaques more common than subcutaneous nodules (purpuric or ecthyma gangrenosum-like); panniculitis
- Treatment: no well-established treatment due to drug resistance (cannot treat with caspofungin); localized disease amenable to surgical debridement and systemic antifungal therapy (e.g., voriconazole, posaconazole)

Penicilliosis

- Species: ***P. marneffei*** is only pathogenic species
- Geography: **Southeast Asia**
- Microscopy: intracellular parasitic phase in macrophages
- Pathogenesis: acquired by inhalation or possibly abrasions; **bamboo rat exposure** may be risk factor
- Clinical presentation: similar to histoplasmosis: fever, weight loss, LAD, cough, and hepatosplenomegaly
  - Cutaneous manifestations: papules with central necrosis and **molluscum-like lesions**; face, arms, and trunk are most common sites
- Treatment: polyenes (amphotericin B and terbinafine) and azole antifungals

V. Uncommon fungal, protozoal, and algae pathogens

Zygomycosis (mucormycosis)

- Species:
  - Order *Mucorales*, genera *Rhizopus, Rhizomucor, Mucor, Absidia,* and others—**systemic and cutaneous** disease
  - Order *Entomophthorales* (e.g., *Conidiobolus coronatus*)—rare, chronic, **cutaneous, and subcutaneous** infection in tropics
- Geography: ubiquitous in soil and decaying vegetation
- Microscopy (Fig. 5.21): **broad ribbon-like nonseptate** hyphae with **90° angle** branching, angioinvasive with thrombosis
- Pathogenesis: most commonly enter via respiratory tract (though there are other portals of entry like skin), and can **invade blood vessels → thrombosis/infarction/necrosis**
  - More common in immunosuppressed patients, but also nonimmunodeficient (e.g., severe diabetes and severe burns)
- Disease manifestation—subtypes include: **rhinocerebral** (most common subtype; usually in **diabetes** patients with DKA), pulmonary, GI, **primary cutaneous** (from surgery, catheterization, or burns), and disseminated
  - All forms are rapidly progressing and **commonly fatal**
  - Cutaneous lesions (can be primary or secondary) typically indurated, **necrotic black plaques/eschars** most commonly seen on face (nasal and oral in rhinocerebral type)
  - Rhinocerebral type may have epistaxis, facial pain, periorbital cellulitis, proptosis, and loss of extraocular muscle movement (2° to cranial nerve palsies)
- Treatment: **aggressive surgical resection** of all necrotic areas (crucial to survival of patient) and **amphotericin B** (lipid formulation); posaconazole, isavuconazole may be alternatives

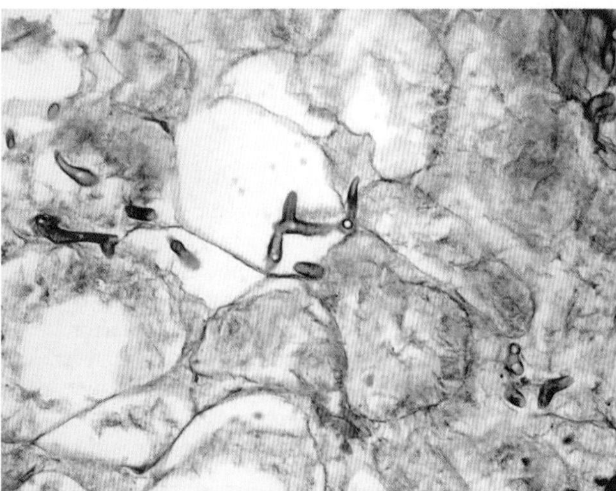

Fig. 5.21 Zygomycosis. Nonseptate thick hyphae (H&E, 40x). (Courtesy of Dr. Derek Marsee, Diagnostic Pathology Medical Group.)

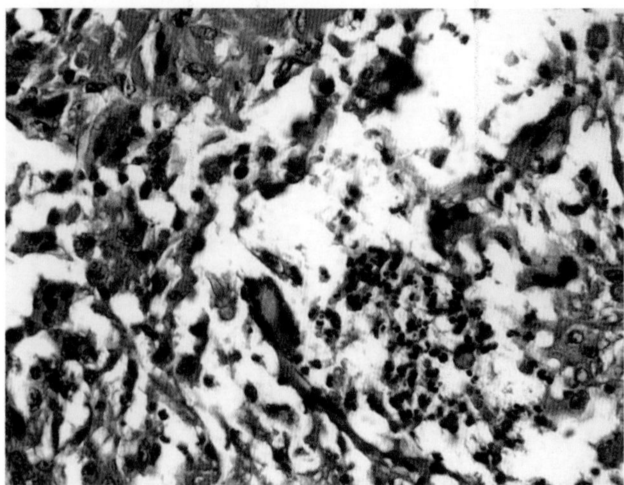

Fig. 5.22 Phaeohyphomycosis. Brown hyphae (H&E, 40x). (Courtesy of Dr. Derek Marsee, Diagnostic Pathology Medical Group.)

Phaeohyphomycosis

- Due to **dematiaceous** (pigmented) fungi: ***Exophiala jeanselmei* (#1 cause)**, *Wangiella dermatitidis, Alternaria, Bipolaris, Phialophora,* and *Curvularia*
- Geography: tropics and temperate zones
- Microscopy: **cyst** composed of macrophages and short hyphae, with a fibrous capsule
  - **Hyphae are pigmented/brown**, and stain positive with Fontana-Masson (Fig. 5.22)
- Pathogenesis: immunosuppressed patients
- Clinical presentation: **subcutaneous, possibly draining, inflammatory abscesses/cysts** (may mimic Baker cysts)
- Treatment: **excision** and itraconazole

Protothecosis

- Species: *Prototheca wickerhamii*, not a fungus but an **algae**
- Geography and pathogenesis: introduced into skin via trauma in **contaminated water**
- Microscopy: organisms have a **morula-like appearance** on H&E
- Clinical presentation: nodules/ulcers/plaques and/or **olecranon bursitis**
- Treatment: excision and systemic antifungals (e.g., amphotericin B)

Rhinosporidiosis

- Species: *Rhinosporidium seeberi*, not a fungus but a **protozoa**
- Geography: tropics (southern India and Sri Lanka)
- Pathogenesis: likely caused by **contaminated water** contact as this is a fish parasite
- Microscopy: **Very large** (up to 300 μm sporangia containing trophozoites in dermis
- Clinical presentation: slow-growing **friable, red-purple, soft, lobulated, mucosal polyps**, particularly on **nose** (associated with epistaxis), and conjunctivae; young men most commonly
- Treatment: excision

5.5 PARASITES AND OTHER CREATURES

Parasitic infestations

Scabies

- *Sarcoptes scabies* var. *hominis*
- Most consistent factor associated with scabies is overcrowding
- Host-species restricted (each species lives only on its natural host)
- 30-day lifecycle within stratum corneum; 1-week survival off human; classically affects **interdigital webspaces**, postauricular, axillae, wrists, **genitals** (a/w chronic, reactive inflammatory nodules), feet, nipples/areolae and umbilicus; **mineral oil scraping** demonstrates scabies mite (dermoscopy can help visualize mites and burrows)
- Crusted **(Norwegian) scabies in immunosuppressed/ HIV**/elderly patients
  - Most common complication is secondary bacterial infections
- Treatment of choice = **permethrin 5% cream (two treatments 1 week apart)**; other treatment options = ivermectin (200–400 mcg/kg × 2 [1 week apart]), sulfur or lindane; after treatment, postscabetic pruritus/ dermatitis up to 4 weeks

Lice

- Head louse—*Pediculus humanus capitis*
  - Active infection only if within 5 mm from scalp; most commonly located in occipital and **postauricular** areas
  - Mites can survive 36 hours w/o blood meal; nits are **strongly adherent** to hair shaft and can survive 10 days w/o blood meal
- Body louse—*Pediculus humanus corporis*
  - Larger, but similar shape to head louse
  - Not seen on skin but usually on clothing
  - Vector in **epidemic typhus (*R. prowazekii*), louse-borne relapsing fever (*B. recurrentis*), and trench fever (*B. quintana*)**
  - Live and lay eggs on clothing; more common in **homeless** population (since unable to change/wash clothes regularly)
- Pubic louse—*Pthirus pubis*
  - Identify by four frontal crab-like appendages and short/ broad body
  - **Maculae ceruleae** (blue-gray macules on thighs/trunk 2° to bilirubin → biliverdin) may be seen on surrounding skin
  - Can occur on **eyelashes** as well as pubic hairs
- Treatment—permethrin 1%, pyrethrins, lindane 1%, ivermectin 0.5%, spinosad 0.9%, benzyl alcohol 5%, or malathion (**flammable**, only for age > 2 years old)

Tungiasis

- Burrowing flea—*Tunga penetrans*
  - Female burrows head-first into skin (usually **feet/toes**) and extrudes eggs from punctum before dying and being sloughed with epidermis; nodules with crusts in periungual toes (#1), soles, toe webs (Fig. 5.23); can → gangrene
  - Most common: **Caribbean**, Central/South America, and sub-Saharan Africa
  - Treatment: surgical removal or ivermectin (do **tetanus prophylaxis**)

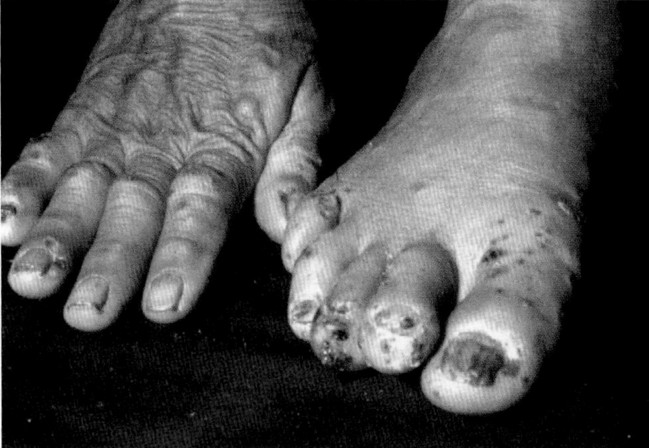

Fig. 5.23 Tungiasis—massive infestation of hand and feet in a cattle handler. (Courtesy of Dermatology Service, Santa Casa de Misericordia, Porto Alegre, Brazil.)

Myiasis

- Infection with dipterous larvae
  - ***Dermatobia hominis* (human botfly**; most common)
    - Eggs can be transmitted by mosquito via exposed skin → larval maturation (see furuncle)
  - Tumbu (*Cordylobia anthropophaga*)
    - Larva are deposited on damp clothing and penetrate skin when clothes are worn (see on non-exposed areas of body)
  - Wound myiasis (*Cochliomyia hominivorax, Chrysomyia bezziana*)—larvae cannot penetrate intact skin; once laid within open wound, penetrate subcutaneous structures and can continue to penetrate through cartilage and bone (leading to cranial penetration if developing near nose)
- Treatment: surgical debridement of larvae + antibiotic for superinfection; ivermectin; tetanus vaccination

Protozoa

Leishmaniasis

- Chronic infection due to **obligate intracellular protozoan**, *Leishmania spp.*
  - Exist in two forms: promastigote and amastigote
  - **Vector**: **sandflies (*Phlebotomus or Lutzomyia*)**
  - Reservoirs: mainly canines and rodents
- Pathogenesis: Within gut of sandfly, organisms proliferate into flagellated promastigotes → migrate to sandfly proboscis → sandfly bites human and transfers promastigotes → histiocytes engulf promastigotes, which then transform into amastigotes and multiply → develop clinical manifestations within weeks (cutaneous

leishmaniasis [CL]) or many months-years later (mucocutaneous and visceral leishmaniasis)
  - Stronger host Th1 response (IL-2, **IFN-γ**) → resolution of disease versus poor Th1 w/ development of Th2 response → progression
- Leishmaniasis may be classified by geographic region (Old World vs. New World), or clinical presentation (cutaneous, diffuse cutaneous, mucocutaneous, or visceral)
- Geographic classification:
  - Old World
    - ***L. major, L. tropica* > *L. aethiopica***, *L. infantum,* and others
    - Vector: ***Phlebotomus*** sand flies
  - New World
    - *L. mexicana, L. braziliensis, L. amazonensis,* and others
    - Vector: ***Lutzomyia*** sand flies
      - Also the vector of *B. bacilliformis* (→ verruga peruana, Carrion disease, bartonellosis, Oroya fever)
- Clinical classification (four major forms):
  - Cutaneous: restricted to skin; more common in Old World (90% occur in Middle East, Brazil and Peru; Texas is the only endemic area in the United States)
    - Old World cutaneous
      - Most common agents: ***L. major, L. tropica*** (>*L. infantum, L. aethiopica*)
      - Begins as a **solitary**, small, erythematous edematous nodule at bite site (usually **exposed skin sites**—arms, face, legs) that ulcerates or becomes verrucous (Fig. 5.24) → may later develop **sporotrichoid spread** with satellite lymphatic nodules and lymphangitis → heals with **scarring** over months to years
    - New World cutaneous
      - Most common agents: ***L. mexicana*** (> *L. braziliensis*)
      - More varied presentation: ulcerations (**Chiclero ulcer** = ear lesion in workers who harvest chicle gum in forest), impetigo-like, lichenoid, sarcoid-like, nodular, vegetating, and miliary
  - Diffuse cutaneous: more widespread cutaneous lesions; usually arises in immunosuppressed patients
    - Most common agent: ***L. amazonensis* (Americas)**, ***L. aethiopica* (Africa)**
    - Multiple keloidal lesions of face (esp. nose) and extremities
  - Mucocutaneous: affects skin and mucous membranes; almost always in New World
    - Predominantly New World subspecies: ***L. braziliensis*** (> *L. amazonensis, L. panamensis,* and *L. guyanensis*)
    - Present with lip, nose, and oropharyngeal infiltration and ulceration
    - Progressive nasopharyngeal destruction → airway obstruction, mutilation of mouth and **perforation of nasal septum** (aka "**tapir face**" or **espundia**)
  - Visceral (Kala-azar, "black fever"): most severe form; due to systemic infection of bone marrow, liver, spleen; Old World > New World; incubation time = months-years
    - Most common agents: ***L. donovani*** (India, Sudan, Bangladesh; most common cause in adults), ***L. infantum*** (Europe; often a/w HIV), ***L. chagasi***
    - Present with fever, weight loss, diarrhea, abdominal tenderness, LAD, hepatosplenomegaly, nephritis, intestinal hemorrhage, and **death within 2 years** (if not treated)
    - Skin changes:
      - Specific: papules, ulcers at bite site
      - Non-specific: purpura, **hyperpigmentation** ("black fever"), kwashiorkor changes (brittle hair w/ discoloration), purpura
  - **Post-kala-azar dermal leishmaniasis**: lesions arising up to 20 years after presumed recovery from untreated visceral leishmaniasis (nodules, verrucous papules, hypopigmented macules)
- Diagnosis
  - PCR is most sensitive and specific test
  - Culture: **Novy-McNeal-Nicolle medium**
  - Histology: amastigotes with **kinetoplasts** are arrayed around periphery of parasitized histiocyte cytoplasm ("**Marquee sign**") (Fig. 5.25); organisms are best seen on **Giemsa**
  - Montenegro delayed-skin reaction test is positive in majority of CL; remains positive after cure and is negative in febrile phase of visceral leishmaniasis
- Prognosis: most cases of Old World CL self-resolve within 15 months; New World CL due to *L. Mexicana* self-resolves in 75%; mucocutaneous leishmaniasis (*L. braziliensis* and *L. panamensis)* does NOT self-resolve and requires treatment to prevent progressive destruction

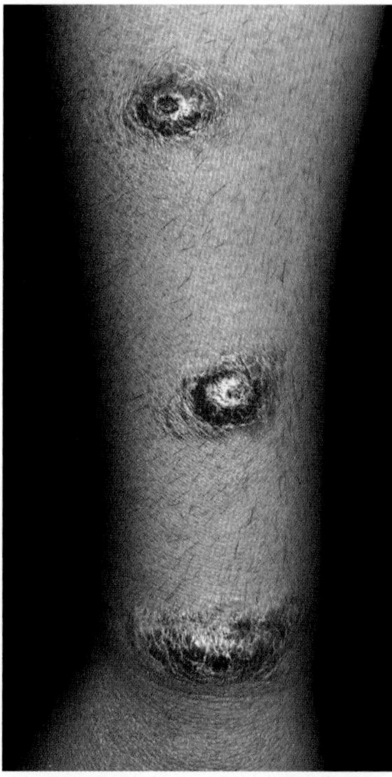

Fig. 5.24 Ulcerated nodules of Old World leishmaniasis in a sporotrichoid pattern. (Courtesy of Dr. Anwar Qais Saadoon, Senior Dermatologist, Basra, Iraq.)

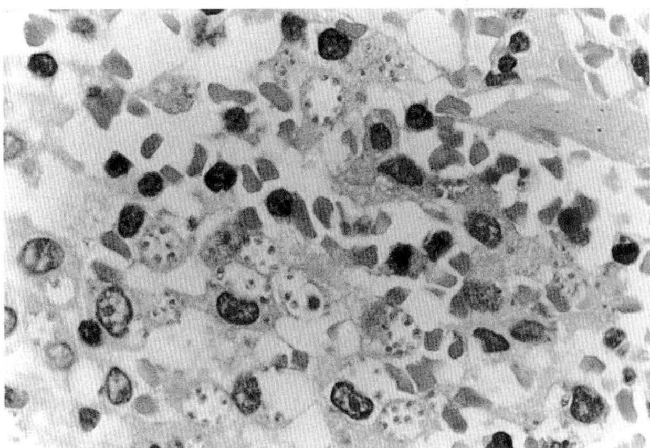

Fig. 5.25 Leishmaniasis. H&E section of skin with several Leishmania organisms inside histiocytes. (From Machado-Pinto J, Laborne L. Leishmaniasis. In: Tyring SK, Lupi O, Hengge UR, eds. *Tropical Dermatology.* 2nd ed. Philadelphia: Elsevier; 2017:42–49.)

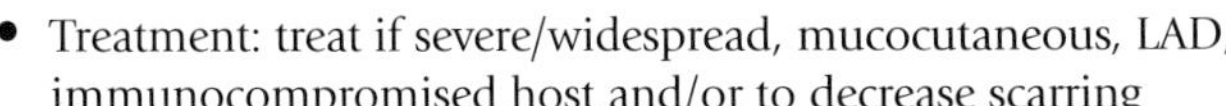

- Treatment: treat if severe/widespread, mucocutaneous, LAD, immunocompromised host and/or to decrease scarring
  - Cutaneous and mucocutaneous leishmaniasis: **pentavalent antimony** (e.g., sodium stibogluconate), miltefosine, pentamidine, intralesional 0.2% ciprofloxacin + long-pulsed Nd:YAG
  - Visceral leishmaniasis: **amphotericin B** (ToC)

Trypanosomiasis

- African trypanosomiasis (sleeping sickness)
  - Species: *T. brucei* ***gambiense*** **(West Africa)**/*T. brucei* ***rhodesiense*** **(East Africa)**
  - Vector: **tsetse fly (*Glossina*)**
  - Clinical presentation:
    - Trypanosomal **chancre (earliest sign:** local pruritic inflammatory reaction at the site of inoculation [48 hours]) → local LAD and ulcerates → **eschar**
    - Fever, headache, and joint pain at irregular intervals
    - **Winterbottom's sign** (posterior cervical LAD) (2–3 weeks) → **trypanids** (erythematous, urticarial or macular diffuse eruptions [6–8 weeks]) → neurologic changes and **Kerandel's deep delayed hyperesthesia, daytime sleepiness (late stage)**
  - Disease course: progressive over weeks to months (East Africa), months to years (West Africa)
  - Treatment: suramin or **pentamidine** (early); melarsoprol (E. African) or eflornithine (W. African) (CNS involvement)
- American trypanosomiasis (Chagas disease)
  - Species: ***T. cruzi***
  - Vector: **triatomine bug (*Reduviidae*)**
    - **Central/South America**
  - Clinical presentation: local inflammatory lesion (often on face) at site of entry (chagoma) → **Romaña sign** (Fig. 5.26) (unilateral eyelid edema and conjunctivitis at site of inoculation) → rapid unilateral painless bipalpebral edema → late **heart, esophagus, and intestinal enlargement (megacolon)**
  - Diagnosed with PCR; Treatment: benznidazole or nifurtimox

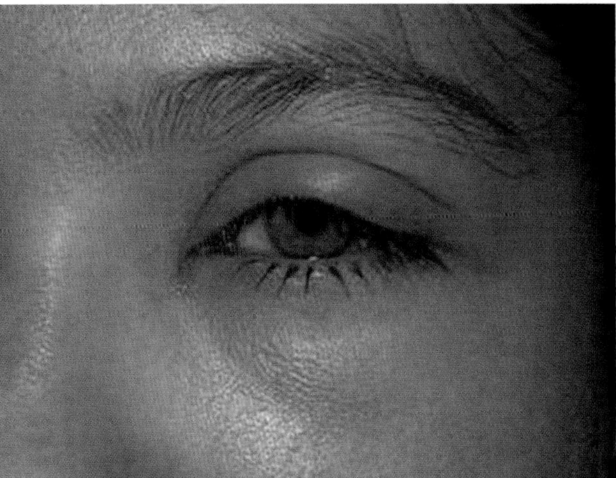

Fig. 5.26 Romaña sign. Acute Chagas disease in a young girl with Romaña sign present in the left eye. (From Lupi O. Bartlett BL, Haugen RN, et al. Tropical dermatology: tropical diseases caused by protozoa. *J Am Acad Dermatol.* 2009;60[6]: 897–925.)

Toxoplasmosis

- Species: ***Toxoplasma gondii***
- Geography: worldwide
- Vector: intestinal parasite of **cats** (human can acquire from cat feces) and raw/undercooked meat pork/lamb/venison meat
- Clinical presentation:
  - Acquired cutaneous disease: LAD + fever, but if immunocompromised can → encephalitis, hepatitis, pericarditis; skin: non-specific urticarial or maculopapular eruption
  - **Congenital disease (TORCH syndrome)** – hemorrhagic papules + possible seizures, deafness, chorioretinitis, HSM, thrombocytopenia (see Chapter 4, Pediatric Dermatology)
- Treatment: sulfadiazine and pyrimethamine

Helminths

Cutaneous larva migrans

- Most common tropical parasite dermatosis; found in animal feces
- Species—***Ancylostoma braziliense*** (most common); also *A. caninum*
- Clinical presentation: erythematous **serpiginous** cutaneous eruption (usually on **feet**) as a result of larva penetrating intact epidermis, but unable to penetrate human basement membrane zone (therefore **unable to cause systemic disease**)
  - Moves **1 to 3 cm/day**
- Treatment: albendazole, ivermectin, topical/oral **thiabendazole**, and liquid nitrogen

Larva currens

- Moves **faster (5–10 cm/hr)**
- *Strongyloides stercoralis*
- Often indurated serpiginous papule on **buttocks/thighs**

- If disseminated, may get **periumbilical (thumbprint) purpura** and petechiae on trunk/proximal extremities
  - **Loeffler's syndrome** = chronic strongyloidiasis (affects **lungs** and GI tract; **eosinophilia**)
- Caused by contact with contaminated soil (e.g., sitting on beach)
- ELISA can help with diagnosis
- Treatment: ivermectin or thiabendazole

Onchocerciasis ("River blindness")

- Species: *Onchocerca volvulus*
- Vector: **Simulium fly (black fly**; also vector for tularemia; has also been implicated in Fogo selvagem form of pemphigus; present **near fast-flowing rivers)**
  - Geography: sub-Saharan **Africa**, South America, and Yemen
- Pathogenesis: nodules of female microfilariae; male microfilariae migrate between nodules to mate
- Clinical presentation: pruritic papules (can be acute, chronic, or **lichenified**) → **leopard skin** (depigmentation and atrophy); nodules (**onchocercomas**) over bony prominences; red to purpule faces → leonine appearance; may develop **Mazzotti reaction** if given **diethylcarbamazine** (itchy eruption develops shortly after giving med in infected paitent)
  - Can → **blindness**
- Treatment: **ivermectin (treatment of choice)**; doxycycline kills symbiotic *Wolbachia* bacteria; **surgical excision of onchocercomas**

Loiasis

- Species: ***Loa***
- Vector: ***Chrysops*** **(Mango/deer flies**; also transmit tularemia)
  - Geography: West and Central Africa
- Clinical presentation: **calabar swellings** (recurrent migratory focal angioedema on limbs); **visible migration of adult worm across eyes**
- Treatment: **diethylcarbamazine**

Filariasis

- Species: *Brugia malayi/timori* and ***Wuchereria bancrofti***
- Vectors: multiple mosquito spp. of ***Culex*** (also West Nile virus vector), ***Aedes*** (also vector of chikungunya fever, Dengue fever, and yellow fever), **and** ***Anopheles*** (also vector of malaria and yellow fever) mosquitoes
- Clinical presentation:
  - Acute—lymphangitis (inguinal nodes #1 site)
  - Chronic—granulomatous reaction in lymphatics → **lymphedema**, elephantiasis, hydrocele
- Treatment: **diethylcarbamazine** (ToC) + doxycycline (for *Wolbachia* endosymbiont)

Swimmer's itch and seabather's eruption

- Swimmer's itch ("cercarial dermatitis")
  - Species: ***Schistosoma***, during the cercarial stage (snails are a vector)
    - Northern United States and Canada **fresh water**

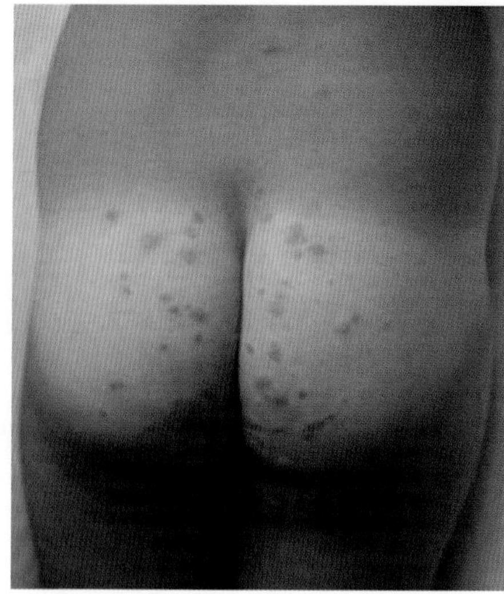

Fig. 5.27 Classic lesions of seabather's eruption in covered areas. The disease is caused by larvae of *Linuche unguiculata*. (Courtesy, Vidal Haddad Jr., MD, PhD, São Paulo, Brazil.)

  - Clinical presentation: papules and papulovesicles on **uncovered skin** 10 to 15 hours postexposure, lasts 5 to 7 days
- Seabather's eruption (NOT a helminthic infection)
  - Species: ***Edwardsiella lineata*** (sea anemone) and ***Linuche unguiculata*** (thimble jellyfish) during larval stage
    - Southern United States and Caribbean **salt water**
  - Clinical presentation: pruritic papules and wheals in **covered areas** within hours with new lesions for days (Fig. 5.27)

Trichinosis

- Species: *Trichinella spiralis*
- Geography: worldwide with domestic and sylvatic infection cycles
  - Most common reports are rural Asia and Latin America
- Vectors:
  - Domestic cycle—**pigs**, which are then **eaten undercooked** (eating undercooked bears = less common cause)
  - Sylvatic cycle—scavengers and carnivorous animals (wild canines and felines, birds, raccoons, boars, and walruses) eat infected rodents, and are themselves eaten undercooked by humans
- Pathogenesis: humans eat animal meat (muscle) that contains larval cysts → these encyst in GI tract and mature into adults → reproduction occurs and larvae are produced, which leaves the GI tract and encyst in skeletal muscle
- Clinical presentation:
  - Primary dermatologic manifestation is **periorbital edema** (as a result of type I allergic reaction) and petechiae during parasite migration (esp. **splinter hemorrhages**)
- Diagnosis: peripheral eosinophilia and IgE are clues; **muscle biopsy is diagnostic**
  - ↑ IgE may persist years after disease resolution

- Treatment: mebendazole or albendazole; may use systemic steroids for moderate to severe hypersensitivity reactions

Dracunculiasis (Guinea worm)

- Species: ***Dracunculus medinensis***
- Vector: **Cyclops water flea** at copepod stage
- Clinical presentation: **nodules and ulcers on lower extremity** (after ingestion of infected Cyclops, the organism travels from intestines to subcutaneous tissue, where adult worms emerge from lesion when reexposed to water)
- Prevention: drinking filtrated/boiled water prevents ingestion of copepods that contain larva
- Treatment: **removal of worm** (ToC), wound care, and metronidazole

Gnathosomiasis

- Species: ***Gnathostoma spinigerum***
- Vector: **raw freshwater fish** (humans get disease by eating—e.g., sushi)
- Clinical presentation: GI symptoms + fever early on; **nodular migratory panniculitis** (can look like cutaneous larva migrans or single tender nodule that moves around skin); CNS (mortality = 25%)
- Treatment: **albendazole** or ivermectin

Cysticercosis

- Species: ***Taenia solium*** (pork tapeworm), ***Taenia saginata*** (beef tapeworm), ***Diphyllobothrium latum*** (fish tapeworm)
- Vector: poorly cooked meat (humans can be intermediate [eggs ingested → larva/oncospheres → encyst → cysticerci] or definitive host [ingest adult worms → travel to intestinal mucosa])
- Clinical presentation: peripheral eosinophilia and minimal symptoms if definitive host; in intermediate hosts, cysts can travel → nodules in skin, and systemic symptoms (brain, heart, etc.—may be seen on CT/MRI/X-ray)
- Treatment: albendazole, praziquantel

Cutaneous amebiasis

Free-living amoeba

- *Acanthomoeba*—subacute granulomatous amebic encephalitis; skin lesions → **chronic ulcers**
- *Balamuthia*—painless, red, and granulomatous plaque on **central face** > trunk/extremities, which precedes **CNS involvement**; treatment: multiagent w/ miltefosine
- *Naegleria*—fulminate, **fatal** acute necrotizing **meningoencephalitis**

GI-associated amoeba

- *Entamoeba histolytica*
  - Usually associated with **amebic colitis** and/or liver/lung involvement
  - Cutaneous lesions may spread to **perianal region** from GI involvement, or be **sexually transmitted** with a painful, ulcerating, ovaloid, erythematous plaque (with a lot of necrosis) near the site of inoculation
  - ToC: metronidazole

Bites and stings

Biting and stinging insects

- Immediate reactions are as a result of histamine, serotonin, formic acid, or kinin release
  - One fourth of cases of **anaphylaxis** are as a result of stings from insects (order **Hymenoptera**)
  - Secondary infection of bites typically from *Staphylococcus*
  - Exaggerated bite reactions: CLL, chronic EBV
- Fire ants (*Solenopsis*): bites→ 5 mm to 1 cm sterile pustules on lower extremities
  - Toxin = **solenopsin D** (piperidine alkaloid)
- Bees/wasps/hornets (*Hymenoptera*): toxin = **phospholipase A**; can → anaphylaxis; myoglobinuria, hemoglobinuria, acute tubular necrosis from wasps/killer bees
- Bed bugs
  - Species: ***Cimex lectularius*** (Fig. 5.28)—nocturnal
  - Nitrophorin is one of its salivary products responsible for human immune reaction; p/w grouped "**breakfast, lunch, and dinner**" urticarial papules at bite sites
- *Lytta vesicatoria*/Spanish fly (blister beetles)
  - **Cantharidin** derived from heme-lymph discharge; p/w blisters at sites of contact
- Fleas
  - Rat flea (*Xenopsylla cheopis*) is vector for *R. typhi* → **endemic typhus** and *Y. pestis* → **bubonic plague** (treatment: streptomycin and gentamicin)
  - Cat flea (*Ctenocephalides felis* and *Ctenocephalides canis*) is vector for ***B. henselae*** (→ cat scratch disease, bacillary angiomatosis), AND ***B. quintana*** (→ bacillary angiomatosis)
  - *Pulex irritans* is the human flea; also affects dogs
- Lepidopterism (caterpillar dermatitis)
  - Direct contact with hairs and toxin-mediated reactions (not allergy)

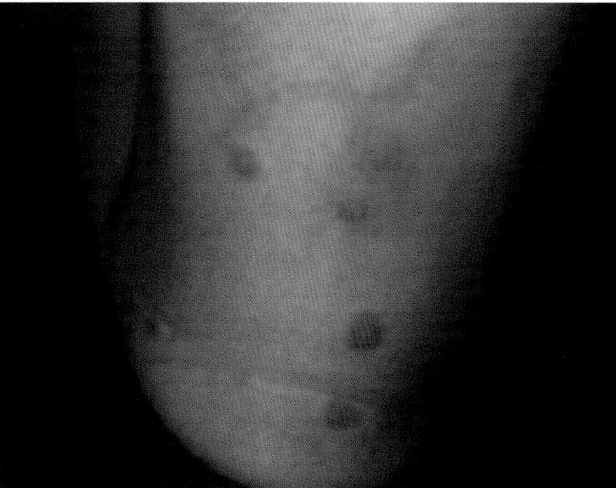

Fig. 5.28 *Cimex* spp. The bites from bedbugs are not accompanied by severe manifestations in nonsensitized persons, but they can cause notable erythema, edema, and itching in those persons allergic to the bites (esp. atopic individuals). (From Haddad V. Tropical dermatology: venomous arthropods and human skin. *J Am Acad Dermatol.* 2012;67[3]:e1–e14.)

- **Train-track appearance of urticaria or hemorrhage**
- Ophthalmia nodosa are ocular reactions as hairs tend to migrate inward
- Specific types of caterpillars:
  - Puss (*Megalopyge opercularis*): lightly brown and wooly appearance; results in painful, **linear petechiae**
  - Io (*Automeris io*): green with adjacent longitudinal red and white stripes
  - Gypsy (*Lymantria dispar*): histamine in hair, which can become airborne
  - Saddleback (*Sibine stimulea*): green saddle-like area on back
- DEET (N,N-diethyl-3-methylbenzamide) is overall the most effective insect repellant

Arachnids (ticks, mites, spiders, and scorpions)

- **Ticks** (Fig. 5.29)
  - *Ornithodorus*
    - Soft-bodied tick
    - Identification: warty/rough, gray, and soft appearance
    - Transmits *B. duttonii* (tick-borne relapsing fever)
  - *Dermacentor*
    - Identification: alternating light and dark bands on body with brown legs
    - Transmits **RMSF** (#1 cause), **tularemia**, tick paralysis, and **human granulocytic anaplasmosis/ ehrlichiosis**, Q fever, Colorado tick fever
  - *Ixodes pacificus, I. ricinus, I. scapularis*, and *I. dammini*
    - Identification: dark legs and solid-colored body with darker scutula
    - Transmits **Lyme disease** (#1 cause; *B. burgdorferi*), acrodermatitis chronica atrophicans (*B. garinii* and *B. afzelli*), **babesiosis** (#1 cause), and **human granulocytic anaplasmosis**
  - *Amblyomma*—lone star tick
    - Identification: white dot on back (female)
    - Transmits human monocytic ehrlichiosis; tularemia; southern tick-associated rash illness; African tick-bite fever; Brazil spotted fever

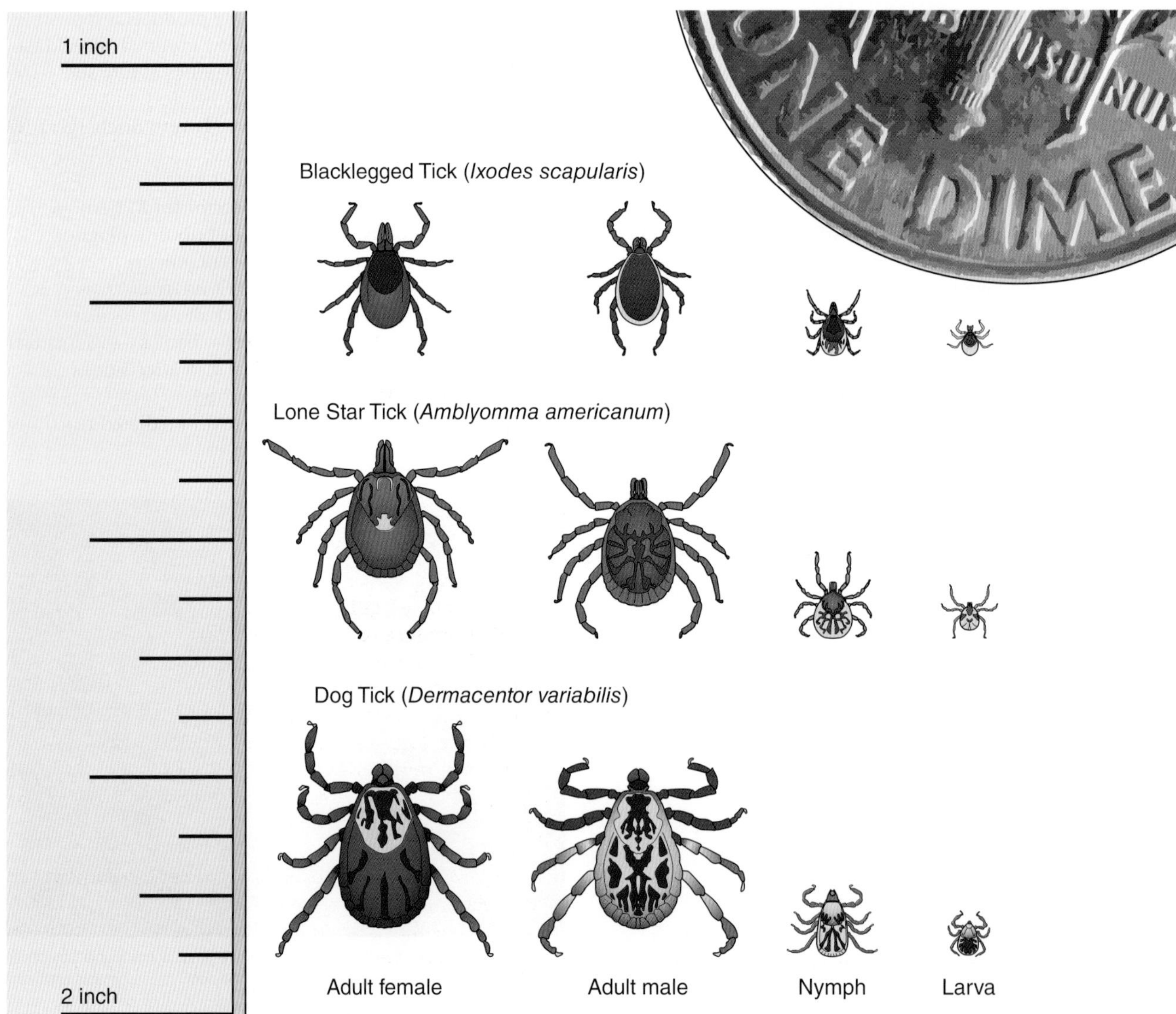

Fig. 5.29 Tick life cycle and size comparison. (From Centers for Disease Control and Prevention, www.cdc.gov.)

- *Rhipicephalus*—dog tick
  - Identification: brown with brown legs
  - Transmits boutonneuse fever, RMSF
- Ticks should be removed with gentle traction; **DEET repellant** + **permethrin-treated clothing** is very effective for prevention

- Mites
  - *Demodex (Demodicidae)*
    - Live in hair follicles of humans
    - Possible association with rosacea/perioral dermatitis/blepharitis
  - Free-living mites
    - Chigger/harvest mite (*Trombicula alfreddugesi*)
      - Vector for *R. tsutsugamushi*, which → scrub typhus
      - Causes grouped pruritic papules on lower extremities/ankles and waistband
      - Causes summer **penile syndrome** in boys
  - House mouse mite (*Allodermanyssus sanguineus*)
    - Vector for *R. akari* → rickettsialpox
  - Dust mite (*Dermatophagoides*)
    - Involved in indoor allergies in atopic patients
  - Fowl mite (*Dermanyssus* and *Ornithonyssus*)
    - Vector for western equine encephalitis
  - Walking dandruff (*Cheyletiella*)
    - Caused by contact with dogs/cats—asymptomatic in dogs/cats but itchy eruption in humans
  - Grain mite (*Acarus siro*)
    - Agent of Baker's itch
  - Cheese mite (*Glyciphagus*)
    - Agent of Grocer's itch
- **Spiders**
  - *Latrodectus mactans*—**black widow** spider; has characteristic **red hourglass** on body
    - Acute pain and edema at site
    - Systemic symptoms: chills, **abdominal pain/rigidity**, rhabdomyolysis, chest pain, sweating, hypertension, and shock, muscle spams
    - **a-Lactotoxin** depolarizes neurons
    - Treatment: IV calcium gluconate; antivenin; **benzodiazepine** supportive
  - *Loxosceles reclusa*—**brown recluse** (Fig. 5.30) spider; characteristic dark brown-black **violin/fiddle**-shaped marking
    - **Necrosis with eschar** formation at site of bite (which is painless; erythema → ischemia → thrombosis)
    - Toxins: **sphingomyelinase D** and hyaluronidase (allows eschars to spread)
    - Can have **hemolytic anemia/thrombocytopenia, shock, DIC and death**
    - Treatment: do not debride; supportive; antivenin; prednisone
  - *Phidippus formosus*—jumping spider
    - Dark and hairy with four eyes (two larger centrally and two smaller ones laterally)
    - Toxin: **hyaluronidase**
    - Is aggressive and bites, but no systemic symptoms
  - *Lycosidae*—wolf spider
    - Large brown spider with black patterns and eight eyes
    - Toxin: **histamine**

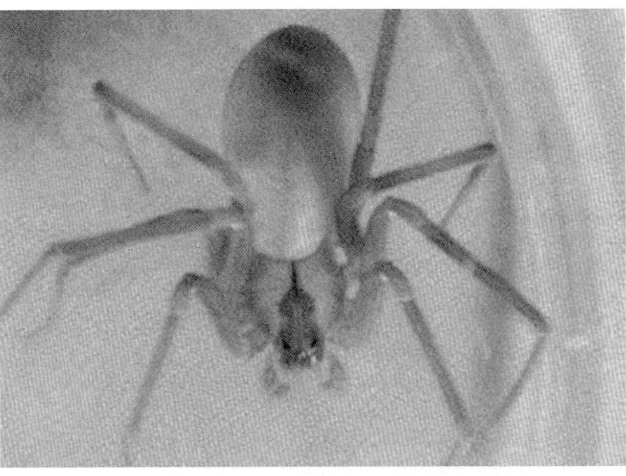

Fig. 5.30 *Loxosceles reclusa* (brown recluse spider). A characteristic "violin" or "fiddle" marking appears on the head and thorax. (Courtesy, Dr. Robert G. Breene, American Tarantula Society, South Padre Island, Texas.)

  - *Chiracanthium*—sac spider
    - Yellow-colored
    - Toxin: **lipase**
  - *Tegenaria agrestis*—hobo spider
    - **Herringbone pattern** on abdomen
    - Painless bite → local necrosis/eschar
    - Web is funnel-shaped
  - *Peucetia viridans*—green lynx spider; has unique neon green color with red spots
    - Green colored with red spots
    - Painful bite without systemic symptoms
  - *Theraphosidae*—tarantula
    - **Urticating hairs** ejected when threatened; can → **ophthalmia nodosa** (chronic granulomatous reaction in eyes; may result in blindness)
- <u>**Scorpions** (*Centruroides sculpturatus* and gertschi)</u>
  - Pain and paresthesia out of proportion to skin lesions
  - Systemic symptoms: convulsions, hemiplegia, temperature instability, tremor, arrhythmia, pulmonary edema, and hypertension

Millipedes and centipedes

- Centipedes (*Chilopoda* class; *Scolopendra* spp.)
  - One pair of legs per segment
  - Bites produce pain and paresthesia
    - **Two puncture wounds**
- Millipedes (*Diplopoda*)
  - Two pairs of legs per segment
  - Chemical irritant contact dermatitis from secretions → **burn and blistering**

Snake bites

- *Viperidae/Crotalidae* (copperhead and rattlesnake): **triangular head** with deep nostril pits
  - Multiple toxins, including thrombin-like glycoproteins
  - **Thrombocytopenia and DIC**
- *Elapidae* (coral snake) round eyes, characteristic **red, yellow and black** banding (mnemonic: "red on yellow kills a fellow")

- α-Neurotoxin—causes neurologic symptoms, nausea, headache, abdominal pain, and paresthesia
- Phospholipase A2 causes wound effects

Marine injuries

- Cnidarians (jellyfish, Portuguese man of war, coral, and anemones)
  - Produces specialized cells—nematocysts
  - **Flagellate eruption in affected areas** (Fig. 5.31)
  - Physical or osmotic trigger releases a coiled filament that discharges toxins
    - **Vinegar (dilute acetic acid) denatures** nematocysts in some, but not all species
  - ***Chironex fleckeri*** (Pacific box jellyfish) stings can → shock and associated fatality
  - Portuguese man of war (*Pysalia* spp.) contain a heat-labile toxin that produces cardiac disturbances and paralysis
    - **Skin lesions are hemorrhagic and vesicular**
- Echinoderms
  - Sea urchins have fragile spines that break off in wounds → foreign body reaction
  - Sea cucumbers eject an irritating liquid (holothurin) → conjunctivitis

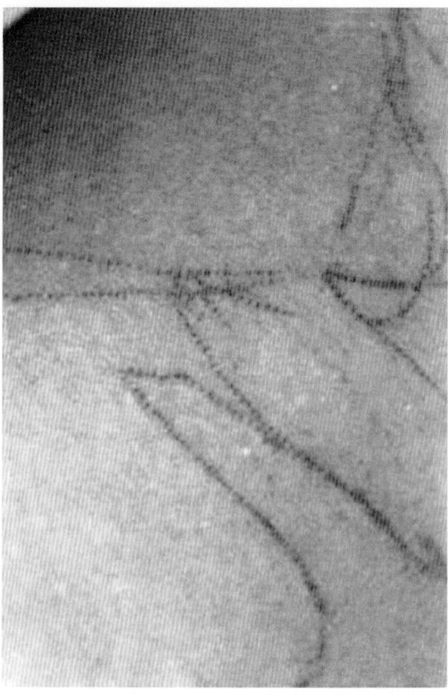

Fig. 5.31 Linear plaques, erythema, and edema in a girl following contact with the tentacles of a Portuguese man of war. (Courtesy, Dr. Vidal Haddad, Jr.)

6 Neoplastic Dermatology

Monisha N. Dandekar, Roberto A. Novoa, Phillip C. Hochwalt, and Spyros M. Siscos

CONTENTS LIST

6.1 KERATINOCYTIC NEOPLASMS
6.2 CYSTS
6.3 MELANOCYTIC NEOPLASMS
6.4 ADNEXAL NEOPLASMS AND HAMARTOMAS
6.5 HAIR FOLLICLE NEOPLASMS/HAMARTOMAS
6.6 SEBACEOUS PROLIFERATIONS
6.7 NEURAL NEOPLASMS
6.8 SMOOTH MUSCLE NEOPLASMS
6.9 HEMATOLYMPHOID NEOPLASMS
6.10 FIBROHISTIOCYTIC NEOPLASMS
6.11 VASCULAR PROLIFERATIONS
6.12 NEOPLASMS OF ADIPOCYTIC LINEAGE
6.13 DERMOSCOPY

NEOPLASTIC DERMATOLOGY

- General features of a benign neoplasm:
  - Clinically: well-demarcated, uniform color, unchanged for years, and lack of concerning symptoms (bleeding, ulceration, and pain)
  - Histologically: **well-circumscribed**, **bland cytology**; lacks all of the following: architectural disorder, necrosis, cytologic atypia, and atypical mitotic figures
- General features of a malignant neoplasm:
  - Clinically: rapid growth or new-onset lesion with concerning features, such as pigment variegation, ulceration, pain, and bleeding
  - Histologically: **poorly-circumscribed** proliferation of cells with **atypical cytology** (nuclear pleomorphism, hyperchromatic cells, ↑ N:C ratio, prominent nucleoli, and abnormally shaped nuclei); **architectural disorder** (infiltrative, destroys neighboring structures, and perineural/intravascular invasion); **signs of hyperproliferative state** (↑ mitotic figures for given tissue type and tumor necrosis), **atypical mitoses** (do not resemble any normal phase of cell division)

6.1 KERATINOCYTIC NEOPLASMS

Seborrheic keratosis (SK)

- Very common, benign; onset fourth decade
- Familial predisposition, autosomal dominant (AD) inheritance w/ incomplete penetrance
- a/w **sun exposure** (↓ incidence on "double-clothed areas" such as buttocks and genitalia), *FGFR3* and *PIK3CA* activating mutations
- Well-demarcated, waxy/verrucous **brown "stuck-on" papules** on hair-bearing skin; spares mucosal sites
- Histology: acanthosis, papillomatosis, hyperkeratosis with **pseudohorn cysts**, **flat base ("string sign")**, bland keratinocytes without atypia or many mitotic figures (if present will be mild and a/w irritation/inflammation); many histologic variants exist (Table 6.1)

Table 6.1 Seborrheic Keratosis Histologic Variants

Acanthotic	**Most common type**; presents as a dome-shaped papule; mostly acanthotic with less papillomatosis/hyperkeratosis; small basaloid keratinocytes with increased melanin, prominent horn pseudocysts
Hyperkeratotic	Prominent hyperkeratosis/papillomatosis ("**church spires**") w/ less acanthosis/pseudocysts/pigmentation
Reticulated	**Thin interlacing strands** of basaloid cells, often pigmented, with horn pseudocysts, +/– lentigo at edges (these may evolve from lentigo)
Irritated	Less sharply demarcated base with lymphoid infiltrate; whorls of pink keratinocytes ("**squamous eddies**")
Clonal	Well-defined nests of paler/monotonous cells (Borst-Jadassohn phenomenon) **mimicking Bowen's** disease, melanoma, or hidroacanthoma simplex
Melanoacanthoma	Heavy pigment mostly in **dendritic melanocytes** (>keratinocytes)

- **Sign of Leser-Trelat**: widespread eruption of SKs on trunk; a/w underlying adenocarcinoma (GI #1)
- Multiple clinical variants (Table 6.2)

Porokeratosis

- Subtypes
  - Porokeratosis of Mibelli: onset in infancy or childhood; **extremities**; large (often > 3 cm) **circinate plaque** with keratotic border
  - Disseminated superficial actinic porokeratosis (DSAP): **most common** subtype; onset in **middle age**; F > M; numerous brownish-red macules w/ keratotic borders in sun-exposed areas; most common on **legs** (rare on face); immunosuppression is risk factor; some inherited cases linked w/ mevalonate kinase mutations
  - Linear porokeratosis: onset in newborns; linear lesion on extremities, follows lines of Blaschko (Fig. 6.1); **highest risk** of progression to squamous cell carcinoma (SCC)
  - Punctate porokeratosis: onset in adolescence; 1- to 2-mm "seed-like" papules on palms/soles
  - Porokeratosis palmaris, plantaris, et disseminata: onset in childhood/adolescence; occurs on palms/soles initially
  - Porokeratotic eccrine ostial and dermal duct nevus: clinically resembles a nevus comedonicus of palm or sole, but histology shows abundant **cornoid lamellae arising from acrosyringium**
- Histology: **cornoid lamella** (angled column of parakeratosis w/ underlying hypogranulosis and dyskeratotic cells); centrally between two cornoid lamellae the epidermis may be atrophic, hyperplastic, normal, or benign lichenoid keratosis-like
  - Boards tip: cornoid lamellae may be at edge → **MUST look at entire slide!**
- SCC can develop in any subtype except **punctate porokeratosis (0% risk)**; second lowest risk in DSAP; **highest risk in linear porokeratosis**

Epidermal nevus

- Hamartoma of epidermis and papillary dermis; onset in first year of life
- **Papillomatous, pigmented, linear plaques along Blaschko's lines**
- Variants:
  - Nevus unius lateris: extensive unilateral plaques on trunk
  - Ichthyosis hystrix: extensive bilateral lesions on trunk
  - Inflammatory linear verrucous epidermal nevus (ILVEN): along lines of Blaschko without associated neurologic defects
  - Epidermal nevus syndrome (Schimmelpenning syndrome): a/w developmental abnormalities (**neurologic** and **musculoskeletal** most commonly)

Table 6.2 Seborrheic Keratosis Clinical Variants and Other Benign Keratoses

Dermatosis papulosa nigra	Darkly pigmented individuals, often **African Americans**; onset in young adulthood; F > M; familial tendency; hyperpigmented keratotic papules on face; histology identical to SK, except horn pseudocysts are not common
Stucco keratosis	White scaly variant of SK; onset after 40 years old; M > F (4:1); white to gray hyperkeratotic papules/plaques symmetrically distributed on **lower legs, ankles, feet**; a/w **HPV-23b**, HPV-9, HPV-16, and HPV-37
Lichenoid keratosis	Often represents an **inflamed/regressing lentigo/SK**; clinically **mimics BCC** or SCCIS; solitary pink/brown scaly papule on trunk or forearms; fourth to seventh decade; F > M; histologically resembles lichen planus (but may have parakeratosis), often adjacent lentigo or SK
Inverted follicular keratosis	**Endophytic** variant of irritated SK; white-pink firm solitary papules on face/neck (especially **cheek and upper lip**); middle-aged/older adults; histology: endophytic SK with **prominent squamous eddies**
Large cell acanthoma	Likely represents an early macular SK/solar lentigo; flesh-colored to brown patch/plaque on sun-exposed areas in older individuals; histology: papillomatosis, hyperkeratosis, elongation of epidermal rete with **large** and **slightly atypical keratinocytes** +/– basal pigmentation
Acrokeratosis verruciformis of Hopf	Tan-flesh colored warty papules on **dorsal hands/feet**; **Autosomal dominant** disorder of keratinization often **a/w Darier disease**; ***ATP2A2* mutations**; histology: "**church spire**" hyperkeratosis and papillomatosis (identical to stucco keratosis)
Clear cell acanthoma (Degos acanthoma)	Solitary erythematous papule on **lower leg** with "wafer-like scale" at the periphery; histology: sharply demarcated zone of **pale keratinocytes** (**PAS+**; as a result of **phosphorylase deficiency → glycogen** accumulation), **psoriasiform hyperplasia**, parakeratosis, loss of granular layer, and intraepithelial neutrophils **Mnemonic**: "looks like a well-demarcated papule of psoriasis composed of clear keratinocytes"

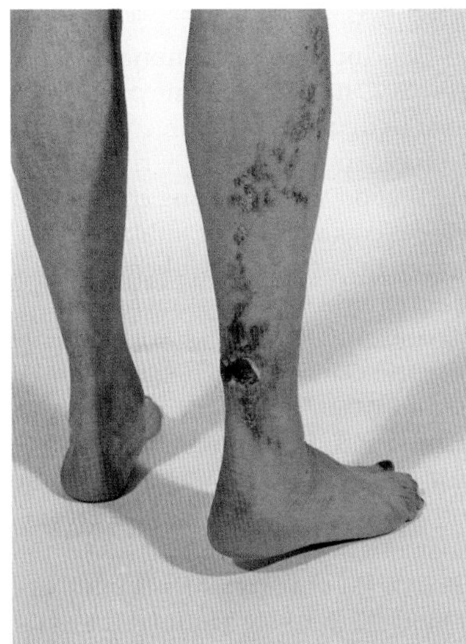

Fig. 6.1 Linear porokeratosis with squamous cell carcinoma. (From James WD, Elston DM, Treat JR, Rosenbach MA, Neuhaus IM. Genodermatoses and congenital anomalies. In: *Andrews' Diseases of the Skin*. 13th ed. Philadelphia: Elsevier; 2020:547–586.)

- Histology: epidermal papillomatosis; orthohyperkeratosis
  - May see **epidermolytic hyperkeratosis** due to genetic mosaicism (defects in **keratins 1 and 10**) → ↑ risk of **bullous congenital ichthyosiform erythroderma in offspring**
- Mutations in *FGFR3, KRAS, NRAS,* and *PIK3CA* have also been identified

Nevus comedonicus

- Hamartoma; onset in childhood; worsens during puberty
- Comedones in a **linear array on face** > trunk
- ***FGFR2* mutations** involved
  - *FGFR2* also involved in Alagille syndrome, Apert syndrome, cardiocranial syndrome, and Crouzon syndrome
- Histology: dilated epidermal invaginations filled w/ cornified debris

Flegel disease (hyperkeratosis lenticularis perstans)

- Rare disorder with AD inheritance; adult onset
- **Absent/altered lamellar granules (Odland bodies;** important for normal desquamation) on electron microscopy → a decrease/absence of these membrane-coating granules → ↓ desquamation of the stratum corneum → retention hyperkeratosis
- Small (1–5 mm), **disc-shaped** keratotic papules in symmetric distribution; **distal extremities (dorsal foot** > lower legs, dorsal hands)
- Histology: discrete orthohyperkeratosis overlying atrophic epidermis; lichenoid dermal inflammation

Warty dyskeratoma

- Onset in fifth to seventh decade; M > F
- Solitary verrucous papulonodule w/ central keratotic plug usually on **head/neck**

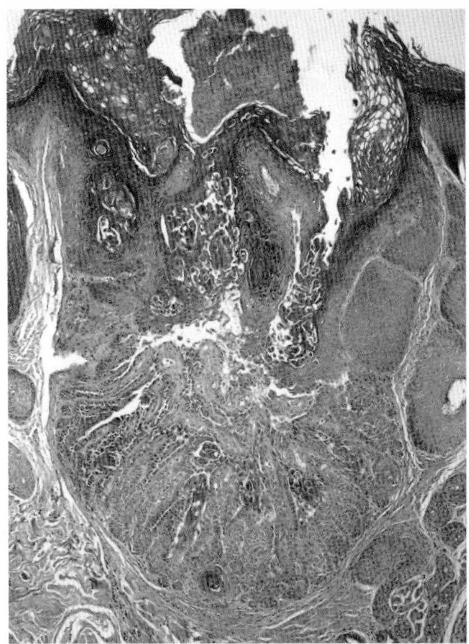

Fig. 6.2 Warty dyskeratoma. The outward growth is verrucoid. The inward-growing component shows suprabasilar acantholysis. (From Wyatt AJ, Busam KJ. Tumors of the epidermis. In: Busam KJ, ed. *Dermatopathology: A Volume in the Series: Foundations in Diagnostic Pathology*. 2nd ed. Philadelphia: Elsevier; 2016:339–387.)

- Histology: **cup-like epidermal invagination** with **acantholytic dyskeratosis** and corps ronds/grains (Fig. 6.2)
  - "Cup-shape" and solitary nature distinguishes from Darier's

Premalignant/malignant

Actinic keratosis (AK)

- Scaly, red papules/plaques on sun-damaged areas; a/w chronic sun exposure, male sex, older age, and fair skin phenotypes
- **UVB** responsible for AK development → induces **thymidine dimers** (C→T or CC→TT)
  - **p53 mutations** within keratinocytes → impaired apoptosis
- Histology: basal layer atypia (lower 1/3 of epidermis) with budding/finger-like projections into dermis; **"Flag sign"**: overlying parakeratosis (pink) alternating with orthohyperkeratosis (blue); atypia and parakeratosis often spares adnexal structures; solar elastosis in dermis
- Treatment: destructive measures (cryotherapy, ED&C, CO_2 ablation, topical 5-FU +/− calcipotriene, imiquimod, photodynamic therapy, tirbanibulin, ingenol mebutate, topical diclofenac, and TCA peel)
  - Topical 5-FU +/− calcipotriene appears most effective in recent head-to-head trials
- Rate of transformation to SCC = 0.075%–0.096% per year

Bowen's disease *(squamous cell carcinoma in situ)*

- Can progress from AK or occur *de novo*
- Risk factors: elderly, chronic sun exposure, lightly pigmented skin, immunosuppression, arsenic exposure, ionizing radiation, human papillomavirus (HPV), and chronic irritation

- Hyperkeratotic erythematous patch or plaque; may affect any site
- Histology: acanthosis with **full-thickness keratinocytic atypia**, disorganized ("**windblown**") architecture, ↑ mitoses, dyskeratotic keratinocytes, and parakeratosis
- Variants: pigmented, pagetoid, verrucous, **Bowenoid papulosis** (multiple hyperpigmented penile/vulvar papules, 2% progress to invasive SCC, HPV-16 and HPV-18 are #1 causes), and **erythroplasia of Queyrat** (juicy red, erosive plaque on glans penis; >30% progress to invasive SCC, HPV-16 is #1 cause)
- Treatment: destructive therapies (e.g., C&E), 5-fluorouracil (off-label), excision, and Mohs

Invasive cutaneous squamous cell carcinoma (cSCC, "SCC")

- **Second most common** skin cancer after basal cell carcinoma (BCC)
- Traditional teaching: "SCC accounts for 20% of NMSCs and is much less deadly than melanoma"
- New Teaching: "SCC is more prevalent and more dangerous than previously recognized!"
  - SCC incidence has increased by 263% since 1970s → current ratio of BCC:SCC is now closer to 1:1
  - SCC mortality rate now approximates that of melanoma!
- Clinical presentation: erythematous scaly papulonodule/ plaque; most commonly on **head/neck** and **dorsal extremities**
  - Oral SCC: most common sites are posterior lateral **tongue** > floor of mouth > soft palate
- Risk factors: chronic sun exposure, M > F (3:1), older age, fair skin phenotypes, genetic syndromes, **immunosuppression** (degree/duration → ↑ risk), solid-organ transplant recipient (65x–250x ↑ incidence; **heart/lung > liver > renal**; switching to sirolimus may help), HPV-16 and HPV-18, ionizing radiation (→ more aggressive course w/ ↑ recurrence and 10%–30% metastatic rate), CLL (↑ incidence and severity), chronic nonhealing wound (**Marjolin** ulcer → 25% metastatic rate), **hypertrophic LE/LP**, **arsenic** exposure, **chronic lichen sclerosus et atrophicus (LS&A; genital)**, RA patients on treatment, TNF-α inhibitors, **azathioprine**, tobacco use, **vemurafenib** (wart-like appearance common), long-term **voriconazole** usage, **vismodegib** (8x ↑ SCC risk)
- Molecular:
  - Mutations: ***TP53 (most common) >CDKN2A, RAS,*** *NOTCH1*
    - UVB → **thymidine dimers** (C→T or CC→TT)
    - Cutaneous SCC has a **very high mutational burden** compared with most malignancies (5x higher than lung cancer and melanoma) → may be more sensitive to immunotherapy-based treatment approaches
- Histology: full-thickness keratinocytic atypia w/ dermal invasion; tumor often "paradoxically differentiated" (tumor cells are MORE eosinophilic/keratinizing than surrounding keratinocytes)
  - High-risk subtypes: **desmoplastic, poorly-differentiated,** adenomatous, sarcomatous, spindle cell
  - Low-risk subtypes: verrucous carcinoma, keratoacanthoma (KA)
- Staging
  - Due to ↑ SCC incidence and mortality rates → tumor staging for SCC has become one of the "hottest" areas of research in dermatologic surgery
  - Goal of cancer/tumor staging = **risk stratification**
    - We need good tumor staging criteria to predict which patients w/SCC are at high risk of morbidity and mortality → allows for better clinical decision-making, clinical trial enrollment, etc.
  - Two major staging systems for SCC: American Joint Committee on Cancer (AJCC; 8th edition) and Brigham and Women's Hospital (BWH)
  - **AJCC staging system (8th edition)**
    - Only applies to SCC located on **head, neck, and vermillion lip** → cannot be used for staging SCC on other anatomic locations
    - All three TNM characteristics (tumor, nodes, metastatic disease) are required for cancer staging (vs. only T for the BWH staging system) → ↓ ease of use, especially for dermatologists
    - T stage scoring system
      - T1 = tumor diameter **< 2 cm**
      - T2 = tumor diameter between **2** and **4 cm**
      - T3 = tumor diameter **≥ 4 cm** *or* any **high-risk feature** (minor bone erosion, perineural invasion [PNI] of nerves ≥ 0.1 mm in caliber or PNI beneath the dermis, deep invasion [≥ 6 mm or beyond subcutaneous fat])
      - T4 = strictly reserved for **major bone involvement** or invasion of skull base
  - **BWH staging system**
    - Shown to be **more effective at risk stratification** than AJCC staging system (higher specificity [93%] and positive predictive value [30%] for identifying cases at risk for metastasis and death)
    - **T (tumor) staging only**! → very easy for dermatologists to use
      - Staging does not require any information about the status of the lymph nodes (N) or presence of metastatic disease (M)
    - Four high-risk features (each counts as 1 point): **PNI** (≥ 0.1 mm caliber nerve), **diameter ≥ 2 cm, invasion beyond SQ fat,** and **poorly differentiated** histology
    - T stage scoring system
      - T1 = zero high-risk features
      - T2a = one high-risk feature
      - **T2b = two to three high-risk features** (metastatic rate ~35%; **mortality rate** ~**20%)**
      - T3 = all four high-risk features *or* **bone invasion** (automatically upgrades stage to T3, regardless of other features)
    - **Stage T2b are *"rare but deadly!"***
      - Only 5% of all SCC are classified as **BWH stage T2b**
      - However, these 5% of tumors (T2b) account for **72% of ALL nodal metastases and 83% of ALL deaths from cSCC** → very important to identify T2b lesions!
- **NCCN Treatment Guidelines** (important for Mohs Board Exam)
  - Low-risk

- Treatment
  - Curettage and electrodesiccation (except terminal hair-bearing areas) → transition to excision if C&E (curettage and electrodessication) extends beyond dermis
  - Excision with 4 to 6 mm clinical margins
    - If margin positive → Mohs or other peripheral and deep en face margin assessment (PDEMA), re-excision, or radiation therapy (RT)
  - Mohs or other PDEMA
  - RT for non-surgical candidates
- High-risk
  - Treatment
    - Mohs or other PDEMA
    - Excision with wider margin
      - If margin positive → Mohs or other PDEMA, re-excision, or RT
    - RT +/− systemic therapy for non-surgical candidates or systemic therapy alone if RT not feasible
- If positive margins with Mohs or excision and re-resection not feasible → multidisciplinary consult → RT +/− systemic therapy or systemic therapy alone if RT not feasible
- If extensive perineural, large, or named nerve involvement, or other poor prognostic features → consider adjuvant RT even with negative margins
- Lymph node (LN) metastasis +/− distant metastasis
  - Palpable or abnormal LNs on imaging → fine-needle aspiration (FNA) or core biopsy
    - If negative FNA or core biopsy → consider excisional LN biopsy
    - If positive FNA or core biopsy → further imaging (CT with contrast or PET/CT)
      - If operable → excision of primary tumor and LN dissection as indicated **AND** often RT (especially if multiple nodes or large node or extracapsular extension [ECE])
        - If ECE or incompletely excised nodal disease → RT and consider concurrent systemic therapy
        - Regional LN recurrence or distant mets → multidisciplinary consultation
  - If inoperable → multidisciplinary consultation → RT +/− systemic therapy or systemic therapy alone if RT not feasible
- Systemic therapy
  - Systemic therapy options for use **with** RT:
    - Cisplatin preferred
    - Useful in certain circumstances:
      - Epidermal growth factor receptor (EGFR) inhibitor (cetuximab)
      - Cisplatin + 5-FU
      - Carboplatin +/− paclitaxel
  - Options for systemic therapy alone:
    - **Cemiplimab** or **pembrolizumab** preferred (if curative RT or surgery not feasible for locally advanced, recurrent, or metastatic disease)
      - If ineligible for (i.e., SOTR) or progressed on immune checkpoint inhibitors and clinical trials → carboplatin + paclitaxel

- Prognosis: metastatic rate (all-comers with SCC) = 5%; mortality rate = 3.5%
  - ↑ Risk of metastasis: immunosuppressed state, location on **lip/ear**, diameter > **2 cm**, Breslow **depth > 2 mm**, extension beyond SQ fat, SCC arising in **burn/scar (Marjolin ulcer)**, PNI (≥0.1 mm), and poorly differentiated histology
  - LN metastases from head and neck SCC have a high cure rate when identified and treated early
  - High stage SCC (BWH T2b/T3) has ≥ 30% metastatic rate → management requires greater consideration
  - **Oral mucosal SCC has a worse prognosis than SCC of the lip which has a worse prognosis than cSCC**
- **Additional Boards Fodder**
  - **Which factor is most strongly associated with ____?"**
    - **Disease-specific death?** ***Diameter** > 2 cm*
      - *Mnemonic: "Die = DIE-ameter"*
      - 19-fold ↑ mortality rate, compared with tumors < 2 cm
    - **Recurrence and metastasis?** ***Depth** > 2 mm*
      - Breslow depth < 2 mm → ~0% metastasis rate
      - Breslow depth = 2.1 to 6.0 mm → 4% metastasis rate
      - Breslow depth > 6.0 mm → 16% metastasis rate
      - Also, extension beyond SQ fat → high rates of local recurrence (28%) and nodal metastasis (27%)
  - **Genetic syndromes associated with SCC:**
    - Oculocutaneous albinism
    - Xeroderma pigmentosum
    - Dystrophic epidermolysis bullosa (DEB; SCC is **#1 cause of death**)
    - Epidermodysplasia verruciformis
    - Dyskeratosis congenita
    - Porokeratosis, linear type
    - Keratitis, ichthyosis, deafness (KID) syndrome
    - Rothmund-Thompson syndrome
    - Werner syndrome
    - Chronic mucocutaneous candidiasis
    - Bloom syndrome

Verrucous carcinoma

- Low-grade, locally destructive SCC a/w **HPV-6 and HPV-11**
- Large exo-endophytic nodule; three clinical variants:
  - Epithelioma cuniculatum: slow-growing mass on **plantar** foot (Fig. 6.3)
  - Buschke-Lowenstein tumor (giant condyloma): large cauliflower-like growth in **anogenital** region
  - Oral florid papillomatosis: widespread oral lesions
- Histology: **very well-differentiated** (minimal to no cytologic atypia); bulbous/**pushing border**, massive size and ↑ depth of base = clues to malignancy

Keratoacanthoma

- Variant of SCC with unique features: **initial rapid growth** over weeks → **self-resolves/involutes** over months
  - **Subungual KAs** are the exception (do NOT involute)

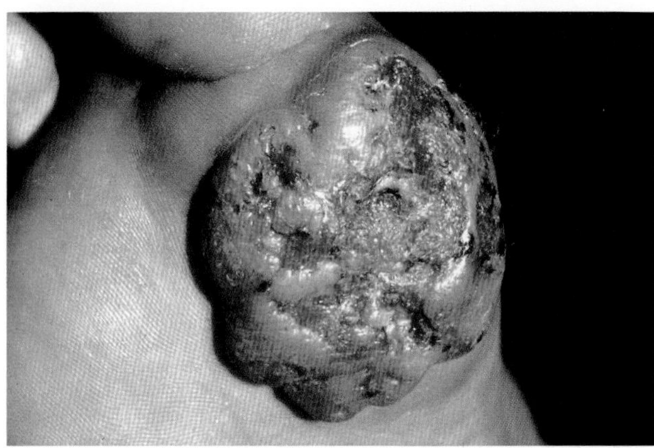

Fig. 6.3 Verrucous carcinoma of the foot (epithelioma cuniculatum). Verrucous carcinomas often reach large sizes before diagnosis because they are often treated as warts.

- Clinical variants: solitary, multiple, giant, intraoral, subungual, and KA centrifugum marginatum (can reach several centimeters)
- KA syndromes:
  - Ferguson-Smith: **AD inheritance**; rapid onset of multiple KAs; onset **third decade**, sun-exposed areas, and **resolves** spontaneously
  - Grzybowski: sporadic; 1000s of milia-like KAs in **later adulthood**; can involve **airway**; a/w **scarring**, **ectropion**, and mask-like facies. **Mnemonic**: "Old (later onset) **Grizzlies** Growl (airway affected)"
- Other associations: **Muir-Torre syndrome** (classic KAs, or KAs w/ sebaceous differentiation), immunosuppression, and HPV
- Histology: **crateriform**, endophytic nodule w/ **well-differentiated** keratinocytes (lacks significant atypia), central keratin plug, and peripheral inflammation w/ eosinophils
- Treatment: excision or Mohs; may observe if certain involuting

Basal cell carcinoma

- THE **most common** human malignancy!
- Onset typically 50s to 60s, but can occur earlier; slow/indolent growth; locally destructive (esp. morpheaform, infiltrative, and micronodular subtypes)
- Due to UV exposure (intermittent and intense > chronic and cumulative); certain medications (e.g., sphingosine 1-phosphate receptor modulators for multiple sclerosis) may increase risk
- **Boards Fodder: *PTCH* mutations (chromosome 9q; most common) > *TP53* mutations** (p53 tumor suppressor; second most common) (Fig. 6.4; Box 6.1)
- Sun-exposed skin; rare on palms, soles, and mucous membranes
- Numerous clinicopathologic variants (Table 6.3)
- General histologic features: nests of basaloid, uniform cells w/ high N:C ratio, peripheral palisading, epidermal connection (at least focally), myxoid stroma, stromal–epithelial retraction, and mitotic/apoptotic activity
  - High-risk subtypes: infiltrative, micronodular, morpheaform, basosquamous, sclerosing, carcinosarcomatous
  - Other high-risk features: poorly defined borders, recurrent, site of prior RT, immunosuppressed patient, perineural involvement, mask areas of face/genitals/hands/feet, >10 mm on cheeks/forehead/scalp/neck/pretibial, >20 mm on trunk/extremities
- Very low metastatic potential (<0.1%; dependent on stroma for growth)
  - Basosquamous subtype may behave more like SCC → ↑ metastatic potential
- **Niacinamide 500 mg BID reduces BCC and SCC risk by 23%**
- **NCCN treatment guidelines**
  - Low-risk
    - Treatment
      - C&E (except terminal hair-bearing areas) → transition to excision if C&E extends beyond dermis

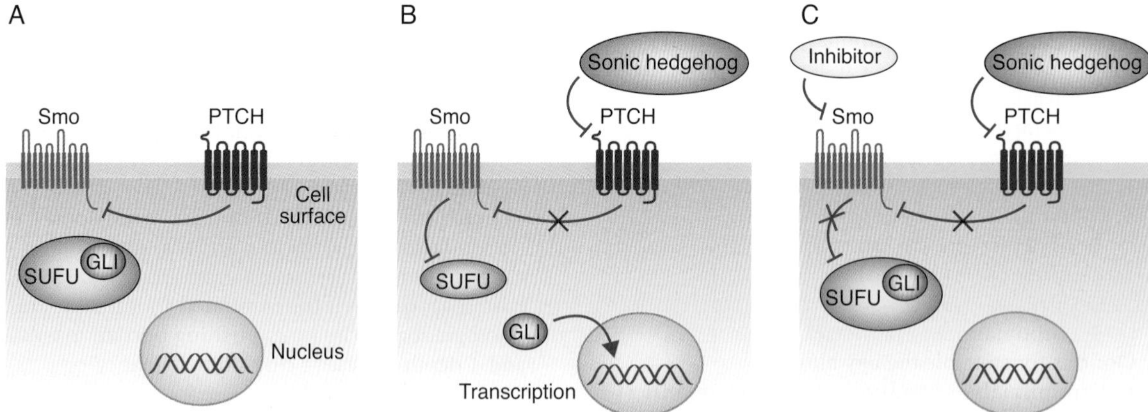

Fig. 6.4 The hedgehog inhibitor pathway. (A) Non-proliferative state: patched receptor **(PTCH) inhibits the activity of smoothened *(Smo)***, allowing suppressor of fused (SUFU) to bind to and inactivate GLI transcription factors. (B) Binding of the sonic hedgehog ligand to PTCH allows activation (dis-inhibition) of Smo → activated Smo inhibits the binding of SUFU to GLI → GLI transcription factors are then free to enter the nucleus and modulate transcription of hedgehog pathway-associated genes. (C) Vismodegib and Sonidegib act like "artificial PTCH" by inhibiting Smo activation → SUFU is free to to bind to and inactivate GLI transcription factors. (Redrawn from Lear JT, Corner C, Dziewulski P, et al. Challenges and new horizons in the management of advanced basal cell carcinoma: a UK perspective. *Br J Cancer*. 2014;111[8]:1476–1481: From Fitzpatrick JE, Morelli JG. *Dermatology Secrets Plus*, 4th ed. Philadelphia: Elsevier, 2011)

Box 6.1 Mnemonic: Genetic Syndromes a/w Multiple BCCs

"Green Berets Rarely Buy eXtra Shoes ... but they get a lot of BCCs from being in the sun!"

- **G**orlin's
- **B**azex-Dupré-Christol
- **R**ombo
- **B**rooke-Spiegler
- **X**eroderma pigmentosum
- **S**chöpf-Schulz-Passarge

Table 6.3 Basal Cell Carcinoma Variants

Nodular	Favors **head/neck**; histology: large nests (centrally +/– necrosis, cystic spaces); cells lack organization centrally, prominent peripheral palisading, and may be ulcerated
Superficial	Erythematous scaly patch, most common type in younger patients, **trunk and extremities** (>head/neck); histology: multiple buds from epidermis do not extend beyond papillary dermis
Morpheaform	Scar-like pink to white plaque; histology: small angulated nests and cords within a sclerotic stroma; retraction not prominent; may be more deeply invasive
Micronodular	Smaller nests than nodular type; micronodules are separated by normal intervening collagen, and does not form a circumscribed contour at the deep aspect
Fibroepithelioma of Pinkus	Pedunculated, "soft/fleshy" lesion on **lower back**; histology: thin anastomosing strands form a network within pinker stroma; retraction and myxoid material are less prominent
Pigmented	Nodular pattern BCC with aggregates of melanin in the nests and dermal melanophages
Infundibulocystic (keratotic, follicular)	Well-circumscribed, comprised of basaloid and squamoid cells in anastomosing cords, w/ horn cysts → **resembles benign follicular tumors** (trichoepithelioma and basaloid follicular hamartoma)
Basosquamous	Ambiguous term w/ variable meanings; may refer to: (1) BCCs with "squamoid appearance" (pinker cells, more cytoplasm, and keratinization); (2) carcinomas with features indeterminate between BCC and SCC; or (3) collision lesions of BCC + SCC

- Excision with 4 mm clinical margins
  - ➔ If margin positive → Mohs or other PDEMA, re-excision, or RT
- RT for non-surgical candidates

- High-risk
  - Treatment
    - **Mohs** or other PDEMA
    - Excision with wider margin
      - ➔ If margin positive → Mohs or other PDEMA, re-excision, or RT
    - RT or systemic therapy (vismodegib, sonidegib, cemiplimab) for non-surgical patients
- If positive margins with Mohs or excision and re-resection not feasible → RT and multidisciplinary consult (systemic therapy if curative RT not feasible)
- Primary or recurrent nodal metastasis: multidisciplinary consult
  - Surgery if feasible
  - RT or systemic therapy with hedgehog inhibitors (vismodegib >> sonidegib) or cemiplimab if surgery not feasible
- Distant metastasis: multidisciplinary consult
  - Systemic therapy with **vismodegib (NOT sonidegib)** or **cemiplimab**
  - RT or surgery for limited metastasis
  - Palliative/supportive care

6.2 CYSTS

Epidermoid cyst (epidermal inclusion cyst)

- Clinical features
  - Firm dermal nodule with **central punctum**; any site, but most commonly head/neck/upper trunk
- Pathogenesis/histopathologic features
  - Derived from follicular infundibular epithelium; may arise primarily, or secondary to follicle disruption/traumatic implantation; lined by stratified squamous epithelium w/ **intact granular layer** and **no adnexal structures** in the wall (vs. vellus hair cyst and dermoid cyst); **laminated/flaky keratin** centrally
- Comments
  - Multiple epidermoid cysts may be a/w **Gardner syndrome** (often have pilomatricoma-like areas histologically)

Trichilemmal (pilar) cyst

- Clinical features
  - Firm dermal nodule; **90% on the scalp**; usually multiple (70%); subset **AD inheritance**
- Pathogenesis/histopathologic features
  - Derived from isthmic follicular epithelium; stratified squamous epithelium **lacking granular layer; dense pink homogenized keratin** with frequent calcification centrally

Proliferating trichilemmal cyst/tumor

- Clinical features
  - Slow-growing dermal nodule; **scalp (90%)**; usually **elderly women**
- Pathogenesis/histopathologic features
  - Resembles trichilemmal cyst but more **proliferative centrally** w/ areas of multicystic architecture; well-circumscribed at periphery; variable cytologic atypia and mitotic activity
- Comments
  - Small percentage behave aggressively → complete removal recommended

Dermoid cyst

- Clinical features
  - **Infants**; occur **along embryonic fusion lines** (most commonly **lateral eyebrow**)

- Pathogenesis/histopathologic features
  - Derived from entrapment of epidermis during embryogenesis; lined by stratified squamous epithelium with **granular layer** and **adnexal structures (hair follicles and sebaceous glands) in cyst wall**
- Comments: be careful if biopsying b/c may have intracranial connection

Vellus hair cyst

- Clinical features
  - Multiple ("eruptive") domed and flesh-colored or **hyperpigmented papules**; trunk; subset AD inheritance
- Pathogenesis/histopathologic features
  - Same histology as epidermoid cyst, but has **multiple vellus hairs** in cyst cavity (flip condenser to see)
- Comments
  - Can occur as part of **Lowe syndrome** (XLR inheritance, Fanconi-type renal failure, mental retardation, various eye issues)

Steatocystoma

- Clinical features
  - Single or multiple (**multiplex; AD inheritance**) lesions; chest/axilla/groin; drain oily fluid if punctured
- Pathogenesis/histopathologic features
  - Lined by thin stratified squamous epithelium with no granular layer and **thin bright pink corrugated ("shark-tooth" or "dragon scale") cuticle; sebaceous glands in wall**
- Comments
  - Multiplex form with ***KRT17* mutations**; a/w **pachyonychia congenita type 2**

Hidrocystoma

- Clinical features
  - Translucent **bluish cysts**; face (eyelids #1); solitary or multiple
- Pathogenesis/histopathologic features
  - Unilocular or multilocular cyst with low cuboidal lining +/− decapitation secretion (if apocrine); lumen appears empty
- Comments
  - May be a/w **Schöpf-Schulz-Passarge** (multiple hidrocystomas, syringofibroadenomas, palmoplantar keratoderma, hypodontia, and hypotrichosis)

Bronchogenic cyst

- Clinical features
  - Solitary; present at birth; **suprasternal notch**/anterior neck
- Pathogenesis/histopathologic features
  - Sequestration of respiratory epithelium during embryogenesis; pseudostratified, ciliated columnar cells with **goblet cells**; +/− **smooth muscle**/mucous glands/**cartilage** in wall
- Comments
  - Main clues for Boards: **cartilage, smooth muscle, and ↑↑ goblet cells**

Thyroglossal duct cyst

- Clinical features
  - Children/young adults; **midline anterior neck; moves w/ swallowing**
- Pathogenesis/histopathologic features
  - Columnar, cuboidal, or stratified squamous lining with **thyroid follicles** in the wall (low cuboidal epithelium with bright pink contents)
- Comments
  - Main clue for Boards: **pink thyroid follicles** (pathognomonic)

Median raphe cyst

- Clinical features
  - Men; **ventral penis** between urethral meatus and anus; pain during intercourse
- Pathogenesis/histopathologic features
  - Variable lining of cyst; **"dirty debris"** within cyst; genital skin features (e.g., smooth muscle and small nerves)

Branchial cleft cyst

- Clinical features
  - Second or third decades; **lateral neck** (anterior sternocleidomastoid, preauricular, and mandibular)
- Pathogenesis/histopathologic features
  - Pseudostratified columnar or stratified squamous epithelium with surrounding dense lymphoid tissue including **lymphoid follicles w/ germinal centers (main clue for Boards!)** → Mnemonic: "You can see the immune system's **'branches'** in a branchial cleft cyst"

Pseudocyst of the auricle

- Clinical features
  - Middle-aged men; scaphoid fossa
- Pathogenesis/histopathologic features
  - Cystic space in cartilage with fluid, no epithelial lining and no inflammation in cartilage
- Comments
  - a/w chronic **trauma from cell phones** or wrestling

Omphalomesenteric duct cyst

- Clinical features
  - Umbilical polyp in children
- Pathogenesis/histopathologic features
  - Occurs as a result of a failure to obliterate the connection between midgut and yolk sac during embryogenesis; ectopic columnar gastrointestinal mucosa

6.3 MELANOCYTIC NEOPLASMS

Ephelides (freckles)

- 1- to 3-mm macules of ↑ pigmentation; darken w/ sun-exposure; **sun-exposed** areas of body, mainly face, dorsal upper extremities, and upper trunk

- More common in blonde or red-haired individuals; absent at birth, but appear in first 3 years of life
- ↑ Melanogenesis and ↑ melanin transfer to keratinocytes
- Histology: ↑ basilar keratinocyte pigmentation +/– enlarged melanocytes without increased melanocyte density
- No propensity for malignant transformation, however are a marker of UV damage

CALM (café au lait macule)

- Discrete uniform tan to brown macules or patches; may be seen in infants, children, and young adults; isolated finding in 10%–20% of normal population
- Multiple CALMs may be a/w numerous genodermatoses:
  - **Neurofibromatosis type 1 (NF1) > type 2 (NF2)**
  - **McCune-Albright syndrome**
  - Russell-Silver
  - Noonan syndrome
  - Bloom syndrome
  - **Tuberous sclerosis**
  - **MEN-I**
  - **Fanconi anemia**
  - Ataxia-telangiectasias
- Histology: ↑ melanin deposition in basilar keratinocytes

Solar lentigo

- Multiple pigmented macules on sun-exposed areas; most common in Caucasians (essentially ubiquitous after 60 years of age) > light-skinned Asians
- Histology: elongated bulbous rete ridges with hyperpigmentation ("**dirty socks**"); +/– mild increase in melanocyte density; solar elastosis in dermis

Lentigo simplex

- Well-demarcated, evenly pigmented brown to black macule; any age and any anatomic site
- Histology: basal layer hyperpigmentation; elongated rete ridges with mild ↑ melanocyte density
- Conditions a/w multiple lentigines:
  - **LEOPARD (most heavily "spotted" appearance)**
  - **Carney complex (LAMB/NAME)**
  - **Peutz-Jeghers (especially oral/perioral)**
  - Laugier-Hunziker
  - Cowden syndrome
  - **Bannayan-Riley-Ruvalcaba (penile)**
  - Xeroderma pigmentosum
  - Cronkhite-Canada

Mucosal melanotic macule

- Compared with lentigo simplex can be more irregular and mottled
- Oral lesions usually occur in **adults > 40 years old** on **vermilion lip** > gingiva, buccal mucosa, or palate; genital lesions most common on labia minora
- Histology: acanthosis; mild basilar hyperpigmentation +/– subtle increase in melanocyte density

Dermal melanocytosis

- <u>Congenital (Mongolian/cerulean spot)</u>: present at birth in most **Asians and Blacks**; **lumbosacral** region; p/w gray-blue patch (as a result of the **Tyndall effect** where shorter light wavelengths are reflected by melanocytes); often **resolves** during childhood
  - Histology: sparsely distributed elongated dendritic melanocytes in lower 2/3 of dermis, lying parallel to epidermis
- <u>Nevus of Ota</u>: presents in first year of life or around puberty; ↑ incidence in pigmented individuals (Asians and Blacks); p/w coalescing gray-blue macules in **V1/V2 distribution** and frequent **scleral involvement** (60%); unilateral (90%) > bilateral; persists for life; may **enlarge under hormonal influences**; **10% develop glaucoma;** rare malignant degeneration to **uveal melanoma** (perhaps higher risk in nevus of Ota lesions with activating mutations in *GNAQ*)
  - Histology: elongated dendritic melanocytes more numerous than in congenital dermal melanocytosis; involves upper dermis
- <u>Other clinical variants:</u>
  - **Nevus of Ito:** located on the shoulder, supraclavicular, and scapular regions; essentially no risk of progression to melanoma
  - **Hori's nevus**: acquired nevus of Ota-like macules of the **bilateral** zygomatic region; East Asian females
  - **Sun's nevus:** acquired, **unilateral** variant of Hori's nevus
    - Mnemonic: "There is only **1 Sun**, but the (w)**HO**le face is affected in **HO**ri's"
- Histologically, dermal melanocytoses are **distinguished from blue nevi** by their ↓ **cellularity**, poor circumscription, and **lack of dermal sclerosis**

Blue nevus

- Onset in childhood/adolescence, but can also occur in older patients; 25% of cellular blue nevi (CBN) are congenital
- Most common sites: **scalp**, **sacral area**, and **distal extensor extremities**
- Derived from dermal melanocytes (persist during embryogenesis rather than populating epidermis)
- Activating mutations in ***GNAQ*** and ***GNA11*** seen in 83%; results in downstream MAPK pathway activation
  - Same mutations are the most common mutations in **uveal melanoma** (46%; concomitant *BAP-1* loss in uveal melanoma leads to increased risk of metastasis and death)
- Multiple blue nevi and epithelioid blue nevi (much more specific) a/w **Carney complex**
- Variants:
  - <u>Common blue nevus</u>:
    - Blue/gray macules or papules usually less than 1 cm
    - Elongated, dendritic melanocytes containing melanin pigment usually in the upper 2/3rd of dermis with associated **sclerotic collagen**; no junctional component

- Cellular blue nevus:
  - Blue/gray/black plaques or nodules; often **larger** (1–3 cm); favor **buttocks or scalp**
  - **Dense proliferation of plump/fusiform pale gray melanocytes** containing little pigment + admixed dendritic melanocytes resembling common blue nevus cells; characteristically bulges into subcutis ("**dumbbell configuration**")
- Epithelioid blue nevus:
  - Heavily pigmented; strongly a/w **Carney complex**
  - Demonstrates ***PRKAR1A*** and ***PRKCA*** mutations (inherited or somatic)
  - Sometimes called pigmented epithelioid melanocytoma
  - If significant **atypia/cellularity/mitoses** → **"animal-type melanoma"**
- Malignant blue nevus (= melanoma): often arises **within CBN**; **scalp** (#1); commonly see benign precursor within specimen; deep tumor extension + necrosis + mitoses; frequently have **concomitant** ***GNAQ/GNA11*** mutations + ***BAP-1*** **loss** (a/w more aggressive behavior; tumorigenesis similar to uveal melanoma)

Recurrent melanocytic nevus

- Repigmentation **confined to the scar** (vs. pigment extending beyond biopsy site = melanoma); usually **arises within 6 months** of initial biopsy
- Histology (3 key features)
  - Dermal scar
  - Atypical junctional melanocytic proliferation (resembles melanoma in situ) confined to area above dermal scar
  - Bland dermal nevus remnants below/adjacent to scar (#1 Boards clue)

Balloon cell nevus

- Clinically indistinguishable from ordinary nevi
- Histology: **>50% dermal melanocytes are "balloon cells"** (large, pale, and polygonal melanocytes with foamy/vacuolated cytoplasm and variable pigmentation); balloon cell change is a result of **melanosome degeneration**
  - Boards tip: can always identify conventional nevus somewhere within lesion

Halo nevus (Sutton nevus)

- Pigmented nevus with surrounding hypopigmented zone; most commonly second decade; most commonly on the **back**; most commonly benign
  - May be **a/w vitiligo or melanoma** (rarely) at another site (perform full skin exam if seen)
- Multiple lesions can occur idiopathically or w/ various monoconal antibodies (e.g., infliximab, tocilizumab, pembrolizumab)
- Histology: bland nevus w/ **lymphocytes intertwined ("mingling") with melanocytes**
  - In contrast, lymphocytes form a lichenoid band (**"riot police barrier"**) under and around melanoma

Spitz nevus

- Clinical
  - Acquired, usually solitary lesions in **first two decades** (use caution in diagnosing a patient in the fourth decade and older); most common on **head/neck** > extremities
  - Rapidly growing pink-red papulonodule; usually < 1 cm
- Pathogenesis
  - ***HRAS*** mutations/**11p gain**
    - Most Spitz nevi **lack** ***BRAF*** **mutations** (vs. conventional nevi and melanomas)
  - **Gene fusions:** *ALK, NTRK1, NTRK3, MET, ROS*
  - **"BAPoma:"** distinctive subset of **atypical epithelioid spitzoid nevi** with **loss of** ***BAP-1*** tumor suppressor gene; have unique histology, and unlike most Spitz nevi, have activating ***BRAF*** **mutations**
    - Two cell populations: **conventional** nevus cells + **epithelioid** cells (large, rounded, melanocytic population w/ nuclear inclusions)
    - Big cells are negative for *BAP-1* on immunohistochemistry (IHC)
- Histology (Fig. 6.5):
  - **Symmetric and circumscribed**; most often compound
  - **Epidermal hyperplasia** (vs. consumption of epidermis in melanoma)

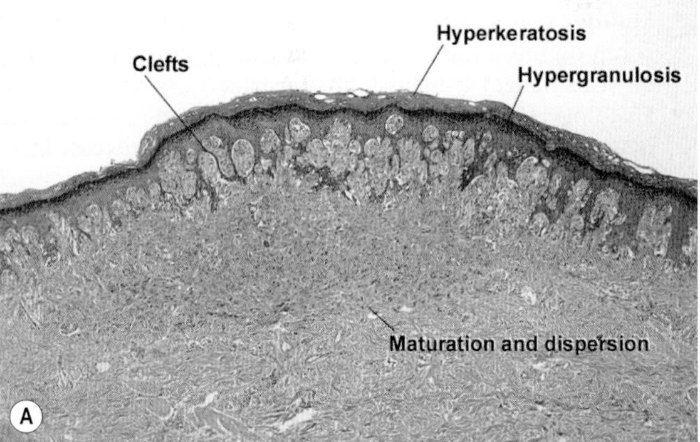

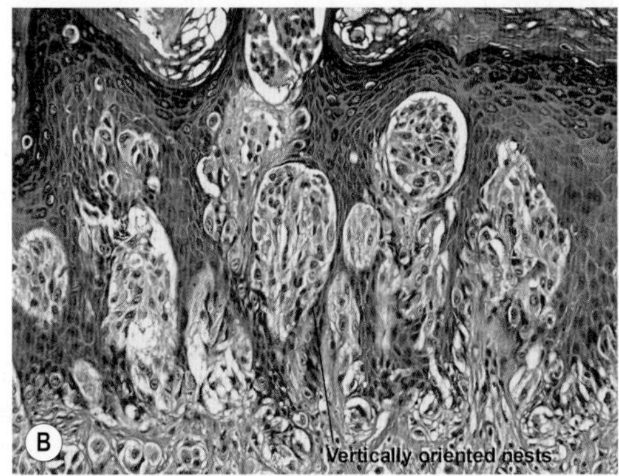

Fig. 6.5 (A) and (B) Spitz nevus histology. Note the pseudoepitheliomatous hyperplasia of the epidermis with vertically oriented spindled and epithelioid nests ("bananas on the tree") and clefts around the nests. (From Elston DM. Melanocytic neoplasms. In: Elston DM, Ferringer T, eds. *Dermatopathology*. 3rd ed. Philadelphia: Elsevier, 2019:101–131.)

- Large junctional nests with **clefting** around entire nest (vs. discohesion of nests in melanoma, where the nest itself becomes fragmented)
- Parallel "**raining-down**" orientation of nests and cells
- **Kamino bodies**: pink clumps of basement membrane zone **(BMZ) material (collagen IV)** within epidermis
- "Spitzoid" cytology: large epithelioid and spindled cells w/ abundant **pink-purple (amphophilic)** cytoplasm and prominent **lilac-colored nucleoli** (vs. cherry red nucleoli in melanoma); usually not pigmented
- Dermal component "**matures**" with depth (reduction in density and cell size)
- **Superficial mitoses** allowable, especially in young patients → if numerous (>2–3), deep or atypical mitoses are present, raises concern for melanoma

- Immunostains: **S100A6+**, S100+, Melan-A+, and **p16+**
  - **p16 is frequently lost/diminished in atypical Spitz tumors and spitzoid melanoma**
- Treatment: controversial, but complete excision often recommended, especially if biopsy transected
- **Boards fodder: fluorescence in situ hybridization (FISH) analysis and comparative genomic hybridization (CGH) very helpful in risk stratification** of atypical Spitzoid lesions
  - **Homozygous loss of 9p21** (most predictive gene locus; corresponds to p16/CDKN2a gene) → ↑ **risk of metastasis and death**
  - Multiple gains and losses on CGH = melanoma
  - On sequencing, ***TERT* promoter mutations** → predictive of **poor outcomes**

Pigmented spindle cell nevus of Reed

- Heavily pigmented variant of Spitz nevus **comprised ~exclusively of spindled spitzoid melanocytes**
- **Young** F > M; **thigh** most commonly (> other extremities and trunk)
- Darkly pigmented macule/papule, usually < 6 mm
- Histology: **junctional or superficial compound**, symmetric, circumscribed proliferation of **spindled melanocytes** arranged in vertically oriented fascicles + **numerous melanophages** (much more than in conventional Spitz nevi) in superficial dermis +/− **pigmented parakeratosis**
  - Architecture: similar to Spitz nevus but almost always **confined to junction** (or very superficial dermis)
  - Cytology: spindled melanocytes are same as in Spitz nevi, but PSCN **lacks the epithelioid cells** seen in conventional Spitz nevi

Deep penetrating nevus (DPN)

- Most commonly is a component of combined nevus (overlaps w/ clonal nevus, and inverted type A nevus)
- Activating **β-catenin mutations** in a pre-existing nevus → increased nuclear cyclin D1
- Distinct from blue nevus family based on lack of *GNAQ/GNA11* mutations
- Face, upper trunk and extremities; usually **second and third decades**
- Well-circumscribed blue to black papule; <1 cm in size
- Histology: compound melanocytic proliferation with small but nearly-ubiquitous **junctional component**, superficial **dermal nests resembling ordinary nevus nests** (very helpful clue in distinguishing from CBN), and prominent **wedge-shaped dermal component**, which **extends deep** into the dermis or subcutis, tracks along adnexal structures or neurovascular bundles; **epithelioid pigmented melanocytes** in loose nests with a lot of **melanophages** (Fig. 6.6A and B); **β-catenin** nuclear positivity in epithelioid pigmented melanocytes on IHC
  - Versus CBN: DPN has **junctional component** (always absent in CBN), **superficial dermal nests resembling ordinary nevus nests** (not seen in CBN), **more pigment** within melanocytes (CBN melanocytes are amelanotic → pigment is predominantly in surrounding melanophages), melanocytes are larger and have more cytoplasm; nuclear β-catenin+ on IHC

Congenital melanocytic nevus

- ***NRAS* mutations** in majority of cases (>*BRAF* mutations)
- Divided into small (<1.5 cm), medium (1.5–19.9 cm), and **large (≥20 cm)**
  - Small congenital nevi have same low risk of developing melanoma as conventional nevi
  - Large congenital nevi (>20 cm) have ↑ **melanoma risk** (~2%–3%; majority develop in **first decade**)

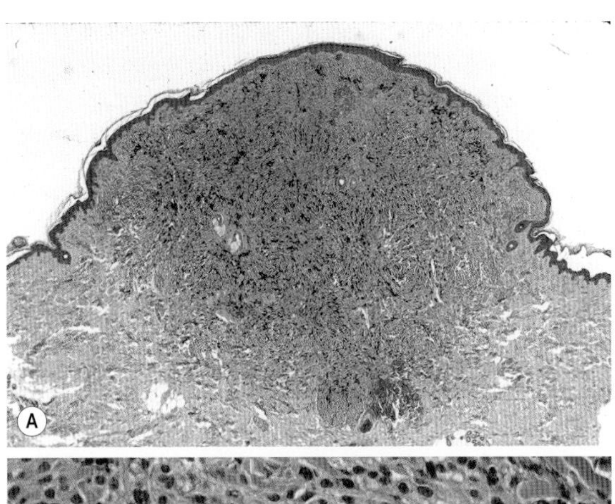

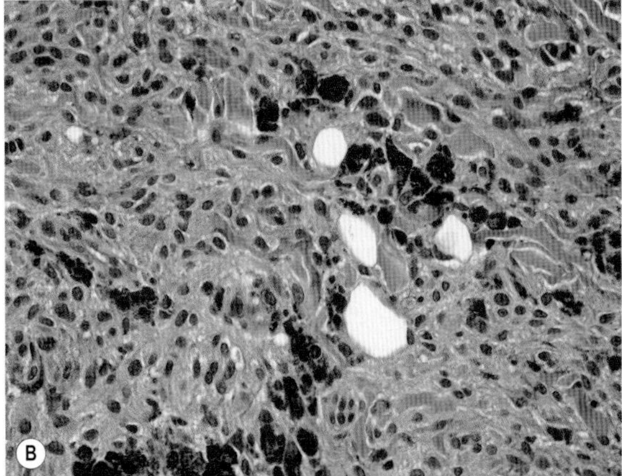

Fig. 6.6 Deep penetrating nevus. (A) A pigmented melanocytic nevus with a wedge-shaped silhouette is seen. (B) Pigmented spindle and epithelioid melanocytes are present, as well as melanophages. (From Busam KJ. Melanocytic proliferations. In: *Dermatopathology: A Volume in the Series: Foundations in Diagnostic Pathology*. 2nd ed. Philadelphia: Elsevier; 2016:447–512.)

- Initially raised tan lesions that may darken over the first year of life; +/– hypertrichosis
- Often develop "**proliferative nodules**" → mimic melanoma clinically and histologically
- **Neurocutaneous melanosis/melanocytosis** = large congenital nevus in association with melanocytic proliferation (benign or malignant) within leptomeninges and brain parenchyma
  - Affects various sites in CNS → variable clinical presentation; **high mortality** in symptomatic patients due to mass effect
- Histology: compound or intradermal melanocytic proliferation; dermal component extends deeper than common acquired nevi; dermal component displays single cell dispersion in deeper dermis, **surrounds/ infiltrates vessels, adnexal structures, muscle, and nerve** (not concerning)
- Treatment (large congenital nevi):
  - Surgical resection should be attempted when possible after 6 months of age; if not possible or only partial resection → serial examinations, early biopsies of nodular areas
  - If **large posterior axial congenital nevi** or **multiple satellites** (>4, particularly if at least one is at least a medium congenital nevus) → recommend **MRI screening** for neurocutaneous melanosis

Nevus spilus/speckled lentiginous nevus

- Presents within the first year of life
- Homogeneous tan patch within which develops small pigmented macules and papules
- Trunk and extremities most commonly affected sites
- May be a/w **phakomatosis pigmentovascularis** and phakomatosis pigmentokeratotica
- Risk of melanoma is low
- Confused w/ **agminated nevus**, but the latter occurs in teenage years and with a cluster of nevi over a skin-colored (rather than tan) background; significant subset of lesions due to activating *HRAS* mutation

Common acquired melanocytic nevus

- Most prevalent in Caucasians; may see **eruptive acquired nevi** at affected sites in **EB** (**"EB nevi"**; benign, but often confused for melanoma because of atypical clinical and histologic features) and **LS&A**
- Any site; increase in number over first three decades, then decrease
- "Abtropfung hypothesis": nevus cells start as junctional proliferation → subsequently migrate into dermis (compound nevus) → later become entirely intradermal → may involute
- UV exposure, immunosuppression, hormonal influences implicated; ***BRAF*** **mutations** in up to 80% (>*NRAS* mutations)
- Clinically well-circumscribed, symmetric, small (<6 mm), and evenly pigmented
- Histology: symmetrically junctional, compound or dermal proliferations w/ small regular nests, and dermal component shows "maturation" with depth (melanocytes become smaller and less nested)

Atypical (dysplastic) melanocytic nevus

- Occur sporadically or in the setting of familial atypical multiple mole melanoma syndrome (FAMMM)
  - FAMMM: AD inheritance; characterized by multiple melanocytic nevi (50+), family history of melanoma, and mutations in *CDKN2A* gene (encodes p16 and $p14^{ARF}$)
- Any site (**trunk and scalp** most common); wide age range
  - Potential pitfall: new "atypical/dysplastic nevi" on sun-damaged sites of elderly are most likely well-nested lentigo maligna!
- Solitary or multiple; asymmetric, irregularly bordered, and variably pigmented nevi ranging in size (often > 6 mm)
  - When multiple, patients tend to have clinically (and histologically) similar **"signature nevi"** → melanomas in these patients often appear as **"ugly duckling"** lesions (different appearance than their signature nevi)
- Histology: classic features of dysplastic (Clark) nevus:
  - **Asymmetry**, lack of circumscription
  - Junctional "**shoulder**" (extends three or rete ridges beyond dermal component)
  - Irregular size and placement of junctional nests with **bridging** or **lentiginous pattern** (single-cell junctional growth)
  - Papillary dermal **concentric** and/or **lamellar fibrosis**
  - **Cytologic atypia**: nuclei enlarged (+/– prominent nucleoli), **"dirty" gray cytoplasm**
  - Significant interobserver variability in grading degree of atypia!
- Treatment: controversial; recent studies support clinical observation of mild and moderately atypical nevi; **severely atypical nevi should be re-excised**
- Prognosis: risk of melanoma directly related to the number of atypical/dysplastic nevi; however, individual dysplastic nevi have **extremely low rate of malignant degeneration**

Becker melanosis (NOT a true melanocytic disorder)

- 0.5% prevalence, more common in adolescent and **young adult males**
- May be as a result of androgen-mediated hyperplasia
- Onset around **puberty**
- Hyperpigmented plaque with thickening, irregularity, and/ or hypertrichosis on **upper torso** most commonly
- **Ipsilateral breast hypoplasia** seen in some patients (Poland syndrome), rarely a/w skeletal defects and/or limb asymmetry
- Histology: **increased basal melanocytes**, epidermal thickening, elongation of the rete ridges, and dermal **smooth muscle hamartoma-like** changes (very difficult to histologically distinguish from smooth muscle hamartoma)

Melanoma

Epidemiology

- Most cases in Caucasians; rare cases in dark-skinned individuals (typically acral lentiginous)
- Incidence is increasing; currently the most rapidly rising cancer in Caucasians; trend toward early detection and therefore thinner melanomas (vs. over-diagnosis)
- Wide age range, but mostly fourth decade onward

Risk factors

- Genetic:
  - **Inherited *CDKN2A* mutations** (FAMMM syndrome; dysplastic nevus syndrome):
    - Protein products **p14**^{ARF} and **p16** modulate cell cycle progression via p53 and retinoblastoma (Rb) pathways, respectively
    - Detectable mutations in 25% of familial melanomas
  - Other familial mutations: *POT, TERT, TP53, BAP-1*
- Other: lightly pigmented skin, UV exposure (cumulative and short intermittent bursts), organ transplant recipient; large number of acquired common and atypical melanocytic nevi, ephelides, and solar lentigines

Pathogenesis (Boards favorite!)

- *BRAF* (V600E is most common mutation): **non–chronic sun-damaged (non-CSD) sites, superficial spreading melanomas**
- *NRAS*: Chronic sun-damaged (**CSD**) skin sites, nodular melanomas
- *C-KIT*: **CSD sites**, **acral** and **mucosal** melanomas
- *CCND1/CDK4*: amplifications common on **CSD sites, acral** and **mucosal** melanomas
- *GNAQ/GNA11*: **uveal melanoma**, **blue nevi**, and nevus of Ota
- *BAP-1* (BRCA1-associated protein 1, a histone deubiquitinase): germline loss-of-function mutations in this tumor suppressor gene lead to increased risk of cutaneous melanoma, **uveal melanoma and malignant CBN** (both have concomitant *GNAQ/GNA11* mutations; in this context, ***BAP-1* loss is strongly a/w worse prognosis**), **epithelioid spitzoid nevi ("BAPomas"**; benign, possess concomitant activating *BRAF* > *NRAS* mutations), and **internal malignancies** (mesothelioma, renal cell carcinoma [RCC], and others)

Subtypes

- Superficial spreading: **most common** subtype; may arise *de novo* or in association with a nevus; peak onset 40 to 60 years old; predilection for **trunk (men)** and **legs (women)**; irregularly shaped/variably pigmented macule during radial growth phase → becomes papulonodular during vertical growth phase
- Nodular: onset around sixth decade; most commonly on **head/neck** and back; M > F; rapidly growing blue-black nodule; often ulcerated; **lacks horizontal growth phase**; tends to present at a more advanced stage
- Lentigo maligna: onset seventh decade and older; **CSD sites** particularly head and neck; presents as an irregularly pigmented brown macule; long horizontal growth phase precedes invasion
- Acral lentiginous: less common variant; onset around the seventh decade; **most common type seen in darkly pigmented races**; overall incidence is equal across Caucasians and darkly pigmented races; nail matrix lesions appear as longitudinal melanonychia w/ **Hutchinson sign**; usually presents at an advanced stage because of delayed clinical detection
- Other less common subtypes:
  - Desmoplastic melanoma (**Melan-A and HMB-45 negative, S100+ and SOX10+**); often amelanotic on head and neck
  - Mucosal melanoma: most common oral site is **hard palate**; most important prognostic factor = early diagnosis; metastasis in up to 50%
  - Spitzoid melanoma (**homozygous loss of 9p21 detected by FISH → poor outcome**)
  - Uveal melanomas (***GNAQ/GNA11* mutations** = most important driver mutations; very high risk of metastasis if also have concomitant *BAP-1* loss)
  - Malignant blue nevus (***GNAQ/GNA11* mutations** = most important driver mutations; often have concomitant *BAP-1* loss)

Histologic features

- General features: asymmetry, poor circumscription, and irregularly sized and shaped junctional nests with **discohesion** (nest fragments into individual cells); lentiginous/confluent growth along dermoepidermal junction (DEJ) predominates over nests; pagetoid scatter; "**epidermal consumption**" (melanoma effaces epidermis → epidermal thinning, ulceration); extension down adnexal epithelium; **lack of maturation** of dermal component (sheets of melanocytes and large nests at the base); dermal mitoses; cytologic atypia (irregular, large nuclei w/ **prominent red nucleoli**)
- Staging parameters:
  - **Most important**: Breslow thickness, ulceration
  - Others: mitoses, subtype, regression, lymphovascular invasion, host response, microsatellites, and associated nevus (Tables 6.4 and 6.5)

Prognosis

- Variable, depending on stage: >95% 10-year survival for stage IA disease, versus <50% for stage IIIC; algorithm using the 31-gene expression profile (31-GEP) may help to identify risk of sentinel node positiviey, recurrence, metastasis, and survival
- Factors a/w poor prognosis: Breslow > 1 mm, ulceration, ↑ mitotic rate, ↑ age, male sex, palpable LN metastases, head/neck/trunk location, and visceral metastases; treatment delays

NCCN treatment guidelines

- Localized melanoma
  - Treatment
    - Stage 0 *in situ* → wide excision with 0.5 to 1 cm margins
    - Stage IA (T1a) (<0.8 mm thick, no ulceration) → wide excision with 1 cm margins
    - Stage IB (T1b) (<0.8 mm thick with ulceration or 0.8–1.0 mm thick +/– ulceration) → discuss and **consider** sentinel lymph node biopsy (SLNB) → wide excision with 1 cm margins +/– SLNB
    - Stage IB (T2a) and stage II (T2b or higher) → discuss and **offer** SLNB + wide excision (1–2 cm

Table 6.4 Melanoma TNM Classification (AJCC 8th Edition)

T Classification	Thickness	Ulceration Status/Mitoses
Tis	NA	N/A
T1	≤1.0 mm	a: <0.8 mm without ulceration b: <0.8 mm with ulceration, 0.8–1.0 mm with or without ulceration
T2	>1.0–2.0 mm	a: without ulceration b: with ulceration
T3	>2.0–4.0 mm	a: without ulceration b: with ulceration
T4	>4.0 mm	a: without ulceration b: with ulceration
N Classification	**Number of involved nodes**	**In-transit or satellite metastases[a]**
N0	0 nodes	N/A
N1	N1a: 1 node (clinically occult) N1b: 1 node (clinically detected) N1c: 0 nodes	No No Yes
N2	N2a: 2–3 nodes (clinically occult) N2b: 2–3 nodes (1+ clinically detected) N2c:1 node (clinically occult or detected)	No No Yes
N3	N3a:4+ nodes (clinically occult) N3b: 4+ nodes (clinically detected)/matted nodes N3c: 2+ nodes (occult or detected) and/or matted nodes	No No Yes
M Classification	**Site**	**Serum Lactate Dehydrogenase**
M0	No distant metastases	N/A
M1a	Distant skin, soft tissue or non-regional node	M1a(0): Normal M1a(1): Elevated
M1b	Lung metastases	M1b(0): Normal M1b(1): Elevated
M1c	All other non-CNS visceral metastases	M1c(0): Normal M1c(1): Elevated
M1d	CNS metastasis	M1d(0): Normal M1d(1): Elevated

[a]In-transit metastases are > 2 cm from the primary tumor, but not beyond the regional lymph nodes; satellite lesions are within 2 cm of the primary.
Adapted from Amin MB, ed. AJCC Cancer Staging Manual. *8th ed. Chicago: American College of Surgeons; 2018.*

Table 6.5 Stage Groupings for Cutaneous Melanoma

	Clinical Staging[a]			Pathologic Staging[b]		
	T	**N**	**M**	**T**	**N**	**M**
0	Tis	N0	M0	Tis	N0	M0
IA	T1a	N0	M0	Tla/1b	N0	M0
IB	T1b T2a	N0	M0	T2a		
IIA	T2b T3a	N0	M0	T2b T3a	N0	M0
IIB	T3b T4a	N0	M0	T3b T4a	N0	M0
IIC	T4b	N0	M0	T4b	N0	M0
III[c]	Any T	N1 N2 N3	M0			
IIIA				T1a/1b-T2a	N1a/2a	M0
IIIB				T1a/b-T2a T2b/3a	N1b/c/2b N1a-N2b	M0
IIIC				T1a-T3a T3b/4a T4b	N2c or N3 N1-3 N1a-2c	M0
IIID				T4b	N3	
IV	Any T	Any N	Any M1	Any T	Any N	Any M1

[a]Clinical staging includes microstaging of the primary melanoma and clinical/radiologic evaluation for metastases. By convention, it should be used after complete excision of the primary melanoma with clinical assessment for regional and distant metastases.
[b]Pathologic staging includes microstaging of the primary melanoma and pathologic information about the regional lymph nodes after partial or complete lymphadenectomy. Pathologic stage 0 or stage IA patients are the exception.
[c]There are no stage III subgroups for clinical staging.
Adapted from Amin MB, Ed. AJCC Cancer Staging Manual. *8th ed. Chicago: American College of Surgeons; 2018.*

margin if 1.0–2.0 mm thick or 2 cm margin if > 2.0 mm thick)
  - Note: Microscopic satellites on biopsy or excision specimen are beyond the scope of this chapter. Please refer to detailed NCCN flowcharts for further information.
- Sentinel node positive
  - Workup
    - Imaging for baseline staging (consider in IIIA, recommended for IIIB and above) and to evaluate specific signs or symptoms
    - *BRAF* mutation testing (consider in IIIA, recommended for IIIB and above)
  - Primary treatment
    - Nodal basin ultrasound surveillance (generally preferred) or completion LN dissection
  - Adjuvant treatment
    - Systemic therapy
      - Preferred systemic options: nivolumab, pembrolizumab, dabrafenib/trametinib (for *BRAF* V600-activating mutation)
    - Observation based on risk of recurrence
- Clinically node positive
  - Workup
    - Core biopsy (preferred) or FNA
      - If needle biopsy not possible, excision LN biopsy acceptable
    - Imaging for baseline staging and to evaluate specific signs or symptoms
    - *BRAF* mutation testing
  - Primary treatment
    - If resectable → wide excision of primary tumor and therapeutic lymph node dissection
      - Consider neoadjuvant therapy (preferably in the context of clinical trial)
  - Adjuvant treatment
    - Systemic therapy **and/or** locoregional therapy with RT to nodal basin in selected high-risk patients **versus** observation based on risk of recurrence
      - Preferred systemic options: nivolumab, pembrolizumab, dabrafenib/trametinib (for *BRAF* V600-activating mutation)
  - Note: Clinical satellites or in-transit disease is beyond the scope of this chapter. Please refer to detailed NCCN flowcharts for further information.
- Stage IV metastatic disease
  - Workup
    - Imaging for baseline staging and to evaluate specific signs or symptoms
    - LDH
    - *BRAF* mutation testing
  - Treatment
    - Oligometastatic → systemic therapy +/− metastasis-directed therapy (resection or stereotactic ablative therapy)
    - Widely disseminated → systemic therapy +/− palliative resection or RT or intralesional t-vec
    - Preferred systemic options: **nivolumab or pembrolizumab**
      - Other recommended regimens: nivolumab + ipilimumab or *BRAF*+*MEK* inhibitors (for *BRAF* V600-activating mutation)
      - Useful in certain circumstances: ipilimumab if prior exposure to anti-PD-1 agents

6.4 ADNEXAL NEOPLASMS AND HAMARTOMAS

- High-yield subject area for dermatology examinations, because of classic histopathologic features

Poroma

- Benign sweat gland neoplasm that presents as a **solitary, vascular-appearing** papule/nodule +/− ulceration and **bleeding**; classically surrounded by a **thin moat**; most common sites = **palms/soles** (because of ↑ density of eccrine glands) > head/neck/scalp; may be a/w nevus sebaceus
  - Poromatosis: widespread or acral eruption of poromas
- Histology: circumscribed **endophytic** proliferation with **broad, multifocal epidermal connections** (Fig. 6.7); composed of monomorphous **"poroid cells"** (small cuboidal cells with intercellular desmosomal bridges; mnemonic: "poroid cells look like a cute, miniature version of a keratinocyte"); variably sized **sweat ducts** containing a **pink cuticle** encircling luminal aspect of duct; **highly vascularized stroma** resembling granulation tissue
- Immunostains: **CEA, EMA**, and **PAS** highlight ducts and intracytoplasmic lumina
- Poroma variants:
  - Wholly intraepidermal poroma (hidroacanthoma simplex): clinically mistaken for SK or squamous cell carcinoma in situ (SCCIS); most common on **distal extremities**; histology: multiple well-demarcated nests of small poroid cells within the epidermis; ducts may not be easily visualized
  - Juxtaepidermal poroma ("classic poroma"): described previously
  - Wholly dermal poroma (dermal duct tumor): well-circumscribed, "blue balls/nodules within dermis" composed of poroid cells w/ ducts; lacks epidermal connection
- Malignant counterpart: porocarcinoma
  - **Most common sweat gland malignancy**; elderly (avg. 70 years old); most commonly on **lower extremity**; arises within longstanding poroma (11%), *de novo*, or within nevus sebaceus; **frequent metastasis** (20% to regional LN and up to 10% widespread); **10% mortality**
    - Histology: resembles classic poroma, but has cytologic atypia, ↑ mitoses, atypical mitoses, and **infiltrative** growth pattern at tumor base

Hidradenoma

- Benign sweat gland (apocrine > eccrine) neoplasm that presents as a **solitary nodule** (often multilobulated) with a **deep red-purplish hue** and **cystic** quality
- Histology: circumscribed, **large** tumor nodules +/− **large areas of cystic degeneration**; occupies entire dermis; scattered **sweat ducts** within the tumor nodules;

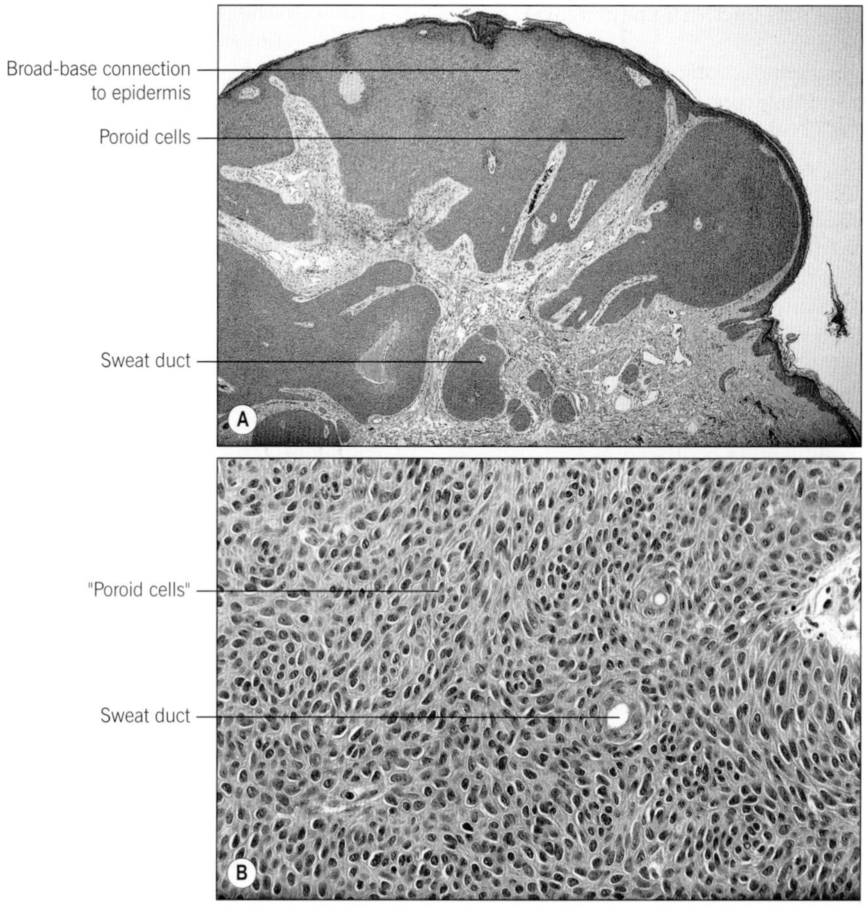

Fig. 6.7 (A) Eccrine poroma (low mag). (B) Eccrine poroma (high mag). (From Rapini RP. Sweat gland neoplasms. In: *Practical Dermatopathology*. 2nd ed. Philadelphia: Elsevier; 2012:321–330.)

prominent **dermal sclerosis with keloidal collagen (most useful clue!)**; very focal epidermal connection (never has broad epidermal connections)

- Tumor nodules are composed of **three main cell types** (Fig. 6.8): (1) **squamoid** cells, (2) **poroid** cells, and (3) **clear cells**
  - Any of these three cell types may predominate in a given tumor, but all three are present to some degree
  - Variants: clear cell hidradenoma (clear cells predominate), poroid hidradenoma (poroid cells predominate), and solid-cystic hidradenoma (prominent cystic degeneration)
- Malignant counterpart: hidradenocarcinoma
  - Aggressive tumor w/ significant metastatic and death risk; **head/neck (#1 site)**; histology: similar to hidradenoma, but has atypia, numerous mitoses, atypical mitoses, comedo-like necrosis, and lymphovascular invasion; treatment: Mohs (study from Mayo Clinic reported 0% recurrence and 0% metastatic rate), or wide local excision (WLE; up to 75% local recurrence rate and 20%–50% metastatic rate)

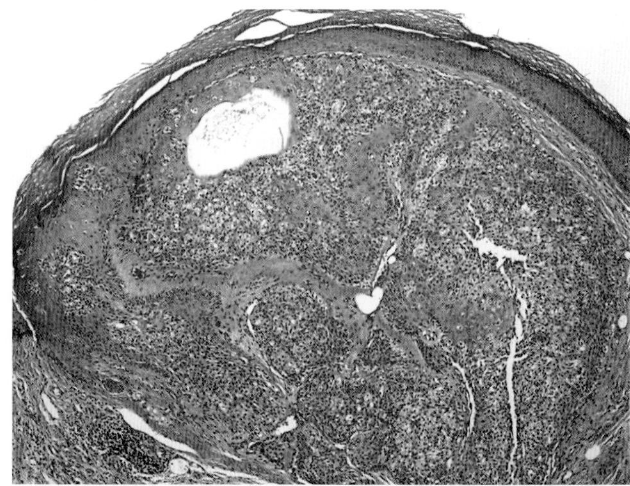

Fig. 6.8 Hidradenoma. Superficial dermal nodulocystic tumor with connections to the epidermis, clear cell features, and squamous metaplasia. (From Prieto VG, Shea CR, Celebi JT, Busam KJ. Adnexal tumors. In: Busam KJ, ed. *Dermatopathology: A Volume in the Series: Foundations in Diagnostic Pathology*. 2nd ed. Philadelphia: Elsevier; 2016:388–446.)

Syringoma

- Benign tumor consisting of translucent-skin colored papules; **periorbital region (eyelids #1), cheek >**

anterior trunk, genitals; ↑ incidence in **females**, **Asians**, and in **Down syndrome**
  - Eruptive syringomas (clinical variant): p/w 100s of hyperpigmented small papules on **anterior trunk/neck**; most commonly in **Africans/Asians** and in **Down syndrome**
  - **Clear cell syringoma** (histologic variant): a/w **diabetes mellitus**
- Histology: circumscribed proliferation of small **tadpole** or **comma-shaped** sweat ducts lined by a thin two cell layer of cuboidal cells; **eosinophilic cuticle** within sweat ducts + **amorphous sweat** within lumen; surrounding **sclerotic stroma**; confined to **upper half of dermis**
- Malignant counterpart = syringomatous carcinoma (eccrine ductal carcinoma and syringoid carcinoma); rare sweat gland malignancy w/ infiltrative growth and minimal cytologic atypia; **always arises *de novo***

Mixed tumor (MT; chondroid syringoma)

- Nonspecific, slow-growing, solitary nodule seen on head/neck (**nose, cheek, and upper lip** > other facial sites); middle-aged adults; M > F; clinically mistaken as cyst
- ***PLAG1* rearrangements** in significant subset of cases (present in 90% of apocrine MT; rare in eccrine MT); *PLAG1* rearrangements also seen in pleomorphic adenoma (a salivary gland tumor)
- Probably arise from the myoepithelial cells lining the sweat glands, which can differentiate toward epithelial or stromal cells
- Composed of ~50/50 mixture of **epithelial** (ectodermal) and **stromal** (mesodermal) components → hence the name, "mixed tumor"; appearance of each component is variable:
  - Epithelial component: usually **eccrine** or **apocrine** (> follicular, sebaceous, or plasmacytoid)
  - Stromal component: **myxoid** or **chondroid** (> collagenous > osteoid or lipoid)
- Histology: **circumscribed** dermal/SQ tumor consisting of **glandular structures, ducts**, and epithelial strands with **myxoid/chondroid stroma** (Fig. 6.9)
  - IHC: + for keratins in epithelial cells; SMA+, S100+, SOX10+ in myoepithelial cells
- Pleomorphic adenoma: salivary tumor w/ similar *PLAG1* rearrangements and histology as cutaneous MT; may undergo malignant degeneration with subsequent metastasis
- Treatment: benign; excision is curative
- Malignant counterpart = malignant MT: extremely rare; very aggressive (50% metastatic rate and 25% mortality); usually arises *de novo* on distal extremities/foot (uncommon sites for benign MT); histology: epithelial and/or stromal component appears malignant, w/ infiltrative growth, ↑ mitoses, and atypical mitoses

Spiradenoma ("eccrine spiradenoma")

- Benign sweat gland neoplasm; controversial cell of origin, likely **apocrine** (despite historical name of "eccrine spiradenoma")
- Solitary, **painful** dermal or subcutaneous nodule with blue-purple hue; favors **upper half of body**
- Histology: well-circumscribed proliferation of "blue balls in the dermis" w/ **ductal formation** (including **cystically dilated ducts**); tumor nodules are composed of **biphasic** epithelial cell population: (1) peripheral small blue cells with hyperchromatic nuclei and minimal cytoplasm, and (2) larger, pale-staining inner cells w/ ↑ cytoplasm; **intratumoral lymphocytes** (**"lymphocytes peppered in the tumor"** = classic finding!); **PAS+ eosinophilic hyaline droplets** composed of **BMZ material** (**type IV collagen**) found **within** tumor (same material is found in cylindromas, but typically *encircles* the tumor to form separate jigsaw pieces); very vascular appearance because of the **widely ectatic vessels** around periphery of tumor and cystically dilated ducts w/ hemorrhage (Fig. 6.10)
- **Brooke-Spiegler syndrome: AD** inherited condition cause by ***CYLD* mutation**; p/w multiple spiradenomas, cylindromas, trichoblastomas, and trichoepitheliomas
  - *CYLD* (tumor suppressor): normally **binds NEMO** component of I-kappa-B kinase (IKK) complex → inhibits NF-κB–mediated resistance to apoptosis
  - In absence of *CYLD*, get ↑ NF-κB signaling → resistance to apoptosis

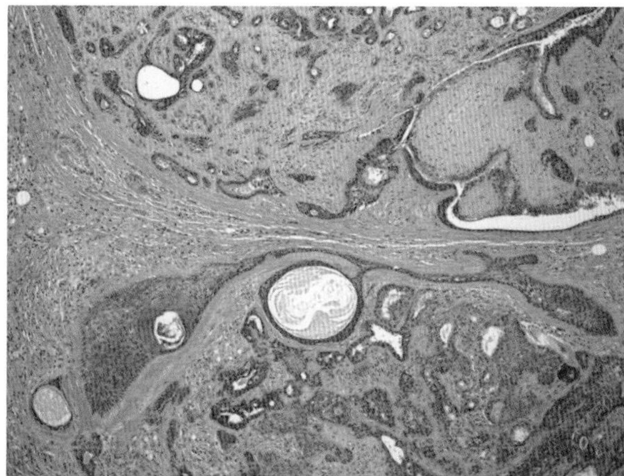

Fig. 6.9 Benign mixed tumor. A combination of ducts, keratocysts, myoepithelial cells, and myxoid stroma changes are present. (From Prieto VG, Shea CR, Celebi JT, Busam KJ. Adnexal tumors. In: Busam KJ, ed. *Dermatopathology: A Volume in the Series: Foundations in Diagnostic Pathology*. 2nd ed. Philadelphia: Elsevier; 2016:388–446.)

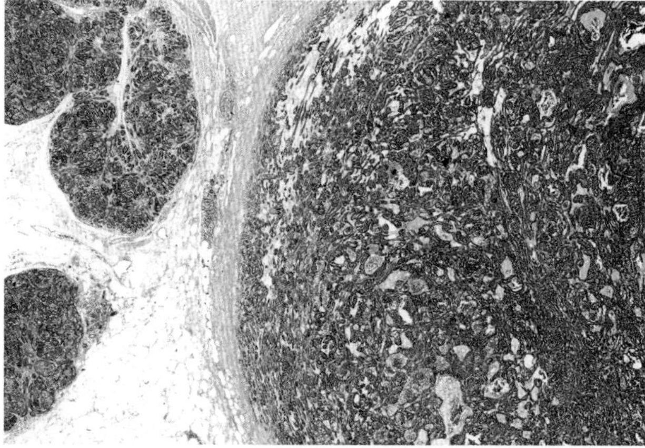

Fig. 6.10 Eccrine spiradenoma: in this example, there are three discrete tumor lobules. The largest appears encapsulated. (From Calonje E, Brenn T, Lazar AJ, Billings SD. Tumors of the sweat glands. In: *McKee's Pathology of the Skin*. 5th ed. Philadelphia: Elsevier; 2020:1611–1679.)

- Malignant counterpart = spiradenocarcinoma: very rare, poorly differentiated tumor with aggressive behavior (30% metastatic rate and 20% mortality); **arises within benign spiradenoma**; more common in patients with **Brooke-Spiegler syndrome**; histology: resembles spiradenoma, but **loses its biphasic nature**, **lacks the characteristic intratumoral lymphocytes;** has ↑ mitotic rate; atypical mitoses

Cylindroma

- Benign sweat gland neoplasm (**apocrine**) existing on a spectrum w/ spiradenoma; **solitary erythematous-purple nodule** with telangiectasias; 90% occur on head/neck (**scalp #1**)
- Multiple cylindromas may coalesce to form multinodular plaques on scalp ("**turban tumor**") in **Brooke-Spiegler syndrome**
- Histology: well-circumscribed basaloid proliferation composed of multiple smaller tumor **lobules encircled by thick hyaline BMZ material (type IV collagen)** → multiple small lobules fit together like a **"jigsaw puzzle"**; **biphasic** cell population (same as spiradenoma) with **small ducts** (Fig. 6.11)
- Malignant counterpart = cylindrocarcinoma: very rare, poorly differentiated tumor with aggressive behavior (45% metastatic rate); **usually seen in Brooke-Spiegler syndrome**; arises within a benign cylindroma; scalp (#1); histology: resembles cylindroma, but **loses biphasic nature**, has ↑ mitotic rate, atypical mitoses, infiltrative growth pattern, and neurovascular invasion

Hidradenoma papilliferum (HPAP)

- Benign, painless 1- to 2-cm skin colored nodule; almost exclusively on vulva (**labia majora #1**) of **young adult women**
- Histology: well-circumscribed cystic proliferation in dermis with numerous **papillary projections** with apocrine differentiation invaginating into central cyst-like spaces → **"maze-like"** appearance (Fig. 6.12); **lacks epidermal connection** (major distinguishing feature from syringocystadenoma papilliferum (SPAP) → "HPAP Hides in the dermis whereas SPAP Slides in from the epidermis")

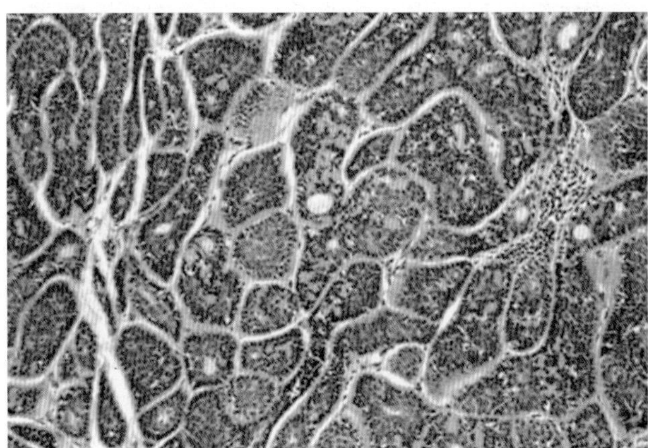

Fig. 6.11 Cylindroma. The jigsaw pattern is well developed in this example. Note also the hyaline droplets within the tumor lobules. (From Brinster NK, Liu V, Diwan H, McKee PH. Cylindroma. In: *Dermatopathology: A Volume in the High Yield Pathology Series*. Philadelphia: Elsevier; 2011:423.)

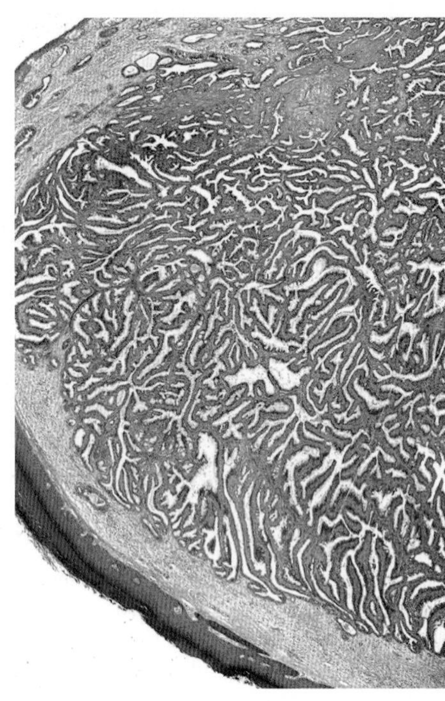

Fig. 6.12 Hidradenoma papilliferum: low-power view of an exophytic ulcerated nodule. The epidermal collarette is seen in the lower left of the field. (From Calonje E, Brenn T, Lazar AJ, Billings SD. Tumors of the sweat glands. In: *McKee's Pathology of the Skin*. 5th ed. Philadelphia: Elsevier; 2020: 1611–1679.)

Syringocystadenoma papilliferum (SPAP, SCAP)

- Benign apocrine neoplasm; presents at **birth or early childhood** with a **solitary**, **warty papule**/plaque on **scalp** (> other sites on head/neck > trunk and extremities); usually **a/w nevus sebaceus**
- Histology: **exo-endophytic papillary glandular** proliferation w/ apocrine differentiation; opens onto skin surface; **abundant plasma cells** in peritumoral stroma (Fig. 6.13)
- Malignant transformation is exceptionally rare

Papillary eccrine adenoma (PEA)

- Benign; **legs (#1)**; favors **Black women**
- Histology: well-circumscribed proliferation of **small- to medium-sized sweat ducts** w/ **papillary projections** (Fig. 6.14) that are often elongated (vs. syringoma)

Tubular apocrine adenoma (TAA)

- Benign; most commonly on **scalp** a/w **nevus sebaceus**
- Histology: often **indistinguishable from PEA except for decapitation secretion** and ↓ papillary projections

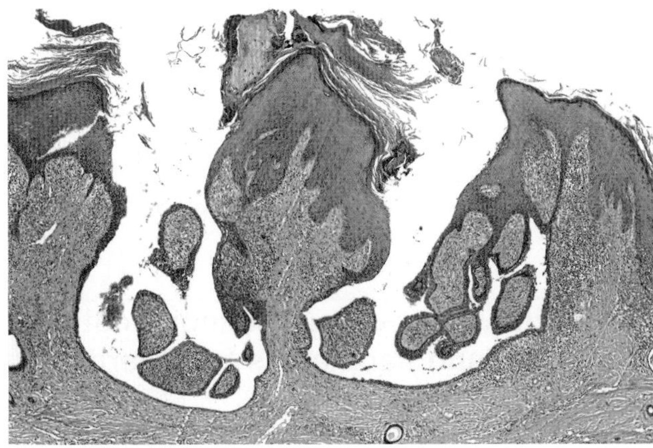

Fig. 6.13 Syringocystadenoma papilliferum: this exophytic lesion developed within a nevus sebaceus. Note that the surface is covered with squamous epithelium. (From Calonje E, Brenn T, Lazar AJ, Billings SD. Tumors of the sweat glands. In: *McKee's Pathology of the Skin*. 5th ed. Philadelphia: Elsevier; 2020:1611–1679.)

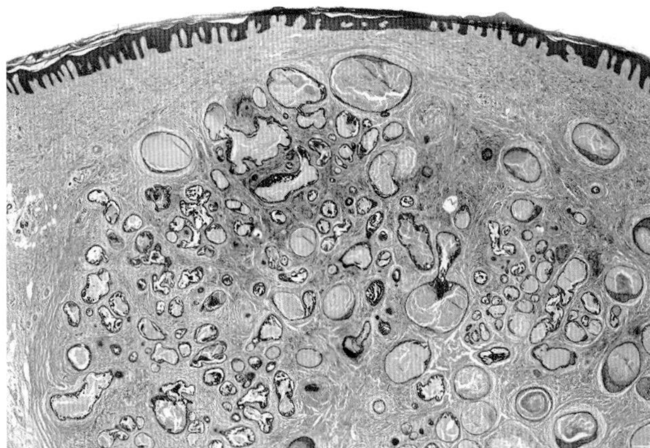

Fig. 6.14 Papillary eccrine adenoma: the lesion is composed of dilated ducts and cysts dispersed in a fibrous stroma. (From Calonje E, Brenn T, Lazar AJ, Billings SD. Tumors of the sweat glands. In: *McKee's Pathology of the Skin*. 5th ed. Philadelphia: Elsevier; 2020:1611–1679.)

Syringofibroadenoma

- Rare, benign sweat gland proliferation (unclear if true neoplasm or reactive); **legs (#1)**
- May be a/w:
  - **Schöpf-Schulz-Passarge**
  - **Clouston syndrome**
  - **Chronic stasis dermatitis** (reactive process), **burns, scarring**
- Histology: **thin, anastomosing strands of sweat duct-containing epithelium** projecting downward from epidermis into mid dermis; rich fibrovascular stroma (similar to poroma)

Microcystic adnexal carcinoma (MAC, sclerosing sweat duct carcinoma)

- **Locally aggressive** adnexal carcinoma with **divergent/bi-lineage differentiation** (follicular + sweat gland)
- **Firm, indurated plaque** on **lip** (>**chin and cheek**) of **middle-aged women** (Fig. 6.15)

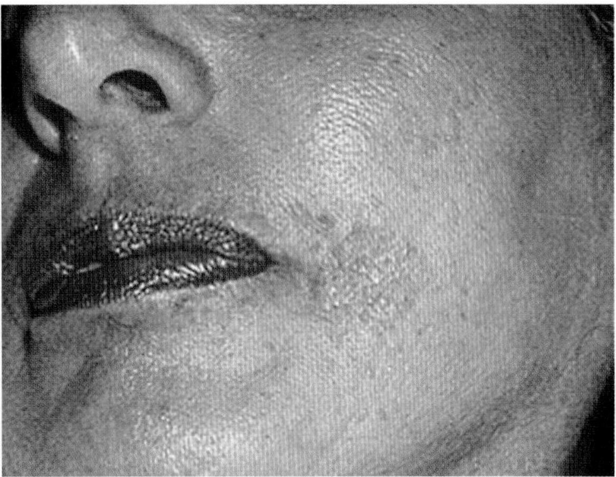

Fig. 6.15 Middle-aged woman with a typical microcystic adnexal carcinoma. (From Prado R, Mellette JR. Uncommon malignant tumors of the skin. In: Fitzpatrick JE, Morelli JG, eds. *Dermatology Secrets Plus*. 5th ed. Philadelphia: Elsevier, 2016:425–433.)

- Treatment: **Mohs** (ToC) >> WLE (high recurrence rate)
- Histology: poorly-circumscribed, **deeply-infiltrative** sclerosing basaloid proliferation with **divergent/bi-lineage differentiation** (mixture of small sweat ducts + keratinizing "microcysts"); typically has **PNI** and prominent **lymphoid aggregates** (most helpful clues on examination); cytologic atypia is minimal

Aggressive digital papillary adenocarcinoma (ADPA)

- Rare, **highly aggressive** malignant sweat gland neoplasm (14% metastatic rate even w/ amputation); affects **volar digits** of middle-aged adults; **M** » F (7:1)
- Treatment: **amputation**
- Histology: solid and cystic proliferation with papillary projections, deeply infiltrative growth pattern, cytologic atypia, and ↑ mitotic rate; may appear quite bland but all cases should be treated aggressively

Primary cutaneous mucinous carcinoma (PCMC)

- Very rare malignant sweat gland neoplasm; presents as a slow-growing, soft nodule; most commonly on **eyelid/periocular region**; average age = 60 years old
- Two subtypes: **non-neuroendocrine** PCMC (**aggressive**; 30% recurrence rate, 11% overall metastatic rate with 4% distant metastasis) and **neuroendocrine** PCMC (much less aggressive; ~0% metastatic rate; strongly associated with endocrine mucin-producing sweat gland carcinoma)
- Treatment: **Mohs** (lower recurrence rates) recommended over WLE
- Histology: basaloid epithelial tumor nodules "**floating in lakes of mucin**" (**sialomucin**); intratumoral ducts give rise to **cribriform appearance** (Fig. 6.16); **CK7+, CK20-**
- **Clinical pearl:** mucinous carcinomas on the **face** are **almost always primary**, whereas lesions arising on **trunk** may represent metastasis of visceral malignancy (GI, breast, lung, or ovarian); may be indistinguishable from mucinous breast cancer metastasis

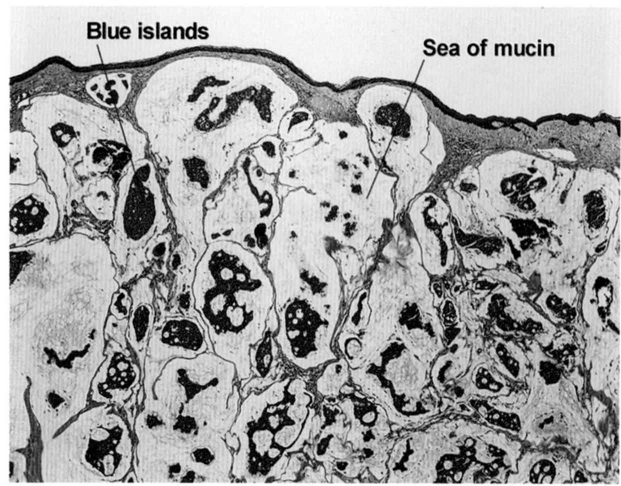

Fig. 6.16 Mucinous carcinoma. (From Elston DM. Sweat gland neoplasms. In: Elston DM, Ferringer T, eds. *Dermatopathology*. 3rd ed. Philadelphia: Elsevier; 2019:83–100.)

Endocrine mucin-producing sweat gland carcinoma (EMPSGC)

- Rare, low-grade sweat gland carcinoma that presents as a slow-growing nodule/cyst; ~exclusively **eyelid/periocular region;** F > M (2:1); average age = 60 to 70 years
- Often **occurs in conjunction with primary cutaneous mucinous carcinoma (neuroendocrine subtype)** → thought to be a **precursor lesion** (mucinous carcinoma *in situ*)
- Histology: dermally based, multilobular tumor with solid, cystic, cribriform, and papillary areas; small mucinous pseudocysts (vs. "LARGE lakes of extracellular mucin" in PCMC); bland cytology; **expresses neuroendocrine markers**
  - Mnemonic: "essentially looks like the epithelial areas of PCMC but without huge lakes of mucin"
  - **IHC:** must be positive for **one or more neuroendocrine marker** (synaptophysin, chromogranin, NSE, or CD57); usually positive for low-molecular cytokeratins (Cam5.2 and CK7), EMA (luminal cells), and **ER/PR**; negative for CK20 and S100. Myoepithelial markers (SMA, calponin, p63/p40, SOX10, and S100) may be used to identify the periphery of *in situ* component → if present, supports a primary cutaneous (vs. metastatic) origin
- Prognosis/treatment: excision is curative; rarely recurs and never metastasizes; may progress to mucinous carcinoma (specifically, neuroendocrine PCMC)

Adenoid cystic carcinoma (ACC)

- May arise as a primary adnexal carcinoma or cutaneous metastasis from **salivary gland**
  - Primary cutaneous ACC: **indolent tumor**; most commonly on the **scalp** of middle-aged adults; minimal metastatic risk, but up to **70% local recurrence rate** (as a result of extensive PNI)
  - Salivary gland ACC: **highly-aggressive** (50% metastatic rate and high mortality)
- Histology: poorly-circumscribed proliferation of small- to medium-sized **basaloid cuboidal tumor nodules w/ cribriform appearance**; extends into SQ fat w/ **prominent PNI**; lacks epidermal connection
  - May have fibrotic or mucinous stroma (but **no large "lakes of mucin"**)
  - Contains myoepithelial cells (lining ducts; stains positive for SMA, calponin, p63/p40, SOX10, and S100)
  - Fusions/mutations in *MYB, NFIB, and MYBL1* seen in nearly all cases

Comparative dermatopathologic features of sweat gland neoplasms for Board Exam purposes

Poroma (classic juxtaepidermal type)

- **Critical histologic features**
  - Circumscribed endophytic proliferation with **broad, multifocal epidermal connections**; monomorphous "poroid cells"; variably sized **sweat ducts**; **highly-vascularized stroma**
  - Immunostains: **CEA**, **EMA**, and **PAS** highlight ducts and intracytoplasmic lumina
- **Most commonly encountered differential diagnosis (DDx)**
  - Trichilemmoma: similar endophytic growth pattern, but has **peripheral palisade** with **thick pink BMZ**, prominent **clear cell change**, and lacks small poroid cells and sweat ducts
  - Hidradenoma: almost entirely confined to dermis, w/ **minimal epidermal connection** (vs. broad multifocal connection in poroma); has **three cell types** (poroid + clear cells + squamoid cells); has prominent **stromal sclerosis w/ hyalinized or keloidal collagen**

Hidroacanthoma simplex

- **Critical histologic features**
  - Wholly intraepidermal poroma variant; multiple well-demarcated nests of small poroid cells within the epidermis; sweat ducts may not be easily visualized
- **Most commonly encountered DDx**
  - **Clonal SK, or SK with Borst-Jadassohn effect**: cells are at least same size as (often larger than) surrounding keratinocytes
  - **Bowenoid SCCIS:** keratinocytes are highly atypical, ↑ mitoses, and ↑ dyskeratotic keratocytes

Dermal duct tumor

- **Critical histologic features**
  - Wholly dermal poroma variant; well-circumscribed **"blue balls within dermis"**; tumor nodules composed of rounded poroid cells with same appearance as classic poroma; **lacks epidermal connection**
- **Most commonly encountered DDx**
  - Hidradenoma: both may look like "big blue balls" in the dermis with sweat ducts; however, hidradenoma is composed of **three cell types** (poroid + squamoid + clear cells), has prominent **stromal sclerosis/ keloidal collagen** around tumor, and has **dilated cystic spaces**

- Trichoblastoma: both may look like "big blue balls" in the dermis and are composed of small blue cells, but trichoblastoma has **hair follicle differentiation** with rudimentary **hair shafts**, **papillary mesenchymal bodies**, **keratin debris**, and **dystrophic calcification** (none of which are seen with dermal duct tumor); trichoblastoma **lacks sweat ducts**
- Cylindroma: both appear as blue balls in dermis with sweat ducts, but cylindroma has **thick pink BMZ** material around tumor lobules, **hyaline deposits** within tumor lobules, and **biphasic cell types** (Dermal duct tumor is composed only of small blue poroid cells)
- Spiradenoma: both appear as blue balls in dermis with sweat ducts, but spiradenoma has **hyaline deposits** within tumor lobules, and **biphasic cell types** (Dermal duct tumor is composed only of small blue poroid cells), and **large cystic spaces**

Hidradenoma

- **Critical histologic features**
  - Circumscribed, large tumor nodules composed of **three main cell types:** (1) **squamoid** cells, (2) **poroid** cells, (3) **clear** cells; +/– **large cystic spaces** ("solid-cystic hidradenoma"); lesion occupies entire dermis; scattered **sweat ducts**; prominent **dermal sclerosis w/ keloidal collagen** (major clue!); minimal to no epidermal connection
- **Most commonly encountered DDx**
  - Classic poroma (see above)
  - Dermal duct tumor (see above)
  - Trichoblastoma: both may look like "big blue balls" in the dermis, but trichoblastoma has **hair follicle differentiation** w/ rudimentary hair shafts, papillary mesenchymal bodies, keratin debris, and dystrophic calcification; **lacks sweat ducts**
  - Cylindroma: both appear as blue balls in dermis with sweat ducts, but cylindroma has **thick pink BMZ** material around tumor lobules, **hyaline deposits** within tumor lobules, and **biphasic cell types**; cylindroma **lacks the three cell types** characteristic of hidradenoma; also **lacks stromal sclerosis/ hyalinization/keloidal** collagen
  - Spiradenoma: both appear as blue balls in dermis with sweat ducts and dilated cystic spaces; but spiradenoma has **hyaline deposits** within tumor lobules, **biphasic cell types**, **"lymphocytes peppered"** within tumor; spiradenoma **lacks the three cell types** (squamoid, poroid, and clear cells) of hidradenoma and **lacks stromal sclerosis/keloidal** collagen
  - Mixed Tumor: both tumors have ducts, a mixture of epithelial cell types, and stromal changes; however, MT has **much more chondroid/myxoid stromal changes** (vs. sclerotic collagen/keloidal stroma in hidradenoma)

Spiradenoma

- **Critical histologic features**
  - Well-circumscribed, nodulo-cystic proliferation of "blue balls in the dermis" with **ductal formation** (often **cystically dilated**); **biphasic** epithelial cell population; intratumoral lymphocytes (**"lymphocytes peppered in the tumor"**); **PAS+ eosinophilic hyaline droplets** composed of **BMZ material** (**type IV collagen**) found **within** tumor (same material as in cylindromas, but usually located *within* the tumor, rather than *encircling* the tumor to form separate jigsaw pieces); very **vascular-appearing** because of the **widely ectatic vessels** around periphery of tumor
- **Most commonly encountered DDx**
  - Cylindroma: **thick hyaline BMZ** material predominantly ***encircles*** nodules (vs. droplets found *within* nodules, as in spiradenoma) and separates them into small **jigsaw puzzle** pieces; **lacks "lymphocyte peppering,"** also lacks large cystically dilated ducts and ectatic vascular spaces of spiradenoma
  - Hidradenoma (see above)
  - Dermal duct tumor (see above)

Cylindroma

- **Critical histologic features**
  - Well-circumscribed proliferation of multiple small- to medium-sized **blue tumor lobules** encircled by thick **hyaline BMZ material (type IV collagen** mainly) → leads to **"jigsaw puzzle"** pattern; scattered **small ducts**; **biphasic** cell population
- **Most commonly encountered DDx**
  - Spiradenoma (see above)
  - Dermal duct tumor (see above)
  - Hidradenoma (see above)

Syringoma

- **Critical histologic features**
  - Circumscribed proliferation of small **tadpole** or **comma-shaped** sweat ducts w/ **eosinophilic cuticle** and **amorphous sweat** within lumen; sclerotic stroma; confined to **upper half of dermis**
  - Boards fodder: you should never see **follicular differentiation** or multiple **horn cysts** in a syringoma → if you see either → more likely desmoplastic trichoepithelioma (DTE) or MAC!
- **Most commonly encountered DDx**
  - DTE: **follicular differentiation,** lots of **horn cysts,** and dystrophic **calcification; lacks sweat ducts**
  - Morpheaform BCC: follicular differentiation, +/– horn cysts (fewer than in DTE), atypical cells w/ ↑ mitoses, and apoptotic cells; lacks sweat ducts
  - MAC: like syringoma has sweat ducts, but has concomitant **follicular differentiation** w/ horn cysts (**divergent/bi-lineage differentiation** is a key feature of MAC!), **more deeply infiltrative** into deep dermis/ SQ, **PNI w/ lymphoid aggregates** (not seen in syringoma)

Mixed tumor (MT; "chondroid syringoma")

- **Critical histologic features**
  - Tumor of **mixed** epithelial and mesenchymal derivation (hence the name); circumscribed dermal/SQ tumor consisting of **glandular structures,**

ducts, and epithelial strands with **myxoid/chondroid stroma**
- **Most commonly encountered DDx**
  - Hidradenoma (see above)
  - Syringoma: lacks chondroid/myxoid stroma

Hidradenoma papilliferum (HPAP)

- **Critical histologic features**
  - Well-circumscribed cystic proliferation in dermis with innumerable **papillary projections** invaginating into central cyst-like spaces; has **"maze-like"** appearance; **lacks epidermal connection**
- **Most commonly encountered DDx**
  - SPAP (SCAP): has broad epidermal connection; ↑ plasma cells in peritumoral stroma; lacks maze-like quality of HPAP
  - Nipple adenoma/erosive adenomatosis: arises on nipple rather than vulva; typically has connection to overlying epidermis; less maze-like
  - TAA/PEA: dermal-based proliferation of multiple small ducts w/ papillary projections into lumen; lacks maze-like appearance of HPAP

Syringocystadenoma papilliferum (SPAP, SCAP)

- **Critical histologic features**
  - Verrucous epidermal hyperplasia w/ endophytic growth into dermis; **broadly opens onto epidermis**; papillary projections lined by two cell layers (inner myoepithelial and outer apocrine layer with decapitation secretion); **abundant plasma cells** in peritumoral stroma
- **Most commonly encountered DDx**
  - HPAP: **maze-like quality**; lacks epidermal connection

Papillary eccrine adenoma (PEA)

- **Critical histologic features**
  - Favors **legs of Black women**; well-circumscribed proliferation of **small- to medium-sized sweat ducts w/ papillary projections** extending into the lumen
- **Most commonly encountered DDx**
  - TAA: nearly identical appearance, but favors scalp; has **decapitation secretion** and ↓ papillary projections
  - ADPA: more infiltrative growth pattern; solid and cystic architecture; ↑ mitoses and atypia; occurs on digits

Tubular apocrine adenoma (TAA)

- **Critical histologic features**
  - Similar to PEA, but favors scalp; **apocrine differentiation** w/ decapitation secretion and **fewer papillary projections**
- **Most commonly encountered DDx**
  - PEA: see above
  - ADPA: occurs on fingertips; more infiltrative; solid and cystic architecture; ↑ atypia and mitoses

Porokeratotic eccrine ostial and dermal duct nevus

- **Critical histologic features**
  - Punctate epidermal hyperkeratosis with **cornoid lamellae** arising from **acrosyringium**
- **Most commonly encountered DDx**
  - Porokeratosis: cornoid lamellae arise from epidermal epithelium, not acrosyringium

Syringofibroadenoma

- **Critical histologic features**
  - **Thin, anastomosing strands** of sweat duct-containing epithelium extending down from the epidermis into the mid dermis; **rich fibrovascular stroma** surrounds tumor
- **Most commonly encountered DDx**
  - Tumor of follicular infundibulum: **follicular** differentiation (lacks sweat ducts); grows laterally in superficial dermis in a **"plate-like"** fashion; multiple connections to overlying epidermis with fibrotic stroma (architecture resembles superficial BCC)
  - Fibroepithelioma of Pinkus: endophytic, bulbous architecture, w/ multiple connections to the overlying epidermis and BCC-like stromal changes; **lacks sweat ducts**

Microcystic adnexal carcinoma (MAC)

- **Critical histologic features**
  - Sclerosing **basaloid** proliferation with **divergent/bi-lineage differentiation** (follicular and sweat), giving rise to proliferation of **small sweat ducts** and "**follicular microcysts**"; minimal cytologic atypia; **deeply infiltrative** throughout dermis, SQ and into muscle; typically has **PNI** and **lymphoid aggregates**
  - Boards fodder: mixture of sweat and follicular differentiation (divergent/bi-lineage differentiation) is a very useful clue for MAC; typically do not see this w/ syringoma, DTE, or BCC!
- **Most commonly encountered DDx**
  - Syringoma: both have basaloid tadpole appearance, but syringoma is **circumscribed** (vs. infiltrative), **confined to upper half of dermis**, only has **sweat duct differentiation** (lacks follicular elements)
  - Morpheaform BCC: cells more atypical, w/ ↑ mitoses, apoptosis, and **myxoid stroma** (vs. sclerotic in MAC); only demonstrates follicular differentiation **(lacks sweat ducts)**
  - DTE: **follicular differentiation** only (lacks sweat ducts)

Aggressive digital papillary adenocarcinoma (ADPA)

- **Critical histologic features**
  - Solid and cystic proliferation w/ papillary projections; deeply infiltrative, cytologic atypia, and ↑ mitotic rate

- **Most commonly encountered DDx**
  - PEA, HPAP, and TAA: may have similar low-power appearance, but infiltrative growth pattern and **anatomic site** is critical to diagnosis of ADPA!

Primary cutaneous mucinous carcinoma (PCMC)

- **Critical histologic features**
  - Mnemonic: **"blue tumor islands floating in lakes of mucin"**
  - Immunostaining pattern:
    - Positive: AE1/AE3, CAM5.2, EMA, CEA, **CK7, ER, PR,** and +/– neuroendocrine markers (neuron-specific enolase [NSE], chromogranin, and synaptophysin)
    - Negative: **CK20**
  - Important note: PCMC frequently has an ***in situ*** component that is identified by finding a **myoepithelial layer (p63/p40+, SMA+, calponin+, SOX10+, and S100+)** surrounding the tumor → this **confirms primary cutaneous origin** (rules out metastatic adenocarcinoma from internal organs, since a myoepithelial layer is never present in metastatic tumors)
- **Most commonly encountered DDx**
  - Metastatic mucinous carcinoma from breast: can be ruled out if *in situ* component of PCMC is found (unfortunately, not always present); otherwise, appears **identical to PCMC** by histologic and immunohistologic studies → need history, examination, and imaging studies; most likely to arise on **trunk** (vs. face, which is highly suggestive of PCMC)
  - Metastatic mucinous carcinoma from colon: $CK7^-$/**$CK20^+$** (vs. $CK7^+$/$CK20^-$ in PCMC); GI tumors also have a different mucin type than PCMC → can distinguish with mucin histochemistry:
    - **GI tumors = sulfomucin** (Alcian blue positive at pH 1.0 and 0.4)
    - PCMC = sialomucin (Alcian blue positive at pH 2.5)
      - Also may be ruled out if *in situ* component of PCMC is found

Adenoid cystic carcinoma (ACC)

- **Critical histologic features**
  - Poorly circumscribed, infiltrative proliferation of multiple small- to medium-sized **cribriform "blue balls in dermis"** with intratumoral ducts; typically has extension into SQ fat and **PNI**; lacks large "lakes of mucin"
- **Most commonly encountered DDx**
  - Mucinous carcinoma: epithelial tumor nodules are **floating in huge lakes of mucin**
  - Trichoblastoma: also appears as "blue balls within dermis" and may also have cribriform appearance, but has **follicular differentiation**; **lacks sweat ducts** and PNI
  - Dermal duct tumor: also appears as "blue balls within dermis," but the proliferation is well-circumscribed; lacks PNI and cribriform appearance

6.5 HAIR FOLLICLE NEOPLASMS/ HAMARTOMAS

Folliculo-sebaceous-apocrine hamartomas

Trichofolliculoma

- **Clinical and histopathologic features**
  - Benign follicular hamartoma; skin colored papule w/ **central follicular punctum** from which **numerous tufted vellus hairs** emerge
  - Histology: **dilated central cystic follicle** connected to multiple **fully formed** vellus follicles (Fig. 6.17); background fibrous stroma
  - Sebaceous trichofolliculoma (variant): radiating follicles are accompanied by sebaceous glands
  - Folliculosebaceous cystic hamartoma: likely same entity as sebaceous trichofolliculoma; often embedded in a stroma containing superficial fat
- **Histologic DDx**
  - Fibrofolliculoma: both have a large central follicle with numerous emanating epithelial attachments; however, fibrofolliculoma only has **thin strands** of primitive follicular epithelium (**lacks hair shafts**)
  - Pilar sheath acanthoma: cystically dilated central follicle with radiating **acanthotic epithelium**; no hair shafts in acanthotic buds
- **Other high-yield facts/comments**
  - **Mnemonic**: "multiple baby hairs connected to a large mama hair"

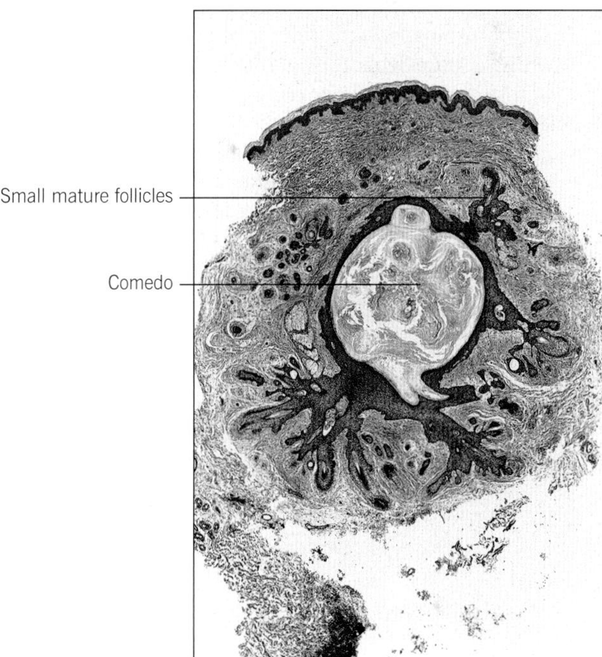

Fig. 6.17 Trichofolliculoma (low mag). (From Rapini RP. Follicular neoplasms. In: *Practical Dermatopathology*. 2nd ed. Philadelphia: Elsevier; 2012: 311–319.)

Fibrofolliculoma

- **Clinical and histopathologic features**
  - Benign hamartoma; nondistinctive, small, skin-colored papules involving **head/neck**; treatment: none required but may try dermabrasion or CO_2 laser ablation
  - Histology: central follicle/cyst with numerous **thin strands of follicular epithelium** radiating from it; lacks hair formation; lesion surrounded by delicate, loose **fibromyxoid stroma** (Fig. 6.18)
  - Variants (perifollicular fibroma, trichodiscoma, and acrochordons): likely same entity, just viewed in different histologic sections; may not visualize the thin strands of follicular epithelium
- **Histologic DDx**
  - Trichofolliculoma: has similar central cyst, but attached structures are **fully formed vellus hairs w/ hair shafts**
- **Other high-yield facts/comments**
  - Birt-Hogg-Dubé syndrome: Mutation in ***FLCN*** (encodes folliculin, a tumor suppressor), **AD inheritance**; **triad** of skin lesions (fibrofolliculomas, trichodiscomas, and acrochordons); a/w **RCC** (oncocytic or chromophobe), spontaneous **pneumothorax**, **pulmonary cysts**, and **medullary carcinoma of thyroid**

Nevus sebaceus

- **Clinical and histopathologic features**
  - Benign hamartoma with follicular, apocrine, and sebaceous components; present **at birth** along **Blaschko lines**; becomes more yellow and verrucous after puberty; scalp/face most common sites (>trunk and neck); **alopecia** of affected area
  - Histology: verrucous epidermis with malformed, diminutive hairs, **lacks fully formed terminal hairs** within lesion; **sebaceous glands open directly** onto skin surface; **dilated apocrine glands**
- **Histologic DDx**
  - Epidermal nevus: appears similar histologically
  - Sebaceous hyperplasia: **nodular** architecture; lacks dilated apocrine glands and malformed/diminutive hairs
- **Other high-yield facts/comments**
  - If extensive, may be a/w **Schimmelpenning syndrome** or phakomatosis pigmentokeratotica
  - Secondary adnexal neoplasms arising within nevus sebaceus: **trichoblastoma (#1)** > **SPAP** > trichilemmoma, poroma, TAA, and **BCC**

Neoplasms with follicular germinative differentiation

Trichoepithelioma

- **Clinical and histopathologic features**
  - Benign; **solitary or multiple** (a/w inherited syndromes) smooth, skin-to-pearly colored, dome-shaped papules w/ telangiectasias; **central face** (**nose** #1, nasolabial folds, upper cutaneous lip, and scalp)
  - Histology: well-circumscribed follicular **basaloid proliferation**; well-organized nodules with epithelial fronds, **reticulated strands**, and **cribriform nodules** ("Swiss cheese") (Fig. 6.19); **numerous horn cysts** (much more than BCC); peripheral palisading; **papillary mesenchymal bodies**; **highly-cellular fibrotic pink stroma** (fibroblasts account for ~50% of tumor's overall cellularity); almost entirely intradermal w/ **minimal to no epidermal connection**; rarely ulcerates; **no clefting** between tumor cells and stroma (stroma is tightly attached to epithelial cells; may have stromal-stromal retraction)
  - IHC: scattered **CK20+ Merkel cells** within tumor; **PHLDA1+**; **stroma is CD34+ and CD10+**; BCL-2 only stains **periphery** of trichoepithelioma (vs. diffuse in BCC); androgen receptor negative (vs. AR+ in most BCC)
- **Histologic DDx**
  - BCC: ↑ cytologic atypia, ↑ apoptosis, and ↑ mitoses; **myxoid stroma** (vs. collagenous w/ ↑ fibroblasts); **lacks cribriform or reticulated architecture**; **retraction** from surrounding stroma; lacks papillary mesenchymal bodies; far fewer horn cysts; has more connection to epidermis; stains: **BCL-2+** (diffuse), **CK20 negative**, **PHLDA1 negative**; stroma is CD10 negative
  - Trichoblastoma: may refer to **large** trichoeps or follicular neoplasms w/ exclusively bulbar differentiation (immature blue cells)

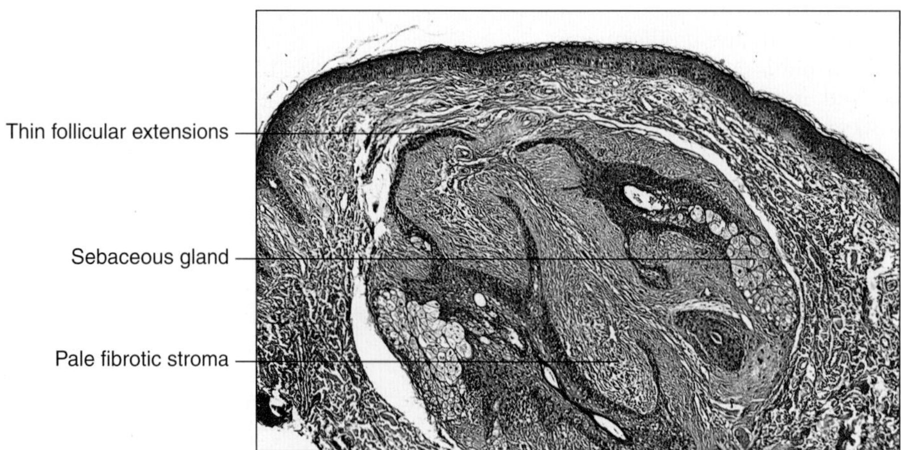

Fig. 6.18 Fibrofolliculoma histology—hair follicle with thin extensions of epithelium into surrounding mucinous stroma. (From Rapini RP. Follicular neoplasms. In: Rapini RP, ed. *Practical Dermatopathology*. 3rd ed. Philadelphia: Elsevier; 2021:321–329.)

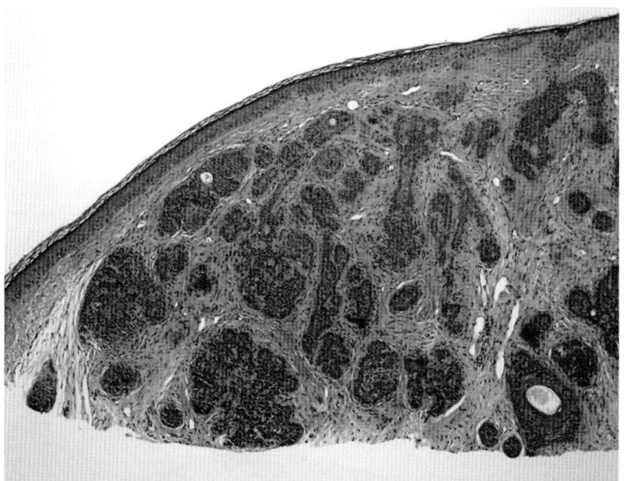

Fig. 6.19 Trichoepithelioma. Groups of basaloid cells surrounded by fibroblasts forming a fibroepithelial lesion. (From Prieto VG, Shea CR, Celebi JT, Busam KJ. Adnexal tumors. In: Busam KJ, ed. *Dermatopathology: A Volume in the Series: Foundations in Diagnostic Pathology*. 2nd ed. Philadelphia: Elsevier; 2016:388–446.)

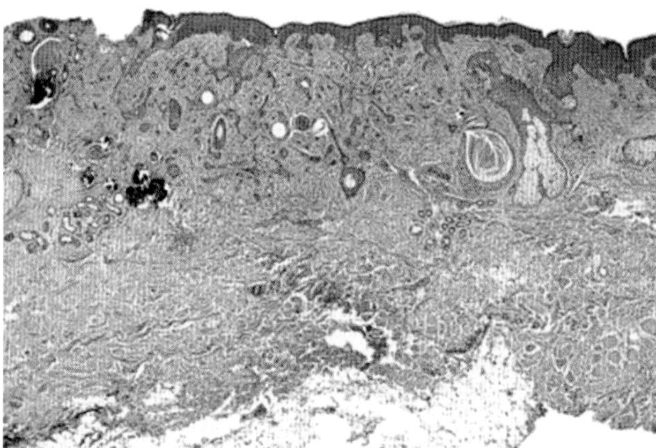

Fig. 6.20 Desmoplastic trichoepithelioma. Characteristic low-power view showing epithelial strands, cysts, and foci of calcification. There are multiple points of continuity within the epidermis. (From Brinster NK, Liu V, Diwan H, McKee PH. Desmoplastic trichoepithelioma. In: *Dermatopathology: A Volume in the High Yield Pathology Series*. Philadelphia: Elsevier; 2011:390.)

- **Other high-yield facts/comments**
  - Benign follicular tumors are **CK20+** and **PHLDA1+** (new stain) → distinguishes from BCC
  - Syndromes a/w multiple trichoepitheliomas:
    - **Brooke-Spiegler syndrome:** *CYLD* mutation, multiple trichoepitheliomas, trichoblastomas, spiradenomas, and cylindromas
    - **Rombo syndrome:** atrophoderma vermiculatum, hypotrichosis, acro-facial vasodilation and cyanosis, milia, and multiple BCCs

Desmoplastic trichoepithelioma (DTE)

- **Clinical and histopathologic features**
  - **Young adult** F > M; always solitary; almost always on face (**cheek** #1); **firm annular plaque w/ central dell**
  - Histology: well-circumscribed proliferation contained within upper half of dermis; **thin cords** of basaloid cells (two to three cell layers thick) within **sclerotic/thickened collagenous stroma;** numerous **horn cysts, keratin granulomas** (from ruptured microcysts) and **dystrophic calcification** (Fig. 6.20)
- **Histologic DDx**
  - Morpheaform BCC: atypical cells w/ ↑ mitoses, ↑ apoptosis, sharply angled nests, and fewer horn cysts
- **Other high-yield facts/comments**
  - Not a/w inherited syndromes
  - **CK20+** and **PHLDA1+** (vs. negative in morpheaform BCC)

Neoplasms with follicular matrix differentiation

Pilomatricoma (calcifying epithelioma of Malherbe)

- **Clinical and histopathologic features**
  - Solitary, **firm**, flesh-colored nodule with **white-chalky hue** from calcification; **cheek (#1)**; **children** > adults; caused by a mutation in the ***CTNNB1* gene (encodes β-catenin**, involved in WNT pathway)
  - Histology: well-circumscribed; complex cystic proliferation with internal **"rolls and scrolls"** appearance (Fig. 6.21); **matrical (basaloid) cells** w/ abrupt transition to fully keratinized, **anucleate**

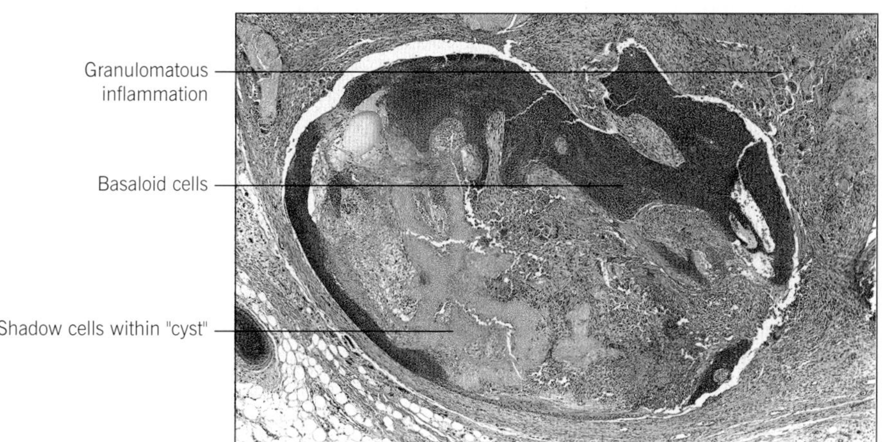

Fig. 6.21 Pilomatrixoma (low mag). (From Rapini RP. Follicular neoplasms. In: *Practical Dermatopathology*. 2nd ed. Philadelphia: Elsevier; 2012:311–319.)

"**shadow/ghost cells" (eosinophilic)**; keratin production leads to intense **granulomatous inflammation**; **calcification** in 80% (ossification in 20%)

- **Histologic DDx**
  - Proliferating pilar tumor: similar convoluted cystic architecture ("rolls and scrolls"), but has **dense eosinophilic trichilemmal keratin** in cyst cavity rather than ghost cells; **lacks basaloid matrical cells**
  - Pilomatrical carcinoma: **adults** on head/neck; **basaloid cells predominate** over ghost cells; numerous mitoses and infiltrative architecture
- **Other high-yield facts/comments**
  - Old pilomatricomas may be composed entirely of ghost cells, with calcification and ossification
  - **Conditions a/w multiple pilomatricomas:**
    - Myotonic dystrophy
    - Turner syndrome
    - Gardner syndrome (usually multiple hybrid epidermoid cysts w/ pilomatrical differentiation)
    - Rubinstein-Taybi (broad thumbs)

Neoplasms with follicular sheath (trichilemmal) differentiation

Trichilemmoma

- **Clinical and histopathologic features**
  - Benign; smooth, skin-colored, **verrucous** papule on **central face (nose or upper lip** most commonly); may arise within nevus sebaceus
  - Histology: circumscribed **lobular** proliferation of **pale to clear staining cells** containing **abundant glycogen** (resemble outer root sheath cells); **broad epidermal connection, warty surface** w/ hypergranulosis, and **peripheral palisading** with **eosinophilic/hyalinized BMZ (PAS+)** (Fig. 6.22)
  - Immunostains: pan-keratin+ and **CD34+** (marker of outer root sheath differentiation)
- **Histologic DDx**
  - Clear cell acanthoma: both are clear cell proliferations arising from epidermis; however, CCA is **not endophytic/lobular** → instead, has regular **psoriasiform hyperplasia** + **neutrophils** in stratum corneum (mnemonic: "looks like **psoriasis w/ clear cells**")
  - Poroma: similar endophytic/lobular architecture, but is composed of small blue **poroid cells w/ rounded nuclei, + sweat ducts + highly vascular stroma**
  - Verruca vulgaris: lacks clear cells and hyalinized BMZ
- **Other high-yield facts/comments**
  - Multiple trichilemmomas → diagnostic of **Cowden syndrome**

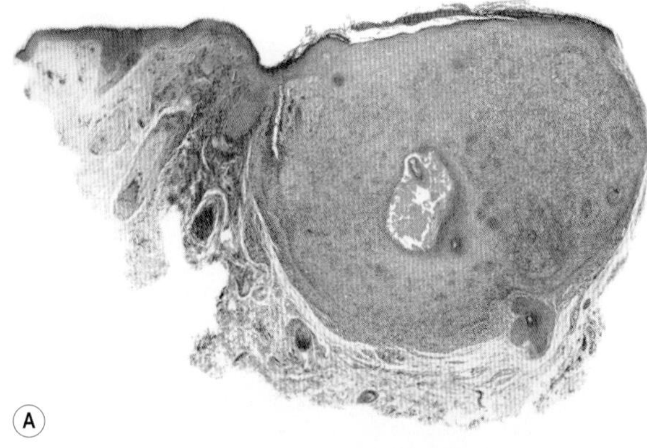

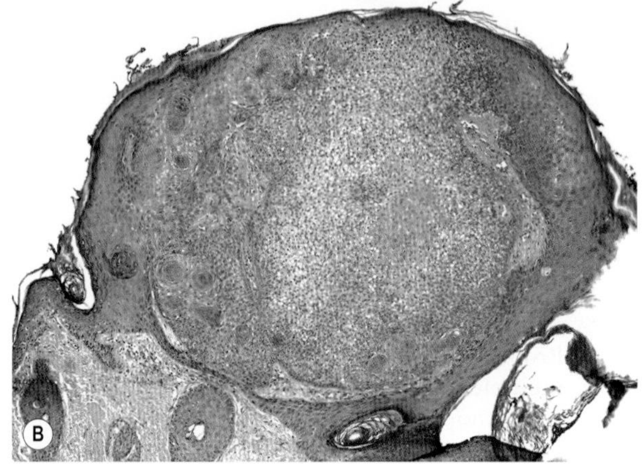

Fig. 6.22 Trichilemmoma. A superficial dermal nodule of small cuboidal keratinocytes with a lobular growth pattern is associated with a follicle. (A) Low power (B) high power. (From Prieto VG, Shea CR, Celebi JT, Busam KJ. Adnexal tumors. In: Busam KJ, ed. *Dermatopathology: A Volume in the Series: Foundations in Diagnostic Pathology*. 2nd ed. Philadelphia: Elsevier; 2016:388–446.)

Desmoplastic trichilemmoma (DTL)

- **Clinical and histopathologic features**
  - **Always solitary**; slow-growing flesh-colored papule on **face** (#1 site); often arises within nevus sebaceus
  - Histology: mistaken for invasive SCC because has angulated, **pseudoinfiltrative epithelial strands in center** of lesion, accompanied by **sclerotic/desmoplastic stroma**; conventional trichilemmoma almost always present at periphery (key to Dx!); tumor is pan-keratin+ and **CD34+** (marker of outer root sheath differentiation)
- **Histologic DDx**
  - Invasive SCC/BCC: lacks conventional trichilemmoma at periphery, cells appear atypical, w/ ↑ mitoses, pleomorphism, and apoptosis
- **Other high-yield facts/comments**
  - **Boards relevance**: they mostly want to see if you can differentiate from SCC
  - Hint: look at periphery to identify conventional trichilemmoma features

Neoplasms with superficial follicular (isthmus and infundibular) differentiation

Tumor of the follicular infundibulum (TFI)

- **Clinical and histopathologic features**
  - Benign; scaly plaque on head/neck
  - Histology: **plate-like proliferation** of eosinophilic isthmic keratinocytes arranged in a reticulate fashion in

superficial dermis; has broad but intermittent epidermal connections; peripheral palisading, fibrous stroma

- **Histologic DDx**
  - Superficial BCC: both have broad, intermittent epidermal connections and peripheral palisade, but BCC has clefting, mucinous stroma, and single-cell necrosis
  - Eccrine syringofibroadenoma: both have anastomosing or reticulated architecture, but ES has prominent sweat ducts, highly vascular stroma, and deeper extension into dermis
- **Other high-yield facts/comments**
  - Boards: not commonly tested; only the histology is testable

Trichoadenoma (TA; of Nikolowski)

- **Clinical and histopathologic features**
  - Benign follicular neoplasm on spectrum with DTE: whereas DTEs have a 50/50 mixture of basaloid **follicular epithelial structures** and keratin-filled **microcysts**, TAs are composed almost entirely of the **small, keratin-filled microcysts**, with minimal to no basaloid follicular epithelial structures
  - Histology: well-circumscribed, superficial dermal proliferation composed of **small keratinizing milia-like cysts** ("microcysts") + **sclerotic stroma** (similar to DTE stroma)
- **Histologic DDx**
  - DTE: (see above)
  - Milia: the microcysts of TA individually look identical to milia, but simple milia lack the sclerotic stroma of TA
- **Other high-yield facts/comments**
  - Mnemonic: **"trichoadenomas look like DTEs that are composed purely of keratin microcysts"**
  - Mnemonic: "trichoadenoma looks like dozens of small milia crammed together in a small biopsy"

Proliferating pilar (trichilemmal) tumor

- Discussed in Cyst section

6.6 SEBACEOUS PROLIFERATIONS

Sebaceous hyperplasia

- **Clinicopathologic features**
  - Common, benign enlargement of normal sebaceous glands; p/w multiple **yellow papules with central dell** on face and upper trunk
  - Histology: enlarged sebaceous glands with **normal internal architecture** (peripheral thin layer of immature basaloid **seboblasts** surrounding central, mature, white sebocytes); enlarged sebaceous lobules circumferentially surround a central infundibulum
- **Histologic DDx**
  - Sebaceous adenoma: thicker layer of immature, peripheral, basaloid **seboblasts**; the central sebocytes have cytoplasm that is slightly pinker and more granular than would be expected for a mature sebocyte (should be very white)
- **Other high-yield facts/comments**
  - May assume a linear configuration on clavicle/neck → "**juxtaclavicular beaded lines**"

Sebaceous adenoma

- **Clinicopathologic features**
  - Benign, small **yellowish papule** on **head/neck**
  - Histology: well-circumscribed, endophytic proliferation with **dilated, direct opening that dumps sebaceous debris onto skin surface** → debris forms impetiginized crust; tumor confined to superficial dermis; tumor is composed of sebaceous glands w/ ↑ **peripheral basaloid seboblasts** (30%–50% of tumor) + slightly immature central sebocytes (cytoplasm is pinker and more granular than fully mature, white sebocytes); lacks necrosis, atypical mitoses, and infiltrative growth (Fig. 6.23)
- **Histologic DDx**
  - Sebaceous carcinoma: ↑ seboblasts, ↑ mitoses, atypical mitoses, infiltrative growth, necrosis
  - Sebaceoma: purely **intradermal in almost all cases** (limited to no connection to skin surface); **well-circumscribed nodule** composed of ↑↑ seboblasts (>50%); **lacks normal sebaceous gland architecture** (vs. sebaceous adenoma, which has the same architecture as normal sebaceous glands, but just too many seboblasts)
- **Other high-yield facts/comments**
  - Most common sebaceous neoplasm a/w Muir-Torre syndrome
  - **Muir-Torre**: AD inheritance; mutation in ***MSH2* > *MLH1*** > *MSH6*, and *PMS2*; characterized by multiple sebaceous neoplasms; multiple KAs; ↑ risk of **colon (#1)** and GU (#2) cancer

Sebaceoma (sebaceous epithelioma)

- **Clinicopathologic features**
  - Benign; more **deeply-seated** than sebaceous adenoma

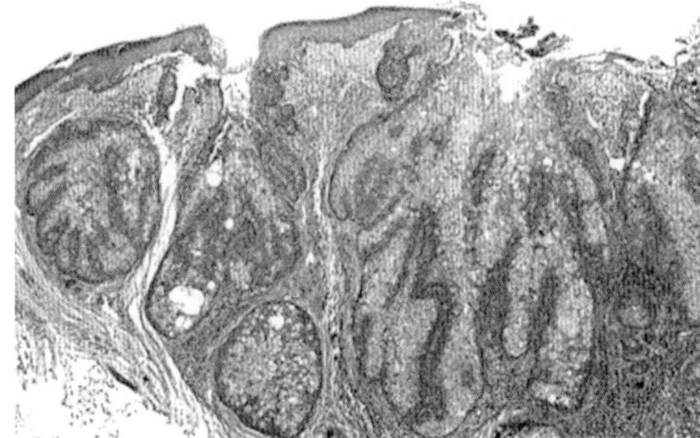

Fig. 6.23 Sebaceous adenoma. Part of a well-circumscribed tumor with surface continuity. (From Brinster NK, Liu V, Diwan H, McKee PH. Sebaceous adenoma. In: *Dermatopathology: A Volume in the High Yield Pathology Series*. Philadelphia: Elsevier; 2011:410.)

- Histology: **well-circumscribed**, ~entirely **intradermal nodule** with minimal to no connection to overlying skin surface (vs. sebaceous adenoma which dumps open to skin surface); **seboblasts are the predominant cell type (»50%)**, with a small number of randomly scattered mature sebocytes; **lacks the normal sebaceous gland architecture** (mature white sebocytes are randomly scattered rather than concentrated centrally); **lacks** malignant features (cytologic atypia, mitoses, necrosis, and infiltrative growth)
- **Histologic DDx**
  - Sebaceous adenoma: **opens broadly onto skin surface**, dumping its contents/debris onto skin surface; retains normal architecture of a sebaceous gland
  - Sebaceous carcinoma: malignant cytologic (nuclear atypia, numerous/atypical mitoses) and architectural (poorly circumscribed, infiltrative) features
- **Other high-yield facts/comments**
  - Boards tip: if a sebaceous neoplasm has > **50% basaloid** cells (seboblasts) → must either be **sebaceous carcinoma** or **sebaceoma**

Sebaceous carcinoma

- **Clinicopathologic features**
  - Malignant; **significant metastatic potential**; separated into **ocular** and **extraocular** types; most commonly presents as a nonspecific red nodule +/– ulceration; most common sites: **periorbital area > other sites on head/neck** > trunk
  - Histology: asymmetric, **infiltrative** basaloid proliferation (often > **50% seboblasts**) w/ ↑ mitotic rate, atypical mitoses, and tumor necrosis; arises from epidermis, w/ extension into dermis; ocular sebaceous carcinoma often has prominent **pagetoid scatter** within epidermis (Fig. 6.24)
    - Can lose MSH2/MSH6, MLH1/PMS2 expression on IHC, either as part of Muir-Torre syndrome or sporadically
- **Histologic DDx**
  - Sebaceous adenoma: see above

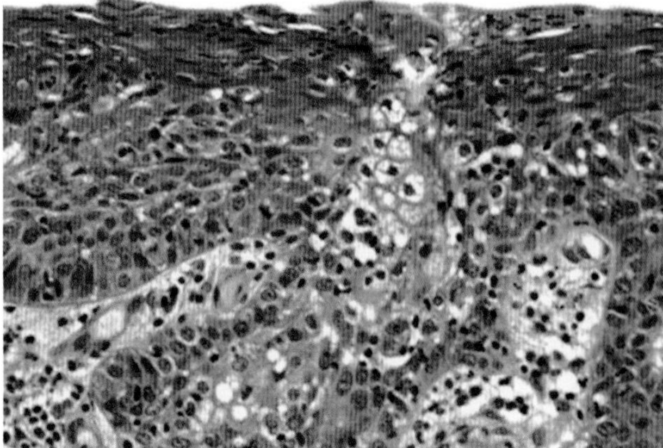

Fig. 6.24 Sebaceous carcinoma. There is extensive epidermal involvement with conspicuous sebocytes. (From Brinster NK, Liu V, Diwan H, McKee PH. Sebaceous carcinoma. In: *Dermatopathology: A Volume in the High Yield Pathology Series*. Philadelphia: Elsevier; 2011:412–413.)

  - Sebaceoma: although it also appears very basaloid with ↑ N:C ratio, sebaceoma lacks other malignant features
- **Other high-yield facts/comments**
  - May be a/w Muir-Torre syndrome or arise *de novo*
  - Ocular form most commonly misdiagnosed as **chalazion** or blepharitis

6.7 NEURAL NEOPLASMS

Traumatic neuroma

- Reactive proliferation of nerve fibers at sites of trauma → arises from attempted regeneration of nerve
- Flesh-colored firm papule or nodule; **painful**
- Histology: variably sized/shaped, **haphazardly distributed small nerve bundles** (resemble normal nerves, in that Schwann cells and axonal components are present in a 1:1 ratio); background **scar**
  - S100+ and neurofilaments+ (stains axons)

Palisaded encapsulated neuroma (PEN; solitary circumscribed neuroma)

- Adults; most common on **face** (90%)
- Flesh-colored firm papule
- Histology: **circumscribed dermal nodule w/ clefting at the periphery** (but lacks a true capsule); nodule composed of tightly packed, fascicular bundles of plump, wavy spindle cells (recapitulates normal nerve; **Schwann cells: axons = 1:1**)
  - S100+ and neurofilaments+ (stains axons)
- Histologic DDx:
  - **Schwannoma**: both are fascicular, but PEN is way more superficial (schwannomas arise in deep fat/muscle near large nerves), has axons (neurofilament stain is negative in schwannoma), and lacks a true capsule (schwannoma has EMA+ perineurial capsule)
  - **Neurofibroma**: individual cells are similar, but PEN is much more sharply circumscribed and organized as discrete fascicles
- **Multiple mucosal neuromas of MEN 2B (similar histologically)**: multiple pink papules in oral cavity, conjunctiva, and nasal and laryngeal mucosa

Schwannoma (neurilemmoma)

- Benign proliferation composed almost entirely of **Schwann cells (S100+)** with **perineurial capsule (EMA+)**
- Solitary pink nodule most commonly on flexural extremities (>head/neck)
- Histology: **deep** (arises in SQ near large nerves), well-circumscribed, **encapsulated** proliferation of plump wavy cells (Schwann cells) with **hypercellular (Antoni A)** areas containing **Verocay bodies** (palisaded nuclei around acellular pink material), and **hypocellular (Antoni B)** myxoid areas; **lacks axons** (vs. NF, PEN, traumatic neuromas); may see large nerve from which it arose at periphery (Fig. 6.25)
  - **S100+** (stains Schwann cells), **EMA+** (stains perineurial capsule); **negative for neurofilaments** (lacks axons)

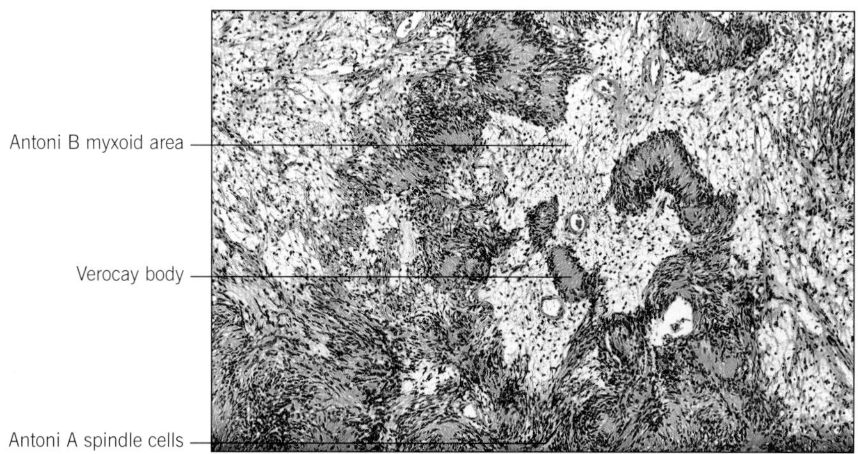

Fig. 6.25 Schwannoma (high mag). (From Rapini RP. Neural neoplasms. In: *Practical Dermatopathology*. 2nd ed. Philadelphia: Elsevier; 2012:367–377.)

- Degenerative atypia is present in "ancient schwannomas" (benign)
- **Boards tip**: almost **never see epidermis** in biopsy specimen since so deeply seated (typically appears "shelled-out")
- 10% of cases are bilateral acoustic neuromas seen in NF2 patients

Neurofibroma (NF)

- Benign proliferation of Schwann cells + other nerve components (fibroblasts, perineurial cells, intermediate cells, and axons)
- Flesh-colored soft nodule w/ "**buttonhole sign**"
- Histology: dermal location; not as well-circumscribed as PEN; **wavy "buckled" nuclei**; cells haphazardly arranged; **loose, myxoid stroma** with ↑ **mast cells** and thin, **wavy collagen fibers**
  - **S100+, neurofilaments+**
- 10% have multiple lesions → raises concern for NF1
- **Plexiform neurofibromas ("bag of worms"): pathognomonic of NF1**; ↑ risk of transformation to malignant peripheral nerve sheath tumor (MPNST)

Nerve sheath myxoma ("neurothekeoma")

- Formerly called "neurothekeoma" or "myxoid neurothekeoma" → terms have been abandoned and replaced by "nerve sheath myxoma" (preferred current name)
- Soft skin-colored nodule; most commonly **hands/fingers** of 40- to 50-year-old adults
- Histology: **plexiform** proliferation of discrete **myxoid lobules** containing bland spindle cells
  - **S100+** (unlike cellular neurothekeoma) (Fig. 6.26)

Cellular neurothekeoma

- Benign neoplasm; uncertain histogenesis
- Firm, pink papules on **face** of **young adults** (20–30 years old); **F > M**

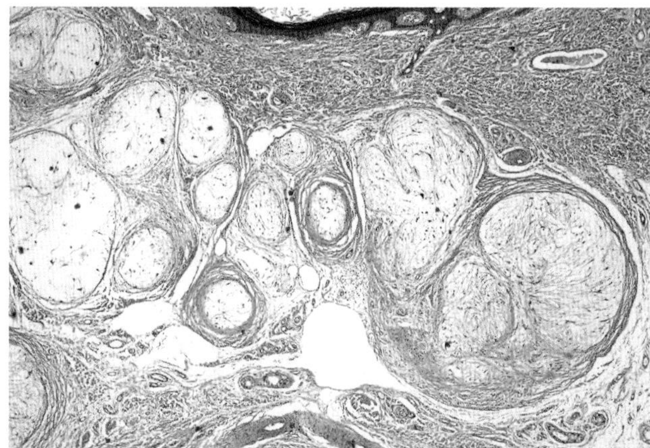

Fig. 6.26 Nerve sheath myxoma: the tumor is composed of discrete lobules separated by fibrous septa. (From Calonje E, Damaskou V, Lazar AJ. Connective tissue tumors. In: Calonje E, Brenn T, Lazar AJ, Billings SD, eds. *McKee's Pathology of the Skin*. 5th ed. Philadelphia: Elsevier; 2020:1698–1894.)

- Histology: dermal proliferation; nests and fascicles of **epithelioid cells** (cells resemble Spitz nevus cells or sarcoidal histiocytes)
  - **Boards favorite**: always **S100 negative** (vs. classic "neurothekeoma"); but **S100A6+, NKI/C3+**, and **PGP 9.5+**

Granular cell tumor

- Benign (malignant in 1%); **neural-crest/Schwann cell derived**
- Most common in adults (particularly females and African Americans)
- 90% solitary; firm asymptomatic nodule; **tongue (#1)**, but any site affected
- Histology: **pseudoepitheliomatous hyperplasia** overlying an ill-defined dermal proliferation of large polygonal cells with **abundant pink, granular cytoplasm** and a small

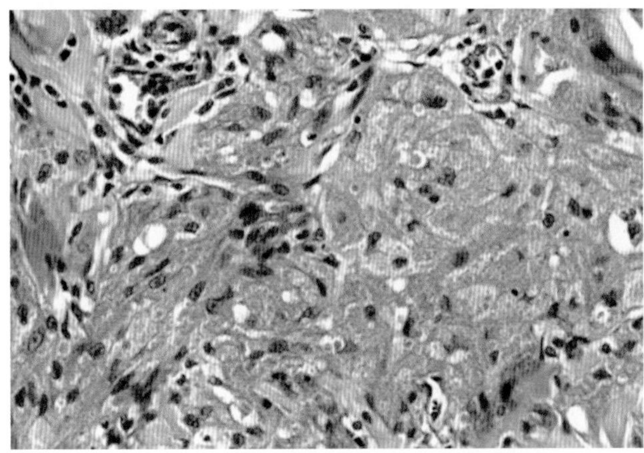

Fig. 6.27 Granular cell tumor. The tumor cells are large with abundant eosinophilic cytoplasm and uniform vesicular nuclei. (From Brinster NK, Liu V, Diwan H, McKee PH. Granular cell tumor. In: *Dermatopathology: A Volume in the High Yield Pathology Series*. Philadelphia: Elsevier; 2011:510–511.)

nucleus, pink cytoplasmic inclusions (**pustulo-ovoid bodies of Milian** = aggregated **lysosomes**) (Fig. 6.27)
- **S100+**
- Boards favorite: if see SCC-like epidermal changes → look in dermis for granular cell tumor!

Malignant peripheral nerve sheath tumor (MPNST)

- Presents as a **rapidly growing nodule within a plexiform neurofibroma** (lifetime risk = 2%–13%); may have a large overlying CALM
- Histology: densely cellular proliferation of atypical spindle cells often with large areas of necrosis ("**geographic necrosis**") and a high mitotic rate
  - Often **only focally S100+**

Merkel cell carcinoma (MCC)

- Aggressive malignant neoplasm (deadlier than melanoma); most common in **elderly** on **head/neck**; UV exposure is major risk factor; ↑ risk w/ **immunosuppression**
- Erythematous to **violaceous papulonodule** which grows rapidly and has high propensity for metastasis **(LN metastasis = 50%; distant metastasis = 33%)**
- Pathogenesis: Merkel cell polyomavirus (**MCPyV**) **implicated in 80%** of cases in the United States and Europe; UVR also plays a major role
  - MCPyV integrates into host genome → oncogene expression, Rb inhibition → cell proliferation
    - MCPyV^{+}: ↓ mutational burden and ↓ UV-signature mutations (vs. MCPyV^{-} tumors, which have higher recurrence risk)
  - UVR → inactivating mutations in p53 and other tumor suppressor genes
- Histology: infiltrative or nodular dermal/subcutaneous mass composed of sheets of uniform basaloid cells with high N:C ratio and finely **speckled "salt-and-pepper" chromatin** (usually without prominent nucleoli); **numerous mitoses** (often > 30/mm^2) and apoptotic cells
  - Positive stains: **CK20 (paranuclear dot pattern**, highly sensitive), **neurofilaments** (paranuclear dot pattern, highly sensitive), **chromogranin/synaptophysin, NSE,** EMA, and CD56; **MCPyV+ (80%)**
  - Negative stains: **TTF-1**, CK7, S100, and CEA
- Histologic DDx
  - Small cell lung carcinoma (main consideration!): **TTF-1+** and CK7+; **negative for CK20** and neurofilaments (lacks dot pattern)
  - Lymphoma: caution because MCC usually expresses PAX-5+ (80%–90%) and TdT+ (70%)
- Prognostic factors a/w poor outcomes
  - Clinical: male, immunosuppression, older age, head/neck location, **diameter > 2 cm, SLNB+**
  - Histological: **p63+, infiltrative** (vs. nodular) growth pattern, **lymphovascular invasion** (detected via H&E or D2-40 immunostain), ↑ mast cell burden on histology, MCPyV^{-} (debatable)
- **NCCN Workup and Treatment Guidelines**
  - Initial workup
    - Given the high risk of MCC, additional **initial** workup warranted and includes:
      - H&P, complete skin and LN exam
      - Imaging is encouraged in most cases (whole-body PET with fused axial imaging may be most sensitive for detecting metastasis at baseline)
      - Consider quantification of serum MCPyV oncoprotein antibodies
      - If immunosuppressed, consider modification/reduction of immunosuppression
  - Clinically node negative (N0)
    - Treatment
      - No baseline risk factors → excision with 1 to 2 cm margins and SLNB
        - ➔ If clear margins, negative SLNB, and no adverse risk factors → observe
        - ➔ If positive margins or other adverse risk factors on excision specimen → re-excision or RT
      - One or more baseline risk factor → excision with individualized margins, SLNB, and adjuvant RT with multidisciplinary consultation
        - ➔ Baseline risk factors for MCC include:
          - ◇ Tumor size > 1 cm
          - ◇ Chronic T-cell immunosuppression, HIV, CLL, SOTR
          - ◇ H/N primary site
          - ◇ Lymphovascular invasion
      - SLNB negative
        - ➔ Observe if low risk
        - ➔ Consider RT to nodal basin in high-risk patients at increased risk for false-negative SLNB
      - SLNB positive
        - ➔ Node dissection and/or radiation AND adjuvant systemic therapy (preferably in a clinical trial, typically PD-1/PD-L1 inhibitors)
      - Recurrent locally advanced MCC → consider pembrolizumab

- Clinically node positive (N+)
  - Workup
    - Imaging
    - FNA or core biopsy
      - If negative → excisional biopsy of LN or radiographic surveillance
  - Treatment
    - If node positive (N+) and no disseminated metastasis (M0) on workup:
      - Node dissection and/or radiation AND adjuvant systemic therapy (preferably in a clinical trial, typically PD-1/PD-L1 inhibitors)
- Disseminated MCC (M1)
  - Treatment (clinical trial preferred)
    - Consider any of the following therapies or combinations of:
      - Systemic therapy
        - Typically, PD-1/PD-L1 inhibitors such as avelumab, pembrolizumab, nivolumab
      - RT
      - Surgery
      - Palliative/supportive care

Primitive neuroectodermal tumor (neuroblastoma)

- Third most common childhood malignancy
- Tumor of primitive neural crest cells of sympathetic nervous system → adrenal gland or **retroperitoneum** most common sites
  - In skin, usually metastatic although rarely can be primary
- Clinical:
  - **75% have metastatic disease** at the time of diagnosis
  - Cutaneous metastases are presenting sign in 30% w/ metastatic disease → p/w multiple **blue nodules** on trunk and extremities
  - Peripheral blanching after stroking lesion, due to catecholamine release
  - **"Raccoon eyes"** (periorbital darkening/purpura) from orbital metastases
  - ↑ **Urinary catecholamines (>90%)**
  - Infants < 1 year old → favorable prognosis; older children → poor prognosis
- Histology: dermal or subcutaneous nodule composed of **small, round, blue cells**
  - NSE+ and neurofilaments+ → favors neuroblastoma over other small round blue cell tumors (lymphoma, MCC, small cell lung carcinoma, Ewing sarcoma)
  - FISH for n-Myc aids in diagnosis and is a/w worse prognosis

6.8 SMOOTH MUSCLE NEOPLASMS

Pilar leiomyoma

- Benign proliferation of smooth muscle arising from **arrector pili**
- **Red-brown papules** on **trunk** or **extremities**
  - **Painful**, especially with cold exposure
  - **Pseudo Darier sign**: stroking of lesion → becomes red, painful, and elevated (as a result of contraction of smooth muscle)
- Multiple lesions can occur as part of **Reed syndrome** (AD inheritance, **fumarate hydratase mutations,** multiple cutaneous and **uterine leiomyomas** and **RCC**) (Fig. 6.28)
- Histology: ill-defined dermal proliferation of haphazardly arrayed, **intersecting fascicles of smooth muscle cells** (spindle cells with **bright pink cytoplasm** and **"cigar-shaped" nuclei**); lacks mitotic activity (Fig. 6.29)
  - Stains: **desmin+**, **SMA+**, and caldesmon+; smooth muscle fibers are pink-red with Masson trichrome stain

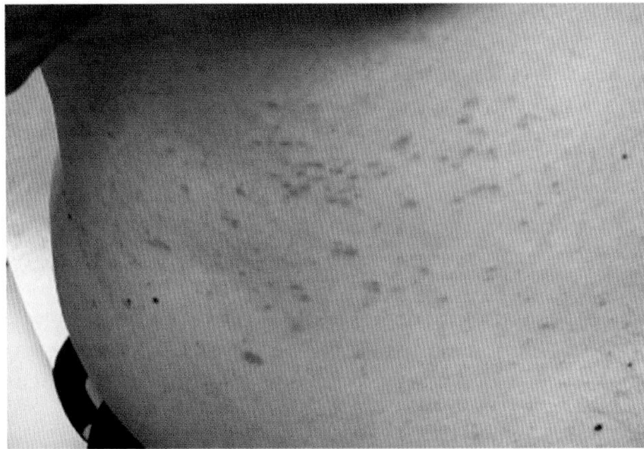

Fig. 6.28 Leiomyoma. Numerous grouped leiomyomata in a middle-aged woman manifesting as tender erythematous papules on the trunk. (From Brinster NK, Liu V, Diwan H, McKee PH. Leiomyoma and angioleiomyoma. In: *Dermatopathology: A Volume in the High Yield Pathology Series*. Philadelphia: Elsevier; 2011:523–524.)

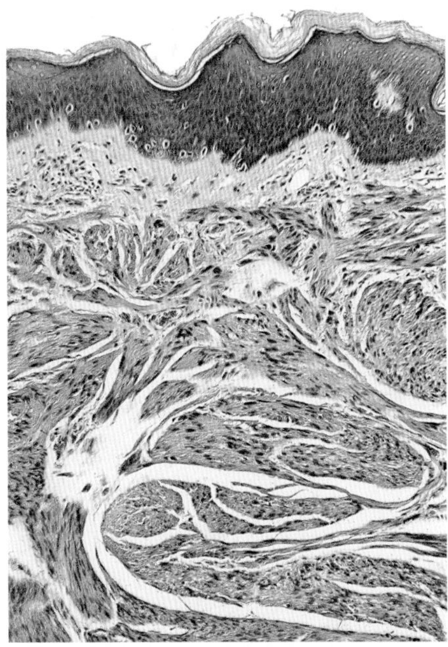

Fig. 6.29 Pilar leiomyoma. The reticular dermis is replaced by interlacing bundles of smooth muscle cells (H&E). (From Patterson JW. Tumors of muscle, cartilage, and bone. In: *Weedon's Skin Pathology*. 4th ed. Philadelphia: Elsevier, 2016: 1029–1040.)

- Histologic DDx:
  - Smooth muscle hamartoma/Becker's nevus: fewer and more discrete smooth muscle bundles interspersed in normal dermal collagen
  - Angioleiomyoma: larger and deeper; smooth muscle bundles circumferentially arrayed around collapsed vessels
- Treatment: excision if solitary; if multiple → gabapentin or nifedipine (reduces smooth muscle contraction)

Genital Leiomyoma

- Solitary lesions on the vulva, scrotum, and areola arising from superficial network of smooth muscle found at these sites; asymptomatic
- Histology: similar to pilar leiomyomas, but often **larger**, less sharply circumscribed, and may have mitoses

Angioleiomyoma

- Benign proliferation derived from smooth muscle in wall of subcutaneous vessels
- Most commonly **middle-aged females** on **lower extremity**; frequently **painful** (Box 6.2)
- Histology: **subcutaneous, well-circumscribed nodule** w/ compact fascicles of **smooth muscle cells circularly arrayed** around vessels with collapsed ("**slit-like**") **lumens** (Fig. 6.30)
  - Is a proliferation of muscle in vessel wall, not a proliferation of endothelial cells → central **vascular lumens are compressed** by muscular wall → "slit-like" lumens surrounded by a ton of circularly arrayed smooth muscle
  - Stains: **desmin+** (differentiates from myopericytoma), **SMA+**, calponin+ and h-caldesmon+

Box 6.2 Mnemonic: Painful Skin Lesions

"BANGLE(S)"
Blue rubber blebs
Angiolipoma
Neuroma
Glomus tumors
Leiomyoma
Eccrine **S**piradenoma

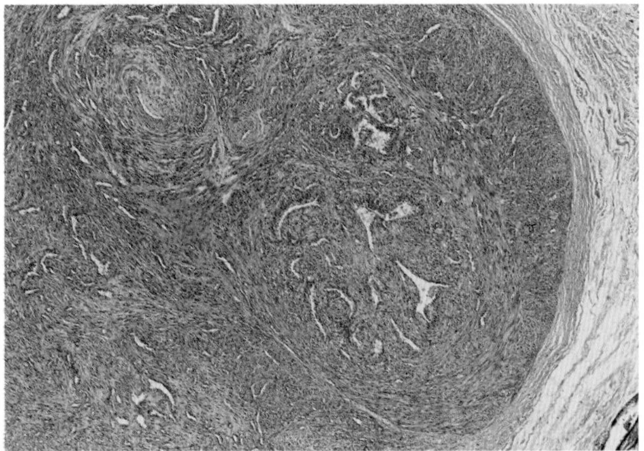

Fig. 6.30 Angioleiomyoma. (From Patterson JW. Tumors of muscle, cartilage, and bone. In: *Weedon's Skin Pathology*. 5th ed. Philadelphia: Elsevier, 2021: 1081–1092.)

Leiomyosarcoma (LMS)

- LMS divided into superficial and deep forms:
  - Deep LMS (subfascial variant): almost never encountered by dermatologists (→ not discussed further); deep soft tissue sarcoma; often arises from smooth muscle walls of large vessels; usually fatal
  - Superficial LMS (suprafascial variant): most relevant variant for dermatologists; arises from arrector pili or genital/areolar smooth muscle; generally **good prognosis**
    - Dermal LMS: most behave in indolent fashion, and some experts have argued they are not true malignancies; however, a 2014 study from Mayo Clinic reported a **10% metastatic rate** with dermal LMS
    - Subcutaneous LMS: arises from vascular smooth muscle; **behaves more aggressively** than dermal LMS → ↑ **risk of metastases** (esp. if diameter > 5 cm)
- **Red-brown nodules or plaques**; most common on **extremities**
- Histology: ranges from low-grade (resemble leiomyoma, but have ↑ cellularity, ↑ mitotic activity, and pleomorphism) to high-grade lesions (AFX-like)
  - Stains: **desmin+** and **SMA+**

6.9 HEMATOLYMPHOID NEOPLASMS

Mycosis fungoides (MF)

Epidemiology

- Accounts for 50% of all primary cutaneous lymphomas
- Most common type of cutaneous T-cell lymphoma
- Onset typically in sixth or seventh decade, but can occur in younger patients including children

Clinical features (Table 6.6)

- Progression though patch, plaque, and tumor stages
- Patch stage: irregular erythematous scaly patches occurring in **non–sun-exposed/bathing suit distribution**; may be pruritic (Fig. 6.31A)
- Plaque stage: well-demarcated variably shaped violaceous to red-brown plaques; may be pruritic
- Tumor stage: rapidly enlarging **nodules with frequent ulceration**; arises in a background of patch and plaque lesions (otherwise unlikely to be MF) (Fig. 6.31B)
- Rare LN and visceral involvement

Histology

- Patch stage: **epidermotropic atypical lymphocytes** (enlarged w/ **cerebriform, hyperchromatic nuclei**) predominantly in the epidermis in clusters (**Pautrier**

Table 6.6 Cutaneous T-Cell Lymphoma Staging

Stage	T	N	M	B
IA	T1: <10% BSA T1a: patches T1b: plaques	N0: no palpable nodes or histologic evidence of MF	M0: no visceral involvement	B0: <5% peripheral lymphocytes atypical B0a: clone-negative B0b: clone-positive B1: >5% of lymphocytes atypical but < 1000/μL B1a: clone-negative B1b: clone-positive
IB	T2: >10% BSA T2a: patches T2b: plaques	N0	M0	B0-B1
IIA	T1 or T2	N1: no dermatopathic histological evidence of MF N1a: clone-negative N1b: clone-positive N2: early involvement with MF, aggregates of atypical cells with preservation of nodal architecture N2a: clone-negative N2b: clone-positive	M0	B0-B1
IIB	T3: tumors (lesions > 1 cm diameter w/ deep infiltration)	N0-N2	M0	B0-B1
IIIA	T4: erythroderma (>80% BSA)	N0-N2	M0	B0
IIIB	T4	N0-N2	M0	B1: >5% of lymphocytes atypical but <1000/μL
IVA1	T1-T4	N0-N2	M0	B2: >1000/μL circulating atypical lymphocytes (Sézary cells)
IVA2	T1-T4	N3: lymph nodes involved w/ loss of normal architecture	M0	B0-B2
IVB	T1-T4	N0-N3	M1: metastasis	B0-B2

B, *Blood;* BSA, *body surface area;* M, *metastasis;* MF, *mycosis fungoides;* N, *node;* T, *tumor.*

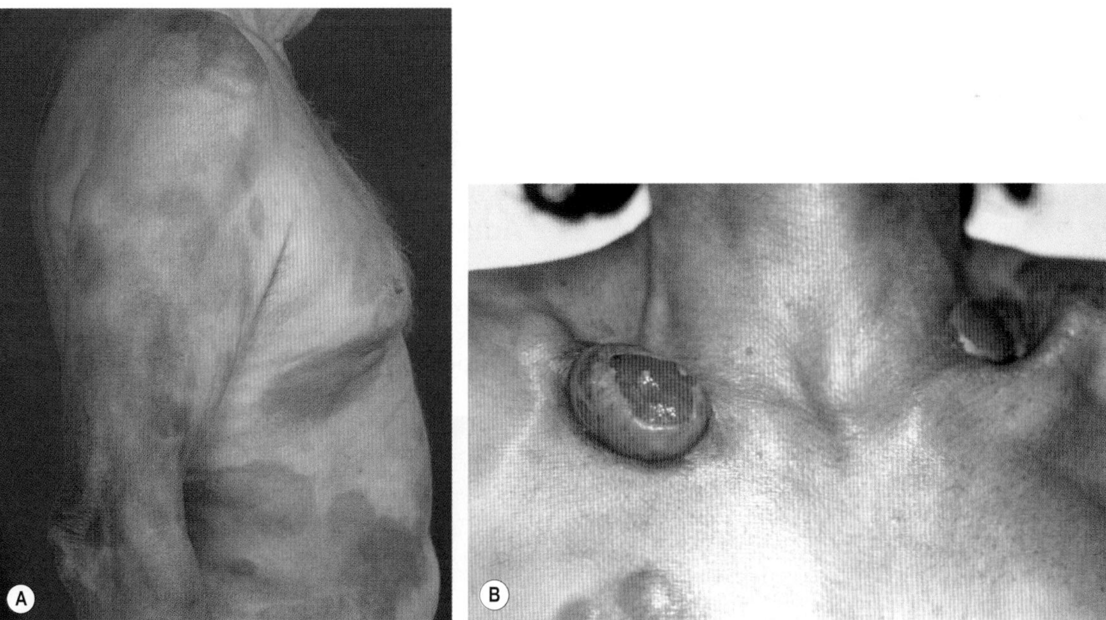

Fig. 6.31 Mycosis fungoides. (A) Patch stage. (B) Tumor stage. (From James WD, Elston DM, McMahon PJ. Cutaneous lymphoid hyperplasia, cutaneous T-cell lymphoma, other malignant lymphomas, and allied diseases. In: *Andrews' Diseases of the Skin Clinical Atlas*. Philadelphia: Elsevier; 2018:501–516.)

microabscesses) and **lined up at DEJ** with clear halos surrounding the cells; superficial dermal **band-like/ "lichenoid" lymphocytic infiltrate** (predominantly reactive lymphocytes); **"wiry" papillary dermal fibrosis** (Fig. 6.32)

- Clue to epidermotropism (vs. exocytosis) = **intraepidermal lymphocytes out of proportion to the degree of spongiosis**

- Plaque stage: **more prominent epidermotropism** w/ more atypical lymphocytes in the dense dermal band-like infiltrate

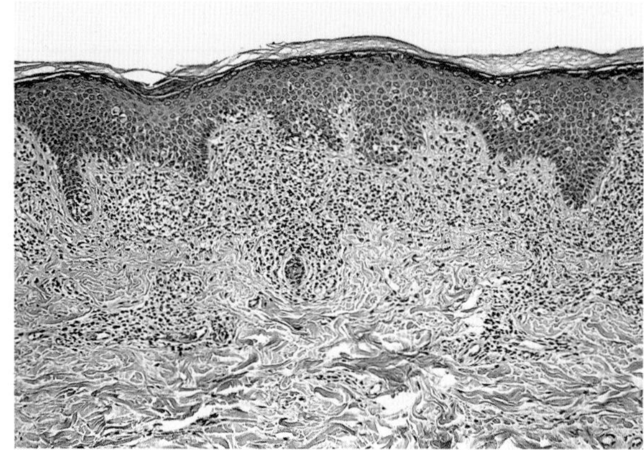

Fig. 6.32 Mycosis fungoides. There is a band-like dermal infiltrate with atypical lymphocytes in the basal epidermis (H&E). (From Patterson JW. Cutaneous infiltrates—lymphomatous and leukemic. In: *Weedon's Skin Pathology*. 5th ed. Philadelphia: Elsevier, 2021:1225–1272.)

- Tumor stage: ↑ density and depth of dermal infiltrate of atypical lymphocytes with **decreased/absent epidermotropism**
  - Large cell transformation defined by > **25% large cells** (>4 times the size of a mature lymphocyte) +/- **CD30 expression** (often present, but not required for diagnosis; CD30 negative a/w poor prognosis)
- Immunophenotype:
  - Typical phenotype: **CD3+/CD4+/CD8−** mature T lymphocytes
  - **Variable loss of pan T-cell markers: CD7 loss (most common**, least specific) > CD5 and CD2 loss (less common, more specific)
- Histologic features are often ambiguous in early patch stage → **molecular testing for T-cell receptor gene rearrangement** (TCR-GR) may be useful, but has pitfalls!
  - False positives: clonal rearrangements detected in some non-neoplastic inflammatory dermatoses (including eczema) → must correlate w/ clinical and histologic findings
  - False negatives: common in very early patch stage
- **Hypopigmented MF (variant)**: favors darkly pigmented patients; more common presentation in young patients; usually **CD4−/CD8+** → cytotoxic phenotype → a/w more interface changes (apoptotic keratinocytes and pigment incontinence) → explains hypopigmentation seen clinically

Treatment

- Patch/plaque stage: topical/intralesional steroids, topical nitrogen mustard/mechlorethamine, topical bexarotene/alitretinoin, and phototherapy, (NB UVB for patch and PUVA)
- Can add methrotrexate (MTX) or pralatrexate, oral acitretin or bexarotene for progressive disease
- More advanced disease: histone deacetylase inhibitors (vorinostat, romidepsin, resminostat), brentuximab vedotin (anti-CD30 antibody) for transformed MF, mogamulizumab (anti-CCR4 antibody; useful because MF homes to skin using CCR4)
- Systemic chemotherapy (e.g., CHOP, gemcitabine, doxorubicin): reserved for advanced/rapidly progressive disease, ↑ risk of secondary infections; radiotherapy (local if few tumors vs. total skin electron beam for generalized plaques/tumors), ECP (for erythrodermic MF), and allogeneic stem cell transplant (effective for some advanced MF and Sezary patients, but a/w high mortality and recurrence) represent other treatment options

Clinical variants

- Folliculotropic: 10% of patients; **head/neck** area a/w papules/acneiform lesions (early) to plaques with alopecia (advanced) (Fig. 6.33); histology: atypical infiltrates **involve follicular epithelium + follicular mucinosis**; ↑ depth makes it more refractory to treatment → **worse prognosis (similar to tumor stage** MF), sustained remission is rare
- Pagetoid reticulosis (Woringer-Kolopp disease): rare, progressive solitary **psoriasiform** plaque on **distal extremities**; histology: **very prominent epidermotropism** in a pagetoid pattern; **good prognosis**
- Granulomatous slack skin: extremely rare; sagging skin folds in the **axilla/groin**; granulomatous inflammation w/ **multinucleated giant cells**, atypical lymphocytes, and **prominent elastophagocytosis** (→ loss of elastic recoil); **indolent course**; usually evolves to classic MF; up to **30% develop Hodgkin lymphoma**

Sézary syndrome

- Erythroderma (**intensely pruritic**); lymphadenopathy and neoplastic Sézary cells in the skin, blood, and LNs; considered distinct from MF
- Must demonstrate a circulating population of CD4+ neoplastic T-cells with an absolute count > **1000 cells/μL** or expanded CD4+ T-cell population → CD4/CD8 ratio ≥ 10, CD4+/CD7- cells ≥ 40% or CD4+/CD26 cells ≥ 30%
- Histologic features may be nonspecific or resemble MF (often more spongiosis, less epidermotropism than typical MF); CD4+/8−, PD-1+, TOX+, KIRDL2+
- Treatment: ECP + systemic therapies (e.g., bexarotene); chemotherapy, mogamulizumab, and alemtuzumab for worse cases; poor prognosis

Adult T-cell leukemia/lymphoma (ATLL)

- a/w **HTLV-1 virus** → endemic in areas with high virus prevalence (Japan, Caribbean, Central Africa)
- p/w leukemia, lymphadenopathy, organomegaly, **hypercalcemia**, and skin lesions; poor prognosis

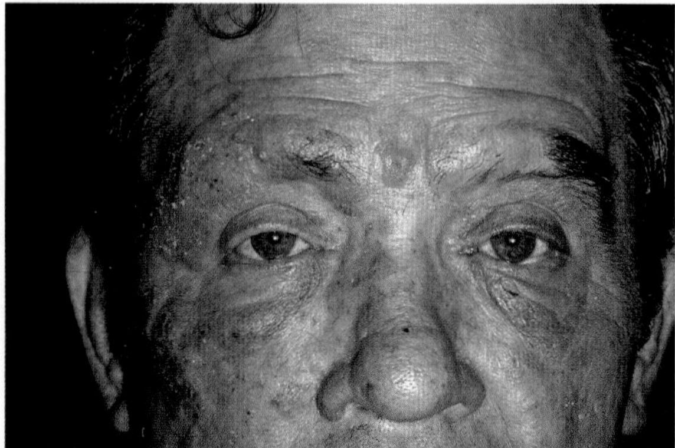

Fig. 6.33 Alopecia mucinosa. (From James WD, Elston DM, Treat JR, Rosenbach MA, Neuhaus IM. Cutaneous lymphoid hyperplasia, cutaneous T-cell lymphoma, other malignant lymphomas, and allied diseases. In: *Andrews' Diseases of the Skin*. 13th ed. Philadelphia: Elsevier; 2020:731–749.)

- Histopathology resembles MF, but has characteristic "**floret**" or "**clover-leaf**" malignant T cells
  - Immunophenotype: $CD4^+/CD8^-/$**$CD25^+$, PD-1$^+$**

Lymphomatoid papulosis (LyP)

- **CD30+ lymphoproliferative disorder, along with ALCL** (see below) and "borderline" cases—this group of disorders are indolent with recurrences but good prognosis overall
- Any age, but favors **adults in 40s** (vs. PLEVA, which favors children); multiple (10–20 lesions usually), **recurrent**, **ulcerative**, and red-brown papulonodules on **trunk and extremities** → individual lesions **self-resolve** in 1 to 2 months → heals w/ **atrophic varioliform scars** (Fig. 6.34A)

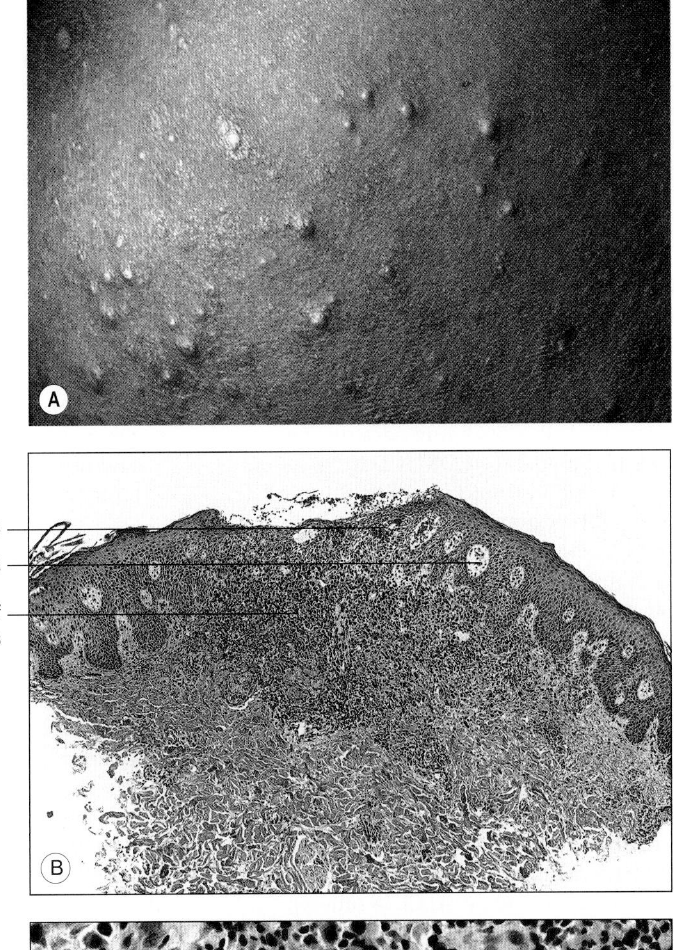

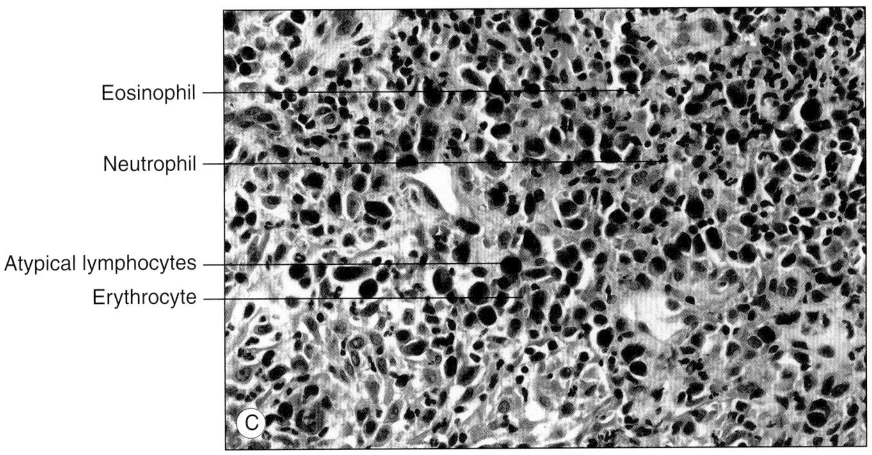

Fig. 6.34 Lymphomatoid papulosis. (A) Clinical presentation with varied skin lesions (e.g., papules, pustules, necrotic lesions) in different stages of evolution. (B) and (C) Diffuse infiltrate, extending into the dermis, with atypical lymphocytes, as well as some neutrophils and neutrophils. (*A*, From James WD, Elston DM, McMahon PJ. Cutaneous lymphoid hyperplasia, cutaneous T-cell lymphoma, other malignant lymphomas, and allied diseases. In: *Andrews' Diseases of the Skin Clinical Atlas*. Philadelphia: Elsevier; 2018:501–516. *B* and *C*, From Rapini RP. Myeloproliferative disorders. In: Rapini RP, ed. *Practical Dermatopathology*. 3rd ed. Philadelphia: Elsevier; 2021:341–364.)

- Histology (all histological variants have the same clinical presentation)
  - Type A (75%; most classic form, most important for Boards): **wedge-shaped** infiltrate with **clusters of large, atypical, Reed-Sternberg-like CD30+ (Ki-1) lymphocytes**, ↑ mitotic activity and atypical mitoses, mixed inflammation (lymphocytes, **eosinophils**, and **neutrophils**); overlying ulceration and parakeratotic scale (see Fig. 6.34B and C)
  - Type B (MF-type, 10%–15%): histologically resembles patch/plaque **MF**; epidermotropic infiltrate of small, hyperchromatic, cerebriform CD4+ cells; CD30 usually negative (rarely see large CD30+ cells in this variant)
  - Type C (ALCL-type, 10%): dense **pan-dermal** infiltrate with sheets of CD4+/CD8−/CD30+ large lymphocytes; histologically indistinguishable from anaplastic large cell lymphoma **(ALCL)** and **large cell transformation of tumor-stage MF** → need clinical correlation
  - Type D (epidermotropic CD8+ variant, <5%): abundant epidermotropic CD4-/**CD8$^+$**/CD30$^+$ cells; histologically resembles aggressive epidermotropic T-cell lymphoma, but has much better prognosis → need clinical correlation to ensure correct diagnosis; also could confuse histologically with pagetoid reticulosis (very different clinical presentation)
  - Type E (angioinvasive LyP; <5%): Angiodestructive clusters of small-medium CD4$^-$/**CD8$^+$/CD30$^+$** lymphocytes, along with fibrinous vasculitis/thrombi; histologically resembles extranodal NK/T-cell lymphoma, γδ-TCL, angioinvasive ALCL
  - Type 6p25.3 (chromosomal rearrangement of DUSP22-IRF4): **Biphasic growth pattern** = small cerebriform lymphocytes in epidermis and dense collections of large, atypical lymphocytes in dermis; CD4$^-$/CD8$^-$/CD30$^+$ immunophenotype
- TCGR clonal rearrangement in 40%–90% (not correlated w/ biologic behavior); identical clones may be demonstrated in peripheral blood of patients with severe disease
- Excellent prognosis **(>99% disease-specific survival; overall survival at 10 years** = **92%)**
- Up to **25% of LyP patients have an associated malignant lymphoma (MF > Hodgkin disease, ALCL >** others); may arise before, during or after LyP diagnosis; recommend Q6-12mo followup to assess for development of malignant lymphoma
  - Fascin, TGF-β pathway, CD30 promotor alterations all a/w ↑risk of associated malignant lymphoma (MF, ALCL, HD, etc.)
  - Editor note (TH): I often wonder if LyP is not truly a disease *sui generis*, but rather a "clinical reaction pattern" or clinical phenotype that arises when a "pre-lymphomatous cell" with some oncogenic driver mutation for lymphoid cells attempts to grow into a full-blown lymphoma but lacks the necessary "second-hit" (may be one of the genes already shown to be a/w ↑risk of developing a secondary malignant lymphoma) → without a second-hit, the lesion regresses/is partially killed off by the patient's immune system → clinical lesion regression. **This could explain why LyP has one common clinical presentation despite having many histological variants** with vastly different immunophenotypes, and why multiple distinct types of malignant lymphomas have been seen to arise in association with LyP. In fact, some experts have recently raised concern that Type B LyP may be better classified as papular MF. I think it is possible that LyP may just be a "common clinical phenomenon" that can be seen during the progression of multiple distinct types of malignant lymphomas early in their tumorigenesis ("lymphomagenesis") when they have enough "juice" to get started (papules, nodules), but not enough to keep it going, so they regress. Over time, perhaps some of these aspiring lymphomas develop the necessary second-hit that allows them to become full-fledged MF or pcALCL. Further research and time will tell!
- Treatment: only treat if symptomatic, because treatment does not prevent secondary lymphomas; **MTX** → dramatic improvement in 90% (recurs within weeks of stopping), phototherapy is also first line; **brentuximab** can be used if the former therapies are ineffective
- **Boards pearls**
  - Type A LyP is distinguished from PLEVA by presence of **large CD30+ cells**, and **"dirty infiltrate"** containing **numerous eosinophils** (never seen in PLEVA) and neutrophils
  - ~**25%** have antecedent, concurrent, or subsequent malignant lymphomas (**MF** > ALCL, Hodgkin lymphoma > others)
  - Dermal hypersensitivity reactions (scabies, bug bites, and drug reactions) often have scattered CD30+ cells → may histologically mimic LyP

Primary cutaneous anaplastic large cell lymphoma (pcALCL)

- Must exclude systemic ALCL!!!
- **Solitary** (>multiple [20%]), growing, ulcerated tumors up to 10 cm (larger than LyP); usually adults, M > F; **unlike LyP, lesions do not rapidly "come and go"**
- Frequently persists/relapses in skin; infrequent nodal involvement (~10%)
- Histology: **sheets** of large, atypical CD30$^+$ lymphocytes comprising > 75% of infiltrate
- Usually **lack ALK translocations** (vs. systemic ALCL); EMA negative as well
- 6p25.3 rearrangements (DUSP22-IRF4) predicts good prognosis in systemic ALCL; found in 25%–30% of pcALCL
- Very good prognosis (90% 5-year survival)
  - Features a/w poor prognosis: older age, **generalized skin involvement**, no spontaneous remission, **leg** involvement/extensive regional single-limb disease, solid organ transplant
- Treatment: surgical **excision or radiation (first-line);** low-dose **MTX** (second-line); **Brentuximab** vedotin (anti-CD30 antibody) is a good option in recalcitrant cases or for spread to lymph nodes

Subcutaneous panniculitis-like T-cell lymphoma (SPTCL)

- Lymphoma composed of CD4–/ **CD8+**/ CD56–/ **TIA1+/ Granzyme B+ (cytotoxic)** T lymphocytes with **α/β phenotype**
  - Category previously included aggressive forms now re-classified as γ/δ-delta T-cell lymphoma (universally fatal)

- Any age affected; generalized **subcutaneous nodules** on **legs and trunk**; lesion regression → focal lipoatrophy; systemic symptoms may occur (e.g., fever, weight loss, ↑ LFTs, cytopenia)
- Histology: subcutaneous lobular infiltrate of **neoplastic T cells that "rim" adipocytes**; prominent necrotic debris and **cytophagocytosis ("beanbag cells")**; lacks interface changes at DEJ and angiodestruction (vs. γ/δ-delta T-cell lymphoma); lacks nodular lymphoid aggregates and germinal center formation (vs. lupus profundus)
- **Good prognosis** (80% 5-year survival), but 15% develop **hemophagocytic lymphohistiocytosis** (high mortality, may be a/w *HAVCR2* mutations);
- Treatment: steroids, MTX, cyclosporine

Primary cutaneous γ/δ T-cell lymphoma

- Aggressive **CD4⁻/CD8⁻** ("double negative") T-cell lymphoma w/ expression of **γ/δ T-cell receptor** and **cytotoxic markers** (CD56+, TIA-1+, granzyme B+, and perforin+)
  - **β-F1 negative** (vs. SPTCL, which is β-F1+), **TCR-δ positive**
- Multiple eroded nodules and plaques + visceral involvement
- Histology: dense dermal and subcutaneous lymphoid infiltrate w/ **epidermotropism**, **lichenoid interface changes (major clue)**, vascular destruction, +/– **fat rimming** (mimicking SPTCL)
  - Lichenoid interface changes distinguish from SPTCL (which never has epidermal involvement)
  - Lupus profundus is extremely hard to distinguish → γ/δ stain is helpful; also lupus tends to have reactive lymphoid follicles with clusters of CD123+ plasmacytoid dendritic cells (not seen in γ/δ TCL)
- Rapidly fatal

Extranodal NK/T-cell lymphoma, nasal type

- **EBV⁺ lymphoma** with **NK phenotype**
- Abrupt onset of **ulcerated tumors**, most commonly on **nasal region**
- Histology: variably sized neoplastic cells with prominent **vascular destruction**, +/– epidermotropism
- CD2+/**CD56+** and CD3+ (cytoplasmic, not surface)
- Usually fatal

Aggressive epidermotropic cytotoxic (CD8+) T-cell lymphoma

- Old name = Ketron-Goodman type of pagetoid reticulosis
- Eruptive ulcerated tumors with visceral involvement
- Histology: malignant, cytotoxic, CD8+ infiltrate with prominent epidermotropism and angiodestruction
  - Histologically indistinguishable from other epidermotropic CD8⁺ lymphomas (MF, pagetoid reticulosis, and type D LyP) → distinction best made clinically
- Usually fatal

Primary cutaneous CD4-positive small/medium pleomorphic T-cell lymphoproliferative disorder

- Presents as a **solitary** plaque or nodule on the **head/neck** (>upper trunk) with an **excellent prognosis**
- Histology: dense dermal/subcutaneous infiltrate of small to medium lymphocytes; minimal to no epidermotropism; **MF-like immunophenotype** (CD4⁺/CD8⁻/CD30⁻)
- **Histology and immunophenotype indistinguishable from tumor stage MF** → need clinical correlation (lacks preceding MF patches/plaques)

CD8+ acral T-cell lymphoma

- Usually 1 or a few nodules on acral sites
- Histology: dense dermal infiltrate of small-to-medium atypical lymphocytes (CD3+, CD8+, TIA-1+) with nuclear atypia; no epidermotropism; perinuclear dot pattern with CD68 stain
- Indolent course with good prognosis; surgical excision or radiotherapy if needed

Primary cutaneous B-cell neoplasms

- B-cell neoplasms limited to the skin after systemic workup (except intravascular B-cell lymphoma); relatively less common than T-cell neoplasms
- IgH clonality studies are useful in differentiating low-grade B-cell lymphomas from cutaneous lymphoid hyperplasia
- Typically **CD20+** and **CD79a+** (Table 6.7)

Leukemia cutis

- Most commonly **acute myeloid leukemia (AML)**
  - Generally there is preceding marrow and peripheral blood involvement, but aleukemic forms can occur
- Violaceous papules and nodules at any location
- Skin involvement is **most common with myelomonocytic and monocytic types**
- Histology: **Grenz zone**, diffuse **dermal infiltrate of myeloid blasts** (monotonous cells with high N:C ratio and fine chromatin); may be seen in sheets, nodules, perivascularly, or as infiltrative cords (**"Indian-filing"**)
- **MPO+, CD117 (c-KIT)+**, CD13+, CD33+, and CD34+
- Boards fodder: **chloromas = green nodules** in the setting of AML, because of myeloperoxidase activity

6.10 FIBROHISTIOCYTIC NEOPLASMS

Dermatofibroma (DF)

- Common benign fibrohistiocytic lesion; favors adults (**F > M**); most commonly on **lower extremities**
- Firm dermal papules w/ **overlying pigmentation** and **"dimple" sign** (moves downward when pinched)
- Unclear pathogenesis, may be related to prior trauma/bug bite

Table 6.7 Cutaneous B-Cell Lymphomas

	Clinical Features	Histopathologic Features
Primary cutaneous follicle center cell lymphoma	Violaceous, usually solitary papule or nodule on the **scalp/forehead** or **back ("Crosti lymphoma")**; **excellent prognosis**	Irregularly shaped neoplastic follicles; lacks a well-defined mantle zone and **tingible body macrophages** -Usually **lacks t(14;18)** IgH-Bcl-2 translocation characteristic of systemic follicular lymphoma **-BCL-6(+)** and BCL-2(–) **-Boards Mnemonic:** Severity of cutaneous B-Cell lymphomas correlates with their "BCL score:" **Marginal zone lymphoma** (least dangerous, lowest "BCL score" = 2, because BCL-2+) < **Primary cutaneous follicle center cell lymphoma** (second least dangerous, second lowest "BCL score" = 6, because BCL-**6+**) < **pcDLBCL** (highest danger level, highest "BCL score" = 8, because BCL-**2+** and BCL-**6+**)"
Primary cutaneous marginal zone lymphoma	Purple to brown nodule on the upper extremities or trunk; **excellent prognosis**	Nodular dermal infiltrate with prominent **monocytoid B cells** (small lymphocytes with clear halo) and often **numerous plasma cells (major clue),** some with **Dutcher bodies** -BCL-6(–) and **BCL-2(+)**
Primary cutaneous diffuse large B-cell lymphoma, leg type	**Elderly**, F > M; red to brown nodule on **distal extremity (leg #1)**, but can occur at other sites; must exclude systemic disease; **less favorable prognosis** (5-year survival = 50%)	**Dense sheets** of large round, **markedly atypical lymphocytes** w/ mitoses and apoptotic debris in dermis and possibly subcutis; Grenz zone **-Bcl-2+, BCL-6+ (most cases), and MUM-1+**
Intravascular B-cell lymphoma	Purple patches and plaques; trunk/thighs; usually **systemic involvement including CNS** (→ **neuro deficits**), but can be limited to the skin	Large atypical **CD20+ B lymphocytes within vessels**

- Histology: **dermal spindle cell proliferation** with whorled/**curlicue pattern**, peripheral **collagen trapping**, admixed inflammatory cells, **Touton-type giant cells** that may contain **hemosiderin, overlying epidermal hyperplasia** ("tabled rete"), basal hyperpigmentation and **folliculosebaceous induction (Boards tip—induction may resemble superficial BCC!!!)**; frequently abuts but **never deeply infiltrates fat**
  - Immunophenotype:
    - Positive: **Factor XIIIa**, CD10 (strong, diffuse), **stromelysin-3** (distinguishes from DFSP)
    - Negative: **CD34,** S100, and pan-keratin
- Key distinguishing features of DF (vs. DFSP):
  - Collagen trapping (**best appreciated at periphery**)
  - Touton-type giant cells and foamy histiocytes (never seen in DFSP)
  - Hemosiderin-laden histiocytes/Touton giant cells (never seen in DFSP)
  - **DF only "flirts" with upper part of fat, but never penetrates it deeply** (Fig. 6.35)
  - Epidermal and folliculosebaceous induction (rarely seen in DFSP)
  - Factor XIIIa+, stromelysin-3+, and CD34 negative
- DF variants:
  - Cellular DF: ↑ cellularity, cells arranged in longer fascicles; more mitoses; most common type to be confused w/ DFSP (see above clues)
  - Hemosiderotic: prominent hemosiderin and small blood vessels
  - Lipidized/xanthomatous: prominent foam cells
  - Aneurysmal: large cavernous vascular spaces; clinically worrisome for melanoma or malignant vascular lesion
  - DF with "monster" cells: contains large, bizarre, and highly pleomorphic cells; mitoses are rare, never see atypical mitoses
- ↑ **Risk of local recurrence** w/ aneurysmal, atypical, and cellular DFs → re-excision recommended

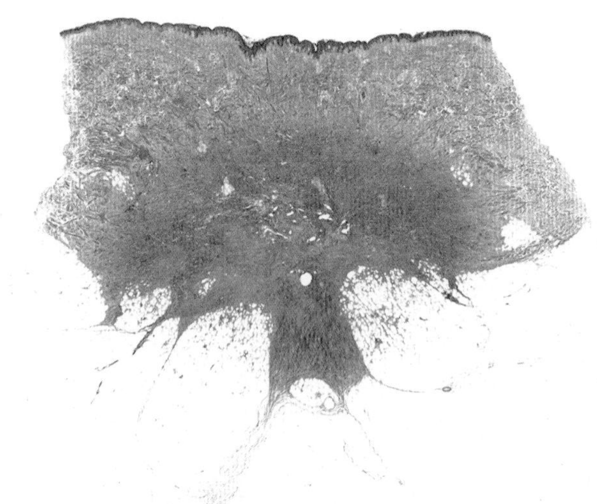

Fig. 6.35 Cellular dermatofibroma (cellular benign fibrous histiocytoma). Stellate-shaped lesion that extends into the superficial subcutis along fibrous septa. (From Buehler F, Billings SD. Soft tissue tumors and tumor-like reactions. In: Busam KJ, ed. *Dermatopathology: A Volume in the Series: Foundations in Diagnostic Pathology*. 2nd ed. Philadelphia: Elsevier; 2016:513–594.)

Dermatofibrosarcoma protuberans

- Tumor of intermediate malignant potential characterized by **t(17;22)** ***COL1A1-PDGFB*** **fusion**
  - Most common abnormality: **supernumerary ring chromosomes** (chr22 most commonly)
- Young to middle-aged adults; M ≈ F; favors **trunk (shoulder #1), proximal extremities,** and **groin** » head/neck
- **Mnemonic**: "**DFSP** affects people **17 to 22** years old Called Pat" → helps remember young age (17–22) and the order of the fused genes (17 = COL1A1; 22 = PDGFB)
- Firm plaque that expands and develops multinodular appearance (Fig. 6.36)

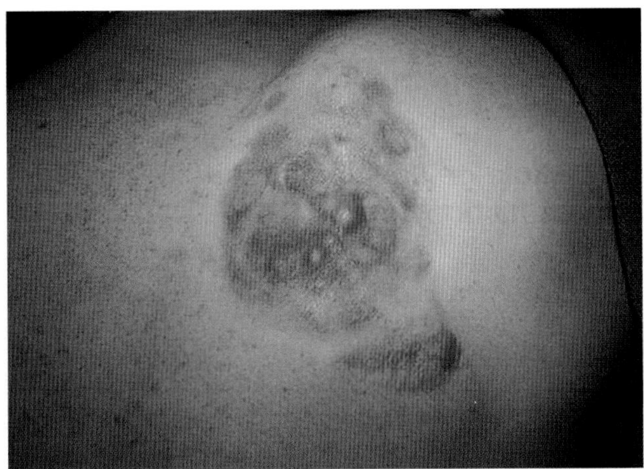

Fig. 6.36 Congenital dermatofibrosarcoma protuberans of the back at presentation in a 16-year-old boy, featuring various morphologic clinical features, including plaques, nodules, atrophy, telangiectasia, and scar-like changes. (From Johnson-Jahangir H, Ratner D. Advances in management of dermatofibrosarcoma protuberans. *Dermatol Clin*. 2011;29[2]:191–201.)

- Histology: **monotonous** spindle cells (cells are more bland and uniform than DF!) with a **storiform** architecture in dermis and throughout SQ fat; characteristic **"honeycomb" infiltration of fat;** 5% with **melanin (Bednar tumor)**
  - **CD34 strongly positive**
  - Negative for Factor XIIIa and stromelysin-3
- **Fibrosarcomatous degeneration:**
  - Occurs in 9%–20% (more common in recurrent DFSP)
  - Histology: ↑ cellularity, ↑ mitoses, ↑ atypia, "**herringbone pattern**," and ↓ **CD34 staining** (weak or lost)
  - Recent study (Hoesly et al., *J Am Acad Dermatol*, 2015) showed ↑ **recurrence rate and** ↑ **metastasis (18% vs. 0%** for conventional DFSP) for lesions with fibrosarcomatous change
- Treatment: **Mohs (ToC) >** WLE w/ 3 cm margins down to deep fascia
  - **Imatinib** is approved for unresectable or metastatic disease (46% partial response rate) → blocks activity of *COL1A1-PDGFB* fusion protein
- Prognosis: propensity for **local recurrence (1% with Mohs;** average of **15% w/ WLE;** up to 50% recurrence with WLE for head/neck lesions); very low risk of metastatic disease (<1%)
  - Multiply recurrent lesions have ↑ risk of fibrosarcomatous transformation → ↑↑ metastatic potential
- **Giant cell fibroblastoma** (pediatric variant): occurs in early childhood; affects **boys** » girls; possesses same ***COL1A1-PDGFB*** **translocation** as DFSP; favors **head/neck**, trunk, and groin; histologically resembles DFSP, but has distinctive **pseudovascular spaces surrounded by giant cells**

Atypical fibroxanthoma (AFX)

- Relatively common low-grade, superficial (**dermally-based**) sarcoma that arises on **CSD** skin (**head and neck #1** > upper trunk and extremities) of **elderly** (70–80 years old); p/w **rapidly-growing, ulcerated red nodule**
- Recurs in up to 5% of cases, but **almost never metastasizes**
- Treatment: **Mohs** > WLE

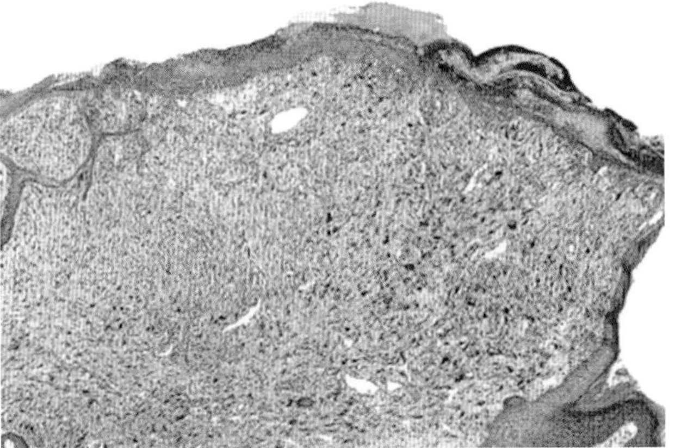

Fig. 6.37 Atypical fibroxanthoma. Low-power view of a pleomorphic, ulcerated tumor. Note the lateral collarette. (From Brinster NK, Liu V, Diwan H, McKee PH. Atypical fibroxanthoma. In: *Dermatopathology: A Volume in the High Yield Pathology Series*. Philadelphia: Elsevier; 2011:474.)

- Histology: fairly well-circumscribed, **overtly malignant** dermal proliferation **slammed** up against an atrophic/ulcerated epidermis; tumor extends down to deep dermis in a "pushing" fashion; tumor is composed of variable mixture of **four main cell types:** (1) **spindle** cells, (2) **histiocyte-like** cells, (3) **xanthomatous** cells, and (4) **bizarre, multinucleated giant cells**; all cell types are notable for hyperchromatic nuclei, pleomorphism, and a **high mitotic rate** w/ numerous **wildly atypical mitoses** (Fig. 6.37)
  - **AFX never extensively infiltrates SQ fat** → if present, should consider "superficial undifferentiated pleomorphic sarcoma" (UPS), or "pleomorphic dermal sarcoma" (PDS; discussed below)
  - Immunostains: **no specific immunostain** to confirm Dx of AFX! Stains positively with **CD10** (nonspecific), procollagen I, CD99, CD68 (histiocyte-like cells), and **SMA in a "tram-track" pattern** (pattern consistent with myofibroblastic differentiation, rather than true smooth muscle)
- **AFX is a diagnosis of exclusion** → must first rule out other entities in the **"SLAM" DDx** (malignant dermal spindle cell neoplasm **SLAMmed** up against the epidermis):
  - <u>S</u>CC (sarcomatoid/spindle cell variant): stains positively with high-molecular-weight keratin (**CK903 and CK5/6**) or broad-spectrum keratin (**MNF-116), p63** and **p40** (newest and most specific marker)
  - <u>L</u>MS: **desmin+** and **SMA+** (diffuse cytoplasmic staining vs. tram-track in AFX)
  - <u>A</u>FX: negative for high-molecular-weight keratin, p63, p40, S100, SOX10, and desmin
  - <u>M</u>elanoma (spindle cell or desmoplastic variants): **S100+ and SOX-10+**
- Lesions related to AFX:
  - <u>Pleomorphic dermal sarcoma (PDS)</u>: recently-described entity; arises on same sites as AFX, but has **deeper subcutaneous invasion**, necrosis, lymphovascular invasion or PNI; a/w ↑ **recurrence** (28%) and ↑↑ **metastases** (10%)
    - **Clinical relevance**: if an AFX-like lesion has significant involvement of fat → would be wise to call it a PDS instead

- Undifferentiated pleomorphic sarcoma (UPS): "UPS" has replaced the old term "malignant fibrous histiocytoma" (MFH); UPS has similar ugly cell types as AFX, but is a deep sarcoma that arises in **deep soft tissues (thigh #1)** of middle-aged adults; **5-year mortality = 50%**

Other fibroblastic proliferations

Angiofibroma

- Clinical features
  - **Fibrous papule:** solitary domed papule; nose/face of adults; mimics BCC
  - **Pearly penile papules:** aggregated pearly papules; corona/sulcus of glans penis
  - **Facial/periungual angiofibromas**: a/w various syndromes
- Histopathologic features
  - Dermal proliferation of stellate (triangular) or multinucleated fibroblasts with **fibrotic stroma** and ectatic thin-walled **vessels**
- **Other high-yield facts/associations**
  - Multiple facial angiofibromas: seen in **TS**, **MEN-1**, and Birt-Hogg-Dubé
  - Periungual fibroma (**Koenen tumor**) is also characteristic of TS

Sclerotic fibroma

- Clinical features
  - Firm/pearly papule or nodule; any site; can be solitary or multiple
- Histopathologic features
  - Sclerotic collagen bundles arranged as intersecting stacks (**"plywood" or "starry night" pattern**); inconspicuous spindle cells between collagen fibers
- Other high-yield facts/associations
  - **Boards tip**: the characteristic histology and association with **Cowden syndrome** are the only two commonly tested points

Pleomorphic fibroma

- Clinical features
  - Domed or pedunculated papules on extremities of adults; F > M; **resemble skin tags clinically**; benign
- Histopathologic features
  - Looks similar to acrochordon, but has scattered hyperchromatic, bizarre, multinucleated, or stellate cells; lacks mitoses
  - CD34+, **loss of RB1**
- Other high-yield facts/associations
  - May simply represent a skin tag with "ancient change"
  - Part of the newly-described **"RB1-deleted soft tissue tumor family"** (spindle cell lipoma, pleomorphic lipoma, pleomorphic fibroma, and other less common entities)

Multinucleate cell angiohistiocytoma

- Clinical features
  - Multiple, grouped red papules on **dorsal hands** or **legs** of women in their 40s; benign
- Histopathologic features
  - Looks like a "cell-poor DF" w/ **characteristic multinucleated giant cells** and prominent proliferation of **dilated vessels** in dermis; stains like DF (Factor XIIIa+ and S100 negative)

Epithelioid cell histiocytoma (epithelioid fibrous histiocytoma)

- Clinical features
  - Solitary, pyogenic granuloma-appearing papules; most common on **thighs** of 50-year-old **women**
- Histopathologic features
  - Well-circumscribed dermal proliferation of **epithelioid cells (resembles Spitz nevus cells)** w/ **epidermal collarette** and dermal sclerosis; stains like a DF
- Other high-yield facts/associations
  - Know the characteristic histology!
  - **ALK gene rearrangement**, ALK+ on IHC

Acral fibrokeratoma

- Clinical features
  - Middle-aged adults; **finger; exophytic keratotic papule** w/ surrounding **collarette**
- Histopathologic features
  - Hyperkeratosis/epidermal acanthosis w/ dermal collagen fibers oriented perpendicular to skin surface; **lacks nerves**
- Other high-yield facts/associations
  - DDx: **supernumerary digit** (has abundant nerve fascicles) and periungual fibroma (more vascular)

Dermatomyofibroma

- Clinical features
  - Young adults; F > M; solitary, well-circumscribed 1 to 2 cm oval **plaque** resembling plaque type DFSP or DF; most commonly on **upper trunk/neck**; benign
- Histopathologic features
  - Reticular dermis has **long fascicles of spindled myofibroblasts** arrayed **parallel** to the skin surface; **respects adnexal structures** (vs. ablated in DF)
- Other high-yield facts/associations
  - Derived from myofibroblasts → **SMA+** (tram-track staining pattern); **CD34 negative** (distinguishes from plaque-type DFSP), S100 negative (distinguishes from NF), Factor XIIIa negative (vs. DF), and desmin negative (vs. pilar leiomyoma)

Inclusion body fibromatosis (infantile digital fibroma)

- Clinical features
  - **Infants**; multiple firm papules on **dorsolateral fingers and toes** (spares thumb/first toe); benign; often spontaneously regress, but can recur after excision (**50% recurrence rate)**
- Histopathologic features
  - Entire dermis filled w/ intersecting **fascicles of plump spindle cells**; on high power can see the **pathognomonic pink-red inclusion bodies** (same size as an RBC) (Fig. 6.38)

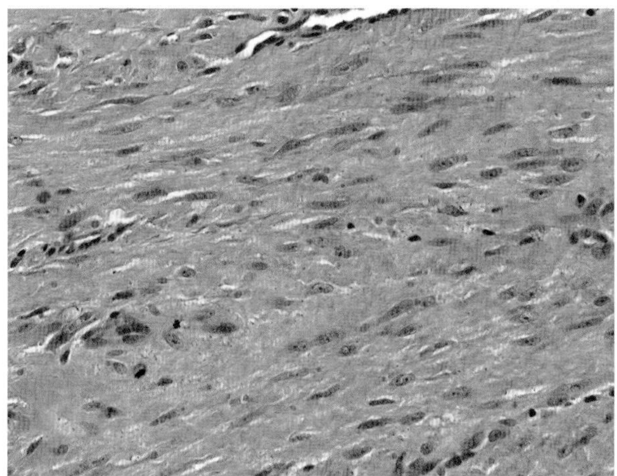

Fig. 6.38 Infantile digital fibromatosis. Infantile digital fibromatosis is composed of fascicles of bland spindle cells that have perinuclear intracytoplasmic eosinophilic inclusions. (Courtesy of Dr. KJ Busam. From Busam KJ, ed. *Dermatopathology: A Volume in the Series: Foundations in Diagnostic Pathology*. 2nd ed. Philadelphia: Elsevier; 2016.)

- **Other high-yield facts/associations**
  - Pink **inclusions** are **composed of actin** filaments → **SMA+**, calponin+, **desmin+**, and stain **red w/ trichrome**

Fibromatosis

- Clinical features
  - Superficial variants:
    - Palmar (**Dupuytren's**)
    - Plantar (**Ledderhose**)
    - Penile (**Peyronie's**)
    - Knuckle pads
  - Deep variants: seen in abdominal wall, intra- and extra-abdominal → all a/w ↑ **morbidity and mortality**
- Histopathologic features
  - Dermal/subcutaneous; **extremely long fascicles** of bland spindled, **wavy fibroblasts** and myofibroblasts; often infiltrates fascia and skeletal muscle
- Other high-yield facts/associations
  - **Deep desmoid** tumors may be a/w **Gardner syndrome**, have **β-catenin mutations**, and stain **β-catenin+**
  - Superficial fibromatoses: benign but locally destructive → **excision + fasciotomy** is ToC

Nodular fasciitis

- Clinical features
  - Young to middle-aged adults; **rapidly growing** 1–5 cm subcutaneous nodule; classically on **upper extremities (#1 site overall)** and **head/neck (#1 site in children)**; may have history of trauma; benign self-limited lesions
- Histopathologic features
  - **Well-circumscribed**, deep **subcutaneous** nodule often a/w fascia; plump spindle cells with "**tissue culture**" appearance and **frequent mitoses** (but none atypical); admixed lymphocytic inflammation; characteristic **myxoid stroma** (early), collagenous stroma (later); numerous small blood vessels with **extravasated RBCs** (Fig. 6.39)
  - **Prototypical "pseudosarcoma"** because of its ↑ cellularity (composed of spindle cells) and frequent mitoses
- Other high-yield facts/associations
  - Boards tip: histology is frequently tested b/c it is a classic "**pseudosarcoma**" → potential medico-legal pitfall
  - Major clues: **myxoid stroma, sharp circumscription, lack of atypical mitoses,** and RBC extravasation
  - ***MYH9-USP6* translocation** (present in >75%; other *USP6* gene fusions present in remainder of cases)

Fibrous hamartoma of infancy

- Clinical features
  - Infants; M > F (3:1); skin-colored subcutaneous nodule; shoulder/arm/axilla; recurrence uncommon after excision
- Histopathologic features
  - Poorly circumscribed hamartoma; benign

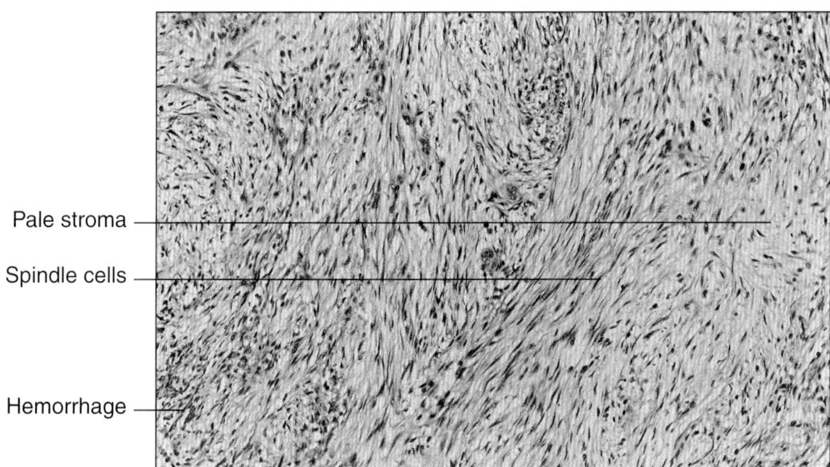

Fig. 6.39 Nodular fasciitis histology. Note the myofibroblasts in the mucinous loose stroma with a "tissue culture" appearance. (From Rapini RP. Fibrohistiocytic proliferations and neoplasms. In: Rapini RP, ed. *Practical Dermatopathology*. 3rd ed. Philadelphia: Elsevier; 2021:393–411.)

- ■ **Triphasic proliferation**:
  - ○ **Plump spindle cells in fascicles** a/w collagenous stroma
  - ○ Small aggregates of **immature mesenchymal cells**
  - ○ Mature **fat**
- • Other high-yield facts/associations
  - ■ Frequently tested on dermpath specialty boards

Myofibroma (infantile myofibromatosis)

- • Clinical features
  - ■ Infantile form: 50% at birth; p/w **multiple** pink-violaceous dermal/SQ nodules on **head** (>trunk); **F >** M; can involve bones and internal organs → ↑ **morbidity and mortality**
  - ■ Adult form: **solitary** 1–3 cm nodules; most commonly on **head/neck**; **benign**
- • Histopathologic features
  - ■ **Biphasic** proliferation:
    - ○ **Hypocellular areas** of blue-pink nodules (may appear cartilaginous, "myoid," or hyalinized) w/ fascicles of bland myofibroblasts
    - ○ **Hypercellular areas** w/ primitive-appearing round, blue cells with ↑ N:C ratio, and ectatic **staghorn ("hemangiopericytoma-like") vessels**
  - ■ Stains confirm myofibroblastic derivation (**SMA+ tram-track** and desmin negative)
- • Other high-yield facts/associations
  - ■ Most common form of fibromatosis in children
  - ■ If limited to soft tissue and bone involvement → self-resolves; good prognosis
  - ■ **Visceral** involvement is a/w **high mortality**
  - ■ Variant: when hypercellular areas predominate → termed infantile hemangiopericytoma

Giant cell tumor of tendon sheath (tenosynovial giant cell tumor)

- • Clinical features
  - ■ Adults; F > M; firm subcutaneous nodule; most common on **fingers**; benign, but 30% recur
- • Histopathologic features
  - ■ Nodular proliferation of round polygonal cells and **osteoclastic giant cells**; variable collagen, inflammation and hemosiderin in the background
- • Other high-yield facts/associations
  - ■ **Boards tip:** this is the only testable neoplasm w/ numerous osteoclastic giant cells

Connective tissue nevus (collagenoma and elastoma)

- • Clinical features
  - ■ Firm papulonodules or plaque; any site
- • Histopathologic features
  - ■ **Collagenoma**: haphazard, thickened collagen bundles
  - ■ **Elastoma**: ↑ elastic fibers; histologic changes may be very subtle → need VVG stain
- • Other high-yield facts/associations
  - ■ **Syndromes a/w connective tissue nevi:**
    - ○ **TS**: Shagreen patch (pebbly plaque on the lower back)

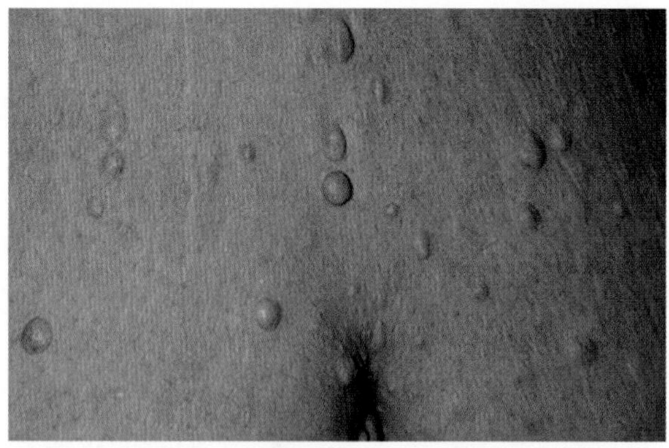

Fig. 6.40 Collagenomas. Periumbilical skin-colored papulonodules. (From Zeller S, Marx SJ, Lungu AO, Cowen EW, Turner ML. Multiple angiofibromas and collagenomas in a 45-year-old man with recurrent nephrolithiasis, fatigue, and vision loss. *J Am Acad Dermatol*. 2009;61[2]:319–322.)

- ○ **MEN-1**: pedunculated collagenomas (Fig. 6.40) + facial angiofibromas + endocrine neoplasia
- ○ **Buschke-Ollendorf** (aka dermatofibrosis lenticularis disseminata): either collagenomas or elastomas + **osteopoikilosis**
- ○ **Proteus syndrome**: cerebriform plantar connective tissue nevi

6.11 VASCULAR PROLIFERATIONS

- • As a general rule, benign vascular lesions:
  - ■ Have: **lobular growth patterns** (multiple lobules/nodules of vessels) and **well-circumscribed** borders
  - ■ May have: mitoses (but lack atypical mitoses) and reactive atypia (enlarged/"revved-up" endothelial cells)
  - ■ Do not have: infiltrative architecture, hyperchromatic nuclei, markedly pleomorphic cells, atypical mitoses, or necrosis

Benign vascular lesions

Vascular malformation (includes "port wine stain," "cavernous hemangioma" old terminology)

- • Present **at birth**; may be capillary, venous, lymphatic, or arteriovenous malformation → **does not rapidly enlarge** (because it is a malformation rather than a true neoplasm), unlike infantile hemangiomas
- • Variable clinical appearances; tend to persist and become more verrucous over time
- • **GLUT-1 negative**
- • Associations: **Maffucci** syndrome, **Klippel-Trenaunay**, **Sturge-Weber**, **Blue Rubber Bleb** (cavernous hemangiomas), Kasabach-Merritt syndrome, and Proteus syndrome

Intravascular papillary endothelial hyperplasia (Masson tumor, pseudoangiosarcoma)

- • **Reactive phenomenon** (organization of a thrombus) most commonly seen **within a vein** (>in a vascular malformation/neoplasm > extravascular hematoma)

- **Slow-growing dusky nodules**; most commonly in veins of **head/neck** or fingers
- Histology: thrombosed vessel with **intraluminal proliferation of endothelial cells** → forms **papillary structures** mimicking angiosarcoma
  - **Major clues = sharply circumscribed** (entirely contained within the thrombosed vessel), lacks multilayering of endothelial cells, and cells are not hyperchromatic

Angiokeratoma

- Superficial keratotic/verrucous vascular lesions
- Five types:
  - Angiokeratoma of Mibelli: 10 to 15 years old; fingers and toes
  - Angiokeratoma of Fordyce: older men (scrotum) or females (vulva)
  - Angiokeratoma corporis diffusum: multiple lesions in childhood/adolescence; bathing suit distribution; seen in **Fabry disease** and other enzyme deficiencies
  - Angiokeratoma circumscriptum: children; F > M; aggregate of lesions forming a plaque
  - Solitary and multiple angiokeratomas: children and adults; arise on any site; may be related to chronic irritation/trauma of superficial dermal vessel
- Histology: dilated superficial dermal vessels with epidermal hyperplasia; rete hug vessels

Infantile hemangioma

- Onset in first couple months of life (usually not obvious at birth) → **rapid growth for 4 to 6 months** → **slow involution** over years
  - Standard teaching—50% involute by 5 years and 90% by 9 years
- ↑ Incidence in: **premature infants, females and placental abnormalities**
- Most are superficial and therefore clinically bright red; arise at any site
  - Deeper lesions are purple-blue
- Histology: dense dermal +/− subcutaneous **capillary proliferation** that is **GLUT-1 positive**
- Treatment for problematic lesions (ulceration, sensitive location): **β-blockers** (first line), corticosteroids, and surgical or laser therapies
  - Airway hemangioma: concern for involvement if a plaque-type hemangioma is present from the preauricular cheek along the mandible, lower lip, chin, or anterior neck (**beard distribution**)
  - Periorbital hemangioma: concern for development of astigmatism (from direct pressure on the globe) and amblyopia (caused by obstruction of the visual axis)
- Rapidly involuting infantile hemangioma (**RICH**): fully developed at birth, no postnatal proliferation, and involutes over 1 year; **GLUT-1 negative**
- Noninvoluting infantile hemangioma (**NICH**): fully developed at birth, grows proportionally with patient; does not involute; **GLUT-1 negative**

Pyogenic granuloma (lobular capillary hemangioma)

- Benign capillary proliferation; a/w **trauma**, **pregnancy**, and medications (**oral contraceptive pills, oral retinoids, indinavir**, BRAF and EGFR inhibitors)
- Most common in children and young adults; rapidly growing, exophytic, and **hemorrhagic papule w/ epidermal collarette**
- Common sites: **gingiva (pregnancy)**/oral cavity, lips, and digits
- Histology: **well-circumscribed**, **lobular** proliferation of small capillaries w/ RBC extravasation; ↑ mitotic activity (no atypical mitoses) and reactive atypia of endothelial cells

Epithelioid hemangioma (angiolymphoid hyperplasia with eosinophils, ALHE)

- Grouped nodules or plaques on head/neck (most commonly **around ear**) of young to middle-aged adults
- Histology: lobular dermal proliferation of capillaries and **larger, thicker vessels w/ large epithelioid endothelial cells** lining the vessel lumen; **intracytoplasmic vacuoles** within endothelial cells (represents primitive vascular lumens); background of **lymphocytic and eosinophilic inflammation** (often intense, with occasional lymphoid follicles); fibrotic stroma (Fig. 6.41)
- *FOS* **rearrangements** by FISH

Targetoid hemosiderotic lymphatic malformation (hobnail hemangioma, targetoid hemosiderotic hemangioma)

- Clinically distinctive, **acquired** lesion; affects children and **young adults**; **legs** (> arms > trunk); red-brown papules with **"target-like" appearance** (dark centrally → pale area is first ring → bruise-like patch in outer ring); often a/w trauma

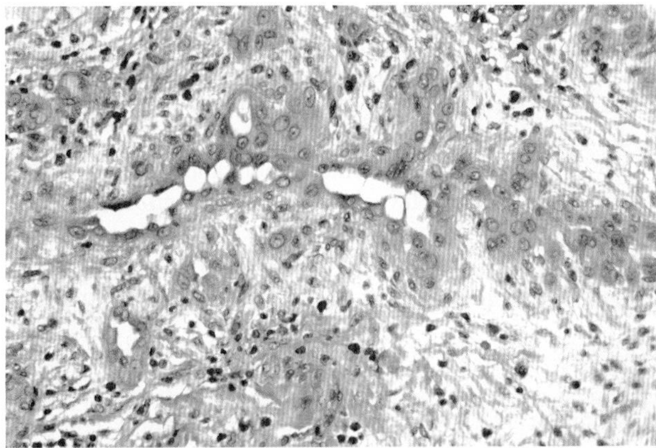

Fig. 6.41 Angiolymphoid hyperplasia with eosinophils (a.k.a., epithelioid hemangioma, ALHE). The vascular channels are lined by plump, partly vacuolated endothelial cells. There are scattered eosinophils in the stroma (H&E). (From Patterson JW. Vascular tumors. In: *Weedon's Skin Pathology*. 4th ed. Philadelphia: Elsevier, 2016:1069–1115.)

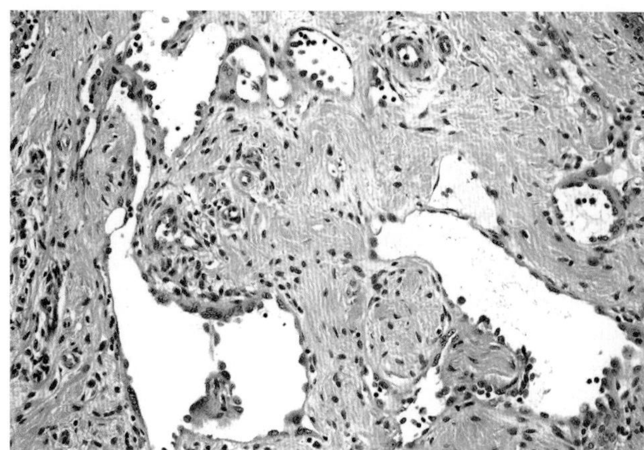

Fig. 6.42 Hobnail hemangioma: the endothelial cells are prominent and protrude into the lumen. Note the papillary processes. (From Calonje E, Damaskou V, Lazar AJ. Connective tissue tumors. In: Calonje E, Brenn T, Lazar AJ, Billings SD, eds. *McKee's Pathology of the Skin.* 5th ed. Philadelphia: Elsevier; 2020:1698–1894.)

- New terminology reflects expression of lymphatic markers by lesional cells
- Histology: biphasic lesion
  - Upper dermis (**Boards favorite**): markedly dilated thin-walled vessels lined by **thin, elongated endothelial cells that protrude** ("**hobnail**") into lumen (Fig. 6.42)
  - Lower dermis: **vessels become more slit-like**; RBC extravasation and **hemosiderin** deposition within dermis

Tufted angioma

- Pink-red macules, plaques located on **neck** or trunk → spreads to involve large areas; may represent a superficial form of Kaposiform hemangioendothelioma (KHE)
- Most commonly appears in **first year of life** (25% congenital); congenital form can be a/w **Kasabach-Merritt** phenomenon (occurs less frequently than with KHE)
- Histology: dermal/subcutaneous tightly packed lobules of capillaries in a "**cannonball" pattern**; a characteristic empty-appearing **"crescent" surrounds the periphery of each lobule** (represents dilated lymphatic channels)

Glomeruloid hemangioma

- Rare vascular proliferation seen in **POEMS syndrome** (>**multicentric Castleman** disease); most common on trunk/proximal extremities; does not clinically appear different than common cherry angiomas
- a/w ↑ **VEGF levels** → vascular proliferation
- **Histology (Boards favorite)**: well-circumscribed dermal proliferation comprised of **dilated vessels** that are **filled centrally with a small ball of well-formed capillary loops** → resultant architecture resembles **renal glomeruli**

Glomus tumor/glomangioma

- Benign proliferations of perivascular epithelioid cells derived from **Suquet-Hoyer canal**
- Glomus tumor (more common):
  - **Solitary**; **painful**; favors young **adults**; **subungual** (most common site)

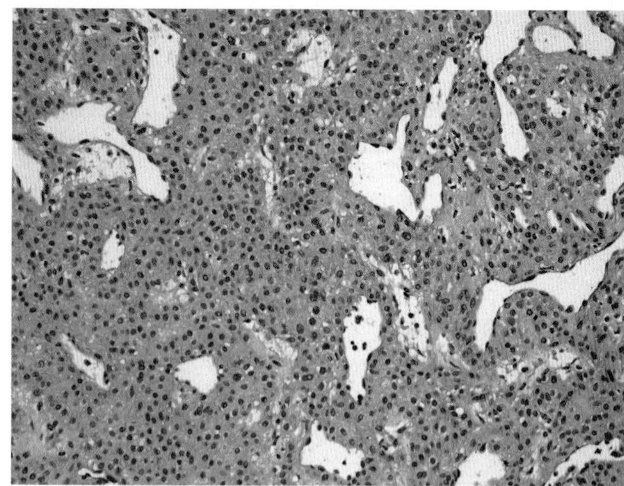

Fig. 6.43 Glomus tumor. Cytologically bland round tumor cells with uniform nuclei and sharp cellular membranes surround blood vessels. (From Buehler D, Billings SD. Soft tissue tumors and tumor-like reactions. In: Busam KJ, ed. *Dermatopathology: A Volume in the Series: Foundations in Diagnostic Pathology.* 2nd ed. Philadelphia: Elsevier; 2016:513–594.)

  - Histology: dense proliferation of glomus cells surrounding small vascular spaces (Fig. 6.43)
- Glomangioma/glomulovenous malformation (less common):
  - Arises in **infancy or childhood**; frequently **multiple lesions, less painful than glomus tumors** (may be tender on palpation, pain may increase with menstruation/pregnancy)
  - Histology: main feature is large, dilated vessels surrounded by a smaller number of glomus cells
- Treatment: surgery is curative

Borderline vascular neoplasms

Kaposiform hemangioendothelioma

- Rare vascular tumor of childhood; a/w **Kasabach-Merritt** phenomenon; **GLUT-1 negative**
- Violaceous plaque; becomes massively engorged when Kasabach-Merritt occurs
  - Usually involves an extremity; can involve subcutis and deeper tissues
  - Can be present in retroperitoneum and present as ecchymoses
- Histology: nodules of densely packed spindle cells with slit-like lumens (resembles nodular Kaposi sarcoma); may resemble tufted hemangioma but has deeper involvement
  - Positive for CD34 and CD31; negative for Factor VIII

Kaposi sarcoma (KS)

- **HHV-8** (present in 100%) induced vascular proliferation w/ variable clinical behavior
- Clinical variants:
  - Classic KS: **Mediterranean**, Ashkenazi **Jewish** descent; **elderly males**; initial lesions on **distal extremities** → some progress to disseminated involvement

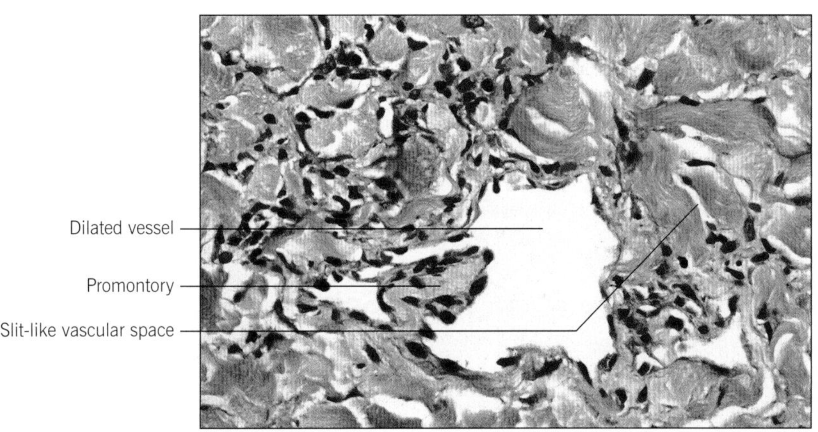

Fig. 6.44 Kaposi sarcoma (medium mag). (From Rapini RP. Vascular proliferations and neoplasms. In: *Practical Dermatopathology*. 2nd ed. Elsevier; 2012:353–365.)

- African endemic: **young African males** in endemic regions; LN involvement and **fulminant/fatal course**
- Iatrogenically immunocompromised: seen in patients with organ transplants, cancer, and autoimmune diseases
- AIDS-associated: most common in **homosexual males**; solitary (trunk and **midface** common) or multiple lesions; may disseminate
- Slowly growing violaceous patches, plaques, or nodules
- Histology:
  - Patch stage: subtle infiltrative small vessels with bland endothelium and associated **plasma cells; RBC extravasation + hemosiderin** +/– **promontory sign** (Fig. 6.44)
  - Plaque stage: proliferation more pronounced and extends deeper into dermis/subcutis with plasma cells
  - Nodular stage: cellular nodules of plump spindle cells with slit-like lumina containing red blood cells (**sieve-like** appearance); **cells are never as atypical as those seen in angiosarcoma**; may have more ectatic vessels in the periphery; plasma cells
- IHC: nuclear positivity for latency-associated nuclear antigen **(LANA-1)** of HHV-8 is very helpful diagnostically (~100% sensitive and specific)
- Treatment: cryotherapy, laser surgery, PDT, topical alitretinoin gel, and RT
  - Rapidly progressive KS w/ visceral involvement is treated w/ systemic chemotherapy

Other borderline vascular neoplasms (rare; not commonly tested)

- Dabska-type hemangioendothelioma, retiform hemangioendothelioma (architecture resembles rete testes), and epithelioid hemangioendothelioma (+vacuoles; t(1;3)(p36;q25) *CAMTA1-WWTR1* rearrangement in 90%)

High-grade malignant vascular neoplasms

Angiosarcoma

- Cutaneous angiosarcoma seen in a variety of clinical settings:
  - **Elderly, sun-damaged sites (head/neck #1)** (Fig. 6.45)

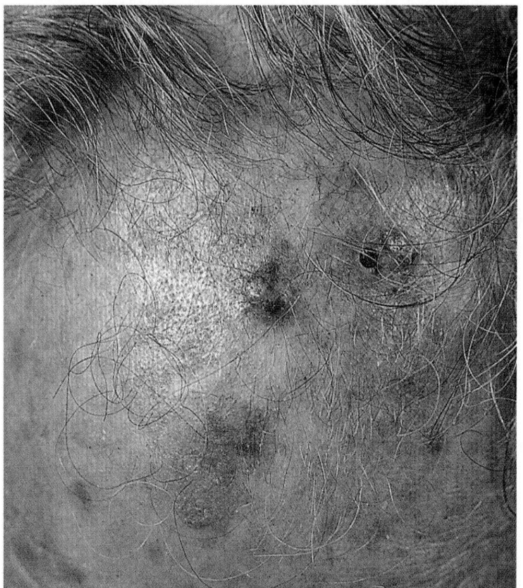

Fig. 6.45 Dark blue-purple plaques and nodules of angiosarcoma on the forehead and scalp of a 70-year-old man. The circular area is the biopsy site. (From Schaffer JV, Bolognia JL. Vascular neoplasms. In: Callen JP, Jorizzo JL, Zone JJ, Piette WW, Rosenbach MA, Vleugels RA, eds. *Dermatological Signs of Systemic Disease*. 5th ed. Philadelphia: Elsevier, 2017:192–204.)

  - **Stewart-Treves syndrome**: chronic lymphedema associated (mostly following breast cancer treatment with axillary LN dissection)
  - **Postradiation**: most commonly on breast; arises after RT for breast cancer
- Histology: large, **hyperchromatic, pleomorphic** tumor cells **dissecting between collagen bundles** → forms **anastomosing vascular networks**; endothelial cells lining the vessels have "**multilayered**" or "**piled-on" architecture** (many malignant endothelial cells crowded on top of each other with some tumor cells floating freely inside the lumen → this is never seen in benign vascular neoplasms!); prominent **hemorrhage** (Fig. 6.46)
  - Poorly differentiated areas may have large epithelioid cells which resemble carcinoma and lack clear vascular differentiation
  - Immunostains: **CD31+, CD34+, ERG+** (most sensitive and specific), and **FLI-1+**

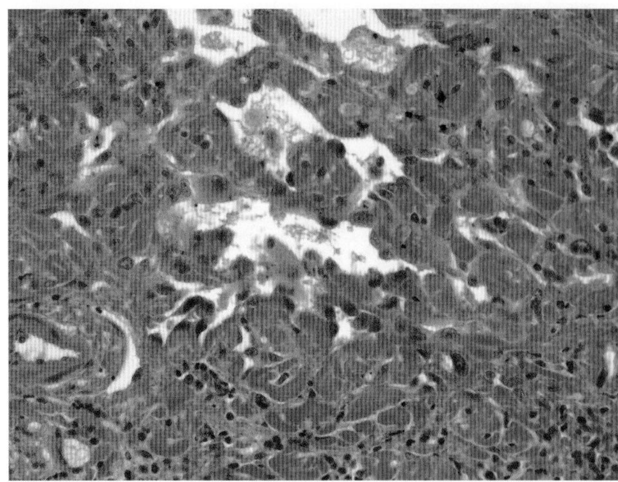

Fig. 6.46 Angiosarcoma histopathology. Anastomosing dilated vessels, lined by crowded endothelial cells, extend between preexisting collagen bundles. (H&E-saffron stain; original magnification: 40x) (From Karkouche R, Kerob D, Battistella M, et al. Angiosarcoma in patients with xeroderma pigmentosum: less aggressive and not so rare? *J Am Acad Dermatol*. 2013;69[3]:e142–e143.)

- Poor prognosis
- Treatment: surgical excision with wide margins, RT
- **Boards fodder**: ***c-MYC*** **amplifications** (detected by immunostaining or FISH) reliably distinguishes between atypical vascular lesions ("AVLs," which are negative) and radiation-induced **angiosarcoma (positive)**

Vascular neoplasm associations

See Fig. 6.47.

6.12 NEOPLASMS OF ADIPOCYTIC LINEAGE

Lipoma

- Benign neoplasm composed of mature adipose tissue; subset with heterogeneous clonal aberrations involving chromosome 12q13-15 region (→ ↑ ***HMGA2*** **gene**) as well as 6p21 and 13q
- Soft subcutaneous nodule; any anatomic site; typically middle-aged adults
- Histology: well-circumscribed sheets of mature adipocytes w/ minimal to no increase in fibrous tissue
- **Conditions a/w multiple lipomas:**
  - Familial multiple lipomatosis: AD; multiple painless lipomas on trunk/extremities
  - Madelung disease: multiple large lipomas around neck/shoulders; generally in middle-aged alcoholic males
  - Gardner syndrome
  - Bannayan-Riley-Ruvalcaba syndrome
  - Proteus syndrome
  - CLOVES syndrome (Congenital Lipomatous asymmetric Overgrowth, Vascular malformations, Epidermal nevi, Skeletal and spinal anomalies)
  - PTEN hamartoma tumor syndrome

Angiolipoma

- Young adults; forearms (#1); often multiple lesions; **painful**
- Small subcutaneous nodules
- Histology: mature fat with areas containing **proliferative capillary lobules** that are characteristically **thrombosed** (→ hence painful) (Fig. 6.48)
- Benign; excision is curative

Spindle cell/pleomorphic lipoma

- Firm, subcutaneous nodule on **posterior neck/shoulder** of adult **males**
- Histology: mature fat, areas of bland spindle cells with a **myxoid background** and characteristic **thick "ropey" collagen** fibers (Fig. 6.49)
  - Pleomorphic lipoma: identical, except it additionally has large **"floret-like" cells** (Fig. 6.50)
- Spindle cells are **CD34+**, w/ **RB1 loss** (differentiates from liposarcoma)
  - Part of the newly-described **"RB1-deleted soft tissue tumor family"** (spindle cell lipoma, pleomorphic lipoma, pleomorphic fibroma, and other less common entities)
- Benign; excision is curative

Hibernoma

- Benign tumors of **brown fat**
- **Young adults**; trunk and neck; slowly growing subcutaneous nodules
- Histology: hibernoma cells (polygonal cells with **eosinophilic, multivacuolated cytoplasm**) admixed with normal appearing adipocytes
- Benign; excision is curative
- **Boards tip**: only the histology is likely to be tested

Well-differentiated liposarcoma (atypical lipomatous tumor)

- Uncommon in the skin; typically involves deep soft tissue or retroperitoneum; large lesions that slowly enlarge
- ***MDM2*** **amplification (12q13-15 ring/giant chr) detected in >99%** → extremely sensitive and specific tool
- Histology: mixture of mature fat and **fibrous bands containing hyperchromatic atypical stromal cells** (most important finding); **lipoblasts** may be seen but are not essential for diagnosis
- Prone to local recurrence; dedifferentiation to a high-grade sarcoma can also occur

Myxoid/round cell liposarcoma

- Rare type of liposarcoma; most testable point is its characteristic histology (**buzzword: "chicken-wire" vessels**)

6.13 DERMOSCOPY

- Synonyms: dermatoscopy, epiluminescence microscopy, skin surface microscopy, and magnified oil immersion diascopy

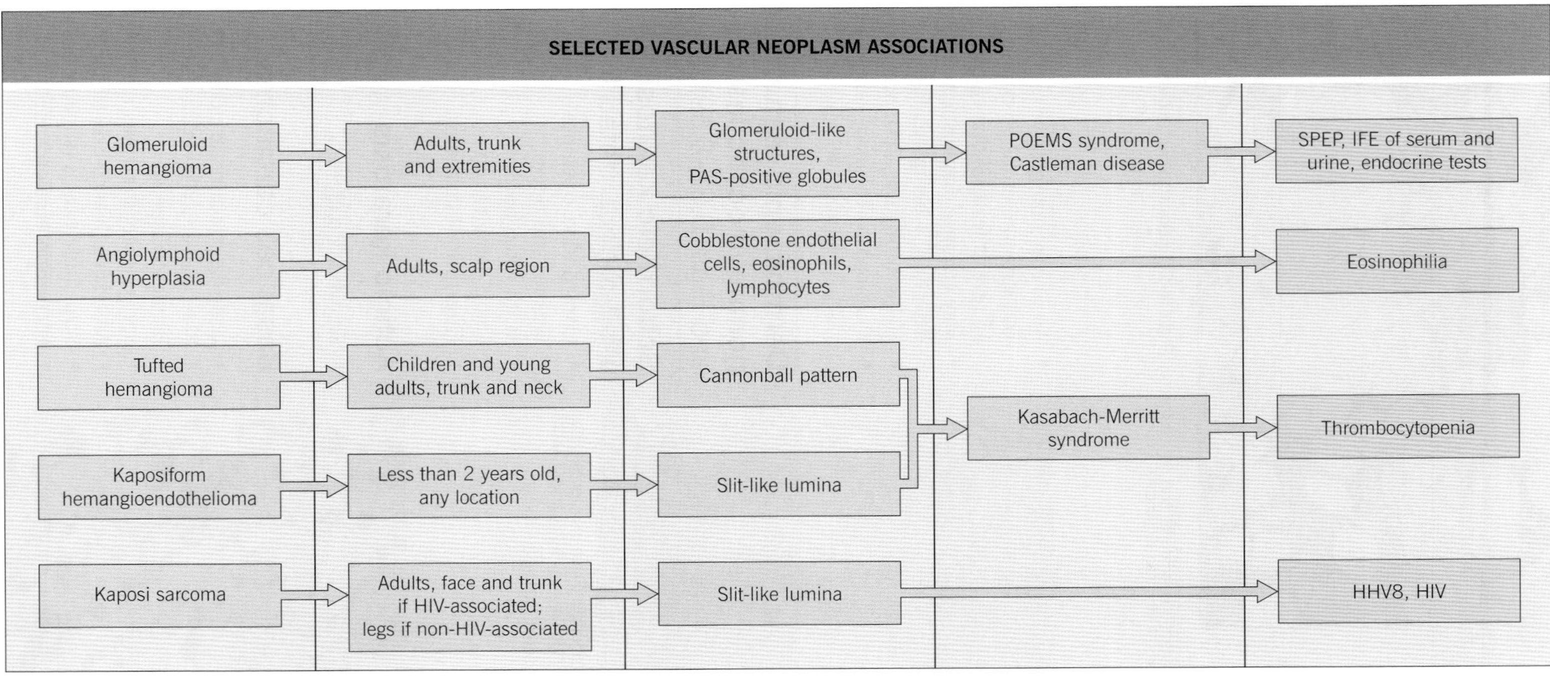

Fig. 6.47 Selected vascular neoplasm associations. *HHV8*, Human herpesvirus 8; *HIV*, human immunodeficiency virus; *IFE*, immunofixation electrophoresis; *PAS*, periodic acid–Schiff stain; *SPEP*, serum protein electrophoresis. (From North PE. Vascular neoplasms and neoplastic-like proliferations. In: Bolognia JL, Schaffer JV, Cerroni L, eds. *Dermatology*. 4th ed. Philadelphia: Elsevier; 2018:2020–2049.)

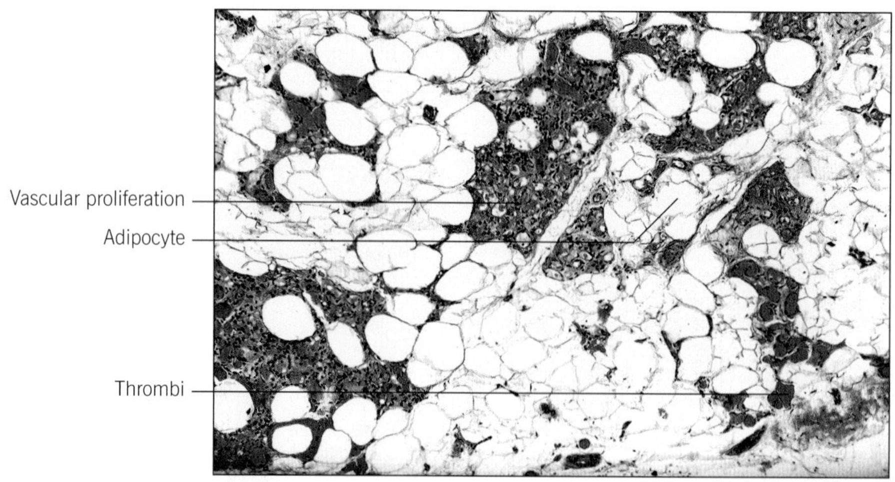

Fig. 6.48 Angiolipoma. (From Rapini RP. Miscellaneous remnants and neoplasms. In: *Practical Dermatopathology*. 2nd ed. Philadelphia: Elsevier; 2012:405–415.)

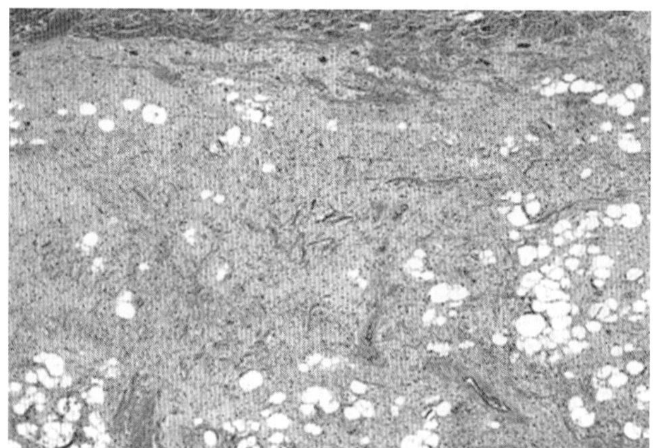

Fig. 6.49 Spindle cell lipoma. Low-power view of an encapsulated tumor composed of spindled cells with admixed foci of adipocytes. (From Brinster NK, Liu V, Diwan H, McKee PH. Spindle cell lipoma. In: *Dermatopathology: A Volume in the High Yield Pathology Series*. Philadelphia: Elsevier; 2011:530–531.)

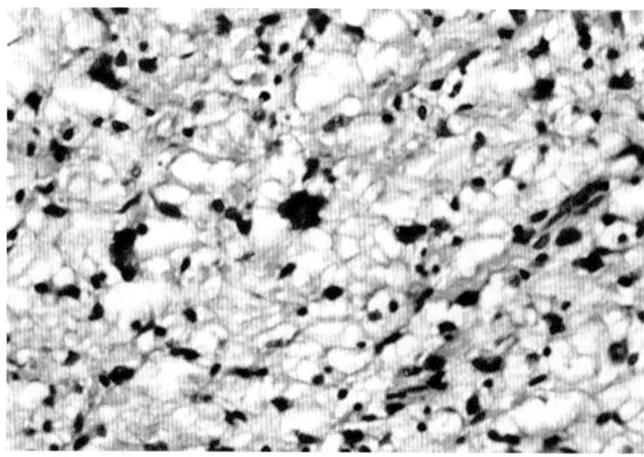

Fig. 6.50 Pleomorphic lipoma. High-power view of floret giant cells. (From Brinster NK, Liu V, Diwan H, McKee PH. Pleomorphic lipoma. In: *Dermatopathology: A Volume in the High Yield Pathology Series*. Philadelphia: Elsevier; 2011:532.)

- An *in vivo*, noninvasive technique to enhance the color and structure of the epidermis, DEJ and superficial dermis → reveals features that cannot be seen with the naked eye
- May enhance diagnostic accuracy (↑ sensitivity skin cancer detection; ↓ benign malignant biopsy ratio)
- Helps distinguish melanocytic from nonmelanocytic lesions
- Dermoscopy colors of keratinizing, melanocytic, and vascular tumors (see Fig. 6.51)

Dermoscopic features of nonmelanocytic lesions (see Table 6.8 and Figs. 6.52–6.59)

Seborrheic keratosis

- Milia-like cysts
- Comedo-like openings
- Fissures and ridges
- Moth-eaten borders
- Sharp demarcation
- Fingerprint-like pattern

Actinic keratosis

- Strawberry pattern

Basal cell carcinoma

- Leaf-like structures at periphery
- Blue-gray ovoid nests and globules
- Pigmented specks
- Spoke-wheel structures/concentric structures
- Arborizing (branch-like) telangiectasias (non-superficial BCCs)
- Serpentine vessels (superficial BCCs)
- Ulceration/erosion

Squamous cell carcinoma *in situ*

- Atypical clusters of glomerulus-like (coiled) vessels
- Dark globules/globules in lines

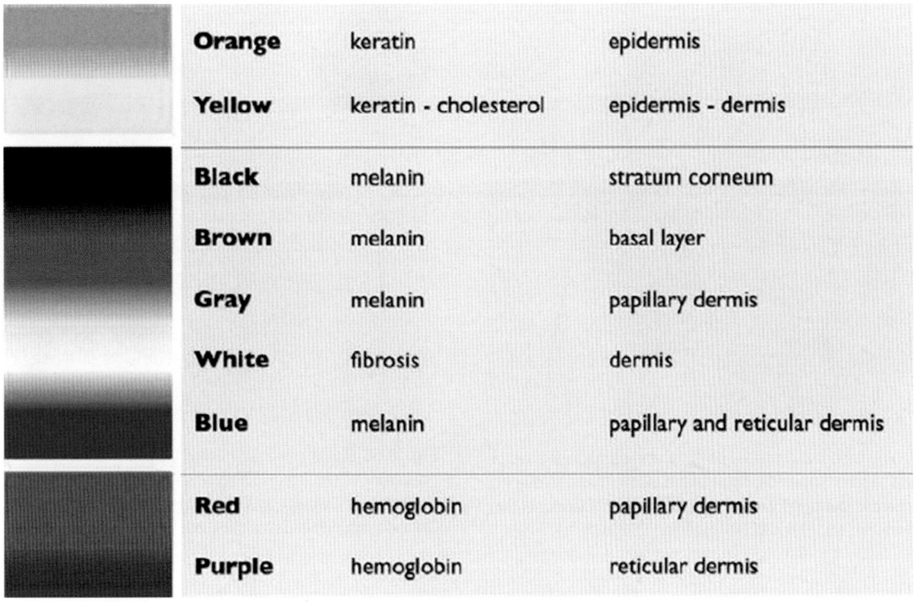

Orange	keratin	epidermis
Yellow	keratin - cholesterol	epidermis - dermis
Black	melanin	stratum corneum
Brown	melanin	basal layer
Gray	melanin	papillary dermis
White	fibrosis	dermis
Blue	melanin	papillary and reticular dermis
Red	hemoglobin	papillary dermis
Purple	hemoglobin	reticular dermis

Fig. 6.51 Dermoscopy colors of keratinizing, melanocytic, and vascular tumors. (From High WA, Tomasini CF, Argenziano G, Zalaudek I. Basic principles of dermatology. In: Bolognia JL, Schaffer JV, Cerroni L, eds. *Dermatology*. 4th ed. Philadelphia: Elsevier; 2018:1–43.)

Table 6.8 Vascular Structures Seen in Various Skin Tumors

Pattern	Definition	Diagnostic Significance
Comma	Coarse vessels that are slightly curved and barely branching	Congenital and dermal nevi (monomorphous); if polymorphous, then consider melanoma
Dotted	Tiny red dots densely aligned next to each other	Melanocytic lesion (often Spitz nevus and melanoma)
Linear-irregular (serpentine)	Linear, irregularly shaped, sized and distributed red structures	Melanoma Superficial basal cell carcinoma
Hairpin	Vascular loops sometimes twisted and bending that can be surrounded by a whitish halo	With white halo: keratinizing proliferation (seborrheic keratosis, squamous cell carcinoma, keratoacanthoma, and viral wart) Without white halo: melanoma
Glomerular	Variation on the theme of dotted vessels; tortuous (coiled) capillaries, often distributed in clusters mimicking the glomerular apparatus of the kidney	Bowen disease
Arborizing	Larger diameter vessels that branch into finer secondary vessels; bright red color; in-focus on dermoscopy as a result of their superficial location	Basal cell carcinoma
Crown	Groups of orderly bending, scarcely branching; vessels located along the border of the lesion **but do not cross center**	Sebaceous hyperplasia
Lacunae	Red, purple, or black clods	Angioma (red, purple) Angiokeratoma (black, blue)
Strawberry	Pink to red "pseudonetwork" around hair follicles of the face, frequently intermingled with fine, linear wavy vessels; often hair follicles are filled with yellowish keratotic plugs	Actinic keratosis
Corkscrew	Linear vessels twisted along a central axis	Thick melanoma or melanoma metastasis
String of pearls	Dotted vessels in serpiginous pattern	Clear cell acanthoma
Milky-red color	Globules and/or larger areas of fuzzy or unfocused milky-red color often corresponding to an elevated part of the lesion	Melanoma
Polymorphous	Any combination of two or more different types of vascular structures. The most frequent is linear-irregular and dotted vessels	Malignant tumor (melanoma, basal cell carcinoma, Merkel cell carcinoma, angiosarcoma, and squamous cell carcinoma) Eccrine poroma

Modified from High WA, Tomasini CF, Argenziano G, Zalaudek I. Basic principles of dermatology. In: Bolognia JL, Schaffer JV, Cerroni L. Dermatology. *4th ed. Philadelphia: Elsevier. 2018:1–43.*

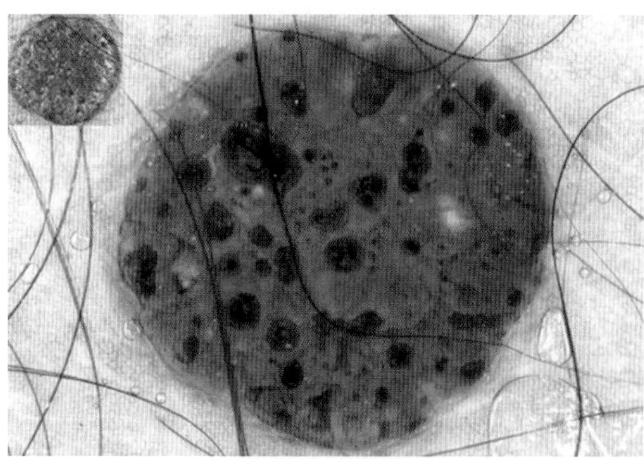

Fig. 6.52 Seborrheic keratosis: milia-like cysts *(white dots)* and comedo-like openings *(black targetoid circles)*. (From Soyer PH, Argenziano G, Hofmann-Wellenhof R, Zalaudek I. Pattern analysis: dermoscopic criteria for specific diagnoses. In: *Dermoscopy: The Essentials*. 3rd ed. Philadelphia: Elsevier; 2020:33–137.)

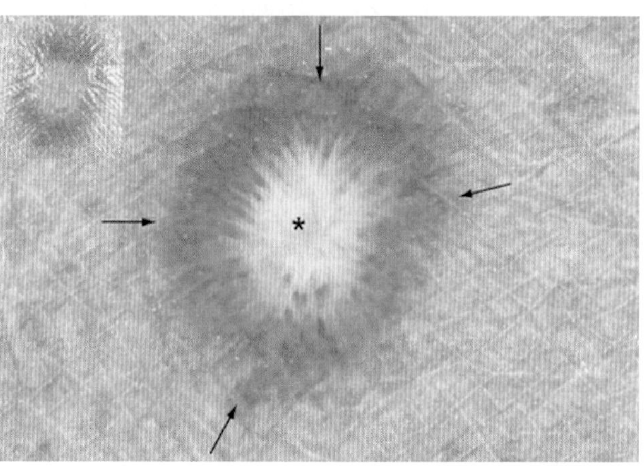

Fig. 6.53 Dermatofibroma: central white patch *(asterisk)* and subtle pigment network *(arrows)*. (From Soyer PH, Argenziano G, Hofmann-Wellenhof R, Zalaudek I. Pattern analysis: dermoscopic criteria for specific diagnoses. In: *Dermoscopy: The Essentials*. 3rd ed. Philadelphia: Elsevier; 2020:33–137.)

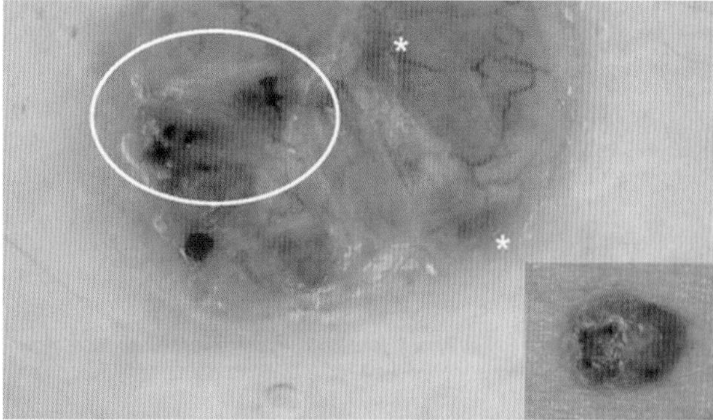

Fig. 6.54 Basal cell carcinoma: arborizing blood vessels, blue-gray blotches *(asterisks)*, and ulceration *(circle)*. (From Soyer PH, Argenziano G, Hofmann-Wellenhof R, Zalaudek I. Pattern analysis: dermoscopic criteria for specific diagnoses. In: *Dermoscopy: The Essentials*. 3rd ed. Philadelphia: Elsevier; 2020: 33–137.)

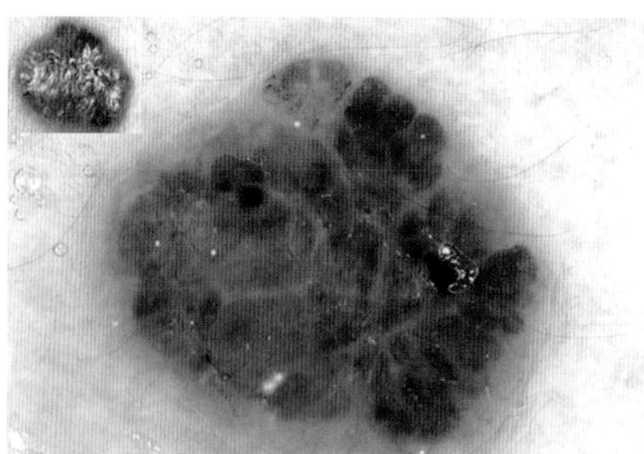

Fig. 6.55 Basal cell carcinoma: Leaf-like areas (3 o'clock to 6 o'clock at the periphery of the lesion). (From Soyer PH, Argenziano G, Hofmann-Wellenhof R, Zalaudek I. Pattern analysis: dermoscopic criteria for specific diagnoses. In: *Dermoscopy: The Essentials*. 3rd ed. Philadelphia: Elsevier; 2020:33–137.)

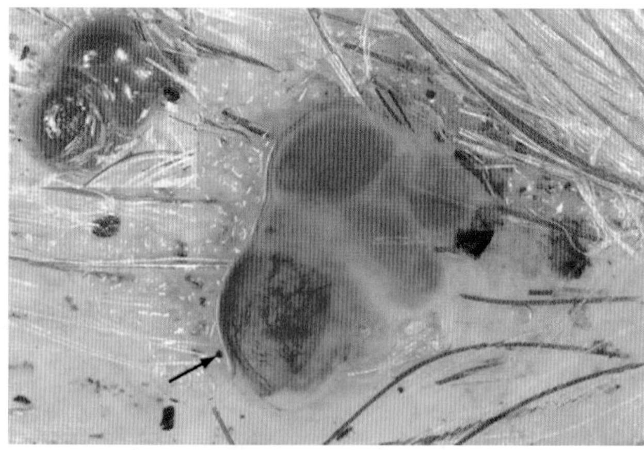

Fig. 6.56 Pyogenic granuloma: homogenous red color with red lacunae. (From Soyer PH, Argenziano G, Hofmann-Wellenhof R, Zalaudek I. Pattern analysis: dermoscopic criteria for specific diagnoses. In: *Dermoscopy: The Essentials*. 3rd ed. Philadelphia: Elsevier; 2020:33–137.)

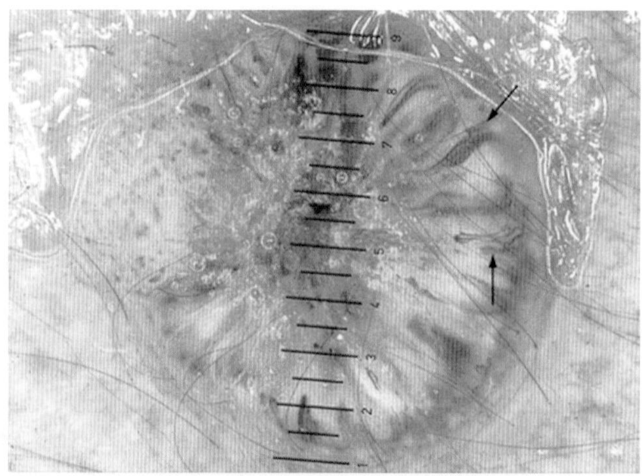

Fig. 6.57 Keratoacanthoma: classic hairpin-shaped vessels *(arrows)*, white background (hyperkeratosis of keratinizing tumor), and central crust. (From Soyer PH, Argenziano G, Hofmann-Wellenhof R, Zalaudek I. Common clinical scenarios: side-by-side comparisons of similar-appearing lesions that are benign or malignant. In: *Dermoscopy: The Essentials*. 3rd ed. Philadelphia: Elsevier; 2020:138–214.)

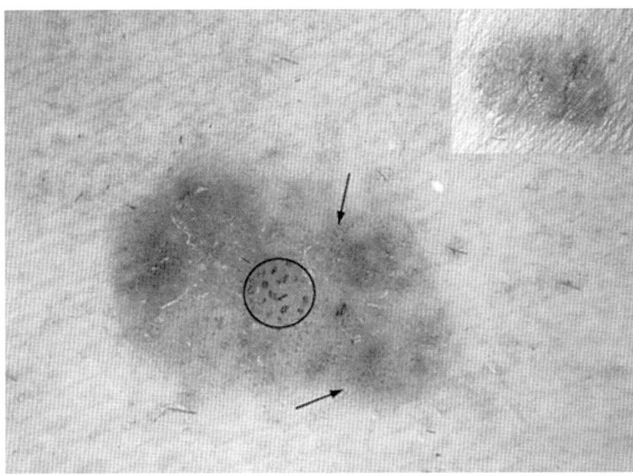

Fig. 6.58 Pigmented Bowen disease: well-circumscribed glomeruloid blood vessels *(circle)* with closely packed tiny brown dots *(arrows)*. (From Soyer PH, Argenziano G, Hofmann-Wellenhof R, Zalaudek I. Common clinical scenarios: side-by-side comparisons of similar-appearing lesions that are benign or malignant. In: *Dermoscopy: The Essentials*. 2nd ed. Philadelphia: Elsevier; 2012.)

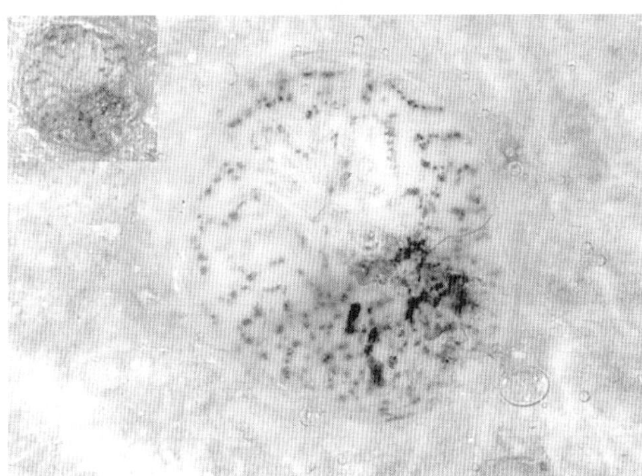

Fig. 6.59 Clear cell acanthoma: this pattern of dotted vessels is rather typical for clear cell acanthoma. (From Soyer PH, Argenziano G, Hofmann-Wellenhof R, Zalaudek I. Common clinical scenarios: side-by-side comparisons of similar-appearing lesions that are benign or malignant. In: *Dermoscopy: The Essentials*. 2nd ed. Philadelphia: Elsevier; 2012.)

Squamous cell carcinoma

- Ulceration may be seen +/– bleeding
- May be pink versus white with possible central crust/scale
- White circles
- Varied-appearing blood vessels (e.g., looped vessels, diffuse)

Dermatofibroma

- Central white patch
- Annular (peripheral) pigment network

Ink spot lentigo

- Dark, bizarre, and sharply demarcated pigment network

Vascular lesions (e.g., cherry angiomas)

- Red or purple lacunae

Hemorrhage

- Peripheral red/purple/blue globules

Porokeratosis

- Cornoid lamella around lesion (seen better w/ marker applied to lesion, then wiped off with ETOH)

Sebaceous hyperplasia

- Yellow lobules in a polygonal pattern around a central follicular opening
- Uniform, regular "crown" telangiectasias

Dermoscopic patterns of melanocytic lesions

- Melanoma findings: atypical pigment network, negative pigment network, blue-whitish veil, atypical vessels, more than four colors, milky red areas, streaks, shiny white streaks (a/w dermal invasion), peripheral streaks, black color, irregular blotches, ulceration w/o pigmented network, granularity/peppering (a/w *BRAF*, *NRAS* mutations), dotted vessels (a/w BRAF wild-type melanomas), dark homogeneous streaks (a/w *KIT* mutations)

See Tables 6.8–6.10 and Figs. 6.60–6.65.

Table 6.9 Melanocytic Global Patterns

Global Pattern/Local Variant	Morphology	Histology	Diagnosis
Reticular	Honeycomb-like network of brownish lines	Elongated, pigmented rete ridges	Melanocytic lesion
Atypical pigment network	Black, brown, and gray reticular pattern with thickened lines and irregular meshing	Irregular and broadened rete ridges	Melanoma
Typical pigment network	Thin, regularly meshed, brown reticular pattern with evenly spaced meshing	Regular and elongated rete ridges	Benign nevus

Continued

Table 6.9 Melanocytic Global Patterns—cont'd

Global Pattern/Local Variant	Morphology	Histology	Diagnosis
Negative pigment network	Thick, interconnected reticular hypopigmented lines around brown curved globules/clods	Possibly hypopigmented elongated rete ridges around melanocyte nests in the dermal papillae	Melanoma Spitz nevus
Globular	Variably sized, round to oval structures	Aggregates of melanin-containing structures located throughout the epidermis and upper dermis	Melanocytic lesion
Irregular dots and globules	Irregular distribution of variably sized round to oval structures	Irregularly distributed melanin-containing structures in the epidermis and upper dermis	Melanoma
Regular dots and globes	Regular distribution of variably sized round to oval structures	Regularly distributed melanin-containing structures in the epidermis and upper dermis	Benign nevus
Homogenous	Diffuse, uniform, and structureless color in the absence of other local criteria	Varies depending on colors	Melanocytic lesion
Irregular blotches	Diffuse hyperpigmentation that varies in size and shape with irregular borders; obscures other dermoscopic features	Histopathologic structures with pronounced melanin throughout the epidermis and upper dermis	Melanoma
Regular blotches	Diffuse hyperpigmentation with uniform shape and color symmetrically located in the lesion	Histopathologic structures with pronounced melanin throughout the epidermis and upper dermis	Benign nevus
Blue-whitish veil	Irregular, confluent, and gray-blue to white-blue pigmentation	Acanthosis and hypergranulosis above pigmentation in dermis	Melanoma
Homogenous blue pattern	Uniform blue color	Dermal melanocytes (high density)	Blue nevus Melanoma
Regression	Bone white scar-like depigmentation with or without gray pepper-like granules	Thickened papillary dermis with fibrosis and variable amounts of melanophages	Melanoma
Starburst	Pigmented streaks, and/or dots and globules in a radial arrangement at the periphery of a melanocytic lesion	Fascicles of pigmented cells running parallel to the epidermis at the dermoepidermal junction	Reed nevus/Spitz nevus
Regular streaks	Pigmented linear structures of variable thickness found regularly dispersed around the periphery of the entire circumference of a lesion (radial streaming)	Fascicles of pigmented cells regularly dispersed running parallel to the epidermis	Reed nevus/Spitz nevus
Irregular streaks	Pigmented linear structures found irregularly dispersed around the periphery of a portion of a lesion (pseudopods)	Fascicles of pigmented cells irregularly dispersed running parallel to the epidermis	Melanoma

Table 6.10 Site-Specific Melanoma-Specific Criteria

Site	Criteria	Morphology
Face, nose, ears	Annular-granular structures	Brown or blue-gray dots surrounding follicular ostia This criterion and the three listed below are seen in lentigo maligna
	Asymmetrically pigmented follicles	Gray circles/rings of pigment asymmetrically distributed around follicular ostia ("circle within a circle" is a variant)
	Rhomboidal structures/angulated lines	Thickened areas of pigmentation surrounding the follicular ostia with a rhomboidal appearance
	Gray pseudonetwork	Confluent annular-granular structures forming gray pigment surrounding follicular ostia
Acral sites	Parallel ridge	Parallel pigmented lines thicker than nonpigmented ones with white dots running along like a string of pearls Of note, parallel furrow pattern is the opposite and is benign
Nails	Irregular pigmented bands	Thick, possibly multicolored, irregularly spaced lines stemming from the proximal nail fold
Mucosal sites	Homogeneous pattern w/ various colors (blue, gray, white)	Diffuse discoloration w/ no clear structures

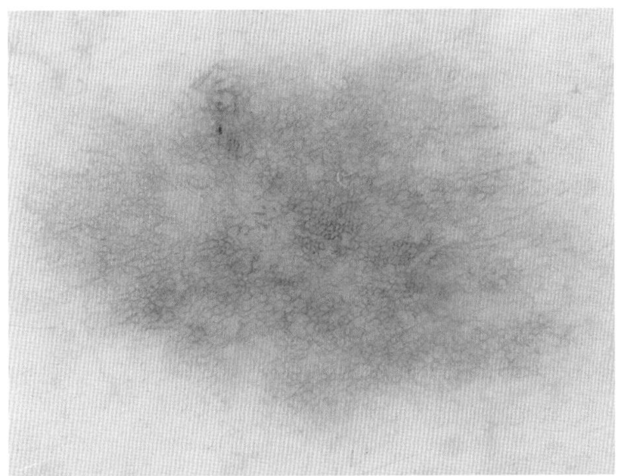

Fig. 6.60 Benign nevus with reticular pattern in dermoscopy. (From Marghoob AA, Usatine RP. Dermoscopy. In: Usatine RP, Pfenninger JL, Stulberg DL, Small R, eds. *Dermatologic and Cosmetic Procedures in Office Practice*. Philadelphia: Elsevier; 2012:384–403. Copyright Ashfaq A. Marghoob, MD.)

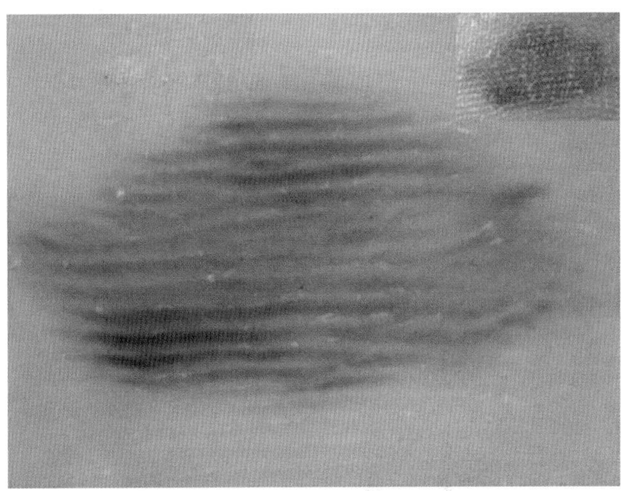

Fig. 6.63 Acral melanoma: parallel ridge pattern.

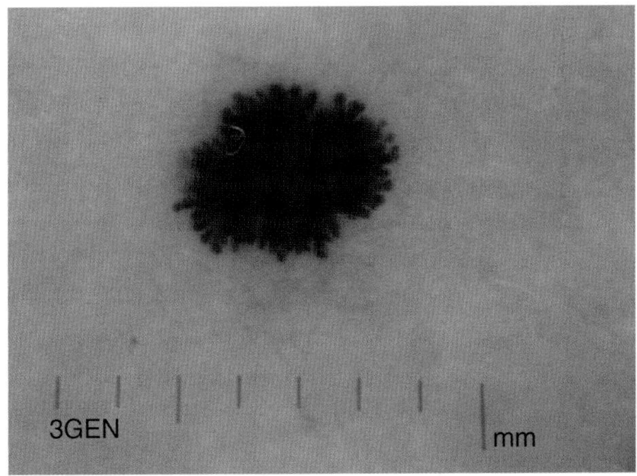

Fig. 6.61 Dermatoscopic patterns of Reed nevus. Starburst pattern in which black, homogeneous, central pigmentation can be seen with regular radial projections at the periphery. (From Sainz-Gaspar L, Sánchez-Bernal J, Noguera-Morel L, Hernández-Martín A, Colmenero I, Torrelo A. Spitz nevus and other spitzoid tumors in children—part 1: clinical, histopathologic, and immunohistochemical features. *Actas Dermosifiliogr*. 2020;111[1]:7–19.)

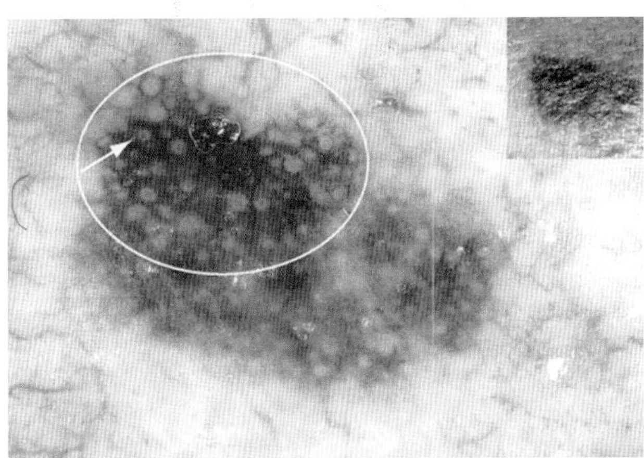

Fig. 6.64 Melanoma: annular-granular structures make up rhomboidal structures *(arrow)*. Confluent rhomboidal structures make up the gray pseudonetwork *(circle)*.

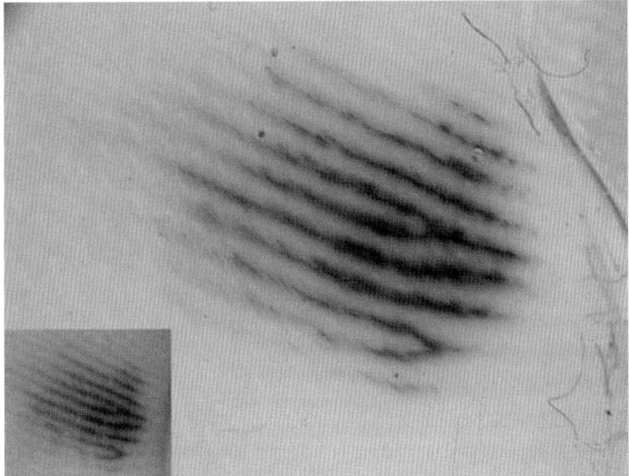

Fig. 6.62 Acral nevus: parallel furrow pattern.

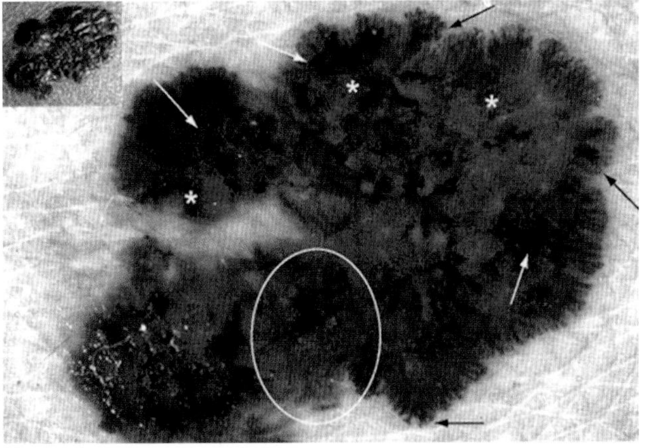

Fig. 6.65 Melanoma: atypical pigment network *(circle)*, irregular dots and globules *(asterisks)*, irregular streaks *(black arrows)*, irregular blotches *(white arrows)*, with blue-white structures centrally.

7 Dermatopathology

Julia S. Lehman and Roberto A. Novoa

CONTENTS LIST

7.1 ESSENTIAL CONCEPTS IN DERMATOPATHOLOGY
7.2 HIGH-YIELD DERMATOPATHOLOGY DIAGNOSES AT A GLANCE
7.3 HIGH-YIELD DERMATOPATHOLOGY DIFFERENTIAL DIAGNOSES

Acknowledgments: We wish to thank Dr. John Griffin and Dr. Rahul Chavan, the authors of the previous edition's Dermatopathology chapter.

7.1 ESSENTIAL CONCEPTS IN DERMATOPATHOLOGY

The microscopic appearance of normal skin varies based on anatomic location, and it is important to understand normal histology (Table 7.1) so as to then recognize pathologic features, particularly those that are so subtle that they comprise the "normal skin" differential diagnosis (see Table 7.12 in Section 7.3).

Various histopathologic changes, including characteristic bodies or cells, may be suggestive of particular diagnoses (Table 7.2). The use of special stains can help identify subtle or ambiguous findings (Tables 7.3–7.5). It is important to differentiate pathologic changes from artifacts and/or the effects of exogenous material (Table 7.6). Certain categories of neoplasms, including spindle cell neoplasms, those showing pagetoid scatter, or epithelial carcinomas, can be challenging to diagnose based on histopathologic changes alone. Immunostaining may be required for accurate diagnosis (Tables 7.8–7.9).

Text continued on p. 400

Table 7.1 Features of Normal Skin

Site	Histopathologic Clues	Comments
Anogenital skin	**Undulating epidermis (papillomatous)**, abundant **smooth muscle** in dermis, and highly vascular	–
Areola	**Smooth muscle** (abundant); may also see lactiferous/mammary **ducts** (modified apocrine glands)	Presence of smooth muscle differentiates from axilla Presence of lactiferous ducts differentiates from genital
Axilla	**Apocrine glands** (abundant)	–
Back	Thick dermis (extends deeper than other sites); broad fascicles of collagen	Most commonly asked to distinguish from scleredema, which has abundant mucin between widely-spaced collagen fibers
Ear	Thin epidermis, **cartilage**, and numerous **vellus hairs** (small caliber hairs with bulbs situated in dermis)	Accessory tragus: domed papule w/ identical histopathologic features
Eyelid	Dermis contains only loosely arranged collagen, lacks subcutaneous fat, and has **superficially located skeletal muscle**	Eyelid skin + foamy histiocytes in dermis = **xanthelasma**
Lip (dry vermillion)	Keratinizing epidermis (has stratum corneum) with granular layer; **skeletal muscle** (main clue)	
Lip (wet mucosa)	**Pale keratinocytes** (glycogen rich), lacks granular layer, **non-keratinizing** (lacks stratum corneum), minor salivary glands (basaloid), and lacks hair follicles (glabrous)	Vulvar mucosa appears similar (but lacks salivary glands and skeletal muscle) Parakeratotic scale on lip is clue to abnormal mucosa (oral LP > other inflammatory dz)
Nose	Abundant **sebaceous glands** Frequent intrafollicular *Demodex*	–
Palms/soles	Massively thickened stratum corneum, **compact orthohyperkeratosis**; **Meissner's corpuscles** in dermal papillae; lacks hair follicles (glabrous)	–
Scalp	**Numerous terminal hairs** w/ deeply situated bulbs (subcutaneous fat)	–

Table 7.2 High-Yield Dermpath Bodies/Cells

Body	Description	Associated Disease(s)/Comments
Antoni A	Cellular area of schwannomas; has abundant **Verocay bodies**	Schwannoma (neurilemmoma)
Antoni B	Hypocellular area of schwannomas; has loose myxoid stroma and low cellularity	Schwannoma (neurilemmoma)
Asteroid bodies	Star-shaped, eosinophilic intracytoplasmic inclusions	**Sarcoid** and other granulomatous disorders
Balloon cells	Clear-appearing cells with vesicular cytoplasm, and small hyperchromatic nucleus w/ pseudonuclear inclusions	Balloon cell nevus, balloon cell melanoma (has classic features of melanoma in junctional component)
Banana bodies	Crescentic golden **yellow-brown (ochre) fibers**, in dermis	Endogenous ochronosis (**alkaptonuria**) > exogenous ochronosis (from **hydroquinone**) Endogenous ochronosis is as a result of deposition of **homogentisic acid** on collagen and cartilage
Beanbag cells	Histiocytes that have engulfed WBCs, RBCs, and nuclear debris (**cytophagocytosis**)	Subcutaneous panniculitis-like T-cell lymphoma, lupus profundus, and **hemophagocytic lymphohistiocytosis** (historical term: cytophagic histiocytic panniculitis)
Birbeck granules	Only seen on electron microscopy; classically appear as **tennis racket** structures or rods	Pathognomonic of Langerhans cells and **LCH cells** **Langerin (CD207)** is the major component of Birbeck granules → Langerin immunostain is the **most specific** stain (>CD1a) for Langerhans cells and LCH cells Histiocytes in Langerhans cell histiocytosis can carry BRAF V600E mutation, a potential therapeutic target
Caterpillar bodies	Eosinophilic material comprised of **BMZ material (PAS+ and collagen IV+)**, found in **roof of blisters** and basal layer of epidermis	**PCT**, EPP Caterpillar bodies are composed of basement membrane proteins including collagen IV; same material as Kamino bodies (Spitz nevi)
Cholesterol clefts	Elongated, needle-shaped clear spaces once occupied by cholesterol (cholesterol, itself, is removed during processing)	Within adipocytes (radiating pattern): **SQ fat necrosis of newborn, sclerema neonatorum, and poststeroid panniculitis** Within dermis: **NXG** (>NL), plane xanthoma, and eruptive xanthoma Within arterioles: **cholesterol embolism** (fibrin thrombus surrounds cholesterol) *Don't confuse cholesterol clefts with keratin granuloma
Cigar bodies	Oval yeast (**PAS+** and GMS+)	Sporotrichosis May also see "**sporothrix asteroid" bodies** = yeast with radiating pink hyaline material (immune complexes on yeast surface)
Civatte/colloid/cytoid bodies	Apoptotic keratinocytes (eosinophilic)	**Lichen planus** classically, but seen in all interface dermatitides
Clover leaf (flower) cells	Atypical T-lymphocytes with a cloverleaf or flower-like nucleus; seen mainly in peripheral blood smear (>tissue)	HTLV-induced adult T-cell leukemia/lymphoma (pathognomonic)
Comma-shaped bodies	Comma-shaped electron dense membranes seen within histiocytes (electron microscopy)	Classically associated with **benign cephalic histiocytosis** (but also seen in juvenile xanthogranuloma)
Corps ronds/grains	Two special types of dyskeratotic keratinocytes: Ronds: single or grouped, round keratinocytes with a **perinuclear halo**, brightly eosinophilic cytoplasm, and pyknotic nucleus; found in **spinous layer** >stratum corneum Grains: smaller, flattened basophilic keratinocytes resembling parakeratosis; found in **granular layer/stratum corneum**	**Darier's disease, warty dyskeratoma**, Grover's, Hailey-Hailey (less prominent), acantholytic dyskeratotic acanthoma (trunk is #1 site), papular acantholytic dyskeratosis (multiple lesions on vulva, mistaken for condyloma), and PRP (focally)
Cowdry A body	Intranuclear inclusions (eosinophilic globules) surrounded by halo	**HSV, VZV**, and CMV ("owl's eye" endothelial cells)
Cowdry B body	Intranuclear inclusions	**Poliovirus** > adenovirus
Donovan bodies	Intracytoplasmic **"safety pin"-shaped bacteria** in macrophages	Granuloma inguinale (Klebsiella granulomatis)
Dutcher body	Pseudo-intranuclear pink collection of immunoglobulin within plasma cells	Classically seen in **malignant B-cell processes**: **B-cell lymphoma**, **multiple myeloma**, and Waldenström macroglobulinemia Mnemonic: Dutcher = Dead (a/w malignant process), versus Russell bodies (a/w benign conditions; "happy, pregnant plasma cells")
Flame figures	**Major basic protein** from eosinophils deposited on collagen	**Wells syndrome**, dermal hypersensitivity reaction (exaggerated arthropod assault, drug), and bullous pemphigoid (rarely) Neutrophilic processes (esp. PNGD, RA) can have **bluish-purple "flame figure-like**" structures as a result of **neutrophilic debris** deposited on collagen
Floret cells	Multinucleated giant cells with peripherally located overlapping nuclei (**resembles flower**) and "smudgy"/indistinct chromatin	**Pleomorphic lipoma**
Gamma-Favre body	Intracytoplasmic basophilic inclusions within endothelial cells	Lymphogranuloma venereum (*Chlamydia trachomatis*)
Gaucher cells	Glucocerebroside-laden histiocytes ("crinkled tissue paper-like histiocytes")	Gaucher disease

Table 7.2 High-Yield Dermpath Bodies/Cells—cont'd

Body	Description	Associated Disease(s)/Comments
Ghost/shadow cells (pilomatricoma)	**Anucleate**, eosinophilic, keratinized cells with a ghost-like outline where the nucleus previously resided; often surrounded by transitional cells and basaloid cells (derived from matrix cells of hair follicle)	**Pilomatricoma** Clinically have a "tent sign" (seen better when skin over tumor is stretched) Usually sporadic but may be associated with certain forms of myotonic dystrophy, Gardner syndrome, Rubinstein-Taybi syndrome (beta-catenin mutation)
Ghost cells (pancreatic panniculitis)	Blue-purple calcium outlines remnants of necrotic lipocytes	**Pancreatic panniculitis**
Globi	Amphophilic, encapsulated collections of mycobacteria	**Lepromatous leprosy** Other leprosy buzzword: **Virchow cells** (pale, foamy histiocytes parasitized by *Mycobacterium leprae*)
Glomus bodies	Specialized A-V shunts that bypass capillaries; mostly found on **fingers and toes**; responsible for **temperature regulation**	Glomus tumor: solid nodular proliferation of glomus cells; favors fingers and toes Glomangiomas: ectatic vascular malformation with fewer glomus cells than glomus tumor; widespread anatomic distribution
Guarnieri body	Eosinophilic cytoplasmic inclusions	Smallpox
Hallmark (horseshoe) cells	Markedly atypical, enlarged T lymphocytes with a horseshoe-shaped nucleus	Anaplastic large cell lymphoma **(ALCL)** and LyP (type C)
Henderson-Paterson bodies	Large, pink-to-purple intracytoplasmic inclusions (Fig. 7.1)	**Molluscum contagiosum**
Kamino bodies	Collections of amorphous eosinophilic/hyaline **BMZ material (PAS+** and **collagen IV+)** in tips of dermal papillae and within epidermis	Spitz nevi Large aggregates of Kamino bodies are rarely (if ever) seen in melanoma!
Koilocytes	Keratinocytes with viral cytopathic changes (**perinuclear halo, shrunken hyperchromatic nucleus**, and irregular nuclear contours)	**HPV** Unlike pap smears, true koilocytes are not always seen in HPV skin infections → may just see **vacuolated keratinocytes** and coarse keratohyalin granules
Langhans giant cells	Histiocytic giant cells with a peripheral ("**horse-shoe**") arrangement of nuclei	Classically associated with **tuberculosis**, but often seen in sarcoidosis and other granulomatous diseases Not to be confused with LangERhans cells!
Mariner's wheel	Central round yeast (60 μm) w/ multiple radiating buds	**Paracoccidioidomycosis** ("South American Blastomycosis", *Paracoccidioides brasiliensis*)
Max-Joseph (Caspary-Joseph) spaces	**Focal clefts at DEJ** formed by extreme damage to basal layer from interface dermatitis	**Lichen planus** Exaggerated Max-Joseph spaces → bullous LP
Medlar bodies	Thick-walled clusters of **brown round yeast** forms ("**copper pennies**")	**Chromomycosis** DDx: **pigmented hyphae** are seen in phaeohyphomycosis
Michaelis-Gutmann body	**Round, calcified**, and laminated bacterial remnants	**Malakoplakia**; bodies can be highlighted with calcium stain (von Kossa)
Miescher's radial granuloma	Small granuloma composed of **radially arrayed histiocytes around a central cleft**; located in **fat septae**	**Erythema nodosum** Do not confuse with "Miescher's granuloma" (aka actinic granuloma of O'Brien, or annular elastolytic giant cell granuloma)
Mikulicz cells	Foamy histiocytes containing gram-negative rods ***(Klebsiella rhinoscleromatis)***	**Rhinoscleroma** Other rhinoscleroma buzzword: Russell bodies
Mulberry cells	Large **pink/red-colored** fat cells with a **central nucleus** (vs. peripheral in normal adipocytes) and a multivacuolated, **granular, eosinophilic** cytoplasm	**Hibernoma** Tumor of **brown fat**; most common in adults on neck and upper back
Morula	Organism (2–11 μm) with numerous internal septations → appears similar to morula stage of embryogenesis or like a "**soccer ball**"; **PAS+** and **GMS+**	**Protothecosis** (an achloric alga)
Negri body	Neuronal inclusion	Rabies
Odland (lamellar) bodies	**Oval granules w/ lamellar organization** seen w/ **electron microscopy**; contain phospholipids, glycoproteins and acid phosphatases; found in upper spinous and granular layer; major role in **barrier function** and keratinocyte cohesion	**Harlequin fetus** (absent), **Flegel** disease (decreased or absent)
Papillary mesenchymal bodies	**Condensed clusters of fibroblasts** adjacent to basaloid epithelial follicular buds; recapitulates appearance of normal hair bulb (dermal papilla-hair matrix)	Present in **trichoepithelioma, DTE**, and trichoblastoma Absent in BCC
Psammoma body	Concentric, calcified laminated spheres	**Meningioma**, mesothelioma, ovarian cancer, **papillary thyroid cancer**, and ovarian cancer
Pustulo-ovoid bodies of Milian	**Round eosinophilic cytoplasmic inclusions** comprised of **lysosomes**/Golgi material **(PAS+** and **diastase-resistant)**	**Granular cell tumor**
Reed-Sternberg cells	Large atypical lymphoid cells derived from germinal center **B cells**; characteristic **bilobed nucleus w/ prominent central nucleolus** within each nucleus → **"owl's eye"** appearance; **CD30+, CD15+**, and PAX-5+ (B-cell origin)	Hodgkin lymphoma
Reed-Sternberg-like cells	Appear similar to Reed-Sternberg cells on H&E but are **T cells**; CD3+, CD4+, **CD30+**, and **CD15–**	**LyP,** ALCL

Continued

Table 7.2 High-Yield Dermpath Bodies/Cells—cont'd

Body	Description	Associated Disease(s)/Comments
Rocha-Lima bodies	Intracytoplasmic inclusions within endothelial cells	Oroya fever, verruga peruana
Russell bodies	Intracytoplasmic immunoglobulin collections (eosinophilic) stuffing the cytoplasm of plasma cells	**Rhinoscleroma, granuloma inguinale** Russell bodies are classically a/w benign diagnoses ("happy, pregnant plasma cells") versus malignant associations for Dutcher bodies
Schaumann bodies	Calcified laminated collections	Sarcoid
Sézary cells	Atypical lymphocytes with **cerebriform** nuclei (seen in peripheral blood smear > tissue)	**Sézary syndrome**, MF
Signet ring cells	Cell with eccentric nucleus and large pool of intracytoplasmic mucin (pushes nucleus to periphery)	Any mucin-producing adenocarcinoma (usually metastatic, if seen in skin)
Sunburn cells	**Dyskeratotic keratinocytes** scattered in upper and mid-epidermis (> basal layer)	Sunburns and **phototoxic drug** eruptions
Touton giant cells	Large, multinucleated histiocytes with **wreath-like** arrangement of nuclei and peripheral cytoplasmic lipid	**JXG** (and other xanthomas), **dermatofibroma** (often contain hemosiderin) Boards pearl: Touton giant cells are ubiquitous in DF but not seen in DFSP!
Verocay bodies	Two stacked rows of elongated **palisading nuclei surrounding amorphous pink material** (cytoplasmic processes of Schwann cells); seen in hypercellular (Antoni A) areas of schwannomas	Schwannoma (neurilemmoma)
Virchow cells	Foamy histiocytes parasitized by acid-fast bacilli	**Lepromatous leprosy** Other boards buzzword: globi (encapsulated amphophilic masses of *M. leprae*)
von Hansemann cells	Large histiocytes with granular eosinophilic cytoplasm; the cytoplasm of these cells contains Michaelis-Gutmann bodies	**Malakoplakia**
Weibel-Palade bodies	Cytoplasmic organelle of endothelial cells seen only with EM; contains **vWF** and P-selectin	von Willebrand disease is caused by qualitative or quantitative vWF deficiency

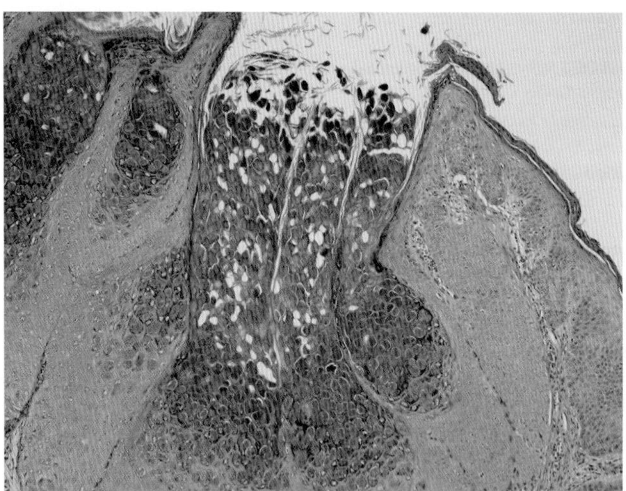

Fig. 7.1 Molluscum contagiosum. Viral inclusions (Henderson-Paterson bodies) are prominent.

Table 7.3 Most Commonly Used Special Stains

Stain	Target	Color(s)	Comments
Collagen/elastic fibers			
Verhoeff-van Gieson (VVG)	Elastic fibers Collagen Rest of connective tissue	Black Red Yellow	Most commonly used collagen/elastin stain Distinguishes between various perforating diseases, can show areas of loss (morphea) or clumping (PXE)
Smooth muscle			
Masson trichrome	Collagen fibers Smooth muscle	Blue or green Red	Stains the **inclusions (red) in infantile digital fibromatosis**; shows dense collagen in collagenoma
Movat's pentachrome	Elastic fibers Collagen Smooth muscle, fibrin	Black Yellow Red	Stains the inclusions (red) in infantile digital fibromatosis
Phosphotungstic acid hematoxylin	Collagen Smooth muscle, fibrin	Red Blue	Stains the inclusions (blue) in infantile digital fibromatosis
Lipids (all stains must be performed on frozen tissue only! → not commonly used); may be helpful in confirming that clear cell changes attributable to sebum in sebaceous neoplasms			
Oil-red-O	Lipids	Red	
Sudan black B	Lipids	Black	–
Scarlet red	Lipids	Red-brown	–
Iron/hemosiderin			
Perls/Prussian blue	Hemosiderin/iron	Blue	Most commonly used in conjunction with Fontana-Masson stain to distinguish between melanin (black w/ Fontana-Masson) and hemosiderin pigment Does not stain iron in intact RBCs → does not work well for talon noir Hemosiderin also a common finding in stasis dermatitis, pigmented purpuric dermatosis, and Kaposi sarcoma
Calcium			
von Kossa	Calcium (salts)	Brown-black	Most commonly used "calcium stain," but actually stains the anions rather than calcium itself → less calcium-specific than Alizarin red
Alizarin red	Calcium	Red-orange	More specific for calcium than von Kossa
Mucin			
Alcian blue pH 0.5	Sulfated acid MPS (heparin, chondroitin, and dermatan sulfates)	Blue	In normal skin, most mucin is sulfated acid MPS Hyaluronic acid (nonsulfated acid MPS) does not stain with Alcian blue at pH 0.5
Alcian blue pH 2.5	Nonsulfated acid MPS (hyaluronic acid)	Blue	In diseases w/ ↑ mucin (lupus, GA, and follicular mucinosis), most mucin is hyaluronic acid Mnemonic: **"HIGH-luronic acid stains with Alcian blue at HIGH pH (pH 2.5) only!"** Sulfated acid MPS stain with Alcian blue at both pH 2.5 and pH 0.5
Colloidal iron	Acid MPS (sulfated and nonsulfated)	Blue	Hyaluronidase may be added to distinguish between hyaluronic acid and other mucin types
Mucicarmine	Epithelial mucin (primarily sialomucin)	Pink-red	Used primarily for adenocarcinoma, **Paget disease**, and ***Cryptococcus*** (capsule) Not a good stain for dermal mucins
Periodic acid–Schiff (PAS)	Neutral MPS (basement membrane), fungi, and glycogen	Pink	Highlights BMZ material, fungal organisms, and glycogen Does not stain acid MPS (hyaluronic acid and other mucins)
Toluidine blue	Acid MPS	Red-purple ("metachromatic staining": stains tissue a different color than blue color of stain)	Rarely used as a mucin stain → more commonly used as mast cell stain

Continued

Table 7.3 Most Commonly Used Special Stains—cont'd

Stain	Target	Color(s)	Comments
Amyloid (Note: Mass spectrometry can be used to subtype amyloid [AA vs. AL])			
Congo red	Amyloid	Pink-red; **apple green birefringence** when polarized	Most commonly used amyloid stain In real world, not always reliable for macular/lichen amyloid
Thioflavin T	Amyloid (fluorescence microscopy)	Yellow-green	Requires fluorescence microscopy
Cresyl violet	Amyloid	Red	Of note, cotton dyes (e.g., Pagoda red or Dylon) also stain amyloid
Melanin			
Fontana-Masson (silver stain)	Melanin	Black	Most commonly used in conjunction with an iron stain (e.g., Perls) to distinguish melanin from hemosiderin. Vitiligo has complete loss of epidermal staining
Silver nitrate	Melanin	Black	May represent artifact from prior treatment with silver nitrate sticks
Mast cell stains (all except Leder stain and c-KIT are unreliable in degranulated skin → use lidocaine without epinephrine to avoid mast cell degranulation and improve staining)			
Leder (chloroacetate esterase)	Mast cell cytoplasm and granules	Red	Unlike most other mast cell stains, it is **NOT dependent on presence of mast cell granules** → effective even in degranulated skin Only Leder and c-KIT (CD117) are reliable in degranulated skin
cKit (CD117) (immunostain, but is discussed here for convenience)	Mast cell cytoplasm	Brown or red (color depends on type of peroxidase used)	**NOT dependent on presence of mast cell granules** Also stains melanocytes and myeloid cells
Tryptase (immunostain, but is discussed here for convenience)	Mast cell granules	Brown or red (color depends on type of peroxidase used)	Dependent on presence of mast cell granules
Giemsa	Mast cell granules	Purple-blue (metachromatic)	Dependent on presence of mast cell granules
Toluidine blue	Mast cell granules	Purple (metachromatic)	Dependent on presence of mast cell granules
Microbial stains			
Periodic acid–Schiff (PAS)	Fungi, neutral MPS (basement membrane), and **glycogen**	Pink	Positive in **clear cell acanthoma** and **trichilemmoma**, as a result of ↑ glycogen → becomes negative if add diastase (PAS-D) Does not stain acid MPS (hyaluronic acid and other mucins)
Periodic acid–Schiff w/ diastase (PAS-D)	Fungi, neutral MPS (basement membrane)	Pink	Helpful for demonstrating BMZ thickening (lupus, DM) and thickened vessel walls of porphyria
Gomori methenamine silver (GMS; a silver stain)	Fungi	Black (stains fungal wall)	Green background (counterstain)
Gram stain (Brown-Hopps and Brown-Brenn)	Gram-positive bacteria Gram-negative bacteria	Blue Red	Gram-negative bacteria not well-visualized in skin biopsies
Fite	*Mycobacterium leprae*, *Nocardia*, and atypical mycobacteria	Red	Stain of choice for "partially acid-fast" organisms (***M. leprae***, *Nocardia*), and **atypical mycobacteria** because these are over-decolorized by Ziehl-Neelsen Peanut oil and gentle decolorization process allows for better color preservation than in Ziehl-Neelsen
Ziehl-Neelsen	Acid-fast bacteria (AFB)	Red	Most commonly used AFB stain **Less effective for *M. leprae* and atypical AFB** → use Fite instead
Auramine-rhodamine	Acid-fast bacteria	Yellow fluorescence	Requires fluorescence microscopy
Warthin-Starry (silver stain)	Spirochetes (syphilis, Borrelia)	Black	Also stains organisms in bacillary angiomatosis, granuloma inguinale (Donovan bodies), and rhinoscleroma Disadvantage: nonspecific ("dirty") staining pattern → has been largely replaced by spirochete immunostain
Steiner (silver stain)	Spirochetes (syphilis, Borrelia)	Black	Same staining pattern as Warthin-Starry
Giemsa	**Leishmania**, Histoplasma, and Rickettsia	Purple-blue	—
Other stains			
Bodian	Nerve axons (filaments)	Black	Positive in neurofibromas, traumatic neuromas, and PEN; **negative in schwannoma** (lacks axons)
Methyl green pyronin	RNA DNA	Pink Blue-green	Requires frozen tissue
Feulgen	DNA	Red-purple	—

Table 7.4 Characteristic Immunostains by Cell Type

Cell Type	Immunostain
B lymphocytes	**CD20** (most commonly used B-cell marker; absent in plasma cells; target for rituximab), **PAX-5** (more sensitive and specific than CD20, can be negative in plasma cells), **CD19** (target for CAR-T-cell therapy; useful in monitoring response to rituximab therapy, because CD20-negative B cells may arise following therapy), **CD79a** (B cells and plasma cells), CD45 (LCA; expressed on all hematopoietic cells except platelets and RBCs), and IgG light chains (κ and λ). When patient has received rituximab, use marker other than CD20 to detect B lymphocytes.
Dermal dendritic cells	Two distinct populations: Type I: **factor XIIIa**$^{+}$; reside in papillary dermis; involved in phagocytosis, antigen presentation, and wound healing; abundant in **dermatofibroma** Type II: **CD34**$^{+}$; reside in reticular dermis; **CD34 expression is lost in scleroderma/morphea**, and ↑ in NSF and scleromyxedema *Notable CD34+ tumors in dermpath: **DFSP**, **spindle cell lipoma**/pleomorphic lipoma, **Kaposi sarcoma** (endothelial cells), **neurofibroma** (diffuse NF can be misdiagnosed as DFSP!), **fibrofolliculoma/trichodiscoma** (spindled stromal cells), **trichilemmoma/DTL** (epithelial cells), **solitary fibrous tumor (STAT6+)**, **leukemia cutis** (less sensitive than CD43, c-KIT, CD68, lysozyme, MPO), Kaposiform hemangioendothelioma (endothelial cells), epithelioid hemangioendothelioma (endothelial cells), sclerotic fibroma, pleomorphic fibroma, superficial angiomyxoma, superficial acral fibromyxoma (and cellular digital fibroma), cellular angiofibroma of vulva/genital region, and ischemic fasciitis
Endothelial cells	**CD31** (**previous gold standard** for endothelial cells → superseded by ERG and FLI-1), **CD34** (less specific than CD31), **ERG** (excellent stain; very sensitive and specific), **FLI-1** (nuclear stain; improvement over CD31 and CD34 but not as good as ERG), *Ulex europaeus* agglutinin 1, factor VIII ag
Fibroblasts	Vimentin, procollagen I (also expressed in DFSP, AFX, NSF, and scleromyxedema)
Histiocytes/ macrophages	**CD68**, **CD163** (more specific than CD68), **lysozyme**, α-1 antitrypsin, HAM-56^{+} (esp. JXG and related xanthogranulomas), CD11b, CD14b, factor XIIIa, MAC-387 (true macrophages), and vimentin
Keratinocytes	**Cytokeratin**, **p63**, and **p40**
Langerhans cells	**S100**, **CD1a**, **Langerin** (**CD207**; stains Birbeck granules→ extremely specific), **BRAF** (in certain malignant Langerhans cell processes such as LCH and Erdheim-Chester disease), peanut agglutinin, and vimentin
Lymphatics	**D2-40** (**podoplanin**), **LYVE-1** (negative in blood vessel endothelium), PROX1 (nuclear) and vimentin
Mast cells	**c-KIT (CD117)** and **tryptase** (conventional/non-immunostains: Giemsa, Leder, toluidine blue)
Melanocytes	**S100, HMB-45** (gp100; less sensitive but more specific than S100; typically negative in desmoplastic melanoma), **MART-1/Melan-A** (less sensitive but more specific than S100; typically negative in desmoplastic melanoma), **MITF** (nuclear stain; positive in only 30% of desmoplastic melanomas and macrophages), **p16** (positive in Spitz nevi; often lost or diminished in spitzoid melanoma and ASTs), **p75/NGFR** (useful in desmoplastic melanoma, esp. when S100 is negative), **Sox10** (nuclear stain; helpful in distinguishing desmoplastic melanoma from scar tissue), tyrosinase, vimentin, and c-Kit
Merkel cells	**CK20 (paranuclear-dot pattern)**, synaptophysin, chromogranin, neurofilament (extremely useful and under-utilized stain; esp. helpful for CK20-negative Merkel cell carcinomas), and NSE. TTF-1 negative
Myofibroblasts	**SMA ("tram-track" pattern)**; myofibroblasts do not express desmin (vs. true smooth muscle cells)
Natural killer cells	**CD56** (most commonly used), **granzyme** A/B, and **TIA-1** (latter two stains are also positive in cytotoxic T cells)
Nerves	Axons: **neurofilament** and NSE Schwann cells: S100, GFAP, and MBP
Neutrophils	**MPO** (myeloperoxidase; esp. useful stain in histiocytoid Sweet's)
Plasma cells	**CD138**, CD79a, and CD45
Plasmacytoid dendritic cells	**CD123, with coexpression of CD4 (but not other T-cell markers)** ↑ Plasmacytoid dendritic cells are present in perivascular clusters **in lupus** (but not in dermatomyositis) and ↑ **in GA** (» NLD, rheumatoid nodules). When present in sheets and with blastoid morphology, may represent **blastic plasmacytoid dendritic cell neoplasm**
Sebaceous glands	**EMA, adipophilin, androgen receptor**, and cytokeratin
Smooth muscle	SMA (diffuse pattern), **desmin**
Sweat glands	CEA, EMA, GCDFP-15 (apocrine > eccrine), and cytokeratin
T lymphocytes	CD2, **CD3** (most specific), CD4, CD5, CD7, CD8, CD45 (LCA), **CD45Ra** (naïve T-cells), **CD45Ro** (memory T cells; positive in MF), and FOX-P3 (T-regulatory cells); T-cell markers often diminished/lost in MF (CD7 most commonly lost) and other neoplastic T-cell processes

Table 7.5 Most Commonly Used Epithelial Immunostains

Immunostain	Description/Staining Pattern	Comments
AE1/AE3	Cocktail of low- (AE1) and high- (AE3) MW keratin antibodies; typically positive in all epithelial tumors	Helps confirm diagnosis of SCC and adnexal carcinomas **Often fails to stain sarcomatoid SCC** → need additional cytokeratin stains (MNF116, CK903, or CK5/6), p63 or p40 to diagnose high-grade/sarcomatoid SCC
MNF116	Newer pankeratin immunostain w/ better sensitivity than AE1/AE3; stains all epithelial tissue	Helps differentiate **high-grade/sarcomatoid SCC** (positive) versus AFX (negative)
CK5/6	High-MW keratin immunostain; stains lower level of epidermis	Positive in primary cutaneous SCCs and adnexal carcinomas, but negative in metastatic adenocarcinomas → distinguishes **primary cutaneous adnexal carcinoma** (positive) versus metastatic adenocarcinomas from internal organs (negative), particularly when used in combination with p63 and/or D2-40 (same staining profile) Helps differentiate **high-grade/sarcomatoid SCC** (positive) versus AFX (negative)
CAM5.2	Low-MW keratin immunostain directed against **CK8**/18; stains **glandular epithelium** (mnemonic: "CAM5.2 = Gland5.2"); negative in squamous epithelium (including epidermis)	Positive in **Paget's and EMPD**, and eccrine glands/neoplasms
CK7	Stains glandular epithelium	Positive in **Paget's and EMPD** Also used in conjunction with CK20 to determine **origin of metastatic adenocarcinoma**: • CK7⁺ = malignancy **above the diaphragm** (breast, lung) • CK20⁺ = malignancy **below diaphragm** (stomach, colon)
EMA (epithelial membrane antigen)	Stains normal skin adnexae	Positive in **Paget's and EMPD**, adnexal neoplasms (including **sebaceous carcinoma**), most SCCs, and **epithelioid sarcoma** (INI-1 loss and EMA positivity are the two classic stains!)
CEA	Stains normal sweat glands (eccrine and apocrine); positive in sweat gland neoplasms	Positive in **Paget's and EMPD**
Ber-EP4	Stains non-keratinizing epithelial cells	Differentiates between **BCC** (positive), SCC (always negative), and sebaceous carcinoma (usually negative)
p63	Homologue of p53 that is positive in normal epidermis and adnexal epithelium	Stains > 90% of adnexal neoplasms (benign and malignant; Notable exception = primary apocrine carcinoma) Differentiates between **primary cutaneous adnexal carcinomas (positive)** and metastatic adenocarcinomas involving the skin (negative) Also stains **high-grade/sarcomatoid SCC** (distinguishes from AFX)

Table 7.6 Artifacts and Effects of Exogenous Materials

Inciting Cause	Histopathologic Features
Cryotherapy/freezing artifact	Keratinocyte vacuolization, subepidermal blister
Electrocautery artifact	Vertically oriented parallel keratinocytes (Fig. 7.2)
Knife/"chatter" artifact	Long parallel cuts in tissue, can be seen near foreign body (Fig. 7.3)
Gelfoam	Purple, angulated foreign material with surrounding granulomatous inflammation (Fig. 7.4)
Suture granuloma	Foreign body granuloma surrounding suture material (polarized light may show birefringence)
Intralesional corticosteroids	Amorphous, homogenous white to pink material +/– surrounding fibrous capsule
Fillers	Features depend on specific filler (see Figs. 7.5–7.8 and corresponding captions for details)

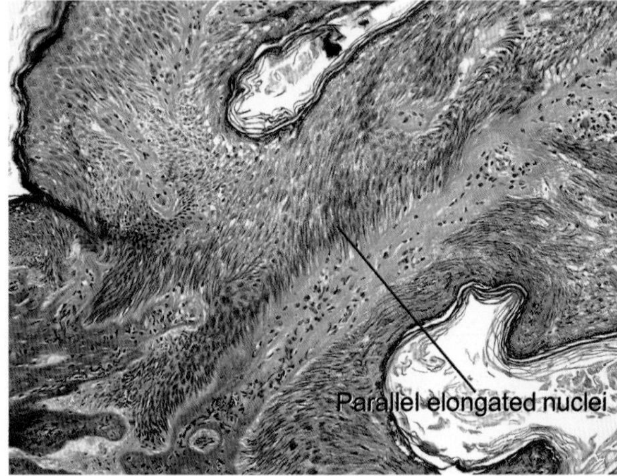

Fig. 7.2 Electrocautery. (From Ferringer T: External agents and artifacts. In: Elston DM, Ferringer T, eds. *Dermatopathology,* ed 3. Philadelphia: Elsevier, 2019:509-516.)

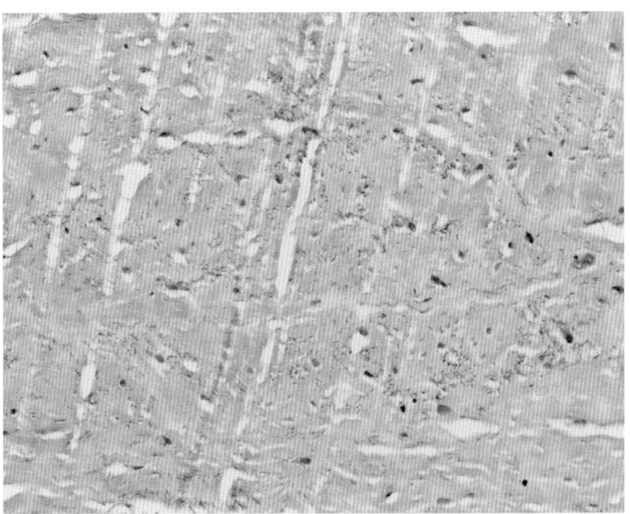

Fig. 7.3 Knife ("chatter") artifact from calcinosis cutis.

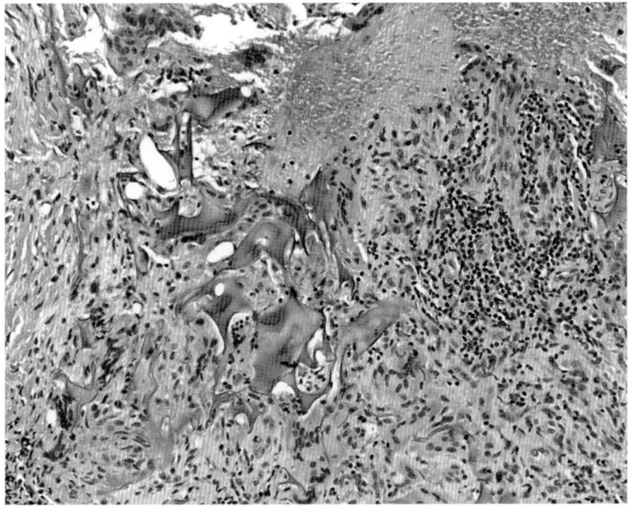

Fig. 7.4 Gelfoam (purple, angled deposits with surrounding host foreign-body response.

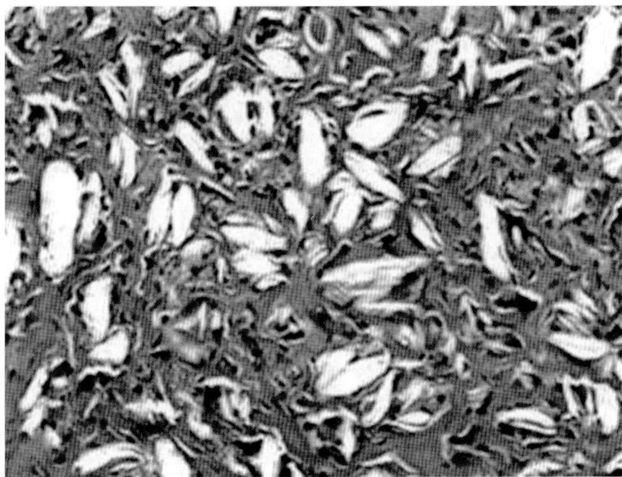

Fig. 7.5 Histopathologic features of granulomatous reaction to New-Fill (L-polylactic acid). Most of the particles show fusiform or oval shape. (From Requena L, Requena C, Christensen L, Zimmermann US, Kutzner H, Cerroni L. Adverse reactions to injectable soft tissue fillers. *J Am Acad Dermatol* 2011;64[1]:1-34).

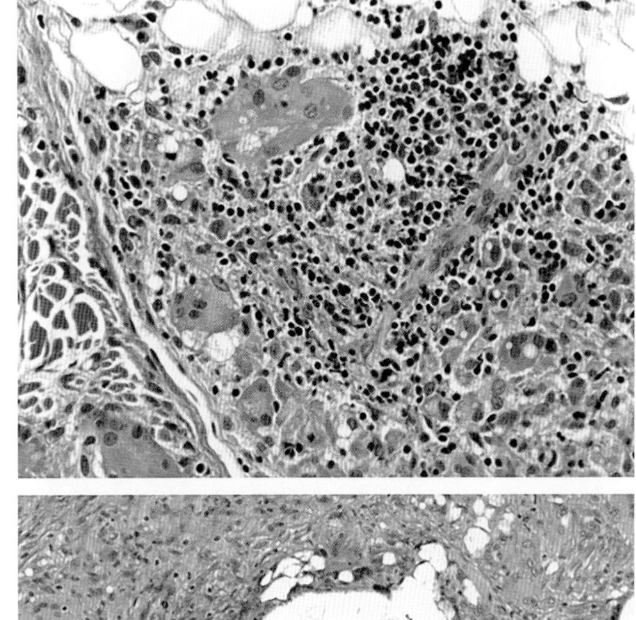

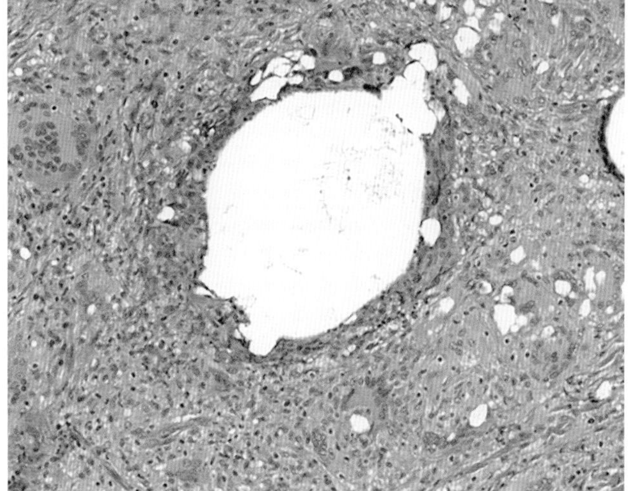

Fig. 7.6 Silicone granuoma, showing variably sized tissue vacuoles with an associated host granulomatous response.

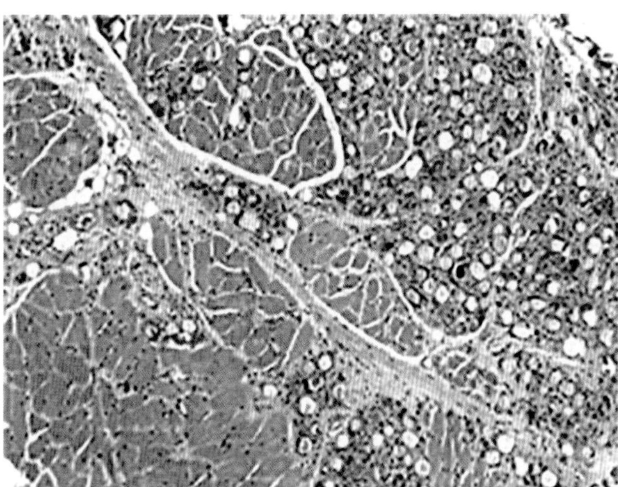

Fig. 7.7 Regularly sized mauve-to-gray or beige spherules of calcium hydroxylapatite in skeletal muscle surrounded by histiocytes and within foreign body giant cells (hematoxylin-eosin, original magnification x100).

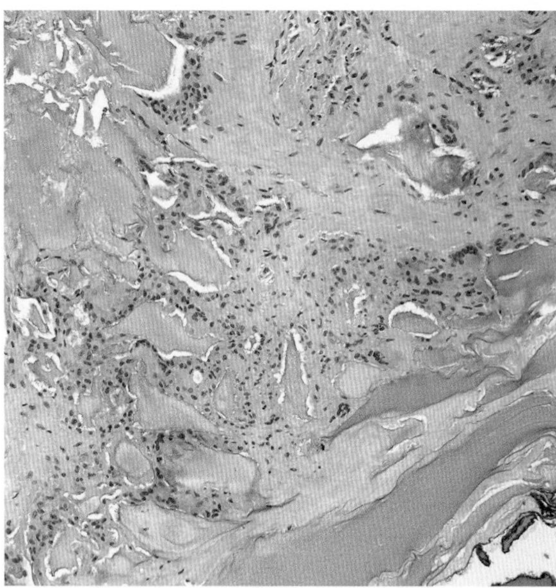

Fig. 7.8 Granulomatous reaction to hyaluronic acid. Basophilic material resembling mucin is surrounded by histiocytes and multinucleated giant cells.

Table 7.7 Spindle Cell Neoplasms

	CK	Vimentin	S100	SMA
SCC	+	–	–	–
Leiomyosarcoma	–	+	–	+ **(also desmin+)**
AFX	–	+	–	–
Melanoma	–	+	+	–

Modified from Ferringer T, Ko CJ. The basics: diagnostic terms, skin anatomy, and stains. In: Elston DM, Ferringer T, eds. Dermatopathology. *3rd ed. Philadelphia: Elsevier; 2019:1–35.*

Table 7.8 Neoplasms With Pagetoid Scatter

	CK	CEA	S100	LCA
Bowen disease	+	–	–	–
Paget's/EMPD	+	+	–	–
MF	–	–	–	+
Melanoma	–	–	+	–
Sebaceous carcinoma	+	+	–	–

Modified from Ferringer T, Ko CJ. The basics: diagnostic terms, skin anatomy, and stains. In: Elston DM, Ferringer T, eds. Dermatopathology. *3rd ed. Philadelphia: Elsevier; 2019:1–35.*

Table 7.9 Epithelial Carcinomas

	Ber-EP4	EMA	Androgen Receptor	Adipophilin
SCC	–	+	–	–
BCC	+	–	+/–	–
Sebaceous carcinoma	–	+	+	+

Immunofluorescence and related studies

Immunodermatology is its own subspecialty within dermatopathology and key details are as follows (summarized in Table 7.10).

- **Direct immunofluorescence (DIF)**
  - Performed on sections obtained from a biopsy of **intact, inflamed perilesional skin**
    - Exception: if dermatitis herpetiformis (DH) is suspected, the DIF should be **1 cm away** from active lesions
  - Requires **Michel's/Zeus transport media** or fresh frozen tissue
  - DIF patterns:
    - Linear (Fig. 7.9)
      - C3 only: pemphigoid gestationis
      - IgG and C3: bullous pemphigoid (BP), lichen planus pemphigoides, epidermolysis bullosa acquisita (EBA), cicatricial pemphigoid, anti-p200, anti-p105, anti-laminin-332, and bullous systemic lupus erythematosus (SLE)
        ➔ NEED further studies to distinguish!
      - IgA: linear IgA bullous dermatosis (LABD)
      - IgM: rarely reported in Waldenström macroglobulinemia; usually spurious
    - Granular
      - IgM, C3, IgG, IgA (in descending order of frequency) along the basement membrane zone (BMZ) = **lupus band** (Fig. 7.10)
      - IgA in dermal papillae +/– along BMZ: DH (Fig. 7.11)
    - Intercellular
      - IgG and C3 ("pemphigus pattern"; [Fig 7.12]): pemphigus vulgaris, pemphigus vegetans, pemphigus foliaceus, pemphigus erythematosus, fogo selvagem, and paraneoplastic pemphigus (paraneoplastic autoimmune multiorgan syndrome)
        ➔ Need clinical correlation and further studies to differentiate
      - IgA: IgA pemphigus
    - Linear to granular BMZ and intercellular: pemphigus erythematosus (Senear-Usher)
    - Linear BMZ and intercellular: paraneoplastic pemphigus (PNP)
      - May also see lichenoid tissue reaction
    - Lichenoid tissue reaction
      - Shaggy BMZ deposition with fibrinogen +/– cytoid bodies with various conjugates
      - Nonspecific finding; may be seen in any lichenoid process (lichen planus, lichenoid drug reaction, erythema multiforme, fixed drug eruption, connective tissue diseases, PNP, etc.) and also following excoriation
    - Vessel wall staining
      - **Stippled, not thickened**: leukocytoclastic vasculitis (LCV), including IgA vasculitis/Henoch-Schonlein purpura **(HSP)** (Fig. 7.13)
      - **Thickened and smooth: porphyrias** with cutaneous involvement and pseudoporphyria; may also see thick linear BMZ staining in these entities!
    - **n-serrated/u-serrated** pattern of linear deposition evaluated on DIF and may be used as a substitute for salt-split skin analysis (Fig. 7.14)
- **Indirect immunofluorescence (IIF): serologic study** where patient serum is incubated with a biologic substrate (salt-split skin; monkey esophagus; rat bladder

Table 7.10 Staining Characteristics of Subepidermal Blistering Diseases

Parameter	BP	EBA	BSLE	LAD	DH
DIF	Linear IgG, C3	Linear IgG > C3	Linear IgG, C3, +/− lupus band (granular IgM > IgA > C3 > IgG; along BMZ)	Linear IgA	Granular IgA (BMZ and in dermal papillae)
IIF (monkey esophagus substrate)	Linear IgG 75%–80%	Linear IgG 25%–50%	Linear IgG 60%	Linear IgA 30%	Antiendomysial antibodies (IgA >> IgG)
IIF (human salt-split skin substrate)	Roof	Floor	Floor	Roof, or floor, or both	N/A
Type IV collagen (immunostain on fixed tissue)	Floor	Roof	Roof	Roof or floor	N/A
EM: site of split	LL	Sub-LD	Sub-LD	LL, sub-LD, or both	Papillary dermis
Western blot	BP180 kD BP230 kD	290 kD (type VII collagen)	290 kD (type VII collagen)	BP180 kD BP230 kD 200/280 kD 285 kD 250 kD 290 kD	Antigen uncertain

BMZ, Basement membrane zone; *BP,* bullous pemphigoid; *BSLE,* bullous systemic lupus erythematosus; *DH,* dermatitis herpetiformis; *DIF,* direct immunofluorescence; *EBA,* epidermolysis bullosa acquisita; *EM,* electron microscopy; *IIF,* indirect immunofluorescence; *LAD,* linear IgA disease; *LL,* lamina lucida; *sub-LD,* sub-lamina densa; *N/A,* not applicable.

Modified from Luzar B, McGrath JA. Inherited and autoimmune subepidermal blistering diseases. In: Calonje E, Brenn T, Lazar AJ, Billings SD, eds. McKee's Pathology of the Skin With Clinical Correlations. *5th ed. Philadelphia: Elsevier; 2020:118–170.*

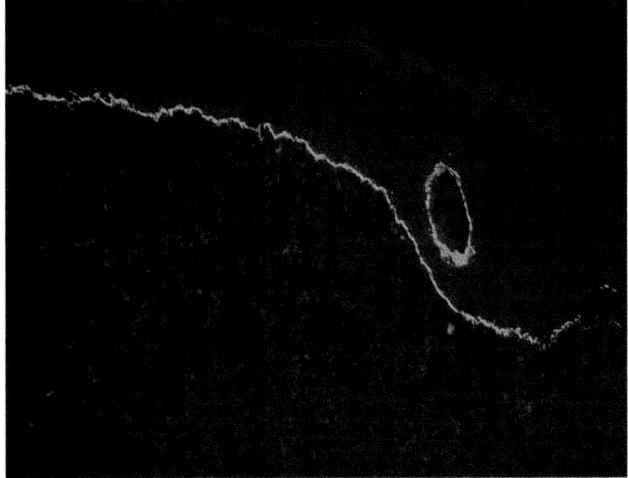

Fig. 7.9 Direct immunofluorescence showing linear IgG along the dermoepidermal junction, as may be seen in pemphigoid, epidermolysis bullosa acquisita, and bullous lupus erythematosus.

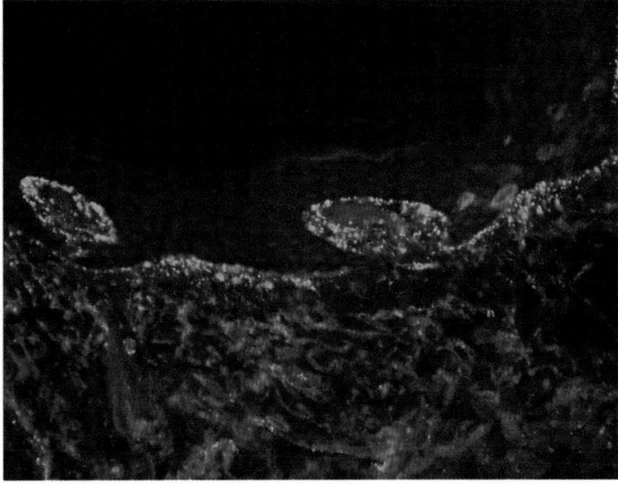

Fig. 7.11 Direct immunofluorescence showing granular deposition of IgA along the basement membrane zone and in the dermal papillae, as is characteristic of dermatitis herpetiformis.

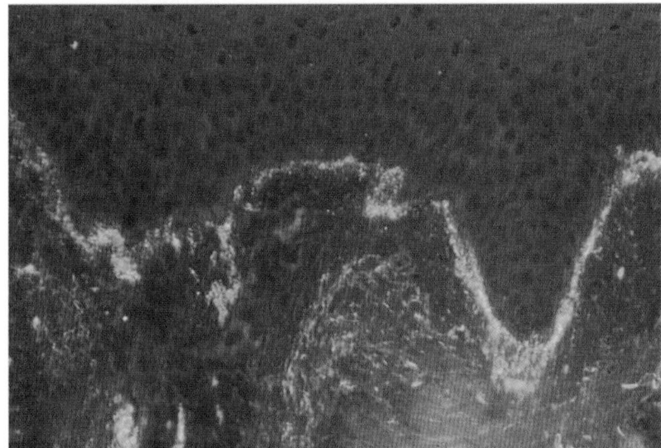

Fig. 7.10 Direct immunofluorescence showing granular IgM deposition along the basement membrane zone, as may be seen as part of a lupus band. (From Brinster NK, Liu V, Diwan AH, McKee PH. *Dermatopathology: A Volume in the High Yield Pathology Series*. Philadelphia: Elsevier; 2011.)

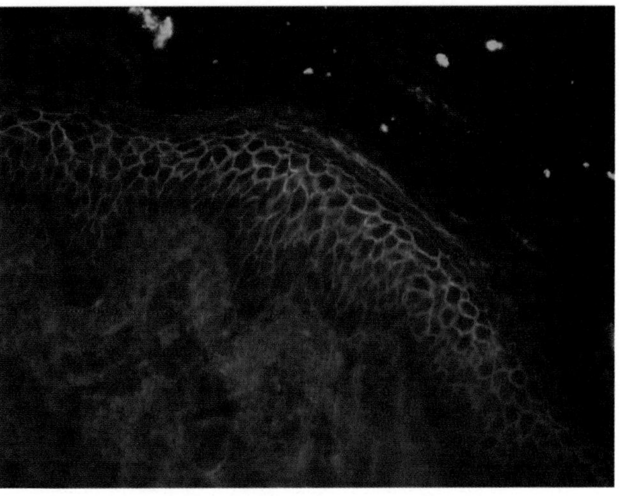

Fig. 7.12 Intercellular deposition of IgG in pemphigus.

Fig. 7.13 Perivascular granular deposition of IgA within walls of multiple superficial dermal blood vessels in IgA vasculitis.

epithelium); staining patterns same as for DIF; generally less sensitive than DIF (Table 7.11).

- **Salt-split skin studies (IIF):** incubation of normal human skin in 1M NaCl → separation of the skin at the dermoepidermal junction (DEJ; at lamina lucida) → visualization of where the immunoreactants are depositing → allows differentiation amongst various subepidermal blistering diseases (see Table 7.11 and Fig. 7.15).
- **Collagen IV immunostaining (lamina densa) of fixed patient tissue**
  - Performed on paraffin-embedded sections to localize the level of the dermal-epidermal separation to above or below the lamina densa
  - An alternative to salt-split skin immunofluorescence (but is not well-validated; mostly used for research purposes)
  - Staining of collagen IV along the **floor** of a blister: **BP**
  - Staining of collagen IV along the **roof** of a blister: diseases targeting collagen VII (**EBA and bullous SLE**)
  - BE CAREFUL! Collagen IV immunostaining patterns are **OPPOSITE of salt-split skin DIF and IIF** patterns!

Text continued on p. 415

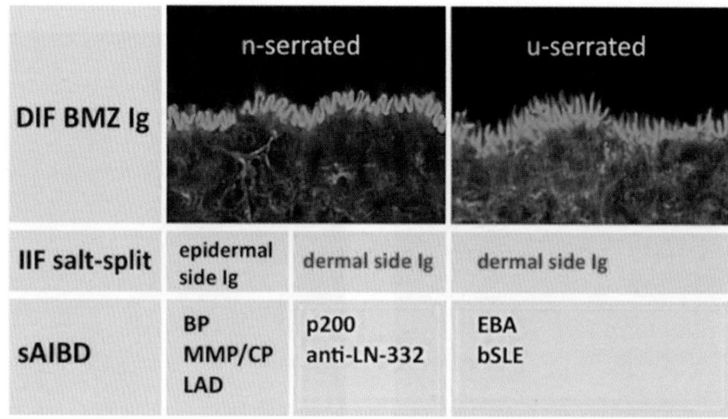

Fig. 7.14 Overview n- and u-serrated pattern and different forms of subepidermal autoimmune blistering diseases (sAIBD). *BMZ*, Basement membrane zone; *BP*, bullous pemphigoid; *bSLE*, bullous systemic lupus erythematosus; *CP*, cicatricial pemphigoid; *DIF*, direct immunofluorescence; *EBA*, epidermolysis bullosa acquisita; *IIF*, indirect immunofluorescence; *LAD*, linear IgA disease; *MMP;* mucous membrane pemphigoid. (From Vodegel RM, Jonkman MF, Pas HH, De Jong MCJM. U-serrated immunodeposition pattern differentiates type VII collagen targeting bullous diseases from other subepidermal bullous autoimmune diseases. *Brit J Dermatol*. 2004;151[1]:112–118.)

Table 7.11 High-Yield Dermatopathology Diagnoses at a Glance

Dx	Buzzwords/Essential Features	Mimics in DDx
Acanthosis nigricans	Epidermal papillomatosis	Microscopically **identical** to CARP, acrokeratosis verruciformis of Hopf, and SK
Accessory digit	Pedunculated papule, **numerous nerve bundles**	Acquired digital fibrokeratoma (lacks nerves, more fibrotic), and accessory tragus (vellus hairs, cartilage, and lacks nerve bundles)
Accessory nipple	Domed papule, papillomatous surface +/− central invagination, ↑ **smooth muscle**, sebaceous glands opening directly onto skin surface, and **mammary ducts/glands**	Becker's nevus (lacks mammary glands and sebaceous glands opening directly onto skin surface), and normal nipple (need clinical Hx)
Accessory tragus	Polypoid, multiple **vellus hairs**, +/− **cartilage**	Accessory digit (nerve bundles; lacks vellus hairs)
Acne keloidalis nuchae	Suppurative folliculitis with **mixed inflammation** (neutrophils, plasma cells, and lymphocytes), **hypertrophic scar**, and naked hair shafts	Folliculitis decalvans (similar, but lacks hypertrophic scar), infection, LPP (lymphocytic inflammation; usually lacks free hair shafts)
Acquired digital fibrokeratoma	Polypoid, massive orthohyperkeratosis, and vertically oriented collagen	Wart (koilocytes), accessory digit (nerves)
Actinomycosis	Light-colored grains of filamentous bacteria, surrounded by Splendore-Hoeppli phenomenon (pink)	Eumycetoma, botryomycosis
Atypical fibroxanthoma	Dense dermal proliferation of spindled cells, histiocyte-like cells, foam cells, and **bizarre multinucleated** cells; **numerous atypical mitoses**; +/− ulceration	Undifferentiated pleomorphic sarcoma (UPS) and pleomorphic dermal sarcoma (PDS): cells appear identical but tumor extends into fat or deeper soft tissue; more aggressive **SLAM DDx**

Table 7.11 High-Yield Dermatopathology Diagnoses at a Glance—cont'd

Dx	Buzzwords/Essential Features	Mimics in DDx
Alopecia areata	**"Swarm of bees"** lymphocytic infiltrate near hair bulb in fat; profound shift to catagen/telogen; **lymphocytes, eosinophils, and melanin in fibrous tracts, +/− pigment casts**	Trichotillomania (has pigment casts but inside follicle, also has trichomalacia; lacks eosinophils and lymphocytes in fibrous streamer tracts), LPP (inflammation much more superficial [infundibulum]), syphilitic alopecia (can show swarm of bees but also contains plasma cells and epidermal/dermal changes of syphilis)
Amalgam tattoo	**Oral mucosa**, dark colored specks along BMZ and scattered throughout dermis (in macrophages or along elastic fibers)	Normal skin DDx
Amyloid (macular and lichen)	Waxy pink globules in papillary dermis, pigment incontinence; **amyloid is keratin-derived (AK)** and stains with **Congo red (weak)** and keratin stains	Normal skin DDx, colloid milium (extends deeper into dermis; adult form has prominent solar elastosis); nodular amyloid (deeper, ↑ inflammation w/ plasma cells, and amyloid is light-chain derived = AL)
Amyloid (nodular)	Large fissured pale pink material in superficial and **deep** dermis, prominent inflammation w/ **plasma cells**, and **amyloid is light chain-derived (AL)**	Macular/lichen amyloid (more superficial, keratin-derived, and lacks inflammation), colloid milium (lacks inflammation)
Angiofibroma (fibrous papule, Koenen tumor, and adenoma sebaceum)	Papule, proliferation of normal and stellate fibroblasts w/ **concentric perivascular fibrosis**	DF (collagen trapping, epidermal hyperplasia)
Angiolipoma	Lipoma w/ lobular capillary proliferations +/− intravascular thrombosis	Lipoma (lacks proliferative collections of capillaries), spindle cell lipoma (myxoid stroma w/ small spindle cells, "ropey" bright pink collagen, lacks capillary proliferations)
Angiosarcoma	Poorly-circumscribed dermal proliferation of anastomosing vessels; atypical, plump, **hyperchromatic** endothelial cells with **multi-layering**, mitoses; Often arises in **irradiated skin,** severely sun-damaged sites **(head/neck)**, or **chronic lymphedema**	Kaposi (cells are **spindled** and not nearly as hyperchromatic nor as mitotically active; slit-like vessels, hemorrhage, **plasma cells**, promontory sign); aneurysmal DF (peripheral collagen trapping; giant cells containing hemosiderin)
Arteriovenous malformation (AV hemangioma)	**Mix of thick** (centrally located) and **thin** (peripherally located) walled vessels in mid-upper dermis	Lobular capillary hemangioma (small thin-walled capillaries and endothelial cells), angioleiomyoma (located much deeper in SQ; concentric pink smooth muscle compresses large vessels to form slit-like vessels)
Balloon cell nevus	Melanocytes w/ abundant **vacuolated clear cytoplasm** arranged in nests that decrease in size with descent into the dermis, dermal melanophages, and **scattered conventional nevus nests (critical clue to diagnosis!)**	Renal cell carcinoma (very vascular w/ hemorrhage; lacks dermal melanophages and conventional nevus nests), clear cell hidradenoma (sweat ducts; foci of keratinizing dermal nests, lacks conventional nevus nests), xanthoma (lacks pigment and conventional nevus nests)
Blastomycosis	**PEH w/ intraepidermal pustules**, dermal granulomatous inflammation, large 8–15 μm round yeast w/ **broad-based budding**	Coccidioidomycosis (much larger spherules with endosporulation; lacks broad-based budding), PEH with pus DDx
Bowen's disease	"**Wind-blown**" architecture, full-thickness atypia, and **dyskeratotic keratinocytes**	Paget's/EMPD (mucin, nests compress basal keratinocytes), melanoma (pigment, lacks dyskeratotic keratinocytes), MF (lacks dyskeratotic keratinocytes, less cytologic atypia)
Branchial cleft cyst	Epidermoid or ciliated pseudostratified cyst lining; **prominent lymphoid aggregates with germinal centers** surrounding cyst	Bronchogenic cyst (smooth muscle and cartilage around cyst; abundant goblet cells), thyroglossal cyst (pink hyaline thyroid follicles)
Bronchogenic cyst	Ciliated columnar/pseudostratified epithelium, **goblet cells**, smooth muscle and **cartilage** around cyst	Branchial cleft cyst (prominent lymphoid nodules/germinal centers), thyroglossal cyst (pink thyroid follicles), and cutaneous ciliated cyst (lacks smooth muscle and cartilage)
Bullous impetigo	**Superficial acantholysis** (PF-like), subcorneal neutrophilic microabscesses +/− bacteria	Pemphigus foliaceus (lacks bacteria and subcorneal neutrophilic microabscesses; positive DIF); IgA pemphigus (can have subcorneal neutrophilic microabscesses and superficial acantholysis but has +DIF)
Bullous pemphigoid/herpes gestationis	**Sub-epidermal blister w/ eos**, eosinophilic spongiosis, and **DIF+ (linear IgG** and **C3** along BMZ) For pemphigoid gestationis, often only C3 is positive on DIF	PCT (pauci-inflammatory, sun-damaged skin), EBA (pauci-inflammatory +/− scattered neuts), bullous EM (apoptotic keratinocytes, lymphocytic, eos uncommon), LABD/DH (neutrophils)
Bullous SLE	**Sub-epidermal blister w/ neuts**, dermal PV/PA lymphocytic inflammation, ↑ mucin, and **DIF+ (granular to linear IgG** (+/− IgA and IgM) along BMZ); Dermal deposition on human salt-split skin indirect IF	PCT (pauci-inflammatory, sun-damaged skin), EBA (more pauci-inflammatory), bullous EM (apoptotic keratinocytes, lymphocytic, eos uncommon), LABD/DH (neutrophilic papillitis)
Calcinosis cutis	Large purple deposits; **Knife artifact** often present, due to dragging of calcium across tissue during tissue processing	PXE (small, wavy calcified fibers), calcified pilomatricoma or epidermoid cyst (epithelium surrounds calcified material)
Calciphylaxis	**Concentric calcification of small to medium sized vessels w/ thrombosis**, extra-vascular calcification (esp. peri-eccrine), +/− ulceration	Thrombotic vasculopathies (lack intra- and extravascular calcification)

Continued

Table 7.11 High-Yield Dermatopathology Diagnoses at a Glance—cont'd

Dx	Buzzwords/Essential Features	Mimics in DDx
Cellular blue nevus	Highly cellular, **purely dermal proliferation** of plump or fusiform pale gray **melanocytes containing minimal pigment** + admixed dendritic melanocytes resembling common blue nevus cells; bulges into subcutis (**"dumbbell configuration"**) Often located on the **buttock**, head, or low back	Deep penetrating nevus (usually has **junctional component** and superficial **dermal nests resembling ordinary nevus nests →** CBN always lacks both these features!)
Cellular neurothekeoma	Fibrohistiocytic neoplasm (despite name); comprised of **dermal nests and fascicles** of spitzoid to histiocytoid appearing cells, S100–, **S100A6+, NKI-C3+, and PGP9.5+**	"Neurothekeoma"/nerve sheath myxoma (nodules are much less cellular and much more myxoid, cells are S100+ and spindled/fibroblast-like rather than epithelioid/spitzoid)
Chondrodermatitis nodularis helicis (CNH)	Central ulceration w/ adjacent epidermal hyperplasia, subjacent healing skin changes, and degenerating (eosinophilic) cartilage	SCC and AK (atypia), relapsing polychondritis (lichenoid lymphocytic infiltrate adjacent to degenerating cartilage)
Chromoblastomycosis	**PEH** + clusters of pigmented round yeast (**"copper pennies/Medlar bodies"**) within granulomatous dermal infiltrate	Blastomycosis (also has PEH, but has broad-based budding; lacks brown pigmentation), phaeohyphomycosis (pigmented hyphae rather than round yeast)
Clear cell acanthoma	**Psoriasiform** hyperplasia with **clear (glycogenated) cells**, intracorneal neutrophils, **sharp demarcation** from surrounding normal skin	Trichilemmoma (large endophytic lobules rather than psoriasiform, peripheral palisading, and thickened pink BMZ), psoriasis (lacks clear cells and is not as sharply demarcated)
Clonal SK	Whorled intraepidermal nests of keratinocytes within SK	Hidroacanthoma simplex (sweat ducts w/ eosinophilic cuticle; smaller monotonous poroid cells), SCCIS (atypical cytology w/ mitoses, dyskeratotic keratinocytes, and "windblown" pattern)
Coccidioidomycosis	**Large spherules (up to 80 μm)** containing smaller endospores	Rhinosporidiosis (gigantic sporangia with central dot-like nuclei and many endospores), blastomycosis (PEH more common; smaller organisms without endospores)
Coma/barbiturate blister	**Paucicellular/noninflammatory subepidermal bulla**, diffuse epidermal necrosis, and **sweat gland necrosis**	SJS/TEN (scattered eos; sweat gland necrosis less common and less pronounced when present)
Congenital nevus	Usually compound nevus with extension down adnexae; melanocytes become singly distributed between collagen in deep dermis	Acquired nevi (do not extend as deeply and do not involve adnexal structures as much)
Cryoglobulinemia type 1	Noninflammatory **intravascular occlusion w/ homogeneous light pink PAS+ material in lumen**	LCV (vessels destroyed, fibrin in vessel walls rather than occluding lumens), thrombotic vasculopathies (very difficult to distinguish, except calciphylaxis which has calcium deposits)
Cryptococcus	**Clear gelatinous capsule (mucicarmine+)** surrounding yeast clusters; entire dermis may be gelatinous appearing ("gelatinous *Cryptococcus*")	Histoplasmosis (much smaller organism, intracellular within histiocytes, and has a pseudocapsule rather than a true capsule), lepromatous leprosy (clear cell changes but also has pink globi +/–perineural granulomatous inflammation)
Cylindroma	See Chapter 6, Neoplastic Dermatology	See Chapter 6, Neoplastic Dermatology
Darier disease	**Acantholytic dyskeratosis, corps ronds, corps grains**	Pemphigus (lacks dyskeratosis, corps ronds/grains), warty dyskeratoma (more endophytic, more circumscribed lesion), herpetic infection (viral cytopathic change and neutrophils)
Deep penetrating nevus	Typically **compound** w/ small junctional component, **superficial dermal nests resembling ordinary nevus nests**, and dense wedge-shaped dermal component of plump **epithelioid pigmented melanocytes** with **abundant melanophages** extending into deep dermis/subcutis, tracks along adnexal and neurovascular structures; may have "dumbbell configuration" like cellular blue nevus. **β-catenin+** (nuclear) in heavily pigmented cells	Cellular blue nevus (**never has junctional component**, never has superficial dermal nests resembling ordinary nevus nests; melanocytes are smaller and much less pigmented), nodular melanoma (severe cytologic atypia w/ mitoses)
Dermal melanocytosis (nevus of Ito/Ota/Mongolian spot)	Paucicellular, spindled dendritic melanocytes scattered randomly throughout dermis; **lacks dermal sclerosis**	Blue nevus (more cellular, more circumscribed, has dermal sclerosis); drug-induced hyperpigmentation
Dermatitis herpetiformis	Abscess-like **neutrophil aggregates in dermal papillae**, small subepidermal bullae, and **DIF+ (granular IgA** in dermal papillae)	BP (eosinophils predominate, bigger bullae), bullous SLE (lymphocytic and neutrophilic inflammation along DEJ and around adnexae, increased mucin), and LABD (neutrophilic infiltrate and blisters are more diffuse along DEJ; DIF easily distinguishes)
Dermatofibroma	Interstitial "fibrohistiocytic" infiltrate in mid-deep dermis, **collagen trapping** (best seen at periphery), follicular and epidermal **induction**, and Touton giant cells containing hemosiderin (**ringed sideroblasts**); **Factor XIIIa+,** stromelysin 3+, **CD34–**	DFSP (infiltrates fat deeply [honeycombing pattern], lacks follicular and epidermal induction, lacks giant cells with hemosiderin; stains: CD34+, factor XIIIa–, and stromelysin 3–)
Dermatofibroma (aneurysmal variant)	DF w/ **abundant hemorrhage** and hemosiderin within giant cells; collagen trapping seen at periphery	Angiosarcoma (lacks multinucleate giant cells and collagen trapping), Kaposi sarcoma (lacks multinucleate giant cells)

Table 7.11 High-Yield Dermatopathology Diagnoses at a Glance—cont'd

Dx	Buzzwords/Essential Features	Mimics in DDx
Dermatofibrosarcoma protuberans (DFSP)	Dense, monomorphous spindle cell proliferation, **storiform** pattern, extensive **honeycombing of fat**, **CD34+**, factor XIIIa–, and stromelysin 3–; may have fibrosarcomatous transformation (monomorphic spindled cells arranged in a herringbone-like distribution) which is a/w poorer prognosis	Cellular DF (abuts, but does not infiltrate and deeply penetrate fat; peripheral collagen trapping, folliculo-epidermal induction, and hemosiderin-laden multinucleate giant cells), diffuse NF (may also be CD34+ but less densely cellular, lacks honeycombing, and is S100+)
Dermatomyositis	**Subtle vacuolar interface**, BMZ thickening, **abundant dermal mucin**, and mild inflammation	Lupus (more robust interface changes, less mucin, dense superficial and deep PV/PA lymphocytic inflammation), GVHD (squamous atypia and metaplasia from chemotherapy effect common, lacks mucin), EM (more robust interface, lacks mucin)
Digital mucous cyst	Circumscribed nodule of mucin on acral skin without a true epithelial lining	Mucocele (mucosal location), nerve sheath myxoma/"neurothekeoma" (multiple small nodules of mucin + spindled cells)
Dysplastic nevus	Junctional or compound nevus with at least one of the following: **asymmetry**, **poor circumscription**, focal pagetoid scatter, **bridging** of melanocyte nests, "**shouldering**" of junctional component, concentric or lamellar **papillary dermal fibrosis**, and **cytologic atypia**	Melanoma (diffuse pagetoid scatter, consumption of epidermis, severe cytologic and/or architectural atypia, and lacks maturation with depth)
Elastosis perforans serpiginosa (EPS)	Narrow, **serpiginous** epidermal channel with perforating **pink-red elastic fibers**	Reactive perforating collagenosis (thicker volcano-like channel and perforating basophilic collagen)
Endometriosis (cutaneous)	Multiple **bland-appearing glands** with surrounding **edematous/fibromyxoid stroma; hemorrhage**	Metastatic adenocarcinoma (lacks fibromyxoid stroma and glandular cells appear malignant)
Epidermodysplasia verruciformis	Pale **gray-blue color** of the upper epidermis	Verruca plana (superficial hypergranulosis w/ clumpy keratohyalin granules +/– koilocytes; lacks pale gray-blue hue), nutritional deficiency (upper half of epidermis is pale/clear colored; psoriasiform hyperplasia)
Epidermolytic hyperkeratosis	**Verrucous** surface, marked **hyperkeratosis**, **coarse keratohyalin** granules, and **epidermolysis** (keratinocytes being ripped apart from each other—can see stretched out spinous connections)	Wart (koilocytes; lacks epidermolysis), acantholytic disorders (keratinocytes rounded, lack spinous connections)
Epithelioid hemangioma/ALHE	Domed papule, large superficial dermal vessels with **large epithelioid endothelial cells, dense lympho-eosinophilic infiltrate;** often on **head and neck**	Granuloma faciale (infiltrate has neutrophils and plasma cells, not dome shaped, and lacks epithelioid endothelial cells), bug bite/dermal hypersensitivity reaction (no increased vessels), Kimura disease (much deeper; very rare in Western countries; not usually tested)
Eruptive xanthoma	Foamy/xanthomatized histiocytes, **extracellular lipid**	GA (mucin, altered collagen, lacks xanthomatized histiocytes), xanthelasma (eyelid skin, lacks extracellular lipid), JXG (often has intermixed eosinophils, Touton giant cells, and many non-lipidized histiocytes)
Erythema annulare centrifugum	**Tight ("coat-sleeve")** lymphocytic perivascular inflammation +/– mild spongiotic dermatitis +/– thin mounds of parakeratosis	Tumid lupus (abundant mucin +/– vacuolar interface), annular erythema (a/w SCLE and Sjögren syndrome; has anti-Ro antibodies; +/– interface), PMLE (massive papillary dermal edema), dermal hypersensitivity reaction (abundant eos), pityriasis rosea (RBC extravasation, less dense inflammation)
Erythema induratum/nodular vasculitis	**Lobular and septal fat necrosis**, granulomatous inflammation ("infection-like"), and **vasculitis of medium-sized vessels** ("PAN-sized vessels")	PAN (targets vessels almost exclusively, with minimal fat necrosis)
Erythema multiforme	**Basket-weave stratum corneum, scattered necrotic keratinocytes in all levels** of epidermis, brisk inflammation comprised almost exclusively of **lymphocytes**; typically **lacks eosinophils**	SJS/TEN (diffuse epidermal necrosis, less inflammatory, and more eos), LP (orthohyperkeratosis, epidermal acanthosis, and necrotic keratinocytes confined to basal layer), lupus (deeper PV/periadnexal infiltrate, mucin), DM (less keratinocyte apoptosis, abundant mucin), GVHD (less inflammatory, epidermal chemo effect/squamous dysmaturation)
Erythema nodosum	**Thickened SQ septae** w/ septal granulomatous inflammation, giant cells, and **Miescher's granulomas**; though granulomatous inflammation can spill into SQ lobules, it should be centered in SQ septae	Lobular panniculitides (involves pannicular lobules), eosinophilic fasciitis/deep morphea (both may have thickened septae but lack granulomatous inflammation; deep morphea may have lymphoplasmacytic clusters)
Fibrofolliculoma	See Chapter 6, Neoplastic Dermatology	See Chapter 6, Neoplastic Dermatology
Fixed drug eruption	**EM-like** epidermal changes + **eosinophils** + **deeper pigment incontinence**	EM (lacks: eosinophils and deep pigment incontinence; lymphocyte predominant), SJS/TEN (less inflammatory), GVHD (lacks eosinophils; more adnexal interface)
Follicular mucinosis (alopecia mucinosa)	**Mucin in follicle** +/– adnexotropic atypical lymphocytes; conspicuous eosinophils	Follicular eczema (spongiosis in follicles; lacks mucin)
Folliculitis decalvans	**Suppurative folliculitis** w/ mixed inflammation (neutrophils, plasma cells, and lymphocytes), **free hair shafts**	LPP (lymphocytic inflammation, typically lacks free hair shafts), acne keloidalis nuchae (similar, but has hypertrophic scar)

Continued

Table 7.11 High-Yield Dermatopathology Diagnoses at a Glance—cont'd

Dx	Buzzwords/Essential Features	Mimics in DDx
Giant cell tumor of tendon sheath	Dense proliferation of **osteoclastic giant cells** and histiocytes, located very deep (near tendon)	JXG (more superficial [dermis], has Touton giant cells, intermixed eosinophils, and xanthomatized histiocytes, lacks osteoclastic GC), giant cell epulis (oral equivalent of GCTTS)
Glomus tumor	Dermal proliferation of monomorphic round blue cells w/ associated vessels; **SMA+**	Mastocytoma ("fried egg" mast cells, more abundant cytoplasm, and lacks vascular component), poroma/dermal duct tumor (sweat ducts, lacks vessels w/ RBCs)
Gout	**Needle-shaped dermal or subcutaneous crystals** w/ surrounding granulomatous inflammation; crystals may dissolve w/ processing (better preserved if skin specimen is collected in **alcohol**)	Intralesional Kenalog deposits (amorphous, bubbly foreign material, rather than needle-shaped)
Granular cell tumor	Dermal proliferation of cells w/ granular cytoplasm and **pustulo-ovoid bodies** of Milian, **pseudoepitheliomatous hyperplasia** (50%), **S100+**	Hibernoma (deeper, large intracytoplasmic vacuoles), xanthoma (foamy histiocytes are whiter, versus pink cytoplasm in GCT), SCC (**Boards Pearl:** always check the dermis underneath an apparent SCC for GCT or deep fungal infection!)
Granuloma annulare (classic type)	Distinct zones of **palisaded histiocytes** encircling altered collagen and **mucin**; areas of normal intervening dermis; frequent **eosinophils**	NL (square biopsy sign, diffuse/pan-dermal necrobiosis [degenerated collagen], plasma cells, lacks eosinophils), rheumatoid nodule (deeper, central pink fibrin rather than mucin, and neutrophilic debris), AEGCG (elastophagocytosis, focal loss of solar elastosis), epithelioid sarcoma (pseudo-palisaded w/ central tumor necrosis and atypical peripheral cells w/ mitoses)
Granuloma annulare (interstitial)	Interstitial histiocytes w/ adjacent **mucin**, mild collagen degeneration, and PV lymphoeosinophilic inflammation	Kaposi sarcoma (spindled cells, hemorrhage, hemosiderin, and abundant plasma cells; lacks mucin), metastatic breast carcinoma (atypical cells with small duct formation; lacks mucin), leukemia cutis/AML (immature neutrophils/band forms, atypical myeloblasts with mitoses; no mucin and no collagen alteration)
Granuloma faciale	**Grenz zone**; perivascular mixed inflammation (**neutrophils, plasma cells, eosinophils,** and lymphocytes); may occasionally see LCV	ALHE/epithelioid hemangioma (dome-shaped, large epithelioid endothelial cells, infiltrate predominantly lymphocytes and eosinophils; much less neutrophils and plasma cells), EED (similar to GF, but has "onion skin" vessel thickening)
Guttate psoriasis	**Thick, mounded parakeratosis adherent** to epidermis; neutrophilic microabscesses; +/– psoriasiform hyperplasia	Pityriasis rosea (thinner, nonadherent mounds of parakeratosis, RBC extravasation, and lacks neuts)
Acute GVHD	Vacuolar (> lichenoid) interface with frequent involvement of hair follicles and adnexae, sparse lymphocytic infiltrate, **"chemo effect"** (dysmaturation of keratinocytes and squamous metaplasia of eccrine ducts), and **"satellite cell necrosis"** (apoptotic keratinocytes abutting lymphocytes)	EM (more inflammatory), DM (more mucin), lupus (denser superficial and deep PV/PA inflammation)
Hailey-Hailey	**Epidermal hyperplasia** (acanthosis), acantholysis ("**dilapidated brick wall**"), and **keratinocytes appear pinker** than normal	Darier's (more corps ronds/grains), pemphigus (lacks acanthosis, involves hair follicles, tombstoning, and DIF+)
Halo nevus	Dense lymphocytic infiltrate mingling with nevus cells **("Cocktail party")**	Melanoma w/ lichenoid regression (band-like lymphocytic infiltrate deep to melanoma = **"Riot Police"**), LP (lacks melanocytic nests)
Hibernoma	Eosinophilic lipocytes w/ multivacuolated **"mulberry cells"** (white vacuoles w pink borders)	Granular cell tumor (more superficial – dermis, smaller cells, pustulo-ovoid bodies of Milian)
Hidradenoma	See Chapter 6, Neoplastic Dermatology	See Chapter 6, Neoplastic Dermatology
Hidradenoma papilliferum	See Chapter 6, Neoplastic Dermatology	See Chapter 6, Neoplastic Dermatology
Hidroacanthoma simplex (intraepidermal poroma)	See Chapter 6, Neoplastic Dermatology	See Chapter 6, Neoplastic Dermatology
Hidrocystoma	Simple cyst with two cell layer thick lining (apocrine or eccrine); frequently contextual clues to periorbital location (vellus hairs, solar elastosis, skeletal muscle from orbicularis oris)	Steatocystoma (eosinophilic "shark tooth" lining and sebaceous glands in cyst wall), PEA/TAA (multiple smaller cysts +/– papillary projections)
Histoplasmosis	Granulomatous inflammation with **parasitized histiocytes** containing small 2–3 μm dots **evenly spaced** throughout cytoplasm; each organism has **pseudocapsule**; narrow-based unequal budding	Leishmaniasis ("marquee sign," kinetoplast, and lacks pseudocapsule)
HSV/VZV	**Acantholysis**, viral cytopathic changes (**M**ultinucleated keratinocytes, chromatin **M**argination, nuclear **M**olding, and steel-gray keratinocytes); accompanying acute sebaceitis and vasculitis may be seen	Pemphigus (lacks multinucleated cells and viral cytopathic changes), acantholytic SCC (chromatin is not marginated to cell edges)
Hyalohyphomycosis (*Aspergillus*, *Fusarium* and *Penicillium*)	**Narrow, septated, blue hyphae** with **bubbly cytoplasm**, **45° branching**; **angioinvasive** with subsequent thrombosis and epidermal/dermal necrosis	Zygomycosis (broad, nonseptated, pink hollow hyphae with 90° branching, angioinvasive—epidermal/dermal necrosis)
Ichthyosis vulgaris	**Compact orthohyperkeratosis** w/ paradoxically **decreased granular layer**	Normal skin DDx

Table 7.11 High-Yield Dermatopathology Diagnoses at a Glance—cont'd

Dx	Buzzwords/Essential Features	Mimics in DDx
Incontinentia pigmenti	Eosinophilic spongiosis; **apoptotic keratinocytes** (most helpful clue to DDx)	Allergic contact dermatitis ("flask-shaped" Langerhans cell microabscesses; lacks apoptotic keratinocytes), bullous pemphigoid (eosinophils line up at DEJ, subepidermal bullae, and lacks apoptotic keratinocytes)
Infantile digital fibromatosis	Dome-shaped nodule; fascicles of **spindled myofibroblasts** with characteristic perinuclear eosinophilic cytoplasmic **inclusion bodies (PTAH+, trichrome+ , SMA+)**	Scar (lacks inclusions), digital fibrokeratoma (lacks spindle cells w/ eosinophilic inclusions)
Intravascular papillary endothelial hyperplasia (Masson's tumor, IPEH)	**Sharply circumscribed**, reorganizing thrombus within large vessel; papillary projections	Kaposi sarcoma (infiltrative architecture, poorly circumscribed; lacks thrombus), angiosarcoma (very atypical hyperchromatic endothelial cells, mitoses)
Inverted follicular keratosis	Endophytic version of irritated SK (squamous eddies; minimal cytologic atypia; smooth tumor base)	SCC (cytologic atypia; infiltrative deep border)
Juvenile xanthogranuloma (JXG, xanthogranuloma)	Domed nodule, dense histiocytic infiltrate with **Touton giant cells**, foam cells, and **eosinophils**	Reticulohistiocytoma (two-toned cytoplasm, less xanthomatized/ Touton cells), xanthoma/xanthelasma (all xanthomatized histiocytes)
Kaposi sarcoma	Bundles and fascicles of relatively bland spindle cells, **thin "sieve-like" vessels** w/ hemorrhage and hemosiderin, conspicuous **plasma cells**; all forms are **HHV8**+	Angiosarcoma (cells typically round rather than spindled, endothelial cells much more atypical and hyperchromatic w/ ↑ mitoses), aneurysmal DF versus nodular KS (cells more atypical, peripheral collagen trapping, and giant cells w/ hemosiderin), interstitial GA versus plaque KS (mucin, collagen alteration; lacks: hemorrhage, hemosiderin, and plasma cells)
Keloid	Large, haphazardly arrayed, thick neon-pink collagen bundles; acellular stroma	Scar (more fibroblastic, horizontal collagen orientation, smaller collagen bundles)
Keratin granuloma	Thin **flecks of keratin** surrounded by **foreign body giant cell +/–** cholesterol clefts	None
Langerhans cell histiocytosis	Dermal aggregates of **reniform cells** +/– epidermotropism, eosinophils, papillary dermal edema	MF (hyperchromatic lymphoid cells w/ minimal cytoplasm, less edema, halos, DEJ tagging), mastocytosis ("fried egg" cells), spongiotic dermatitis (Langerhans cell microabscesses in epidermis but only scattered Langerhans cells in dermis)
LCV	Perivascular **neutrophilic infiltrate** with **leukocytoclasis, fibrin deposition, vascular damage**, and RBC extravasation	Urticaria (lacks RBC extravasation, vessel damage, and leukocytoclasis), Sweet syndrome (neutrophilic infiltrate way more diffuse; massive papillary dermal edema)
Leiomyoma (angioleiomyoma)	**SQ** nodule, concentric nodules of smooth muscle **encircling collapsed/"slit-like" vessels**	Piloleiomyoma (more superficial, haphazardly arrayed fascicles of smooth muscle; lacks vascular component)
Leiomyoma (piloleiomyoma)	Circumscribed **dermal** nodule, **haphazardly arrayed fascicles** of pink smooth muscle resembling arrector pili, cigar-shaped nuclei, and clear perinuclear vacuoles	Angioleiomyoma (deeper—arises in SQ, concentric nodules of smooth muscle encircling collapsed/"slit-like" vessels), smooth muscle hamartoma and Becker nevus (smaller muscle bundles, hyperpigmented and papillomatous epidermis)
Leishmaniasis	Granulomatous inflammation with **parasitized histiocytes** containing 2 μm dots **around periphery** ("**marquee sign**"), **kinetoplast** (generally only visible with oil immersion microscopy)	Histoplasmosis (organisms more evenly spaced throughout cytoplasm and have pseudocapsules)
Leprosy (lepromatous)	**Grenz zone**; PV/PA lymphohistiocytic inflammation, **globi** (clear cells)	"Grenz zone DDx"(granuloma faciale, leukemia cutis, and cutaneous B-cell lymphoma)
Leprosy (tuberculoid)	Horizontal/linear **granulomas tracking along nerves**	Lepromatous leprosy (Grenz zone; PV/PA lymphohistiocytic inflammation; globi), sarcoidosis (lacks horizontal granulomas)
Leukemia cutis (AML, AMML)	**Grenz zone**; **single cell filing** of immature neutrophils, band forms and atypical myeloid cells/myeloblasts	Metastatic breast carcinoma (larger cells, forms ducts), interstitial GA (mucin, collagen alteration)
Lichen nitidus	**"Ball and claw"** (downward projections of epidermis encircle lichenoid-granulomatous infiltrate), atrophic overlying epidermis	LP (lacks granulomatous component, less circumscribed, +sawtoothing)
Lichen planopilaris	Dense lymphocytic inflammation with follicular interface centered around infundibulum, lacks interfollicular epidermal interface, lacks deep PV/PA inflammation and dermal mucin	DLE (interfollicular + follicular interface centered deeper [isthmus], mucin, and denser superficial and deep PV lymphocytic inflammation), folliculitis decalvans (mixed infiltrate of neuts and plasma cells without interface)
Lichen planus	**Orthohyperkeratosis**, wedge-shaped **hypergranulosis**, "**sawtoothed rete**," apoptotic keratinocytes localized to basal layer, lichenoid infiltrate, and lacks eos (except hypertrophic LP and drug-induced LP)	Lupus (less lichenoid, infiltrate extends deeper, and ↑ mucin), GVHD (less inflammatory, chemo-effect), EM (less lichenoid; apoptotic keratinocytes scattered in all levels), drug-induced LP (parakeratosis, eosinophils), lichenoid inflammation a/w melanoma (subtle melanocytic nests!), lichen striatus (deep peri-eccrine lymphocytic inflammation)
Lichen planus (drug)	Like LP, but has **parakeratosis** + **eosinophils**	LP (lacks parakeratosis and eosinophils)
Lichen planus (oral)	Like LP, but has **parakeratosis; lacks granular layer**	LP (hypergranulosis, lacks parakeratosis), syphilis (dirtier infiltrate [neuts, plasma cells, and debris], swollen endothelial cells)

Continued

Table 7.11 High-Yield Dermatopathology Diagnoses at a Glance—cont'd

Dx	Buzzwords/Essential Features	Mimics in DDx
Lichen planus-like keratosis ("benign lichenoid keratosis")	Like LP but solitary, +/– parakeratosis and eosinophils; generally lacks fully-evolved sawtoothing or hypergranulosis	LP (lacks parakeratosis and eosinophils; CPC often required), lichenoid inflammation with melanoma (subtle melanocytic nests)
Lichen sclerosus (LS&A)	**Orthohyperkeratosis**, edematous-**hyalinized superficial dermis** w/ underlying **lichenoid** lymphocytic infiltrate; follicular plugging; +/– subepidermal **hemorrhage**	Radiation dermatitis (entire dermis appears hyalinized "sick"; non-inflammatory, +bizarre fibroblasts, vascular ectasia)
Lichen simplex chronicus	Orthohyperkeratosis, **hypergranulosis**, **irregular epidermal hyperplasia**, and papillary dermal fibrosis (vertical collagen) and angioplasia	Psoriasis (parakeratosis, regular "psoriasiform" epidermal hyperplasia), prurigo nodularis (on spectrum, but more dome shaped)
Lichen striatus	LP-like interface at DEJ + **deep peri-eccrine lymphocytic inflammation**	LP (lacks peri-eccrine infiltrate), perniosis (↑ dermal edema, prominent endothelial cell swelling; lacks prominent interface)
Linear IgA dermatosis/chronic bullous disease of childhood	**Neutrophil-rich subepidermal bullae**, DIF+ (linear IgA along BMZ)	DH (blistering usually more focal, DIF easily distinguishes), bullous SLE (DIF easily distinguishes)
Lipodermatosclerosis	Lipomembranous fat necrosis ("**frost on window pane**"), dermal and pannicular fibrosis, +/– **stasis** changes	Lupus panniculitis/profundus (may have lipomembranous changes but also has "waxy pink" fat hyalinization, dense PV inflammation, and mucin)
Livedoid vasculopathy (atrophie blanche)	Thick pink fibrin ("**pink-red crayon**") deposition in vessel walls	LCV (more inflammatory w/ perivascular neutrophilic infiltrate, vessel destruction and leukocytoclasis); PCT (cell-poor subepidermal bulla, caterpillar bodies, + solar elastosis)
Lobomycosis	Numerous large organisms linked together in chains ("**pop bead-like**"), granulomatous infiltrate	Blastomycosis (similar size, but does not form long chains)
Lobular capillary hemangioma (pyogenic granuloma)	Polypoid or nodular, **lobular proliferation of endothelial cells** and small capillary-sized vessels, noninfiltrative architecture, +/– ulceration	Bacillary angiomatosis (similar, but more PMNs and amphophilic clumps of bacteria, particularly deep and not just at ulcerated surface), angiosarcoma (infiltrative rather than lobular; atypical hyperchromatic endothelial cells w/ atypical mitoses)
Lupus (discoid)	**Orthohyperkeratosis**, vacuolar-to-lichenoid interface dermatitis of hair follicles (> interfollicular epidermis), **dilated follicles** w/ follicular **keratin plugs**, superficial and deep PV/PA lymphoplasmacytic infiltrate, and ↑ **mucin. Thickened BMZ on PAS-D stain**; clusters of **CD123+** plasmacytoid dendritic cells present in majority of cases (comprises up to 20% of infiltrate)	SCLE (more basal vacuolar change, epidermal atrophy and superficial mucin; less orthohyperkeratosis, dermal inflammation, follicular plugging, and BMZ thickening), LPP (interfollicular epidermis not involved; lacks PV inflammation, mucin and follicular plugging)
Lupus (SCLE)	Orthohyperkeratosis, prominent basal vacuolar interface, epidermal atrophy, superficial mucin, mild superficial and deep PV/PA lymphocytic inflammation	DLE (more dermal PV/PA lymphocytic inflammation, interface changes most prominent at follicles, follicular plugging, less basal vacuolar change), DM (less interface, less inflammation, much more mucin), EM (basket weave stratum corneum, lacks deep PV/PA inflammation and mucin), GVHD (chemotherapy-induced epidermal dysmaturation, less deep PV/PA inflammation, lacks mucin), and FDE (basket weave corneum, more eosinophils and pigment incontinence; lacks mucin)
Lupus (tumid)	**Massively increased dermal mucin** (rivaling DM), moderately dense superficial and deep PV/PA lymphocytic inflammation. Typically minimal to no interface changes	Jessner's lymphocytic infiltrate and gyrate erythema (lack mucin), DM (subtle vacuolar interface, lacks significant dermal PV/PA inflammation), perniosis (acral skin, spongiosis and dermal edema; lacks mucin)
Lupus profundus/panniculitis	**Hyaline lobular fat necrosis ("pink wax"** appearance), **nodular lymphoid aggregates w/ plasma cells**, interface changes (20%–50%), +/– mucin, +/– lipomembranous changes; **clusters of CD123+** plasmacytoid dendritic cells present in majority of cases (comprises up to 20% of infiltrate; helps differentiate from SPTCL)	Gamma-delta T-cell lymphoma (close mimic! Has interface dermatitis, fat rimming by atypical lymphocytes, angiotropism/angiodestruction; lacks nodular lymphoid aggregates and plasma cells), SPTCL (fat rimming by atypical lymphocytes, lacks interface, and lacks nodular lymphoid aggregates; lacks clusters of CD123+ cells → useful stain!)
Lymphangioma	Pink lymphatic fluid with widely ectatic lymphatic vessels and intraluminal valves	Venous lake (RBCs within solitary ectatic vessel that lacks valves), Inflammatory metastatic carcinoma (anytime there are dilated lymphatics, check carefully for evidence of metastatic tumor obstructing lymphatics upstream)
Lymphomatoid papulosis (Type A)	Dense **wedge-shaped** infiltrate w/ **neutrophils, eosinophils, and large CD30+ Reed-Sternberg-like cells**; +/– RBC extravasation; lichenoid interface and ulceration	PLEVA (purely lymphocytic, lacks eosinophils), ALCL, and MF w/ large cell transformation (need clinical history) ***Other LyP Types** (less commonly tested)—Type B: MF-like; CD4+, CD8– with few CD30+ cells. Type C: ALCL-like with sheets of large CD4+, CD8–, CD30+ cells. Type D: Epidermotropic infiltrate of CD4–, CD8+, CD30+ T cells; mimics aggressive epidermotropic T-cell lymphoma. Type E: Angioinvasive CD4–, CD8+, CD30+ infiltrate with fibrinous vasculitis and thrombi; mimics Gamma delta T-cell lymphoma. Type 6p25.3: Pagetoid infiltrate of small CD4–, CD8–, CD30+ T cells with dense dermal infiltrate of large atypical lymphocytes; mimics Pagetoid reticulosis

Table 7.11 High-Yield Dermatopathology Diagnoses at a Glance—cont'd

Dx	Buzzwords/Essential Features	Mimics in DDx
Mastocytoma	Tumoral aggregates of monomorphous "**fried egg**" **mast cells** with amphophilic (purple) cytoplasm	Intradermal nevus (lacks fried egg cells, cells are nested), glomus tumor (vessels present, cells have less cytoplasm)
Melanoma (lentigo maligna type)	**Poorly circumscribed lentiginous (single cell) proliferation** of melanocytes along DEJ and follicular epithelium, arises on **solar elastotic skin**, variability of melanocyte nest size and shape, modest pagetoid scatter (less than superficial spreading type), variable degrees of cytologic atypia	Pagetoid DDx (see Table 7.22)
Melanoma (superficial spreading type)	Asymmetric, poorly circumscribed, often trails off as single junctional cells rather than nests, **epidermal consumption/thinning, pagetoid scatter** diffuse throughout lesion, severe cytologic atypia (enlarged irregular nuclei, prominent "**cherry red**" **nucleoli**), increased mitotic rate, and lacks maturation with descent into the dermis	Spitz nevus (symmetric, well-circumscribed, begins and ends in nests, spindled and epithelioid melanocytes with enlarged amphophilic or pink cytoplasm, "raining down" pattern of nests and cells, clefts around junctional nests, epidermal hyperplasia rather than consumption/thinning, Kamino bodies, maturation with descent into dermis, and pagetoid scatter limited to central portion of lesion) Pagetoid DDx (see Table 7.22) Dysplastic nevus (bridging of melanocyte nests, "shouldering" of junctional component beyond dermal component, concentric or lamellar papillary dermal fibrosis, cytologic atypia; distinguished from melanoma mainly by ABSENCE of diffuse pagetoid scatter, severe cytologic atypia, or consumption of epidermis)
Merkel cell carcinoma	Dense basaloid infiltrate (low power), pale/"washed-out" blue nuclei with "**salt-and-pepper" chromatin** (high power), nuclear molding, innumerable mitoses, stains positive for neuroendocrine markers (synaptophysin, chromogranin, NSE, CD56), **CK20+** (**dot-like/paranuclear)**, and TTF-1-; **p63+ portends worse prognosis**; Merkel cell polyomavirus (MCPyV) present in 80%	Metastatic small cell lung cancer (TTF-1+ and CK20-), lymphoma (nuclei more basaloid/hyperchromatic on high power)
Metastatic breast adenocarcinoma	Infiltrative single cells ("**single-cell filing**") and **small glands** with **cytologic atypia**, mitoses and apoptosis, +/– **intralymphatic tumor clusters, CK7+**	Interstitial GA (mucin, altered collagen, lacks atypia and glands), leukemia cutis (often see associated neutrophils, immature myeloid cells and "band forms"; lacks gland formation), primary cutaneous adnexal/adenocarcinomas (p63+ and CK5/6+, unlike metastatic adenocarcinomas)
Metastatic colon adenocarcinoma	Infiltrative glands with cytologic atypia, mitoses and tumor necrosis ("**dirty necrosis**"). **CK20+**	Endometriosis (larger glands lacking atypia, fibromyxoid or edematous stroma surrounds glands, extravasated RBCs), primary cutaneous adnexal/adenocarcinomas (p63+ and CK5/6+, unlike metastatic adenocarcinomas)
Metastatic renal (clear) cell carcinoma	Dense pan-dermal proliferation of **clear cells**; **highly vascular** lesion with dermal hemorrhage, **PAX8+**	Clear cell hidradenoma (in addition to clear cells, also contains squamoid cells, sweat ducts, and a hyalinized/keloidal stroma), balloon cell nevus (can always identify conventional nevus nests elsewhere in lesion, melanophages, lacks hemorrhage and increased vascularity)
Microcystic adnexal carcinoma	See Chapter 6, Neoplastic Dermatology	See Chapter 6, Neoplastic Dermatology
Mixed tumor (chondroid syringoma)	See Chapter 6, Neoplastic Dermatology	See Chapter 6, Neoplastic Dermatology
Morpheaform BCC	Angulated strands and islands of atypical basaloid cells, clefting, numerous apoptoses and mitoses	Desmoplastic trichoepithelioma (small tadpole/"paisley tie" shaped basaloid epithelial islands and nests, fibroblast-rich pink stroma, abundant small horn cysts w/ calcifications), syringoma (basaloid tadpoles with sweat ducts containing eosinophilic cuticle and amorphous pink sweat; sclerotic stroma; lacks horn cysts and calcifications), MAC (mixed follicular and sweat gland differentiation; extends deeper, with perineural invasion and lymphoid aggregates)
Mucinous carcinoma	See Chapter 6, Neoplastic Dermatology	See Chapter 6, Neoplastic Dermatology
Mucocele	Circumscribed nodule of mucin, **mucosal location,** minor salivary glands present; **no true cyst lining** but fibrohistiocytic pseudocyst lining can be present	Digital mucous cyst (acral), nerve sheath myxoma (aka "neurothekeoma"; multiple hypocellular dermal nodules comprised of abundant mucin and scattered spindled/fibroblast-like cells)
Mycosis fungoides	**Epidermotropism**, **Pautrier microabscesses**, hyperchromatic **cerebriform lymphocytes** surrounded by halo, superficial band-like lymphocytic infiltrate, "**bare underbelly" sign**, "wiry" papillary dermal fibrosis), and minimal spongiosis relative to degree of lymphocytes in epidermis	Melanoma in situ (nested pigmented melanocytes), SCCIS (dyskeratotic keratinocytes, solar elastosis), Paget's/EMPD (mucin within nests, ducts), and LCH (reniform cells with increased cytoplasm, papillary dermal edema)

Continued

Table 7.11 High-Yield Dermatopathology Diagnoses at a Glance—cont'd

Dx	Buzzwords/Essential Features	Mimics in DDx
Myofibroma/ myopericytoma	**Biphasic proliferation**: (1) **hypocellular** areas of blue-pink nodules (may appear cartilaginous, "myoid," or hyalinized) with bland myofibroblasts; (2) **hypercellular** areas with primitive-appearing round, blue cells with ↑ N:C ratio, and ectatic "**staghorn**"/"**hemangiopericytoma-like**" vessels	Mixed tumor/chondroid syringoma (has sweat ducts, lacks staghorn vessels), solitary fibrous tumor/hemangiopericytoma (hyalinized vessels, artifactual cracks, STAT6+)
Myxoid liposarcoma	"**Chicken wire**" blood vessels in myxoid background; scattered lipoblasts; p16+, MDM2 amplification by FISH	Spindle cell lipoma (resembles lipoma, but has myxoid zones containing bland spindle cells and scattered thick ("ropey") bright pink collagen fibers; lacks lipoblasts, mitoses and "chicken wire" vascular pattern)
Necrobiosis lipoidica (NL, NLD)	**Square biopsy** sign, diffuse "**cake-layered" necrobiosis** (lacks intervening areas of normal collagen), frequent **plasma cells**, and lacks eosinophils	GA (focal zones of palisaded necrobiosis with **intervening areas of normal collagen**, has **eosinophils**; lacks square biopsy and plasma cells), NXG (cholesterol clefts; large and bizarre-shaped foreign body or Touton giant cells; "dirtier-appearing" [cellular debris])
Necrobiotic xanthogranuloma (NXG)	Broad zones of dermal and SQ necrosis + granulomatous inflammation; Touton giant cells, lipidized histiocytes and **gigantic multinucleated giant cells** (much larger than those seen in NL) with weird **horseshoe or osteoclastic** appearance (up to 50–100 nuclei may be present in a single giant cell!), neutrophilic debris, **cholesterol clefts**, plasma cells	NL (fewer cholesterol clefts and foamy histiocytes, lacks the "dirty" neutrophilic debris and bizarre multinucleated giant cells), plane xanthoma (nearly identical appearance)
Nephrogenic systemic fibrosis (NSF or NFD)	↑ **CD34+ fibrocytes in dermis and SQ** septae, variably thickened collagen fibers, increased cellularity, ↑ **dermal mucin,** and **sclerotic bodies** (oval pink blobs of collagen with trapped elastic fibers)	Scleromyxedema (almost identical, but does not extend as deeply into fat), morphea/scleroderma (thick hyalinized collagen, no increase in cellularity, loss of CD34+ dermal fibrocytes, and lacks mucin)
Nerve sheath myxoma ("neurothekeoma")	Multiple small myxoid nodules w/ bland S100+ spindled cells	Angiomyxoma, myxoma, digital mucous cyst, and mucocele (lack multi-nodular architecture)
Neurofibroma	Superficial nodule, **haphazard proliferation** of wavy spindle cells, pink "**bubble gum**" **stroma**, and **mast cells**, S100+, often CD34+ (do not confuse with DFSP!)	Angioleiomyoma (deep SQ well-circumscribed nodule, dense pink smooth muscle cell proliferation with cigar-shaped nuclei and perinuclear vacuole, and compressed large vessels with slit-like lumens), Piloleiomyoma (haphazard fascicles of dense pink smooth muscle cells w/ cigar-shaped nuclei and perinuclear vacuole, lacks mast cells), PEN (more sharply circumscribed w/ surrounding pseudocapsule, organized as fascicles rather than haphazard), Schwannoma (much deeper SQ nodule, much more organized architecture, Verocay bodies, and large dilated/hyalinized vessels)
Nevus sebaceus	See Chapter 6, Neoplastic Dermatology	See Chapter 6, Neoplastic Dermatology
Nodular amyloid	Large amorphous fractured pink dermal nodules; ↑**plasma cells**	Macular/lichen amyloid (more superficial, lacks plasma cells), lipoid proteinosis (lacks plasma cells), colloid milium (more superficial, more bluish, lacks plasma cells)
Nodular fasciitis	**Circumscribed** nodule in SQ or fascia, "**tissue culture-like"** fibroblasts in **feathery/myxoid stroma**, extravasated **RBCs**, and **lymphocytic inflammation**; mitoses are common but shouldn't be atypical; ***MYH9-USP6 translocation*** (present in >75%; other USP6 gene fusions account for remainder)	Fibrosarcoma (not well-circumscribed, atypical hyperchromatic nuclei with "herringbone" pattern, lacks "feathery" appearance and mucin), low-grade fibromyxoid sarcoma (alternating fibrous and myxoid zones, whorling, atypical hyperchromatic cells, MUC4+), fibromatosis (more uniformly cellular, longer "sweeping" fascicles of fibroblasts/myofibroblasts with wavy nuclei, collagenous rather than myxoid stroma)
Nutritional deficiency (NME and acrodermatitis enteropathica)	**Psoriasiform** hyperplasia; **pallor** of superficial epidermis +/− superficial dyskeratosis	Psoriasis (lacks epidermal pallor), epidermodysplasia verruciformis (upper epidermis keratinocyte nuclei light blue, not clear)
Ochronosis	Yellow-brown banana-shaped bodies in dermis	None
Orf	Intraepidermal blister; **eosinophilic inclusion bodies** in keratinocytes	HSV/VZV (acantholysis, multinucleate cells, nuclear molding and chromatin margination)
Osteoma cutis	Pink bone in dermis (purple if calcified), frequent knife artifact from bone being dragged through tissue by microtome blade	Calcinosis cutis (purple instead of pink)
Paget's disease/EMPD	Intraepidermal nests of **pale bluish cells**, compressed basal keratinocytes, diffuse pagetoid scatter ("**buckshot**" pattern), and transepidermal elimination of tumor cells; **CK7+, CK20−**	Pagetoid DDx (see Table 7.22)
Palisaded encapsulated neuroma (solitary circumscribed neuroma)	**Superficial** dermal nodule; sharply circumscribed w/ **pseudocapsule**; wavy nuclei and **well-organized** nerve fascicles	Schwannoma (much deeper [SQ or deeper] and larger, mixture of Antoni A and B areas, Verocay bodies, has true capsule, and large ectatic/hyalinized vessels), NF (less circumscribed, haphazard rather than organized, and lacks fascicles), angioleiomyoma (much deeper SQ nodule, concentric proliferation of pink smooth muscle cells encircle large vessels with collapsed "slit-like" lumens), piloleiomyoma (not sharply circumscribed, cigar-shaped nuclei)

Table 7.11 High-Yield Dermatopathology Diagnoses at a Glance—cont'd

Dx	Buzzwords/Essential Features	Mimics in DDx
Panfolliculoma	Benign follicular neoplasm with differentiation towards multiple components of the hair follicle apparatus, often with cystic component	Other neoplasms with follicular or cystic differentiation
Pancreatic fat necrosis	Calcified necrotic lipocytes ("**ghost cells**")	SQ fat necrosis of newborn and poststeroid panniculitis (maple leaf-shaped crystals within lipocytes, granulomatous inflammation), sclerema neonatorum (maple leaf-shaped crystals within lipocytes, no granulomatous inflammation)
Paracoccidioidomycosis	Multiple **radially distributed** round yeast arising from central larger yeast ("**mariner's wheel**"); narrow-based budding	None
Pemphigus erythematosus	Indistinguishable from pemphigus foliaceus on H&E; **DIF shows granular to linear deposition along BMZ in addition to intercellular staining**	Pemphigus foliaceus (DIF distinguishes, as well as absence of ANA)
Pemphigus foliaceus	Superficial acantholysis (granular layer or upper spinous layer), DIF+ (intercellular IgG and C3)	Bullous impetigo (subcorneal neutrophilic microabscesses +/− bacteria), SSSS (need DIF), pemphigus vulgaris (deeper acantholysis, tombstoning of basal keratinocytes)
Pemphigus vegetans	**PEH** with intraepidermal **eosinophilic abscesses**/ spongiosis; +/− acantholysis	Chromoblastomycosis, blastomycosis, coccidioidomycosis (fungal organisms present in dermal granulomatous areas; lacks eosinophilic abscess and acantholysis), ALCL (atypical lymphocytes), halogenoderma (neutrophilic abscesses, no bugs)
Pemphigus vulgaris	**Acantholysis**, **tombstoning** of basal keratinocytes, follicular acantholysis, DIF+ (intercellular IgG and C3)	Hailey-Hailey (**epidermal hyperplasia**, keratinocytes appear pinker than normal, scattered dyskeratotic keratinocytes; DIF negative), pemphigus foliaceus (more superficial acantholysis, lacks tombstoning), HSV/VZV (viral cytopathic changes with necrotic keratinocytes, interface dermatitis and sebaceitis/ sebaceous gland necrosis), IgA pemphigus (subcorneal or intraepidermal neutrophilic microabscesses with minimal-no acantholysis), paraneoplastic pemphigus (acantholysis + interface dermatitis with apoptotic keratinocytes, DIF+ in intercellular and BMZ pattern)
Perniosis	**Acral** skin, papillary dermal edema, dense lymphocytic infiltrate, and peri-eccrine involvement	PMLE (lacks peri-eccrine inflammation, non-acral skin), lupus (less edema, more mucin), lichen striatus (also has deep peri-eccrine inflammation, but easily distinguished by presence of lichenoid interface dermatitis)
Pigmented purpuric dermatosis	Mild perivascular lymphocytic infiltrate w/ RBC extravasation and dermal **pigment (hemosiderin)**	Pityriasis rosea (in addition to RBC extravasation, has spongiotic dermatitis and thin mounds of parakeratosis), Nevus of Ota/Ito (diffuse pigmented melanocytes; melanin is less refractile than hemosiderin), LCV (neutrophil-predominant PV infiltrate, vessel wall destruction +/− fibrin in wall)
Pigmented spindle cell nevus (Reed's nevus)	Same as Spitz nevus except more pigmented and almost entirely comprised of **nested junctional spindle cells**, +/− overlying pigmented parakeratosis; has **minimal-to-no dermal involvement** (if present, is confined to superficial dermis), symmetric growth pattern	Spitz nevus (mixture of epithelioid and spindle cells, cytoplasm more pink or amphophilic, less pigmented, and has ability to extend deeper into dermis), melanoma (not sharply circumscribed, often trails off as single junctional cells rather than nests, epidermal consumption/thinning, and diffuse pagetoid scatter throughout lesion)
Pilomatricoma	**Peripheral basaloid cells**, central anucleate "**ghost cells**," and **calcified debris**; "rolls and scrolls" architecture	Trichilemmal/pilar cyst (lacks ghost cells), proliferating pilar tumor (also has "rolls and scrolls" architecture but is more atypical and has no basaloid cells)
Pityriasis rosea	**Thin**, nonadherent mounds of **parakeratosis** ("scale is flying away from epidermis"), **spongiosis**, and **extravasated RBCs**	Guttate psoriasis (**thicker, adherent mounds** of parakeratosis; neutrophilic microabscesses), PPD (minimal or no epidermal changes), EAC (also has nonadherent mounds of parakeratosis and spongiosis, but lacks extravasated RBCs)
Pityriasis rubra pilaris (PRP)	**Checkerboard parakeratosis**, **shoulder parakeratosis, follicular plugging,** psoriasiform or irregular acanthosis, thick suprapapillary plates, lacks neutrophils, and **focal acantholysis**	Psoriasis (confluent parakeratosis, more regular epidermal hyperplasia, thinning of suprapapillary plates, lacks checkerboard and shoulder parakeratosis), seborrheic dermatitis (more spongiotic, lacks checkboard parakeratosis and follicular plugging)
Pleomorphic lipoma	Spindle cell lipoma variant w/ multinucleated **floret cells** ("flower-like" arrangement of nuclei); **CD34+**, **loss of RB1** in ~100% of cases ("RB1-deleted soft tissue tumor family" = spindle cell lipoma/ pleomorphic lipoma, pleomorphic fibroma, atypical spindle cell/pleomorphic lipomatous tumor, and other less common entities; most RB1-deleted tumors are benign)	**Spindle cell lipoma** (well-circumscribed SQ nodule comprised of varying mixture of mature adipocytes, "**ropy collagen**," and bland CD34+ spindle cells with loss of RB1; distinguished from pleomorphic lipoma by lack of floret cells), atypical lipomatous tumor/well-differentiated liposarcoma (ALT/WDL; ~always observe ***MDM2* or *CDK4* amplification** [distinguishes from benign lipomatous lesions], no loss of RB1; atypical hyperchromatic stromal cells in SQ septae, lipoblasts, and mitoses), pleomorphic fibroma (similar appearing multinucleated stromal cells but a superficial dermal process)

Continued

Table 7.11 High-Yield Dermatopathology Diagnoses at a Glance—cont'd

Dx	Buzzwords/Essential Features	Mimics in DDx
Pityriasis lichenoides and PLEVA	**P**arakeratosis, **L**ichenoid interface, **E**xtravasated blood, **V**-shaped ("wedge") dermal lymphocytic infiltrate, and **A**cute epidermal changes (spongiosis +/– ulceration). PEARL: the infiltrate in PLEVA is **almost purely lymphocytic** → most helpful clue for quickly distinguishing from LyP, which typically has conspicuous eos and neutrophils. Pityriasis lichenoides chronica (PLC) has less intense infiltrate	LyP (large, atypical CD30+ cells; mixed infiltrate w/ neuts and eos), lupus (lacks parakeratosis, RBC extravasation, and spongiosis)
PMLE	Dense superficial and deep perivascular lymphocytic infiltrate w/ marked **papillary dermal edema**	Sweet syndrome (dense neutrophilic infiltrate), tumid lupus (less dermal edema, much more mucin, +peri-eccrine inflammation), dermal hypersensitivity reaction (eosinophils admixed w/ lymphs), perniosis (acral skin, infiltrate more diffuse/less angiocentric, peri-eccrine inflammation)
Polyarteritis nodosa (PAN)	Vasculitis affecting an isolated (or a few) medium-sized deep dermal/pannicular arteriole; **minimal to no involvement of fat lobules** away from affected vessel	Erythema induratum (much more extensive lobular involvement with fat necrosis and thickened fibrous septae), LCV (affects more superficial vessels), thrombophlebitis (involves veins, not arterioles)
Porokeratosis	**Cornoid lamellae** +/– lichenoid inflammation and reactive epidermal atypia	AK (lacks angled cornoid lamellae)
Poroma	See Chapter 6, Neoplastic Dermatology	See Chapter 6, Neoplastic Dermatology
Pretibial myxedema	Abundant **mucin** concentrated in mid to lower dermis, **widely spaced wispy collagen**, and no significant increase in fibroblasts	Scleromyxedema and NSF (abundant spindled cells, less mucin), scleredema (milder increase in mucin; mucin more evenly distributed throughout dermis, square biopsy sign)
Proliferating pilar (trichilemmal) cyst/tumor	Complex cyst w/ "rolls and scrolls" pattern, squamoid epithelium, and central dense pink trichilemmal keratin, **lacks granular layer**	Pilomatricoma (also has "rolls and scrolls" architecture, but has basaloid peripheral germinative cells, central anucleate ghost cells, and more frequent calcification and/or ossification)
Protothecosis	**Morulae** ("soccer ball" appearance)	None
Pseudoxanthoma elasticum	Calcified, curly, and purple elastic fibers in dermis ("PXE = Purple Pubes in Dermis")	None
Psoriasis	**Confluent parakeratosis, hypogranulosis**, regular/psoriasiform hyperplasia, neutrophilic **microabscesses** (**Munro and Kugoj**), and thinning of suprapapillary plates	LSC (orthohyperkeratosis, irregular epidermal hyperplasia, and thickened granular layer), PRP (checkerboard parakeratosis, follicular plugging, irregular acanthosis, thickened suprapapillary plates, acantholysis), syphilis (lichenoid infiltrate; abundant plasma cells, endothelial cell swelling)
Pustular psoriasis	**Subcorneal pustule** +/–spongiosis, +/– mild psoriasiform epidermal hyperplasia	AGEP (more dermal edema, eosinophils), Candida/tinea/impetigo (organisms present), IgA pemphigus (acantholysis, DIF+)
Radiation dermatitis	"**Sick dermis**" w/ pale amorphous collagen, dilated superficial vessels (telangiectasias), atypical or stellate ("radiation") fibroblasts	Morphea ("healthy, robust" collagen bundles; lacks atypical fibroblasts and dilated vessels), LS&A (dense lichenoid infiltrate underlying amorphous area, orthohyperkeratosis, + follicular plugging)
Reactive perforating collagenosis (RPC)	**Wide channel ("volcano-like")** w/ perforating **basophilic collagen**	EPS (thinner **pink-red** elastic fibers, **narrow/thin serpiginous channel**)
Recurrent nevus	Atypical junctional melanocytic proliferation overlying dermal scar, +/– benign appearing nevus beneath scar	Melanoma (lacks scar and benign nevus underneath scar, or atypia extends beyond scar), epidermolysis bullosa-associated nevi ("EB nevi" have similar microscopic appearance; history of EB is required for Dx)
Reticulohistiocytoma	**Nodular** dermal infiltrate comprised of **large histiocytes** with **large nuclei**, prominent nucleoli and distinctive **two-toned (pink & purple) cytoplasm** with "ground glass" or "oncocytic" appearance +/– neutrophils	JXG (Touton giant cells with more eosinophils, lacks two-toned histiocytes), Spitz nevus (junctional component, pigment, epidermal hyperplasia, lacks neutrophils)
Rheumatoid papule/nodule	Deep dermal or SQ palisaded granuloma w/ **central pink-red fibrin**, neutrophilic debris	GA (more superficial, central blue mucin, eosinophils, lacks neutrophilic debris), gout (needle-shaped crystals), epithelioid sarcoma (pseudo-palisaded w/ central tumor necrosis and atypical peripheral cells w/ mitoses; loss of INI-1 staining, keratin+)
Rhinoscleroma	Dense pan-dermal plasma cell infiltrate w/ **Russell bodies** and **Mikulicz** cells	Lepromatous leprosy (granulomatous inflammation w/ Grenz zone, globi), granuloma inguinale (PEH w/ neutrophilic abscesses, parasitized histiocytes)
Rhinosporidiosis	**Gigantic sporangia** (up to 300 μm) with **central nucleus** and numerous endospores	Coccidioidomycosis (much smaller spherules [8–80 μm], +/– PEH)
Sarcoidosis	Epithelioid histiocytes aggregate to form "**naked granulomas**" (minimal surrounding lymphocytic inflammation)	Tuberculoid leprosy (linear granulomas along nerve, more lymphocytic inflammation around granulomas), foreign body granuloma (frequently see polarizable material), granulomatous rosacea (perifollicular), cutaneous Crohn disease (usually more tuberculoid but need CPC), zirconium/beryllium granulomas (not polarizable—need spectrography), aluminum granulomas (can be basophilic)
Scabies	Mite and/or scybala (yellow-brown scabies feces) in subcorneal area; perivascular lymphoeosinophilic inflammation; **pigtail-like keratin**	Dermal hypersensitivity reaction as a result of other bug/drug (lacks scabies mite), tungiasis (acral skin, bug is much larger)

Table 7.11 High-Yield Dermatopathology Diagnoses at a Glance—cont'd

Dx	Buzzwords/Essential Features	Mimics in DDx
Scar (cicatrix)	Horizontally arrayed ("**East-West**") collagen and fibroblasts; vertical vessels +/– loss of rete ridges	DF (collagen trapping, epidermal hyperplasia), hypertrophic scar (whorled collagen and fibroblastic nodules), keloid (↓ fibroblasts; keloidal collagen)
Schwannoma (neurilemmoma)	**Very deep (SQ or deeper)** nodular proliferation, peripheral capsule, large dilated/hyalinized vessels, **hypercellular Antoni A areas with Verocay bodies**, and hypocellular/myxoid **Antoni B** areas	NF (more superficial, haphazard proliferation rather than organized, lacks Antoni A and B areas, and lacks capsule), PEN (much more superficial [dermis], has nerve fascicles, and lacks Antoni A and B areas)
Scleredema	**Widely-spaced (but normal-sized) collagen bundles** with **markedly increased mucin**; increased dermal thickness; no increase in dermal spindle cells/fibroblasts	Normal back (no mucin), scleroderma/morphea (thickened/keloidal collagen, perivascular lymphoplasmacytic infiltrate, eccrine gland trapping, lacks mucin), scleromyxedema and NSF (increased spindle cells)
Scleroderma/morphea	**Square biopsy** sign, thickened collagen (sclerotic/keloidal/hyalinized), **loss of peri-adnexal fat**, PV inflammation with **plasma cells**, and **loss of CD34+ fibroblasts**	Scleredema (abundant interstitial mucin, normal-sized but widely spaced collagen bundles), scleromyxedema and NSF (increased CD34+ spindled cells, mucin, less collagen thickening, and no loss of periadnexal fat), radiation dermatitis ("sick" or pale dermal collagen, dilated vessels)
Scleromyxedema (papular mucinosis)	Square biopsy sign, spindle cell proliferation with ↑ **interstitial mucin**	Scleroderma/morphea (lacks spindle cell proliferation and mucin), scleredema (lacks spindle cell proliferation), NSF (similar, but extends deeper in SQ septae), pretibial myxedema (mucin more concentrated in mid dermis, widely spaced wispy collagen fibers, and less spindle cells)
Sclerosing lipogranuloma/paraffinoma	"**Swiss cheese**"-like clear holes in fat and dermis	None
Sebaceous adenoma	See Chapter 6, Neoplastic Dermatology	See Chapter 6, Neoplastic Dermatology
Sebaceous carcinoma	See Chapter 6, Neoplastic Dermatology	See Chapter 6, Neoplastic Dermatology
Seborrheic dermatitis	**Shoulder parakeratosis** + spongiotic dermatitis	Psoriasis (confluent parakeratosis, more epidermal hyperplasia, and less spongiosis), PRP (checkerboard parakeratosis, shoulder parakeratosis, follicular plugging)
SJS/TEN	**Confluent full-thickness epidermal necrosis**, **pauci-inflammatory**, +/– subepidermal bulla	EM (lacks confluent keratinocyte necrosis, more inflammatory, lacks eos), coma bulla (sweat gland necrosis), thermal burn/excoriation/acid burn (more uniform keratinocyte necrosis rather than individual apoptotic cells), epidermal necrosis due to vessel occlusion/vasculitis (vessel damage/occlusion is present)
Spiradenoma	See Chapter 6, Neoplastic Dermatology	See Chapter 6, Neoplastic Dermatology
Spitz nevus	**Symmetric**, **well-circumscribed**, begins and ends in nests, spindled and/or epithelioid melanocytes with enlarged **amphophilic or pink cytoplasm**, "raining down" pattern of nests and cells, **clefts** around junctional nests, epidermal hyperplasia, **Kamino bodies** (PAS+ pink BMZ material), maturation with depth, and central pagetoid scatter is acceptable	Melanoma (asymmetric, poorly circumscribed, often trails off with single junctional cells rather than nests, epidermal consumption, pagetoid scatter throughout lesion, increased mitotic rate, lacks maturation with depth) Atypical Spitz nevus/tumor (somewhat subjective but lacks some of the classically reassuring features of Spitz nevi; FISH or array CGH helpful in predicting aggressive lesions) **FISH defects (especially homozygous 9p21 deletion) or array CGH findings (multiple gains and losses) behavior) help diagnosis of MM. On sequencing, *TERT* promoter mutations predict poor outcome**
Sporotrichosis	**Cigar-shaped yeast** surrounded by granulomatous inflammation	None
Stasis dermatitis	Lobular proliferation of capillaries in superficial and mid dermis, **RBC extravasation, hemosiderin**, +/– epidermal spongiosis	Kaposi (interstitial and infiltrative proliferation rather than lobular, vessels are not well-formed capillaries, +plasma cells), angiosarcoma (infiltrative architecture, hyperchromatic atypical cells with mitoses)
Steatocystoma	Collapsed empty cyst, **pink "shark-toothed"** ("dragon scale") **cuticle**, and sebaceous glands in wall	Epidermoid cyst (central keratin debris, lacks pink cuticle and sebaceous glands in wall), dermoid cyst (also has pink cuticle and sebaceous glands in wall; distinguished by presence of hair follicles in wall and central keratin debris)
Subcutaneous fat necrosis of newborn	**Radiating feathery crystals ("maple leaf-like")** within lipocytes + dense **granulomatous** inflammation	Sclerema neonatorum (lacks granulomatous inflammation), gouty tophus (larger aggregates of needle-shaped crystals)
Subcutaneous panniculitis-like T-Cell lymphoma (SPTCL)	**Fat rimming** by atypical CD8+ T cells that express cytotoxic markers (TIA-1+, granzyme B+, perforin+)	Lupus profundus (nodular lymphoid aggregates w/ plasma cells, +/– mucin ,interface changes), gamma-delta T-cell lymphoma (interface changes, beta-F1 negative, TCR delta positive)
Supernumerary digit	Polypoid, numerous well-formed nerve bundles; may rarely see cartilage or bone in center	Acquired digital fibrokeratoma (lacks nerves), amputation neuroma (scar; nerve bundles not as well-formed)
Supernumerary nipple	Papillomatous epidermis, abundant smooth muscle, +/– lactiferous ducts. Located along milk line	Acanthosis nigricans (lacks smooth muscle); Becker nevus (lacks ducts)

Continued

Table 7.11 High-Yield Dermatopathology Diagnoses at a Glance—cont'd

Dx	Buzzwords/Essential Features	Mimics in DDx
Suture granuloma	Foreign body giant cells surrounding evenly sized, round or thread-like, **polarizable suture** material	None
Sweet syndrome	Diffuse **superficial to mid dermal neutrophilic infiltrate** with leukocytoclasis, marked **papillary dermal edema**; lacks angiocentricity and primary vasculitis	LCV (angiocentric neutrophilic infiltrate w/ vascular damage, RBC extravasation; less dense infiltrate and does not have marked edema), PMLE (lymphocytic infiltrate w/ marked papillary dermal edema), pyoderma gangrenosum (very similar to Sweet syndrome but generally has less edema, deeper dermal/SQ neutrophilic infiltrate and ulceration with undermining neutrophilic inflammation)
Syphilis	Psoriasiform hyperplasia (with slender, **"sexy" long rete ridges**), **lichenoid** interface, superficial and deep "dirty" infiltrate (neuts, **abundant plasma cells**), endothelial cell swelling	LP (lacks plasma cells), psoriasis (lacks interface and plasma cells)
Syringocystadenoma papilliferum	See Chapter 6, Neoplastic Dermatology	See Chapter 6, Neoplastic Dermatology
Syringoma	See Chapter 6, Neoplastic Dermatology	See Chapter 6, Neoplastic Dermatology
Talon noir	**Intracorneal** hemorrhage on acral site (foot #1)	None
Tattoo (lead)	Large pitch-black clumps of dermal pigment	Blue nevus and dermal melanocytoses (melanin is not as dark in color), argyria (pigmented silver particles are much smaller and located preferentially around eccrine coils)
Tinea corporis	Hard to visualize **pale-staining hyphae** located within thin layer of compact eosinophilic stratum corneum immediately above granular layer (**"holes in thickened pink corneum"**), overlying basket weave orthokeratosis, **brisk dermal inflammation**, and occasional **subcorneal pustules**	Tinea versicolor (hyphae much easier to see on H&E; located more superficial in upper stratum corneum; minimal to no dermal inflammation; no pustules)
Tinea versicolor	**Easily-visualized purple hyphae and yeast forms** in superficial stratum corneum, **minimal to no dermal inflammation**	Tinea corporis (hyphae in lower stratum corneum, hyphae much harder to see, brisk dermal inflammation)
Traumatic/amputation neuroma	Multiple small nerve fascicles within scar	PEN (lacks scar; more circumscribed)
Trichilemmoma	See Chapter 6, Neoplastic Dermatology	See Chapter 6, Neoplastic Dermatology
Trichilemmoma (desmoplastic variant)	See Chapter 6, Neoplastic Dermatology	See Chapter 6, Neoplastic Dermatology
Trichoepithelioma	See Chapter 6, Neoplastic Dermatology	See Chapter 6, Neoplastic Dermatology
Trichoepithelioma (desmoplastic variant)	See Chapter 6, Neoplastic Dermatology	See Chapter 6, Neoplastic Dermatology
Trichofolliculoma	See Chapter 6, Neoplastic Dermatology	See Chapter 6, Neoplastic Dermatology
Trichotillomania	**Trichomalacia** (distorted hair shafts), melanin **"pigment casts"** in follicle, massive **catagen/telogen shift**, follicular miniaturization with fibrous streamers	Alopecia areata (also causes catagen/telogen shift, and can have pigment casts, but can be distinguished by "swarm of bees" pattern of peri-bulbar lymphocytic inflammation, eosinophils around bulb, and fibrous streamer tracts containing lymphocytes, eos and pigment incontinence)
Vellus hair cyst	Epidermoid cyst containing multiple vellus hairs	Steatocystoma (cysts have attached sebaceous gland, eosinophilic corrugated lining)
Verruca plana	Smooth acanthotic epidermis, mild hypergranulosis, and koilocytes superficially	EDV (blue-gray haze superficially)
Verruca with myrmecial changes	Hyperkeratotic and hyperplastic epidermis with bright pink to purple inclusions	Conventional verruca (lacks bright pink-purple inclusions), molluscum (lacks warty architecture)
Verruciform xanthoma	**Wart-like epidermal surface** with foamy/**xanthomatized histiocytes stuffed in dermal papillae** +/− neutrophils in epidermis	Wart and trichilemmoma (lack xanthomatized cells)
Verrucous carcinoma	Looks like a huge wart with exo-endophytic architecture, "**pushing**" deep border, and minimal to no cytologic atypia	Condyloma acuminata (smaller, lacks deep "pushing" architecture), conventional SCC (more cytologic atypia, infiltrative rather than "pushing" deep border)
Warty dyskeratoma	**Endophytic** ("**cup-shaped**"), well-circumscribed, acantholytic dyskeratosis, corps ronds/grains	Darier's (less endophytic, less circumscribed), wart (lacks acantholytic dyskeratosis and corps ronds/grains), acantholytic SCC (atypia + atypical mitoses)
Wells syndrome (eosinophilic cellulitis)	**Flame figures** (eosinophil degranulation → deposits on collagen) with numerous eosinophils	None
Xanthelasma	Eyelid skin + foamy histiocytes	Eruptive xanthoma (noneyelid skin, extracellular lipid reminiscent of mucin), JXG (Touton giant cells, granulomatous infiltrate, and eosinophils)
Zoon's balanitis (plasma cell mucositis)	Flattened keratinocytes, band-like **plasma cell infiltrate**, RBC extravasation	LP (more apoptotic keratinocytes, predominantly lymphocytes with only scattered plasma cells), plasmacytoma (atypical or binucleate plasma cells, mitoses)
Zygomycosis	Broad, nonseptated, **pink** hollow hyphae with **90° branching**, **angioinvasive** fungal elements, thickened, irregular walls, **thrombotic vessels** with subsequent epidermal/dermal necrosis	Hyalohyphomycosis (narrow, septated, blue hyphae with bubbly cytoplasm, 45° branching; angioinvasive with subsequent epidermal/dermal necrosis)

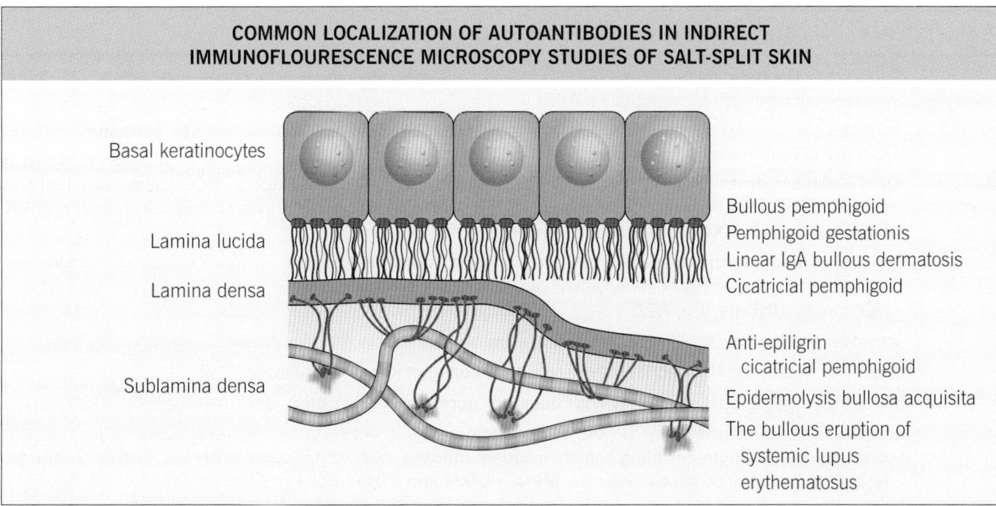

Fig. 7.15 Common localization of autoantibodies in indirect immunofluorescence microscopy studies of salt-split skin. Subregions of salt-split skin commonly bound by circulating autoantibodies in patients with subepidermal immunobullous diseases. (From Yancey KB. The biology of the basement membrane. In: Bolognia JL, Schaffer JV, Cerroni L, eds. *Dermatology*. 4th ed. Philadelphia: Elsevier; 2018:483–493.)

7.2 HIGH-YIELD DERMATOPATHOLOGY DIAGNOSES AT A GLANCE

- Herein, we present an abbreviated summary of the 226 most testable dermpath diagnoses, including their most essential histopathologic features, as well as their mimics (Table 7.11). Because of space constraints, we are unable to include microscopic images of all entities. We encourage the reader to refer to one of the many excellent Elsevier Dermatopathology titles.

7.3 HIGH-YIELD DERMATOPATHOLOGY DIFFERENTIAL DIAGNOSES

- See Tables 7.12 to 7.38.

Table 7.12 "Normal Skin" DDx

Macular amyloid	**Light pink** deposits papillary dermis; pigment incontinence/melanophages
TMEP	Superficial dermal **telangiectasias** + sparse proliferation of **spindled mast cells**; may need **CD117** immunostain or other mast cell stain (Leder, Tryptase, or Giemsa) to confirm (Fig. 7.16)
Tinea corporis	**Pale-staining hyphae** in lower stratum corneum, **brisk dermal inflammation**, +/– subcorneal pustule
Tinea versicolor	**Basaloid spores and hyphae** ("spaghetti and meatballs") in **upper stratum corneum**, much easier to see than tinea corporis on H&E, and **minimal to no dermal inflammation**
Argyria	Small black granules in **sweat glands**
Ichthyosis vulgaris	**Compact orthohyperkeratosis** w/ paradoxically ↓ **granular layer** (almost all other diseases w/ orthohyperkeratosis have ↑ granular layer)
Erythrasma	Organisms one-fifth the size of hyphae; vertical filaments in stratum corneum

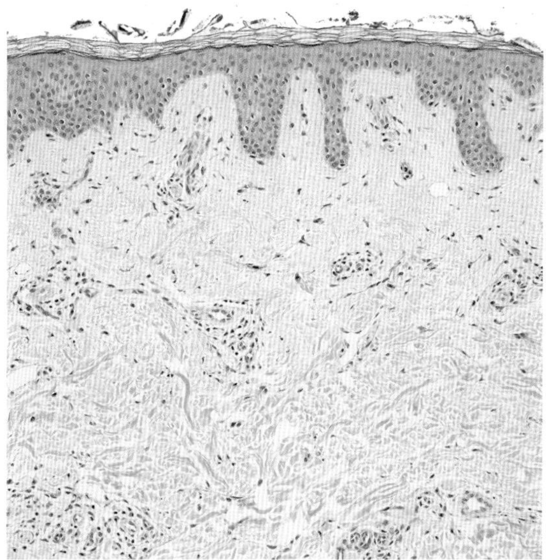

Fig. 7.16 Telangiectasia macularis eruptiva perstans. Microscopic changes are subtle, with a sparse perivascular infiltrate of mast cells that often require demonstration by immunohistochemistry.

Table 7.13 Busy Dermis DDx (Mnemonic: **B**usy **D**ermis **C**an **K**ill **G**randma's **S**weet **N**iece **L**ucy)

Blue nevus	Paucicellular **dendritic melanocyte** proliferation within **sclerotic stroma**, melanophages, and HMB-45 diffusely positive (vs. gradient staining in conventional nevi) (Fig. 7.17)
Dermatofibroma	Interstitial spindle cell proliferation in "curlicue pattern," **collagen trapping**, epidermal/follicular **induction**, hemosiderin-laden histiocytes/**Touton-like GCs**, **Factor XIIIa⁺,** and **CD34⁻** (Figs. 7.18)
Cutaneous metastasis	Most commonly tested: metastatic **breast cancer ("single-cell filing," small ducts)**, **RCC (clear cells, highly vascular)**, colon cancer ("dirty necrosis"); although not always true, a rule of thumb to help determine primary tumor location is: **CK7+** (above diaphragm), versus **CK20+** (below diaphragm) (Figs. 7.19–7.21)
Kaposi sarcoma (plaque stage)	Relatively **bland interstitial spindle cell proliferation**, "**promontory sign**," vascular wrapping, thin **slit-like vascular spaces**, extravasated RBCs, hemosiderin, and increased **plasma cells** (most easily seen in perivascular distribution near tumor); **HHV-8+** (Fig. 7.22)
GA (interstitial)	Interstitial histiocytes w/ foci of altered collagen, ↑ **mucin**, perivascular lymphocytes with eosinophils (Fig 7.23)
Scleromyxedema	Bland dermal spindled fibroblastic proliferation w/ fine **collagen fibers;** ↑ **mucin** (Fig 7.24)
Neurofibroma	Loosely arranged spindle cells with **wavy/ "buckled" nuclei**, **myxoid stroma**, and ↑ mast cells (see Fig. 7.25)
Leukemia cutis	Interstitial infiltrate of atypical cells w/ "**blast" morphology** (fine chromatin, prominent nucleoli, and larger than normal inflammatory cells) arranged in **single-cell filing** pattern; **frequent mitoses**; myeloid/monocytic leukemias typically positive for **CD68 and lysozyme** (two most sensitive markers) > **MPO** > **CD34 and CD117** (see Fig. 7.26)

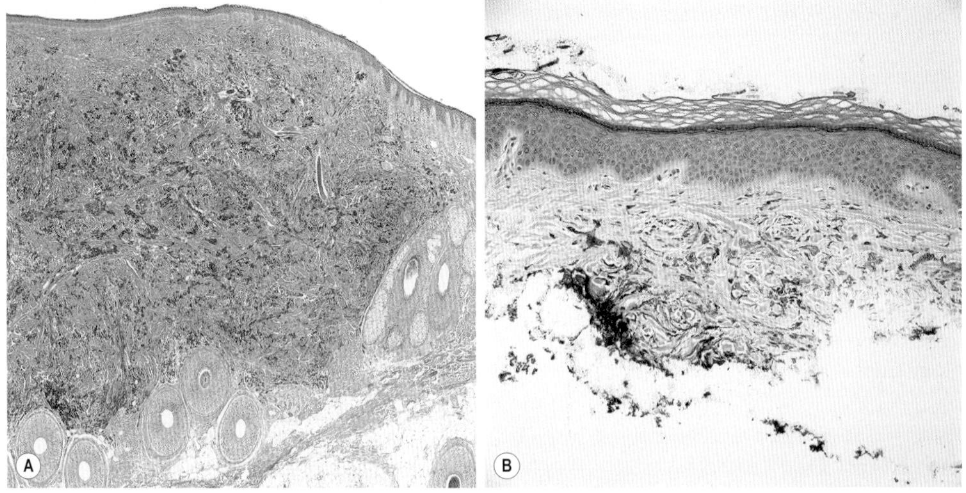

Fig. 7.17 (A) and (B) Blue nevus. Spindled melanocytes with dendritic processes and cytoplasmic melanin are present between the dermal collagen bundles, which are often fibrotic.

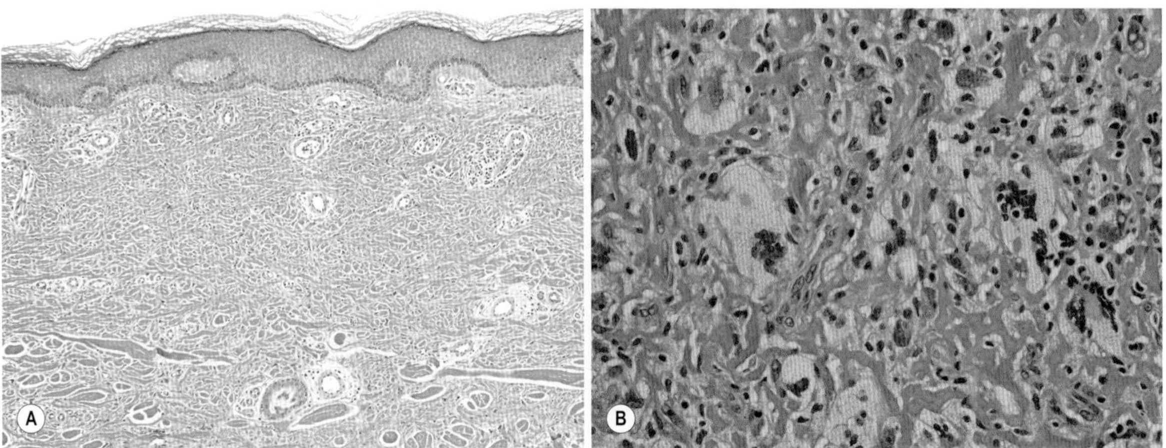

Fig. 7.18 (A) Dermatofibroma. Scanning section shows the characteristic architecture. The lateral borders of the lesion interdigitate with the adjacent dermis (so-called "collagen trapping"). The overlying epidermis often shows induction (either epidermal hyperplasia, epidermal hyperpigmentation, hyperkeratosis, or potentially basaloid or sebaceous differentiation). (B) Dermatofibroma, ankle-type. Hemosiderin-laden Touton giant cells (ringed siderophages) are prominent.

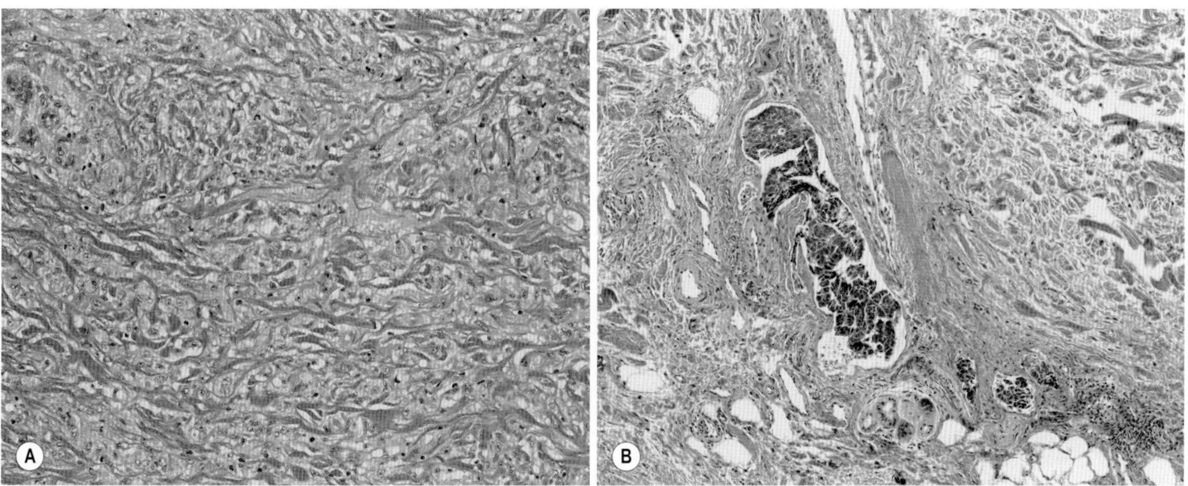

Fig. 7.19 (A) Metastatic breast adenocarcinoma, interstitial type. Atypical cells are seen coursing through the dermis single-file, and duct formation is noted. Breast adenocarcinoma is typically immunoreactive for CK7 stain, with variable expression of ER, PR, and Her2neu. CK20 is usually negative. (B) Metastatic breast adenocarcinoma, inflammatory type. Tumor aggregates are noted within dermal lymphatics.

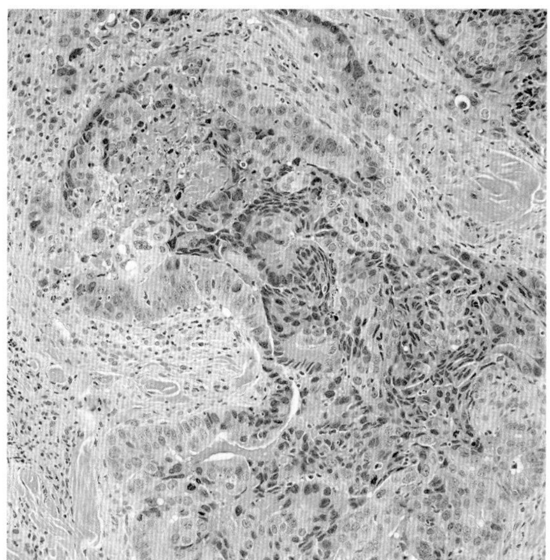

Fig. 7.20 Metastatic colon adenocarcinoma. Dirty necrosis is seen within gland lumina. Colon cancer may stain for CK20 and CDX2; CK7 is usually negative.

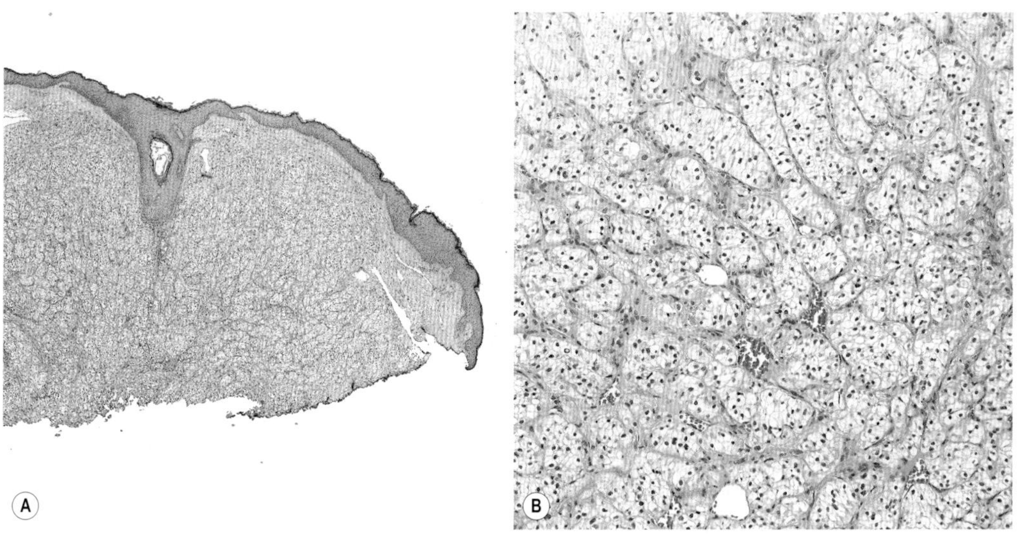

Fig. 7.21 (A) and (B) Metastatic renal cell carcinoma (RCC). Atypical clear cells forming ducts with a highly vascular stroma are noted. RCC may stain with keratin markers such as AE1/AE3, RCC stain, CD10, and PAX8.

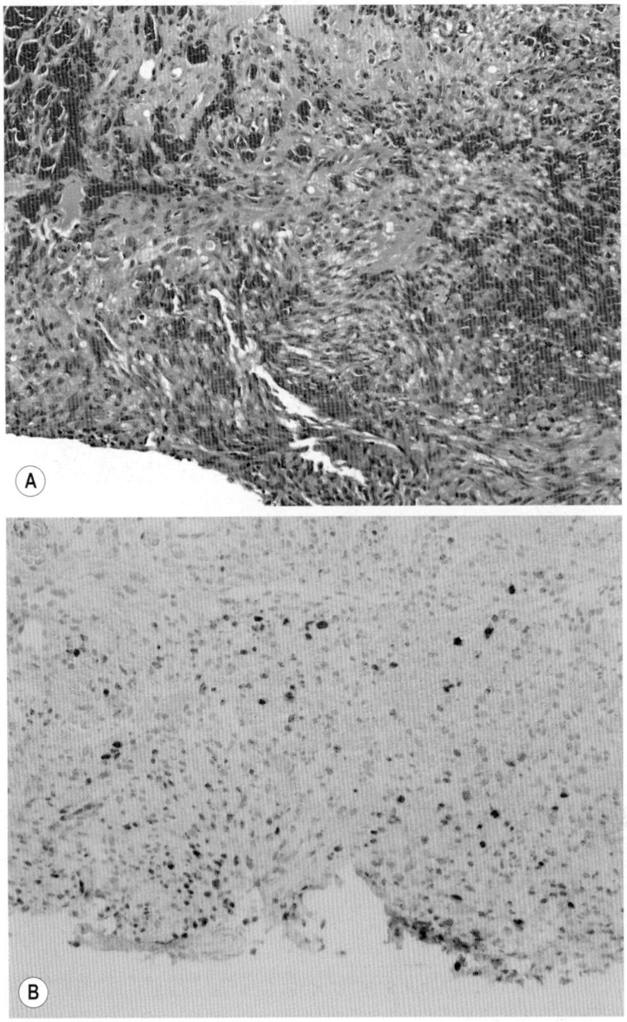

Fig. 7.22 Kaposi sarcoma (KS; patch stage; (A) H&E; (B) HHV-8 immunohistochemistry stain). Increased vascularity, spindled cells with adjacent vascular spaces, hemosiderin deposition, and intermixed plasma cells. The promontory sign, in which new blood vessel formation is observed within larger vessels, may be present. KS is uniformly immunoreactive for HHV-8 by immunohistochemistry.

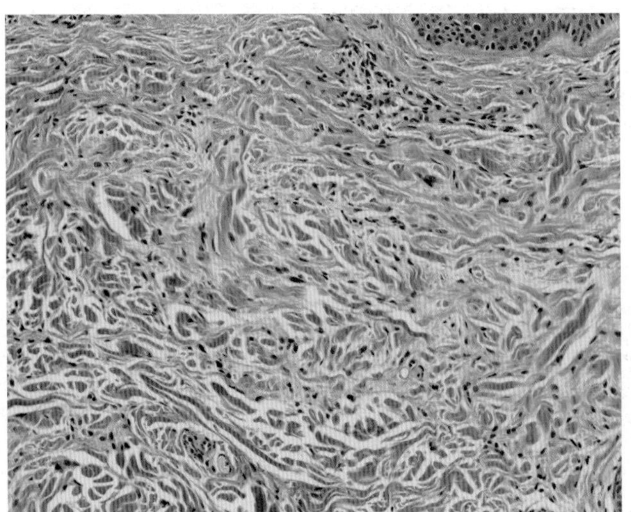

Fig. 7.23 Interstitial granuloma annulare. Increased interstitial histiocytes with abundant interstitial mucin are seen within the dermis (part of the "busy dermis" differential).

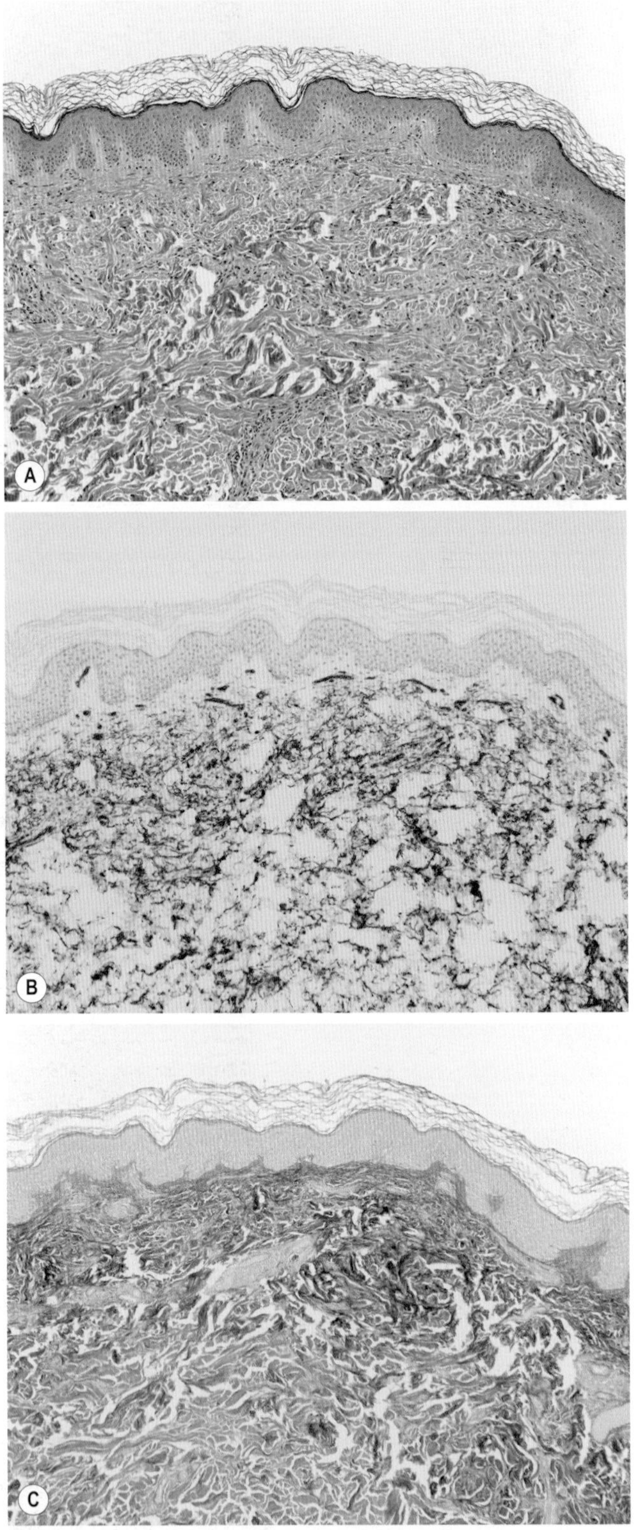

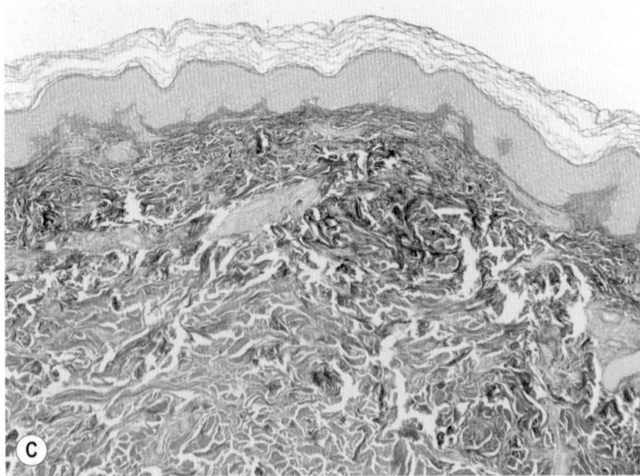

Fig. 7.24 Scleromyxedema (lichen myxedematosus A): Dermal fibrosis with increased fibroblasts (marked with CD34; B) is noted, along with separation of collagen fibers by increased dermal mucin (marked with colloidal iron stain, C).

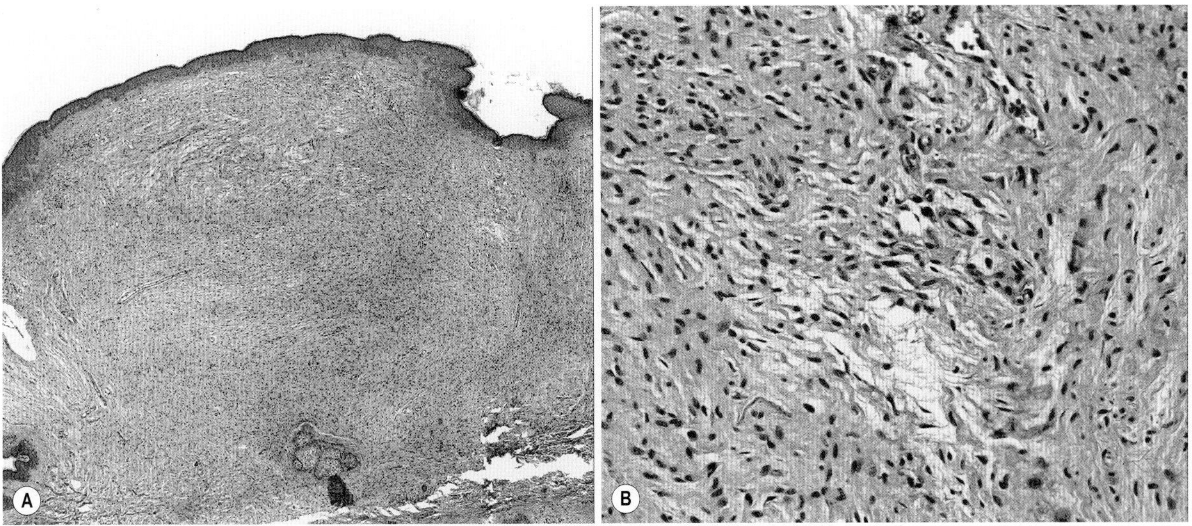

Fig. 7.25 Neurofibroma (NF), shown at low (A) and high (B) power. This neoplasm is composed of spindled cells with "s-shaped" nuclei. The associated collagen has a "shredded carrot" appearance (B). Mast cells are usually scattered within the neoplasm. NF is S100 positive and also may stain with CD34.

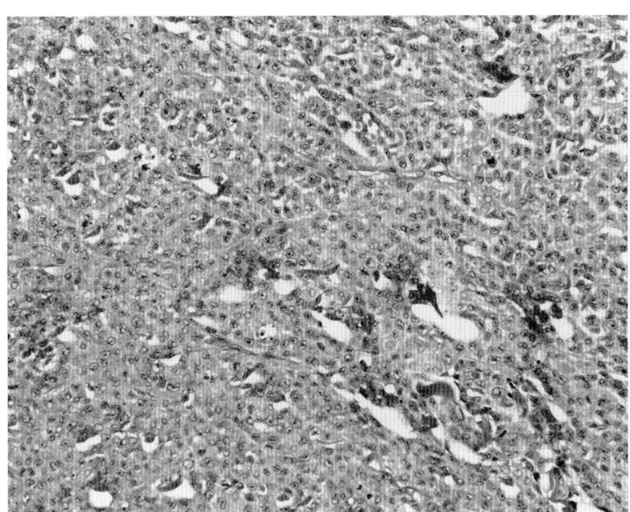

Fig. 7.26 Acute myeloid leukemia involving the skin. There is a dense infiltrate of blasts (dispersed chromatin, nuclear molding), some of which contain conspicuous eosinophilic granules. The blasts usually are immunoreactive for myeloperoxidase, TdT, CD33, CD34, and CD117 (cKit) immunostains.

Table 7.14 Vacuolar Interface Dermatitis DDx

Lupus erythematosus (SCLE)	Orthohyperkeratosis; **brisk vacuolar interface** diffusely affecting epidermis, **superficial (> deep) PV/PA lymphocytic infiltrate**, BMZ thickening, ↑ mucin; lacks eosinophils (Fig. 7.27)
Lupus erythematosus (discoid)	Orthohyperkeratosis; **moderate vacuolar interface centered around follicular epithelium** (> interfollicular epidermis), **hyperplastic follicular infundibulae** (esp. hypertrophic DLE), dilated follicles w/ **follicular plugging**, interfollicular epidermal atrophy, **dermal fibrosis/scar, superficial and deep PV/PA** lymphocytic infiltrate, BMZ thickening, and ↑ mucin; lacks eosinophils (Fig. 7.28)
Dermatomyositis	Orthohyperkeratosis, epidermal atrophy, sparse lymphocytic infiltrate (<LE), **minimal vacuolar interface** (<LE, EM, FDE, and PLEVA), **↑↑↑ dermal mucin (>>LE)** and vascular ectasia (telangiectasias); **lacks deep PV/PA inflammation** (vs. LE), lacks eosinophils (Fig. 7.29)
Erythema multiforme	**Basket-weave** (acute) stratum corneum, prominent apoptotic keratinocytes scattered throughout **all levels** of epidermis, superficial lymphocytic infiltrate w/ lymphocyte exocytosis; **lacks eosinophils** (vs. frequent eosinophils in SJS/TEN and FDE) (Fig. 7.30)
Fixed drug eruption	**Basket-weave** (acute) stratum corneum, **EM-like** vacuolar interface, **chronic dermal changes** (deeper **pigment incontinence**, papillary dermal fibrosis), and mixed dermal inflammation w/ numerous **eosinophils**
Acute GVHD	**Orthohyperkeratosis,** EM-like vacuolar interface, **keratinocyte dysmaturation** (from **chemo effect**), "**satellite cell necrosis**"; frequently involves follicular and other adnexal epithelium (Fig. 7.31)
PLEVA	**P**arakeratosis, **L**ichenoid-to-vacuolar interface, **E**rythrocyte extravasation, **V**-shaped (wedge) lymphocytic infiltrate, **A**cute surface changes (scale crust +/– ulceration); **never has eosinophils** (if more than a few eosinophils present → not PLEVA!) (Fig. 7.32A,B)

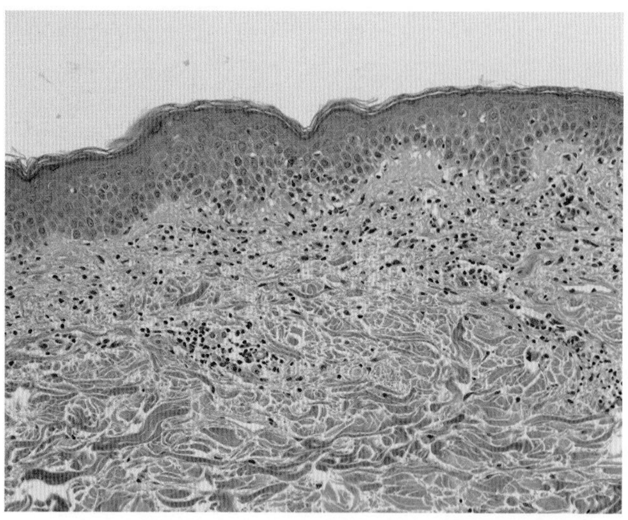

Fig. 7.27 Subacute cutaneous lupus erythematosus. Vacuolar interface inflammation with perivascular mononuclear inflammation. Increased dermal mucin and perifollicular lymphocytic inflammation are often noted. Follicular plugging is a feature seen more frequently in chronic cutaneous lupus erythematosus (discoid lupus; not shown).

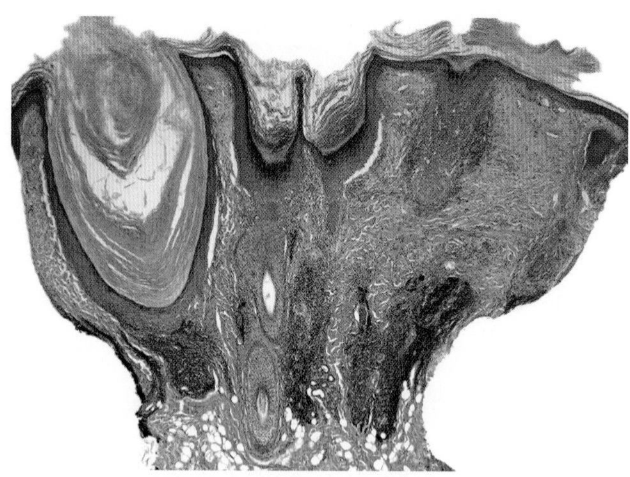

Fig. 7.28 Discoid lupus exhibits follicular plugging, superficial and deep perivascular and perifollicular lymphocytes. There is interfollicular atrophy and interface dermatitis affecting both the epidermis and follicular epithelium. (From Fung MA. Inflammatory diseases of the dermis and epidermis. In: Busam KJ, ed. Dermatopathology: *A Volume in the Series: Foundations in Diagnostic Pathology*, 2nd ed. Philadelphia: Elsevier; 2016, pp 11-78.)

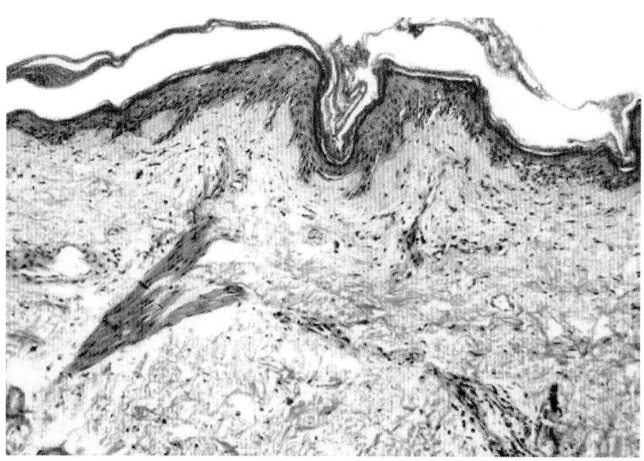

Fig. 7.29 Dermatomyositis: there is hyperkeratosis, epidermal atrophy, mild basal vacuolar change and marked increase in dermal mucin. (From Luzar B, Calonje E. Idiopathic connective tissue disorders. In: Calonje E, Brenn T, Lazar AJ, Billings SD, eds. *McKee's Pathology of the Skin*, 5th ed. Philadelphia: Elsevier; 2020, pp 771-825.)

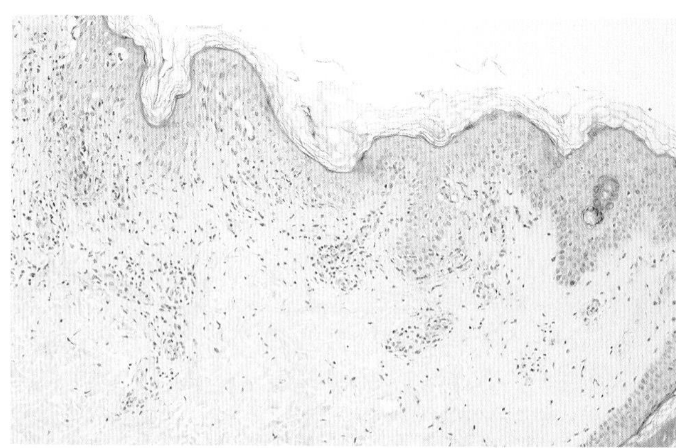

Fig. 7.30 Erythema multiforme. This process is characterized by a basket-weave stratum corneum and brisk interface infiltrate with abundant dyskeratotic keratinocytes scattered throughout the epidermis.

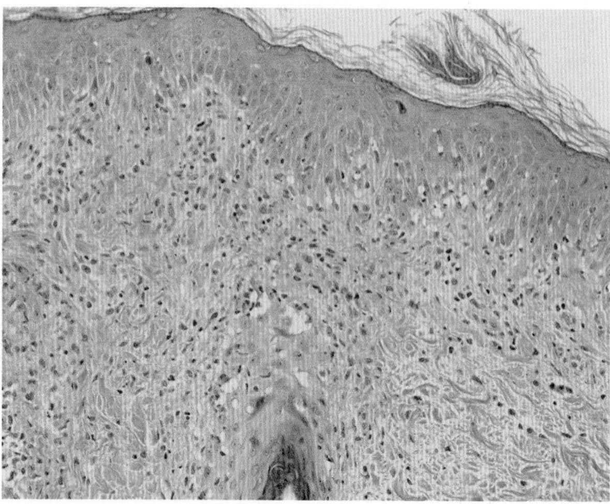

Fig. 7.31 Acute graft-versus-host disease (GVHD), with vacuolar interface changes often extending along the hair follicles and adnexal structures. Though not entirely specific for GVHD, satellite cell necrosis (juxtaposition of a lymphocyte next to a necrotic keratinocyte) may be observed.

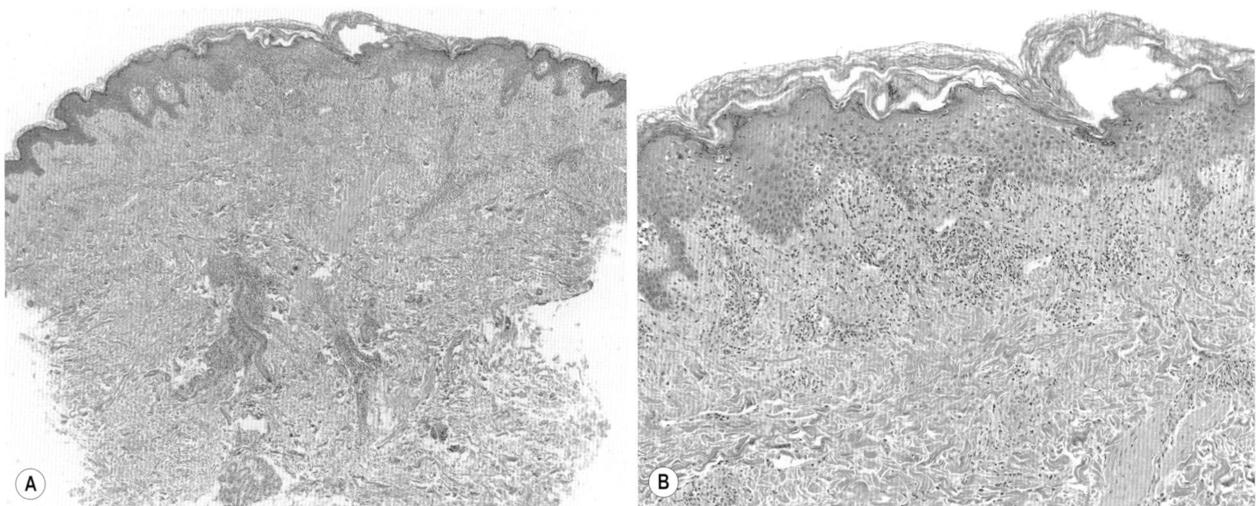

Fig. 7.32 (A) and (B) Pityriasis lichenoides. At scanning magnification, there is a lichenoid lymphocytic infiltrate with scale crust and occasional necrotic keratinocytes. In the acute form (pityriasis lichenoides et varioliformis acuta), the infiltrate is typically more dense and wedge-shaped, includes erythrocyte extravasation, and has parakeratosis.

Table 7.15 Lichenoid Interface Dermatitis DDx

Lichen planus	Orthohyperkeratosis, **irregular acanthosis, V-shaped hypergranulosis**, **"saw-toothed" rete ridges**, and **apoptotic keratatinocytes limited to lower levels of epidermis**; lacks eosinophils (exceptions = hypertrophic LP, drug-induced LP), lacks deep PV/PA inflammation
Lichen planus-like keratosis (BLK)	Like LP, but may have **parakeratosis**, **eosinophils**; frequently see solar lentigo/SK at periphery; often do not have as prominent saw-toothing or hypergranulosis
Lichenoid drug eruption	Looks like LP, but often has **parakeratosis** and deeper PV inflammatory infiltrate **w/ eosinophils**
Lichenoid GVHD	Infiltrate less dense than LP, **satellite cell necrosis**, and epidermis often has **chemotherapy effect/dysmaturation**
Melanoma w/ lichenoid regression	Search periphery for atypical melanocytic lesion; prominent pigment incontinence and plasma cells at regressed area
Lichen nitidus	Small circumscribed papule, **"ball and claw,"** and **epidermal collarette**; dermal infiltrate is more mixed, consisting of lymphocytes, histiocytes, and giant cells
Lichen striatus	Similar to LP, but w/ ↑ **spongiosis** and **deep peri-eccrine inflammation**; usually young patients (solar elastosis rare)
Lichenoid pigmented purpura	Lichenoid and PV lymphocytic inflammation w/ **RBC extravasation and hemosiderin** deposition
Lichenoid secondary syphilis	**"Dirty" infiltrate** (lymphocytes, **neutrophils**, histiocytes, nuclear debris, and **plasma cells**), **slender elongated rete,** swollen endothelial cells, superficial and deep inflammation
Hypertrophic lupus erythematosus	**Mistaken for SCC** because of the hyperplastic follicular epithelium (unlike SCC, the **interfollicular epidermis is typically normal-atrophic**); lichenoid infiltrate resembles LP but has other features of lupus: **deep PV/PA inflammation**, ↑ **mucin**, and BMZ thickening. Clusters of **CD123+ plasmacytoid dendritic cells** on IHC

Table 7.16 Weird Endophytic Neoplasms DDx

Poroma	Uniform small cuboidal ("poroid") cells; multifocal epidermal connections; **eosinophilic cuticle in ducts** (Fig. 7.33)
Trichilemmoma	Lobular architecture, **clear (glycogenated) cells w/ peripheral palisade** and thick **eosinophilic BMZ**, +/– squamous eddies, +/– verrucous surface (see Fig. 7.34)
Clear cell acanthoma	**Psoriasiform** hyperplasia w/ **neutrophils** in corneum, **sharply demarcated** from surrounding normal epidermis ("looks exactly like psoriasis but with clear cells") (Fig. 7.35)
Panfolliculoma (cystic panfolliculoma)	Benign, **cystic** (usually) follicular neoplasm with differentiation toward **multiple components of hair** follicle apparatus (Fig.7.36)
Pilar sheath acanthoma	Acanthotic lobules attached to dilated pore ("dilated pore of Winer on steroids") (Fig. 7.37)
Tumor of follicular infundibulum	Multiple slender connections to epidermis; fenestrated **"plate-like" architecture, fibrous stroma** (Fig. 7.38)
Trichoepithelioma	Basaloid tumor cells within **highly cellular pink (fibroblast-rich) dermis**; minimal to no epidermal attachment (vs. vast majority of BCCs); **papillary mesenchymal bodies and numerous horn cysts** (many calcified) (see Fig. 7.39)
Eccrine syringofibroadenoma	Multiple epidermal connections; anastomosing thin strands of epithelial cells, **ducts**, and fibrovascular stroma (Fig. 7.40)

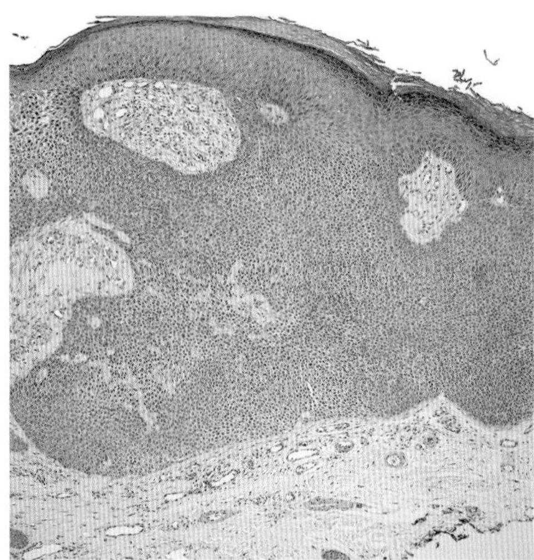

Fig. 7.33 Poroma. This scanning view shows anastomosing tumor islands with eccrine differentiation that demonstrate multiple foci of attachment to the epidermis. Cells are monotonous, with more rounded nuclei than typical keratinocytes.

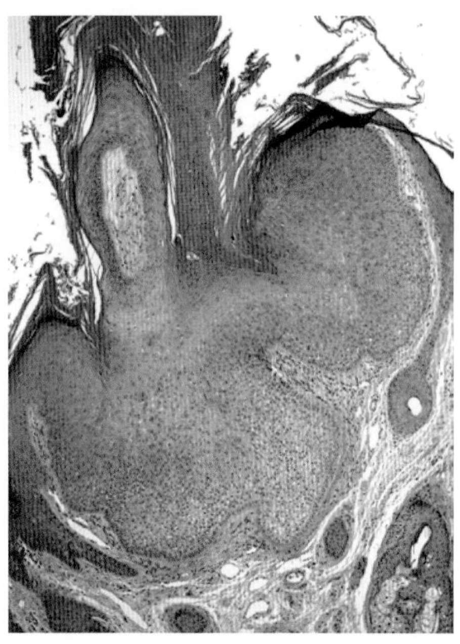

Fig. 7.34 Trichilemmoma. An exophytic verrucous growth pattern is associated with a lobular perifollicular clear cell proliferation at the base of the lesion. (From Prieto VG, Shea CR, Tok Celebi J, Busam KJ. Adnexal tumors. In: Busam KJ, ed. *Dermatopathology: A Volume in the Series: Foundations in Diagnostic Pathology*, 2nd ed. Philadelphia: Elsevier; 2016, pp 388-446.)

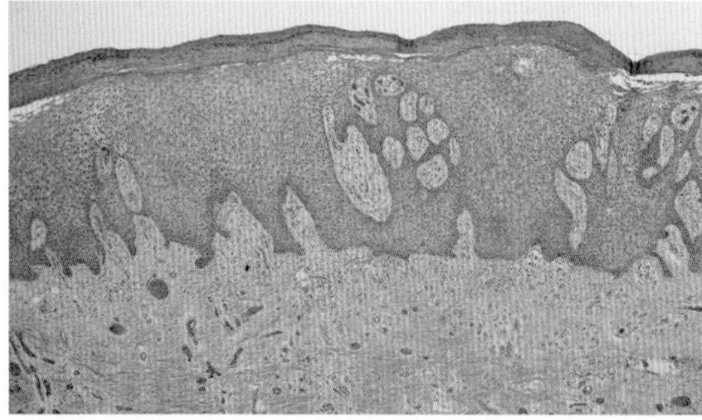

Fig. 7.35 Clear cell acanthoma. Although the basal epithelial cells retain their normal tinctorial properties, most of the epithelium shows marked pallor. Intracorneal neutrophils and loss of the granular layer are frequent findings.

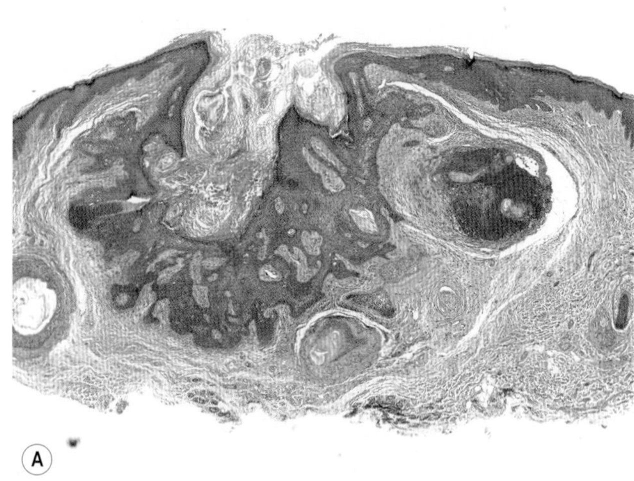

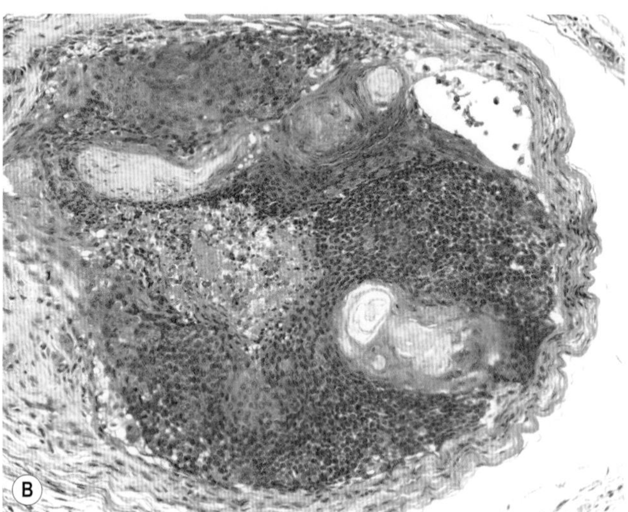

Fig. 7.36 Panfolliculoma. Benign neoplasm with differentiation representing various regions of the hair follicle. (A) Low power. (B) High power.

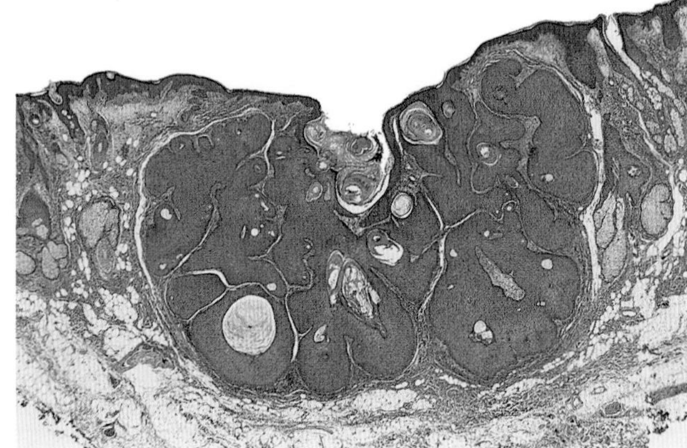

Fig. 7.37 Pilar sheath acanthoma. Tumor lobules, composed of outer root sheath epithelium, radiate from a central depression. (From Patterson JW. Tumors of cutaneous appendages. In: *Weedon's Skin Pathology*, 4th ed. Philadelphia: Elsevier; 2016, pp 903-965.)

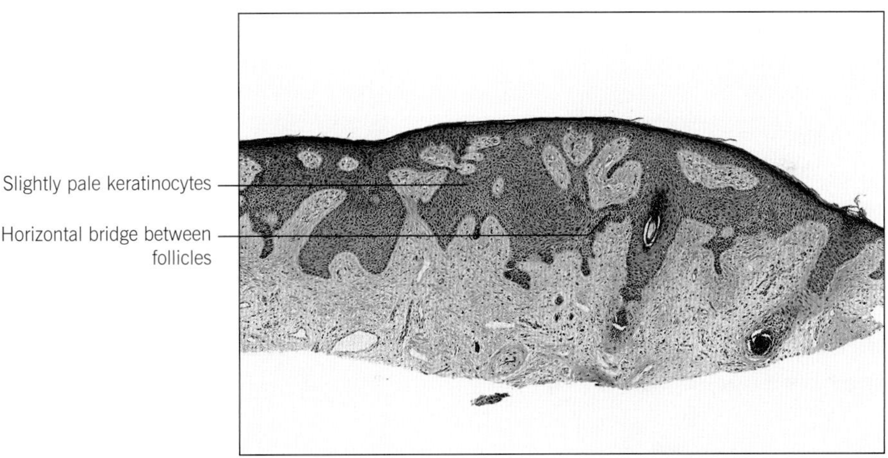

Fig. 7.38 Tumor of follicular infundibulum (From Rapini RP: Follicular neoplasms. In: Rapini RP, ed. *Practical Dermatopathology*, 3rd ed. Philadelphia: Elsevier; 2021, pp 321-329.)

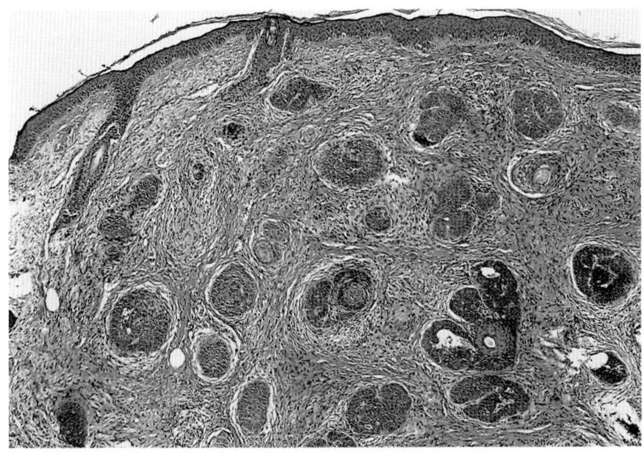

Fig. 7.39 Trichoepithelioma. There are multiple nests of basaloid cells, some showing abortive hair follicle differentiation. (From Patterson JW. Tumors of cutaneous appendages. In: *Weedon's Skin Pathology*. 5th ed. Philadelphia: Elsevier; 2021:951–1016).

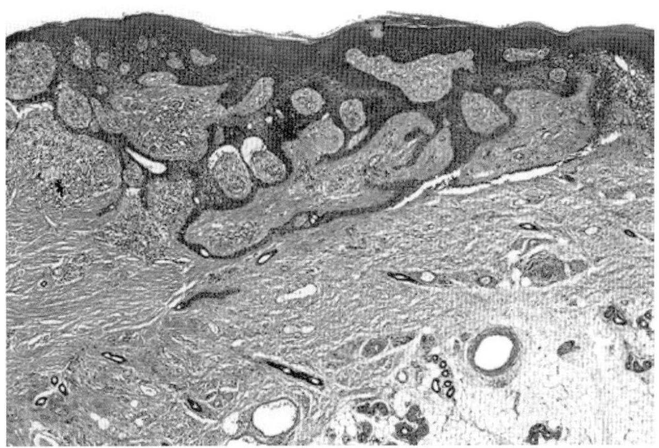

Fig. 7.40 Eccrine syringofibroadenoma: this lesion presented as a solitary tumor. Arising from the epidermis are numerous anastomosing strands of epithelium surrounded by a cellular fibrous stroma. (From Calonje E, Brenn T, Lazar AJ, Billings SD. Tumors of the sweat glands. In: Calonje E, Brenn T, Lazar AJ, Billings SD, eds. *McKee's Pathology of the Skin*, 5th ed. Philadelphia: Elsevier; 2020, pp 1611-1679.)

Table 7.17 Paisley Tie ("Tadpole") DDx

DTC	**Central dell**, bland basaloid epithelial strands, **numerous horn cysts** (many w/ **calcification**), and **fibroblast-rich pink collagenous stroma**; lacks: retraction, myxoid stroma, and perineural involvement (see Fig. 7.41)
MAC	**Deeply infiltrative tumor** (into subcutis/skeletal muscle almost always) with **bi-lineage** differentiation: horn cysts (**follicular**) and small syringoma-like ducts (**sweat**) in superficial dermis + infiltrative epithelial strands in deep dermis/SQ/skeletal muscle; **perineural invasion**; scattered **lymphoid nodules** (see Fig. 7.42)
Syringoma	Basaloid epithelial strands and **ducts** in fibrotic stroma; ducts contain amorphous eosinophilic debris; **lacks follicular differentiation** (vs. MAC, DTE and BCC) (see Fig. 7.43)
Morpheaform BCC	**Sharply angulated** strands of atypical basaloid cells in morphea-like stroma, numerous **mitoses** and **apoptotic cells**; fewer horn cysts and calcifications than DTE; lacks ductal differentiation (vs. MAC and syringoma) and lymphoid nodules (vs. MAC) (Fig. 7.44)

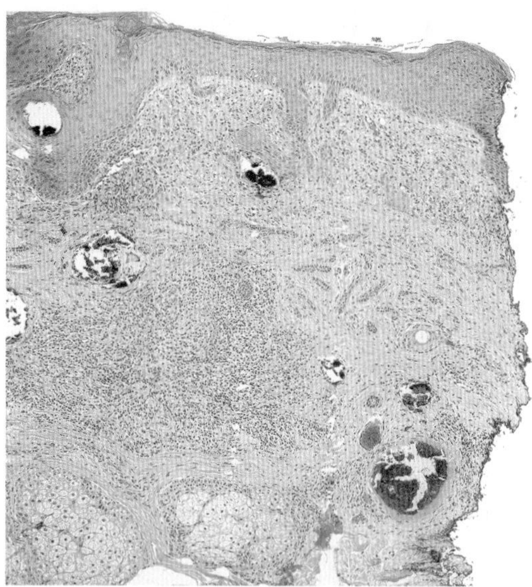

Fig. 7.41 Desmoplastic trichoepithelioma. Central dell, with paisley-tie epithelial cords and epithelial cells demonstrating oval nuclei. Dermal calcium deposits and cysts containing keratin. Usually on the head and neck.

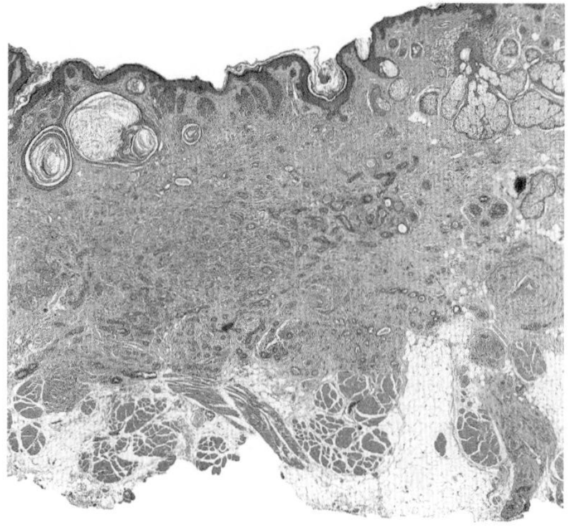

Fig. 7.42 Microcystic adnexal carcinoma. Combination of cysts and ducts, with deep extension into subcutis and underlying structures, as well as perineural invasion, are features.

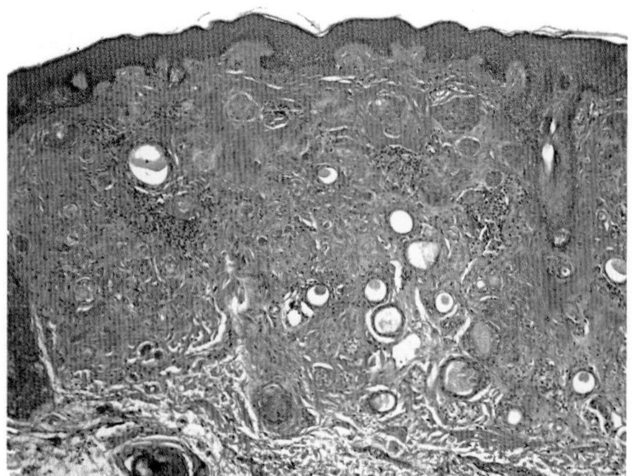

Fig. 7.43 Syringoma. Ducts lined by eosinophilic cuticle and containing proteinaceous, amorphous material. "Tadpoles" with cuboidal nuclei limited to the dermis. (From Patterson JW. Tumors of Cutaneous Appendages. In: *Weedon's Skin Pathology*. 5th ed. Philadelphia: Elsevier; 2021, pp 951–1016.)

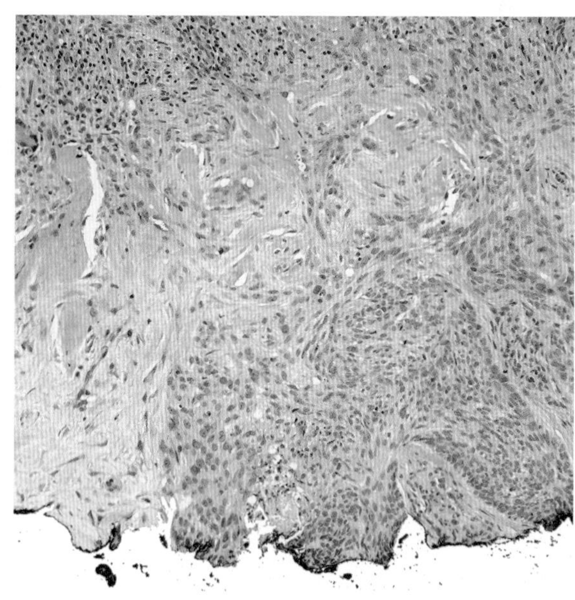

Fig. 7.44 Morpheaform basal cell carcinoma. There is dermal fibrosis and keloidal collagen formation adjacent to the infiltrative islands of tumor. The tumor demonstrates peripheral palisading and single-cell necrosis. Mucinous stroma can be scant. The tumor demonstrates epidermal connection.

Table 7.18 Complex Cystic Proliferations ("Rolls and Scrolls")

Proliferating pilar cyst	Dense pink trichilemmal keratin within cyst cavities; **lacks granular layer**; multilobular proliferations of pink squamous cells; lacks anucleate ghost cells or basaloid germinative cells
Pilomatricoma	Multilobulated dermal tumor; basaloid and pink **ghost cells** within the tumor lobules; **calcification** typically present +/– **ossification**

Table 7.19 Epidermoid Cyst Mimickers

Vellus hair cyst	Small **vellus hairs** within cyst cavity
Dermoid cyst	Complete array of **adnexal structures** (follicles, sebaceous glands, and apocrine glands) inserting in cyst wall
Steatocystoma	Sebaceous glands in cyst wall, **eosinophilic cuticle ("sharktooth"** lining), and cyst cavity appears empty and collapsed

Table 7.20 Blue Balls in Dermis

Cylindroma	Multiple basaloid tumor micronodules fused together in **jigsaw pattern**, small ducts, and thick **hyaline (pink) BMZ material surrounding** each tumor micronodule
Spiradenoma	Larger basophilic dermal nodules with **sweat ducts**, **hyaline droplets within** tumor micronodules, and **lymphocytes "peppered into tumor"**
Dermal duct tumor	Nodule of **monomorphous poroid cells** w/ cuticle-lined sweat ducts. No epidermal connection
Glomus tumor	Monomorphous **glomus cells encircling delicate blood vessels**; lacks sweat ducts (vs. dermal duct tumor)
Hidradenoma	Nodule comprised of a mixture of **squamoid and clear cells** with **sweat ducts**; **keloidal/hyalinized stroma**; +/– cystic degeneration ("solid-cystic hidradenoma")
Trichoblastoma	Dermal/SQ basaloid nodules (solid or cribriform), **fibroblast-rich pink collagenous stroma, papillary mesenchymal bodies**, and horn cysts; lacks stromal mucin and retraction (vs. BCC), lacks ducts (vs. sweat gland neoplasms)

Table 7.21 Clonal SK vs. Hidroacanthoma Simplex vs. Bowen's Disease

Clonal SK	Intraepidermal nests of keratinocytes w/ minimal atypia; cell size ≥ surrounding keratinocytes; lacks ducts
Hidroacanthoma simplex	Acanthotic epidermis w/ intraepidermal nests of **small poroid cells** (smaller than surrounding keratinocytes); **small ducts** present at least focally
Bowen's disease	Full thickness keratinocyte atypia ("**windblown**" appearance) with **atypical mitoses**, **dyskeratotic keratinocytes** (not seen in other two entities)

Table 7.22 Pagetoid DDx

Disease	Essential Features	Immunostaining Profile
Pagetoid Bowen's disease	Clear cytoplasm, intercellular bridges, and involves basal layer	CK5/6+, CK7-(usually), BerEP4–
EMPD/Paget's disease	**Mucin** in cytoplasm; nests of Paget cells compress the healthy basal layer of keratinocytes; +/– ducts (Fig. 7.45)	**Cytokeratin 7+**, **CK20**–, CEA+, BerEP4+ (helps to distinguish from pagetoid Bowen's, which is negative)
Melanoma *in situ*	Pigmented, expect to see some nesting at base of rete	S100$^+$, Melan-A$^+$, HMB-45$^+$
Mycosis fungoides	**Lymphocytes lining up at DEJ**; irregular nuclear contours ("**cerebriform**"), **perinuclear halo** around lymphocytes ("lumps of coal resting on a pillow"), and "**wiry" papillary dermal fibrosis** (abnormally thickened collagen fibers in papillary dermis entrapping lymphocytes) (Fig. 7.46)	CD3+, **CD4+, CD8–** (Exception = hypopigmented MF, which is usually CD8+ and CD4–). Often see **loss of CD5 and CD7** (most common aberrant staining pattern)
Peri-ocular sebaceous carcinoma	**Eyelid skin** (pagetoid spread is rare in extra-ocular sebaceous carcinoma), **pale vacuolated cytoplasm** with indented/**scalloped central nuclei**	**Adipophilin+, AR+**, EMA+, BER-EP4-

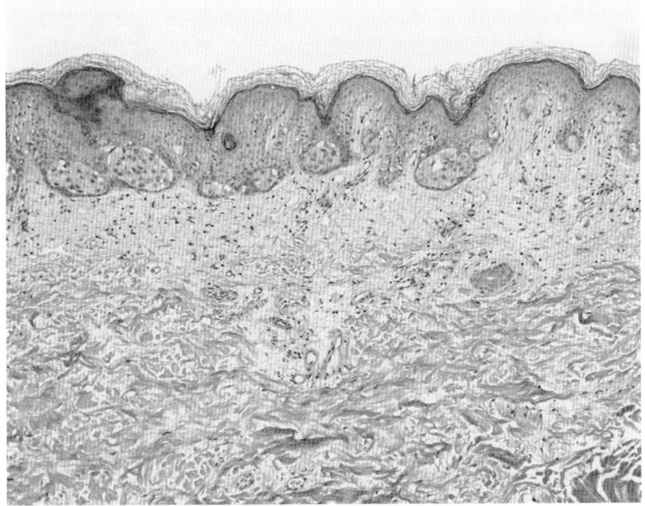

Fig. 7.45 Extramammary Paget disease. Pagetoid cells with ample cytoplasm, sometimes containing vacuoles +/– mucin. Basal keratinocytes are often compressed/crushed by tumor nests (helps to DDx from melanoma, where the tumor nests do not compress the basal layer of epidermis).

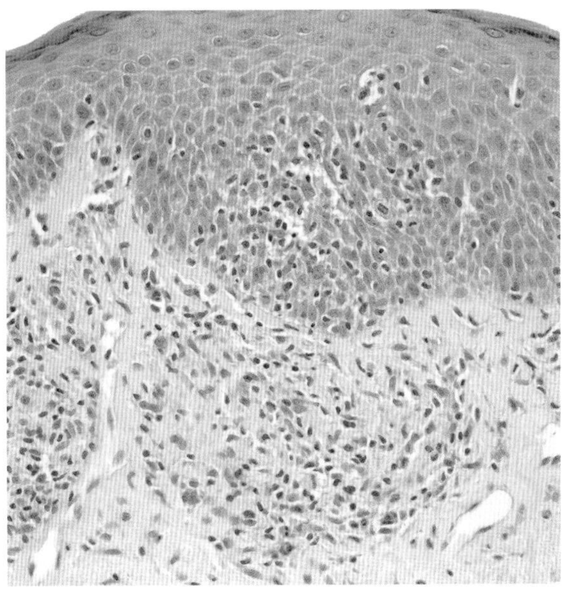

Fig. 7.46 Mycosis fungoides.

Table 7.23 Square Biopsy DDx

Disease	Increased Cellularity?	Essential Features
Chronic radiation dermatitis	No	Homogenized (**"sick-appearing") dermis**, prominent superficial telangiectasias, **stellate fibroblasts**, and **loss of adnexae** (Fig. 7.47)
Necrobiosis lipoidica	**Yes (granulomatous)**	Diffuse granulomatous inflammation w/ **"cake-layered" necrobiosis**, dermal sclerosis (late-stage), **multinucleated GCs**, and ↑ **plasma cells**
Normal skin of the back	No	Normal thickness of collagen bundles—they just extend deeper!.
Scar	**Yes (fibroblasts)**	**"East-West" collagen orientation** with ↑ fibroblast cellularity, vertically oriented blood vessels Hypertrophic scars have "whorled" fibroblastic nodules
Scler**E**dema	No	↑ **Space** and ↑ **mucin** between normal-sized collagen fibers (Fig. 7.48)
Scler**O**derma/ Morphea	No (exception: early/inflammatory morphea has perivascular lymphoplasmacytic inflammation)	**Thick hyalinized (pink) collagen bundles**, loss of perieccrine fat, and deep PV inflammatory infiltrate with **plasma cells** (Fig. 7.49)
Sclerodermoid GVHD	No	Thick collagen bundles, **mild vacuolar interface**, **pigment incontinence**, and loss of adnexae
Scleromyxedema/ NSF	**Yes (fibroblasts)**	↑ **Fibroblasts** in dermis (NSF extends deeper into SQ), mild collagen thickening, and ↑ **mucin** (see Fig. 7.24)

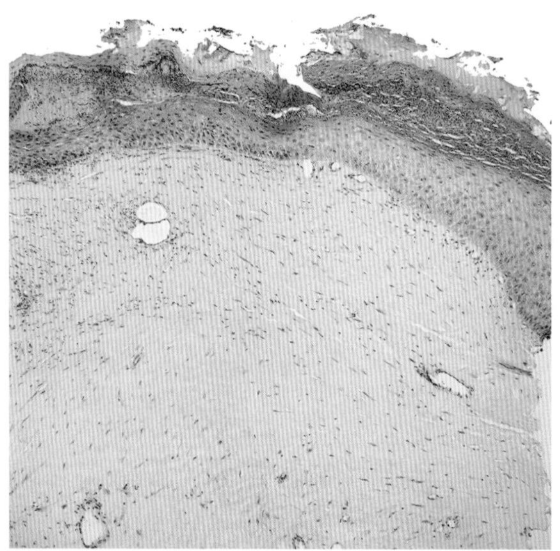

Fig. 7.47 Chronic radiation dermatitis. Dermal sclerosis, with ectatic superficial vessels and bizarre fibroblasts.

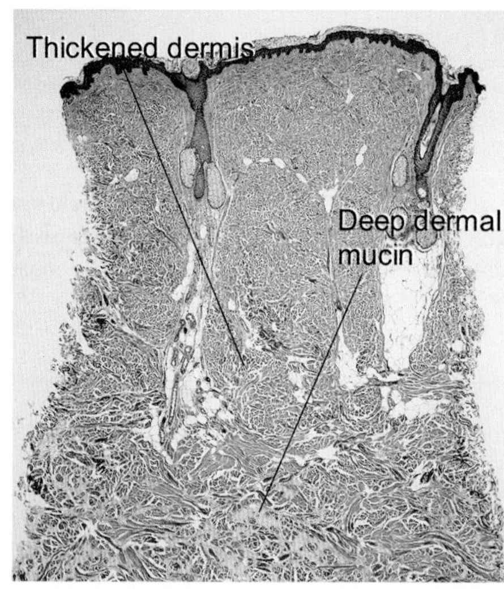

Fig. 7.48 Scleredema. (From Ferringer T: Metabolic disorders. In: Elston DM, Ferringer T, eds. *Dermatopathology*, 3rd ed. Philadelphia: Elsevier; 2019; pp 251-263.)

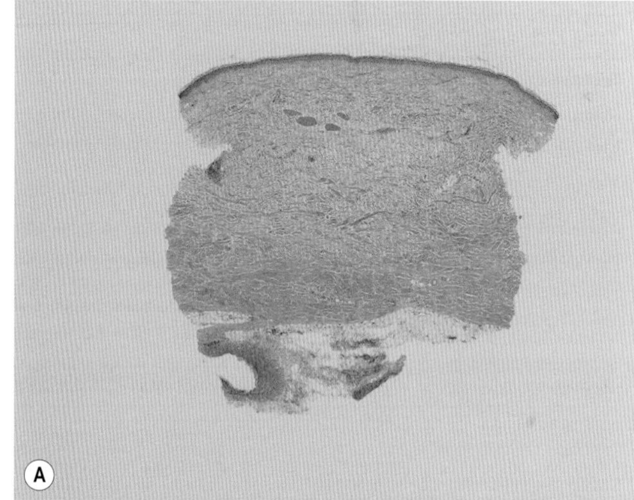

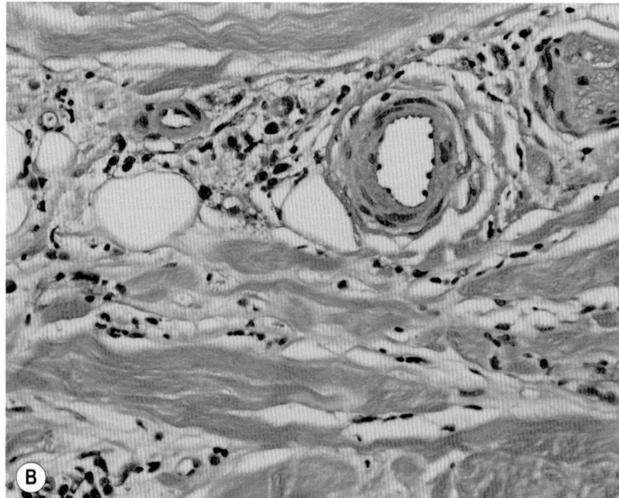

Fig. 7.49 Morphea. Sclerosis of collagen fibers centered in the deep reticular dermis, with trapping/ablation of adnexal structures, and lymphoplasmacytic inflammation in a perivascular pattern (often present at dermo-pannicular junction)

Table 7.24 "SLAM" DDx: Malignant Dermal Spindle Cell Tumor "Slammed" Up Against the Epidermis

Disease	Essential Features	Immunostaining Profile
SCC (spindle cell type)	Overlying epidermal keratinocytic atypia +/− epidermal connection	**Cytokeratin+** (CK5/6, CK903 and MNF116 are most sensitive), **p63+**, **p40+** (most specific marker for SCC vs. AFX)
Leiomyosarcoma	Hyperchromatic spindle cells w/ **fascicular architecture** and **cigar-shaped nuclei** w/ **perinuclear vacuoles (glycogen)**	**SMA+, Desmin+**
AFX	**Bizarre/atypical mitotic figures**; mixture of cell types (**multinucleated GCs**, histiocyte-like cells, foam cells, and **spindle cells**)	AFX is a diagnosis of exclusion! **Most importantly, must be negative for:** Cytokeratin, p63, p40, S100, SOX-10, and Desmin (caution: SMA may have "tram track"/myofibroblast-like staining in AFX) **Most useful positive stains:** **CD10+** (also positive in many spindle cell SCCs), Procollagen-1+ **Other positive stains:** CD68+, CD74+ (weak in AFX, strong in UPS), CD99+ and CD117+ (latter two stains are non-specific)
Melanoma, (desmoplastic/ spindle cell type)	Atypical junctional melanocytic proliferation (often subtle), solar elastosis, **blue-gray myxoid stroma, and nodular lymphocyte aggregates, PNI** (Fig. 7.50)	**S100+, SOX-10+** (differentiates from scar), and **p75/NGFR+** (useful for S100⁻ desmoplastic melanomas)

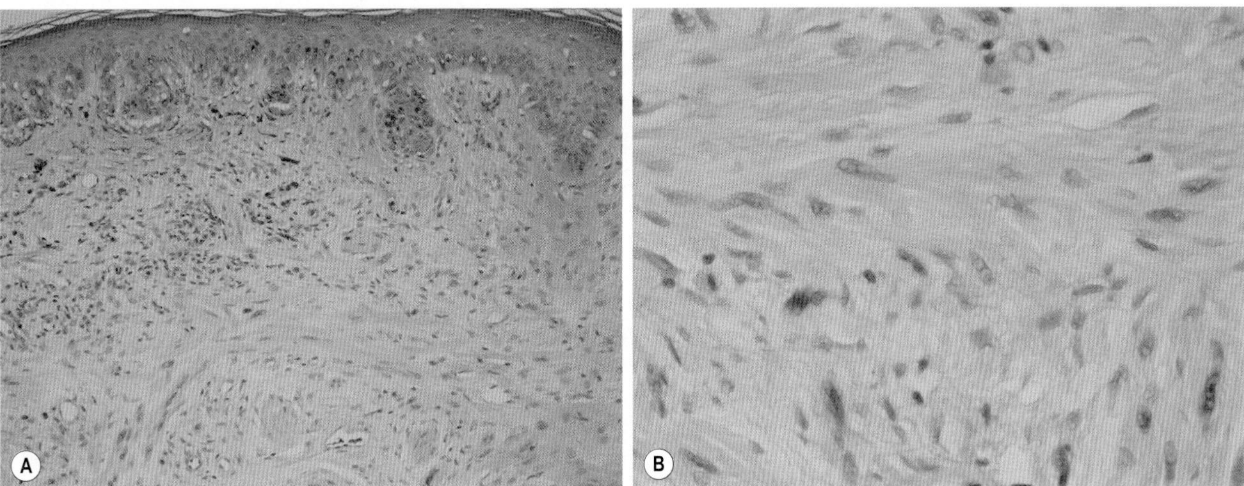

Fig. 7.50 Malignant melanoma with a junctional and desmoplastic component. Dermal lymphoid aggregates may be a clue to the presence of a desmoplastic component.

Table 7.25 Psoriasiform and Spongiotic Disorders

Plaque psoriasis	**Regular ("psoriasiform") acanthosis**, **neutrophil microabscesses** in stratum corneum (Munro) and spinosum (Kugoj), **hypogranulosis**, **confluent parakeratosis**, suprapapillary plate thinning, dilated vessels in dermal papillae, and little or no serum crust
Guttate psoriasis	Minimal acanthosis, +spongiosis, **mounds of neutrophils w/ underlying parakeratosis** (thicker and more adherent than pityriasis rosea) (Fig. 7.51)
Pustular psoriasis	Sub- and intracorneal **neutrophilic abscesses**
Lichen simplex chronicus	**Irregular acanthosis**, **hypergranulosis**, and vertical collagen in dermal papillae; lacks neutrophilic microabscesses
Mycosis fungoides	**Hyperchromatic, cerebriform epidermotropic lymphocytes w/ perinuclear halo** ("lumps of coal on a pillow"); **minimal spongiosis** relative to number of lymphocytes in epidermis, **band-like superficial dermal lymphocytic infiltrate** with minimal to no inflammation deep to superficial vessels (**"bare underbelly sign"**), lymphocytes **"tagging" basal layer of epidermis** ("pigs lining up at the trough"), **wiry papillary dermal fibrosis**, and absence of intraepidermal neutrophils (see Fig. 7.26)
PRP	**Hyperkeratosis** out of proportion to degree of acanthosis, **"checkerboard" parakeratosis** (parakeratosis horizontally and vertically alternating with orthohyperkeratosis), **follicular plugging**, **"shoulder parakeratosis"** (around follicular ostia), **focal acantholysis** (helpful clue), and **thickened suprapapillary plates**; NO NEUTS! (Fig. 7.52)
Secondary syphilis	Psoriasiform hyperplasia (long, **"sexy & slender" rete**); superficial and deep inflammation; **"dirty" lichenoid inflammation** w/ neutrophils and **plasma cells**, lymphocyte exocytosis, and swollen endothelial cells CAUTION: has neutrophils in horn!
Subacute spongiotic dermatitis	Mild to moderate acanthosis +/– parakeratosis, **prominent spongiosis**, **Langerhans cell "microabscesses"** in spinous layer (esp. allergic contact dermatitis) CAUTION: neutrophils may be seen but are limited to areas of serum crust; lacks intraspinous neutrophil microabscesses

Continued

Table 7.25 Psoriasiform and Spongiotic Disorders—cont'd

Pityriasis rosea	Subacute spongiotic dermatitis w/ **thin mounds of parakeratosis** (lacks neutrophils seen in psoriasis), and **extravasated RBCs** around superficial dermal vessels (Fig. 7.53)
ILVEN	**Horizontally alternating** orthokeratosis (WITH granular layer) and parakeratosis (WITHOUT granular layer). Low-power view is helpful.
Tinea	Epidermal changes may resemble psoriasis or spongiotic dermatitis → clue: **"layered" stratum corneum** (compact stratum corneum immediately above granular layer), **"bullet holes"** (hyphae) in compact keratin, and sub/intracorneal neutrophil abscesses
Nutritional deficiency dermatitis	Psoriasiform hyperplasia with confluent parakeratosis AND **pallor of upper 1/3 of epidermis** (Fig. 7.54)

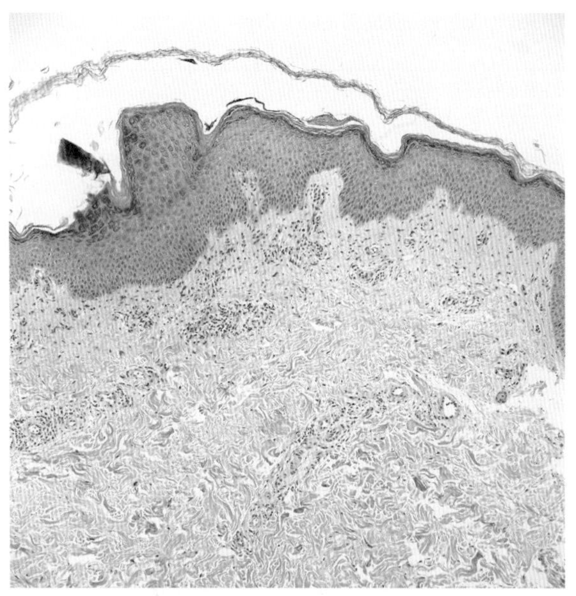

Fig. 7.51 Guttate psoriasis. Adherent mounds of parakeratosis with overlying neutrophilic microabscesses. Only focal hypogranulosis +/– mild spongiosis. Acanthosis is far more subtle than that in classic psoriasis.

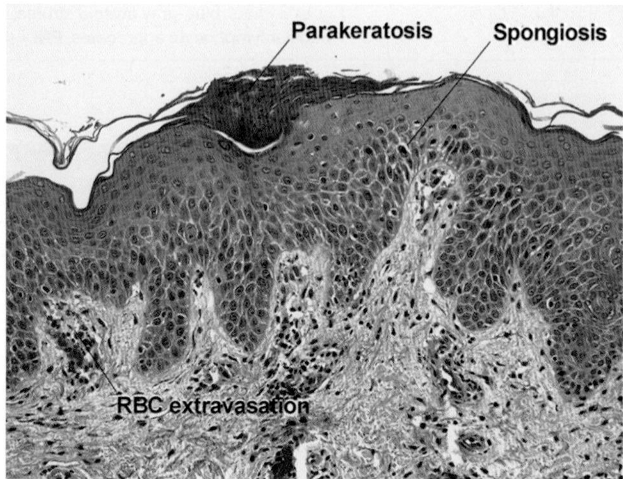

Fig. 7.53 Pityriasis rosea. RBC, red blood cell. (From Elston DM: Psoriasiform and spongiotic dermatitis. In: Elston DM, Ferringer T, eds. *Dermatopathology*, 3rd ed. Philadelphia: Elsevier, 2019; pp 153-164.)

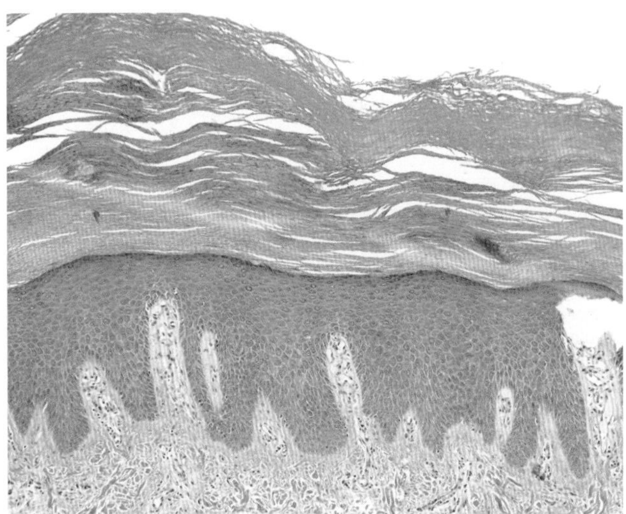

Fig. 7.52 Pityriasis rubra pilaris. Hyperkeratosis out of proportion to degree of acanthosis. Alternating "checkerboard" parakeratosis.

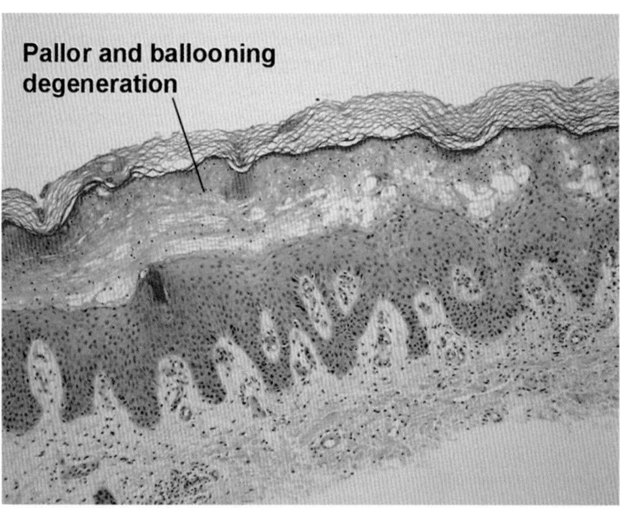

Fig. 7.54 Nutritional deficiency. (From Ferringer T: Metabolic disorders. In: Elston DM, Ferringer T, eds. *Dermatopathology*, 2nd ed. Philadelphia: Elsevier, 2014; pp 224-233.)

Box 7.1 Mnemonic

"Neuts in the horn (stratum corneum) = PTICSS"

Psoriasis, **T**inea, **I**mpetigo, **C**andida, **S**eborrheic dermatitis, **S**yphilis

From Elston DM, Ferringer T, eds. Dermatopathology, 3rd ed. Philadelphia: Elsevier; 2019, p 505.

Box 7.2 Mnemonic

"Subcorneal pustules = CAT PISS"

Candida, **A**cropustulosis of infancy, **T**ransient neonatal pustular melanosis, **P**ustular psoriasis, **I**mpetigo, **S**neddon-Wilkinson (and IgA pemphigus), **S**taph scalded skin

Modified from Elston DM, Ferringer T, eds. Dermatopathology, 3rd ed. Philadelphia: Elsevier; 2019, p 505.

Table 7.26 Acantholytic Disorders

Disease	H&E	DIF	Notes
Pemphigus foliaceus	**Subcorneal split**, acantholysis in granular layer like "shingles blowing off of a roof"	Intercellular IgG and C3	Due to **anti-Dsg1** antibodies Most important Ddx is staph scalded skin → DIF distinguishes
Pemphigus vulgaris	**Suprabasilar split**, "**tombstoning** of basal layer," and **acantholysis extends down hair follicles**	Same as pemphigus foliaceus, but w/ ↑ staining in lower half of epidermis	Due to anti-Dsg1 and **anti-Dsg3** antibodies
Pemphigus vegetans	PEH with **eosinophilic abscesses** in epidermis; subtle suprabasilar clefting	Pemphigus pattern (intercellular IgG and C3)	Clinical variant of PV
Pemphigus erythematosus	Similar to pemphigus foliaceus	**BMZ** (linear to granular) + **intercellular pemphigus pattern**	Overlap of pemphigus foliaceus and cutaneous lupus erythematosus Anti-desmoglein 1 and ANA+
Paraneoplastic pemphigus	Combination of **suprabasilar acantholysis** and **interface dermatitis**	DIF:classically shows combo of intercellular pemphigus pattern + lichenoid changes; appears **similar to pemphigus erythematosus** IIF: positive on **rat bladder** epithelium (because rat bladder contains plakins)	**Antiplakin** family antibodies (including BP-230) detected with immunoblotting or ELISA May be associated with **B-cell lymphoproliferative disorders** (most common), **thymoma, Castleman's** disease, some carcinomas, sarcomas, and even melanoma Associated with **life-threatening bronchiolitis obliterans (#2 cause of death;** #1 is underlying malignancy progression)
Hailey-Hailey	**Epidermal hyperplasia**, full-thickness intraepidermal acantholysis ("**dilapidated brick wall**"), mild dyskeratosis, and keratinocytes have **distinct pink-red cytoplasm** (Fig. 7.55)	Negative	Less dyskeratosis compared with Darier's
Darier's disease	**Acantholytic dyskeratosis** (prominent) with suprabasilar clefting (Fig. 7.56)	Negative	Dyskeratosis manifests as **corps ronds/grains**
Grover's disease	May appear in a pemphigus-like, Darier-like, or Hailey-Hailey-like pattern	Negative	May have mix of all three patterns. If a mix of patterns seen on path, favor Grover's, but CPC required
Warty dyskeratoma	**Endophytic** with either **cup shape** or resembling hair follicle; **prominent acantholytic dyskeratosis** with cells expelled into the center of the crater leaving dermal papillae looking like "villi"	Negative	Solitary nature and **cup-shaped** architecture are the most helpful clues to distinguish from Darier's. Acantholytic acanthoma is not cup-shaped

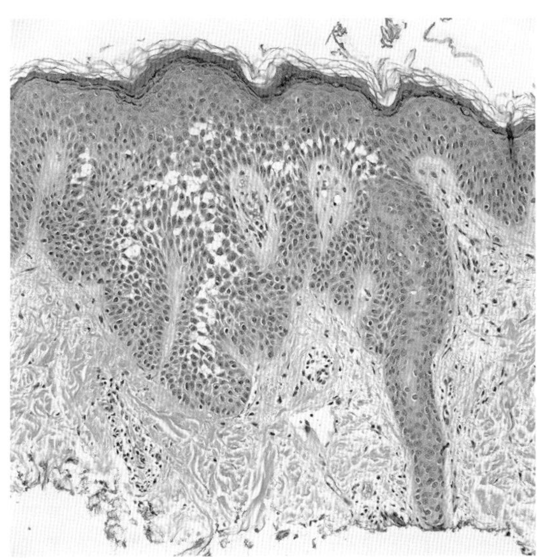

Fig. 7.55 Hailey-Hailey disease. In contrast to Darier disease, dyskeratosis is usually minimal or even absent.

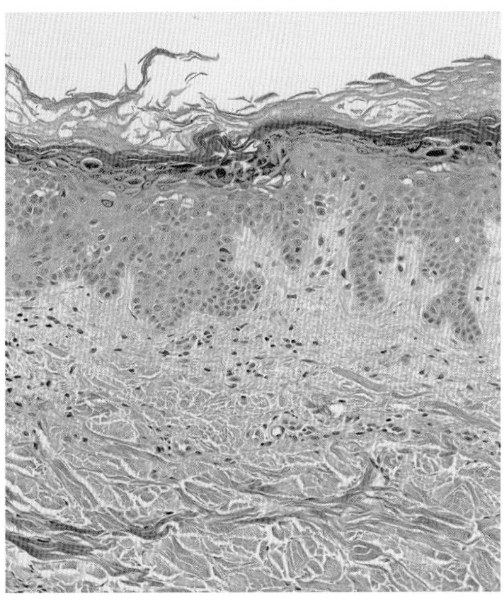

Fig. 7.56 Darier disease. Acantholytic dyskeratosis is seen.

Table 7.27 High-Yield Granulomatous Disorders (Fig. 7.57)	
GA (interstitial)	Patchy interstitial histiocytes, ↑ mucin, lymphocytes, and ↑ eosinophils
GA (palisaded)	Palisaded histiocytes in **superficial-mid dermis** (except deep GA) encircling and degrading collagen fibers; ↑ **mucin**; PV infiltrate with ↑ **eosinophils** (Fig 7.58a and 7.58b)
Gout	Palisaded granuloma around light pink/gray feathery **needle-shaped crystals** (best seen if fixed in ethanol) (Fig. 7.59)
Lupus miliaris disseminatus faciei	Large foci of **caseation necrosis** (amorphic pink debris) surrounded by histiocytes on **facial skin**
Necrobiosis lipoidica	**Layered pan-dermal** granulomatous inflammation and necrobiosis (**"layered lasagna"**), pan-dermal process → entire dermis appears altered, with "square biopsy" sign, and **plasma cells**; lacks eosinophils (vs. GA) (Fig. 7.60)
NXG	**X-shaped** red zones of necrosis w/ nuclear debris within granulomas; **cholesterol clefts** and **bizarre, HUGE multinucleate giant cells** (often with 50–100 nuclei in horseshoe or osteoclast-like pattern)(Fig. 7.61)
Rheumatoid nodule	Deep dermal-SQ **palisaded** granuloma surrounding **pink fibrin**; no mucin (Fig. 7.62)
Sarcoid	**Well-formed epithelioid granulomas** w/ minimal surrounding lymphocytic inflammation ("**naked**"); often difficult to distinguish from Crohn's disease, Melkersson-Rosenthal syndrome, zirconium/beryllium deposition, Blau syndrome, perioral dermatitis, and tuberculoid leprosy. Foreign material may be present ("scar-coid") and does not exclude diagnosis (Fig. 7.63)

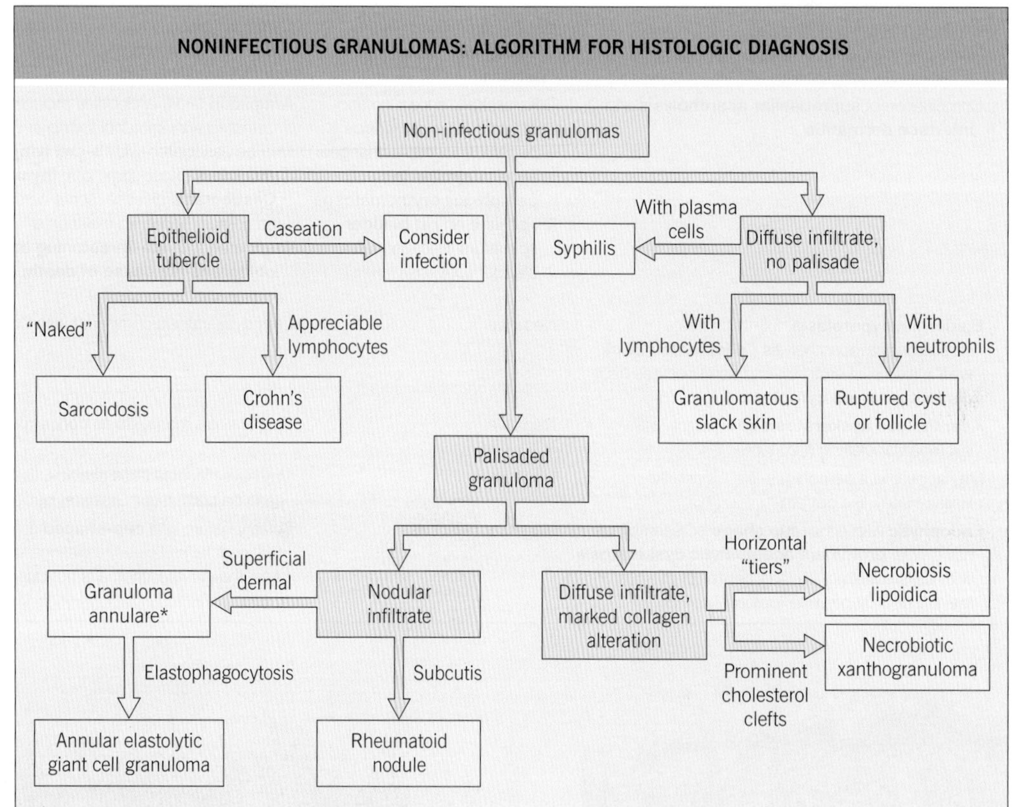

Fig. 7.57 Non-infectious granulomas: algorithm for histopathologic diagnosis. Interstitial granulomatous dermatitis and palisaded neutrophilic and granulomatous dermatitis may represent an additional diagnostic consideration. May also have a patchy dermal interstitial pattern without palisades, or subcutaneous palisades, with more mucin than rheumatoid nodules. (From Rosenbach MA, Wanat KA, Reisenauer A, White KP, Korcheva V, White CR Jr. Non-infectious granulomas. In: Bolognia JL, Schaffer JV, Cerroni L, eds. *Dermatology*. 4th ed. Philadelphia: Elsevier; 2018:1644–1663.)

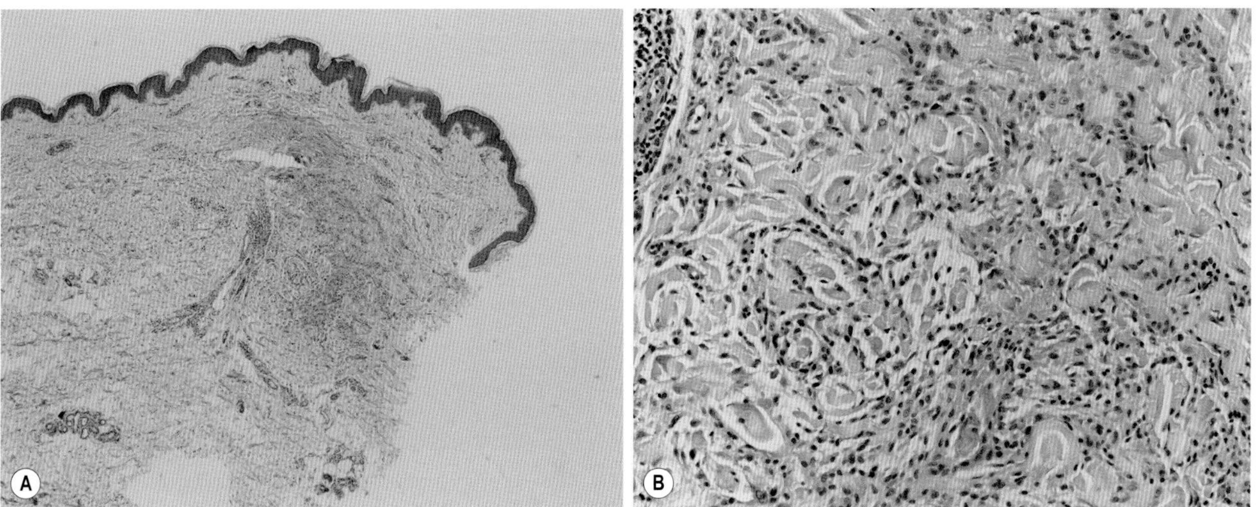

Fig. 7.58 Granuloma annulare (palisaded variant) with palisading granulomatous inflammation, central necrobiosis of collage, and increased mucin. Palisaded appearance is best observed at low power.

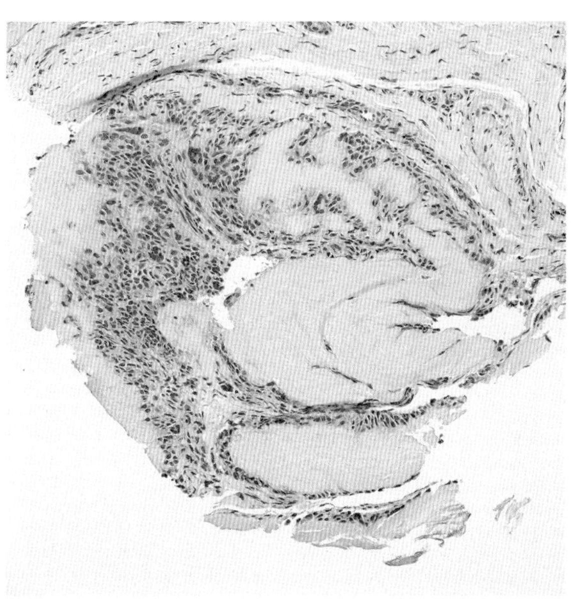

Fig. 7.59 Gout. Granulomatous inflammation surrounding light pink, needle-shaped crystals.

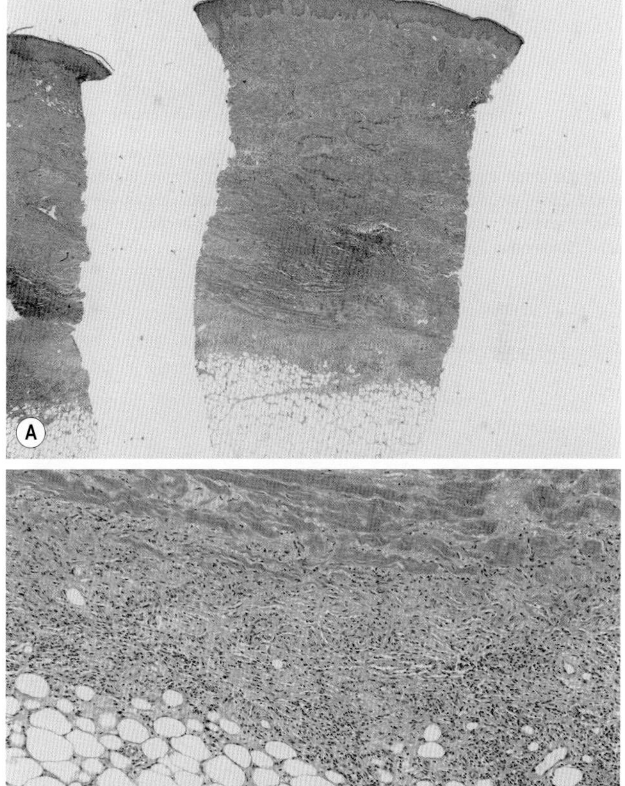

Fig. 7.60 Necrobiosis lipoidica. (A) Low magnification reveals layered pan-dermal granulomatous inflammation with necrobiosis; "wall-to-wall" process with no remaining normal dermis. (B) High magnification.

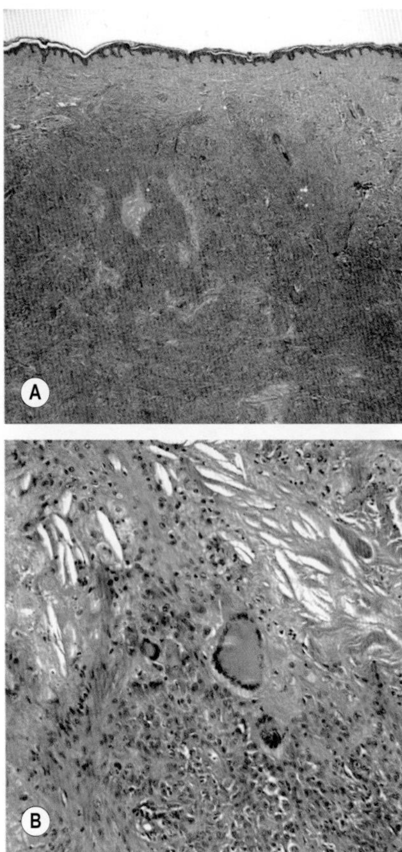

Fig. 7.61 Necrobiotic xanthogranuloma. Low power (A) showing pan-dermal granulomatous inflammation. High power (B) demonstrates cholesterol clefts and bizarre, large multinucleated histiocytic giant cells. (From Johnston RB. Granulomatous reaction pattern. In: *Weedon's Skin Pathology Essentials*, 2nd ed. Philadelphia: Elsevier, 2017, pp 134-162.)

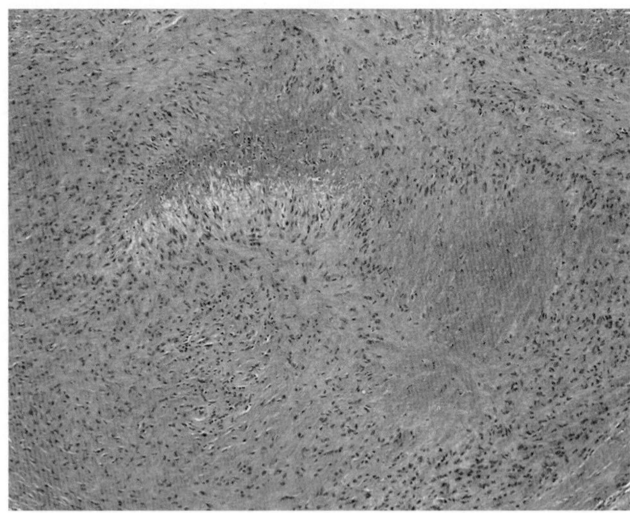

Fig. 7.62 Rheumatoid nodule. Deep and large palisaded granuloma with central pink fibrin; lacks mucin (vs GA)

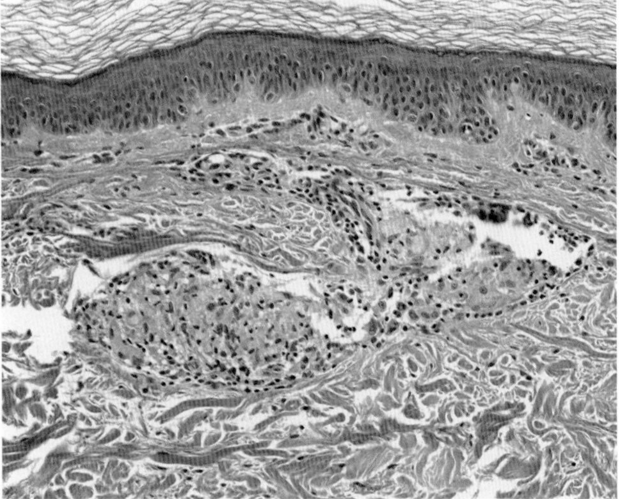

Fig. 7.63 Sacroidosis. "Naked, well-formed granulomas" comprised of discrete balls of granulomatous inflammatory cells (histiocytes and giant cells) with minimal-to-no surrounding lymphocytes.

Table 7.28 Histopathologic Features of the Major Granulomatous Dermatitides (See also Fig. 7.57)

	Sarcoidosis	**Granuloma Annulare**	**Necrobiosis Lipoidica**	**AEGCG**	**Cutaneous Crohn's Disease**	**Rheumatoid Nodule**	**Interstitial Granulomatous Dermatitis**	**Palisading Neutrophilic and Granulomatous Dermatitis**
Typical location	Superficial and deep dermis[a]	Superficial and mid dermis[a]	**Entire dermis**, subcutis	Superficial and mid dermis	Superficial and deep dermis	**Deep dermis**, **subcutis**	Mid and deep dermis	Entire dermis
Granuloma pattern	Tubercle with few peripheral lymphocytes ("naked")	Palisading or interstitial	Diffuse palisading and interstitial; horizontal "tiers"	Palisading, irregular	Tubercle with surrounding lymphocytes	Palisading	Palisading in small "rosettes"	Palisading; **prominent neutrophils and leukocytoclasia**
Necrobiosis (altered collagen)	No	Yes ("blue")	Yes ("red")	No	No	**Yes ("red")**	Yes ("blue")	Yes ("blue")
Giant cells	Yes	Variable	Yes	Yes	Yes	Yes	Variable	Variable
Elastolysis	No	Variable	Variable	**Yes**	No	No	Variable	Variable
Elastophagocytosis	No	No	No	**Yes**	No	No	No	No
Asteroid bodies	Yes	Variable	Variable	Yes	No	No	Variable	Variable
Mucin	No	**Yes**	Minimal	No	No	Variable	**Yes** (but less than palisaded GA)l	Variable
Extracellular lipid	No	Variable	Yes	No	No	Variable	No	No
Vascular changes	No	Variable	**Yes**	No	No	Yes	No	Yes

[a]Subcutaneous variant can also occur.
AEGCG, Annular elastolytic giant cell granuloma.
Modified from Rosenbach MA, Wanat KA, Reisenauer A, White KP, Korcheva V, White CR Jr. Non-infectious granulomas. In: Bolognia JL, Schaffer JV, Cerroni L, eds. Dermatology. *4th ed. Philadelphia: Elsevier; 2018: 1644–1663.*

Table 7.29 High-Yield Inflammatory and Occlusive Vascular Disorders

Vasculitides (Vessel Inflammation and Destruction, Fibrin in Vessel Wall, RBC Extravasation, and Leukocytoclasis)	
Henoch-Schönlein purpura	LCV, **IgA** in vessel walls (DIF)
Mixed cryoglobulinemia	LCV
Granulomatosis with polyangiitis (Wegener's)	LCV involving vessels high up (postcapillary venules) and down low (medium-sized vessels) → may evolve into palisading granuloma with giant cells surrounding **neutrophil-rich** abscess, **+/– granulomatous vasculitis**
Eosinophilic granulomatosis with polyangiitis (Churg-Strauss)	LCV involving vessels up high (postcapillary venules) and down low (medium-sized vessels) → may evolve into palisading granuloma with central degranulating **eosinophils** and **flame figures, +/– granulomatous vasculitis** (Fig. 7.64)
Erythema elevatum diutinum	LCV with numerous eosinophils, **"onion-skin" fibrosis**, and nonfacial location (Fig. 7.65)
Granuloma faciale	LCV w/ numerous eosinophils, plasma cells and histiocytes, **Grenz zone**, mild fibrosis (<EED), and most commonly on face (Fig. 7.66)
Occlusive vasculopathies ("Plugged" Vessels w/ Minimal Primary Vascular Inflammation)	
Thrombotic	**Intravascular thrombus** Causes: cryoglobulinemia type I (intravascular deposits are PAS positive; fluorescence with multiple conjugates on DIF), warfarin necrosis, DIC, lupus anticoagulant, Factor V Leiden mutation, and protein C or S deficiency → all are essentially **indistinguishable histopathologically**
Livedoid vasculopathy	**Bright pink-red hyalinized vessel walls** ("red crayon-like"), **intravascular thrombosis** of superficial dermal vessels, and background **stasis** changes
Calciphylaxis	**Calcified vessel walls w/ thrombosis** deep in the **fat**, +/– extravascular calcium debris (esp. peri-eccrine)
Levamisole-associated vasculopathy	Mixed features of **LCV** + small vessel **thrombosis** high in dermis Patients also have neutropenia and **P- and/or C-ANCA antibodies**

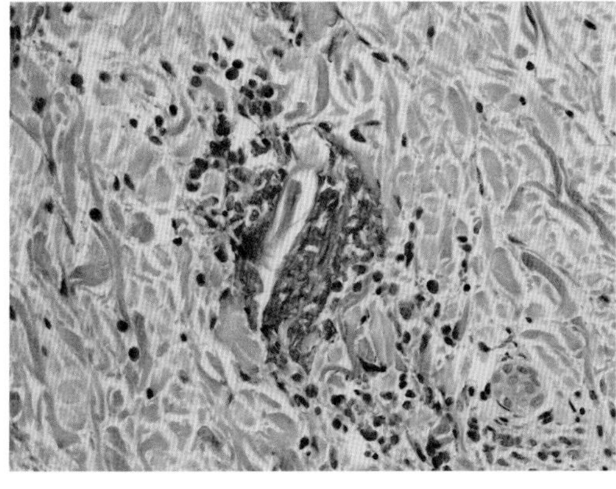

Fig. 7.64 Flame figure, seen in eosinophilic cellulitis (Wells syndrome), Churg-Strauss, and other brisk allergic or dermal hypersensitivity reactions (bug bite, drug, etc). Due to eosinophil degranulation onto collagen fibers.

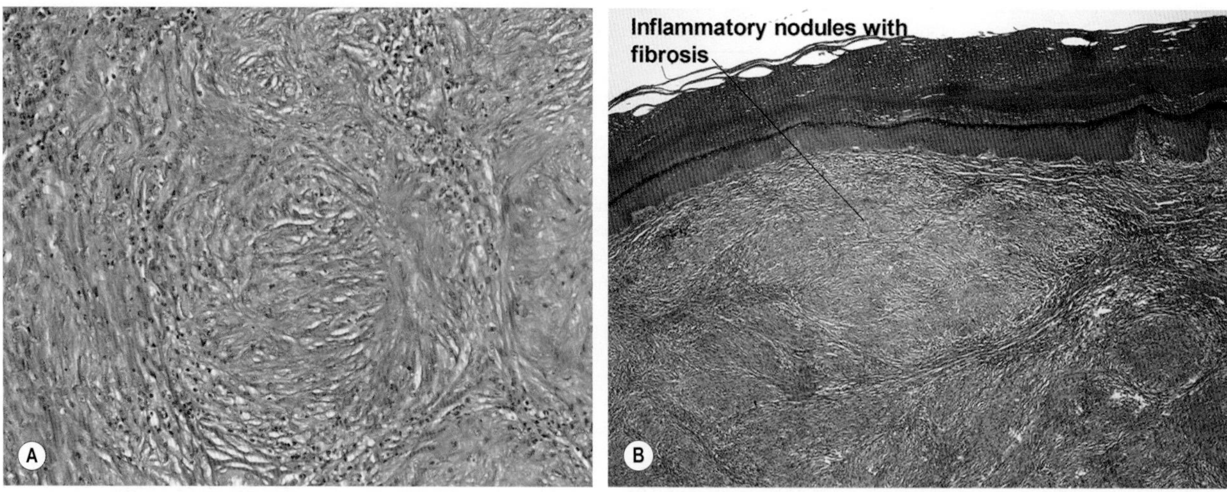

Fig. 7.65 Erythema elevatum diutinum, (A) Low power, (B) High power: Characterized by multiple dermal nodules comprised of nodules of storiform ("onion skin") fibrosis around destroyed vessels, and subtle features of LCV with conspicuous eosinophils. Differentiated from g. faciale by high degree of onion skin fibrosis and non-facial location. (B, from Elston DM: Inflammatory vascular diseases. In: Elston DM, Ferringer T, eds. Dermatopathology, 3rd ed. Philadelphia: Elsevier, 2019; pp 193-219.)

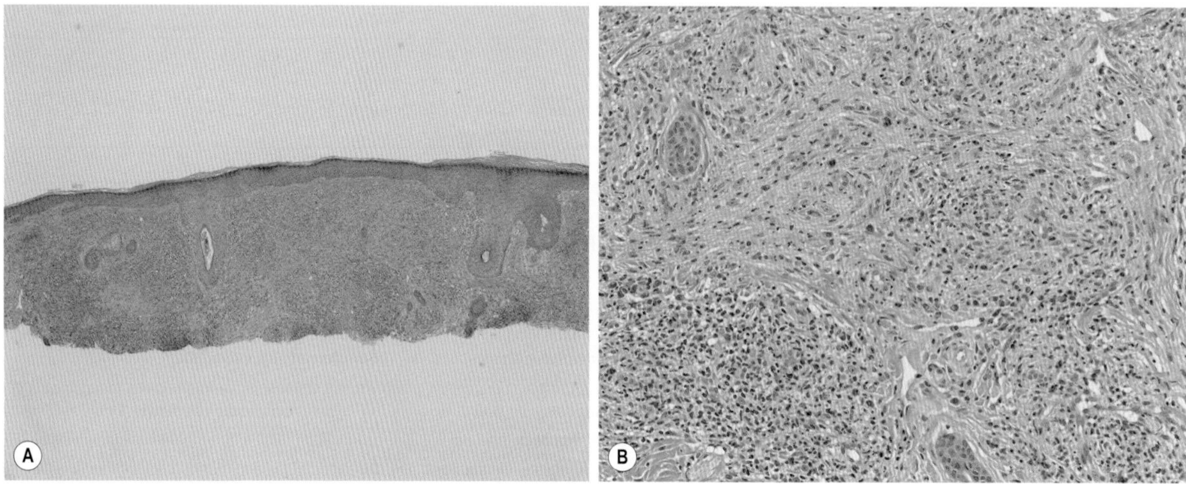

Fig. 7.66 Granuloma faciale. (A) Low power, (B) High power: Characterized by Grenz zone, dense dermal perivascular LCV with numerous eosinophils, plasma cells and histiocytes. Much less onion-skin fibrosis compared to EED.

Table 7.30 High-Yield Panniculitides

Cold panniculitis (deep perniosis)	**Lobular fat necrosis** with lymphocytes, histiocytes, and neuts at dermal-pannicular junction; +/– overlying dermal perniosis
Erythema induratum/nodular vasculitis	**Caseous necrosis of fat lobules** (neutrophil-rich) + **vasculitis** of small and medium (PAN-sized) lobular and septal vessels + **septal thickening** Major clue: involves lobules and septae diffusely, whereas PAN involves one lobule and only damages a small amount of fat immediately surrounding the affected vessel
Erythema nodosum	**Septal panniculitis** with **neutrophils** in septum (early) → progresses to **septal thickening** w/ small granulomas with central clefting (**Miescher's granulomas**) Note: there is only slight spill-over of inflammation into the lobules
Lupus panniculitis	**Lobular** fat necrosis w/ **pink hyalinization** around fat, **nodular PV/PA lymphoplasmacytic aggregates**, +/– clusters **CD123+** plasmacytoid dendritic cells in vast majority of cases (very helpful to DDx from SPTCL, which lacks CD123+ cells) +/– ↑ mucin and interface dermatitis
Sclerema neonatorum	**Lobular** panniculitis w/ **radiating needle-shaped crystals** within adipocytes; lacks surrounding granulomatous inflammation
SQ fat necrosis of newborn (and poststeroid panniculitis)	**Lobular** panniculitis w/ **radiating needle-shaped crystals** within adipocytes w/ associated **brisk granulomatous inflammation**
PAN	**Vasculitis of solitary medium-sized vessel** (artery) in **deep dermis/SQ** tissue with fibrin in vessel wall and obliteration of lumen, +/– very mild **lobular panniculitis** in area immediately adjacent to affected vessel (Fig. 7.67)
Pancreatic panniculitis	**Lobular** panniculitis w/ amorphous purple aggregates in fat lobules representing enzymatic fat necrosis ("**ghost cells**") (Fig. 7.68)
Lipodermatosclerosis (stasis panniculitis)	**Lobular** panniculitis w/ **cystic fat necrosis** and with **lipomembranous** change ("**frost on a window pane**"), septal fibrosis, lipophages, and overlying **stasis changes**

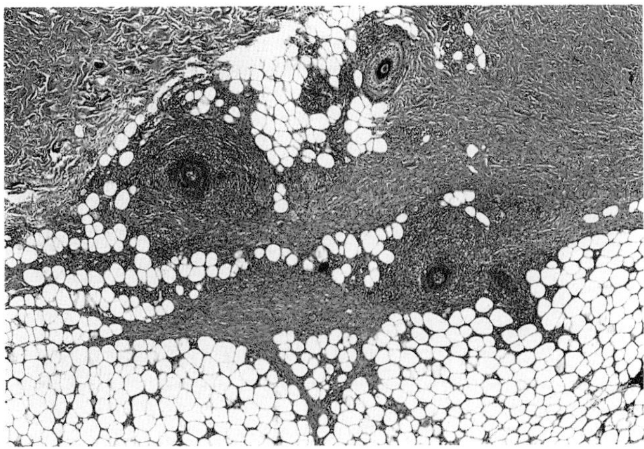

Fig. 7.67 Cutaneous polyarteritis nodosa. The affected small arteries in the upper subcutis show marked fibrin extravasation into their walls. Only a tiny amount of inflammation tends to spill into fat lobules that are in immediate proximity to the affected vessels → very mild lobular panniculitis. (From Patterson JW. The vasculopathic reaction pattern. In: *Weedon's Skin Pathology*. 5th ed. Elsevier. 2021:241–304.)

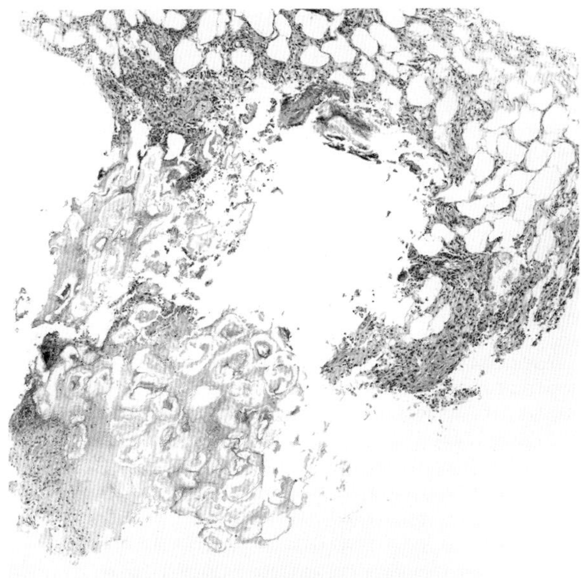

Fig. 7.68 Pancreatic panniculitis. Characteristic "ghost" cells, neutrophils, and basophilic calcification are seen.

Table 7.31 High-Yield Neural Tumors

Neurofibroma (NF)	"Seagull"-shaped **wavy nuclei** in **bubble gum pink stroma**; scattered mast cells
Plexiform neurofibroma	Wavy fascicles of NF embedded in myxoid background of diffuse NF
Schwannoma	**Encapsulated SQ nodule**, **Antoni A/B** areas, **hyalinized ectatic vessels** within tumor
Palisaded encapsulated neuroma (solitary circumscribed neuroma)	Well-circumscribed, pesudoencapsulated **superficial dermal nodule** comprised of **nerve fascicles** separated by clefts
Traumatic neuroma	Small **nerve fascicles** surrounded by **scar** tissue
Nerve sheath myxoma ("Neurothekeoma")	Myxoid lobules of spindled cells in dermis surrounded by fibrous septa

Table 7.32 High-Yield Vascular Tumors

Masson's/IPEH	**Papillary projections** of bland endothelial cells around hyaline cores; **well-circumscribed** (not a feature seen in malignant vascular neoplasms); **arises within large thrombosed vessel** (weird papillary-like appearance is due to re-canalizing of vessel) (Fig. 7.69)
Angiosarcoma	Poorly-formed vessels filled with RBCs and lined by **large, dark, atypical endothelial cells** that protrude into the lumen in a "**piled-on**" fashion; **NOT well-circumscribed** (Fig. 7.70)
Glomeruloid hemangioma	Round nodules comprised of **capillaries contained within a large dilated vascular space** in the dermis → resembles renal glomerulus; part of POEMS syndrome
Angiolymphoid hyperplasia with eosinophilia/epithelioid hemangioma	**Lymphoid nodules** + TONS of **eosinophils** around thick-walled vessels with large "**epithelioid" endothelial cells** often w/ intracytoplasmic vacuoles (Fig. 7.71)
Kaposi sarcoma	**Bloody "busy dermis,"** spindled cells with adjacent **slit-like vessels**, "**promontory sign**" (vessels forming around vessels), ↑ **plasma cells**, ↑ hemosiderin and siderophages (See Fig. 7.22)

IPEH, intravascular papillary endothelial hyperplasia

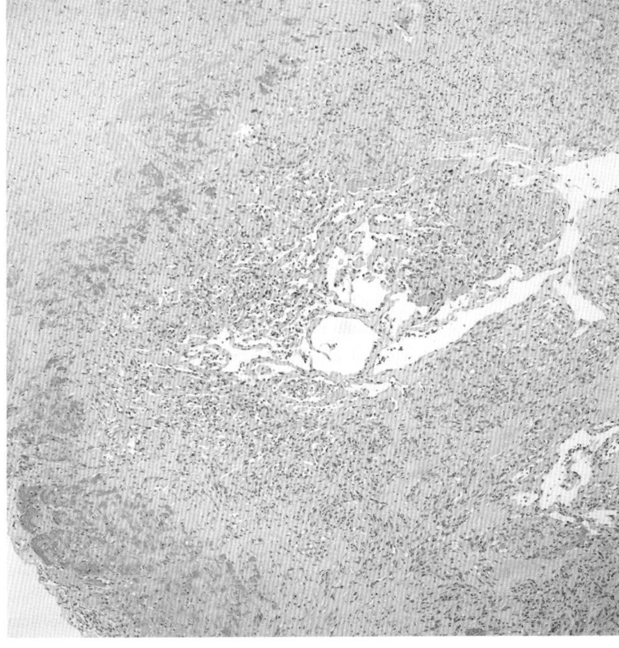

Fig. 7.69 Intravascular papillary endothelial hyperplasia. "Pseudoangiosarcoma" appearance is due to re-canalization of a thrombus within a large vessel (helpful clue = look for the old vessel wall surrounding the well-circumscribed lesion).

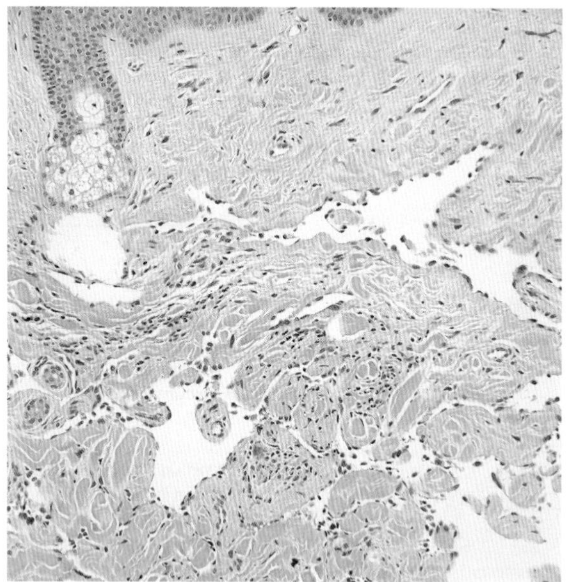

Fig. 7.70 Angiosarcoma. Observe the "dissecting vascular spaces" that appear to be cutting the dermis into multiple pieces. Vascular spaces are poorly-formed and leaky (results in hemorrhagic/bruise-like clinical appearance), and lined by atypical, hyperchromatic endothelial cells with a "piled-on" appearance. Some of the tumor cells appear to be free-floating in the vascular spaces.

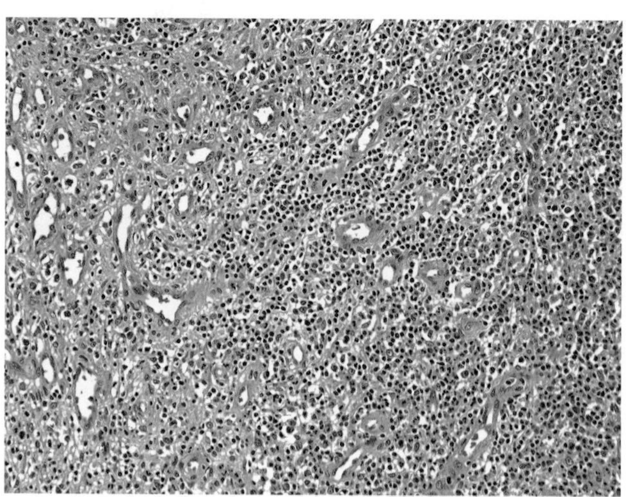

Fig. 7.71 Angiolymphoid hyperplasia with eosinophilia (epithelioid hemangioma). Nodular proliferation of vessels lined by plump epithelioid endothelial cells. A florid inflammatory infiltrate of lymphocytes and eosinophils is present. (From Buehler D, Billings SD. Soft tissue tumors and tumor-like reactions. In: Busam KJ, ed. *Dermatopathology: A Volume in the Series: Foundations in Diagnostic Pathology*, 2nd ed. Philadelphia: Elsevier; 2016, pp 513-594.)

Table 7.33 High-Yield Adipocytic Tumors

Disease	Key Features
Lipoma	Solely mature lipocytes with small eccentric nuclei
Mobile encapsulated lipoma	Lobules of **necrotic** fat enclosed within **fibrous capsule**
Angiolipoma	Lipoma with **capillary proliferation**; capillaries filled w/ **fibrin thrombi**
Pleomorphic lipoma	Mature lipocytes among **myxoid** matrix with interspersed **ropey collagen**, bland spindle cells, and **floret giant cells** (main distinguishing feature from spindle cell lipoma!); **CD34+**, S100 negative, **loss of RB1** in ~100% of cases ("RB1-deleted soft tissue tumor family" = spindle cell lipoma/pleomorphic lipoma, pleomorphic fibroma, atypical spindle cell/ pleomorphic lipomatous tumor, and other less common entities; **loss of RB1 distinguishes from liposarcoma**)
Spindle cell lipoma	Mature lipocytes among **myxoid matrix** containing **spindle cells** and interspersed **ropey collagen**, **CD34**+ S100–, **loss of RB1** in ~100% of cases ("RB1-deleted soft tissue tumor family" = spindle cell lipoma/pleomorphic lipoma, pleomorphic fibroma, atypical spindle cell/pleomorphic lipomatous tumor, and other less common entities; **loss of RB1 distinguishes from liposarcoma**)
Hibernoma	**Multivacuolated** tumor cells, not as pink or grainy-appearing as granular cell tumor. Lipocytes look like **small berries**.
Nevus lipomatosus superficialis	Mature lipocytes infiltrating the superficial dermis; similar, but more extreme features seen in Goltz syndrome

Table 7.34 High-Yield Smooth Muscle DDx

Accessory nipple	Central pore-like structure, deep **mammary** (modified apocrine) **glands** and scattered smooth muscle bundles
Becker's nevus	Looks like **epidermal nevus** + **smooth muscle hamartoma** together with **terminal hairs**
Piloleiomyoma	**Haphazardly arrayed** smooth muscle fascicles in **superficial-mid dermis**
Angioleiomyoma	**Round**, well-circumscribed pink nodule with compressed vascular lumen in **deep dermis/subcutis**
Leiomyosarcoma	Hypercellular proliferation of spindled smooth muscle cells w/ **atypical**, **hyperchromatic nuclei** and **mitoses**. Deep tumors are more aggressive than tumors located entirely within the dermis.

Table 7.35 DF Versus DFSP Versus Fibromatosis

DF	Dermal-based spindle cell neoplasm with "**curlicue" pattern**, **collagen trapping** (most obvious at periphery), overlying **epidermal/ follicular induction**, and **hemosiderin-laden GCs and histiocytes**; +/– significant hemorrhage (aneurysmal DF); **Never infiltrates deeply into fat!**; **factor XIIIa$^+$**, **stromelysin-3$^+$**, and **CD34$^-$**
DFSP	Densely cellular **dermal and SQ tumor w/ storiform** pattern, infiltrates deep into SQ fat enveloping lipocytes in a **"honeycomb" pattern; CD34$^+$, factor XIIIa$^-$, stromelysin-3$^-$, and t(17;22) translocation** (detectable by FISH) (Fig. 7.72)
Fibromatosis	**Long "sweeping"** fascicles of myofibroblasts with **wavy corkscrew nuclei** and wavy collagen Inclusion body fibromatosis (infantile digital fibroma) has characteristic perinuclear eosinophilic inclusions

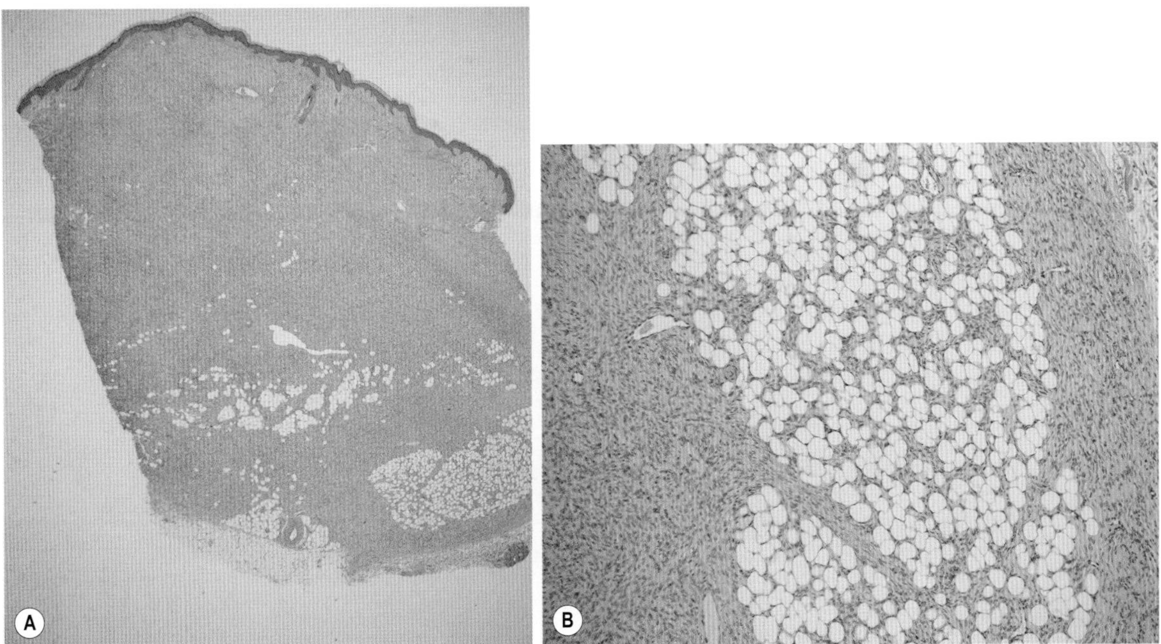

Fig. 7.72 Dermatofibrosarcoma protuberans (DFSP). (A) Low power shows a spindle-cell neoplasm in the dermis. (B) High power shows so-called honeycombing in the fat.

Table 7.36 Amorphous "Pink Stuff in Dermis" DDx

Amyloid (macular/lichen)	Sparse pink deposits of amyloid (**AK type**) in superficial dermis, **melanophages, no inflammation** (Fig. 7.73)
Amyloid (nodular)	**Fissured**, pale pink amyloid (**AL type**) material in superficial to mid dermis, and **abundant plasma cells** (distinguishes from colloid milium) (Fig. 7.74)
Colloid milium	**Fissured**, pale pink deposits **completely filling/expanding superficial-mid dermis** (deeper than macular/lichen amyloid); extensive **solar elastosis (adult form only)**; **no inflammation** (vs. nodular amyloid) (Fig. 7.75)
Erythropoietic protoporphyria	**Dermal deposits of pink material; hyaline cuff** around superficial vessels, no solar elastosis (because patients diligently avoid sun) (Fig. 7.76)
Lipoid proteinosis	Pink **hyaline BMZ material** (type IV collagen; PAS-D+) predominantly centered around superficial and **deep** (deeper than EPP) vessels and adnexae, with "**onion skin"** pattern (Fig. 7.77)

AL, light chain-derived amyloid; BMZ, basement membrane zone; PAS-D, periodic acid-Schiff with diastase; EPP, erythropoietic protoporphyria

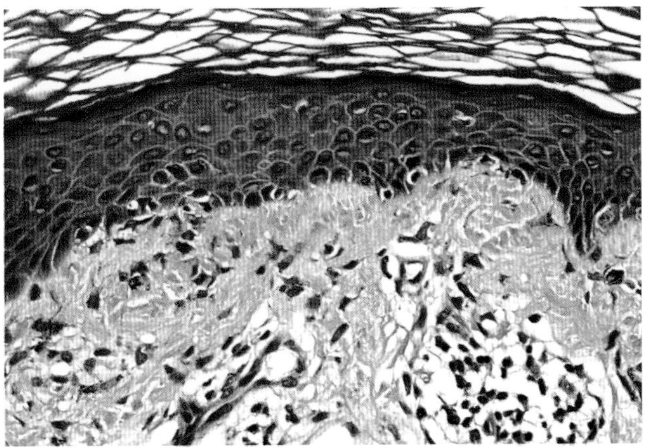

Fig. 7.73 Macular amyloid. (From Brinster NK, Liu V, Diwan AH, McKee PH. Cutaneous amyloidosis. In: *Dermatopathology: A Volume in the High Yield Pathology Series*. Philadelphia: Elsevier, 2011, pp 278-280.)

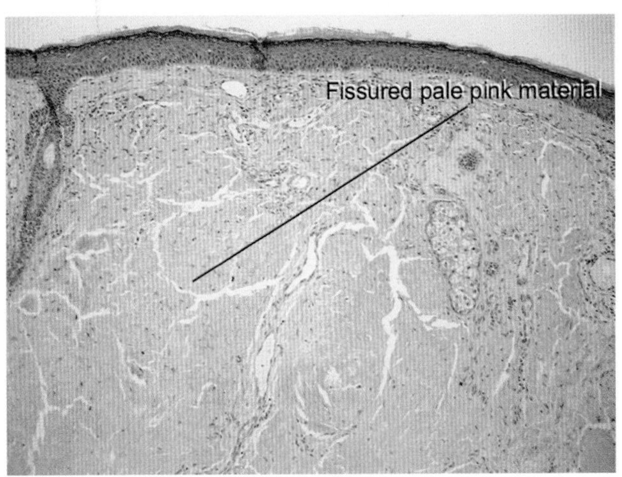

Fig. 7.74 Nodular amyloid. (From Ferringer T. Metabolic disorders. In: Elston DM, Ferringer T, eds. *Dermatopathology*, 3rd ed. Philadelphia: Elsevier, 2019; pp 251-263.)

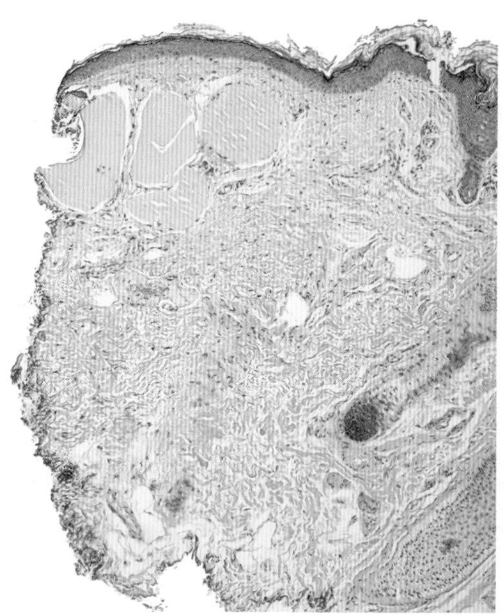

Fig. 7.75 Colloid milium. Fissured pale-pink deposits fill and expand the superficial and mid dermis. Lacks lymphoplasmacytic inflammation (vs nodular amyloid).

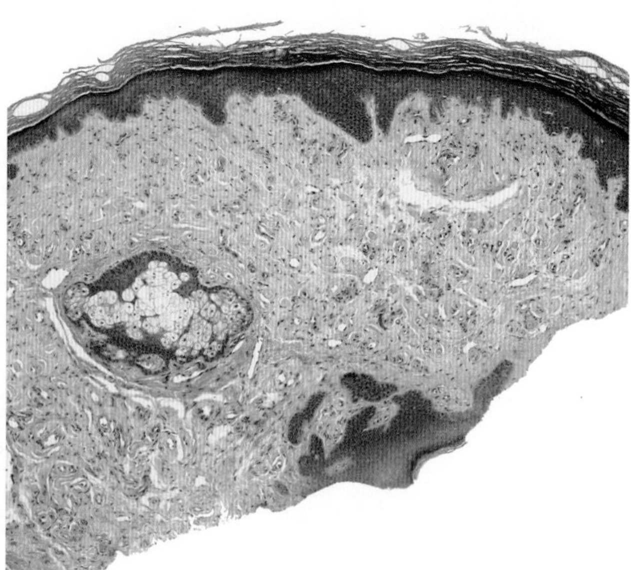

Fig. 7.77 Lipoid proteinosis. Pink, hyaline BMZ material (Type IV collagen) forms "onion skin" deposits around vessels in superficial and deep dermis (deeper than EPP).

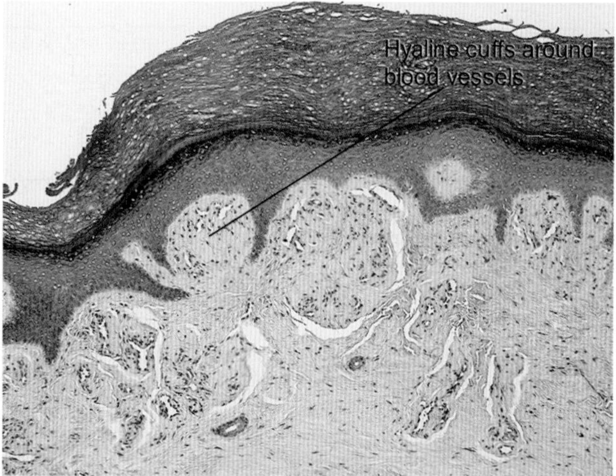

Fig. 7.76 Erythropoietic protoporphyria. (From Ferringer T. Metabolic disorders. In: Elston DM, Ferringer T, eds. *Dermatopathology*. 3rd ed. Philadelphia: Elsevier; 2019:251–263.)

Table 7.37 Immediate Pattern Recognition Diagnoses

Chondrodermatitis nodularis chronicus helicis	**Ulcer** w/ adjacent epidermal acanthosis, **underlying reparative change,** fibrin, vascular ectasia, and eosinophilic **degenerated cartilage**
Coma blister	Paucicellular/noninflammatory subepidermal bulla, diffuse epidermal necrosis → subepidermal bulla, and sweat gland necrosis (differentiates from SJS/TEN) (Fig. 7.78)
Cutaneous endometriosis	Well-formed **glands of varying sizes**, lined by pseudostratified columnar epithelium and surrounded by **endometrial stroma** (basaloid cells in fibromyxoid background); **RBCs and hemosiderin** within and surrounding glands. No atypia (unlike cutaneous mets of endometrial cancer) (Fig. 7.79)
Elastosis perforans serpiginosa	**Elastic fibers** (stains black with VVG) spiraling through **narrow serpiginous channel** in epidermis
Giant cell tumor of tendon sheath	Deep tumor arising from tendon, containing innumerable multinucleate **osteoclast-like giant cells**, and fibrotic pink stroma (Fig. 7.80)
Granular cell tumor	**PEH** + pink cells in dermis w/ **granular cytoplasm** and round **pustulo-ovoid bodies of Milian**
Myofibroma/ myopericytoma	Dermal-SQ tumor w/ multiple **blue-gray (cartilage-colored) hypocellular nodules** surrounded by hypercellular areas containing **"HPC-like" "staghorn" vessels** (Fig. 7.81)
Nevus sebaceus	**Papillomatosis** overlying increased number of **sebaceous glands directly opening** onto epidermis; terminal hairs replaced by **apocrine glands**
Nodular fasciitis	**Circumscribed** nodule located in **deep dermis/SQ**; stellate myofibroblasts w/ **"tissue culture" appearance** set in **loose myxoid stroma** with foci of **hemorrhage and inflammation**
Ochronosis	Yellow-brown "bananas" in superficial dermis
Pseudoxanthoma elasticum	Fragmented purple elastic fibers in dermis (VVG+, von Kossa+)
Sweet syndrome	Dense neutrophilic infiltrate with karyorrhexis in dermis and marked papillary dermal edema; tissue cultures and bug stains MUST be negative!
Verruciform xanthoma	Verrucous hyperplasia with **xanthoma cells stuffed in dermal papillae** and superficial dermis (Fig. 7.82)

PEH, pseudoendothelial hyperplasia; *HPC,* hemangiopericytoma

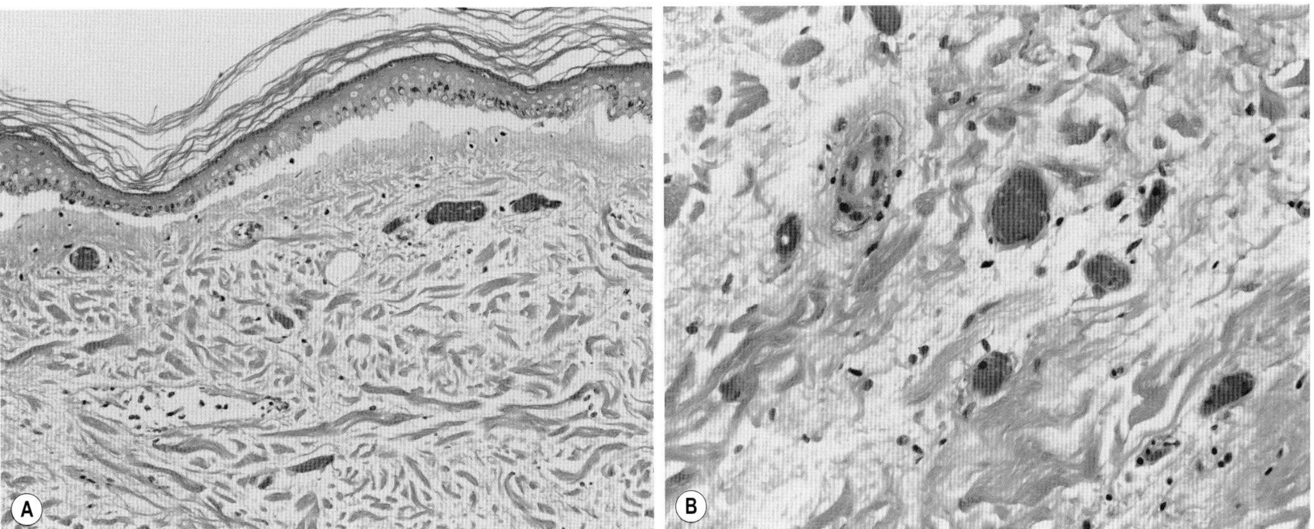

Fig. 7.78 Coma blister. (A) Pauci-inflammatory subepidermal separation. (B) Basophilic necrosis of eccrine glands.

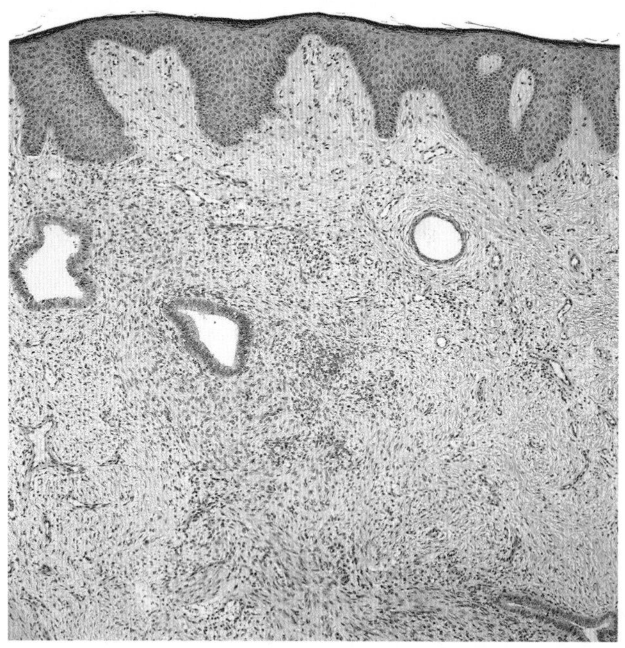

Fig. 7.79 Endometriosis of the umbilicus. Glands and stroma are set in fibrous tissue. The glands are functional with some luminal hemorrhage.

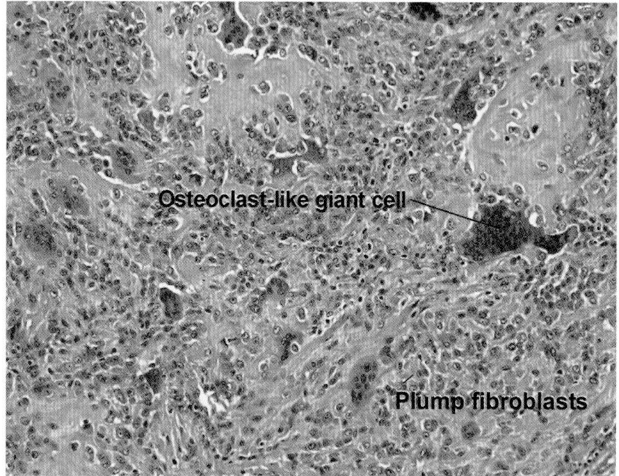

Fig. 7.80 Giant cell tumor of tendon sheath. (From Elston DM, Ko CJ, Ferringer T. Fibrous tumors. In: Elston DM, Ferringer T, eds. *Dermatopathology*, 3rd ed. Philadelphia: Elsevier, 2019; pp 350-392.)

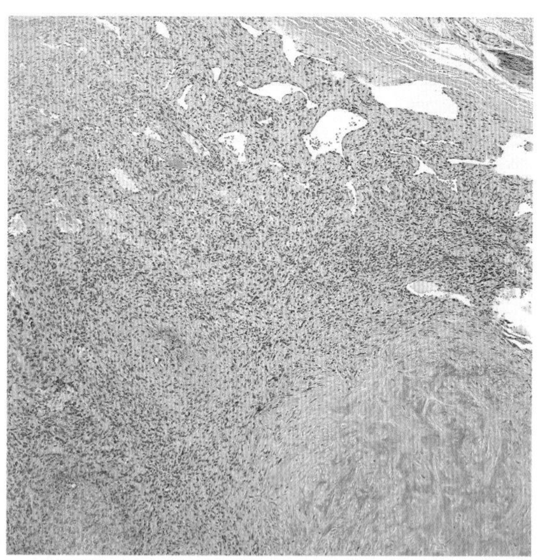

Fig. 7.81 Myofibroma. Biphasic tumor composed of hypocellular, blue-grey myoid nodules surrounded by immature mesenchymal cells and hemangiopericytoma-like vascular spaces.

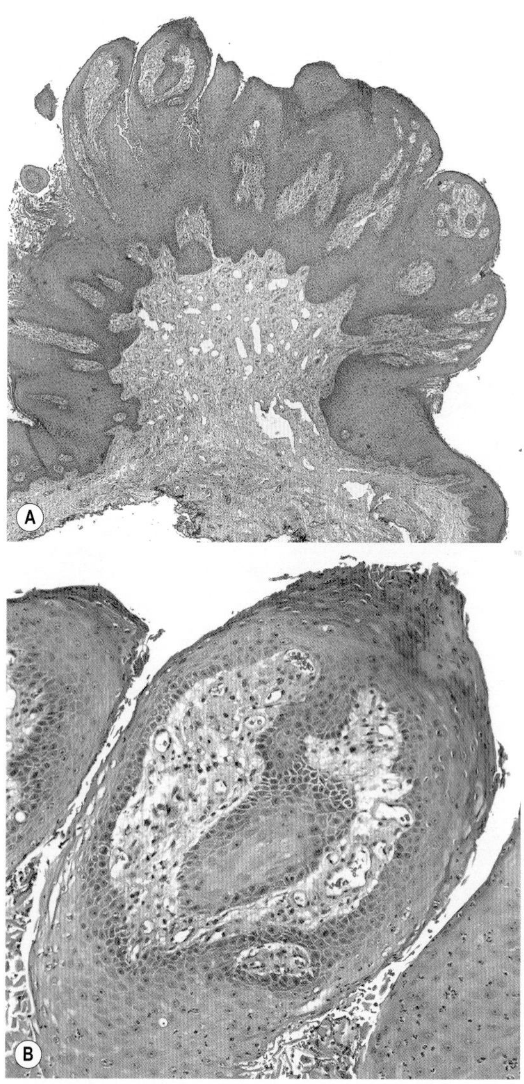

Fig. 7.82 (A) and (B) Verruciform xanthoma. Mnemonic = "wart with foam cells in dermal papillae."

Table 7.38 High-Yield Infectious Diseases

HPV-induced lesions	
	Verruca Vulgaris Myrmecia (Fig. 7.83) Verruca plana (Fig. 7.84) Verruca plana with EDV changes (Fig. 7.85) Verrucous carcinoma (Fig. 7.86)
Histiocytic inclusions	
	"**Hi**s **GIRL** **P**enelope": **Hi**stoplasmosis, **G**ranuloma **I**nguinale, **R**hinoscleroma, **L**eishmaniasis/**L**eprosy, **P**enicillium
Infections with endospores	
	Rhinosporidiosis ("spores as big as a rhino!") (Fig. 7.87) Coccidioidomycosis (Fig. 7.88)

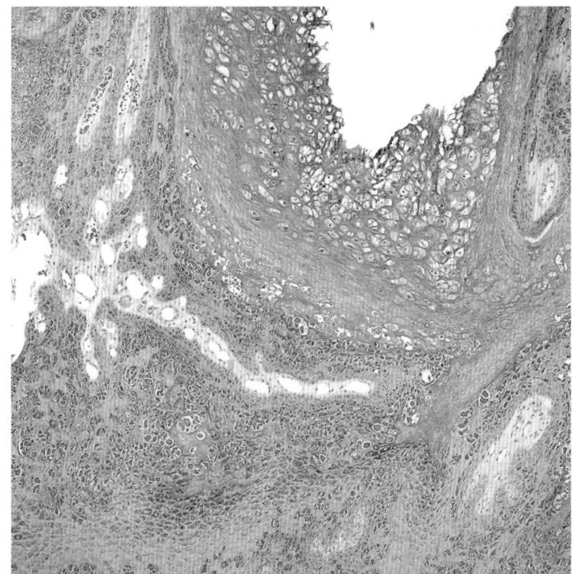

Fig. 7.83 Verruca with myrmecial changes ("myrmecial wart"). Compared with verruca vulgaris, this entity has more extreme hyperkeratosis, epidermal hyperplasia, and bright pink-purple inclusion bodies.

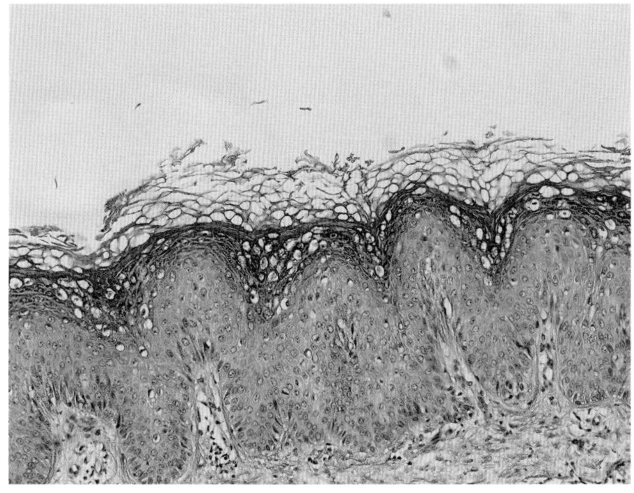

Fig. 7.84 Verruca plana. Minimal papillomatosis (vs VV), mild hypergranulosis, superficial clear-colored koilocytes.

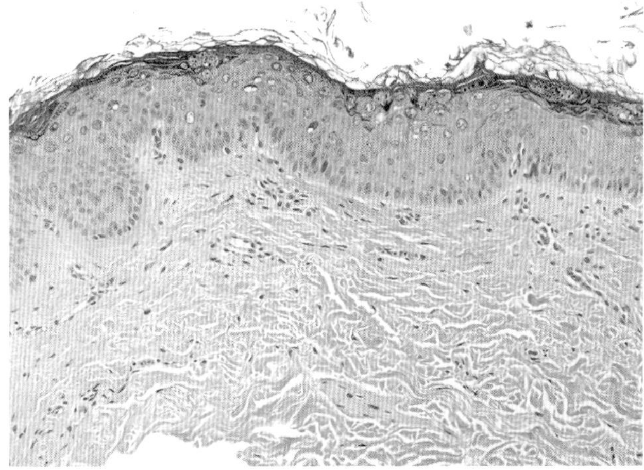

Fig. 7.85 Verruca plana with changes characteristic of epidermodysplasia verruciformis. Distinguished from normal verruca plana by presence of blue-gray color of upper portion of epidermis.

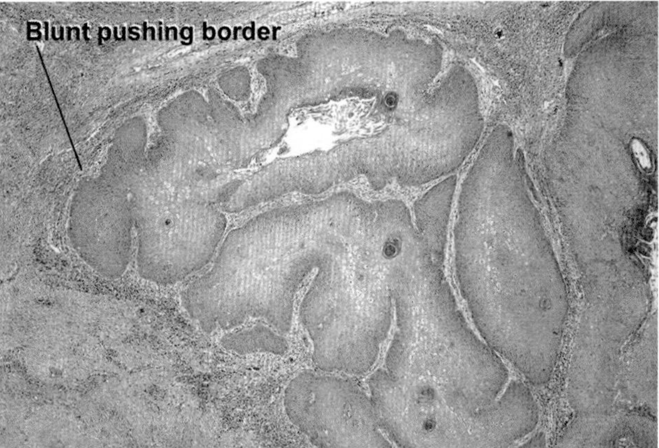

Fig. 7.86 Verrucous carcinoma. (From Elston DM. Malignant tumors of the epidermis. In: Elston D, Ferringer T, eds. *Dermatopathology*. 3rd ed. Philadelphia: Elsevier; 2019:54–67.)

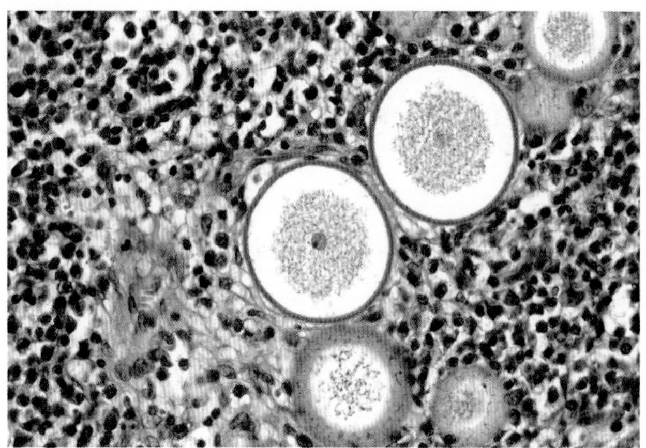

Fig. 7.87 Rhinosporidiosis: individual spores mature to form small trophic cysts. (From Grayson W, Calonje E. Infectious diseases of the skin. In: Calonje E, Brenn T, Lazar AJ, Billings SD, eds. *McKee's Pathology of the Skin with Clinical Correlations*. 5th Ed. Philadelphia: Elsevier; 2020:826–975.)

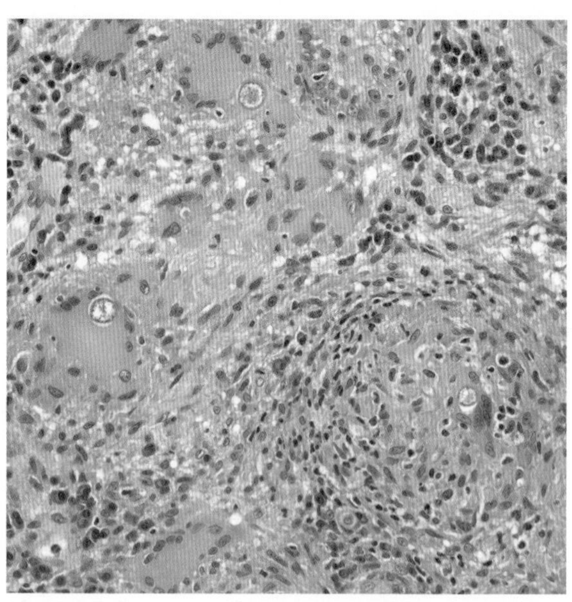

Fig. 7.88 Coccidioidomycosis. Multiple spherules are present with surrounding chronic inflammation.

8 Dermatologic Surgery

Phillip C. Hochwalt and Thomas L.H. Hocker

CONTENTS LIST

8.1 SURGICAL ANATOMY
8.2 LOCAL ANESTHETICS AND PERIOPERATIVE PAIN CONTROL
8.3 SURGICAL INSTRUMENTS AND NEEDLES
8.4 SUTURE TECHNIQUES
8.5 WOUND CLOSURE MATERIALS
8.6 ANTISEPSIS AND STERILIZATION
8.7 ELECTROSURGERY
8.8 CRYOSURGERY
8.9 EXCISIONS
8.10 MOHS SURGERY
8.11 FLAPS
8.12 GRAFTS
8.13 SURGICAL COMPLICATIONS AND MEASURES TO AVOID THEM
8.14 SCAR IMPROVEMENT
8.15 NAIL SURGERY
8.16 WOUND DRESSINGS

8.1 SURGICAL ANATOMY

- Skin lines
  - **Langer's lines**: skin lines that orient in the direction of the natural gape of a wound after puncture with a circular spike; lines run parallel to underlying muscles
    - Different than relaxed skin tension lines (RSTLs); frequently perpendicular to them, in fact
  - **RSTLs** (Kraissl and Borges lines): lines that run perpendicular to underlying muscles; most elective incisions should be made **parallel** to these lines
- Head and neck anatomy
  - Arterial supply (Fig. 8.1)
    - Face supplied by external AND internal carotid:
      - External carotid: supplies **lateral, mid, and lower face**; most important branches include:
        - → **Superficial temporal artery**: anterior and parietal branches; supplies temple, scalp, and lateral forehead
        - → **Maxillary artery**: gives rise to:
          - ◇ Infraorbital artery: exits infraorbital foramen; supplies mid face; anastomoses with the internal carotid-derived arteries (supratrochlear and supraorbital arteries)
          - ◇ Mental artery: exits mental foramen; supplies chin and lower lip
        - → **Facial artery**: gives rise to:
          - ◇ Labial arteries (inferior and superior): supplies lips, columella, and ala
          - ◇ **Angular artery**: extension of facial artery starting near base of ala (**susceptible to intraarterial filler injection**); eventually ends in anastomoses with branches of the internal carotid (**dorsal nasal artery** specifically) near medial canthus
      - Internal carotid: supplies **mid forehead and nasal root;** anastomoses with branches of the external carotid in the area of the medial canthus and dorsal nose
        - → **Ophthalmic artery**: responsible for most of the facial arteries supplied by the internal carotid. It travels through the optic canal into the orbit where it supplies the **retinal**, **supraorbital** and **supratrochlear** (axial artery required for paramedian forehead flap), infratrochlear, **dorsal nasal** (anastomoses with angular artery), **external nasal**, anterior and posterior ethmoidal, and lacrimal branches. These branches supply the retina, forehead, upper dorsal nose, and eyelids
          - ◇ Branches of the ophthalmic artery anastomose heavily with those supplied by the external carotid system

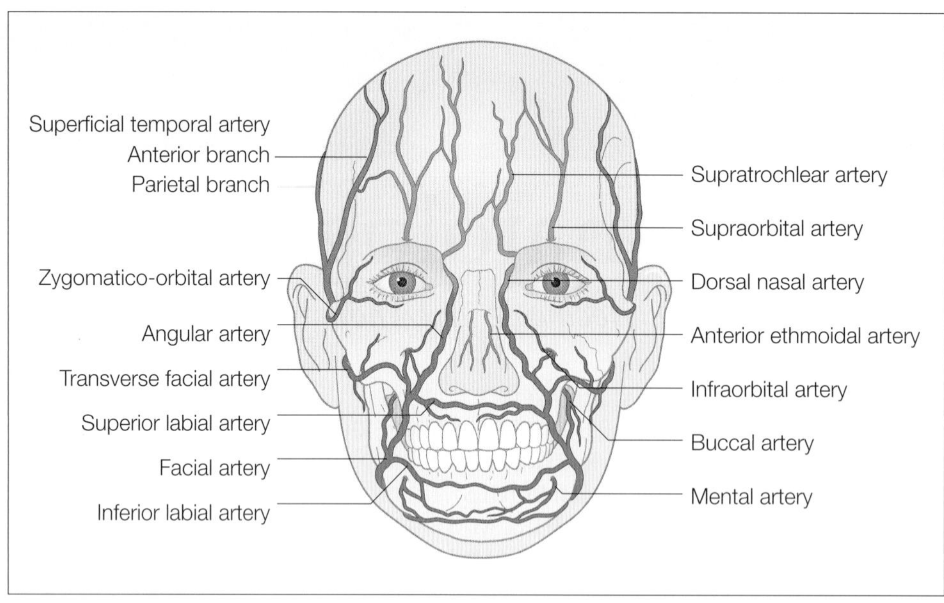

Fig. 8.1 Arterial blood supply of the face. (From Salasche SJ. Anatomy. In: Rohrer TE, Cook JL, Nguyen TH, eds. *Flaps and Grafts in Dermatologic Surgery*. Philadelphia: Elsevier; 2007:1–14.)

        - ◇ These anastomoses are important when **inadvertent intraarterial** injection of steroids or fillers occurs. Inadvertent intraarterial injection of filler (**glabellar area** most commonly) carries risk of **blindness due to retrograde movement of filler** to ophthalmic artery and embolization into retinal artery
- ■ Venous system
    - ○ Veins typically follow their associated arteries
    - ○ Facial vein can communicate w/ cavernous sinus of brain via pterygoid plexus or ophthalmic vein
        - ♦ **Danger triangle**: area extending from corners of the mouth to nasal root; infections in this area can cause **septic cavernous sinus thrombosis**, meningitis, and brain abscesses
- ■ Lymphatic system
    - ○ Important for skin cancer mets; drainage can be variable
        - ♦ Upper and lateral face → parotid, **preauricular**, and infraauricular nodes
        - ♦ Lower and medial face → **submandibular** nodes
        - ♦ Central lower lip and chin → **submental** nodes
        - ♦ Lateral cervical nodes collect from the above areas
- ■ Superficial musculoaponeurotic system (SMAS)
    - ○ Composed of muscles and fascia of the face and neck; allows for coordinated facial movement and helps contain infection and cancer; **contiguous w/ galea**
    - ○ **Motor nerves all run deep to SMAS** (penetrate muscles from undersurface) → staying above SMAS during facial surgery prevents motor nerve damage
    - ○ **Sensory nerves are located superficial to SMAS** → often transected during facial surgery → numbness
- ■ Sensory nerves (Tables 8.1–8.2 and Figs. 8.2–8.4)
    - ○ **Cranial nerve (CN) V (trigeminal nerve)**: almost wholly responsible for sensory innervation of face
        - ♦ **Boards factoids**: Damage to CN V may result in trigeminal trophic syndrome and Frey's syndrome; CN V also supplies motor innervation to muscles of mastication
        - ♦ **Clinical pearl**: injection of anesthetic into the supraorbital, supratrochlear, infraorbital, and mental foramens will result in prolonged anesthesia for vast majority of face (exceptions = parts of nose and angles of mouth)
    - ○ Cervical plexus: supplies sensory innervation to neck and occipital scalp
    - ○ Sensory innervation of ear is complex
- ■ Motor innervation (Tables 8.3 and 8.4; Fig. 8.5)
    - ○ Muscles of facial expression are innervated by **CN VII (facial nerve)**; facial muscles receive motor innervation from their **undersurface**
        - ♦ **Boards factoid**: as a minor function, CN VII also provides *sensory* input for **anterior tongue** (via chorda tympani branch) and a small amount of **external auditory meatus**
    - ○ Facial nerve emerges from stylomastoid foramen, **travels within the parotid gland** and then splits into five branches: **temporal, zygomatic, buccal, mandibular, and cervical** branches ("To Zanzibar By Motor Car")

Table 8.1 Sensory Innervation of Head and Neck

Nerve	Innervation	Comments
Trigeminal nerve		
Ophthalmic (V1; has 3 major branches)	Frontal nerve (2 divisions) Supraorbital (upper eyelid, forehead, and frontal to vertex scalp) Supratrochlear (medial upper eyelid, medial forehead, and medial frontal scalp) Nasociliary nerve (3 important divisions) Infratrochlear (nasal root, medial canthus) Anterior ethmoidal (**distal/inferior half of central nose**: dorsum, supratip, tip, and columella) Ciliary (cornea) Lacrimal nerve: lateral eyelid, conjunctiva, and lacrimal gland	Supraorbital nerve danger zone: nerve courses superficially at vertical distances above the palpable orbital rim of 1.3 cm or greater → nerve easily injured during a deep shave, punch or ED&C of lower to midforehead → paresthesia, traumatic neuroma Supraorbital and supratrochlear nerves are commonly anesthetized via nerve block **Hutchinson's sign**: involvement of **nasociliary branch** by VZV (distal nasal vesicles, ulcers) is almost always a/w **herpes zoster ophthalmicus**; conversely, it is very rare to have ocular involvement in absence of distal nasal skin lesions!
Maxillary (V2)	Zygomaticotemporal nerve (temple and temporal scalp) Zygomaticofacial nerve (malar cheek) **Infraorbital nerve** (medial cheek, lower eyelid, **nasal sidewall**, **nasal ala**, **upper lip**, upper teeth, and maxillary gingiva)	Infraorbital nerve is commonly anesthetized via nerve block
Mandibular (V3)	Auriculotemporal nerve (**superior portion of anterior external ear** and auditory canal, temple, temporoparietal scalp, TMJ, outer aspect of tympanic membrane, and **parasympathetic innervation of parotid**) Buccal nerve (buccal mucosa, angle of mouth, and gingiva) Mental nerve (lower lip and chin) Lingual nerve (**sensation to anterior 2/3 of tongue**)	**Auriculotemporal nerve is frequently injured during TMJ surgery** (→ paresthesia of ear and temple) and **parotidectomy** (→ injured parasympathetic nerves erroneously reattach to sweat glands in area → **Frey syndrome**) Mental nerve is commonly anesthetized via nerve block Mandibular nerve (V3) also provides **motor innervation to muscles of mastication** (masseter, medial and lateral pterygoid, temporalis)
Cervical nerves		
Lesser occipital (C2)	Postauricular neck/scalp	—
Greater occipital (C2)	Occipital scalp (majority)	—
Great auricular (C2, C3)	Infra-auricular neck, mandibular angle, **majority of external ear** (both anterior and posterior portions, including earlobe), and postauricular scalp	—
Transverse cervical (C2, C3)	Anterior and lateral neck	—
Supraclavicular (C3, C4)	Supraclavicular and infraclavicular fossa, upper chest, shoulder	—

Table 8.2 Other High-Yield Sensory Nerve Innervation Facts

Site	Nerves and Innervation	Comments
Ear	In decreasing order of area: **Great auricular**: majority of posterior ear and 3/4 of anterior ear (all except quadrant innervated by auriculotemporal and area innervated by cranial nerves) **Auriculotemporal**: entire "anterior-superior quadrant" of ear (excluding conchal bowl, but including EAM), and superior portion of posterior helix **Cranial nerves VII, IX, and X**: Conchal bowl and EAM (most important!), also contributes to posterior notch innervation **Lesser occipital:** posterior notch	**Ring block around ear anesthetizes everything** (except conchal bowl and EAM = supplied by CN7, CN9, CN10)
Hand	Median, radial, and ulnar	Opposing the thumb and fifth finger makes the palmaris longus tendon apparent; typically use 3–5 mL of anesthetic **Median nerve block**: inject at proximal wrist crease, between palmaris longus and flexor carpi radialis tendons (i.e., inject **radial to palmaris longus tendon** at proximal wrist crease) **Ulnar nerve block**: inject immediately **radial to flexor carpi ulnaris** at proximal wrist crease **Radial nerve block**: inject along the proximal wrist crease, starting immediately lateral to radial artery, extending all the way to dorsal midwrist

Continued

Table 8.2 Other High-Yield Sensory Nerve Innervation Facts—cont'd

Site	Nerves and Innervation	Comments
Foot	Posterior tibial, saphenous, sural, superficial peroneal, and deep peroneal	Sites for foot block are highly testable! Posterior tibial nerve: inject in groove **between medial malleolus and Achilles** tendon; nerve is posterior to posterior tibial artery Sural nerve: inject in groove **between lateral malleolus and Achilles** tendon Deep peroneal: inject lateral to hallucis longus tendon → down to bone (though block rarely needed as local infiltration between first and second toe adequate) Saphenous and superficial peroneal: inject on dorsal foot, subcutaneously, **from malleolus to malleolus**
Fingers, toes	Two dorsal and two ventral nerves per digit	Multiple ways to perform digital block Classic technique: inject immediately distal MCP/MTP, using **1–2 mL on each side** (2–4 mL total per digit); **do NOT exceed 8 mL per digit** (risk of tourniquet effect) Safe to use lidocaine w/ epinephrine, unless patient has underlying PVD
Tongue	**Taste: CN VII** (chorda tympani branch; anterior 2/3) **Sensory: CN V3** (lingual nerve; anterior 2/3) **Glossopharyngeal (CN IX)** provides both taste and somatic sensation to **posterior 1/3**	Motor innervation of tongue: predominantly CN XII (hypoglossal nerve)
Penis	Dorsal nerve of penis bifurcates into major anterior (dorsal) and minor posterior (ventral) branches at the base of the penis	Injecting a ring of lidocaine around the base of penis anesthetizes almost entire penis except periurethral glans

EAM, *External acoustic meatus;* MCP, *metacarpophalangeal;* MTP, *metatarsophalangeal;* PVD, *peripheral vascular disease.*

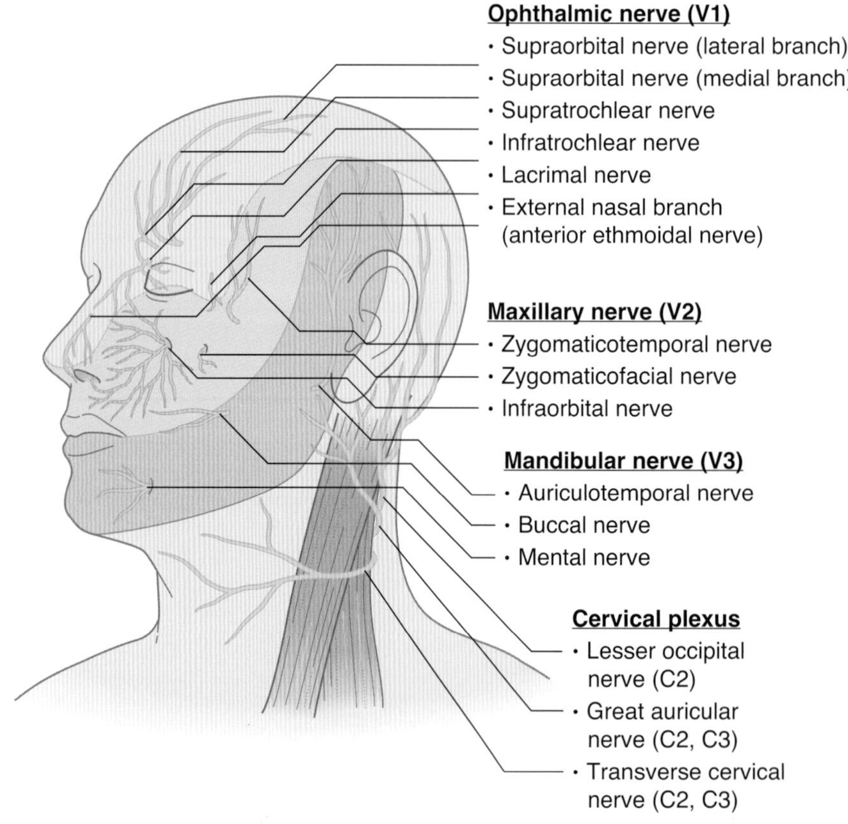

Fig. 8.2 Trigeminal (cranial nerve V) and cervical plexus sensory nerves. (From Salasche SJ, Mandy SH. Anatomy. In: Rohrer TE, Cook JL, Kaufman AJ, eds. *Flaps and Grafts in Dermatologic Surgery*. 2nd ed. Philadelphia: Elsevier; 2018:1–15.)

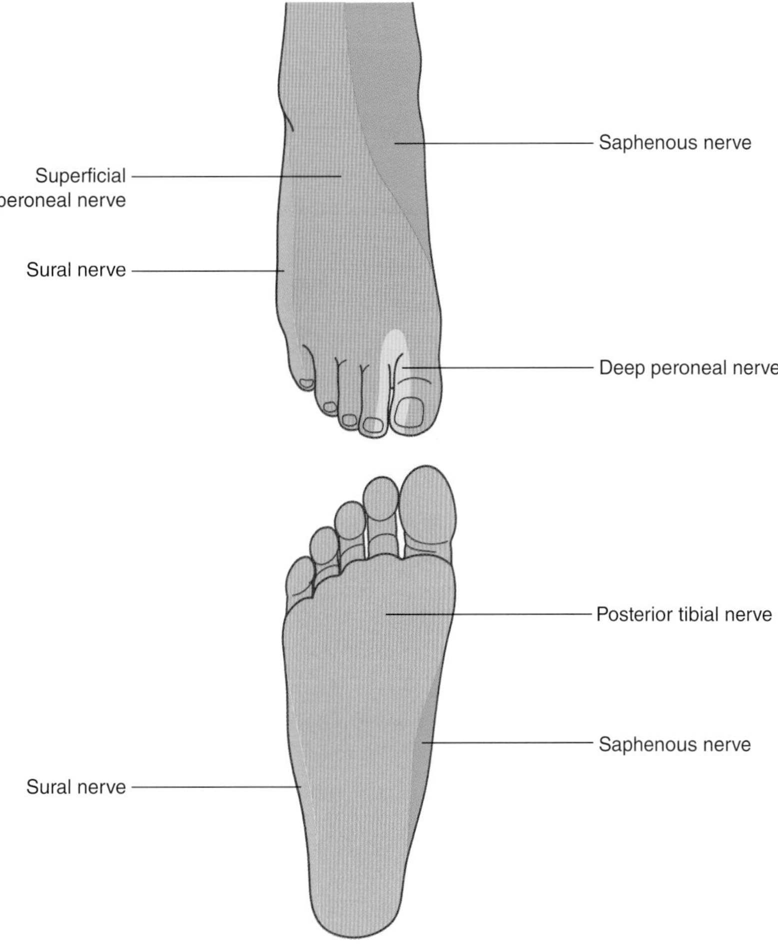

Fig. 8.3 Sensory innervation of the foot. (From Soriano TT, Breithaupt A, Chesnut C. Anesthesia and analgesia. In: Robinson JK, Hanke CW, Siegel DM, Fratila A, eds. *Surgery of the Skin*. 3rd ed. Philadelphia, Elsevier, 2015:43–63.)

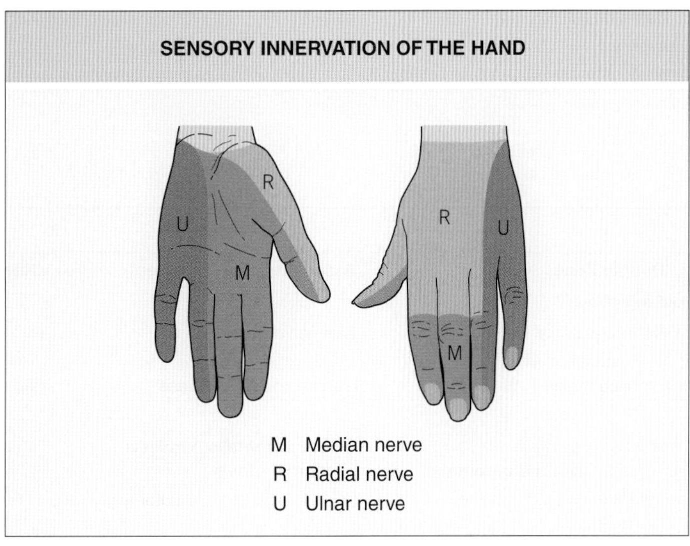

Fig. 8.4 Sensory innervation of the palmar and dorsal surface of the right hand. (From Hruza GJ. Anesthesia. In: Bolognia JL, Schaffer JV, Cerroni L, eds. *Dermatology*. 4th ed. Philadelphia: Elsevier; 2018:2440–2449.)

Table 8.3 Motor Innervation of the Head and Neck

Facial Nerve (CN VII) Branch	Muscles Innervated and Normal Function	Nerve Injury-Related Findings	Other Comments
Temporal	**Frontalis** (eyebrow elevation) **Corrugator supercilii** (pulls eyebrows inferomedially) Upper orbicularis oculi (tight closure of eyelids, blinking)	**Inability to elevate eyebrows** → eyebrow ptosis	Targets for Botox: Frontalis (horizontal forehead wrinkles) Orbicularis ("crow's feet") Corrugator supercilii (vertical glabellar lines, scowling appearance)
Zygomatic	**Orbicularis oculi** (lower portion) **Procerus** (pull eyebrows down, "horizontal glabellar lines") **Nasalis** (transverse—wrinkle nose; alar—flares nostrils) **Lip elevators:** Levator labii superioris alaeque nasi (flares nostril and elevates upper lip) Levator labii superioris (elevates and everts upper lip) Zygomaticus major and minor (mouth angle retractors/elevators, main muscles responsible for smiling)	**Inability to shut eyes** (+/– lower lid ectropion), **flare nostrils, and elevate upper lip**	**Zygomatic and buccal branches have extensive cross innervation** (esp. to nasalis muscle and lip elevators) Targets for Botox: Procerus ("horizontal glabellar lines") Nasalis ("bunny lines" and flared nostrils) Levator labii superioris ("gummy smile")
Buccal	**Buccinator** (flattens cheeks against teeth w/ help of orbicularis oris → prevents food accumulation; high-pressure blowing) **Orbicularis oris** (pursing/puckering of lips, apposition of corners of mouth, pulls lips tight up against teeth, and is required for clear speech) Depressor septi nasi (pulls columella toward lip) **Lip elevators:** Levator labii superioris alaeque nasi, levator labii superioris, zygomaticus major and minor (variable innervation from zygomatic and buccal) **Levator anguli oris** (mouth angle retractor/elevator) **Risorius** (mouth angle retractor, lesser role in smiling)	**Food accumulation** between cheek and teeth **Inability to pucker/purse lips** Drooling as a result of ↓ lip sealing ability **Speech is muffled**, cannot enunciate letters M, V, F, P, and O **Uneven facial expression at rest and w/ smiling** (zygomatic + buccal) vs. only upon smiling with marginal mandibular	Zygomatic and buccal branches have numerous rami and extensive cross innervation, so deficits are often partial and temporary unless extensive damage
Marginal mandibular	Orbicularis oris **Lip depressors:** Depressor anguli oris (lip depressor/retractor) Depressor labii inferioris (lip depressor/retractor) **Mentalis** (lower lip protrusion and elevation) Upper platysma (intercalates with lip depressors/retractors)	Face appears normal at rest but **asymmetric when smiling** Drooling **Inability to evert lower lip**	Marginal mandibular is at **highest risk of causing permanent motor deficits** because has only 1–2 rami and is covered by thin skin and thin platysma Can be injured during neck liposuction or submentoplasty
Cervical	**Platysma** (tenses neck skin, intercalates w/ lip depressors)	↓ Ability to **grimace**	Botox can be used to target platysma ("platysmal bands")

Table 8.4 Cutaneous Danger Zones

Target Structure	Danger Zone	Associated Adverse Event	Other Comments
Vascular occlusion from filler/steroid injections			
Angular artery	Near base of ala	Skin necrosis	Rx: nitroglycerin paste, LMWH, and hyaluronidase (if HA filler)
Supratrochlear artery	Glabellar region	Skin necrosis, **blindness**	Same as above
Motor nerve injury			
Temporal nerve	Most susceptible to injury as it crosses **over the zygomatic arch**	Unilateral **frontalis paralysis, eyebrow ptosis**	Temporal nerve runs a diagonal course from 0.5 cm below the tragus to 1.5 cm above the lateral brow; nerve is superficially located within the fascia as it crosses the zygomatic arch Rx: eyebrow lift
Zygomatic and buccal nerves (less common)	Most significant deficits (i.e., proximal nerve injuries) occur lateral to an imaginary line drawn from lateral canthus to oral commissure	Variable depending on extent of damage (see Table 8.4)	Main trunks of zygomatic and buccal branches of facial nerve lie fairly deep → injuries are uncommon

Table 8.4 Cutaneous Danger Zones—cont'd

Target Structure	Danger Zone	Associated Adverse Event	Other Comments
Marginal mandibular nerve	Most susceptible 2–3 cm inferolateral to oral commissure, as it passes over the mandible (anterior to facial artery)	**Facial asymmetry upon smiling** (normal at rest), inability to protrude lower lip, and drooling	Nerve runs along angle and inferior border of mandible, passing **superficially** over facial artery
Spinal accessory nerve (cranial nerve XI)	Most susceptible to injury at **Erb's point** = site where cervical plexus emerges; located along posterior border of SCM	**Winged scapula**, **inability to abduct arm**, and shoulder pain	**Erb's point** localization: **6 cm inferior** to the midpoint of an imaginary line drawn between the **mastoid** process and **angle of jaw** Great auricular and lesser occipital nerves also emanate from Erb's point
Ulnar nerve	Susceptible to injury around medial epicondyle of humerus	"Claw-hand" deformity; weakness in wrist flexion; loss of sensation and flexion of fourth and fifth digits	—
Other			
Parotid duct	A line drawn from tragus to mid portion of the upper lip approximates its course; duct courses over masseter, pierces buccinator, and drains into the oral vestibule next to second upper molar	Parotid duct fistula; sialocele (distinguished from a seroma by ↑↑ **amylase** levels)	Rx: repair via microsurgery

HA, *Hyaluronic acid;* LMWH, *low-molecular-weight heparin;* SCM, *sternocleidomastoid muscle.*

Branches of facial nerve and danger zones for undermining

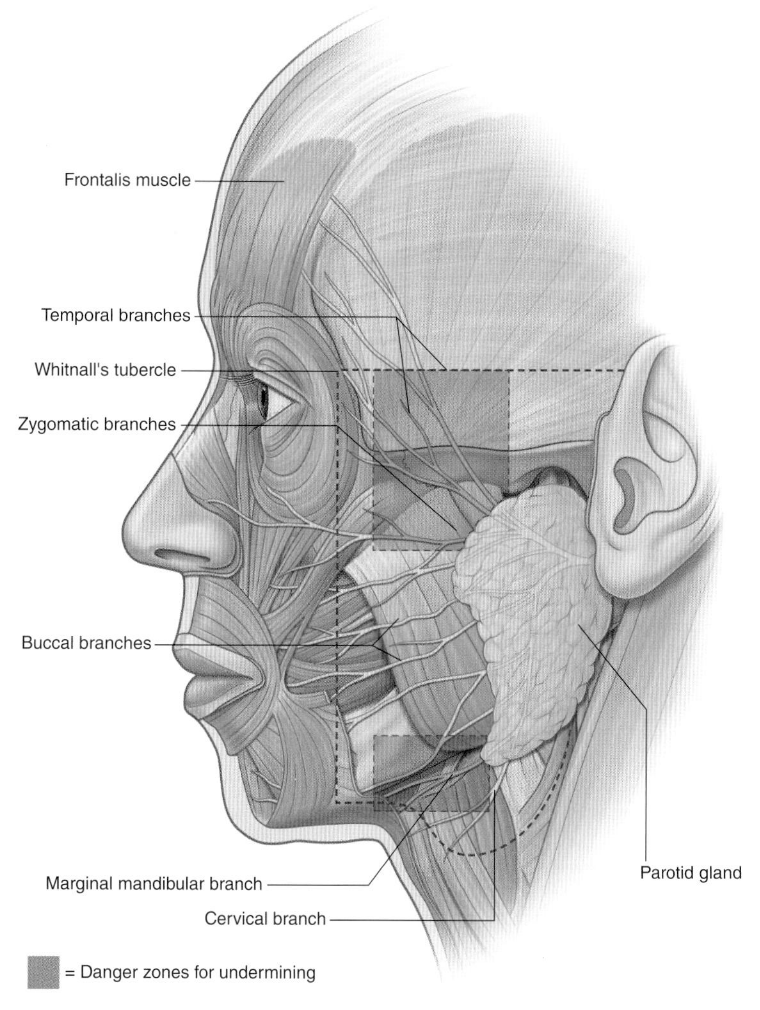

Fig. 8.5 Branches of the facial nerve and danger zones. (From Robinson JK. Anatomy for procedural dermatology. In: Robinson JK, Hanke CW, Siegel DM, Fratila A, eds. *Surgery of the Skin*. 3rd ed. Philadelphia: Elsevier; 2015:1–27.)

8.2 LOCAL ANESTHETICS AND PERIOPERATIVE PAIN CONTROL

- Three major categories of afferent sensory fibers:
  - **C fibers**: small diameter, unmyelinated nociceptors; transmit **diffuse, dull, aching** pain
  - **Aδ fibers**: medium diameter, lightly myelinated fibers; transmit **sharp, localized pain** and **temperature**
  - **Aβ fibers**: fast-conducting, large-diameter, myelinated fibers; detect **vibration and light pressure**; large Aβ fibers respond slowly to local anesthetic → patients continue to "feel something, but not pain" after injection
- Local anesthetics (Table 8.5)
  - Mechanism: reversible **inhibition of sodium ion influx** → prevents depolarization → blocks nerve conduction
  - Chemical structure
    - **Aromatic end**—lipophilic, affects **potency** (more lipid soluble → more potent) and **duration** (more lipid soluble → longer duration because re-lingers longer in tissues)
      - **Clinical** factoid: Bupivicaine is more lipid soluble than Lidocaine →
    - **Intermediate chain**—linkage portion
      - **Amides** (most commonly used)
        - Metabolized via **CYP 3A4** in **liver**
        - **Esters versus amides**: "**two 'I's'** = amIde"
        - Allergic reactions: **very rare** and typically result from **methylparaben or sodium metabisulfite preservatives**, not the anesthetic; if allergy exists, switch to preservative-free lidocaine
        - Caution: **end-stage liver disease**
      - **Esters**
        - Metabolized via **pseudocholinesterases** in **plasma**; renally excreted
        - Less stable in solution
        - **Frequent allergic reactions** to **PABA** metabolite
          - Cross-reacts with multiple contact allergens (Mnemonic "**PPPESTAA**"): Paraphenylenediamine (PPD), PABA, Para-aminosalicylic acid, Ethylenediamine, Sulfonamides, Thiazides, Anesthetics (esters), Azo dyes
        - Contraindications: allergy to PABA or cross-reactors, **pseudocholinesterase deficiency**
        - Caution: renal insufficiency
    - **Amine end**—hydrophilic, binds sodium channel, and determines **onset of action**; more rapid onset when amine group is unprotonated vs. protonated

Table 8.5 Testable Facts Regarding Specific Anesthetics

Anesthetic	Pregnancy Category	Onset (min)	Duration w/o epi (min)	Duration w/ epi (min)	Max Adult Dose (mg/kg) wo/w epi	Most Important Points
Amides						
Lidocaine (Xylocaine)	B	<1	30–120	60–400	4.5 mg/7 mg (safe to use up to 55 mg/kg w/ tumescent anesthesia)	**Fastest onset** of action (<1 min) **Anesthetic of choice in pregnant women**
Prilocaine	B	5–6	30–120	60–400	7 mg/10 mg	**Risk of methemoglobinemia** (↑ risk w/ G6PD deficiency and in children < 1 yo) Component of topical EMLA
Etidocaine	B	3–5	200	240–360	4.5 mg/6.5 mg	—
Ropivicaine	B	1–15	120–360	Same as w/o epi	3.5 mg/NA	Longest duration of action in absence of epinephrine (up to 6 hours)
Mepivacaine	C	3–20	30–120	60–400	6 mg/8 mg	Slowest onset of action Risk of fetal bradycardia
Bupivicaine (Marcaine)	**C**	2–10	120–240	240–480	2.5 mg/3 mg	**Longest duration of action** when combined w/ epinephrine (up to 8 hours) Most common use: added to lidocaine for cases requiring prolonged anesthesia **Highest risk of cardiac toxicity!** Risk of **fetal bradycardia**
Esters						
Procaine (Novocaine)	C	5	15–30	30–90	10 mg/14 mg	Shortest duration of action
Chloroprocaine	C	5–6	30–60	Not known	10 mg/NA	—
Tetracaine	C	7	120–240	240–480	2 mg/2 mg	—

EMLA, *Eutectic Mixture of Local Anesthesia.*
Modified from Soriano TT, Breithaupt A, Chesnut C. Anesthesia and analgesia. Robinson JK, Hanke CW, Siegel DM, Fratila A, eds. Surgery of the Skin. *3rd ed. Philadelphia: Elsevier; 2015:43–63.*

→ alkalinization with bicarbonate speeds onset by decreasing proportion of positively charged/protonated amine groups

- Additives to local anesthetics
  - **Epinephrine** (1:200,000 equally as effective, w/ ↓ toxicity than 1:100,000)
    - Mechanism: vasoconstriction → localization of anesthetic
    - Advantages: ↑ **safety and duration** of anesthetic (because less diffusion and absorption), ↓ **bleeding** (full vasoconstriction takes 7–15 minutes)
    - Disadvantages: ↓ **uterine blood flow (pregnancy category C)**
    - Contraindications: **pheochromocytoma**, uncontrolled HTN, digital anesthesia in severe PVD, and uncontrolled hyperthyroidism
    - Caution: pregnancy (diluting to 1:300,000 considered safe), severe CVD, HTN, narrow-angle glaucoma (periorbital injection), and drugs (nonselective β-blockers, TCAs, and MAO-I)
    - Lidocaine with epinephrine is manufactured to be more acidic (pH 4) than Plain lidocaine (pH 6) because the acidic environment prolongs Epinephrine shelf-life → Lidocaine + Epi is more painful ("burns like acid because it is acid!") than Plain Lidocaine
  - **Sodium bicarbonate** 8.4% (**1 mL per 10 mL** of 1% lidocaine)
    - Mechanism: raises pH to near-physiologic levels → majority of anesthetic remains neutral/uncharged → more rapidly crosses nerve membranes
    - Advantages: ↑ **speed of onset** and ↓ **injection pain** (buffered anesthetic has ~physiologic pH, vs. "injecting acid into skin")
    - Disadvantages: ↑ **epinephrine degradation** → ↓ **shelf life** (must use within 1 week)
    - No need to buffer Plain lidocaine because it is already pH 6
    - Bupivicaine may precipitate if buffered with bicarb; if used, it must be decreased to 0.1mL bicarb per 10mL of Bupivicaine
  - Hyaluronidase
    - Mechanism: digests hyaluronic acid
    - Advantages: ↑ anesthetic diffusion, ↓ tissue distortion
    - Disadvantages: ↓ duration, ↑ toxicity (due to ↑ absorption); contains contact allergen **thimerosal**
- Lidocaine
  - Most commonly used local anesthetic
  - Anesthetic of choice for pregnant women
  - Most commonly used concentrations: **1% (10 mg/mL)**, 2% (20 mg/mL), and 0.1% tumescent (1 mg/mL)
  - Must know the maximum doses!
    - **Without epinephrine** = **4.5 to 5 mg/kg** (31.5–35 mL of 1% lidocaine in a 70-kg patient)
      - ➔ Pediatric = 1.2 to 2 mg/kg (2.4–4 mL of 1% lidocaine in a 20-kg patient)
    - **With epinephrine** = **7 mg/kg** (49 mL of 1% lidocaine in 70-kg patient)
      - ➔ Pediatric = 3 to 4.5 mg/kg (6–9 mL of 1% lidocaine in a 20-kg patient)
    - **Tumescent anesthesia** = **55 mg/kg**
      - ➔ 10-fold dilution of standard 1% lidocaine with 1:100,000 epinephrine (= 0.1% lidocaine with 1:1,000,000 epinephrine)
      - ➔ Advantages: ↓ **bleeding**, ↑ **duration** of anesthesia, and **avoids complications a/w general surgery** (↓ morbidity and mortality)
  - Caution w/ **end-stage liver disease** → ↑ **risk of lidocaine toxicity** (metabolized by liver)
  - Pregnancy class B, lactation safe

- Adverse reactions to local anesthetics (Table 8.6)
  - Must know the presentations of the various adverse reactions to local anesthetics!
  - Mnemonic: lidocaine overdose stages loosely resemble alcohol overdose:
    - **Mild (~"Happily buzzed and tingly feeling")**: restlessness, euphoria, **talkativeness**, lightheadedness,

Table 8.6 Differential Diagnosis of Local Anesthetic Systemic Reactions

Diagnosis	Pulse Rate	Blood Pressure	Signs and Symptoms	Emergency Management
Vasovagal reaction	Low	Low	Excess parasympathetic reaction; diaphoresis, hyperventilation, and nausea	Trendelenburg, cold compress, and reassurance
Epinephrine reaction	High	High	Excess α- and β-adrenergic receptor stimulation; palpitations, muscle tremors, and nervousness	Reassurance (typically short-lived), phentolamine, and propranolol
Anaphylactic reaction	High	Low	Peripheral vasodilation w/ reactive tachycardia; stridor, bronchospasm, urticaria, and angioedema	SQ epinephrine 1:1000 (0.3 mL), antihistamines, corticosteroids, fluids, oxygen, and airway maintenance
Lidocaine overdose				
1–6 mcg/mL	Normal	Normal	Circumoral and digital paresthesias, restlessness, metallic taste, talkativeness, euphoria, and lightheadedness	Observation
6–9 mcg/mL	Normal	Normal	Nausea, vomiting, muscle twitching, tremors, blurred vision, slurred speech, tinnitus, confusion, excitement, and psychosis	Diazepam; airway maintenance
9–12 mcg/mL	Low	Low	Seizures, cardiopulmonary depression	Respiratory support
>12 mcg/mL	None	None	Coma; cardiopulmonary arrest	Cardiopulmonary resuscitation and life support

Modified from Meine JG. Local anesthetics. In: Vidimos AT, Ammirati CT, Poblete-Lopez C, eds. Requisites in Dermatology: Dermatologic Surgery. *Philadelphia: Elsevier; 2009, pp 49–57.*

"funny tingling" around mouth and hands, metallic taste, and **circumoral numbness**
    - **Moderate (~"Hammered! Can't hear or speak well")**: nausea, vomiting, psychosis, **tinnitus**, muscle twitching/tremors, blurred vision, **slurred speech**, and confusion
    - **Severe (~"Severe alcohol poisoning")**: seizures and cardiopulmonary depression
    - **Life-threatening**: coma and cardiopulmonary arrest
  - Easiest way to distinguish between vasovagal (most common), epinephrine reaction, and anaphylaxis (most severe) is to **compare BP and HR**
- Injection techniques to decrease pain (**Boards fodder!**):
  - **Buffer w/ bicarbonate**
  - **Warm anesthetic** to body temperature
  - Pretreat w/ topical anesthetics or ice packs
  - Use **small diameter needle** (30 gauge)
  - Mildly irritate (pinch, rub, Buzzy, ShotBlocker) surrounding skin at the time of injection → decreases transmission of pain signals to brain (**"Gate theory"** of pain)
  - Inject slowly, starting deep in SQ → gradually move superficial
  - Reintroduce needle at previously anesthetized areas and fan out
  - Music and mental distraction also reduce the perception of pain
- **Regional blocks** (see related discussion in Surgical Anatomy section)
  - **Facial**: supraorbital, infraorbital, and mental nerves are the most important (Figs. 8.6 and 8.7)
  - **Feet**: posterior tibial, saphenous, superficial peroneal, and sural nerves (Figs. 8.3, 8.8, and 8.9)
  - **Hand**: median and ulnar nerves (Figs. 8.4 and 8.10)

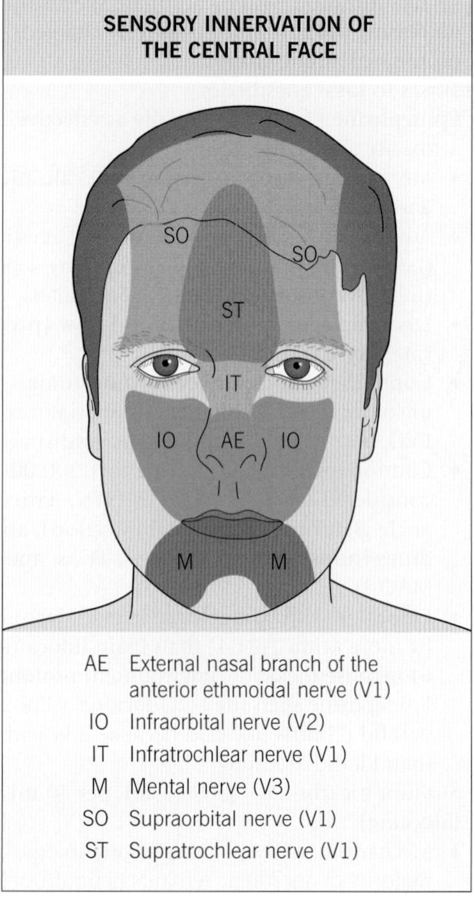

Fig. 8.6 Sensory innervation of the central face. (From Hruza GJ. Anesthesia. In: Bolognia JL, Schaffer JV, Cerroni L, eds. *Dermatology*. 4th ed. Philadelphia: Elsevier; 2018:2440–2449.)

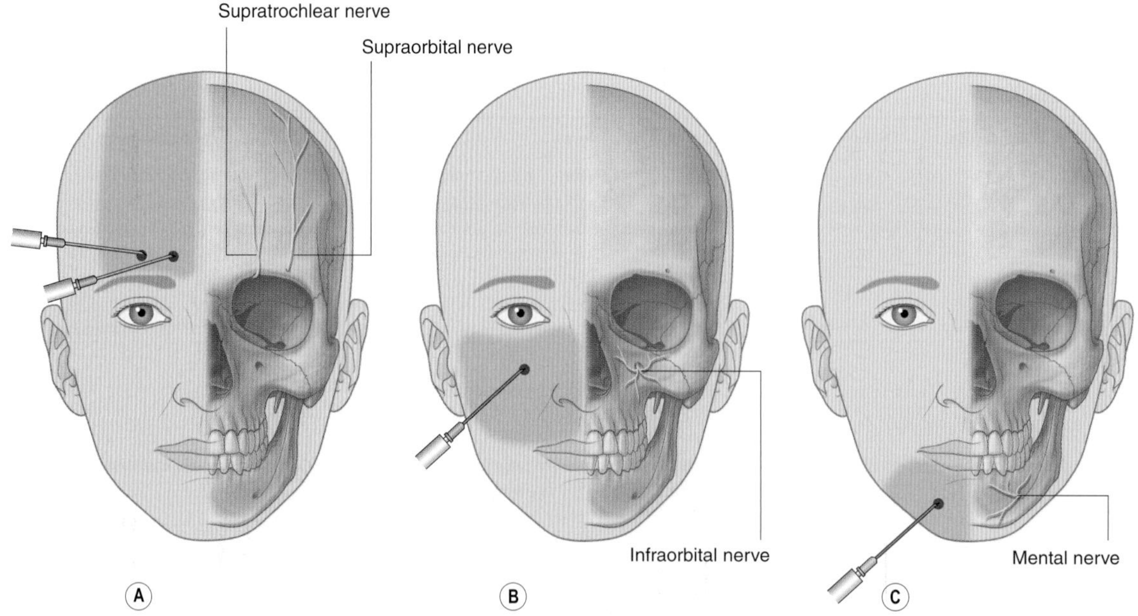

Fig. 8.7 Location and sensory distribution for nerve blocks. (A) Supraorbital and supratrochlear nerve block. (B) Infraorbital nerve block. (C) Mental nerve block. (From Soriano TT, Breithaupt A, Chesnut C. Anesthesia and analgesia. In: Robinson JK, Hanke CW, Siegel DM, Fratila A, eds. *Surgery of the Skin*. 3rd ed. Philadelphia, Elsevier, 2015:43–63.)

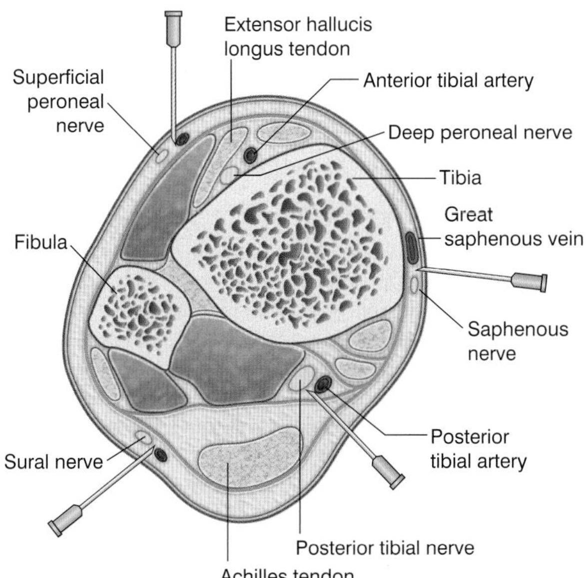

Fig. 8.8 Nerve blocks of the ankle. Transverse section of the right leg above the malleoli. (From Soriano TT, Breithaupt A, Chesnut C. Anesthesia and analgesia. In: Robinson JK, Hanke CW, Siegel DM, Fratila A, eds. *Surgery of the Skin*. 3rd ed. Philadelphia, Elsevier, 2015:43–63.)

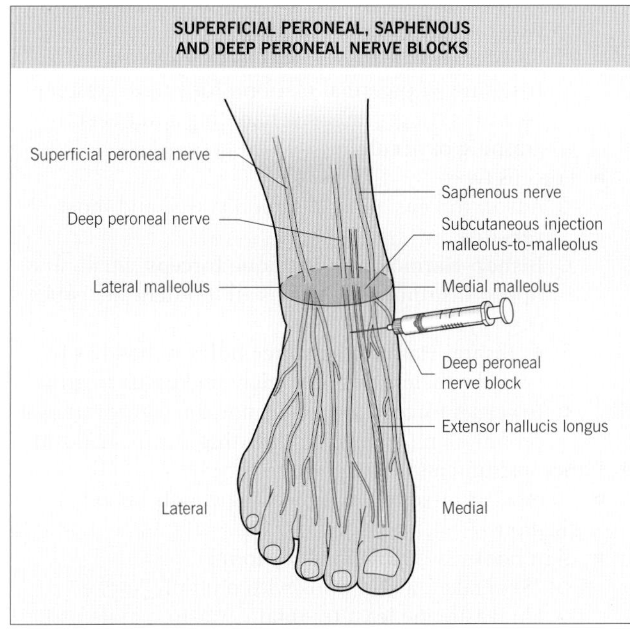

Fig. 8.9 Superficial peroneal, saphenous, and deep peroneal nerve blocks. Great toe dorsiflexion aids in visualizing the extensor hallucis longus tendon. (From Hruza GJ. Anesthesia. In: Bolognia JL, Schaffer JV, Cerroni L, eds. *Dermatology*. 4th ed. Philadelphia: Elsevier; 2018:2440–2449.)

- **Fingers** (digital block): two dorsal and two volar nerves run along sides of finger
  - Lidocaine w/ epinephrine safe **if no history of vascular disease**
  - Proximal block: needle inserted at base of digit, **do not exceed 4 mL total** (risk of tourniquet effect, esp. if >8 mL)
  - Wing block: achieves more rapid anesthesia, but more painful during injection; needle inserted 3 mm

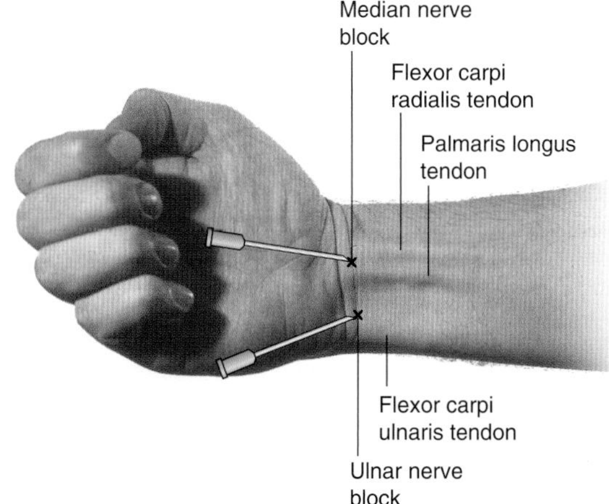

Fig. 8.10 Landmarks for **median and ulnar nerve blocks**. Nerve blocks are delivered by insertion of needles at the proximal crease of the wrist. (Modified from Soriano TT, Breithaupt A, Chesnut C. Anesthesia and analgesia. In: Robinson JK, Hanke CW, Siegel DM, Fratila A, eds. *Surgery of the Skin*. 3rd ed. Philadelphia: Elsevier; 2015:43–63.)

proximal to junction of proximal nail fold (PNF) and lateral nail fold (LNF) → intradermal injection along the PNF → withdraw and redirect along LNF

- **Risks of nerve blocks**: nerve injury, vessel trauma, and intravascular infiltration

- Topical anesthetics
  - Stratum corneum limits penetration → **mucosal sites** benefit more
  - **Boards fodder**:
    - Eutectic mixture of local anesthesia (EMLA): mixture of 2.5% lidocaine + 2.5% prilocaine; **requires occlusion**; risk of **methemoglobinemia in infants** from prilocaine; cannot use near eye (→ corneal injury); on histology, causes **artifactual swelling and vacuolization of upper epidermis + basal layer split**
    - LMX4 (lidocaine 4%): unlike EMLA, does not require occlusion
    - Cocaine: only ester anesthetic to cause **vasoconstriction** (all others → vasodilation); used on nasal mucosa
    - Benzocaine (Anbesol™) and lidocaine jelly: used on mucous membranes
    - Proparacaine and tetracaine: used for ocular/conjunctival anesthesia
- True allergies to local anesthetic are rare!
  - More common: vasovagal reaction (#1) or epinephrine sensitivity
  - Allergic reactions usually due to **preservatives** (**methylparaben** or **metabisulfite** preservatives in amides; or **PABA** in esters)
  - **Amides do not cross-react w/ esters**
- Adjunctive pain/anxiety-control measures:
  - Preoperative anxiolytic
    - **Benzodiazepines** (diazepam and midazolam): generally safe; can reverse overdose w/**flumazenil**
  - Conscious sedation (aka "procedural sedation and analgesia")
    - Short-acting analgesic + sedative → decreased consciousness without need for airway management; requires cardiopulmonary monitoring

- Postoperative pain management
  - **Pain is maximal on night of surgery** → drops dramatically each additional day after surgery
    - Severe pain should not be experienced for >4 to 5 days → if so, consider drug-seeking behavior, infection, or hematoma
  - Rest, Ice, Compression, Elevation (RICE)
  - Acetaminophen
    - Acetaminophen maximum dose/24 hours = **4 g** (<60 yo) or **3 g** (>60 yo)
    - In setting of liver failure, **2 g**/24 hours of acetaminophen alone is safer than either NSAIDs or narcotic
    - **Combining w/ NSAID** superior to either agent alone, but slight ↑ bleeding risk
  - Opioids
    - Occasionally necessary (taut scalp/forehead/large trunk closures)

8.3 SURGICAL INSTRUMENTS AND NEEDLES

- Gold-colored instrument handles: indicates presence of **tungsten carbide**
  - Used in many surgical instruments: needle drivers, forceps, scissors, etc.
  - Tungsten carbide is **harder** and more **durable** than stainless steel
- Scalpel handles
  - Bard-Parker: **standard flat handle (#3, most common)** holds common blades (#15, #15C, #10, #11)
  - Beaver: round or hexagonal; holds smaller, sharper blades; useful for confined spaces or delicate tissue; specific blades (#64, #67)
- Scissors
  - General principles
    - **Short-handled** scissors useful for **delicate work**
    - Long-handled scissors extend the surgeons reach and are useful for undermining
    - Curved blades useful for undermining cysts
    - Straight blades useful for trimming tissue and cutting sutures
    - **Serrated** blades **grab tissue** better
    - Sharp-tipped scissors puncture tissue easily and are best for dissection
    - Blunt-tipped scissors are best for delicate undermining
  - Scissor types
    - **Iris scissors**: sharp-tipped and short-handled; blades may be straight or curved; best for sharp dissection
    - **Gradle scissors**: similar to iris but blades curved and tapered to a fine point at tip; best for delicate tissue (e.g., **periorbital)**
    - **Westcott and Castroviejo scissors**: sharp, fine-tipped, **spring-loaded**; good for **eyelid**
    - **Mayo scissors**: characterized by ~**1:1 handle-to-blade ratio**; primary purpose is coarse dissection
    - **Metzenbaum scissors**: long handles with blunt tips → useful for blunt dissection in **areas that require long reach**
    - O'Brien scissors: angled blade for delicate suture cutting
    - **Supercut scissors**: one blade has a **razor edge**; "supercut" blades are available on most scissor types listed above and often are denoted with **black handles**
- Needle drivers
  - Wide variety; **Webster** and **Halsey** are popular
  - General principles
    - Smaller needle drivers with smooth jaws
      - Ideal for small, delicate needles and work on **face**
      - Advantages: smooth jaws have ↓ **risk of tearing small sutures** (6-0 and smaller) and are **less damaging to fine needles** (P-3 and smaller)
      - Disadvantages: needles not grasped as tightly as with serrated needle drivers → ↑ **needle twisting**
      - Caution: larger needles will ruin small needle drivers
    - Larger, serrated jaws
      - Ideal for larger needles and work on **trunk and extremities**
      - Advantages: serrated jaws hold needles more securely (prevents twisting)
      - Disadvantage: damages delicate needles, shreds small sutures
- Forceps
  - General principles
    - Serrated forceps: **easier to grasp needle**, but results in ↑ **tissue crush injury**
    - Toothed forceps: harder to grasp needle, but handles tissue gently **(↓ crush injury)**
    - Combination forceps: distal teeth for tissue handling w/ proximal platform for suture grasping → allows for gentle tissue handling and easier grasping of needle
  - Forceps types
    - **Adson forceps**: most commonly used and **most versatile**
    - **Bishop-Harmon and Paufique forceps**: small, fine-tipped instruments; most useful for delicate tissues (e.g., **eyelid)**
      - Bishop-Harmon has **three holes** in handles to make them lighter in weight and easier to grip
    - **Jeweler's forceps**: extremely fine tip; suture removal on fine skin (eyelids) and **spitting suture removal**
- Other instruments
  - Hemostats: used to grasp bleeding vessels before ligation
  - Skin hooks: available in many forms;
    - "Skin rake": a skin hook with multiple hooks
    - Hooks are the **least traumatic** way to handle tissue (during electrosurgery and suturing), but are a **sharps hazard**
  - Periosteal elevator: used to remove periosteum or separate nail plate from nail bed
  - Chalazion clamp: useful for eyelid surgery or on the lip to stop bleeding
- Surgical needles
  - Needle is composed of three parts:
    - **Shank (swage)**: swaged portion that attaches to suture; **weakest** part of needle → do NOT grasp here, it will bend or break the needle
      - Size of suture track is determined by shank size, not suture size

- Body: middle portion; **strongest** part of needle → always grasp here; various curvatures (**3/8 circle** most common)
- **Tip**: sharp tip that may be round (tapered) or cutting; minimize grasping of tip → contact w/ other instruments quickly dulls the tip
- Three types of needle tips:
  - Round (tapered): only tip pierces tissue (no sharp edges along arc of needle); **less likely than cutting needles to tear tissues**; used for deep soft tissues (fat and muscle); difficult to pass through skin
  - Cutting: **triangular-shaped** needle point; preferred for skin because it easily passes through tissue; two types:
    - Conventional cutting: cutting surface is on **inner** portion of needle arc; ↑ **risk of suture tearing/ cutting through wound edge** (because cutting edge of needle faces toward wound edge)
    - Reverse cutting: cutting surface is on **outer** portion of needle arc; ↓ **risk of suture tearing/ cutting through wound edge**

8.4 SUTURE TECHNIQUES

- Knots
  - Surgeon's knot: most common; essentially a square knot w/ first knot double thrown to prevent slippage
  - Aberdeen hitch knot: used to tie the end of a running subcuticular suture; **more compact, more secure, and uses less material** than surgeon's knot
- Epidermal ("cuticular") suturing
  - Simple interrupted: used for wounds under **moderate to high tension**; directing the needle away from the wound results in ↑ eversion and ↓ risk of sunken scar
  - Simple running: used for wounds under minimal tension; **faster** to place than interrupted sutures but ↑ risk of dehiscence
  - Running locked sutures: provides **hemostasis** but ↑ strangulation risk
  - **Vertical** mattress: **strongly everts (V**ertical = e**V**ert**)** wound edges; eliminates dead space, and decreases wound edge tension
  - **H**orizontal mattress: provides **H**emostasis **(Horizontal = Hemostasis)**; eliminates dead space, and decreases wound edge tension; significant **strangulation risk** → do not use in poorly vascularized areas
  - Pulley suture: modified vertical mattress suture; used for wounds under **high tension**
  - Running horizontal mattress: same benefits as simple horizontal mattress, but is faster, provides ↑ eversion, and ↓ **strangulation risk;** improved outcomes relative to simple running sutures, but takes longer
  - Tip stitch: half-buried horizontal mattress used for corners (flaps and **M-plasty tips**)
  - High-low (step-off stitch): used to correct imprecise dermal/subcuticular suturing, where one side of the wound edge is higher than the other ("step-off deformity")
- Dermal/subcutaneous ("subcuticular") suturing
  - Simple buried suture: traditional deep suture; minimal eversion; high rate of spitting sutures
  - Buried vertical mattress: **better eversion**; "heart shaped"
  - Set-back suture ("buried butterfly"): suture entry and exit points are both underneath the undermined wound surface; **maximal eversion**; ↓ **spitting sutures** and ↑ **cosmetic outcomes** (vs. buried vertical mattress)
  - Running subcuticular: running sutures in superficial dermis, instead of along epidermal surface; primary advantage = **lack of track marks**; however, ↑ rate of spitting sutures; typically used in combination w/ buried vertical mattress sutures
  - Purse-string: traditionally used to ↓ **wound size** and ↓ **healing time**, relative to second intention; a recent RCT study did not demonstrate any difference in cosmetic appearance or scar size, but there was a trend toward faster healing time
  - Buried pulley suture: essentially just a series of two or more buried sutures; primary advantage = **permits wound closure under high tension**; disadvantage = **tissue strangulation**
  - Fascial plication suture: used to decrease tension on a wound
  - "Figure of 8": used to **tie off bleeding vessels**
- Suture removal recommendations (largely anecdotal): head/neck ≤ 7 days; trunk/extremities = 10 to 14 days; the longer sutures remain in place → ↓ likelihood of dehiscence, but ↑ track-marks
- Suspension sutures: anchor the overlying tissue to periosteum → removes tension from leading edge of flap → **prevents distortion of a free margin** (i.e., tacking cheek rotation flap to lateral orbital rim periosteum to remove tension from leading edge of flap covering lower lid defect); also **prevents flap "tenting" across concavity** (i.e., tacking underside of flap to nasal periosteum when advancing cheek skin medially to cover a nasal sidewall defect)

8.5 WOUND CLOSURE MATERIALS

- Suture types and properties (Tables 8.7–8.11)
- Suture coatings
  - Antifriction coatings present on some multifilament sutures → more easily pulls through tissue
  - Antibiotic (**Triclosan** most common) coating: shown to ↓ **surgery site infection** relative to non-coated
- Barbed sutures
  - New, **knotless** suturing method; barbs hold tissue in place; main benefits = **tension distributed evenly** along entire course of wound, **faster** to use than traditional sutures; most common use = large wounds under ↑ tension
- Tissue adhesives
  - Two categories:
    - **Octyl**: 2-octyl cyanoacrylate (Dermabond)
    - **Butyl**: n-butyl cyanoacrylate (Liquiband)
      - GluSeal is a blend of n-butyl and 2-octyl cyanoacrylate
    - Details:
      - Butyl types **dry faster** than octyl type (30 vs. 150 seconds) but are **more rigid**

Table 8.7 Suture Types

Term	Definition	Comments
Suture type (absorbable vs. nonabsorbable)		
Absorbable sutures	Lose most of their tensile strength within 60 days	Most commonly used as "deep" sutures Tensile strength is lost long before suture is fully absorbed ↑ Absorption rate in moist areas, febrile or protein-deficient patients
Nonabsorbable sutures	Maintains tensile strength for > 60 days	Most commonly used as epidermal sutures
Suture material (absorbable; natural vs. synthetic)		
Natural	Derived from natural proteins (gut, silk)	**Degraded by proteolysis** ↑ Inflammatory reaction and rapidly degraded
Synthetic	Synthetic copolymers	**Degraded by hydrolysis** ↓ Inflammatory reaction and slowly degraded
Configuration (monofilament vs. multifilament)		
Monofilament	Composed of a single filament	Advantages: slide easily through tissue (because of ↓ COF), harbors less bacteria than braided sutures (because of ↓ capillarity), and low-minimal inflammatory reaction Disadvantages: ↓ knot security (because of ↑ memory and ↓ COF); poor "ease of handling" (because of ↓ pliability and ↑ memory)
Multifilament (braided)	Composed of multiple small filaments braided together	Advantages: ↑ ease of handling (because of ↑ pliability and ↓ memory), ↑ tensile strength, and ↑ knot security (because of ↑ COF and ↓ memory) Disadvantages: ↑ **bacterial infections** (because of ↑ capillarity), and ↑ inflammatory reaction

COF, *Coefficient of friction.*

Table 8.8 Specific Suture Properties

Term	Definition	Comments
Tensile strength	Force needed to snap suture	**Synthetic sutures are generally stronger** than natural materials A suture that has been knotted only has 1/3 of its original tensile strength
Size (USP size)	Diameter of suture material necessary to achieve a given tensile strength	**More zeroes = smaller suture diameter** (6–0 suture is smaller than 5–0) Inherent strength of the material also affects USP size (nylon is inherently stronger than gut → 5–0 nylon is smaller in diameter than 5–0 gut)
Coefficient of friction (COF)	Degree of friction encountered when suture is pulled through tissue	**↓ COF → ↓ knot stability** (slippery) Monofilament sutures (particularly polypropylene) have ↓ COF → easily slides through tissue but requires more throws to secure knot Multifilament sutures have ↑ COF → ↑ knot security
Knot security	Strength of the knot	Higher with **multifilament** sutures **Directly proportional to COF** **Inversely related to memory**
Ease of handling	Ease with which suture is used	Multifilament sutures generally have ↑ ease of handling **Directly related to pliability** **Inversely related to memory**
Pliability	Ease with which suture can be bent into a knot; felt as "stiffness" of suture	**Multifilament sutures have ↑ pliability → easier to tie knots/↑ ease of handling** Pliability and memory are the two main determinants of "ease of handling"
Memory	Tendency of suture to retain its original shape; **determined by elasticity, plasticity**, and suture diameter	**↑ Memory → ↓ knot security and ↓ ease of handling** Memory is one of two main determinants of knot security (the other is COF) Memory is one of two main determinants of "ease of handling" (the other is pliability) Monofilament sutures have ↑ memory relative to multifilament sutures
Plasticity	Ability of suture to stretch while maintaining its tensile strength	↑ Plasticity allows suture to **stretch to accommodate postoperative swelling** without cutting into tissue (polypropylene has ↑ plasticity than nylon)
Elasticity	Ability of a suture to return to its original length after being stretched	↑ Elasticity is an **ideal suture property**: elasticity allows suture to stretch to accommodate swelling, and later, resume its original shape → keeps wound edges approximated after edema has resolved **Polybutester** and **poliglecaprone-25** have ↑ elasticity → good for areas that are likely to swell significantly
Capillarity	Ability of suture to absorb fluid	↑ Capillarity → suture wicks more fluid from wound surface into wound (conduit for bacteria) **Multifilament sutures have ↑ capillarity** → ↑ infection
Tissue reactivity	Amount of inflammation incited by suture	Much higher with **natural** sutures (gut, silk) than synthetic

Table 8.9 Absorbable Sutures

Suture	Configuration	Tensile Strength (50%)	Absorption	Ease of Handling	Knot Security	Tissue Reactivity	Comments
Fast-absorbing gut	Virtually monofilament	3–5d	21–42d	Fair	Poor	Low	Often used for skin grafts; pretreated w/**heat** → ↑rate of absorption
Fast-absorbing Polyglactin 910 (Vicryl Rapide™)	Braided	5d	42d	Good	Good	Low	Ionized w/ gamma rays → faster absorption
Plain gut	Virtually monofilament	7d	70d	Fair	Poor	**Moderate-high**	—
Poliglecaprone 25 (Monocryl™)	Monofilament	7–10d	90–120d	Good	Good	**Minimal**	↑ Knot security and ease of handling relative to other monofilaments; **least inflammatory**; **highest initial tensile strength**
Chromic gut	Virtually monofilament	10–14d	90d	Poor	Poor	Moderate (but less than plain gut)	Pretreated w/ chromium salts → collagen cross-linking → slower degradation
Polyglycolic acid (Dexon™)	Braided	14d	90d	Good	Excellent	Low	—
Polyglactin 910 (Vicryl™ and Coated Vicryl Plus Antibacterial™)	Braided	21d	56–70d	Good	Good	Low	↑ Rate of spitting sutures relative to Monocry; coated vicryl plus antibacterial→ ↓pain and ↓ *S.aureus* (MRSA and MSSA) infections; active ingredient = **Triclosan**
Polyglyconate, a copolymer of glycolic acid and polytrimethylene carbonate (Maxon™)	Monofilament	30–40d	180d	Fair	Good	Low	Nearly equivalent to PDS in terms of durability, but has ↑ knot security and is easier to handle
Polydioxanone (PDS II™)	Monofilament	**30–50d**	**180–240d**	Poor	Poor	Low	**Longest lasting absorbable** suture → good for high-tension closures

Modified from Srivastava D, Taylor RS. Suturing technique and other closure materials. In: Robinson JK, Hanke, CW, Siegel DM, Fratila A, eds. Surgery of the Skin. *London: Elsevier, 2015:193–213.*

Table 8.10 Nonabsorbable Sutures

Suture	Configuration	Ease of Handling	Knot Security	Tissue Reactivity	Comments
Silk	Braided	**Gold standard**	Good	**High**	Used on mucosal surfaces Best handling of any suture **Second highest tissue reactivity (#1 is plain gut)**
Nylon (Ethilon™, Dermalon™)	Monofilament (braided form also available)	Good to fair	Poor	Very low	Most common suture used for skin surface closure Clear nylon may be used as a permanent deep suture for periosteal tacking or to prevent scar spread
Polypropylene (Prolene™, Surgilene™)	Monofilament	Good to fair	Poor	**Least**	**Least inflammatory** nonabsorbable suture; has extremely low coefficient of friction → ideal for **running subcuticular suturing** **High plasticity** (**stretches with swelling** rather than cutting into tissue = an ideal suture property), but **low elasticity** (remains stretched when swelling resolves = not an ideal suture property)
Polyester (Ethibond™, Dacron™)	Braided	Very good	Good	Minimal	**Highest tensile strength** of any nonabsorbable suture (excluding stainless steel) Used on mucosal surfaces Similar to silk, but less inflammatory
Polybutester (Novafil™)	Monofilament	Good to fair	Poor	Low	Most useful for skin closure when significant edema is expected (because of ↑ **elasticity**)

Modified from Srivastava D, Taylor RS. Suturing technique and other closure materials. In: Robinson JK, Hanke, CW, Siegel DM, Fratila A, eds. Surgery of the Skin. *London: Elsevier, 2015:193–213.*

Table 8.11 High-Yield Suture Comparisons

Property	Absorbable (Most to Least)	Nonabsorbable (Most to Least)
Tissue reactivity	**Surgical gut** > polyglycolic acid = polyglactin 910 > polydioxanone > **polyglyconate** = **poliglecaprone 25**	**Silk** > nylon > polyester= polybutester > **polypropylene (least)**
Initial tensile strength	**Poliglecaprone 25** > polyglyconate > polydioxanone > polyglactin 910 > polyglycolic acid >> surgical gut	**Stainless steel** (#1 overall) > **polyester** (#1 nonmetal suture) > nylon = polybutester > polypropylene > silk
Time required to decrease to 50% of initial tensile strength	(Longest time to shortest) **Polydioxanone** = **polyglyconate** > polyglactin 910 > polyglycolic acid > chromic gut > poliglecaprone 25 > plain gut > Vicryl Rapide™ > **fast-absorbing gut**	—
Absorption time	(Longest time to shortest) **Polydioxanone** > polyglyconate > poliglecaprone 25 = polyglycolic acid > polyglactin 910 > Vicryl Rapide™ > **fast-absorbing gut**	—

- ♦ All are typically used in combination w/ subcuticular sutures
- ♦ ↑ **Dehiscence rate** and ↓**eversion** (vs. sutures)

- Adhesive strips
  - Applied in combination w/ subcuticular sutures, often w/ topical skin adhesive (Mastisol)
  - Studies demonstrate similar cosmetic outcomes for the combination of subcuticular sutures + adhesive strips (vs. standard bilayered suture closure)
- Staples
  - Traditional staples: typically used on scalp; advantages = **quick**, **easy** application, lower risk of strangulation and ↓ **infection rates** compared w/ sutures; disadvantages = possible ↑ pain after closure
  - Absorbable staples: recently introduced; staples are buried; ↓ pain, ↑ cosmesis compared w/ traditional transcutaneous staples

8.6 ANTISEPSIS AND STERILIZATION

- Hair removal
  - Do NOT shave! Old dogma states that shaving introduces microscopic abrasions → theoretical increase in bacterial access into wound and subsequent infections
    - Recent study by Shaffer (JAAD 2022) found very low risk of infection with razor hair removal → old dogma saying not to shave may be false!
  - DO use clippers and/or chemical depilatories
- Hand hygiene
  - Skin flora is divided into two groups:
    - **Transient bacteria (bad)**: reside superficially; easy to remove w/ hand washing; responsible for most surgical site and nosocomial infections
    - **Resident bacteria (ok)**: reside deeper; difficult to remove; not commonly a/w surgical site infections; for example, *Staphylococcus epidermidis* and diphtheroids
  - Hand hygiene agents: **alcohol or alcohol + chlorhexidine reduces bacterial counts most**, followed by: chlorhexidine only > iodophors > triclosan > soap
- Antiseptic skin preparations (Table 8.12)
  - Activity of these agents is the same as for the hand hygiene products above
  - Important considerations:
    - Alcohol: flammable → may lead to fires, especially in hair-bearing areas
    - **Chlorhexidine: should never be used around the eye (→ severe corneal damage) or ears (ototoxic)**; *Serratia* may colonize chlorhexidine bottles → infection
- Sterilization methods
  - Steam autoclave: most common in office; steam under pressure; **may dull instruments**
  - Chemical autoclave: heated chemical vapor; **lower humidity →less dulling**
  - Dry heat (oven): high temperature, longer time; no humidity → no dulling; **cannot use for cloth, paper, plastic**
  - Gas sterilization: good for large volumes (used primarily in hospitals); expensive, prolonged times and mutagenic gas; effective for heat- and moisture-sensitive instruments
  - Cold sterilization (chemical immersion): not considered adequate for surgical instrument sterilization

8.7 ELECTROSURGERY

Introduction

- Electrocautery and electrosurgery often incorrectly used interchangeably (differences shown in Table 8.13)
  - Electrosurgery: high-frequency **alternating current** to conduct energy via an **unheated** (cold-tipped) electrode
    - High resistance of human tissue (a poor conductor of electricity) to the passage of current causes **conversion of electrical energy to thermal energy** → specific surgical effect (cutting or coagulation)
    - High-frequency current prevents the depolarization of muscles and nerves
    - Types: electrosection, electrocoagulation, electrodesiccation, and electrofulguration
  - Electrocautery: **direct current** → **hot** metallic probe
    - **No flow of current through patient** (vs. electrosurgery); hemostasis is achieved by the direct application of heat

Monopolar versus bipolar

- Terms traditionally used to describe the number of tissue contact tips at the end of an electrode (i.e., "bipolar" forceps have two tips)
- Best to abandon these two terms because "...polar" implies polarity (and unlike direct current, the alternating

Table 8.12 Antiseptics

Agent	Mechanism	Onset	Advantages	Disadvantages	Residual Activity	Comments
Alcohol (isopropyl and ethanol)	Denatures cell walls; 100% alcohol is less effective than **70% (optimal strength)**	Very rapid **(fastest)**	**Broad spectrum**: G(+), G(–), mycobacteria, and many viruses	**Inactive against spores**, protozoan oocysts, and certain nonenveloped viruses; **not effective for soiled hands**	None	**Flammable** → caution w/ electrosurgery and lasers
Chlorhexidine (2%–4%)	Disrupts cell membranes	Rapid	**Broad spectrum**: G(+), G(–), viruses, fungi, and mycobacteria; not inactivated by organics (blood and sputum)	**Inactive against spores**; **ototoxicity**, **keratitis**, and conjunctivitis	**#1 overall** (>6 hours; remains bound to stratum corneum)	**Longest acting** **Often avoided around eyes/ears** Chlorhexidine + alcohol combo antiseptics are **most effective** at preventing SSI
Iodine and iodophors	Oxidation → disruption of protein synthesis and cell membranes	Rapid	**Broad spectrum**: G(+), G(–), **bacterial spores**, mycobacteria, viruses, and fungi	**Skin irritation** and **discoloration** (less w/ iodophors); **inactivated by blood and sputum**	Minimal	**Must wait for it to dry** to be effective Higher risk of SSI compared with chlorhexidine
Chloroxylenol (parachloro-metaxylenol)	Deactivates enzymes and alters cell walls	Slow	Reasonably broad spectrum: G(+) > G(–), mycobacteria, and viruses	Not as broad spectrum, fast-acting, or long-lasting as chlorhexidine; ↓ efficacy in presence of organics	Good	**Ineffective against pseudomonas** unless combined w/ EDTA
Hexachlorophene	Inactivates enzymes	Slow	Effective against staph	Ineffective against G(–), fungi, and mycobacteria; **neurotoxicity**; **teratogenic**	Modest	No longer used Highly absorbed through skin → infants bathed w/ this agent developed **neurotoxicity**
Quaternary ammonium compounds (Benzalkonium)	Induces leaks in cytoplasmic membranes	Slow	G(+) and lipophilic viruses	Ineffective against G(–), mycobacteria and fungi; **inactivated by organic materials and cotton gauze**	Good	Used in **eyedrops**
Triclosan	Alters cytoplasmic membrane and synthesis of RNA, fatty acids, and proteins	Rapid	G(+), mycobacteria, and candida; not inactivated by organics (blood and sputum)	Ineffective against G(–) and filamentous fungi	Good	Not as effective as chlorhexadine, iodophors, or alcohol; Binds **enoylacyl carrier protein reductase** in bacteria; primary agent used in **antibacterial suture coating**
Soap and water	Detergent; removes dirt and organic substances	Very rapid	Highly effective against ***Clostridium difficile*** and **Norwalk** virus	Inconvenient; skin irritation	None	Most appropriate for soiled hands

G(+), *Gram-positive;* G(–), *gram-negative;* SSI, *surgical site infection.*

Table 8.13 Summary of Methods of Electrical Hemostasis

Type	Current	Voltage	Amperage	Terminal	Waveform	Tissue Destruction
Electrocautery	Direct	–	–	N/A	None	++++
Electrodesiccation	Alternating	High	Low	Monoterminal	Markedly damped	+++
Electrofulguration	Alternating	High	Low	Monoterminal	Markedly damped	++
Electrocoagulation	Alternating	Low	High	Biterminal	Moderately damped	++++
Electrosection	Alternating	Low	High	Biterminal	Undamped	Minimal

current used in electrosurgery does not have set positive and negative poles)

Monoterminal and biterminal devices

- Monoterminal and biterminal: refers to the **absence or presence of a grounding electrode** (Table 8.14)
  - Monoterminal circuits (**electrodesiccation** and **electrofulguration**) employ an active electrode **without a grounding pad**
    - Because there is no dispersive electrode to dissipate the accumulated current, **higher voltages** are needed to reach the desired level of effective tissue destruction

Table 8.14 Monoterminal Versus Biterminal

Term	Definition
Monoterminal	No grounding electrode; electrons from patient disperse to table, floor, walls, and air
Biterminal	Presence of a grounding electrode (either grounding pad or biterminal forceps)

- Only electrical difference between electrofulguration and electrodesiccation is that the probe does not directly contact the skin in electrofulguration
  - Biterminal circuits (**electrocoagulation** and **electrosection**) always employ a **dispersive electrode** to recycle current
    - Current travels from the active electrode to the dispersive electrode; if grounding pad is used → current travels through the body, whereas if biterminal forceps are used → current travels between tips of forceps; dispersive electrode provides an outlet of return of current to electrosurgical device, permitting **increased amperage and reduced voltage**
    - Only electrical difference between electrocoagulation and electrosection is the degree of damping

Waveforms

- Waveforms are used to describe the characteristics of a wave's amplitude, frequency, and continuity (**continuous waveforms** result in ↑ **heating** compared to discontinuous waveforms)
- "Undamped" waveform (may be continuous or discontinuous): amplitude remains unchanged throughout sine wave → **pure cutting, no hemostasis**
  - Example: pure **electrosection**
- "Damped" waveform (may be continuous or discontinuous): amplitude decreases with time and eventually reaches zero; the more rapidly the wave's amplitude diminishes to zero, the more damped the current; increased damping results in **greater coagulation/destruction** and **less cutting**
  - Examples: electrodesiccation, electrofulguration, and electrocoagulation

Electrocautery

- **Direct current** supplies energy to device tip → generates heat → **red-hot tip** is applied directly to tissue
  - Mnemonic: "Cautery is Hotery"
  - Electrocautery is distinguished from electrosurgery by its absence of alternating current
- **Current does not pass through the patient**; destruction is achieved solely by heat conducted to the tissue → **safe in patients w/ implantable cardioverter-defibrillators** (ICDs) and pacemakers
- Additional advantages: portable and effective in a wet field

Electrodesiccation

- **Monoterminal** device
- **Low amperage, high voltage**, markedly damped
- **Probe directly contacts tissue** → slowly heats tissue → water loss w/ superficial skin dehydration and mummification, but no significant protein loss

Electrofulguration

- **Monoterminal** device (e.g., hyfrecator)
- **Low amperage, high voltage**, markedly damped
- **Probe held at a distance** (1–2 mm from tissue) → ionized current between probe and tissue ("**spark gap**") → superficial tissue ablation, but underlying tissue protected from heat spread by superficial carbonization → more limited, superficial tissue destruction
- Similar to electrodesiccation in most respects, with the exception that the spark gap and resultant superficial carbonization result in **more limited, superficial tissue destruction**

Electrocoagulation

- **Biterminal** device
- **High amperage, low voltage**, moderately damped
- Probe directly contacts tissue → slow cellular heating → intracellular fluid evaporation, coagulum formation, and resultant protein denaturation
- ↑ **Current (amperage) penetrates more deeply** than in electrodesiccation → ↑ deep tissue destruction and hemostasis

Electrosection

- **Biterminal** device
- **High amperage, low voltage**
- **Undamped** → pure cutting
- Vaporization of tissue without hemostasis; majority of energy dissipates during vaporization → minimal collateral tissue damage
- If used on a "blended mode" with electrocoagulation → provides a **mixture of hemostasis and cutting**

Complications

- Thermoelectric burns at site of current exit may occur if the patient is not properly grounded
- Unwanted current flow through patient
  - Minimize distance a current travels in a patient's body by applying grounding pad to a highly vascularized surface in proximity to operative site
  - Avoid positioning any implantable monitoring devices between the active and dispersive electrodes
- Corneal damage (↑ risk w/ metal eye shields) → be careful around eyes

Fire hazards

- Bowel gas (methane) → exercise caution when using electrosurgery in perianal area

- **Aluminum chloride (flammable)** → must wash off
- **Oxygen should be temporarily disabled** if operative site is in close proximity to the oxygen source
- **Avoid alcohol preps**; use chlorhexidine or povidone-iodine instead

Implantable electronic devices

- Pacemakers and ICDs
  - Most modern (1980s and on) implantable devices have shielding that guards from external electrical interference, though caution still advised
  - **ICDs are more sensitive than pacemakers** to electromagnetic interference (because of the presence of sensing circuits)
  - Electrocautery has 0% risk of electromagnetic interference but is less effective
  - **Biterminal** (often erroneously referred to as "bipolar") **forceps** are effective and very unlikely to cause interference
    - Most surgeons prefer this approach (vs. electrocautery)
  - **Magnet application** can be used to:
    - Temporarily deactivate ICD
    - Switch pacemaker to a preset pacing rate that ignores all electrical signals
  - In cases in which biterminal forceps cannot be used or are unavailable, caution should be taken:
    - Direct the path of current away from implantable devices
    - Do not position implantable devices between the active and dispersive electrodes
    - Use short bursts of energy (<5 seconds and spaced >5 seconds apart)
    - Use lowest effective power settings
    - **Avoid electrosection** (highest risk!)
    - Do not use within 5 cm of implantable device
    - Have a crash cart and ACLS-trained staff ready
  - In cases of uncertainty → cardiology consultation
- Noncardiac implanted electronic devices
  - Examples: deep brain stimulators, spinal cord stimulators, vagal and phrenic nerve stimulators, gastric stimulators, and cochlear implants
  - In contrast to ICDs, patients are usually equipped with an external remote control to power these devices off

8.8 CRYOSURGERY

- Application of low temperature substances → cellular injury → sloughing of damaged tissue
- Mechanism of action (in order):
  - Formation of **ice crystals first in the extracellular space** causing hyperosmotic gradient that pulls water out of cell → intracellular dehydration → membrane damage
  - Further freezing → **intracellular ice crystal formation** → further membrane damage
  - Extracellular thawing reverses gradient and draws water back into cell → cellular swelling and rupture
  - Vasoconstriction from freezing → further damage through anoxia
  - Vasodilation after thawing → release of harmful free radicals into affected tissue → further tissue damage
- Specific cryogens:
  - **Liquid nitrogen (boiling point: −196 °C)** is preferred cryogen due to low boiling point and ease
  - Solid carbon dioxide (boiling point: −79 °C): occasionally used for chemical peels
- Temperature required for cell death (Boards favorite!):
  - By cell type:
    - **Melanocytes (most sensitive): −5 °C**
    - Keratinocytes: −20 °C to −30 °C
    - Fibroblasts (least sensitive): −35 °C to −40 °C
  - Benign versus malignant
    - **Benign: −25 °C**
    - **Malignant: −50 °C**
- Optimal freezing technique = **rapid freezing** + **slow thawing** (favors **intracellular** ice formation)
- Delivery techniques
  - Open technique: most common; liquid nitrogen is released through tips, needles, cannulas, or cones
  - Chamber technique: modification of "open technique"; typically used only for malignancies; cryogen is released into a chamber → turbulence within the chamber → **lower temperatures achieved**, and in shorter amount of time than w/ open technique
  - Closed technique: **cooled probe** is attached to cryogen line in closed system → direct application → tissue destruction
  - Intralesional technique: cryogen injected directly into tissue via cannula or needle

8.9 EXCISIONS

- Indications: biopsy, removal of benign and malignant lesions, and scar revision
- Design: closure of a circle results in large standing cones on each side of the closed wound → therefore, most excisions are executed in a fusiform fashion
  - Apical angles: angles at either end of the excision; **ideally ≤ 30 degrees** in order to avoid formation of standing cones
  - **Length-to-width ratio** should be **≥3:1**
  - Generally, place excisions **parallel to RSTLs**
- Variations:
  - Crescent excision: when one side of excision is designed longer than the other, a curved/crescent shape will result; common uses: sites where RSTLs are curvilinear (**cheek and chin**)
  - M-plasty (Fig. 8.11): used to **shorten length** of excision such that the incision does not extend into an undesired location; common uses: **near free margins** (perioral and periocular regions)
  - S-plasty ("lazy S"): ↑ **total length of scar**, but the linear distance between two apices remains same as linear closure; **redistributes tension** along different vectors → ↓ tension in central portion of scar → ↓ risk of centrally depressed scar, ↓ dehiscence, and ↓ **contraction of scar**; common uses: **convex surfaces (forearm** and shin) and excisions that cross over a joint (elbow and knee)

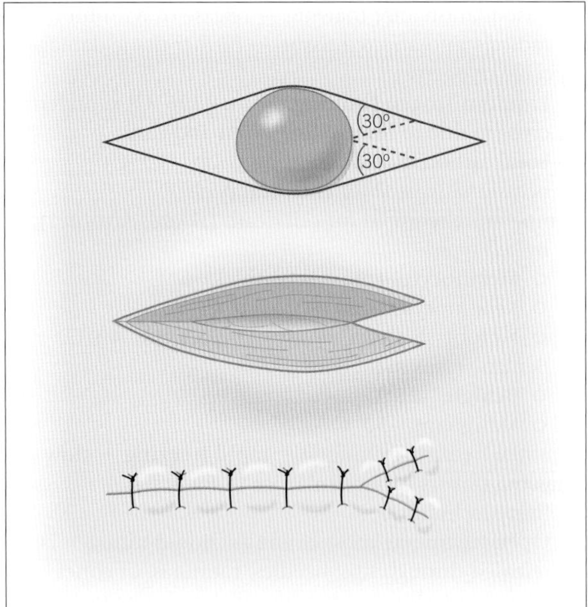

Fig. 8.11 M-plasty. Instead of completing the ellipse, the dashed lines are incised as shown, reducing the length of the scar. (From Cosulich M, Etzkorn J, Shin TM, Miller CJ. Second intention healing and primary closure. In: Rohrer TE, Cook JL, Kaufman AJ, eds. *Flaps and Grafts in Dermatologic Surgery.* 2nd ed. Philadelphia: Elsevier. 2018:34–49.)

  - Lip wedge excision: full-thickness excision of the lip with layered repair; may be used to repair defects up to one third of **the length of lower lip**; must **mark vermillion border before anesthetizing** → ensures precise realignment; close lip in layered fashion in the following **order (high yield!)**:
    - Mucosal layer: use silk or braided polyester
    - Orbicularis oris muscle: use polyglactin 910; re-approximation is critical to maintain competence of oral sphincter
    - Dermis and subcutaneous tissue: start by re-approximating vermilion border
    - Epidermis: hyper-eversion to prevent depressed scar
- Standing cones ("dog ears"):
  - Causes: apical angles that are too wide (>30 degrees), length-to-width ratio <3:1, unequal lengths on each side of wound, convex surfaces, and insufficient undermining at wound apices
  - Repair options ("dog ear repairs"):
    - Extending incision: ↑ excision length allows for redistribution of excess skin
    - M-plasty: removes standing cones
    - Rule of halves: standing cone is redistributed along entire excision length by "halving" it throughout
    - Excision of a Burow's triangle: a triangle of tissue removed from the side of the wound with the standing cone
- Closure types:
  - Simple closure: one layer of sutures (epidermal closure only)
  - Layered closure: two or more layers (epidermal + dermal, SQ or fascia) of sutures → ↓ tension on wound edges (improved cosmesis), ↓ dead space (results in ↓ hematoma and seroma risk)
- **Undermining planes (Boards favorite!):**
  - Trunk/extremities: mid-deep SQ (for small or superficial defects), or just above deep fascia (larger excisions and invasive melanomas)
  - Head/neck: varies by subunit, but generally superficial SQ on face (**superficial to SMAS**); **preserves motor nerves**, which are all deep to SMAS
    - Cheek: mid SQ plane → avoids transecting parotid duct, buccal and zygomatic branches of CN7, and vascular structures
    - Ear: given the near lack of adipose tissue, dissection is always just above **perichondrium**
    - Eyebrow: subcutis, **deep to hair bulbs** → minimizes eyebrow hair loss
    - Eyelid: immediately above orbicularis oculi muscle (because there is minimal SQ tissue)
    - Forehead: deep SQ plane, just **above frontalis (small,** superficial defects); occasionally undermine in avascular **subgaleal plane (large or deep** defects); if desired, superficial SQ undermining may preserve sensory nerves
    - Lateral neck: superficial SQ plane, above spinal accessory nerve → avoids Erb's point
    - Lip: immediately above orbicularis oris muscle → avoids cutting into vascular orbicularis muscle and branches of labial artery
    - Mandible: superficial SQ plane, above marginal mandibular nerve
    - Nose: **submuscular plane immediately above periosteum/perichondrium** (deep to SMAS/nasalis muscle) → relatively avascular plane
    - Scalp: **subgaleal** → avascular plane
    - Temple: **superficial SQ plane** → avoids transection of **temporal branch** of facial nerve and artery
- Wound healing (see Chapter 1, Basic Science)
- **Wound strength following surgery never returns to 100%**; dehiscence risk is highest at the time of suture removal (1–2 weeks)
  - 1 week = 5%
  - 2 weeks = <10%
  - 1 month = 40%
  - 1 year and beyond = **80% (maximum strength)**
- Surgical margins:
  - Melanoma:
    - Melanoma *in situ* → **0.5** to **1 cm** (upper end of range if broad or ill-defined such as lentigo maligna (LM); recent studies by Zitelli et al. recommend 0.9 cm)
    - Breslow depth ≤ 1 mm → **1 cm** wide local excision (WLE) to deep fat or fascia (variable)
    - Breslow depth 1.01 to 2 mm → **1** to **2 cm** WLE to fascia
    - Breslow depth > 2 mm → **2 cm** WLE to fascia
  - Basal cell carcinoma (BCC): **4 mm** margins for most tumors; **0.6** to **1 cm** margins or Mohs for high-risk BCC (high-risk BCC described in Box 8.1)
  - Squamous cell carcinoma (SCC): **4 mm** margins for most low-risk SCC; ≥0.6 cm margins or Mohs for high-risk SCC (high-risk features described in Box 8.1)
  - Dermatofibrosarcoma protuberans (DFSP): **2** to **3 cm** margins extending at least to fascia is recommended, but is a/w ↑ recurrence compared to Mohs

Box 8.1 Mohs Appropriate Use Criteria

BCC/SCC with following features generally considered appropriate for Mohs

Tumors involving:
- **Area H** ("H-zone" or "mask areas" of face, hands/feet, genitalia, nipple/areola): especially if ≥ 0.6 cm
- **Area M** (remaining face, neck, scalp, pretibial): especially if > 1 cm
- Area L: only if > 2 cm or other high-risk features

Recurrent

Perineural/perivascular invasion

Aggressive histologic features:
- BCC: morpheaform, infiltrative, micronodular, or metatypical/basosquamous
- SCC: poor differentiation; depth ≥ 2 mm or ≥ Clark IV; sclerosing, small cell, spindle cell, infiltrating, clear cell, lymphoepithelial, or sarcomatoid subtypes

At site of prior radiation/scar

Immunosuppressed status (CLL, organ transplant, HIV, hematologic malignancy, or pharmacologic immunosuppression)

Genetic syndromes (Gorlin's, XP, etc.)

Lentigo maligna/MMIS with following features generally considered appropriate for Mohs

Area H or Area M

Recurrent

Other rare tumors generally considered appropriate for Mohs

Adenoid cystic carcinoma, adnexal carcinoma, apocrine/eccrine carcinoma, AFX/PDS/UPS, DFSP, EMPD, LMS, MCC (not generally recommended), MAC, mucinous carcinoma, sebaceous carcinoma

Data from Ad Hoc Task Force, Connolly SM, Baker DR, et al. AAD/ACMS/ASDSA/ASMS 2012 appropriate use criteria for Mohs micrographic surgery: a report of the American Academy of Dermatology, American College of Mohs Surgery, American Society for Dermatologic Surgery Association, and the American Society for Mohs Surgery. J Am Acad Dermatol. *2012;67(4):531–550.*

8.10 MOHS SURGERY

- Mohs micrographic surgery (MMS): specialized method of skin cancer removal that provides complete **360° (circumferential) microscopic margin control**; by definition, both the surgery and microscopic evaluation **must be performed by same provider**
- Advantages:
  - Allows for microscopic evaluation of 100% of the excision margins (vs. <1% with "breadloafing" technique used for standard elliptical excisions) → ↑ **cure rates** due to ↓ false-negative margins
  - **Tissue sparing** (smaller margins can be taken w/ confidence that the tumor is clear)
  - Compares favorably in terms of **cost effectiveness** relative to other treatments
- MMS offers superior cure rates for most skin cancers, including rare forms:
  - **BCC/SCC:** 97%–99% for primary lesions (vs. 93% for conventional excision) and 90%–95% for recurrent lesions (vs. 80% for conventional excision)
  - **DFSP (treatment of choice)**: >98%
  - MMIS, including lentigo maligna: >98%
  - AFX: >95%
  - Microcystic adnexal carcinoma: 90%–95%
  - EMPD: 85% (potentially higher if intraoperative CK7 immunostain is used)
  - Leiomyosarcoma (superficial): >90%
  - Sebaceous carcinoma: >90%
  - Erythroplasia of Queyrat: >90%
  - Others: verrucous carcinoma, various adnexal carcinomas, Merkel cell carcinoma (not generally recommended), and angiosarcoma (not generally recommended)
- Tumor must have a contiguous growth pattern to be amenable to Mohs
- Essential steps of Mohs technique:
  - Clinically apparent residual tumor/biopsy site is debulked with curette or scalpel
  - **Beveled** excision (**scalpel held at 45° angle**) of tumor plus a small (1–2 mm) margin of normal-appearing skin
  - Hash marks ("notches") are placed on excision specimen and surrounding nonexcised skin to assist w/ orientation
  - Excised specimen may be divided into two or more pieces (optional)
    - Central **relaxing incisions** (or "**Pac Man**" incision of undivided specimen), and/or dividing into two or more pieces helps flatten tissue to ensure epidermis lies in same plane as deep tissue
  - Excised specimen is inked with two or more colors
  - Histotechnician flattens tissue to ensure that the **epidermis lies in the same plane as the deep tissue** → allows for horizontal processing of slides (stain = **H&E or Toluidine blue**) → enables simultaneous microscopic evaluation of superficial and deep margins
  - Surgeon evaluates slides for residual tumor
  - If tumor is present, the site is marked on the Mohs map, and steps two to seven are repeated until tumor has been eradicated
  - Once tumor is cleared, surgeon discusses reconstructive options w/ patient
- Mohs Appropriate Use Criteria (AUC): criteria established in 2012; developed to guide decision-making, not to establish the standard of care (see Box 8.1)

8.11 FLAPS

- **Indications**:
  - Defects that will heal poorly by secondary intention
  - When linear repair would compromise function, result in excessive tension, or distort a free margin
  - To maintain three-dimensional contour when there is significant tissue loss
- **Advantages**:
  - Excellent color, texture, and thickness match, as the skin is recruited from adjacent tissue reservoirs

- Ability to redirect tension vectors
- Can be used to cover cartilage/bone because of reliable blood supply
- Rapid healing
- Replaces volume when there is significant tissue loss

- **Disadvantages**:
  - Geometric scar lines if not concealed in RSTLs
  - Poor design can lead to functional compromise, free margin distortion, poor esthetics, or flap necrosis
- **Definitions** (Fig. 8.12):
  - Primary defect: defect following tumor extirpation that requires repair
  - Secondary defect: defect created by flap elevation and closure of primary defect
  - Body: tissue that is being shifted ("flapped") onto the defect
  - Pedicle (flap base): vascular base of flap → provides blood flow to flap
  - Flap tip: portion of flap furthest away from the blood supply/pedicle → area at **highest risk for necrosis**
  - Primary lobe (for multi-lobed flaps): portion of flap intended to cover primary defect
  - Secondary lobe (for multi-lobed flaps): portion of flap intended to cover secondary defect
  - Primary flap movement: motion of flap movement required to close primary defect
  - Secondary flap movement: motion of flap movement required to close secondary defect
  - Primary tension vector: direction of force resisting the movement of the flap body
  - Secondary tension vector: direction of force created by closure of donor site defect
  - Pivot point: point on the base of the flap around which the flap transposes/rotates → critical to **undermine this area to obtain optimal flap movement**
  - Flap size (required measurement for billing purposes): entire surface area of flap elevation + surface area of primary defect
  - **Key stitch**: critical **initial stitch** required to move the flap onto the primary defect
  - **Axial pattern flap**: flaps based on a named vessel → most reliable; includes **paramedian forehead flap** (supratrochlear artery), **dorsal nasal rotation "Rieger" flap** (angular artery), and **Abbe cross-lip flap** (labial artery)
  - **Random pattern flap**: flaps with unnamed musculocutaneous arteries within pedicle; elevated portion of flap is perfused by **anastomotic subdermal and dermal vascular plexuses**; includes all flaps not listed above
- There are many ways to classify flaps (primary motion, blood supply, shape, and eponymous name); however, they are **best classified according to primary motion**:
  - Sliding: flap slides into place with linear or curvilinear motion; redundant tissue can be excised anywhere along length of flap; **main tension vector = opposite direction of flap movement**; key stitch closes ***primary*** defect (approximates flap edge to opposite edge of primary defect)
    - Advancement flap (Table 8.15):
      - Mechanics: **does not redirect** primary tension vector
      - Goal: **redistribute Burow's triangle to a more functionally or cosmetically desirable location** (e.g., **away from free margins** [eyelid, ear, lip, and alar rim])

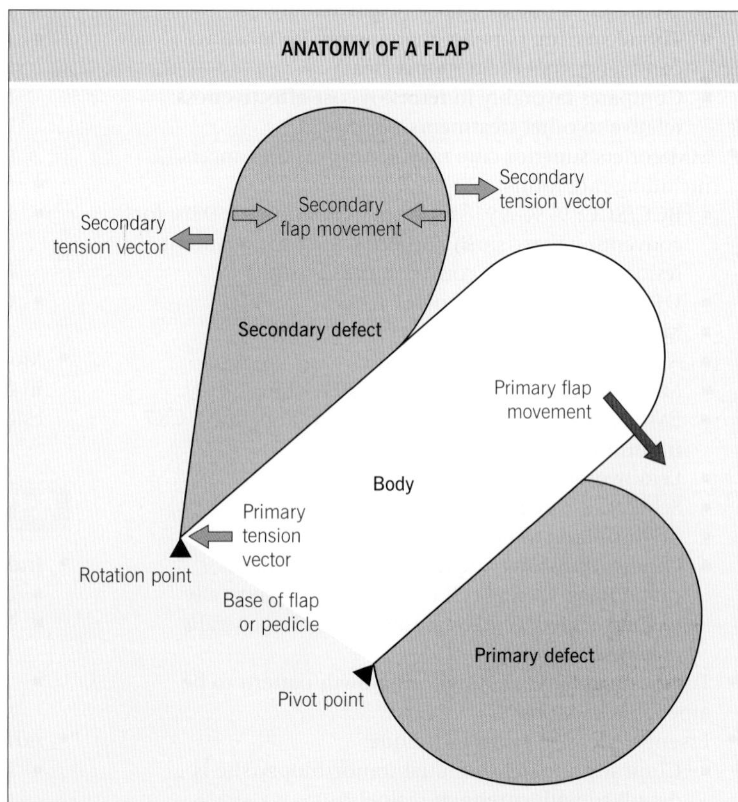

Fig. 8.12 Anatomy of a flap. (From Brodland DG. Flaps. In: Bolognia JL, Schaffer JV, Cerroni L, eds. *Dermatology*. 4th ed. Philadelphia: Elsevier; 2018:2495–2516.)

Table 8.15 Advancement Flaps

Flap Category (Variants/Other Names)	Design	Common Uses	Comments
Unilateral Burow's advancement (A → L, O → L)	Displaces one of the Burow's triangles to a more cosmetically or functionally desirable location (away from free margins or hidden between cosmetic subunits)	Suprabrow (displaces Burow's lateral to eyebrow) Off-center nasal dorsum/tip ("East-to-West" flap; maintains nasal symmetry) Lateral upper cutaneous lip (displaces Burow's into NLF)	Does not provide much added laxity relative to linear closure
Unilateral crescentic advancement (perialar crescentic)	Variant of A → L where a crescentic standing cone is removed within flap body → eliminates need to remove one of the two Burow's triangles	Suprabrow (hides incision above eyebrow hairline) **Cheek-to-nose perialar crescentic advancement**: defects immediately superior to alar crease (hides incision in alar crease +/− NLF)	Cheek-to-nose flap may require suspension/tacking suture from body of flap to nasal periosteum to recreate the nasofacial sulcus and prevent "tenting"
Unilateral O →U advancement	Incisions and Burow's triangles oriented in same direction away from defect → a square or rectangle-shaped flap is advanced onto defect	Helical rim advancement (useful for deeper defects that are not amenable to FTSG or second intention healing) Eyebrow (used to preserve continuity of brow; hides incision lines above and below browline)	**Hyper-evert** helical rim flaps → prevents notching Smaller pedicle → more prone to ischemia
Bilateral A → T advancement (O → T)	Divides one of the two standing cones into two smaller Burow's triangles; two opposing flaps are bilaterally advanced onto defect	Similar to A → L, but can cover larger defects Chin (hides flap incisions in mental crease) Suprabrow (when unilateral is not enough)	—
Bilateral O → H advancement	Essentially a double O → U flap, w/ mirror-image flaps on either end of primary defect	Eyebrow, forehead	Disadvantages: multiple incision lines, **forehead numbness** (as a result of long horizontal incisions)
V →Y advancement flap (formerly island pedicle flap)	Unlike other advancement flaps, **area under flap body is not undermined** (serves as random-pattern pedicle); periphery is undermined widely, then V-shaped island w/ deep pedicle is advanced onto defect; **key stitch**: connects midpoint of leading edge of flap to midpoint of defect's wound edge	Small defects on nasal tip or immediately above alar crease Small, deep alar defects (includes "shark IPF", which can re-create alar crease) **Medium to large defects on lateral upper cutaneous lip** (particularly those involving the nose-lip-cheek junction) Eyebrow defects Repair of ectropion	In reality, a portion of pedicle must be undermined to allow for movement, but **must ensure that ≥ 40% of pedicle remains intact** Tissue-efficient flap (no tissue discarded) Disadvantages: triangular-shaped scar (often prominent); **trap-door effect**
Mucosal advancement	Essentially a linear flap of lip mucosa; **undermine deep to minor salivary glands, but superficial to orbicularis muscle**; undermine to gingival sulcus; flap is advanced onto vermilion defect	Vermilion lip	Disadvantages: **lip numbness** (improves over time); thinning of lip

NLF, *Nasolabial fold.*

- Disadvantages: **limited by degree of elasticity of surrounding tissue** → suboptimal for large defects that lack abundant adjacent tissue reservoir/laxity
- Rotation flap (Table 8.16):
  - Mechanics: **redirects primary tension vector** along an arc adjacent to primary surgical defect while simultaneously creating a secondary defect along the flap arc
  - Goal: take advantage of tissue reservoir/laxity at a distance from primary defect
  - Disadvantages: there is a **functional loss of flap length and height** when flap is rotated onto defect → **length of flap arc must be much longer** than width of primary defect and **height of flap must be taller** than height of primary defect; is a **heavy flap** and prone to causing **unwanted secondary tension vectors** → may result in distortion of free margins (ectropion) if not carefully executed → may require tacking sutures to periosteum to minimize risk
  - Main uses: large defects on medial cheek; large defects on inelastic skin (scalp); areas w/ curved RSTLs (chin and along mental crease); **redistribute tension away from free margins** (lower eyelid, nasal tip, and upper lip)
- Lifting: flap is **lifted and transposed** ("leapfrogged") over normal intervening skin; has both **pivotal and rotational** movements; **redirects primary tension vector** to donor site; goal is to use nearby, but **"nonadjacent," tissue reservoir** ("nonadjacent": intervening normal skin is present between flap donor site and primary defect) in order to **close primary defects at sites that have minimal inherent laxity** (nose, medial canthus, and ear); key stitch varies depending on specific flap
  - Transposition (single-stage) flaps (Table 8.17)
    - Mechanics: **redirects primary tension vector** onto donor site → results in loose flap of skin that can be "plopped onto" primary defect → primary defect closed under minimal to no tension

Table 8.16 Rotation Flaps

Flap Category (Variants/Other Names)	Design	Common Uses	Comments
Unilateral rotation	Curvilinear incision w/ arc length > defect width, and arc height > defect height to compensate for loss of length as flap rotates; **area of pivotal restraint must be undermined** extensively to allow movement; **back-cuts** ↑ mobility, but ↓ blood flow	Upper cutaneous lip (hides incision in melolabial fold) Chin (hides incision in mental crease)	On face, **flap pedicle should be inferior-lateral to ↑ lymphatic drainage** → ↓ flap lymphedema
Unilateral rotation, Rieger variant (dorsal nasal rotation, Hatchet flap, and glabellar turn-down)	**Axial flap** (**angular artery)** w/ **back-cut in glabella**; undermine just above perichondrium; maximal points of **pivotal restraint** = **medial canthal tendon** and nasofacial sulcus	Medium to large (up to 2.5 cm) midline defects on lower 2/3 of nose (tip/supratip)	Disadvantages: **transposition of thick glabellar skin onto medial canthus,** long incision lines, potential **"pig-nose" deformity** (as a result of inadequate undermining and unwanted secondary tension vectors)
Unilateral rotation, Mustarde/Tenzel variant	Laterally based rotation flap of cheek/temple; Mustarde flaps utilize entire cheek/temple reservoir; Tenzel flaps are smaller (partial-cheek)	Mustarde: larger lower lid defects (≥50%) Tenzel: smaller defects of mid to lateral lower lid (<50% of lid)	**Tacking sutures to lateral orbital rim periosteum → ↓ ectropion risk**
Bilateral rotation (O → Z)	Double rotation flap with yin-yang shape	Large defects involving inelastic skin (mainly used for **scalp**)	Disadvantages: long, prominent incision lines (minimize w/ good galeal suturing, eversion)

Table 8.17 Transposition Flaps

Flap Category (Variants/Other Names)	Design	Common Uses	Comments
Rhombic flap	Classic design (Limberg flap): **parallelogram-shaped flap** w/ two 60-degree angles and two 120-degree angles; flap takes off from defect at 90-degree angle; Burow's triangle removed at pivot point; **secondary defect is closed first (key stitch)**	Medial canthus Cheek Temple Upper lateral 1/3 of nose	Final suture line looks like a **question mark** **Eight rhombic flaps possible** for any rhombic-shaped defect **Dufourmental** and **Webster modifications:** ↓ angle of flap tip → **shorter arc of rotation** → easier to close secondary defect, ↑ **tension sharing** between 1° and 2° defect, ↓ reorientation of tension vectors, and ↑ risk of ischemia (as a result of a narrower pedicle)
Bilobed flap (Zitelli modification)	Multilobed transposition flap that **redistributes tension to areas of greater tissue laxity** (i.e., nasal dorsum/sidewall); tension is shared between all lobes; **1° lobe diameter = primary defect diameter; 2° lobe diameter** = **1° lobe diameter** (or slightly smaller); flap takeoff point = midpoint of defect at a 45-degree angle; angle between 1° and 2° lobe also = 45 degrees → flap has **overall angle of 90 degrees**; remove standing cone at pivot point; **undermine flap in submuscular plane to nasofacial sulcus** to achieve adequate movement; **order of closure** = **tertiary defect** (2° lobe donor site; **key stitch**) → secondary defect (1° lobe donor site) → primary defect closed last	Distal 1/3 of nose	May use as many lobes as necessary (trilobe, tetralobe) to reach a tissue reservoir where tension will not cause distortion Risk of **pincushioning (trapdoor)** → may be due to oversizing flap, insufficient undermining, ↑ bulkiness on underside of flap, flap lymphedema (self-resolves), peripheral contraction (↑ risk w/ rounded flaps), or insufficient tacking of flap to wound base Original bilobed flap design was inferior to Zitelli's: used 180-degree overall angle (vs. 90 degrees) and did not remove standing cone at pivot point → ↑ pincushioning of 1° lobe, ↑ standing cone at pivot point
Banner transposition flap	Long, narrow transposition flap w/ **high length:width ratio** (3:1 to 5:1); flap is raised along RSTLs and transposed onto primary defect	Upper helical rim Medial canthus and nasal bridge (donor site: glabella) Lateral lower lid (donor: upper lid) Medial lower lid (donor: nasofacial sulcus)	Narrow pedicle → must ensure flap has robust blood supply to prevent necrosis Prone to **pincushioning (trapdoor) effect** → must undermine recipient site widely, undersize flap or deepen recipient bed, and use tacking sutures to ↓ dead space between flap and recipient site

Table 8.17 Transposition Flaps—cont'd

Flap Category (Variants/Other Names)	Design	Common Uses	Comments
Nasolabial/melolabial transposition flap	Variant of banner flap w/ 60° angle of transposition; tack pivot point to **pyriform aperture** (near junction of lateral ala/ isthmus of upper lip); must thin distal portion of flap extensively	Medium-sized, deep defects of nasal ala	Disadvantages: **blunting of alar crease (almost all cases), pincushioning** → minimized w/ tacking sutures, flap thinning, and wide undermining of recipient site Many cases require revision **Spear flap (variant)**: used for full-thickness alar defects; same general design, but flap is folded on itself to provide internal nasal lining + external coverage
Z-plasty	Transposition flap primarily used for lengthening a contracted scar and redirecting tension; may use various angles: ↑ **angle size** → ↑ **length gain and** ↑ **reorientation** of tension		30° angle → 25% ↑ length and 40° tension reorientation 45° angle → 50% ↑ length and 65° tension reorientation **60° angle → 75% ↑ length and 90° tension reorientation**

RSTLs, *Relaxed skin tension lines.*

- ♦ Goal: utilize nearby tissue reservoirs in order to close defects at sites that have minimal inherent laxity
- ♦ Disadvantages: prone to **pincushioning/"trapdooring" (→ must widely undermine to prevent)**; technically challenging

- o Staged interpolation flaps (Table 8.18)
    - ♦ Mechanics: similar to single-stage transposition flaps but base of flap (pedicle) is not adjacent to defect and must be divided in a second stage; thick vascular pedicle (either **random pattern or axial**) provides ↑ blood flow → allows for **↑↑↑ flap length-to-width ratio** (>4:1 maximum ratio seen w/ most other flaps), and coverage of very large defects; **pedicle typically divided and inset at 3 weeks**
    - ♦ Goal: utilize nearby tissue reservoirs in order to close defects at sites that have minimal inherent laxity or limited blood supply
    - ♦ Main uses: large defects on nose, large helical rim defects, and large lip defects

- Sliding flaps (noteworthy **key stitches** marked with star)
    - Unilateral advancement flap ("O to U" or "U-plasty") (Fig. 8.13)
    - Bilateral advancement flap ("H-plasty") (Fig. 8.14)
    - Bilateral advancement flap ("A-to-T" or "O-to-T") (Fig. 8.15)
    - Burow's advancement flap, crescentic advancement flap (Fig. 8.16)
    - V-to-Y advancement flap (formerly, "island pedicle flap"): vascular supply derived from non-undermined subcutaneous pedicle (Fig. 8.17)
    - Rotation flap (Mustarde type) (Fig. 8.18)
- Lifting flaps
    - Rhombic flap (and variants) (Fig. 8.19)
    - Bilobed transposition flap (Fig. 8.20)
    - Single-stage nasolabial/melolabial transposition (modified banner) flap (Fig. 8.21)

Table 8.18 Staged Interpolation Flaps

Flap Category (Variants/Other Names)	Design	Common Uses	Comments
Paramedian forehead flap (PMFF)	**Axial flap** based on supratrochlear artery; **maximum length of flap = distance between orbital rim to frontal hairline** (if longer, will transplant hair onto nose); pedicle arises at medial brow **contralateral** to the predominant side of nasal defect (minimize twisting); pedicle oriented in vertical fashion; ideal **pedicle width = 1.0–1.5 cm**; flap body elevated from cephalad to caudad in plane just above periosteum; flap tip must be extensively thinned before suturing to nasal tip; **pedicle is divided and inset at 3 weeks**	Large nasal defects	Pedicle too narrow → fails to incorporate artery → ischemia Pedicle too wide → kinking of artery → ischemia and ↓ rotational ability
Abbe lip switch	**Axial flap** based on labial artery; transfers both skin, mucosa and orbicularis oris muscle to recipient site; **pedicle divided and inset at 3 weeks**	Large (>1/3 of lip), full-thickness defects of upper or lower lip	Most commonly used for upper lip defects, because defects involving **up to 1/3** of lower lip can be repaired via **lip wedge** Risk of microstomia and oral incompetence

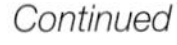
Continued

Table 8.18 Staged Interpolation Flaps—cont'd

Flap Category (Variants/Other Names)	Design	Common Uses	Comments
Nasolabial/melolabial interpolation flap	**Random pattern flap** perfused by small perforators of angular artery; similar in design to single-stage nasolabial transposition flap, but retains a thick vascular pedicle; extensively debulk flap tip before suturing onto primary defect; **pedicle divided and inset at 3 weeks**	Nasal ala (primary use) Large defects of upper cutaneous lip	Advantage: **does not blunt alar crease** (unlike single-stage transposition) Disadvantage: vascularity less reliable than PMFF
Retroauricular ("book") flap	**Random pattern flap**; a rectangular-shaped flap is raised in subcutaneous plane from retroauricular sulcus to the hairline; flap tip is thinned and sutured onto helix; **pedicle divided at 3 weeks**	Large defects of helical rim +/– loss of cartilage	Donor site often left to heal by second intention

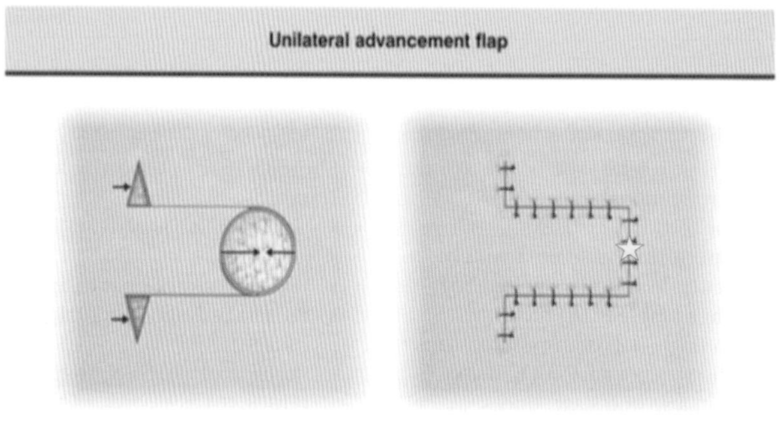

Fig. 8.13 Unilateral advancement flap. Key stitch indicated by yellow star. (Modified from Cook JL, Goldman GD, Holmes TE. Random pattern cutaneous flaps. In: Robinson JK, Hanke CW, Siegel DM, Fratila A, eds. *Surgery of the Skin*. 3rd ed. Philadelphia: Elsevier; 2015:252–285.)

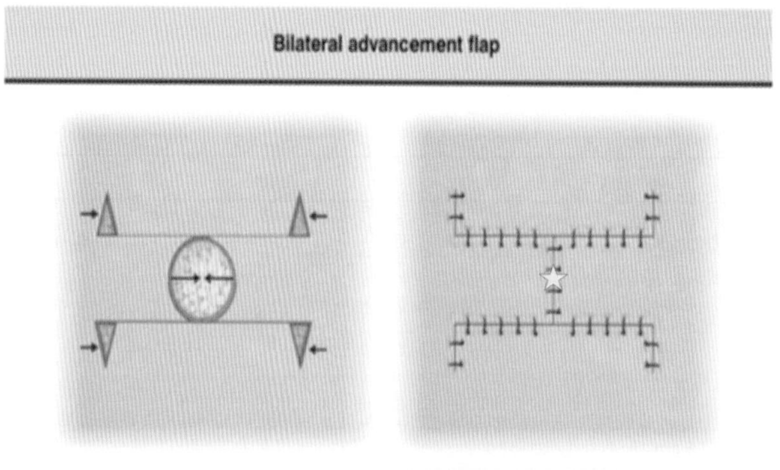

Fig. 8.14 Bilateral advancement flap. Key stitch indicated by yellow star. (Modified from Cook JL, Goldman GD, Holmes TE. Random pattern cutaneous flaps. In: Robinson JK, Hanke CW, Siegel DM, Fratila A, eds. *Surgery of the Skin*. 3rd ed. Philadelphia: Elsevier; 2015:252–285.)

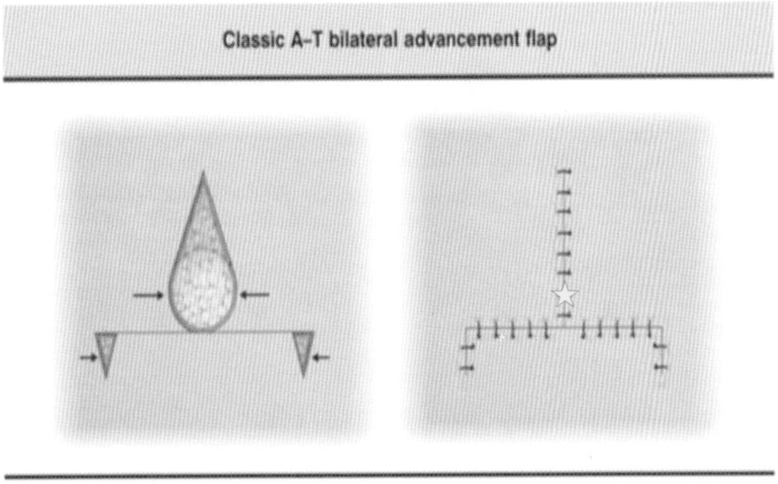

Classic A–T bilateral advancement flap

Fig. 8.15 Bilateral advancement flap ("A-to-T"). Key stitch indicated by yellow star. (Modified from Cook JL, Goldman GD, Holmes TE. Random pattern cutaneous flaps. In: Robinson JK, Hanke CW, Siegel DM, Fratila A, eds. *Surgery of the Skin*. 3rd ed. Philadelphia: Elsevier; 2015:252–285.)

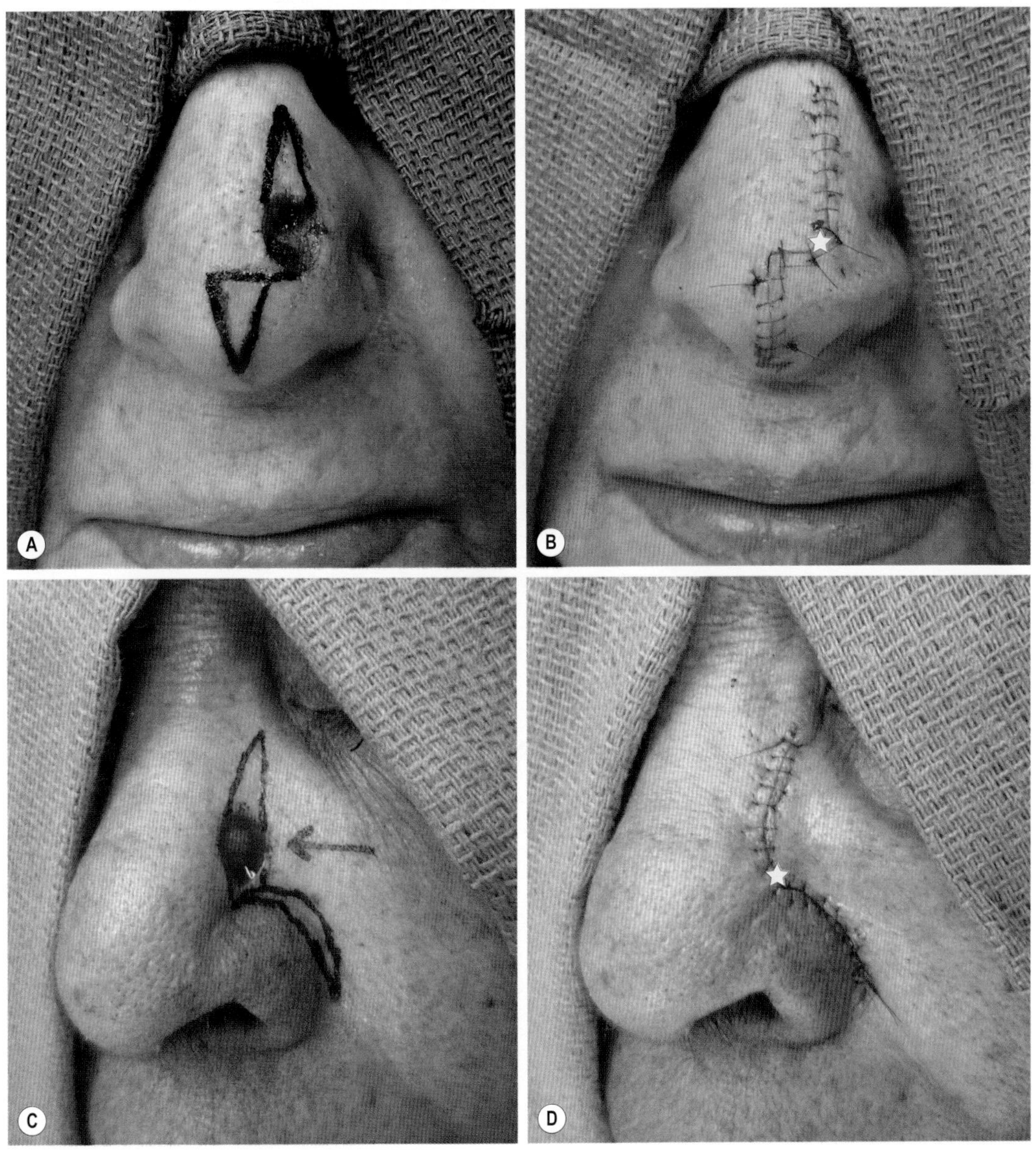

Fig. 8.16 Burow's advancement flap (A and B); crescentic advancement flap (C and D). Key stitches indicated by yellow star.

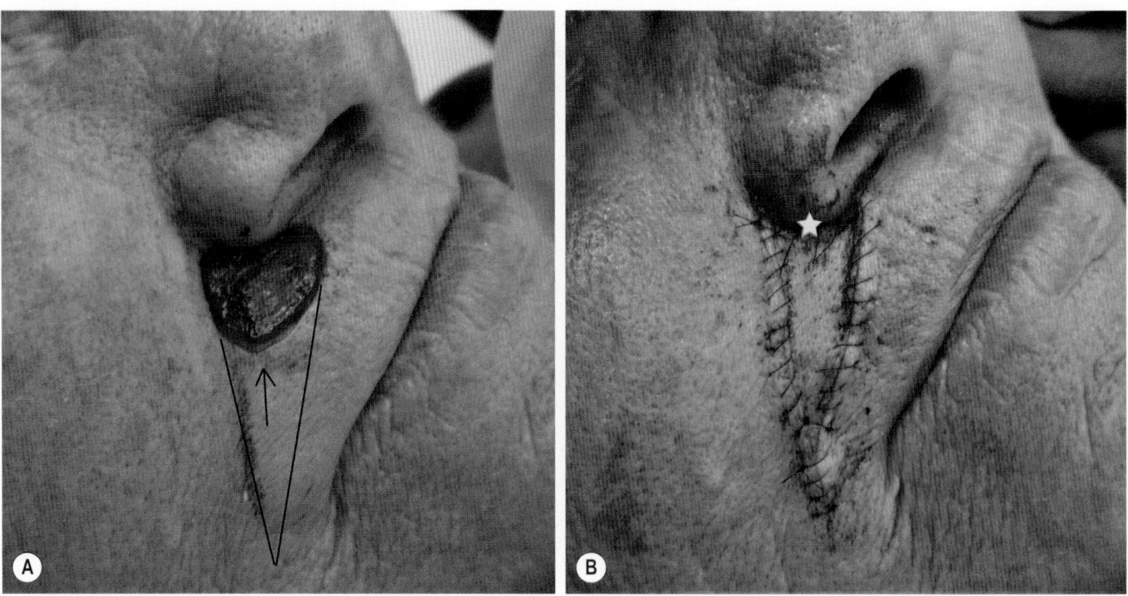

Fig. 8.17 (A) and (B) V-to-Y advancement flap (formerly, "island pedicle flap"). Key stitch indicated by yellow star.

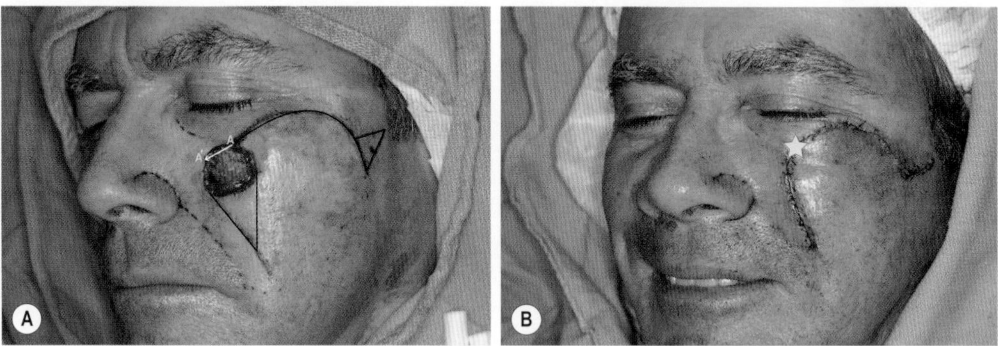

Fig. 8.18 (A) and (B) Rotation flap. Key stitch indicated by yellow star. (Modified from Chen TM, Wanitphakdeedecha R, Nguyen TH. Flaps. In: Vidimos AT, Ammirati CT, Poblete-Lopez C, eds. *Requisites in Dermatology: Dermatologic Surgery*. Philadelphia: Elsevier; 2009:163–180.)

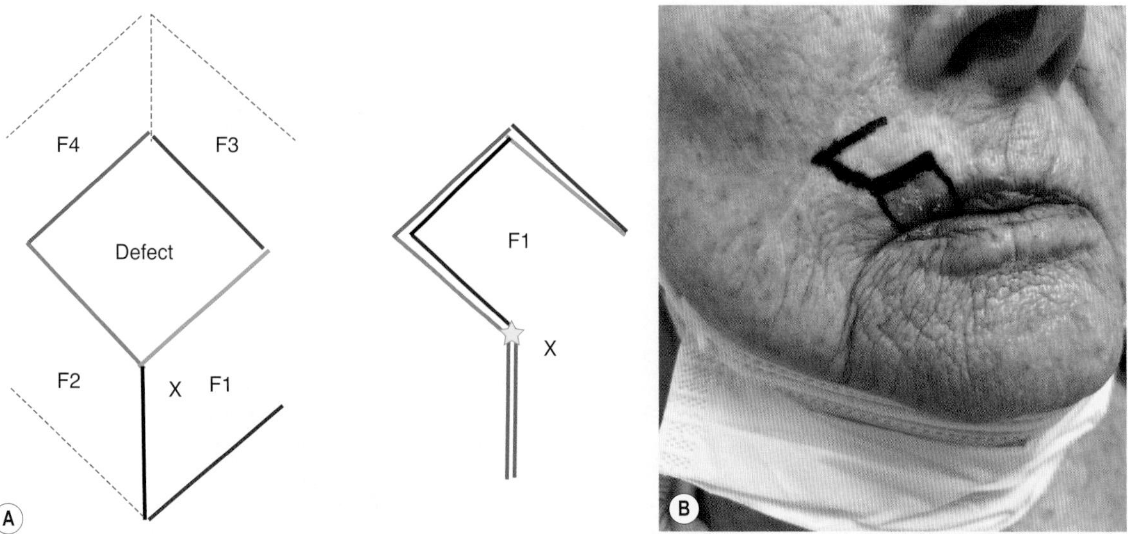

Fig. 8.19 (A) to (D) Rhombic transposition flap. Key stitch indicated by yellow star. (Modified from Kang AS, Kang KS. Rhomboid flap: indications, applications, techniques and results. A comprehensive view. *Ann Med Surg*. 2021;68:102544.)

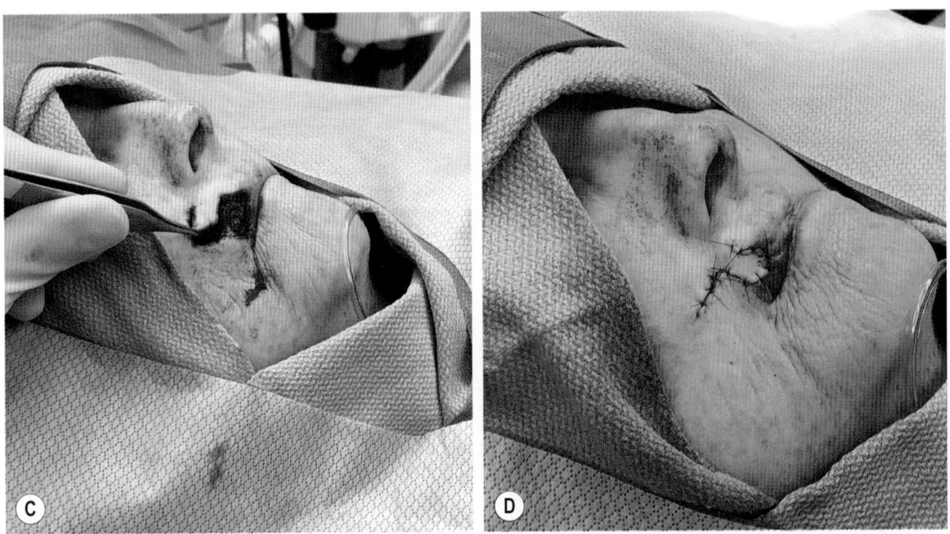

Fig. 8.19, cont'd

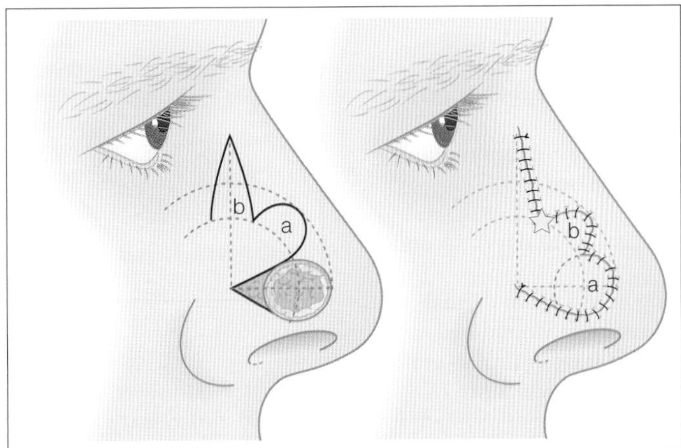

Fig. 8.20 Bilobed transposition flap using Zitelli's modification. Key stitch indicated by yellow star. (Modified from Bhatia AC, Overman J, Rohrer TE. Transpositions flaps. In: Rohrer TE, Cook JL, Kaufman AJ, eds. *Flaps and Grafts in Dermatologic Surgery.* 2nd ed. Philadelphia: Elsevier. 2018:99–115.)

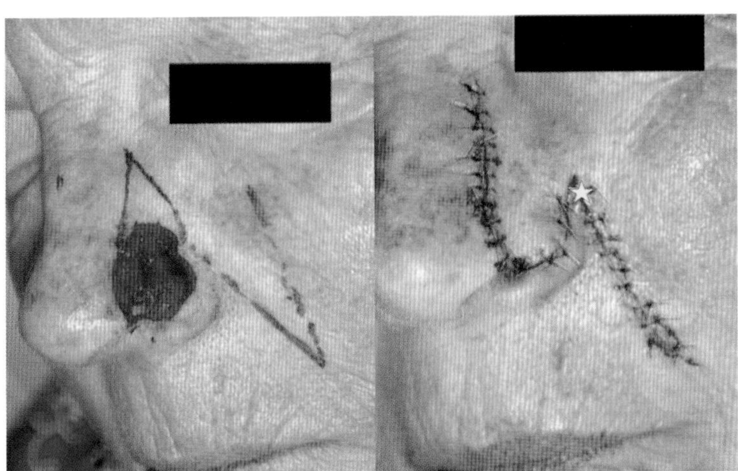

Fig. 8.21 Single-stage nasolabial/melolabial transposition (modified banner) flap. Key stitch indicated by yellow star. (From Cook JL, Goldman GD. Random pattern cutaneous flaps. In: Robinson JK, Hanke CW, Siegel DM, Fratila A, eds. *Surgery of the Skin.* 2nd ed. Philadelphia: Elsevier; 2010:251–287.)

Table 8.19 Comparison of Graft Types Used in Soft Tissue Reconstruction

Graft Type	Tissue Match	Nutritional Requirements	Requirement for Recipient Bed Vascularity	Infection Risk	Graft Contraction Risk	Durability	Sensation	Adnexal Functions
FTSG	Good to excellent	High	High	Low	Low	Good to excellent	Good	Excellent
STSG	Poor to fair	Low	Low	Low	High	Fair to good	Fair	Poor
Composite	Good	Very high	Very high	Moderate	Low	Fair	Fair	Good
Free cartilage	N/A	Moderate	High	Moderate	Migration or deformation possible, with subsequent resorption	Good	N/A	N/A

FTSG, *Full-thickness skin graft; STSG, split-thickness skin graft.*
From Ratner D, Nayyar PM. Grafts. In: Bolognia JL, Schaffer JV, Cerroni L, eds. Dermatology. *4th ed. Philadelphia: Elsevier; 2018:2517–2530.*

8.12 GRAFTS

- Skin grafts often utilized when defect is not amenable to primary or flap closure
- Four main categories of skin grafts are commonly used, each w/ their own pros and cons (Table 8.19)
- Physiology
  - **Imbibition (24–48 hours)**: first stage, ischemic period
    - Fibrin attaches graft to bed
    - Graft is sustained by passive diffusion of nutrients from plasma exudate of wound bed
    - Graft becomes edematous
  - **Inosculation (48–72 hours, lasts 7–10 days)**: second stage
    - Revascularization resulting in linkage of dermal vessels between graft and recipient wound bed
  - **Neovascularization (day 7)**: last stage critical to graft survival, occurs in conjunction w/ inosculation
    - Capillary and lymphatic ingrowth from recipient to graft → revascularization complete by day 7
    - Edema begins to resolve
  - **Reinnervation/Maturation (starts within 2 months)**: slow process that is not completed for many months to years
- Types of grafts
  - Full-thickness skin graft (FTSG):
    - Composed of epidermis and full-thickness dermis
    - Primary goal: match donor skin w/ recipient site based on skin color, texture, thickness, degree of photo damage, and presence/absence of hair (Table 8.20)
    - Advantages: better overall appearance than split-thickness skin graft (STSG), **retains adnexal structures** (and function), better contour and texture match; greater thickness → ↓ **wound contracture**
    - Disadvantages: ↑ metabolic demand → ↑ rate of graft failure
    - **Oversize graft by 10%–20%** to account for graft shrinkage after harvesting
    - **Defatting (classic teaching)**: leaving fat on underside of graft has long been thought to reduce survival → **most books recommend complete removal of adipose tissue on graft**

Table 8.20 Donor Sites for Full-Thickness Skin Grafts

Defect Sites	Donor Sites
Nasal tip, ala	Preauricular, postauricular neck, nasolabial fold, conchal bowl, Burow's graft (particularly at junction of nasal tip and dorsum)
Nasal dorsum, sidewalls	Preauricular, postauricular neck/lateral neck, supraclavicular region (if large)
Lower eyelid, medial canthus	Upper eyelid, postauricular sulcus (slightly thicker than upper eyelid donor site)
Ear	Preauricular, postauricular sulcus, postauricular neck/lateral neck
Face, scalp	Burow's graft (usually saved during partial closure of defect with flap), lateral neck, supraclavicular region, medial upper arm
Dorsal hand and fingers	Ulnar wrist (smaller grafts), ventral forearm, medial upper arm (larger grafts)

      - However, recent studies suggest defatting is not necessary and skin-fat composite grafts survive extremely well, especially on nose
    - Bolster dressing
      - **Purpose: graft immobilization** → ↑ graft adherence to wound bed
      - Technique: Xeroform™ gauze or equivalent bulky nonadherent dressing secured w/ tie-over sutures
    - Delayed grafting
      - Useful for:
        - ➔ Deep defects that cannot be adequately filled by FTSG alone
        - ➔ Defects w/ significant amount of exposed bone or cartilage (>25% of periosteum or perichondrium is lacking)
      - Wound is allowed to **granulate for 1 to 3 weeks before delayed grafting** is performed → granulation tissue provides well-vascularized bed to promote graft survival
    - Burow's graft (commonly used type of FTSG)
      - FTSG derived from skin *adjacent to* the defect (donor skin = discarded Burow's triangle skin resulting from partial primary closure of defect) → provides excellent tissue color and texture match compared with grafts harvested from distant sites
      - Most often utilized when primary repair does not fully close the defect or if complete closure would

result in distortion of free anatomic margin (e.g., alar rim, perioral, and periorbital area)
    - Also useful for defects that span two cosmetic units (nasal dorsum and tip) as it allows primary closure of one unit and graft of the second unit
  - Refinement of FTSG w/ **dermabrasion or dermasanding** (~**4–6 weeks** postop) may ↑ cosmesis
  - **Graft necrosis**: indicated by **black color** (do not confuse w/ purple venous congestion phase, which is normal) → do NOT remove, serves as **biologic dressing**
- Split-thickness skin graft (STSG):
  - Composed of full-thickness epidermis and variable amount of dermis
  - Advantages: **covers larger defects** (>5 cm), ↑ **graft survival** (as a result of ↓ demand for nutritional support), and **easier detection of tumor recurrence**
  - Disadvantages: ↓ **cosmesis**, ↑ **contraction** (→ not recommended near free margins), **lacks adnexal structures**, ↓ anchoring to BMZ (→ bullae within graft site), requires specialized instruments, and painful donor site
  - Classified by overall thickness:
    - Thin (0.005–0.012 in)
    - Medium (0.012–0.018 in) → head and neck
    - Thick (0.018–0.030 in) → trunk and extremities
  - Instruments
    - Weck blade: specialized free-hand knife with accompanying templates for various graft thicknesses
    - Zimmer: electric dermatome used to harvest large STSGs of various thickness and width
    - **Mesher**: flat bed with roller that compresses STSG on plastic template with grid-like etched pattern that puts fine fenestrations into the graft
      - ➔ Meshing enlarges size of STSGs by 25%–35% and increases flexibility
      - ➔ Allows serosanguineous drainage from recipient bed, which may otherwise interfere with graft adherence and survivability
      - ➔ Disadvantage: fenestrations often permanent → ↓ **cosmesis**
- Free cartilage graft:
  - Composed of cartilage and overlying perichondrium
  - Used to restore structural integrity, especially of nasal ala; often used in conjunction with well-vascularized flap
  - Common donor sites include antihelix (thinner, flatter) and conchal bowl (thicker, curved)
- Composite grafts: modified FTSG that contains more than one tissue component, most often cartilage or fat; dependent on bridging phenomenon (rapid revascularization) for survival
  - Skin + cartilage graft
    - Cartilage is used to **restore structural integrity**, especially of the nasal ala, to prevent anatomic distortion and alar collapse during inspiration; very high metabolic demand → **very high risk of necrosis**
    - **Cartilage portion needs to be oversized** (10%–15%) to tuck into subdermal space (the "pocket") of recipient site
  - Skin + fat graft
    - More tenuous survival than FTSGs because of reduced access to vascular supply; graft size should be 1 to 2 cm in maximal diameter to minimize risk of necrosis; consider delayed graft to increase likelihood of survival
    - Caution in elderly patients, smokers, and those with conditions of vascular compromise (diabetes, vasoocclusive disease, and h/o ionizing radiation at graft recipient site)
- Xenografts:
  - Temporary grafts, usually harvested as STSG from swine; function as biologic dressings and **promote granulation**; remain in place for 7 to 14 days; most commonly utilized in secondary intention healing or delayed repairs
  - Advantages: ↓ wound care demands for patient; protect/preserve bone, cartilage, tendons, and nerves; ↓ postoperative pain at granulating site
  - Disadvantages: must be replaced for continued benefit after 2 weeks, contraindicated in patients with pork allergy, and is malodorous after 10 to 14 days

8.13 SURGICAL COMPLICATIONS AND MEASURES TO AVOID THEM

- Infection
  - Vast majority of wounds created during cutaneous surgery are classified as "clean" → low infection rates (1%–2%) (Table 8.21)
  - A recent study (*Derm Surg.* 2020) refuted the commonly-held dogma that "second intention wounds have a LOWER rate of infection than sutured wounds"; in their study, second intention wounds after Mohs surgery had **>2x increased rate of infection** compared to sutured wounds (6.8% vs 3.2%)
  - Presents 4 to **8 days postoperatively**
  - Symptoms: **rubor** (erythema, often extending asymmetrically from suture line), **dolor** (pain), **calor** (warmth), and **tumor** (swelling); may also have

Table 8.21 Wound Classification

Class	Infection Rate (%)	Consider Antibiotic Prophylaxis for Dermatologic Surgery
I. Clean—non-contaminated skin, sterile technique	5	No
II. Clean contaminated—Minor breaks in sterile technique, or GI/GU/respiratory tracts entered without gross contamination	10	Rarely; case-by-case basis
III. Contaminated—Major breaks in sterile technique, or gross contamination from GI/GU/respiratory tracts	20–30	Yes
IV. Infected—wound with acute bacterial infection +/− pus; devitalized tissue	30–40	Antibiotics therapeutic, not prophylactic

From Mariwalla K. Antibiotics. In: Robinson JK, Hanke CW, Siegel DM, Fratila A, eds. Surgery of the Skin. *3rd ed. Philadelphia, Elsevier, 2015:85–94.*

purulent discharge, lymphangitic streaks, fevers, and chills
- *Staphylococcus aureus* = **#1 culprit overall**
  - *Pseudomonas* **is common on ear**
- Always obtain wound culture!
- Treatment:
  - Abscesses: traditional dogma is to incise, drain, and pack the infected wound until it heals by second intention; recent studies suggest that wound may be sutured immediately following drainage
  - Surgical site infection without abscess: start antibiotics (first-generation cephalosporin or β-lactamase-resistant penicillin); consider clindamycin, doxycycline or TMP-SMX if high index of suspicion for MRSA; fluoroquinolone if *Pseudomonas* suspected
- Differential diagnosis: normal inflammation a/w healing and tension (presents earlier); contact dermatitis (pruritic); inflammatory suture reaction (epidermal sutures—erythema surrounding each suture; dermal/SQ sutures—inflammatory papule/pustule, usually presents later)
- Prevention:
  - Surgical site infections: use sterile technique, minimize wound tension, and consider antibiotic prophylaxis if operating on inflamed skin or high-risk areas (lower legs and groin)
  - Perioperative antibiotic prophylaxis recommendations for prevention of infective endocarditis and prosthetic joint infections (Table 8.22 and Fig. 8.22)

- Bleeding
  - Bleeding may lead to hematoma → ↑ risk of infection, ↑ wound tension, and dehiscence
  - Highest risk = first 48 hours postoperatively **(majority within first 24 hours, after epinephrine wears off)**
  - Patient risk factors:
    - Aspirin: irreversibly affects platelet throughout its lifespan of 6 to 10 days; **aspirin should not be held in patients taking for secondary prevention**; if taking aspirin for primary prevention, may consider withholding for 10 days before and 5 to 7 days after surgery (BUT only if it does not pose a risk for cardiac or neurologic event!)
      - Other NSAIDs such as ibuprofen and naproxen also affect platelets, but not as severely/irreversibly

Table 8.22 Antibiotics for Prevention of Surgical Site Infections

Method of Administration	Effect Based on Available Data
Topical antibiotics (postoperative)	No difference compared with white petrolatum
Topical antibiotics (preoperative nasal mupirocin for *Staphylococcus* carriers)	↓ Infection rate
Topical chlorhexidine (preoperative)	↓ Infection rate
Intralesional antibiotics (clindamycin solution mixed into local anesthetic)	("effect based on available data"), ↓ Infection rate
Postoperative systemic antibiotic prophylaxis	Cohort studies suggest a minor benefit (best data is for grafts), but no large RCTs
Preoperative systemic antibiotic prophylaxis (single dose)	Effective; recommended for patients at risk of infective endocarditis or prosthetic joint infection

    - Thienopyridine antiplatelet agents (e.g., clopidogrel and ticlopidine): do NOT stop
    - Novel Oral Anti-Coagulants / Direct Oral Anti-Coagulants (NOAC / DOAC): includes **dabigatran (Pradaxa), rivaroxaban (Xarelto), apixaban (Eliquis),** edoxaban (Savaysa), and betrixaban (Bevyxxa); current AAD recommendations = continue these agents perioperatively
      - Recent study by Siscos et. al (JAAD 2021) found that stopping DOAC/NOAC perioperatively is **NOT** associated with an increased risk of thrombotic complications or mortality; holding NOAC/DOAC perioperatively for 24-48hrs may ↓hematoma risk
    - Warfarin: check INR to ensure it is not supratherapeutic (generally prefer < 3.0) before proceeding w/ surgery
    - Herbs and supplements that enhance anticoagulation effects of warfarin and/or inhibit platelet adhesion: **feverfew, fish oil, garlic, ginger, ginkgo, ginseng, bilberry, chondroitin, vitamin E, licorice, devil's claw, danshen, dong quai, alcohol**
  - Prevention: consider minimizing undermining; consider linear closure rather than flap; drain placement; apply pressure dressing immediately after procedure and leave on for ≥ 24 hours

- Hematoma
  - Gelatin-like clots formed by blood collecting in "dead space" of wound; presents with **pain, swelling, and red-purple discoloration**
  - Hematomas may lead to dehiscence, necrosis, and infection
  - Small hematoma → **pressure sensation**
    - Small and stable hematomas resolve on their own; no intervention needed but may use warm compresses to hasten resolution
  - Large expanding hematoma → **acute throbbing pain**
    - Requires evacuation
    - Expanding hematomas in **periorbital region** (→ blindness), and **neck** (→ airway compromise) are considered **medical emergencies**
  - Hematomas evolve through **four stages**:
    - Early: **first 48 hours postop**; fluctuant; active hemorrhage and blood accumulation → **easy to aspirate** with a 16- or 18-gauge needle
    - Gelatinous: spongy w/ purplish hue
    - Organized: **>1 week postop**; thick, fibrous, and adherent to surrounding tissue (evacuation possible, but more difficult; **cannot be aspirated** via needle)
    - Liquefaction: begins at 7 to 10 days after organization phase (~2 weeks postop); organized hematoma becomes liquefied → **can now be aspirated**, or left alone to self-resorb over many months
  - Bromelain: oral concentrate of proteolytic enzymes derived from the pineapple plant → expedites hematoma resolution

- Ischemia/necrosis
  - Earliest sign of ischemia is **pallor**
    - **Arterial insufficiency**: ↓ skin temperature, lack of bleeding following pinprick test; flaps can remain viable for up to 12 to 14 hours

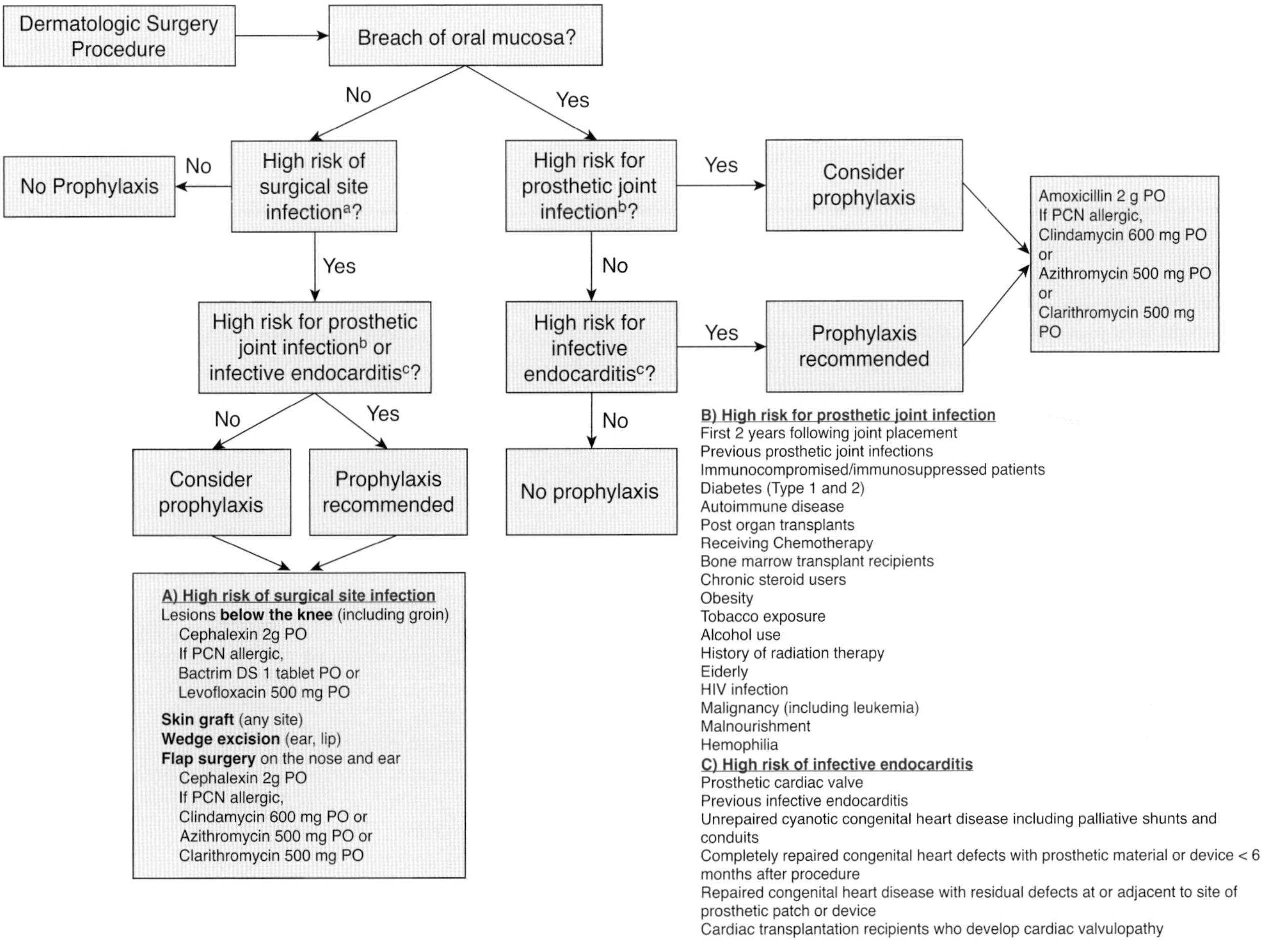

Dermatologic Surgery Procedure → Breach of oral mucosa?

No → High risk of surgical site infection[a]?
- No → No Prophylaxis
- Yes → High risk for prosthetic joint infection[b] or infective endocarditis[c]?
  - No → Consider prophylaxis
  - Yes → Prophylaxis recommended

Yes → High risk for prosthetic joint infection[b]?
- Yes → Consider prophylaxis
- No → High risk for infective endocarditis[c]?
  - Yes → Prophylaxis recommended
  - No → No prophylaxis

Amoxicillin 2 g PO
If PCN allergic,
Clindamycin 600 mg PO
or
Azithromycin 500 mg PO
or
Clarithromycin 500 mg PO

A) High risk of surgical site infection
Lesions **below the knee** (including groin)
Cephalexin 2g PO
If PCN allergic,
Bactrim DS 1 tablet PO or
Levofloxacin 500 mg PO
Skin graft (any site)
Wedge excision (ear, lip)
Flap surgery on the nose and ear
Cephalexin 2g PO
If PCN allergic,
Clindamycin 600 mg PO or
Azithromycin 500 mg PO or
Clarithromycin 500 mg PO

B) High risk for prosthetic joint infection
First 2 years following joint placement
Previous prosthetic joint infections
Immunocompromised/immunosuppressed patients
Diabetes (Type 1 and 2)
Autoimmune disease
Post organ transplants
Receiving Chemotherapy
Bone marrow transplant recipients
Chronic steroid users
Obesity
Tobacco exposure
Alcohol use
History of radiation therapy
Eiderly
HIV infection
Malignancy (including leukemia)
Malnourishment
Hemophilia

C) High risk of infective endocarditis
Prosthetic cardiac valve
Previous infective endocarditis
Unrepaired cyanotic congenital heart disease including palliative shunts and conduits
Completely repaired congenital heart defects with prosthetic material or device < 6 months after procedure
Repaired congenital heart disease with residual defects at or adjacent to site of prosthetic patch or device
Cardiac transplantation recipients who develop cardiac valvulopathy

Fig. 8.22 Updated prophylaxis algorithm for dermatologic surgery. (From Bae-Harboe YS, Liang CA. Perioperative antibiotic use of dermatologic surgeons in 2012. *Dermatol Surg*. 2013;39[11]:1592–1601.)

- ○ **Venous congestion:** cyanotic-purple skin color, ↑ dark purple bleeding following pinprick test; flaps undergo rapid necrosis (<3–4 hours)
- ■ Risk factors:
  - ○ **Hematoma, infection, ↑ wound tension**, tight sutures ("edge necrosis"), extensive superficial undermining (→ damage subdermal plexus), insufficient or excessive electrocoagulation, poor flap planning (narrow pedicle), **smoking**/nicotine
- ■ Prevention: appropriate intraoperative hemostasis, minimize wound closure tension
- ■ Treatment: suture replacement (↓ tension), elevation (↓ edema), heat application (↑ circulation), and hyperbaric oxygen (↑ oxygenation)
  - ○ **Do NOT debride necrotic tissue** (unless shows signs of infection) since it serves as a biologic dressing

- Dehiscence
  - ■ Separation of wound edges as a result of excessive tension, hematoma, infection, or necrosis
  - ■ Highest risk = time of **suture removal** (1–2 weeks)
    - ○ Consider removing sutures in stages if prolonged support is needed
  - ■ Treatment:
    - ○ Classic teaching: **re-suture if within 24 hours**; if ≥ 24 hours → let it granulate on its own
    - ○ Recent literature supports re-suturing if no infection, hematoma, necrosis, or after underlying complication has been treated
- Abnormal healing
  - ■ Chondritis: **painful** (test by "flicking" ear); may occur after any ear procedure involving cartilage; may be a/w *Pseudomonas* infection; treat w/ **NSAIDs + quinolones** (if infected)
  - ■ Contour irregularities: treated w/ **dermabrasion/ dermasanding (6 weeks postoperatively)**, ablative laser, or excision
  - ■ Ectropion:
    - ○ Cause: downward tension on lower lid
    - ○ Risk factors: poor recoil on "**snap test**"
    - ○ Prevention: **tacking sutures** to periosteum and Frost suspension sutures
  - ■ Eyebrow elevation: avoid closures that elevate brow > **3 mm** (classic teaching)
    - ○ Recent studies have actually shown that any brow asymmetry from horizontal forehead closures self-resolves over time
  - ■ Free margin distortion: avoided w/ proper surgical design
  - ■ Keloids: often patient- and site-specific (anterior neck, chest, shoulders, and scars crossing jawline); treat w/ intralesional corticosteroids

- Pincushioning/trapdoor deformity:
    - Risk factors: frequently due to **concentric contractile forces** → flaps w/ curved incision lines have highest risk (e.g., **bilobed flaps**, **nasolabial transposition/interpolation flaps**)
    - Prevention: **wide undermining**, appropriate sizing of flap, remove excess SQ fat on flap, ensure flap adherence to wound base
    - Treatment: intralesional corticosteroids (into SQ) +/– scar revision
- Spitting sutures: ↑ risk w/ Vicryl, larger caliber sutures, or **sutures placed superficially in dermis**; occurs **1 to 3 months postop**; remove if possible (use Jeweler's forceps if suture not visible on surface)
- Suture granuloma: ↑ risk w/ Vicryl, occurs 1 to 3 months postop; self-resolves without sequelae, but may treat w/ intralesional steroids
- Telangiectasias (neovascularization): common after repairs on nose and central cheeks; treated w/ pulsed dye laser
- Thickened scars: treated w/ massage or intralesional corticosteroids
- "Track marks": do not tie sutures too tightly or leave in place for too long; consider running subcuticular epidermal closure
    - More common on trunk/extremity closures since sutures typically left in longer and under greater tension compared to face
- Webbed or contracted scars: consider **Z-plasty** revision

- Motor nerve damage
    - Most severe if nerve transected at its proximal portion → frequently permanent
    - **Avoided by staying above SMAS**
- Sensory nerve damage
    - Generally improves with time
    - Minimize by avoiding transection of multiple sensory nerve branches (e.g., orienting linear repairs on forehead vertically rather than horizontally)

8.14 SCAR IMPROVEMENT

Overview

- Scars mature over at least **2 years**, but if not exhibiting favorable characteristics, may consider intervention after 60 to 90 days
- Manage expectations
    - Goal is to improve, not erase
- Result depends on
    - Size
    - Location
    - Patient's predisposition for appropriate wound healing
- Favorable scars
    - Positioned along aesthetic subunit borders
    - Parallel with RSTLs

Nonsurgical modalities

- Watchful waiting
- Massage
    - Efficacy greatest in postsurgical scars
    - Often best for subtle imperfections
        - Mild webbing, scar depression, or pincushioning
- Pressure therapy
    - Efficacy greatest during scar maturation (first year) and limited thereafter
    - Mechanism of action
        - Pressure → ↓ blood flow and oxygen → ↑ collagen breakdown
- Topical scar therapies
    - Silicone sheeting and gel
        - Mechanism unclear
        - Side effects: skin maceration and rash
    - Vitamin E
        - Efficacy not proven in clinical trials
        - Noted to cause allergic contact dermatitis
    - Steroids
        - Mechanism of action
            - Binding of nuclear steroid receptor
            - Decrease activity of fibroblasts and decreases collagen production
        - Clinical activity
            - Softens scars, ↓ hypertrophy, ↓ pincushioning
        - Group I steroids most efficacious, but ↑ risk of side effects
    - Imiquimod
        - Mechanism of action
            - Stimulates IFN-α → ↑ collagen breakdown, ↓ TGF-β (note: **↑ TGF-β levels are a/w keloid** formation)
        - Clinical activity
            - Prevention of keloid recurrence after excision
            - Results of studies have been mixed
        - Cream is applied nightly for 8 weeks
- Intralesional therapies
    - Steroids
        - Primarily used for hypertrophic and keloidal scars
        - Mechanism of action and clinical activity: same as for topical steroids
        - Consider intraoperative injection if patient has a history of keloids
    - 5-FU
        - Primarily used for hypertrophic and keloidal scars
        - Can be used in combination w/ steroids
        - Mechanism of action
            - **Blocks TGF-β2** gene in fibroblasts → ↓ collagen production → softens scars and ↓ hypertrophy
- Lasers
    - Pulsed dye laser (585–595 nm)
        - Laser of choice for red, hyperemic, pigmented, or hypertrophic scars and keloids
        - Patient phototype important as melanin competes for laser absorption. Must use lower energy densities in darker skin tones
        - Mechanism of action
            - Keloids: nonspecific heating of dermal collagen promotes scar remodeling
            - Redness: destruction of dermal vessels
    - Nd:YAG (1064 nm)
        - Noted to improve pigmentation, vascularity, pliability and height of keloids and hypertrophic scars

- Resurfacing lasers
  - Mechanism of action
    - Dermal heating leads to scar remodeling
  - Types
    - Ablative (CO_2 10,600 nm; Erb:YAG 2940 nm)
      - Destroys stratum corneum (→ recontouring surface irregularities) and deeper structures (dermal heating → scar remodeling)
      - Uses: recontouring atrophic scars → reported equivalent cosmesis to dermabrasion w/ faster clinical recovery
    - Nonablative
      - Preserves stratum corneum with destruction of deeper structures
- Radiotherapy
  - Reserved for scars that are unresponsive to other treatments
  - Not adequate as monotherapy for keloids
  - Frequently combined with surgical resection
  - Mechanism of action
    - ↓ Collagen synthesis due to ↓ fibroblast proliferation and ↑ apoptosis
  - Best results reported w/ 15 to 20 Gy over 5 to 6 sessions in early postoperative period; typically started 24 to 48 hours after surgery

Surgical modalities

- Dermabrasion/electrobrasion
  - Dermabrasion
    - Mechanism of action: epidermis and papillary dermis are removed → allows wound to reepithelialize from surrounding epithelium and underlying adnexa
    - Best performed ~**6 to 8 weeks postoperatively**
    - Re-wounding during fibrillogenesis → ↑ epidermal cell migration into wound → improved appearance of scar
    - Variants:
      - Wire brush
        - Creates microscopic lacerations
        - Less forgiving than diamond fraise
      - Diamond fraise with hand engine
        - Should **rotate in the direction of free margin**
        - Feathering used to avoid demarcation between treated and untreated regions
      - Dermasanding
        - Manually performed with medium-grade drywall sanding screen, sandpaper, or surgical scratch pad (presterilized, equivalent to ~80 grit sandpaper)
        - No aerosolization of infectious particles or blood splatter
    - Side effects
      - Hyper/hypopigmentation
      - Milia formation
      - Persistent erythema
      - Paradoxical worsening of scars
  - Electrobrasion
    - Mechanism of action: controlled skin ablation w/ hyfrecator (low power)
    - Similar results to dermabrasion
    - ↓ Procedure and bleeding time (vs. dermabrasion)
- Subcision
  - Utilized on depressed facial scars
  - 20-gauge tri-beveled hypodermic needle inserted in the skin and sharp edges are maneuvered to release fibrotic scar bands within dermis and subcutaneous tissue
- Scar excision procedures
  - Linear excision of scar
  - W-plasty
    - Irregularization technique; typically followed by dermabrasion
  - Geometric broken line
    - Irregularization technique; incise connected random geometric figures (squares, rectangles, and triangles); typically followed by dermabrasion
- Scar reorienting/lengthening techniques
  - V to Y
    - Can push (V–Y) or pull (Y–V) a free margin into place
    - Less dramatic lengthening than Z-plasty
  - Z-plasty
    - Used to lengthen scar or release contractions
    - Angle of the lateral arms relative to the central limb determines the amount of lengthening
    - **Greater angles → more lengthening** (though flaps become harder to transpose over one another)
      - 30° lengthens by 25%
      - 45° lengthens by 50%
      - 60° lengthens by 75% (Fig. 8.23)

8.15 NAIL SURGERY

- Nail avulsion: typically undertaken for treatment of onychomycosis, onychomadesis, nail biopsy, nail matrix ablation, or nail unit excision
  - Distal nail avulsion (most commonly used technique): entire nail is separated from distal nail bed to PNF
  - Proximal nail avulsion: less traumatic than distal nail avulsion; undertaken when there is **thick subungual hyperkeratosis,** prominent distal subungual damage or no distal free edge
  - Partial nail avulsion: used for onychocryptosis or when the exact location of the subungual lesion is already known
- Nail biopsies (Fig. 8.24):
  - Nail bed:
    - **Longitudinal excision**; excision extends down to periosteum; +/− suturing of defect (not required if defect width ≤ 3 mm); **minimal risk of nail dystrophy**
  - Nail matrix:
    - **Horizontal excision;** make diagonal **5 mm incision** from PNF (extending proximally on finger) to allow visualization of matrix → biopsy carried down to periosteum
    - Matrix biopsies have ↑ **risk of nail dystrophy/ thinning;** highest risk w/ proximal matrix biopsies and if > 3 mm width

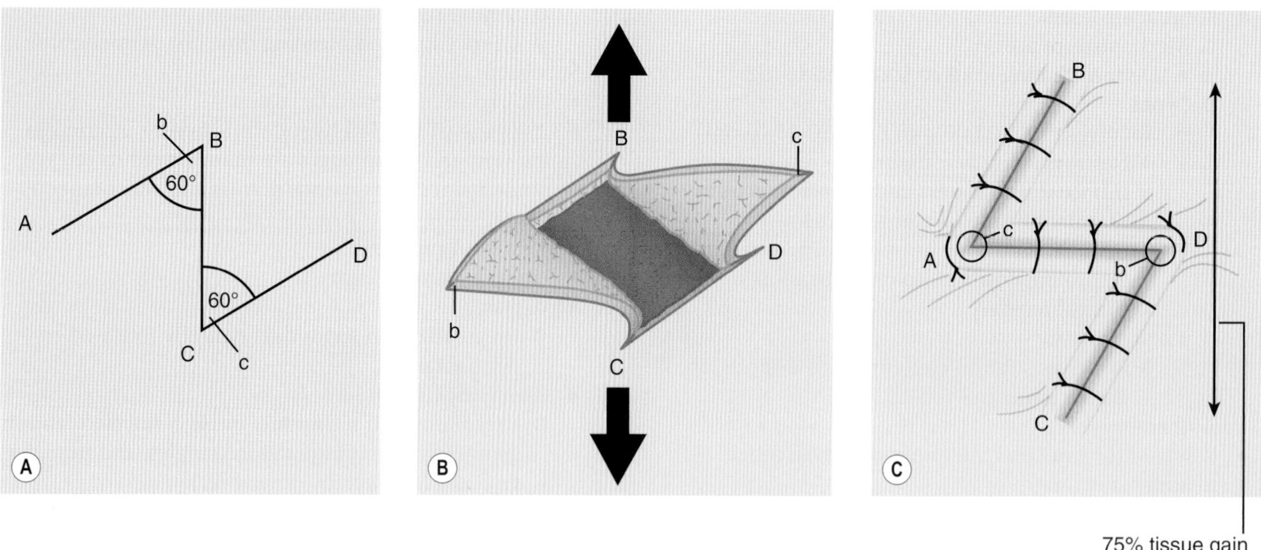

Fig. 8.23 Single Z-plasty, 60 degrees. (A) Central scar is the common diagonal. (B) Two triangular flaps are lifted and transposed. (C) Result is approximately 75% increased tissue length. (From James WD, Elston DM, Treat JR, Rosenbach MA, Neuhaus IM. Dermatologic surgery. In: *Andrews' Diseases of the Skin*. 13th ed. Philadelphia: Elsevier; 2020:881–908.)

Nail biopsies

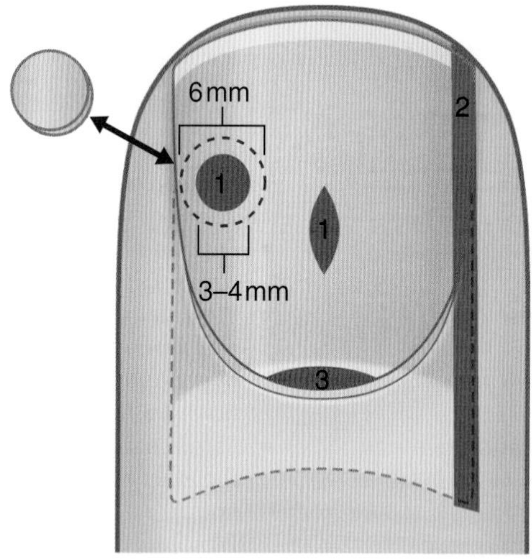

Fig. 8.24 Nail biopsies. Nail bed biopsy (1), lateral longitudinal biopsy (2), and fusiform matrix biopsy (3). (From Haneke E. Nail surgery. In: Robinson JK, Hanke CW, Siegel DM, Fratila A, eds. *Surgery of the Skin*. 3rd ed. Philadelphia, Elsevier, 2015:755–780.)

        - Most nail **melanomas arise from matrix** → matrix biopsy required → ↑ risk of nail dystrophy
    - Lateral longitudinal nail biopsy:
        - Longitudinal excision of entire length of lateral nail unit (nail matrix, folds, bed, plate and hyponychium)
        - Useful for lateral nail pathology or inflammatory conditions in which nail matrix, folds, bed, and plate are concurrently involved
        - Main risks = **spicule or cyst** formation
- Nail unit excision:
    - En bloc excision is typically used for removal of malignancy such as subungual melanoma; aggressive procedure that may result in permanent stiffness of joint, but may be preferable to amputation
    - Excision must be taken back to DIP tendon insertion to remove entire matrix
- Matricectomy
    - Removes nail matrix → inability to form new nail
    - Indications: **ingrown nail/onychocryptosis (#1)** and intractable onychogryphosis
    - Typically only the part of the matrix causing problems needs to be removed
    - Phenol matricectomy
        - After avulsion, phenol (88%) applied to matrix w/ cotton tipped applicator (2–3 passes) for 3 minutes total
            - Attention to lateral matrix horns to avoid spicule formation
        - Nail folds and nail bed should be protected from phenol (w/ petrolatum) and **phenol is neutralized after final pass w/ isopropyl alcohol**
        - ECG monitoring is not necessary
    - Excision and electrodesiccation of the nail matrix have been advocated by some authors as alternatives to phenol; limited data exist on its benefits and harms relative to other forms of nail matricectomy
    - Subungual hematoma:
        - **Trephination** indicated if **hematoma > 50% of nail**
        - May occur in combination w/ fractured distal phalanx → **X-rays recommended**

8.16 WOUND DRESSINGS

- See Table 8.23.

Table 8.23 Types and Characteristics of Occlusive/Moisture-Retentive Wound Dressings

Type	Advantages	Disadvantages	Indications	Examples
Foams	Absorbent, conform to body contours	Opaque, require secondary dressing	Partial-thickness wounds, **moderately to heavily exudative wounds,** pressure relief	Allevyn Flexzan Hydrasorb Lyofoam Vigifoam
Films	Transparent, create bacterial barrier, adhesive without secondary dressing	May adhere to wounds, can cause fluid collection	Donor sites, superficial burns and ulcers, partial-thickness wounds with minimal exudates	Tegaderm Bioclusive BlisterFilm Omniderm Transeal
Hydrocolloids	**(+) Autolytic debridement,** enhance angiogenesis, absorbent, create bacterial and physical barrier	Opaque, gel has unpleasant smell, expensive	Partial- or full-thickness wounds, mildly to **moderately exudative wounds,** pressure ulcers, venous ulcers, donor sites, acute surgical wounds	Duoderm Nu-Derm Comfeel Cutinova Replicare
Hydrogels	Semitransparent, **soothing,** do not adhere to wounds, hydrating	Require secondary dressing, frequent dressing changes	**Painful wounds,** partial-thickness wounds, wounds after laser, dermabrasion or chemical peel, donor sites	Vigilon Tegagel Curagel ClearSite Curafil Elasto-Gel SoloSite wound gel 2nd Skin
Alginates	**Highly absorbent, hemostatic,** do not adhere to wounds, fewer dressing changes	Require secondary dressing, gel has unpleasant smell	**Highly exudative wounds,** partial- or full-thickness wounds, after surgery	AlgiDerm AlgiSite Algisorb Kaltostat Curasorb Polymem SeaSorb Sorbsan

From Levin Y, Brown KL, Phillips TJ. Wound healing and its impact on dressings and postoperative care. In: Robinson JK, Hanke CW, Siegel DM, Fratila A, eds. Surgery of the Skin. *3rd ed. Philadelphia: Elsevier; 2015:114–133.*

9

Cosmetic Dermatology

Ronda S. Farah

CONTENTS LIST

9.1 LASERS
9.2 BOTULINUM TOXIN
9.3 DERMAL FILLERS
9.4 LIPOSUCTION AND FAT REDUCTION
9.5 SCLEROTHERAPY AND VEIN MANAGEMENT
9.6 COSMECEUTICALS, NUTRACEUTICALS, AND OTHER SUPPLEMENTS
9.7 HAIR TRANSPLANTATION
9.8 CHEMICAL PEELS
9.9 OTHER ESTHETIC PROCEDURES AND SCALES

Acknowledgments: With acknowledgments to Addison Demer MD, Lori Fiessinger MD, Seaver Soon MD, Kaichu Lee MD, Neil Sadick MD, and the original author, Raja K. Sivamani.

9.1 LASERS

- LASER = Light Amplification by Stimulated Emission of Radiation (Table 9.1)
- Lasers are characterized by the "3 Cs"
  - Coherence: light waves travel together in-phase in time and space
  - Collimation: light waves travel together in a parallel fashion
  - (mono) Chromatic: light waves are all the same wavelength
- Three different media exist (determine laser wavelength):
  - Gas: CO_2, xenon chloride (excimer laser), krypton, argon, copper vapor, helium-neon
  - Liquid: rhodamine dye (pulsed dye laser [PDL])
  - Solid: two classes exist
    - Crystal: alexandrite, Er-YAG, Nd-YAG, potassium titanyl phosphate (KTP), and ruby
    - Semiconductor: diode
- **Selective photothermolysis**: using a laser to achieve selective destruction of the target structure(s); depends on three factors (Table 9.2):
  - **Wavelength** must target the desired chromophore and reach an appropriate anatomic depth to destroy the desired target tissue. **Medium** determines wavelength of laser.
  - **Pulse duration should be ≤ thermal relaxation time (TRT)** → minimizes diffusion of heat and resultant "collateral damage" to surrounding tissues
  - **Fluence** must be high enough to damage target tissue, but not so high as to nonspecifically damage bystander tissue
- Four different types of laser wave forms:
  - Continuous: emit light **continuously; low power** (e.g., CO_2 laser, and argon)
  - Pulsed: light is emitted periodically, with **short pulse durations (millisecond [ms] range)**, and **high power** (e.g., PDL, ruby, alexandrite, diode, Erbium:glass, and Erbium:YAG)
  - Quality switched (Q-switched [QS]): variant of pulsed lasers with **extremely short pulse durations (nanosecond range)**; **extremely high power** (example: all QS lasers)
    - For **pigmented lesions**, **tattoos**, and **drug deposits** because target molecules are very small → very short TRT (nanoseconds)
  - Quasicontinuous: emits multiple rapid bursts of low-energy light → simulates continuous wave lasers (e.g., KTP and copper vapor)
- Treated skin will have at least one of the following four interactions with emitted laser light particles:
  - Reflection: **4%–7% of light is reflected** ("bounced away") by skin surface, as a result of the difference in refractive index between air and stratum corneum; the **remaining 93%–96% of light enters skin** and will subsequently interact in one of three following ways:
    - Scattering: light bounces off fibers within dermis/SQ → **limits depth of penetration**
    - ↑ Spot size → ↓ scatter → ↑ depth of penetration
    - Transmission: light passes straight through the tissue without interacting with anything → lack of any effect
    - Absorption (desired effect): light is absorbed by its intended target → tissue effects

Table 9.1 Laser Terminology

Term	Definition	Unit	Comments
Energy	Fundamental unit of work	Joules (J)	—
Fluence	Energy delivered per cm^2	J/cm^2	↑ fluence → ↑ energy of treatment per unit area
Power	Rate of energy delivery	Watts (W) = J/s	—
Irradiance	Power delivered per cm^2	W/cm^2	—
Pulse width (pulse duration)	Duration of laser exposure (seconds)	Seconds (or fractions of seconds)	↑ Pulse duration = longer exposure to the laser → ↑ energy/heat delivered to tissue Ideally, pulse duration should be ≤ TRT to prevent collateral damage to bystander tissues
Spot size	Diameter of the laser beam hitting the skin surface (mm)	mm	Larger spot size → ↓ **scatter** → ↑ **depth of penetration**
Wavelength	Length of a specific laser's light wave <u>Four categories</u>: **UV (10–400 nm)** **Visible (400–700 nm)** **Infrared (700 nm–1 mm)** **Radiofrequency/**microwaves (>1 mm)	nm (most commonly)	**Longer wavelengths penetrate deeper** (rule holds true until 1300 nm, at which point penetration decreases as a result of water absorption; Figure 9.1) Most deeply penetrating wavelengths = 650–1200 nm Least penetrating wavelengths = far UV and far IR
Chromophore	Absorptive target tissue of laser	—	Major chromophores in skin (boards favorite): **melanin**, **hemoglobin** (oxyhemoglobin and deoxyhemoglobin), and **water** A laser/light source may target multiple chromophores to differing degrees
Thermal relaxation time (TRT)	The time required for heated tissue to dissipate 50% of its heat	Seconds (or fractions of seconds); proportional to the diameter of target squared	**TRT (seconds) is proportional to the square of the target's diameter** (in mm) Ideally, **pulse duration should be ≤ TRT** If pulse duration > TRT → ↑ undesired damage to surrounding tissues (Table 9.2)
Photomechanical effect	Sudden heating produces thermal expansion with acoustic and/or shock waves → waves produce cavitation (steam bubbles)	—	**Cavitation** is the **primary mechanism of vessel rupture w/ PDL**, and also is responsible for skin whitening during QS laser treatment of tattoos

Table 9.2 Thermal Relaxation Times of Chromophore

Chromophore	Diameter	Thermal Relaxation Times	Typical Pulse Duration
Tattoo ink particle	0.1 micrometer	10 nanoseconds	a. 0.6–10 **nanoseconds** (if Q-switched lasers) b. Picosecond laser
Melanosome	0.5 micrometers	250 nanoseconds	10–100 **nanoseconds** (requires Q-switched lasers)
PWS vessels	30–100 micrometers	1–10 milliseconds	0.4–20 milliseconds
Terminal hair follicle	300 micrometers	100 milliseconds	3–100 milliseconds
Leg vein	1 millimeter	1 second	~0.1 seconds

Modified from Sakamoto FH, Avram MM, Anderson RR. Lasers and other energy-based technologies—principles and skin interactions. In: Bolognia JL, Schaffer JV, Cerroni L, eds. Dermatology. *4th ed. Philadelphia: Elsevier; 2018:2354–2363.*

   - Epidermal damage is minimized via skin cooling (three commonly used methods):
   - **Precooling: most aggressive, most effective** method (e.g., **cryogen [tetrafluoroethane] spray**)
     - Main side effect (SE) = **hyper/hypo-pigmentation**
   - Parallel cooling: only effective for pulses > 5 ms in duration (e.g., solid cold sapphire window pressed against skin)
   - Postcooling: used primarily to ↓ **pain, erythema, and edema** (e.g., ice packs and cold air)
- Photobiomodulation (aka low level light therapy):
  - Mechanism unknown but chromophore thought to be **mitochondrial cytochrome c oxidase**; sources of light include lasers, light emitting diodes, broadband light (within the visible and near infrared spectrum)
  - Used for **androgenetic alopecia** (typically 655–678 nm and available as home or in-office devices), **acne vulgaris** (blue light ~415 nm and red light ~633 nm) and **reduction of periorbital rhytides;** anti-aging/photorejuventation applications exist (red light ~633 nm and near-infrared light ~800–830 nm)
- A variety of lasers exist, each with specific wavelengths, target chromophores, and depths of penetration (Figs. 9.1 and 9.2)
- Non-laser light-based energy sources:
  - Intense pulsed light (IPL):
    - **Xenon flashlamp** (light source) emits **noncollimated, noncoherent**, and polychromatic light (broad wavelength range: 500–1200 nm)
    - A variety of **filters** are utilized to narrow down the range of wavelengths to target the same chromophores that lasers do
    - **Less selective** and **less powerful** than lasers; can be risky in patients with skin types IV–VI
    - Targets lentigines, vascular lesions such as telangiectasias; caution when treating men on the face as it also removes hair

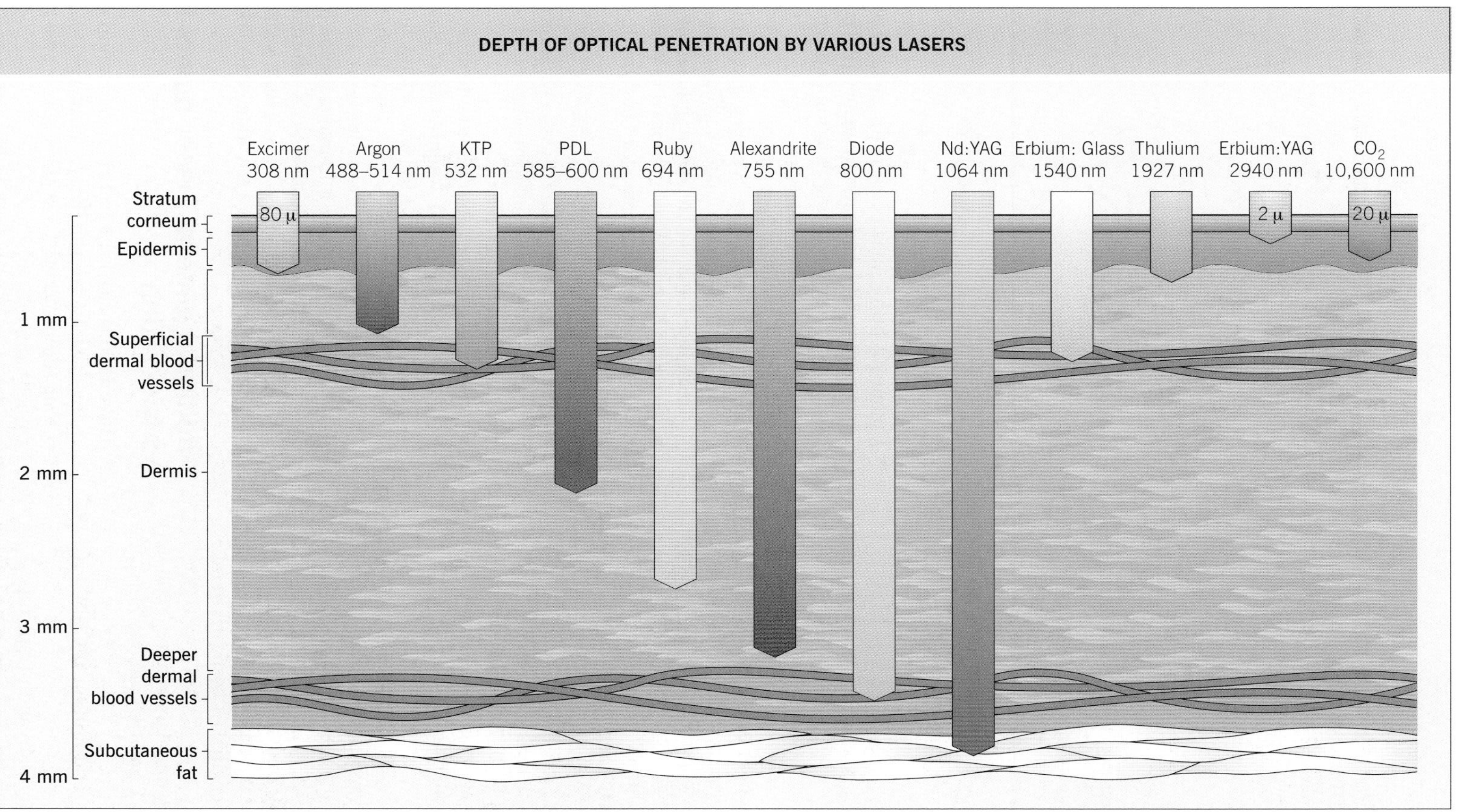

Fig. 9.1 Depth of optical penetration by various lasers. It should be noted that the treatment depth can greatly exceed the optical penetration depth for ablative lasers. On the face, fat can be present at a depth of 2 to 3 mm. For example, the depth of optical penetration for CO_2 lasers is only ~20 microns, but fractional CO_2 lasers can vaporize nearly full-thickness microchannels through the dermis. *KTP*, Potassium titanyl phosphate; *Nd*, neodymium; *PDL*, pulsed dye laser; *YAG*, yttrium aluminum garnet. (From Sakamoto FH, Avram MM, Anderson RR. Lasers and other energy-based technologies—principles and skin interactions. In: Bolognia JL, Schaffer JV, Cerroni L, eds. *Dermatology*. 4th ed. Philadelphia: Elsevier; 2018:2354–2363.)

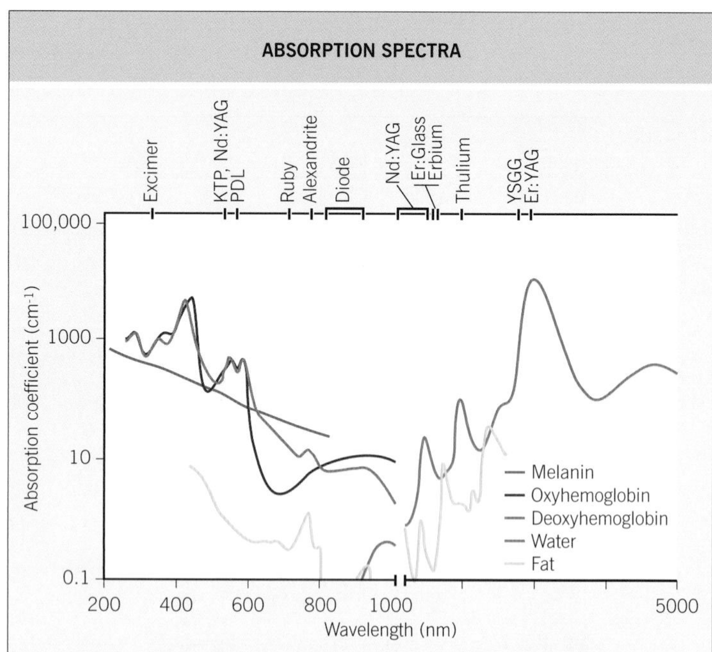

Fig. 9.2 Absorption spectra. The heterogeneous absorption spectra of chromophores allow selective photothermolysis to work. *Er*, Erbium; *KTP*, potassium titanyl phosphate; *Nd:YAG*, neodymium-doped yttrium aluminum garnet; *PDL*, pulsed dye laser; *YSGG*, yttrium scandium gallium garnet. (From Sakamoto FH, Avram MM, Anderson RR. Lasers and other energy-based technologies—principles and skin interactions. In: Bolognia JL, Schaffer JV, Cerroni L, eds. *Dermatology*. 4th ed. Philadelphia: Elsevier; 2018:2354–2363.)

Laser safety

- Four main concerns: blindness, fire hazards, cutaneous burns, and inhalation of biohazardous plume
- Blindness
  - Up to 7% of emitted laser light is reflected by the stratum corneum → reflected light can cause eye damage/blindness (may occur if even 1% of the beam is reflected into eye!)
  - Blindness is **rapid and painless**
  - Any laser/light source in **UV range** (10–400nm) → **lens damage, cataracts**
    - Example: excimer laser (308 nm)
  - Any laser/light source that targets **melanin or hemoglobin** (visible light [400–700nm] and near-infrared [700–1400nm] wavelengths) → **retinal damage** (retina is highly pigmented); also damages **uvea and iris**
    - Examples: KTP (532 nm), PDL (585–600 nm), ruby (694 nm), IPL (various wavelengths), alexandrite (755 nm), diode (800 nm), and Nd:YAG (532 and 1064 nm)
    - Highest risk = **near-infrared** and **QS lasers**
  - Any laser/light source that targets **water** (near-IR [upper end], mid-IR, far-IR wavelengths) → **corneal/scleral damage**
    - Examples: Nd:YAG (1320 nm), Erbium:glass (1550 nm), Erbium:YAG (2940 nm), and CO_2 (10,600 nm)
- Fire hazard
  - Greatest fire risk with **CO_2** and **Erbium:YAG** ablative and fractionated lasers
  - Risks: drapes, clothing, dry hair, and plastic tubes (endotracheal tubes, especially if **oxygen** is being administered)
  - Prevention: moisten hair near treatment field, ensure that any alcohol/acetone skin cleanser has fully dried before using laser, and reduce intraoperative O_2 concentration < 40%
- Cutaneous burns: may occur with any laser or nonlaser energy source (IPL and radiofrequency [RF]); as a result of operator error or device malfunction (e.g., epidermal cooling mechanism fails)
- Inhalation of biohazardous plume
  - **HPV** viral particles have been detected in carbon dioxide laser plumes → cases of laser-surgeons developing HPV-16–induced oral SCC related to inhalation
  - Hepatitis B and HIV also reported in plume
  - Prevention: **smoke evacuator (first line)**; also recommend N95 mask
- Other safety facts:
  - QS lasers can eject tissue due to cavitation
  - Beware of diseases that koebnerize with lasers (e.g., psoriasis and lichen planus)
  - Lasers can damage tooth veneers/dentures
  - Optical density (O.D.): found on laser glasses; is a logarithmic measure of the laser energy that will pass through a filter; higher O.D. value = higher energy attenuation → greater eye protection
    - Each unit represents a 10-fold reduction in transmitted laser light (O.D. 1 = 10% energy transmittance; O.D. 2 = 1%; O.D. 3 = 0.1%, etc.) → there is a 10-fold increase in eye protection for each additional O.D. unit

Additional general lasser points for consideration

- There are increased risks of dyspigmentation with some energy-based devices in darker skin types
- Strong sun protective counseling is key; avoid treating tanned skin
- Decrease laser settings to avoid complications (consider fewer passes, lower joules, decreased surface area treated, and nonablative procedures)
- Isotretinoin and dermatologic procedures:
  - New data suggests insufficient evidence to delay treatment with hair removal lasers, vascular lasers, and

nonablative/ablative fractional devices in those receiving isotretinoin or who have recently received it
    - However, fully ablative treatment of the entire face or areas off the face should generally be avoided
- "Acne laser" targets sebaceous gland at 1726nm for those with mild to severe acne

Vascular lasers

- Commonly treated vascular lesions: blood vessels as a result of photoaging, redness associated with (a/w) rosacea, spider angiomas, Poikiloderma of Civatte, hemangiomas, vascular malformations, redness in striae, redness in scars, verruca vulgaris, and Kaposi sarcoma (less common)
- Utilize selective photothermolysis to damage blood vessels via coagulation of vessel contents → vessel collapse or destruction
- **Target: hemoglobins (oxyhemoglobin >** deoxyhemoglobin > methemoglobin**)**
    - Absorption peaks = 418, 542, and **577 nm**
- Main SE = **purpura** (primarily **PDL**)
    - Other SEs: **dyschromia** (↑ risk in darker skinned patients) and **blistering** (↑ risk with shorter pulse widths, higher fluences, and skin of color)
- Skin cooling via **precooling** is critical → prevents epidermal damage
    - Also allows for greater patient comfort and allows physician to treat at higher, more efficacious fluences
- General anesthesia is recommended for larger pediatric lesions
- Site of eye damage: **retina**
- Consider herpes simplex virus (HSV) prophylaxis for perioral lesions, or larger facial malformations
- Desired treatment endpoints:
    - **PDL—purpura** (due to cavitation and vessel rupture)
        - Nonpurpuric regimens utilize pulse durations of ≥ 20 ms → do not get cavitation or vessel rupture → do not get immediate purpura (but frequently get delayed purpura days later)
    - KTP, Nd:YAG—immediate disappearance of vessel
- Complex vascular lesions typically require several treatments
- <u>Boards fodder</u>:
    - **PDL** (585–600 nm) is the treatment of choice for **most vascular lesions** (port wine stain [PWS], telangiectasias, **cherry angiomas,** erythematous scars, and hemangiomas); may also be effective for **granuloma faciale**
    - **IPL** can be used to treat most **Poikiloderma of Civatte cases** (treats both the vessels and dyschromia)
        - PDL is a second option
    - **Long-pulsed Nd:YAG (1064 nm)** is utilized for most vascular ectasias on the lower leg (venulectasias, telangiectasias, and reticular veins) because it penetrates deeper than other vascular lasers
        - **Venous lake can be treated with this laser or a 755-nm alexandrite**.
        - Diode (800 nm) is another option for legs
    - **IPL** or **long-pulsed PDL** (nonpurpuric) are utilized for **erythematotelangiectatic rosacea**
    - **Topical vitamin K** can reduce the severity of **post-PDL purpura**

Hair reduction lasers and light sources

- Common laser hair reduction uses: removal of unwanted hair, pseudofolliculitis barbae, hidradenitis suppurativa, and pilonidal cyst disease
- Laser hair reduction utilizes selective photothermolysis to damage the hair follicle (Table 9.3).
- **Target: melanin** within hair shaft, outer rooth sheath, and matrix
    - Absorption peaks: broad range (~300–1000 nm)
- Destruction of **bulge and bulbar stem cells** → improved hair removal
- Dark, thick, terminal anagen hairs respond best
    - Thinner, lighter hair is hard to remove
    - **White hair is impossible to remove** (lacks target chromophore) → other epilation techniques recommended
        - In contrast, **electrolysis (not a laser)** uses an electrical current to damage hair follicle and may be used for white/red hair
- For **vaginoplasty** preparation, hair may be removed on penile shaft to base of phallus/mons pubis junction and scrotum to avoid formation of "hair ball," in the neovaginal cavity which has been proposed to possibly trap moisture, ejaculate, and lubricant and act as an infectious nidus
- For **phalloplasty** preparation, hair removal varies based on graft site but may include distal arm and thigh; aim is to avoid urine retention within urethra, dribbling post-void, stones and waxy hair deposits that cause urinary obstruction and may lead to urinary tract infections
- Adverse effects:
    - **Post-inflammatory hyperpigmentation (PIH; ↑ in skin of color)**
        - Recommendation: treat test spot and follow up in 1 to 2 weeks
    - Leukotrichia
    - Blistering/burning (↑ risk in skin of color) may → scarring
    - Reports of vision injury when treating brow/unibrow (site of eye damage: **retina)**
    - **Paradoxical hypertrichosis**

Table 9.3 Laser/Visible Light Sources for Hair Removal

Laser	Wavelength	Skin Type	Comments
Alexandrite	755 nm	Skin types I–III	—
Diode	810 nm; 940 nm	Skin types I–III	**Most effective**
Nd:YAG	1064 nm	All skin types	**Safest in skin of color**
Intense pulsed light	Varying filters	Unsafe in skin types IV–VI	—

- Requires multiple treatment sessions, spaced 4–6 weeks apart; treatments often not permanent → goal is "reduction, rather than removal"
- Recommend shaving before treatment in order to shorten hairs → ↓ skin burns from hairs on skin surface
- **Do NOT fully remove hair shafts** by chemicals, waxing, plucking, or threading for at least 6 weeks before treatment (eliminates target chromophore)
- **Desired treatment endpoint = transient perifollicular edema**
- Use wavelength-specific eyewear to protect **retina**
- Use parallel cooling to protect the epidermis during treatment
- Boards Fodder:
  - **Diode** has been reported to cause **reticulate erythema**
  - **Nd:YAG (1064 nm) = safest hair removal laser in darker skin types**, but slightly less effective (see Table 9.3)

Resurfacing lasers (Table 9.4)

- Common indications: rhytids, photoaging and actinic damage, acne scars, keloid, hypertrophic and burn scars, postsurgical scars, benign skin lesions (seborrheic keratoses [SKs]/warts/syringomas), striae, and rhinophyma
- **Target: water**
  - Absorption peaks: **1450, 1950, and 3000 nm (IR wavelengths)**
- May be ablative or nonablative (Fig. 9.3)
  - Ablative lasers function by removing skin via **vaporization of target tissue** (Fig. 9.4)
  - Nonablative lasers work via subtle **thermal effects on dermis** → stimulates a wound healing response
- May be fractional or nonfractional
  - Fractional: creates thousands of microscopic thermal zones of injury **(MTZ)** → stimulates turnover/remodeling of epidermis and dermis.
    - Advantages: ↓ **downtime and** ↓ **duration of erythema** compared with nonfractional resurfacing
    - Disadvantages: less efficacious; requires more treatment sessions
- Site of eye damage: **cornea, sclera** (burns)
- **Consider HSV** (valacyclovir)/**bacterial prophylaxis**
- Adverse effects:
  - Erythema (often persists for months)
  - Hyperpigmentation
  - Relative hypopigmentation (↑ risk if deeper injury; may arise months after treatment)
  - Milia
  - Secondary infections
    - **HSV: highest risk in first week**
    - Bacteria (*Staphylococcus aureus, Pseudomonas*)
  - Scarring
  - For post-procedure laser complications (esp. face), culture and consider coverage for HSV, bacteria, and/or yeast
  - **Laser-assisted drug delivery:** laser pretreatment is followed by application of a topical agent with aim of improving efficacy of treatment (topicals delivered through laser channels); ablative lasers are more effective than nonablative lasers
    - For example, topical steroid following ablative fractionated CO_2 for hypertrophic scars (Fig. 9.5)
    - Weakened barrier → ↑ risk for infection, systemic absorption, and hypersensitivity

Tattoo removal lasers (Table 9.5)

- Tattoo pigments are very small in diameter → very short TRT (nanoseconds) → **QS lasers** traditionally, but newer **picosecond lasers** which deliver sub-nanosecond pulses (medium may be Nd:YAG or alexandrite) are also an option (more efficient at removing tattoo pigment compared with nanosecond QS lasers)
- **Immediate tattoo whitening (desired endpoint)** is a result of cavitation (Fig. 9.6)

Table 9.4 Resurfacing Lasers/Energy-Based Sources

Laser	Wavelength	Comments
Ablative		
Erbium:yttrium scandium gallium garnet (Er:YSGG)	2790 nm	Less thermal injury → poor coagulation, ↑ bleeding, and ↓ collagen retraction
Erbium:yttrium aluminum garnet (Er:YAG)	2940 nm	Less thermal injury → poor coagulation, ↑ bleeding, and ↓ collagen retraction Targets the 3000 nm absorption peak of water more effectively than CO_2 laser Advantages compared with CO_2 laser: ↓ recovery time, ↓ PIH, and erythema resolves more quickly
Carbon dioxide (CO_2)	10,600 nm	More thermal injury → good coagulation, minimal to no bleeding, and ↑ collagen retraction Depth of ablation is increased by performing more passes
Nonablative		
Vascular lasers (PDL)	585–600 nm	Best for vascular lesions such as port wine stains and spider angiomas; may combine PDL w/ amino-levulinic acid to treat AKs and actinic cheilitis
Infrared lasers	Nd:YAG (1064, 1320 nm) Diode (1450, 1470 nm) Er:glass (1540 nm)	All achieve mild dermal tightening, but do not help with epidermal sun damage Diode is more effective at treating acne scarring than others
Intense pulsed light (IPL)	515–1200 nm	Leads to mild dermal tightening and also treats epidermal photodamage Broad spectrum *Not a laser
Radiofrequency (see Section 9.9)	NA	Electrical current heats dermis → mild skin tightening; can cause atrophy *Not a laser

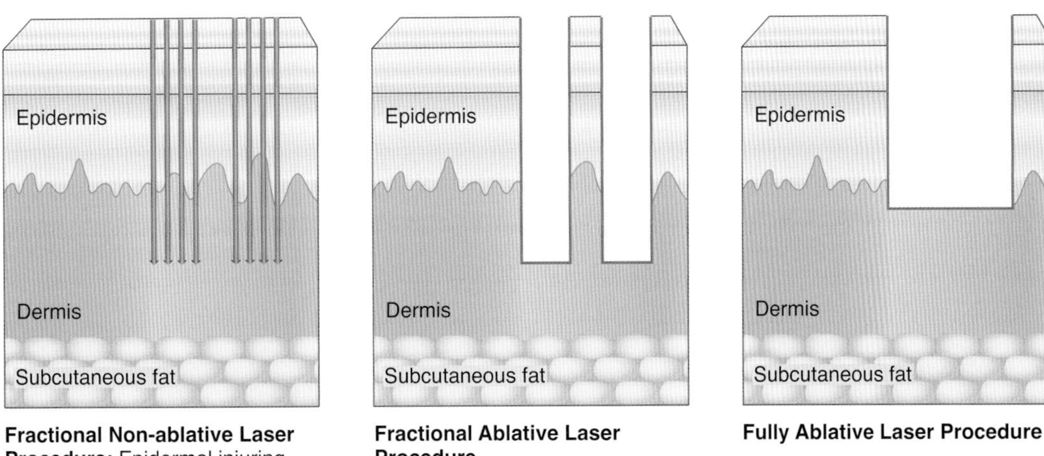

Fig. 9.3 Depiction of non-ablative fractional (A), ablative fractional (B), and fully ablative (C) laser resurfacing concepts. Traditional fully ablative laser resurfacing does not allow for spared zones of tissue. Fractional laser technology allows the clinician to leave islands of untreated tissue. (Courtesy of Ronda S. Farah, MD, University of Minnesota, and Kellen Bodell, MS, Minneapolis, MN.)

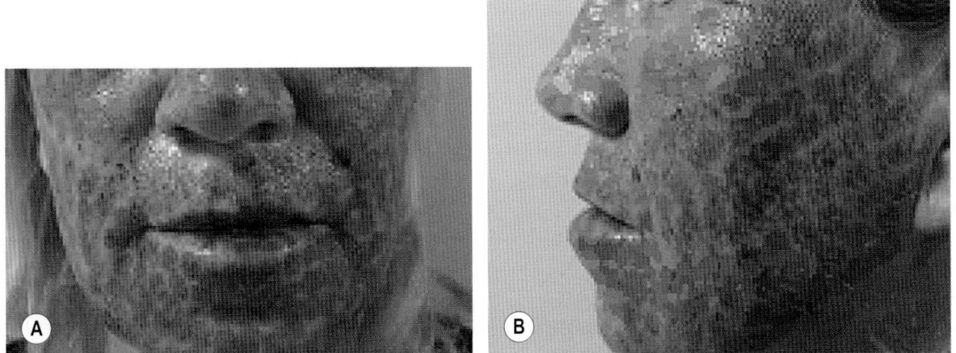

Fig. 9.4 Anterior (A) and lateral (B) views of patient post-CO_2 fractional laser. (Courtesy of Ronda S. Farah, MD, University of Minnesota.)

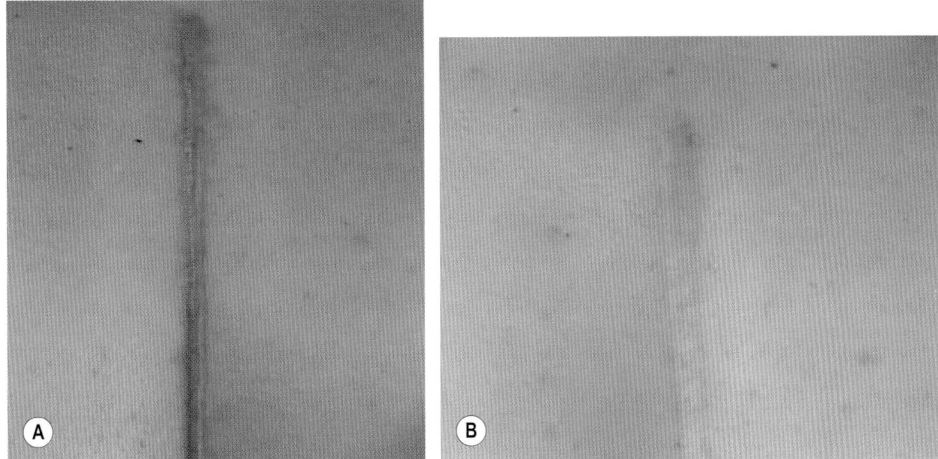

Fig. 9.5 Depiction of hypertrophic scar before (A) and after (B) laser-assisted drug delivery of triamcinolone acetonide via CO_2 fractional laser. Pulsed dye laser was preformed just prior to this procedure. (Courtesy of Ronda S. Farah, MD, University of Minnesota.)

Table 9.5 Tattoo Removal Lasers

Tattoo Color	Pigment	Laser (All are Q-switched)	Wavelength (nm)
Black	Iron oxide, carbon, India ink, lead, and gunpowder	**Ruby** Alexandrite **Nd:YAG**	694 755 1064
Blue	Cobalt	Ruby Alexandrite Nd:YAG	694 755 1064
Brown	Ochre	Ruby Alexandrite Nd:YAG (frequency-doubled) Nd:YAG	694 755 532 1064
Green	Chromium oxide, malachite green	Ruby **Alexandrite**	694 755
Yellow	Cadmium sulfide, ochre	**Nd:YAG (frequency-doubled)**	**532**
White	Titanium dioxide, zinc oxide	**Nd:YAG (frequency-doubled)**	**532**
Red	**Mercuric sulfide (cinnabar)**, azo dyes, cadmium selenide, and sienna	**Nd:YAG (frequency-doubled)**	**532**
Violet	Manganese violet	**Nd:YAG (frequency-doubled)**	**532**

- Amateur tattoos and black tattoos are the most responsive to treatment (usually <5 treatment sessions)
- Professional tattoos and multicolored tattoos are the most difficult to treat (>10 treatment sessions)
- Boards fodder:
  - Mnemonic: "The 3 **Bs** (black, brown, blue tattoos) **RAN** away when they saw the 3 **lasers**" → all 3 colors are treated with Ruby, Alexandrite, or Nd:YAG
  - Mnemonic: "If you have a **Y**ellow, **W**hite, **R**ed, or **V**iolet tattoo, **Y**ou **W**ill **R**eturn **V**isit for **2** or more treatments with frequency-**(2)doubled** Nd:YAG"
  - Only ruby and alexandrite (694nm and 755nm; "red light lasers") treat **green** tattoos
  - **Red** tattoos (cinnabar [**mercuric sulfide**]) → most likely to cause **allergic reactions/lichenoid reactions**
  - **Yellow** tattoos (**cadmium sulfide**) → most likely to cause **phototoxic reaction**
  - Laser treatment in patient allergic to tattoo dye → possible **anaphylaxis**
  - **White** tattoos may undergo **immediate paradoxical darkening** (turns black or blue) with laser because of reduction of $Ti^{4+} \rightarrow Ti^{3+}$
  - **Pink, flesh-toned, or light red tattoos** (classically, permanent lip liner) may undergo **immediate paradoxical darkening** (turns brown-black) with laser because of reduction of **ferric oxide (Fe^{3+})** → **ferrous oxide (Fe^{2+})**
    - For **paradoxical tattoo darkening** management consider numerous repeat QS or picosecond laser therapy sessions and/or CO_2 or Er:YAG to vaporize unwanted pigment

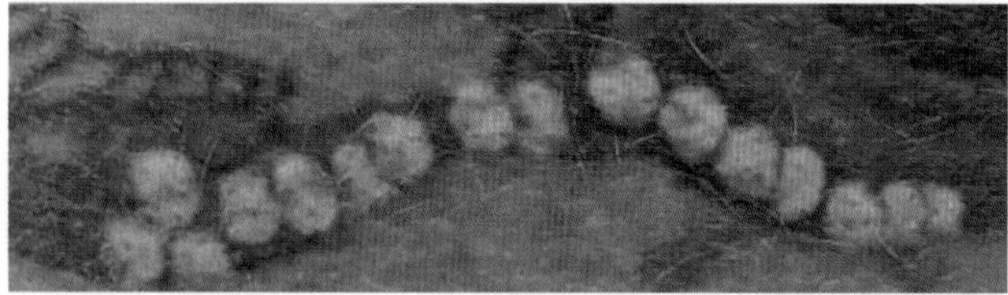

Fig. 9.6 Example endpoint for Q-switched laser tattoo removal. (Courtesy of Ronda S. Farah MD, University of Minnesota.)

  - Traumatic tattoos from gunpowder/fireworks → may explode with laser
  - **Pigmented lesions** (lentigines, ephelides, or nevus of Ota) are treated with the same lasers as black tattoos ("**RAN**" **lasers**)
    - **Ruby** is classically the laser of choice for nevus of Ota/Ito
  - Minocycline hyperpigmentation → treated with the same lasers as black tattoos (**"RAN" lasers)**
  - **Amiodarone**-induced hyperpigmentation → managed with **QS ruby laser**

Excimer laser

- 308 nm; increases expression of apoptotic proteins in T cells
- Utilized for psoriasis, atopic dermatitis, and vitiligo

9.2 BOTULINUM TOXIN

- Botulinum toxin is a neurotoxin derived from the anaerobic gram-positive bacilli *Clostridium botulinum*
- Mechanism: Botulinum toxin inhibits the function of nerve terminals through **presynaptic blockade of SNARE** complex → **prevents acetylcholine (ACh) release** → chemical denervation of muscle → over time, the muscle undergoes atrophy (Fig. 9.7)
- FDA-approved for the temporary improvement in the appearance of glabellar lines, forehead lines, and lateral canthi lines, as well as severe primary axillary hyperhidrosis
  - Numerous off-label cosmetic uses have been reported, particularly on the lower face
  - Takes up to 2 weeks to demonstrate full effect; the effect typically lasts 3 months, but the novel **daxibotulinum toxin median duration is approximately 6 months**
  - Post-injection facial exercises result in shorter time to onset of action
  - Remember, rhytides are perpendicular to muscle fibers

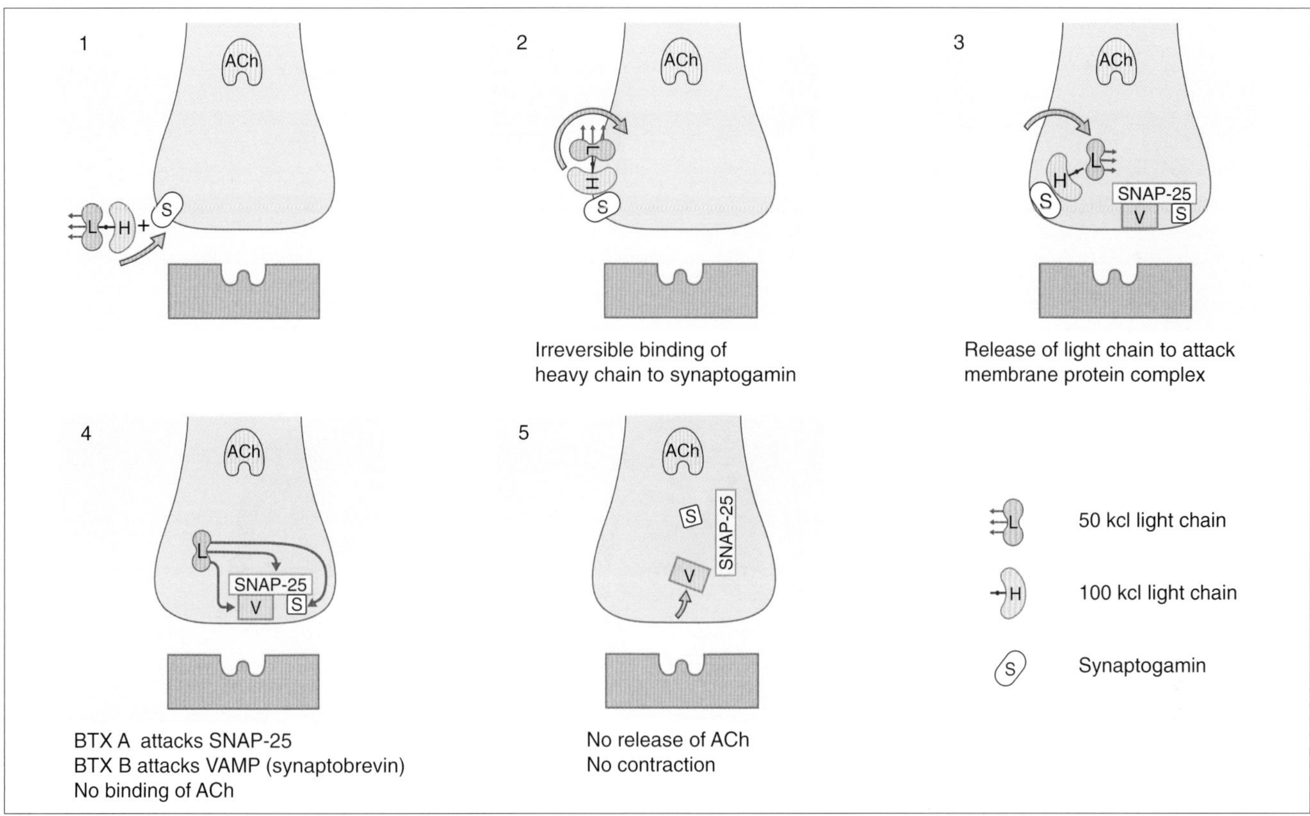

Fig. 9.7 Mechanism of action for botulinum toxin. (From Coleman K. Botulinum toxin: mode of action and serotypes. In: *Botulinum Toxin in Facial Rejuvenation*. 2nd ed. Philadelphia: Elsevier; 2020:2–7.)

Table 9.6 Different Forms of Botulinum Toxin in the United States

	Onabotulinumtoxin A	Abobotulinumtoxin A	Incobotulinumtoxin A	Prabotulinumtoxin A	Rimabotulinumtoxin B	Daxibotulinumtoxin A
Brand name	Botox	Dysport	Xeomin	Jeuveau	Myobloc	Daxxify
Toxin subtype	A	A	A	A	B	A
Target protein	Snap-25	Snap-25	Snap-25	Snap-25	**Synaptobrevin**	Snap-25
Molecular composition	Neurotoxin with complexing proteins	Neurotoxin with complexing proteins	**Neurotoxin**	Neurotoxin with complexing proteins	Neurotoxin with complexing proteins	Neurotoxin without complexing proteins
Storage before/after reconstitution	2°C–8°C/2°C–8°C	2°C–8°C/2°C–8°C	**<25°C/2°C–8°C**	2°C–8°C/2°C–8°C	2°C–8°C/2°C–8°C	Room temp/2°C–8°C

Modified from Frevert J. Pharmaceutical, biological, and clinical properties of botulinum neurotoxin type A products. Drugs R D. *2015;15(1):1–9.*

- Five forms of botulinum toxin type A and one form of botulinum toxin B are currently marketed in the United States (Table 9.6)
  - Abobotulinumtoxin A should be avoided in patients with cow's milk protein allergy
  - Use of preserved saline for dilution reduces patient discomfort (off-label)
- Typical botulinum toxin injection points are shown in Fig. 9.8, and injection doses are shown in Table 9.7 and Fig. 9.9
- **Contraindicated with neuromuscular disorders** (e.g., myasthenia gravis, Lambert-Eaton syndrome, or amyopathic lateral sclerosis)
- **Do not give with aminoglycoside antibiotics** (e.g., gentamycin) or muscle relaxants → may potentiate effects; other medications which may potentiate effects are quinidine, magnesium sulfate, cholinesterase inhibitors, cyclosporine, calcium channel blockers, linocosamides, and polymyxins
- One of the possible SEs of botulinum toxin injections is **eyelid ptosis** (do NOT inject lateral to mid-pupillary line); **Treatment: α-agonist** (**apraclonidine** 0.5%, naphazoline 0.05%, or phenylephrine 2.5%) → **stimulates Müller's muscle** → improves eyelid ptosis
  - Other SEs (depend on site injected): blurred/double vision, mouth droop (depressor labii inferioris), difficulty speaking (orbicularis oris), cheek drooping (zygomaticus—be careful when injecting crow's feet), swallowing difficulties (platysma), bruising (arnica and bromelain can help with bruising), lower eyelid **festooning** after infraorbital injection

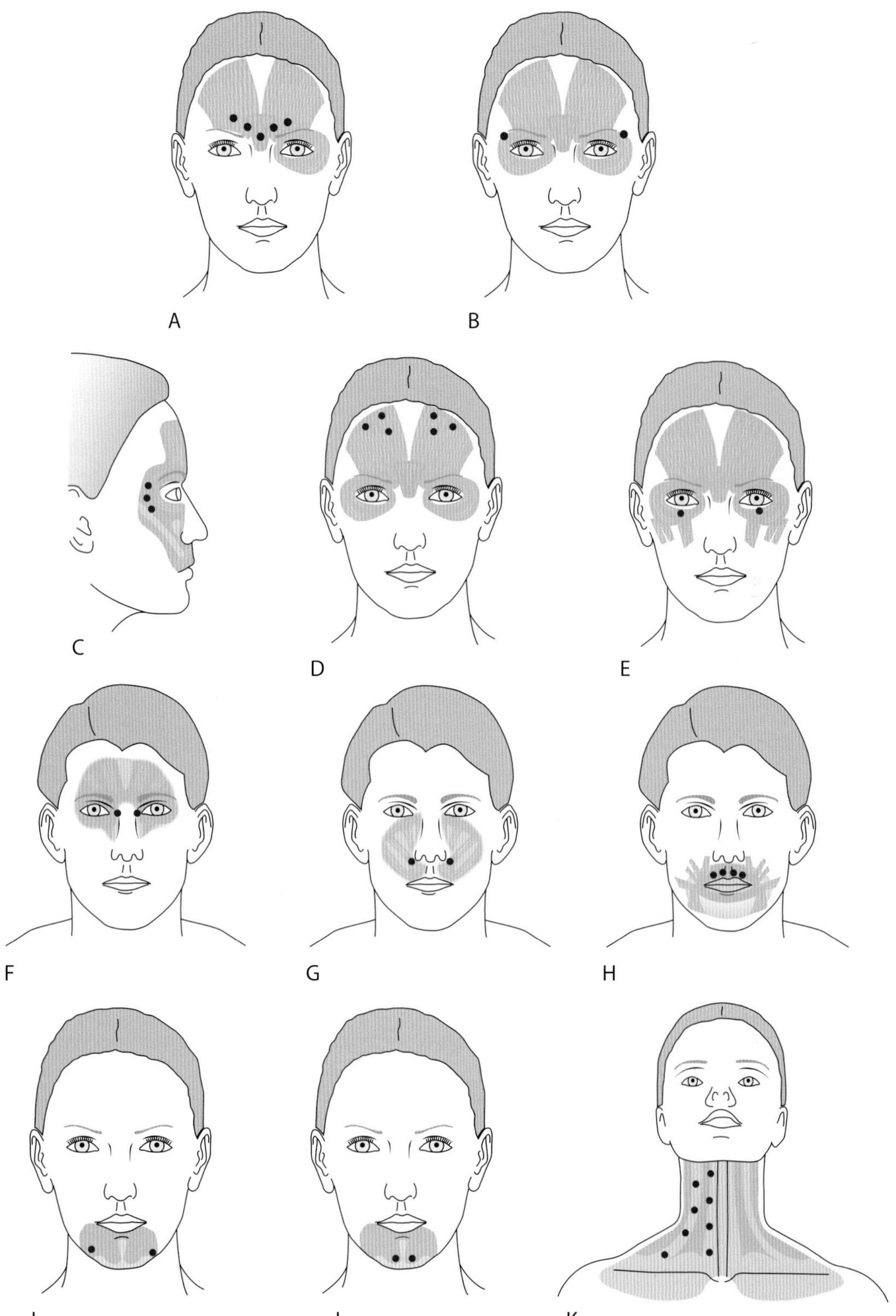

Fig. 9.8 Botulin toxin injection sites: (A) glabella, (B) lateral eyebrow lift, (C) lateral canthal lines, (D) forehead, (E) lower eyelid, (F) bunny lines, (G) gummy smile, (H) upper lip, (I) Depressor anguli oris, (J) mentalis, and (K) platysma.

Table 9.7 Examples of Botox Use

Site/Indication	Target	Significant Complications	Avg. Dose (onabotulinum units)
Treatment of Cosmetic Structural Abnormalities			
Forehead rhytides	Frontalis	Brow ptosis	10-20
Glabellar frown	Procerus, corrugator supercilii, depressor supercilii, orbicularis oculi	Eyelid ptosis	20–40
Lateral canthus/crow's feet	Orbicularis oculi	Diplopia, ectropion, eyelid ptosis, lip ptosis	9–15 per side
Nasal dorsum/bunny lines	Nasalis	Lip ptosis	3–5 per side
Mental/chin dimpling	Mentalis	Asymmetric smile, drooling	5–10, central chin
Perioral/smoker's lines	Orbicularis oris	Difficulty: kissing, forming 'p', 's' and 'b' sounds, sucking, wind instruments, whistling, spitting. May cause drooling.	1–2 total/each lip, 4–6 lip locations total
Neck bands	Platysma	Dysphagia	20–40
Lip/gummy smile	Levator labii superioris alaeque nasi	Lip ptosis, lengthened lip can give an edentulous appearance	1–2, each nasofacial groove
Masseteric hypertrophy	Masseter	Asymmetric smile	20–40/side
Labiomental/marionette lines	Depressor anguli oris	Lower lip protrusion, predisposition to bite the buccal mucosa	1–5, each lateral mentum at jaw angle
Treatment of Hyperhidrosis			
Axillary hyperhidrosis	Eccrine glands	Rare	50–100/axilla
Palmar hyperhidrosis	Eccrine glands	Intrinsic hand weakness	50–200/palm
Plantar hyperhidrosis	Eccrine glands	Rare	50–200/sole
Forehead and scalp hyperhidrosis	Eccrine glands	Brow ptosis	50–100

The ranges listed represent different practice styles as well as variations related to patients. The authors generally suggest beginning at the lower end of the dosing range and increase as required. However, patients with particularly strong muscular rhytides will probably require dosing above the low end of the range. From Murray C & Solish N. Botulinum toxin injections. In: Wolverton SE & Wu JJ (Eds.): Comprehensive Dermatologic Drug Therapy, *4th ed. Philadelphia: Elsevier, 2021, pp 656-664.*

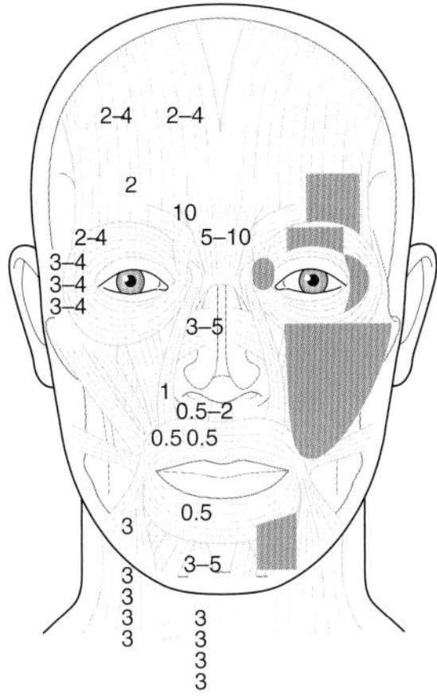

Fig. 9.9 Common Botox injection units per location. (From Murray C & Solish N. Botulinum toxin injections. In: Wolverton SE & Wu JJ (Eds.): *Comprehensive Dermatologic Drug Therapy*, 4th ed. Philadelphia: Elsevier, 2021, pp 656-664.)

9.3 DERMAL FILLERS

- Dermal fillers are used primarily to provide volume augmentation → more youthful appearance of face
- Filler components have changed over time and the use of fillers has expanded rapidly with the development of hyaluronic acid (HA)-based fillers
- HA is a commonly used temporary filler (Table 9.8)
  - HA fillers are usually derived from bacterial (*Streptococcus*) fermentation; avoid in those with hypersensitivity to *Streptococcus*/gram-positive bacteria; there are older-generation products derived from rooster comb
- Differences between various HA fillers is due to differences in the following variables:
  - Concentration: refers to the concentration of HA and includes both the free and cross-linked HA
    - Free HA does not contribute to the firmness of the filler, only cross-linked HA contributes
  - Particle size: larger sizes = longer lasting; typically used for deeper injections; harder to push through small needle bore
  - Degree of cross-linking: refers to the % of the HA that is engaged in cross-links, including incomplete and complete cross-links
    - Natural HA is degraded within days; cross-linking of HA fillers results in macromolecules that are more resistant to degradation
    - ↑ **Cross-linking** → ↑ **durability** of HA fillers (increased stiffness of gel)
    - Proprietary Vycross (VYC) stabilizing technology uses cross-linking of both high- and low-molecular-weight HA; commercial product names start with the prefix "**Vol**" (e.g., Volbella, Voluma, Vollure); the effect is longer-lasting; reports of increased incidence of delayed nodules and granulomas particularly when utilized on lip and perioral areas
  - Filler rheology: influenced by particle size, HA concentration, and cross-linking
    - Effective HA fillers are viscoelastic, demonstrating viscosity during injection while depositing from the needle/cannula, and demonstrating elasticity once implanted by easily recovering shape when shear forces are applied

Table 9.8 Hyaluronic Acid (HA) Fillers Available in the United States

Filler	Juvaderm Ultra	Juvaderm Ultra Plus	Juvaderm Voluma	Juvaderm Vobella	Juvaderm Vollure	Belotero	Restylane	Restylane Silk	Restylane Lyft
Indication	Moderate to severe facial wrinkles and folds	Moderate to severe facial wrinkles and folds	Age-related volume loss in the midface	Lip augmentation Correction of perioral rhytides	Moderate to severe facial wrinkles and folds	Moderate to severe facial wrinkles and folds	Moderate to severe facial wrinkles and folds Lip augmentation	Lip augmentation Correction of perioral rhytides	Moderate to severe facial wrinkles and folds Age-related volume loss
HA Concentration (mg/mL)	24	24	20	15	17.5	22.5	20	20	20
G'	76	148	307	159	273	41	544	344	545
Duration	12 months	12 months	24 months	12 months	18 months	<6 months	6 months	6 months	6 months

Data from Gold M. The science and art of hyaluronic acid dermal filler use in esthetic applications. J Cosmet Dermatol. *2009;8:301–307; Edsman K, Nord LI, Ohrlund A, Lärkner H, Kenne AH. Gel properties of hyaluronic acid dermal fillers.* Dermatol Surg. *2012;38:1170–1179; Fagien S, Bertucci V, von Grote E, Mashburn JH. Rheologic and physicochemical properties used to differentiate injectable hyaluronic acid filler products.* Plast Reconstr Surg. *2019;143:707e–720e.*

- Viscosity: rates the flow of the filler (↑ viscosity → more force required to push it through a syringe)
  - G′: measures elastic properties of the filler in response to shear forces
  - ↑ G′ → ↑ resistance to movement, ↓ spread after placement, ↑ volume support after injection; fillers with high G′ are typically firmer and require deeper placement
- Cohesivity: measures adhesion forces and characterizes the fillers' resistance to vertical compression and spreading; increases with HA concentration and cross-linking degree; low cohesivity fillers are used for shallow (fine) rhytides—easier to mold and spread evenly

- **Non-HA fillers of significance**
  - Bovine (Zyderm®, Zyplast®) and human collagen (Cosmoderm®, Cosmoplast®) fillers **no longer available**
    - Advantages: natural appearance, little swelling/pain
    - Disadvantages: short lived; bovine collagen required two hypersensitivity skin tests prior to use due to risk of **anaphylaxis** (highest risk with bovine collagen [Zyderm, Zyplast])
  - Polymethacrylate (ArteFill®): permanent filler for deep wrinkles (deep dermal injection); Bellafill® is FDA-approved for acne scars
    - Polymethacrylate suspended in bovine collagen—thus skin testing required 30 days before procedure; **elevated risk of allergic reactions**
    - Advantages: long-lasting/permanent
    - Disadvantages: skin testing, avoid on lips, permanent SE (e.g., nodules, granulomas)
  - Calcium hydroxyapatite (Radiesse®): used in deep wrinkles and HIV lipoatrophy, hand rejuvenation
    - 9–18 months of duration
    - **Radio-opaque**—seen on imaging
    - Avoid use on lips and infraorbital areas → increased risk of nodules
    - Nodules often persistent but may respond to hyaluronidase
  - Poly-L-lactic acid (Sculptra®): used in **HIV lipoatrophy**, as well as deep wrinkles
    - FDA-approved for correction of shallow/deep nasolabial contour deficiencies and other facial wrinkles where deep dermal grid pattern (cross-hatch pattern) injections are appropriate
    - Advantages: long-lasting (18–25 months)
    - Disadvantages: suspension preparation requires hour-days, and multiple sessions required for correction; occasionally long-lasting palpable, but not visible, papules/nodules; idiopathic immunologic responses may occur immediately or up to 1 year after injection; of note, massage (5 minutes × 5 times/day × 5 days) initially recommended post-injection but unclear if necessary
  - Silicone: permanent, not cleared by FDA for esthetic indications and has FDA warning
    - Disadvantages: difficult to inject, multiple sessions, permanent nodules, infection, reports of embolism, stroke, disfigurement and death
  - Autologous fat
    - Advantages: good for large areas of volume loss; permanent in some patients
    - Disadvantages: less predictable effects, performance is technique-/user-dependent, more instrumentation required
- **Complications** (may occur with all fillers):
  - Ecchymosis → avoid platelet inhibitors and vitamin E for 10 to 14 days before procedure; cannulas may minimize bruising; manage with ice, pressure, and consider PDL
  - Nodules/biofilms/granulomas (Tables 9.9 and 9.10):
    - May be due to poor technique (too superficially placed/migration/large volume)
    - Vycross fillers may have increased risk of nodules compared with others (Fig. 9.10)
    - **HA fillers → "blue nodules"** from Tyndall effect (see Fig. 9.10); consider massage, aspiration, or **hyaluronidase**
    - Infectious nodules → acute or delayed, erythematous, indurated, +/– constitutional symptoms; consider culture, incision and drainage, macrolide/quinolone

Table 9.9 Timing and Presentation of Filler Complications

Type	Timing	Presentation
Early	<14 days	Erythema, edema, purpura, immediate lumps/bumps, hypersensitivity reaction/anaphylaxis, vascular occlusion/necrosis
Late	>14 days to 1 year	Persistent erythema, erythematous, fluctuant or inert nodules, cellulitis, abscesses, draining sinuses, persistent discoloration, solid edema
Delayed	>1 year	

From Ibrahim O, Overman J, Arndt KA, Dover JS. Filler nodules: inflammatory or infectious? A review of biofilms and their implications on clinical practice. Dermatol Surg. *2018;44(1):53–60.*

Table 9.10 Treatment of Delayed, Inert Filler Granulomas

Initial Therapy	Subsequent Therapy for Resistant Nodules	Final Options
Hyaluronidase[a]	Intralesional corticosteroids	Surgical excision
Dual antibiotic therapy (quinolone and macrolide) for at least 2 weeks	Intralesional 5-fluorouracil	

[a]Hyaluronidase should be administered if the filler is a hyaluronic acid, and may also be considered for other fillers as well.
From Ibrahim O, Overman J, Arndt KA, Dover JS. Filler nodules: inflammatory or infectious? A review of biofilms and their implications on clinical practice. Dermatol Surg. *2018;44(1):53–60.*

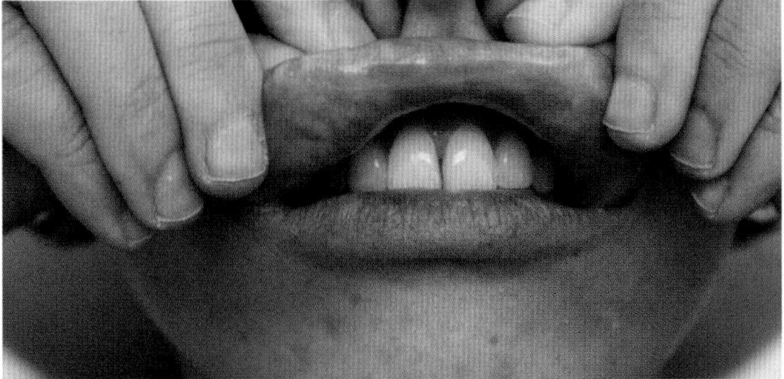

Fig. 9.10 Nodules secondary to injection of Vycross filler in lips. (Courtesy of Neil Sadick MD, New York, NY.)

- Biofilms → may be pyogenic, inert or tender papules/nodules; classic presentation is the recurrence of an infection after antibiotic treatment
  - Culture, biopsy, consider PCR/FISH for bacteria/fungus
  - Treatment: may self-subside, macrolide/quinolone, and excision
- Foreign body granulomas → exclude infection!; Consider massage, hyaluronidase (if appropriate for filler type), oral/IL steroids or IL 5-fluorouracil (FU)
- Low-grade hypersensitivity to filler product → often delayed-onset; rule out infection, consider hyaluronidase, oral/IL steroids, IL 5-FU, surgical excision

- Arterial occlusion/cutaneous necrosis (Fig. 9.11):
  - Findings: immediate, severe, and disproportionate pain and color changes; subsequent necrosis
  - Highest risk in **glabellar region**
  - Prevention: aspirate prior to injection, inject small aliquots (<0.1–0.2 cc), consider blunt cannula, manual occlusion of vessels during injection
  - Treatment (blanching): inject **hyaluronidase (high dose)** for HA fillers
    - Use of aspirin may be helpful; the roles of topical vasodilators and massage remain unclear; prophylactic antibiotic/antivirals have been utilized
  - Treatment (necrosis): wound care

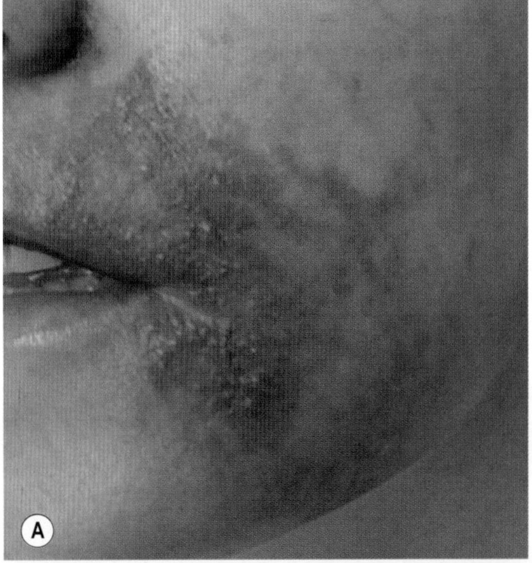

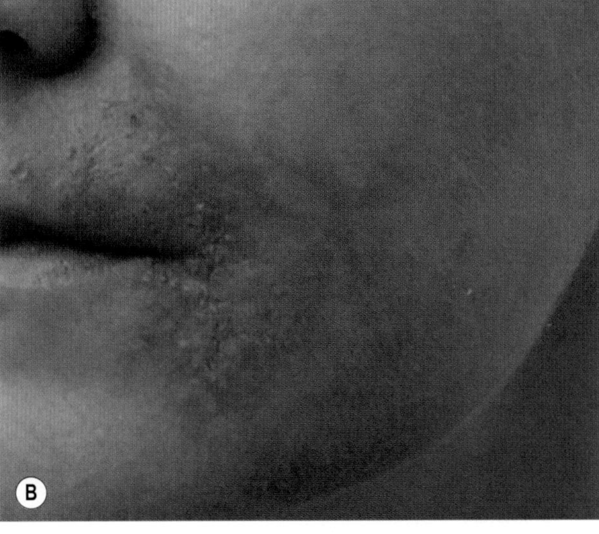

Fig. 9.11 Vascular occlusion 24 hours (A) and 48 hours (B) after hyaluronidase injection. (Courtesy of Neil Sadick, MD, Sadick Dermatology, New York.)

- Blindness:
  - Blindness from occlusion of the ophthalmic/retinal artery branches; occurs via retrograde flow through the internal carotid system (**supraorbital/ supratrochlear/infratrochlear/dorsal nasal arteries → ophthalmic artery → retinal/ciliary arteries**)
  - Highest risk with HA fillers: **nose > glabella > forehead**
  - Acute treatment:
    - 60- to 90-minute window intially proposed (but may be as little as 10 minutes) where blindness may be reversible
    - No generally agreed upon regimen, but consider:
      - ➔ Stop treatment, evaluate vision before intervention, STAT ophthalmology consult, retrobulbar/vascular hyaluronidase, "rebreathing" in paper bag, ocular massage, topical timolol, and oral acetazolamide
- **Anaphylaxis** (rare)
  - Highest risk with **bovine collagen** (Zyderm, Zyplast; all currently off the market) → must perform **two skin tests before treatment** with bovine collagen
  - Patients with history of hymenoptera allergy are at increased risk of allergic reaction to hyaluronidase
  - Consider antihistamines, steroids, and dissolve product if possible
- Prophylaxis against HSV may be indicated based on history and location of injection
- Dermal filler reactions have been reported after SARS-CoV-2 mRNA vaccination

• **Boards fodder**: know the histologic features of the various fillers (see Chapter 7, Dermatopathology) and their reactions

9.4 LIPOSUCTION AND FAT REDUCTION

Liposuction

- Liposuction involves the targeted removal (adipocyte extraction) of fat, whereas many other methods rely on targeted destruction of the fat
- Used for cosmesis, gynecomastia, lipomas, axillary hyperhidrosis
- Performed from the deep to the superficial fat layers with a cross-tunneling technique
- Not recommended for weight reduction or cellulite
- **Tumescent anesthesia** technique allows liposuction to be performed under **local anesthesia → ↓ risk of major SEs** (e.g., bleeding, bowel perforation, death, respiratory failure, pulmonary embolism) compared to general anesthesia
- **Liposuction complications** (Table 9.11)
  - Factors associated with increased complications:
    - Tobacco, anticoagulants, **systemic anesthetics** (general anesthesia and IV sedation), and combining with other procedures
  - Contraindications: cardiac implants and bleeding disorders
  - Local SEs:
    - Edema, ecchymosis, seroma, hematoma, necrosis, asymmetry, over- or under-correction, neurologic, infectious (*Staphylococcus* and *Streptococcus* if superficial and *Mycobacterium* if deep)
  - Systemic SEs:
    - Loss of blood, acute pulmonary edema, hypothermia, visceral perforation, infections (toxic shock syndrome), DVT, fat embolism syndrome

Table 9.11 Adverse Events Associated With Liposuction by Location

Location	Adverse effects
Abdomen	• Overhang of upper abdomen (when only lower abdomen treated) • Skin dimpling (results of over-suction) • Inaccessible fat (intra-abdominal fat) • Abdominal wrinkling due to poor skin quality (low elasticity) • Post liposuction edema
Hips, lateral thighs, buttocks	• Ptosis of buttock due to over-suction • Ligament injury • Dimpling (secondary to superficial treatment)
Knees and medial thighs	• Circumferential thigh suction causing **lymphostasis** • Medial knee nerve injury • Reticulated hyperpigmentation
Upper extremities	• **Compartment syndrome** as a result of fluid compression distal to the area that has been treated with tumescent anesthesia • Anterior flexors should be avoided

Modified from Mariwalla K, Leffell DJ. Primer in Dermatologic Surgery: A Study Companion. *2nd ed. Rolling Meadows, IL: American Society for Dermatologic Surgery; 2011.*

Other fat reduction techniques

- Cryolipolysis—utilized for fat reduction; works well on small areas of localized fat
  - Mechanism over 8 to 12 weeks: cooling → crystallization of lipids within adipocytes → apoptosis → inflammation in subcutaneous layer (lobular panniculitis) → lipid phagocytosis → smaller adipocyte size and wider fibrous septae
  - Manual massage post-treatment and multiple treatments may lead to improved efficacy
  - SEs: bruising, pain, numbness, altered sensation, and paradoxical fat hypertrophy
- *Clostridium histolyticum* (Qwo, Endo International) is the first FDA-approved treatment for moderate to severe cellulite in the buttocks of adult women. Contains two collagenases (AUX-I and AUX-II which degrade collagen types 1 and 2)
- See Table 9.12 for comparison of liposuction and other fat reduction techniques

9.5 SCLEROTHERAPY AND VEIN MANAGEMENT

- Superficial telangiectatic, reticular, and varicose veins of the lower legs constitute a common cosmetic problem for patients (Table 9.13)
- Risk factors: genetic predisposition, hormones (estrogen and progesterone), obesity, and pregnancy

Table 9.12 Fat Reduction Techniques

Technique	Mechanism of Action	Advantages	Side Effects	Notes
Cryolipolysis	Cold-induced apoptosis of adipose cells	Minimally invasive	Numbness and bruising Paradoxical adipocyte hyperplasia, morphea, atrophy	After application of cold stimulus, the treatment area is massaged → this can be the most painful part for the patient
Deoxycholic acid injections (Fig. 9.12)	Degradation of adipose cells (adipocytolysis)	Minimally invasive	Erythema, bruising, alopecia, edema, pain, numbness, temporary marginal mandibular nerve injury (manifesting as inability to depress lower lip and smile)	**Deoxycholic acid** (ATX-101) is FDA-approved for treatment of **submental fat contouring**; off-label use includes jowl reduction
Radiofrequency devices	Heat-induced apoptosis of adipose cells	Minimally invasive	Redness and edema May induce focal atrophy	Need multiple (6 or greater) sessions of treatment
Tumescent liposuction	Direct removal of subcutaneous adipose	Performed under local anesthesia → ↓ **major complications (bowel perforation and ↓ bleeding)** Local vasoconstriction from tumescent anesthesia → ↓ blood loss Does not require general anesthesia (vs. conventional liposuction)	**Breast enlargement** (temporary) Abdominal pain Transient abdominal distention Infection/hematoma/seroma Skin puckers/lumpiness Panniculitis Compartment syndrome Lidocaine toxicity	With tumescent method, **lidocaine limit is 55 mg/kg** (adjust down for lean or elderly; concentration = 0.05%–0.1%) Limit fat removal to 4500–5000 mL of total aspirate—done via cannula Autologous fat transfer—fat harvested from patient (via liposuction or specifically for the procedure; usually from abdomen/thighs/buttocks) and injected into deep wrinkles or hands
Mesotherapy injections	Degradation of adipose cells using various pharmacologic, plant-based and vitamin-derived ingredients	Minimally invasive	Infections, panniculitis, scarring	Not FDA-regulated and may be ineffective and unsafe; thus far deoxycholic acid appears to be the only safe agent

Table 9.13 Classification of Vessels by Size

Vessel Classification	Size (mm)
Telangiectasias	<1
Venulectasias	1–2
Reticular veins	2–4
Non-saphenous varicose veins	3–8

Modified from Mariwalla K, Leffell DJ. Primer in Dermatologic Surgery: A Study Companion. *2nd ed. Rolling Meadows, IL: American Society for Dermatologic Surgery; 2011.*

- Lower extremities have superficial and deep venous systems
  - Most important veins of the superficial venous system = **small** and **great saphenous veins**
    - These veins are typically the most cosmetically disturbing
    - Superficial varicosities located on the medial thigh → suggests great saphenous insufficiency
  - Most important veins of the deep venous system = **femoral** and **popliteal veins**
- Myriad modalities are employed to treat cosmetically undesirable leg veins: sclerotherapy (Table 9.14), ambulatory phlebectomy, endovenous RF ablation, and laser ablation (**Nd:YAG [long-pulsed 1064 nm]**, IPL, and PDL); postprocedural compression stockings required for all forms of treatment
  - For varicose veins, disease-specific quality of life 5 years post-treatment was greater for laser ablation or surgery than for foam sclerotherapy
- Endovenous RF and endovenous laser ablation
  - Treat **sapheno-femoral junction reflux**

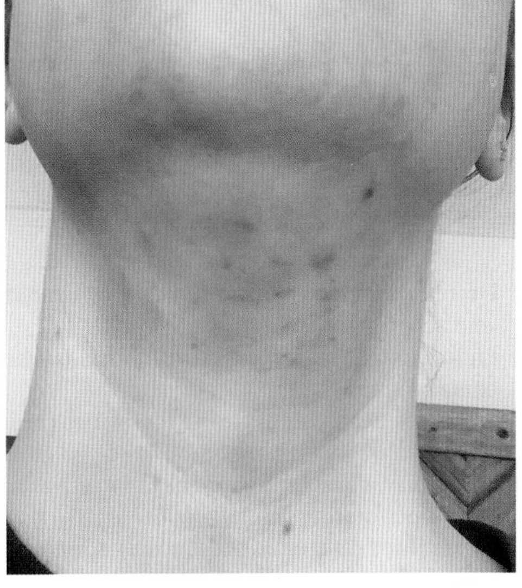

Fig. 9.12 Ecchymosis and edema 1 day post deoxycholic acid injection. (Courtesy of Ronda S. Farah, MD, University of Minnesota.)

  - Use tumescent anesthesia
  - Endovenous laser ablation
    - 810 to 1064 nm (deoxygenated **hemoglobin** is the target)
    - 1320, 1440, and 1500 nm (**water** is the target within vascular wall)
  - RF laser ablation
    - RF catheter is inserted with ultrasound guidance and heat energy is applied to vein wall resulting in collagen shrinkage

Table 9.14 Important Characteristics of Sclerosing Solutions

Sclerosing Solution (Brand Name)	Class	Allergenicity	Risks	FDA Approval	Dose Limitation
Hypertonic saline (11.7%–23.4%)	Hyperosmotic	None	Pain[a] and cramping **Necrosis of skin** Hyperpigmentation	Yes, as abortifacient (18%–30%)	6–10 mL
Hypertonic saline (10%) and dextrose (25%) (Sclerodex®)	Hyperosmotic	Low (due only to added phenethyl alcohol)	Pain[a] (much less than with hypertonic saline alone)	No (sold in Canada)	10 mL of undiluted solution
Sodium tetradecyl sulfate (Sotradecol® [USA], Fibrovein®, Thrombojects®)	Detergent	Very rare anaphylaxis	Pain[a] with perivascular injection Necrosis of skin (with higher concentrations) **Hyperpigmentation**	Yes	10 mL of 3%
Polidocanol (Asclera® [USA], Asklerol®, Aethoxysklerol®, Aetoxisclerol®, and Sclerovein®)	Detergent	Very rare anaphylaxis	Lowest risk of pain Necrosis usually from arteriole injection Hyperpigmentation (with higher concentrations) **Disulfiram-like reaction**	Yes	5 mL of 3% (depends on body weight)
Sodium morrhuate (Scleromate®)	Detergent	**Anaphylaxis**, highest risk	Pain[a] Necrosis of skin Hyperpigmentation	Yes	10 mL
Ethanolamine oleate	Detergent	**Urticaria**, anaphylaxis	Pain[a] Necrosis of skin Hyperpigmentation Viscous, difficult to inject **Acute renal failure** **Hemolytic reactions**	Yes (used primarily for esophageal varices)	10 mL
Polyiodide iodide (Varigloban®, Variglobin®, and Sclerodine®)	Chemical irritant	Anaphylaxis, iodine hypersensitivity reactions	Pain[a] Necrosis of skin Dark brown color makes intravascular placement more difficult to confirm	No	5 mL of 3%
Glycerin (72%) with chromium potassium alum (8%) (Chromex®, Scleremo®); glycerin (72%) diluted 2:1 with 1% lidocaine, with or without epinephrine)	Chemical irritant (plain glycerin may be an osmotic agent as well)	**Very rare anaphylaxis** (none for glycerin alone)	Pain[a] and cramping Low risk of hyperpigmentation Viscous, difficult to inject Hematuria with injections > 10 mL	Yes (for treatment of acute intracerebral edema and acute angle glaucoma)	10 mL

Sclerosing agents are classified into three groups: hyperosmotic agents, detergents, and chemical irritants.
[a]*Includes burning.*
From Goldman MP, Weiss RA. Phlebology and treatment of leg veins. In: Bolognia JL, Schaffer JV, Cerroni L, eds. Dermatology. *4th ed. Philadelphia: Elsevier; 2018:2610–2626.*

   - Decreased pain and quick recovery compared to vein stripping
   - Endovenous heat-induced **thrombosis** is a known complication
- Sclerotherapy is treatment of choice for telangiectasias and reticular veins
  - Foaming may allow for treatment of larger varicose veins and perforating veins
  - There are three categories of sclerosing solutions, each with different mechanisms:
    - **Hyperosmotic agents**: stimulate endothelial damage via dehydration (most common = **hypertonic saline** +/− dextrose)
    - **Chemical irritants**: injure endothelial cells via corrosive action (most common = **glycerin**)
    - **Detergents**: induce vascular injury by altering the surface tension around endothelial cells (most common = **sodium tetradecyl sulfate (STS), polidocanol,** sodium morrhuate, and ethanolamine oleate)
      - Sodium morrhuate and ethanolamine oleate can produce **severe necrosis** with extravasation and harbor a risk for allergic reactions → not recommended for routine sclerotherapy
  - **Foaming** of sclerosing agents, ideally in a ratio of 1:4 (liquid air), is advantageous as it can ↓ number of needed treatments, ↑ efficacy when treating larger veins, and can be applied over a longer segment of a given vein
  - Contraindications to sclerotherapy:
    - Allergy to sclerosants
    - DVT
    - Advanced arterial occlusive disease
    - Symptomatic patent foramen ovale (contraindication to foam sclerosant)
  - **Complications**:
    - Urticaria (very common; Rx: topical steroids or antihistamines; **highest risk of generalized urticaria with ethanolamine oleate**)
    - PIH (due to extravascular hemosiderin; Rx: QS lasers)
    - Telangiectatic matting (↓ risk by using appropriate volume and concentration, and using low pressure when injecting; **highest risk with detergents and lowest with glycerin**)
    - Pain—worse with **hypertonic saline**
    - Swelling—important to use **graduated compression stockings postprocedure**

- Ulceration/cutaneous necrosis—**highest risk on dorsal foot and ankle**
- Systemic allergic reaction—anaphylaxis (**highest with sodium morrhuate and lowest with polidocanol and glycerin)**
- Inadvertent injection of an artery; most common sites: **posterior medial malleolus (posterior tibial artery; superficial injections) and popliteal fossa (deep injections)**

9.6 COSMECEUTICALS, NUTRACEUTICALS, AND OTHER SUPPLEMENTS

- See Table 9.15

Table 9.15 Cosmeceuticals, Nutraceuticals, and Supplements

Ingredients	Other Important Information/Benefits
Aloe vera	Uses: acute frostbite, lichen planus, wound healing, psoriasis, venous leg ulcers, burns, seborrheic dermatitis Classification: anti-inflammatory SE: **allergic contact dermatitis**, hypoglycemia in diabetics taking orally with hypoglycemic agents
Arnica	Uses: **reduces bruising and purpura** Classification: sesquiterpene lactones SE: toxicity with orally ingestion, contact dermatitis
Azelaic acid (10% over the counter and up to 20% prescription)	Uses: acne, melasma, rosacea Classification: free radical scavenger, keratoyltic, comedolytic, reduced *Propionibacterium acnes* SE: irritant dermatitis
Bearberry	Uses: melasma, post-inflammatory hyperpigmentation, decreased UV-related tan SE: oral ingestion can cause green urine, tinnitus, nausea, and vomiting
Bimatoprost	Uses: eyelash hypotrichosis Classification: prostaglandin analog SE: skin discoloration, iris darkening
Biotin (vitamin B7)	Uses: marketed for hair and nail health; evidence for biotin replacement for alopecia is lacking unless related to biotin deficiency/disorder of biotin metabolism; may be helpful for brittle nails SE: caution with biotin supplementation which may cause **thyroid and troponin testing abnormalities**
Brimonidine and oxymetazoline	Uses: facial redness in rosacea; ophthalmic oxymetazoline solution is approved for acquired ptosis Classification: Topical alpha-adrenergic agonists SE: side effects include contact dermatitis, rebound erythema (more so with brimonidine)
Bromelain	Uses: **reduces bruising and purpura**, can potentiate antibiotics Classification: proteolytic enzymes derived from stem of **pineapples**
Ceramides	Uses: atopic dermatitis Other: used in numerous emollients
Chamomile	Uses: can be used to enhance the color of blonde hair Classification: emollient
Cysteamine	Uses: **melasma,** hyperpigmentation Classification: antioxidant Other: initial formulations with sulfur **odor**
Ferulic acid (4-hydroxy-3- methoxy-cinnamic acid)	Uses: may help with photoprotection Classification: antioxidant. Decreases lipid peroxidation, free radical scavenger Other: synergizes with vitamins C and E
Hydroquinone (1.5%–2% over the counter and 4% and above prescription)	Uses: decreases appearance of photo-related skin discoloration and other hyperpigmentation disorders Classification: bleaching agent—inhibits tyrosinase SE: ochronosis, hypopigmentation; avoid use with benzoyl peroxide and hydrogen peroxide due to risk of hyperpigmentation Other: concerns regarding topical toxicity/carcinogenesis have been raised, but are not validated
Kojic acid	Uses: **melasma, lightens pigment** Classification: tyrosinase inhibitor
Licochalcone (licorice extract, glabridin)	Uses: rosacea, lightens pigment Classification: mechanism is via dispersion of melanin and tyrosinase inhibition
Micellar water	Uses: cleansing solution, removes cosmetics, especially those with sensitive skin Classification: surfactant made up of small beads, termed micelles composed of hydrophobic centers with hydrophilic rims, allow sebum to be dissolved
Niacinamide	Uses: acne, rosacea Classification: anti-inflammatory; inhibits mast cells, increases ceramide and collagen, and lightens pigment Uses: decreases nonmelanoma skin cancer incidence, used in high-risk groups
Resveratrol	Uses: keloid scars, antiproliferative effects
Selenium	Uses: may protect against skin cancer and UV-related erythema Classification: antioxidant; glutiathione peroxidase and thioredoxin reductase cofactor SE: toxicity may cause hair loss
Soy	Uses: often combined with sodium sulfacaetamide; used for acne, seborrheic dermatitis, rosacea, scabies, tinea versicolor Active ingredient: phytoestrogens

Continued

Table 9.15 Cosmeceuticals, Nutraceuticals, and Supplements—cont'd

Ingredients	Other Important Information/Benefits
Tranexamic acid	Uses: off-label use in **melasma** (325 mg orally BID; can also be compounded topically); also used for hereditary angioedema Classification: possibly decreases dermal vasculature and melanin synthesis (through altered keratinocyte and melanocyte interaction and decreased tyrosinase activity) Other: not for patients with coagulopathy, thromboembolic disease or other clotting risk factors
Urea	Uses: xerosis, psoriasis, atopic dermatitis, keratosis pilaris, keratodermas, icthyosis Classification: humectant
Vitamin B5	Classification: humectant, emollient
Vitamin C	Uses: lightens pigment and benefits skin texture and tone Classification: antioxidant; ascorbic acid is a cofactor for prolyl hydroxylase and lysyl hydroxylase; L-ascorbic acid is a free radical scavenger which can stimulate collagen Other: L-ascorbic acid combined with vitamin E can protect form UVA and UVB
Vitamin E (Alpha tocopherol)	Uses: some evidence it could decrease skin cancer risk Classification: antioxidant; free radical scavenger and stops lipid peroxidation SE: not for acute wounds to due inhibition of clotting
Vitamin K	Use: ↓ **bruising/purpura**
Zinc	Uses: photoprotective, acne, seborrheic dermatitis; low serum levels may play a role in alopecia Classification: antioxidant

9.7 HAIR TRANSPLANTATION

- Traditionally for non-scarring alopecias
  - Male pattern baldness is typically classified along the Hamilton-Norwood system
  - Female pattern hair loss has been graded along the Ludwig, Savin, and Olsen patterns
  - Most patients require two sessions for desired results
- Surgical intervention involves hair transplantation (Table 9.16)
  - Based on theory of **donor dominance** (transplanted hair retains characteristic of where it was taken from)
  - Grafts harvested from "safe zone" in **occipital scalp** (unaffected by androgenetic alopecia)
  - Usually greater than 25 follicular units/cm^2 for transplant to look natural
  - Typically 150 to 300 grafts per procedure versus mega sessions of 750 to 2000 grafts (achieve desired results in fewer visits but may result in lower graft survival)
  - Two methods to harvest grafts:
    - Strip (elliptical) excision—cannot exceed 30 cm
      - Typically 100 follicular units/cm^2 in donor strip
      - Leaves linear scar in occipital scalp
      - Grafts divided from strip
    - Follicular unit extraction
      - Punch removal of follicular units using manual, motorized, or robotic tools
      - Each follicular unit typically consists of 2 to 3 hair shafts
      - Less visible scarring
      - Preferred in individuals with short hair, risk of hypertrophic/keloid scar, and in younger patients
  - **Post-transplant telogen effluvium** occurs 2 to 3 weeks later (self-resolves)
  - **New hair growth 8 to 20 weeks posts-surgery**, but overall effect apparent at 6 to 9 months
  - Selected SEs: lidocaine toxicity, ingrown hairs, hypoesthesia/numbness (usually resolves within a few weeks), cobblestoning, postoperative edema of forehead (resolves within 1–2 weeks generally), infection, and hypertrophic/keloidal scarring at donor site

Table 9.16 Basic Criteria for Assessment of Candidates for Hair Transplantation

Criteria	More Favorable	Less Favorable
Age	>25 years old is preferable	15–25 years of age
Caliber of hair shaft	Large caliber (>70 microns)	Small caliber hair
Donor hair characteristics	>80 follicular units/cm^2	<40 follicular units/cm^2
Degree of baldness	Baldness primarily affecting frontal scalp	
Hair color	"Salt-and-pepper," red, or blonde hair	Black hair

Modified from Avram MR, Keene SA, Stough DB, Rogers NE, Cole JP. Hair restoration. In: Bolognia JL, Schaffer JV, Cerroni L, eds. Dermatology. *4th ed. Philadelphia: Elsevier; 2018:2637–2648.*

- Poor or no hair growth after transplant most likely due to over-handling, overzealous graft cleaning, or desiccation

9.8 CHEMICAL PEELS (TABLE 9.17)

- Depth of peel correlates volume of solution and friction and pressure of application. For peels associated with clinical frost, peel depth correlates generally with intensity of frost.
- Peel depth is defined by depth of histologic injury: superficial (epidermis) versus medium (papillary to upper reticular dermis) versus deep (mid reticular dermis) peel
- Retinoids enable more efficient penetration of chemical peeling agents by thinning the stratum corneum, visualized by more even and more rapid frost formation
- Depth of penetration, however, is dependent on volume and concentration of solution and friction/pressure of application
  - Consider HSV prophylaxis in those with history of HSV for medium and deep chemical peels on clinically relevant sites
  - Medium depth chemical peels include: TCA 50%, solid CO_2 + TCA 35%, Jessner's solution + TCA 35%, and glycolic acid 70% + TCA 35%

Table 9.17 Chemical Peel Agents

Chemical Peel	Depth of Peel	Use	Neutralization Required?	Frost Level[a]	High-Yield Facts
Salicylic acid	Superficial (epidermal)	**Acne (comedonal, papulopustular)**, Dull skin tone, melasma, hyperpigmentation	No	Minimal (white salicylic acid precipitate)	• **β-Hydroxy** acid • Keratolytic and comedolytic → most commonly used for **acne** • Immediate white frost represents salicylic acid precipitation on skin • May cause **tinnitus** and **salicylism** if use over broad surface areas • **Safe in Fitzpatrick III–VI skin** • **Avoid with strawberry allergies/aspirin allergies**
Glycolic acid	Superficial (epidermal)	Hyperpigmentation, dull skin tone, melasma	Yes (**sodium bicarbonate**) typically after 2 minutes or once erythema is obtained	None	• **α-Hydroxy** acid • Erythema is the endpoint; no frosting (frosting or focal pain suggests over-penetration and requires immediate neutralization), peeling can occur
TCA 10%–35%	Superficial (epidermal)	Dull skin tone, dyspigmentation, melasma, acne	No	Minimal to none (patchy white frost with erythema showingthrough)	• Frosting represents keratin protein coagulation
Jessner's peel *(14% salicylic acid, 14% lactic acid, and 14% resorcinol in ethanol)*	Superficial (epidermal)	Fine wrinkles, melasma, dull skin tone, hyperpigmentation	No	**Minimal (reticulate frost represents precipitation of salicylic acid = "pseuodofrost")**	• Know the components comprising Jessner's (Mnemonic: "**JESNR is LESR**" = **L**actate, **E**thanol, **Sal**icylic acid, **R**esorcinol") • Salicylic acid component may cause **tinnitus** • **Resorcinol** may cause contact dermatitis, **syncope, and hypothyroidism** • Combined Jessner's-TCA (35%) peel has been shown to be as effective as 5-fluorouracil in treating AKs
TCA 50%	Medium (papillary to upper reticular dermis)	Fine to medium wrinkles, actinic keratoses, dyspigmentation, seborrheic keratoses	No	I–II	• TCA 50% has unpredictable penetration and should not be used as a medium depth peel • It has been associated with scarring • Frosting occurs within 2 minutes (self-resolves in 15–20 minutes) • **Post-peel erythema** may last up to 1 month
TCA 90%–100%	Deep (mid-reticular dermis)	Warts, crateriform and icepick type scars	No	III	• Most common side effect is **depigmentation** • **Scarring** is common → high concentration TCA peels (>50%) are not generally recommended (phenol croton oil peels are preferred)
Phenol-croton oil peel, such as Baker-Gordon or Hetter formulas ***(Phenol,** hexachlorophene, tap water, **croton oil)***	Deep (mid-reticular dermis)	Fine to deep wrinkles, scars	No (but use copious amounts of saline or water to flush eyes if contact occurs)	III (gray frost with epidermolysis and petechial hemorrhage)	• Contraindications: Dark skin, history of cardiac arrhythmias, history of renal or liver disease • **Hypopigmentation** is common side effect with higher concentration of croton oil (as in Baker Gordon formula 2.1% croton oil) → contraindicated in dark-skinned patients • **Scarring** and/or **milia** formation may occur • **Cardiac monitoring** required for full face phenol-croton oil peels during, and 1 hour postop, due to **arrhythmia risk** → ↓risk by treating the entire face over 60–90 minutes with a 15-minute interval between each cosmetic unit (decreases systemic absorption) • ↑Risk of **renal toxicity** if inadequately hydrated → **IV hydration** recommended to reduce risk • Post-peel erythema lasts up to 6 months • Boards Fodder: Efficacy correlates with concentration of **Croton oil, Larygneal edema** has been reported

TCA, Trichloroacetic acid

[a]Frost Levels: I, minimal frosting with minimal erythema; II, significant frosting with moderate erythema; III, enamel-like whitening with no erythema.

- Risks: dyspigmentation, infection (bacterial, viral, candida), scarring, delayed healing, milia. Medium and deep peels done off the face increases these risks.

9.9 OTHER ESTHETIC PROCEDURES AND SCALES

- RF (monopolar, unipolar, bipolar, or multipolar) (Fig. 9.13):
  - Electrodes deliver alternating electric current → **locally heats tissue** → stimulates collagen production
  - **Much less selective** and less powerful than lasers and IPL, but does have some specificity for fat (hence, RF is used primarily for **cellulite** and **skin tightening**); safe for darker Fitzpatrick skin types
    - **Unipolar:** transmit around one electrode
    - **Monopolar:** uses grounding plate
    - **Bipolar:** uses two electrodes
    - **Multipolar:** alternates which electrode is the positive pole, with the other electrodes acting as negative poles
    - **Vacuum-assisted RF:** combines RF with vacuum system to target a specific volume of tissue, allowing for lower level of energy use; additionally, the vacuum may stimulate collagen production
  - Risks: erythema, edema, overheating, burns, blistering
- Microwave technology: directs energy to the level of the dermo-subcutaneous junction which non-selectively heats and destroys sweats glands and hair follicles
  - Used to treat axillary hyperhidrosis—two treatments 3 months apart
  - Risks: swelling, bruising, redness, hair loss, altered sensation, brachial plexus injury, compensatory sweating, weakness in limb
- Dermabrasion: a mechanical resurfacing to the level of the papillary **dermis** (endpoint is pinpoint bleeding) used for acne scars, surgical scars, and rhytides
  - Prophylaxis with antibiotics particularly if history of *staphylococcus* colonization
  - HSV prophylaxis, if indicated
  - Methods for dermabrasion (Fig. 9.14)
    - Sandpaper: manual treatment
    - Diamond fraise, wire brush, and serrated wheel: motorized treatment
  - Risks: dyspigmentation, pseudohypopigmentation (due to abraded vs. non-abraded skin being adjacent), milia, acne, scarring
- **Microdermabrasion**: exfoliation procedure utilizing mild mechanical abrasion to resurface the superficial **epidermis**
  - Crystal devices: inert crystals (e.g., aluminum oxide or sodium chloride) are propelled onto the skin, causing corneocyte detachment; known risk of particle inhalation, corneal abrasion
  - Crystal-free devices: abrasive handpiece directly exfoliates and disrupts skin surface
  - Hydradermabrasion: exfoliation utilizing an oxygen- and water-based solution to exfoliate the superficial epidermis
- **Microneedling**: an array of small needles create microscopic punctures within the skin (Figs. 9.15 and 9.16); fibroblast activation with subsequent collagen/elastin deposition leads to improved cosmetic appearance (some are FDA cleared for **wrinkles** and **acne scarring**)
  - May be performed with manual rollers or electric-powered "pens"
  - Risks include foreign body granulomas when used in conjunction with some topicals and scarring
- **High-intensity focused ultrasound**: used for skin tightening and body contouring (FDA-cleared for waist circumference reduction and noninvasive rejuvenation of the face and neck)
  - Mechanism: positive and negative pressure (resonance) causes localized tissue destruction at a precise depth
    - Destruction occurs via three avenues: cavitation, mechanical destruction of cell membranes, and thermal damage

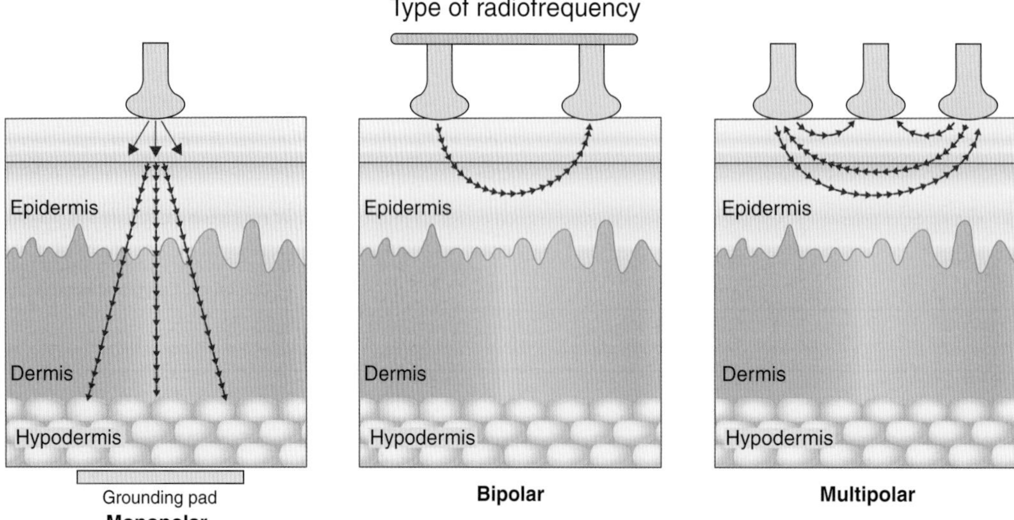

Fig. 9.13 An illustration displaying probes and radiofrequency waves in monopolar, bipolar, and multipolar radiofrequency devices. (Redrawn from Voller LM, Gupta R, Hussain NS, et al. Miscellaneous aesthetic procedures. In: Council ML, ed. *Guide to Minimally Invasive Aesthetic Procedures*. Philadelphia: Wolters Kluwer; 2021. Courtesy Ronda S. Farah, MD, University of Minnesota, Department of Dermatology.)

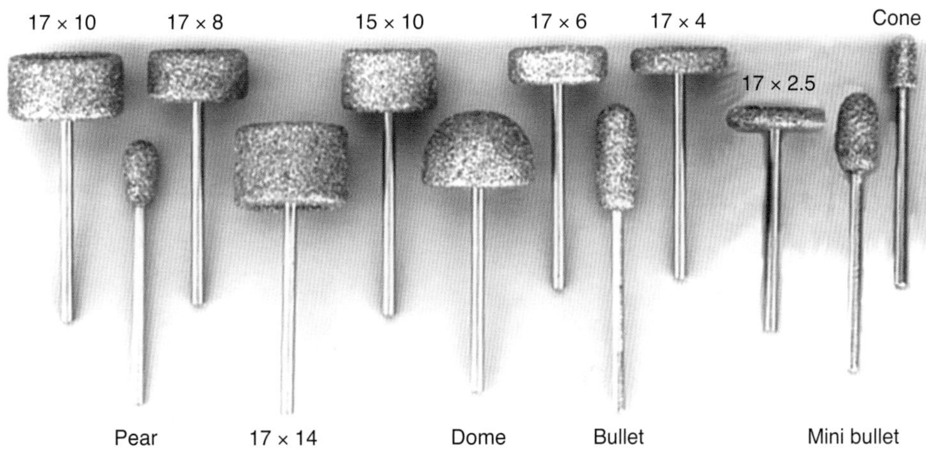

Fig. 9.14 Diamond fraises in various sizes and shapes. (Courtesy of Chuck Ellis, Ellis Instruments, Madison, NJ.)

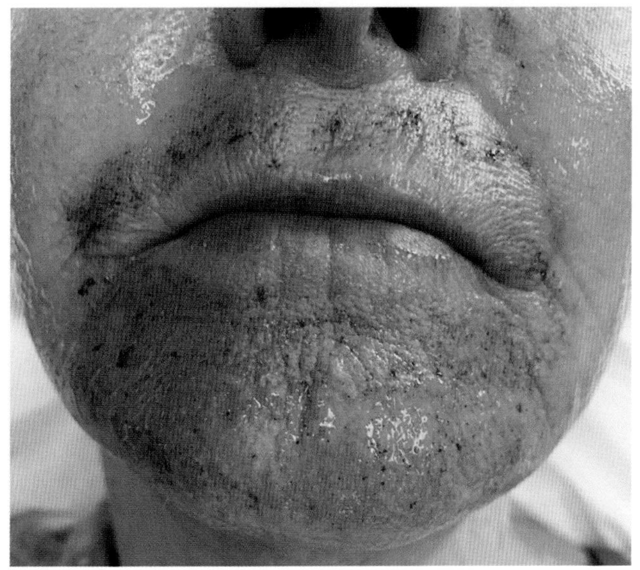

Fig. 9.15 Depiction of patient post-microneedling with pinpoint bleeding as the endpoint. (Courtesy of Ronda S. Farah MD, Univeristy of Minnesota.)

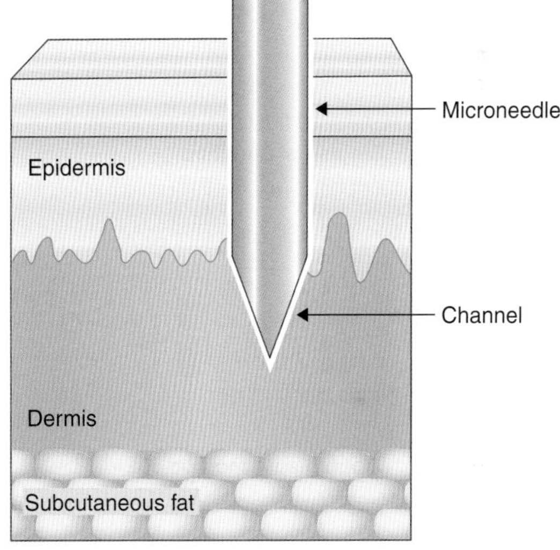

Fig. 9.16 Depiction of microneedle penetrating the skin. (Courtesy of Ronda S. Farah, MD and Sarika Uppaluri, BA, Department of Dermatology, University of Minnesota.)

- SEs: avoid bony areas to prevent thermal injury, erythema, swelling, pain, sensory or muscle discomfort
  - Optimal body contouring results when used on BMI < 30
- Platelet-rich plasma (PRP) is autologous plasma with a platelet count higher than whole blood after centrifugation (Figs. 9.17 and 9.18); the mechanism of action is unknown but proposed to be platelet activation and release of growth factors that activate downstream signaling pathways
  - In dermatology, PRP is utilized for **androgenetic alopecia**; there is limited data for use in photoaging, texture, tone, revolumization, and scarring; of note, PRP is not FDA approved for hair loss
- High-intensity focused electromagnetic technology: induces supramaximal muscle contractions of striated muscle (e.g., abdominal muscles), improving tone; also for strengthening, toning, and firming of buttocks, thighs, and calves
- Thread lifts: use threads to lift ptotic facial or body tissue by grasping and suspending sagging tissue (Fig. 9.19):
  - Silhouette Instalift (Sinclair Pharma): Poly-L-lactic acid (PLLA) (monofilament) that is **bidirectional** (i.e., ends of the thread are both attached to a needle) with polylactide/glycolide (PLGA) **cones**; indicated for mid-face suspension for temporary fixation of the cheek subdermis in an elevated position
  - NovaThreads (Sutura Medical Technology LLC, Miami, FL): polydioxanone absorbable threads that come as barbed, smooth, or twisted; these dissolve in 4 to 6 months

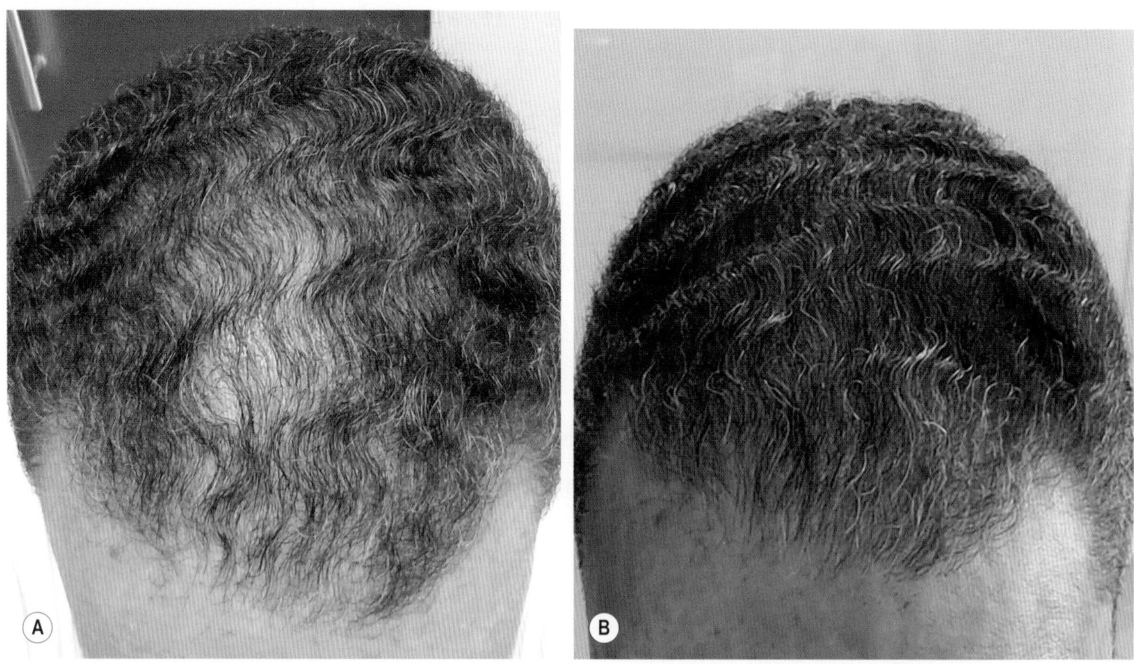

Fig. 9.17 Depiction of androgenetic alopecia before (A) and after (B) use of platelet-rich plasma. (From Crutchfield CE 3rd, Shah N. PRP: what dermatologists should know. *Pract Dermatol*. 2018;55–60. Courtesy of Charles Crutchfield MD, Cruthfield Dermatology, Minnesota.)

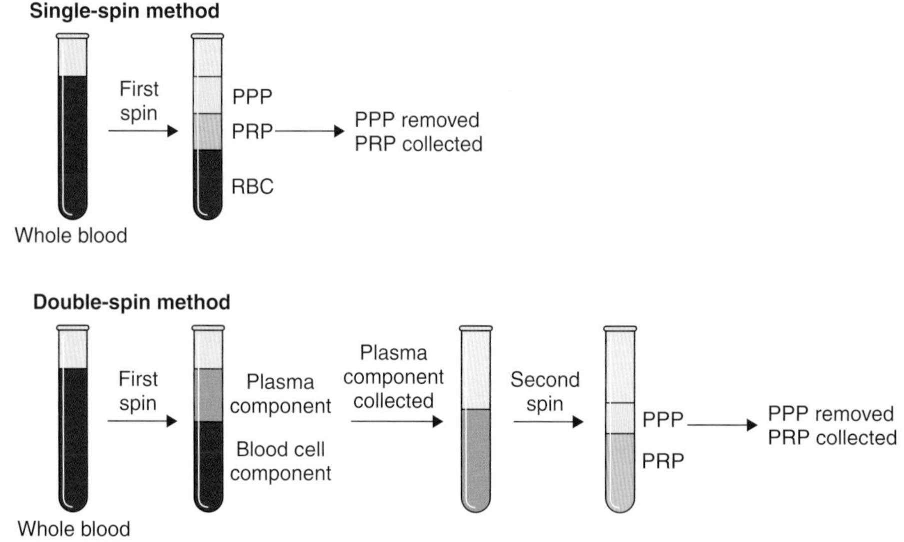

Fig. 9.18 Depiction of platelet-rich plasma *(PRP)* preparation with removal of platelet-poor plasma *(PPP)*. (Redrawn from Voller LM, Gupta R, Hussain NS, et al. Miscellaneous aesthetic procedures. In: Council ML, ed. *Guide to Minimally Invasive Aesthetic Procedures*. Philadelphia: Wolters Kluwer; 2021. Courtesy Ronda S. Farah, MD, University of Minnesota, Department of Dermatology.)

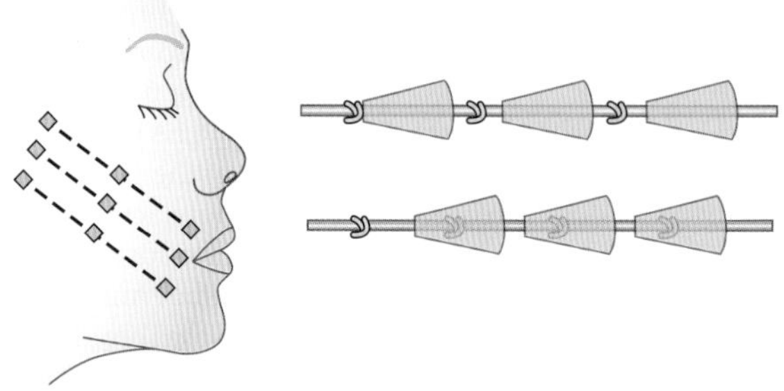

Fig. 9.19 Depiction of thread lift mid face suspension (A) and thread with cones (B).

Table 9.18 Discoloration of Skin With Appropriate Corresponding Recommend Camouflage Color

Discoloration	Camouflage
Red	Green
Brown	White
White	Brown
Yellow	Purple

- Risks: swelling, bruising, dimpling

- **Plasma skin regeneration**: energy from nitrogen gas creates cutaneous thermal effect; removes rhytides
- **Hydrogen peroxide 40% topical solution (Eskata):** initially indicated for the treatment of SK; possible SEs include stinging, erosion, ulceration, vesiculation, and scarring; **removed from market**
- **Camouflage/Foundation**: may use camouflage makeup to hide skin discoloration disorders (Table 9.18)
- **Glogau's photoaging scale** used to assess the severity of cutaneous photodamage (Table 9.19)

Table 9.19 Glogau's Photoaging Scale

Group (Classification)/Age (years)	Wrinkle Description	Exam Characteristics
I (mild)/25–35	None	• Mild change in pigment • No keratosis • Minimal wrinkles • Minimal/no makeup
II (moderated)/35–50	Seen in motion	• Early brown lesions • Palpable keratosis • Appearance of smile lines • Wearing makeup/foundation
III (advanced)/50–65	Seen at rest	• Skin discoloration • Telangiectasias • Keratoses • Heavier makeup
IV (severe)/60–75	Wrinkles only	• Yellow-gray skin tone • Skin cancer history • No wrinkle-free skin

10 Cutaneous Manifestations of Internal Disease and Metastases

Nada Elbuluk

CONTENTS LIST

10.1 CARDIOVASCULAR/CARDIOPULMONARY
10.2 ENDOCRINE
10.3 GASTROENTEROLOGY
10.4 NEUROLOGY
10.5 RENAL
10.6 PARANEOPLASTIC SYNDROMES

- Many of the diseases discussed in this section involve more than one organ system; however, in the interest of conserving space, we have made an attempt to categorize the diseases with their predominant affected organ system
- KEY: *AD*, autosomal dominant; *AR*, autosomal recessive

10.1 CARDIOVASCULAR/ CARDIOPULMONARY

Behçet disease

Cutaneous findings

- **Recurrent orogenital ulcers, acral and facial vesicopustules, palpable purpura, erythema nodosum-like lesions (favor women on legs/buttocks), and pathergy**

Genetics

- Associated with HLA-B51 (80%+ in Asians 15% in Caucasians)

Associations/comments

- A/w pericarditis, **coronary arteritis**, valve disease, **CNS** vasculitis, and ocular disease (e.g., retinal vasculitis, uveitis [panuveitis > posterior uveitis > anterior uveitis], vitritis, retinitis), arthritis, glomerulonephritis, abdominal ulcerations

Birt-Hogg-Dubé syndrome

Cutaneous findings

- **Fibrofolliculomas**, **trichodiscomas**, perifollicular fibromas, and **acrochordons** (Fig. 10.1); lesions most commonly affect the **head/neck**; lesions tend to present in 30s to 40s

Genetics

- Autosomal dominant Folliculin (**FLCN**) gene mutation on chromosome 17 (involved in mTOR pathway)

Associations/comments

- Fibrofolliculoma, trichodiscoma, perifollicular fibroma, and acrochordons are identical lesions just viewed in different histologic planes
- Important associated findings:
  - **Pulmonary cysts** (most common; up to 90%) lead to **spontaneous pneumothorax** (30%)
  - **Renal tumors (higher in men over 40), including renal carcinomas (15%**, most commonly chromophobe renal carcinoma and oncocytoma)
  - Medullary thyroid carcinoma

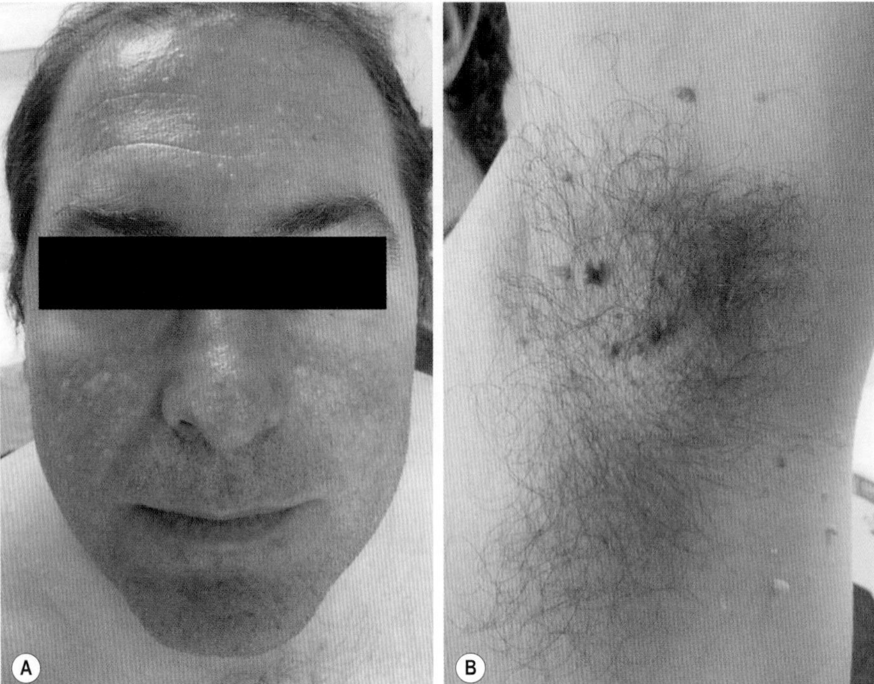

Fig. 10.1 (A) Trichodiscomas and (B) fibrofolliculomas and acrochordons in a patient with Birt-Hogg-Dubé. (From López V, Jordá E, Monteagudo C. [Birt-Hogg-Dubé syndrome: an update.] *Actas Dermosifiliogr*. 2012;103[3]:198–206.)

- Connective tissue nevi
- Colonic adenomas (inconclusive association)

Cardiofaciocutaneous (CFC) syndrome

Cutaneous findings

- **Coarse facies** (long and broad), generalized ichthyosis-like scaling, keratosis pilaris, café-au-lait macules (CALMs), **nevi**, sparse curly and brittle hair, sparse/absent eyebrows, low posterior hairline, patchy alopecia, eczema, palmoplantar keratoderma (PPK)

Genetics

- AD; one of the RASopathies; mutations in **BRAF** (most common), KRAS, and MAP2K1/2 pathway genes

Associations/comments

- A/w psychomotor and intellectual disability, **pulmonic stenosis**, atrial septal defect, **hypertrophic cardiomyopathy**, and short stature
- All **RASopathies** (CFC, NF1, Noonan, Costello syndromes, and LEOPARD) affect RAS/MAPK pathway and have similar clinical presentations → often need genetic tests to distinguish

Carney complex (LAMB and NAME syndromes)

Cutaneous findings

- Also known as cutaneous lentiginosis with atrial myxoma
- LAMB = Lentigines, Atrial myxoma, Mucocutaneous myxomas, Blue nevi (classically **epithelioid blue nevi**)
- NAME = Nevi, Atrial (and cutaneous) myxomas, Myxoid neurofibromas, Ephelides

Genetics

- AD, mutations in **PRKAR1A** gene (encodes type I A regulatory subunit of protein kinase A) on chromosome 17

Associations/comments

- A/w variety of **endocrine neoplasms**
  - **Adrenal gland** (most common); p/w primary pigmented nodular adrenocortical disease → **Cushing syndrome**
  - Other endocrine abnormalities: thyroid tumors, pituitary adenomas, and testicular cancer (Sertoli type)
- A/w **psammomatous melanotic schwannoma and myxoid mammary fibroadenomas**

Carvajal syndrome

Cutaneous findings

- **Striate** epidermolytic PPK; **wooly scalp hair**

Genetics

- AR, **desmoplakin** mutations

Associations/comments

- A/w dilated **left** ventricular cardiomyopathy
- Mnemonic: "CarvajaL = Linear/striate PPK + Left ventricular cardiomyopathy"

Churg-Strauss syndrome (allergic granulomatous angiitis)

Cutaneous findings

- Skin involvement in 60%; leukocytoclastic vasculitis (**LCV**), urticaria, solar urticaria, livedo reticularis, subcutaneous nodules on extensor extremities and scalp (30%), firm **papules on fingertips**, palisaded neutrophilic granulomatous dermatitis, and extravascular granulomas

Associations/comments

- Three phases: first phase involves allergic rhinitis, asthma, and nasal polyps; second phase includes fever, eosinophilia, pneumonia, and gastroenteritis; third phase involves diffuse angiitis of multiple organs
- Classic presentation: **allergic rhinitis, severe asthma, peripheral eosinophilia** of ≥ 10%, sinusitis, transient pulmonary infiltrates, and mononeuritis multiplex
- ↑ **IgE** levels
- Most common causes of mortality: myocarditis and coronary arteritis
  - ANCAs less frequently positive compared with Wegener's (~60% vs ~100%)
- ANCAs detectable in ~60% (**p-ANCA** [anti-MPO] > c-ANCA [PR-3]) and correlate with disease severity
- May be a/w **leukotriene inhibitors** (montelukast and zafirlukast)

Costello syndrome

Cutaneous findings

- **Lax/redundant skin** on the neck, hands and feet, **coarse facies**, low-set ears, deep palmoplantar creases, periorificial papillomas, acanthosis nigricans (AN), and curly hair

Genetics

- AD, one of the RASopathies; mutations in **HRAS** (85%) > KRAS (15%)

Associations/comments

- A/w mental and growth retardation, failure to thrive, **pulmonic stenosis**, hypertrophic cardiomyopathy, arrhythmias, nasal papillomata
- Can have hydrocephalus, brain atrophy, chiari malformation, and syringomyelia
- ↑ Risk of rhabdomyosarcoma and transitional cell (bladder) CA
- All **RASopathies** (CFC, NF1, Noonan, Costello syndromes, and LEOPARD) have similar clinical presentations → need genetic tests to distinguish

Cutis laxa

Cutaneous findings

- Loose, **pendulous** skin of **face** (esp. periocular and cheeks → **"bloodhound facies"**), neck, axillae, and thighs; skin **lacks elastic recoil** (vs. EDS)

Genetics

- Multiple forms:
  - AR: **most common** and most severe; **Fibulin-5 (FBLN5) > Fibulin-4**
  - AD: benign course; **Elastin (ELN)** > FBLN5
  - XLR: ATP7A (copper transporter)

Associations/comments

- **Occipital horn syndrome (OHS)** is the current name for XLR cutis laxa, (which was also formerly called EDS type IX); OHS is a mild variant of **Menkes kinky hair** syndrome
- AR cutis laxa is most frequently a/w internal organ dysfunction and death:
  - Pulmonary: bronchiectasis, pulmonary stenosis, emphysema → **right-sided heart failure**
  - Cardiac: **aortic dilation/rupture**; right-sided heart failure (cor pulmonale)
  - GI: **diverticulae, hernias**
  - Large fontanelles, osteoporosis

Dermatomyositis (DM)

Cutaneous findings

- Gottron papules, heliotrope rash, **shawl sign**, **holster sign**, photodistributed poikiloderma, and psoriasiform dermatitis of scalp

Associations/comments

- A/w ECG changes and pericarditis
- **Cardiac** involvement = poor prognostic sign; a/w **anti-SRP autoantibodies, pericarditis, and congestive heart failure (CHF)**
- **Pulmonary fibrosis** a/w **antisynthetase syndrome (Jo-1, PL7, and PL-12**; autoantibodies target tRNA synthetase)
- Amyopathic (AM) is DM with subclinical or absent myopathy

Ehlers-Danlos syndrome (classic form)

Cutaneous findings

- **Skin hyperelasticity** and fragility, "cigarette paper" and **"fish mouth" scars**, ecchymoses, **Gorlin sign**, and molluscoid pseudotumors

Genetics

See Table 4.13 Ehlers-Danlos Syndrome Classification in Chapter 4, Pediatric Dermatology

Associations/comments

- A/w aortic root dilation, **mitral and tricuspid prolapse** or regurgitation
- Identical cardiac findings may also be seen in **hypermobility** type of EDS (traditionally, EDS type III)

Ehlers-Danlos syndrome (vascular form; formerly type IV EDS)

Cutaneous findings

- **Thin, translucent skin** w/ **visible veins** (most prominent on chest), diffuse bruising

Genetics

- AD; caused by mutations in **collagen III** (COL3A1)

Associations/comments

- **Most dangerous form of EDS** because of the risk of death from rupture of internal organs (**arterial rupture** > GI tract [esp. sigmoid colon], uterus [particularly in pregnancy])
  - Arterial rupture sites: thorax/abdomen > head/neck > extremities
- Most important feature is **vascular fragility → arterial aneurysms, dissection, and rupture** (Mnemonic: "**IV** = **vascular**")

Endocarditis (*Staphylococcus aureus* usually)

Cutaneous findings

- Purpura, **Janeway lesions** (macules/papules; **not painful**; palms and soles; septic emboli w/ microabscess), **Osler nodes** (**painful**; "Osler's = Oww!"; red papules/nodules w/ white centers; finger pads and thenar eminence; immune complex deposition and small vessel vasculitis), nail-fold infarction

Associations/Comments

- A/w **cardiac vegetations** and valvular dysfunction

Erythroderma

Cutaneous findings

- Diffusely red skin, exfoliative dermatitis

Associations/comments

- A/w **high-output cardiac failure, sepsis, acute respiratory distress syndrome, capillary leak syndrome, extensive telogen effluvium, severe itching, fever chills, secondary infections**
- May be as a result of multiple dermatoses, cutaneous T-cell lymphoma, or drug eruptions

Fabry disease

Cutaneous findings

- **Angiokeratoma corporis diffusum** (angiokeratomas in "bathing suit distribution"), macular angiomas on extremities, palms, soles, and vermillion border, hypohidrosis and anhidrosis, episodic pain in hands/feet (**acroparesthesia**), and **whorled corneal opacities** (cornea verticillata) and cataracts, lower extremity edema and lymphedema, scant hair

Genetics

- **XLR**; **GLA** gene mutation → **α-galactosidase** deficiency
  - α-Galactosidase deficiency leads to ↑ **globotriaosylceramide** deposits in tissues → end-organ damage

Associations/comments

- Lysosomal storage disease
- Most serious complications: atherosclerotic disease of CV and CNS → **MI** and **stroke**; chronic proteinuria → **renal failure; GI:** nausea, vomiting, diarrhea; **neuropathic pain**
- "**Maltese crosses**" (birefringent lipid globules) seen on polarization of urine sediment

Hereditary hemorrhagic telangiectasia (pulmonary disease in type I > type II)

Cutaneous findings

- Multiple macular/"**mat-like**" **telangiectasias** most commonly on **lips, oral mucosa**, and extremities (Fig. 10.2)

Genetics

- AD, mutations in genes involved in **TGF-β** transduction pathway:
  - HHT1 = **endoglin** (ENG)
  - HHT2 = **Alk-1** (ACVRL1)
  - HHT with juvenile polyposis = **SMAD4**

Associations/comments

- **Epistaxis** (often the initial symptom), telangiectasias, AV malformations of **lungs (HHT-1** most commonly),

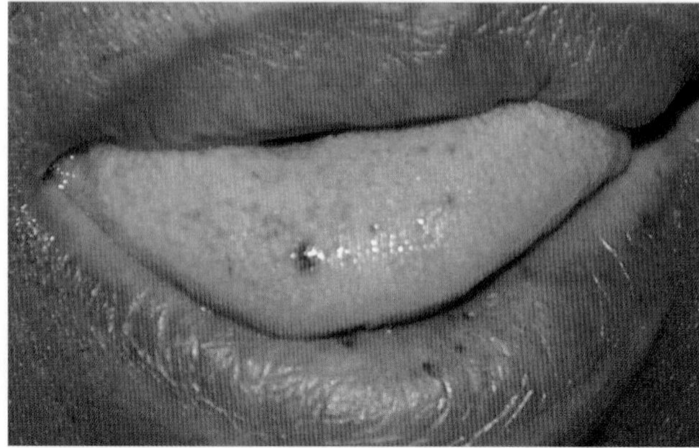

Fig. 10.2 Patient with hereditary hemorrhagic telangiectasia (HHT) and multiple telangiectasias on tongue and lip. (From Irani F, Kasmani R. Hereditary hemorrhagic telangiectasia: fatigue and dyspnea. *CMAJ*. 2009;180[8]:839.)

liver (**HHT-2** most commonly) and CNS, and affected first-degree relative; recurrent upper GI hemorrhage
- Mnemonic: "**Alk-1** is a/w **liver**" (think of **Alk**aline phosphatase, which is found in liver)

Homocystinuria

Cutaneous findings

- **Livedo reticularis, malar rash**, tissue-paper scars, diffuse pigment dilution, tissue paper-like scars, **Marfanoid** habitus, and **ectopia lentis** (downward lens dislocation)

Genetics

- AR; caused by a variety of mutations leading to ↑ homocysteine levels in blood and urine; most common = **cystathionine β-synthase** (**CBS** gene)
- Other gene mutations: **MTHFR**, MTR, MTRR, and MMADHC

Associations/comments

- A/w atherosclerosis, **vascular thrombosis** (arterial + venous), genu valgum
- A/w intellectual disability, seizures, frequent fractures

Hyperlipoproteinemias

Cutaneous findings

- Type I (familial lipoprotein lipase [LPL] deficiency and hyperchylomicronemia): **eruptive xanthomas**
- Type II (familial hypercholesterolemia): **tendinous, tuberous,** tuboeruptive, **interdigital** xanthomas (pathognomonic), and plane xanthomas
- Type III (familial dysbetalipoproteinemia, "broad beta disease"): tendinous, tuberous, tuboeruptive xanthomas, and **plane xanthomas of palmar creases (pathognomonic)**
- Type IV (endogenous hypertriglyceridemia): **eruptive** xanthomas
- Type V: **eruptive** xanthomas

Genetics (hyperlipoproteinemia phenotypic and genetic subtypes)

- Type I: ↑ chylomicrons; **LPL deficiency** and ApoC-II deficiency
- Type IIa: ↑ β-lipoprotein; **LDL receptor** defect and ApoB-100 defect
- Type IIb: ↑ β-lipoprotein with slightly elevated VLDLs
- Type III: ↑ intermediate-density (remnant) lipoprotein; **ApoE** abnormality (results in ↓ hepatic clearance)
- Type IV: ↑ VLDL, due to diabetes, alcoholism, and/or obesity
- Type V: ↑ chylomicrons and VLDL, due to **diabetes**

Associations/comments

- Associated systemic findings:
  - Types I, IV, and V: **acute pancreatitis** (due to ↑ triglycerides)
  - Types II and III: atherosclerosis → **MI and stroke**

Kawasaki disease

Cutaneous findings

- "**Strawberry tongue**," fissuring **cheilitis**, polymorphous skin eruption (favors trunk), **acral erythema/edema** (w/ subsequent desquamation), stomatitis, **conjunctival injection**, periorbital edema, desquamating perianal eruption (early finding), pincer nail deformity, and anterior uveitis

Associations/comments

- A/w **coronary artery aneurysms** (potentially fatal)
- **High fever lasting ≥ 5 days,** cervical lymphadenopathy, truncal rash, hand edema/desquamation, oral findings, and conjunctival injection are diagnostic features
- Can have incomplete/atypical Kawasaki disease (prolonged fever + coronary artery disease [CAD])
- Rx: **high-dose ASA** + **IVIG** are essential to prevent coronary disease

LEOPARD syndrome

Cutaneous findings

- **Lentigines** (upper half of body; appear in childhood), **CALMs**, ocular hypertelorism (widely spaced eyes), **low-set ears**

Genetics

- AD; is one of the RASopathies; most common mutation is **PTPN11 gene** (90%)
  - Less common mutations in MAPK pathway (10%): BRAF and RAF1

Associations/comments

- **L**entigines, **E**CG abnormalities (conduction defects and hypertrophic cardiomyopathy), **O**cular hypertelorism, **P**ulmonary stenosis, **A**bnormalities of genitalia (cryptorchidism #1, hypospadias), **R**etardation of growth, and **D**eafness
- Hard to clinically distinguish from other RASopathies (CFC, NF1, Noonan, and Costello syndromes)

Lymphomatoid granulomatosis

Cutaneous findings

- Dermal or SQ nodules +/– ulceration on trunk and extremities

Associations/comments

- **Frequently fatal** (60% 5-year mortality), **EBV–induced angiodestructive** B-cell lymphoma
- Classically p/w **skin** + **pulmonary (cough, dyspnea, chest pain)** involvement; can also affect brain, kidney, GI tract

Marfan syndrome

Cutaneous findings

- **Striae**, long and narrow face, **elastosis perforans serpiginosa**, **ectopia lentis (upward** lens dislocation), myopia, arachnodactyly, ↓ subcutaneous fat on extremities, and pectus excavatum

Genetics

- AD; gene mutation in **Fibrillin-1**

Associations/comments

- A/w mitral valve prolapse and regurgitation, **aortic root dilation**, and **dissection of ascending aorta**
- Rx: **β-blockers** and **ACE inhibitors** to prevent aortic root dilation

Neonatal lupus erythematosus (NLE)

Cutaneous findings

- Nonscarring, nonatrophic subacute cutaneous lupus erythematosus (SCLE)-like **annular plaques** (most commonly **periocular** and **extremities**), dermal mucinoses, and **prominent telangiectasias (on sun-protected sites)**

Associations/comments

- NLE a/w **congenital heart block** in up to 30% of patients (often irreversible; up to 30% mortality)
- Caused by transplacental passage of maternal **anti-Ro/SSA** antibodies (>anti-La/SSB > anti-U1RNP)
- Thrombocytopenia and hepatic disease can occur in those with cutaneous disease
- Mothers who have one child w/ NLE have **25% recurrence rate** in subsequent pregnancies

PHACES syndrome

Cutaneous findings

- Segmental infantile hemangioma (most commonly **frontotemporal**), typically on face and neck

Associations/comments

- A/w coarctation of the aorta, atrial septal defect, and ventricular septal defect
  - P: posterior fossa malformations
  - H: hemangiomas
  - A: arterial anomalies
  - C: **cardiac defects and coarctation of the aorta**
  - E: eye anomalies
  - S: sternal defects and supraumbilical raphe

Naxos syndrome

Cutaneous findings

- **Diffuse** nonepidermolytic PPK (vs. Linear/striate PPK in CarvajaL syndrome), **wooly scalp hair**

Genetics

- AR, **plakoglobin** mutation

Associations/comments

- A/w arrhythmic **right** ventricular cardiomyopathy (vs. Left ventricular in CarvajaL syndrome); onset in infancy

Neurofibromatosis type 1 (NF-1)

Cutaneous findings

- **CALMs (≥6)**, axillary freckles (**"Crowe sign"**; seen in 30%; may involve neck and other intertriginous sites), multiple neurofibromas (≥2), plexiform neurofibroma, and **Lisch nodules** (iris)

Genetics

- AD; mutation in **NF1** gene (neurofibromin)

Associations/comments

- A/w **HTN** (essential HTN and 2° to pheochromocytoma), optic gliomas, bony defects, acromegaly, cretinism, myxedema, hyperparathyroidism, precocious puberty, intellectual disability, dementia, epilepsy
- Increased risk of **juvenile myelomonocytic leukemia** (esp. in children with both NF1 and JXG)

Primary systemic amyloidosis (AL amyloidosis)

Cutaneous findings

- Petechiae/**pinch purpura/ecchymoses** most common skin finding; bullae more rarely, may also see shiny, translucent **waxy papulonodules** or plaques, **alopecia**, and **macroglossia**

Associations/comments

- A/w **restrictive cardiomyopathy**, conduction abnormalities, GI bleeds, arthropathy, proteinuria, myeloma
- Due to deposition of immunoglobulin **light chains (AL)** in skin and internal tissues; deposits stain **pink-red w/ Congo red (apple-green birefringence** on polarized light)

- Primary systemic amyloidosis a/w skin findings in 30%; **secondary systemic amyloidosis does NOT produce clinical skin changes**

Progeria (Hutchinson-Gilford progeria)

Cutaneous findings

- **Sclerodermoid** changes, accelerated aging with **characteristic facies** (prominent eyes, thin enlarged head with prominent veins, **beaked nose**, protruding ears, and micrognathia), mottled hyperpigmentation, ↓ **SQ fat with atrophy of skin and nails**, and **alopecia**

Genetics

- AD; mutations in **LMNA gene (encodes for lamins A and** C; component of **nuclear lamina**)

Associations/comments

- Most important association: premature death due to **atherosclerosis**, **MI**, or **stroke**

Psoriasis

Associations/comments

- ↑ Risk of **cardiovascular**, **cerebrovascular**, and **peripheral arterial diseases**; ↑ risk of metabolic syndrome

Relapsing polychondritis

Cutaneous findings

- Intense erythema/swelling/pain of cartilaginous portion of ears (**spares earlobes**) **+** inflammation of other cartilaginous tissues (nose and trachea)

Associations/comments

- A/w **tracheal and nasal collapse; nasal chondritis → saddle nose deformity; arthralgia of chest → atypical chest pain; conductive deafness**
- A/w aortic insufficiency and dissecting aortic aneurysm, ocular, and renal manifestations
- **MAGIC syndrome** = relapsing polychondritis + Behçet disease

Rheumatic fever

Cutaneous findings

- **Erythema marginatum**, **subcutaneous nodules**, polyarthritis, chorea, and fever

Associations/comments

- Acute phase: pericarditis
- Chronic: **mitral and aortic valve disease**

Sarcoidosis

Cutaneous findings

- Red-brown papules, nodules, and plaques w/ **"apple jelly"** color on diascopy (can also present as verrucous, icthyosiform, hypomelanotic, psoriasiform, and alopecic); may arise in **preexisting scars; lupus pernio** (strongly a/w lung disease), **EN** (a/w acute bilateral hilar adenopathy and arthritis of ankles = Lofgren syndrome)

Associations/comments

- Pulmonary: pulmonary artery HTN and **interstitial lung disease**
- Cardiac: **pericarditis** and conduction defects; cardiac involvement a/w poor prognosis
- Can also be a/w polyarthralgias, ocular, hepatic, renal, and neurologic manifestations

Systemic lupus erythematosus

Cutaneous findings

- Transient malar erythema +/− edema; photosensitivity +/− DLE and SCLE lesions; rare bullous variant, periungual telangiectasias, diffuse nonscarring hair loss, red lunulae, multiple eruptive dermatofibromas, mucous membrane involvement
- If antiphospholipid antibodies present: necrotizing livedo reticularis, widespread cutaneous necrosis, and leg ulcers

Associations/comments

- A/w **Libman-Sacks endocarditis** (nonbacterial), pericarditis, CAD, arthritis, proteinuria, neurologic disease, hematologic abnormalities

Wegener granulomatosis (granulomatosis with polyangiitis, GPA)

Cutaneous findings

- Skin involvement in 50%; **LCV**, necrotizing cutaneous granulomas, pyoderma gangrenosum (PG)-like lesions ("malignant pyoderma"), **friable ulcerative gingivae ("strawberry gingivae"), mucosal ulcerations, and "saddle nose"**

Associations/comments

- Severe (>90% mortality if untreated) multisystem **necrotizing vasculitis**
- Most common systemic manifestations: **respiratory tract** (**chronic sinusitis** is most common presenting symptom of GPA); **renal** (segmental crescentic necrotizing glomerulonephritis)
- **c-ANCA** (anti-Proteinase-3) autoantibodies in ~**100%** of patients by ELISA and IIF; detectable ANCAs more common in GPA than in Churg-Strauss (~60%)

Yellow nail syndrome

Cutaneous findings

- Thick, **slow-growing**, highly curved, and yellow or **yellow-green nails** w/ onycholysis; absent cuticles and lunulae

Associations/comments

- **Classic triad**: yellow nails, lymphedema, and **pulmonary disease** (bronchiectasis and pleural effusions)

10.2 ENDOCRINE

DIABETES

Bullous diabeticorum

Cutaneous findings

- Tense, noninflammatory, painless bullae on upper and/or lower extremities (Fig. 10.3)

Associations/comments

- A/w peripheral neuropathy, usually heals in 2 to 4 weeks; M > F; treat with supportive care

Benign acanthosis nigricans

Cutaneous findings

- Velvety, brown, digitate plaques on neck and in axillary and inguinal folds; can have overlying acrochordons

Associations/comments

- Slow onset, usually manifests earlier in life
- Can indicate insulin resistance and/or diabetes
- More common in darkly pigmented individuals

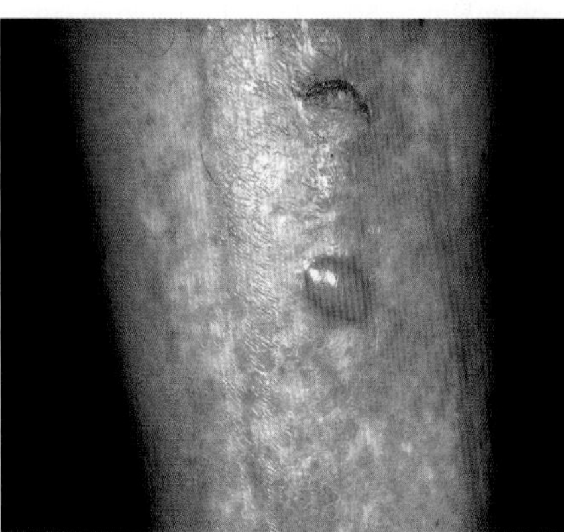

Fig. 10.3 Bullous diabeticorum on the lower extremity. (Courtesy of Jeffrey P. Callen. In: Bolognia JL, Schaffer JV, Duncan KO, Ko CJ, eds. *Dermatology Essentials*. Philadelphia: Elsevier, 2014.)

- Treatment includes improvement of insulin resistance, topical retinoids, keratolytics (e.g., ammonium lactate), and calcipotriene

Granuloma annulare

Cutaneous findings

- Often **affects trunk and extensor limbs**, or may be generalized and eruptive; p/w **nonscaly**, flesh-colored, pink, violaceous, or reddish brown papules that can be grouped in an arcuate or **annular** pattern (patchy, subcutaneous, perforating are rarer subtypes); may resolve with atrophy

Associations/comments

- Usually asymptomatic and spontaneously resolves over months to years; F > M
- Rx: observation, topical steroids, intralesional steroids, cryotherapy, and phototherapy
- May be a/w anterior and chronic uveitis (localized granuloma annulare), hyperlipidemia, HIV, malignancies, medications (IFN-α, TNF-α inhibitors)

Carotenemia

Cutaneous findings

- Diffuse **orange-yellow** discoloration

Associations/comments

- Secondary to increase in serum carotene level; can be seen in hypothyroidism and anorexia nervosa

Neuropathic ulcers

Cutaneous findings

- Nonpainful ulcerations at pressure sites with keratotic rim, commonly on sole of foot

Associations/comments

- Due to sensory neuropathy; commonly a/w diabetes

Scleredema diabeticorum (adultorum of Buschke)

Cutaneous findings

- Erythematous or skin-colored induration of **upper back/neck**

Associations/comments

- Due to glycosaminoglycan deposition; M > F; not related to control of DM
- Histology: **square biopsy** sign, **pauci-cellular** dermis (vs. ↑ cellularity in scleromyxedema), and **widely spaced**

collagen bundles separated by mucin (best seen w/ colloidal iron)
- May also be associated with ***Streptococcus*** infections and **IgG-kappa** monoclonal gammopathy

Acral erythema

Cutaneous findings

- Erysipelas-like erythema of the hands and/or feet

Associations/comments

- May be secondary to small vessel occlusive disease with compensatory hyperemia

Diabetic dermopathy

Cutaneous findings

- Small, oval, red-brown, atrophic macules and patches that are usually on the **lower limbs, can resolve with hyperpigmentation**

Associations/comments

- Due to minor trauma and/or decreased skin perfusion from microangiopathy; seen in up to 40% patients with DM; M > F
- Early recognition can help detect early presence of **renal and retinal microangiopathy**

Necrobiosis lipoidica diabeticorum (NLD)

Cutaneous findings

- Early changes of **small red papules w/ sharp borders → atrophic yellow-orange patches w/ red borders and telangiectasias** +/− central ulceration, often on **pretibial** skin (Fig. 10.4); lesions may ulcerate and heal with **atrophic** scars

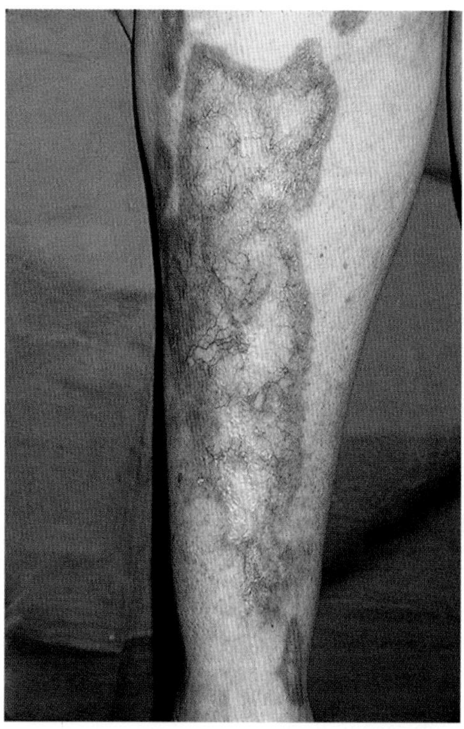

Fig. 10.4 Necrobiosis lipoidica diabeticorum. (From Jones SK. Skin manifestations of systemic disease. *Medicine.* 2004;32[12]:40–43.)

Associations/comments

- A/w diabetic **nephropathy**, **retinopathy**, and **smoking**
- 30% of NLD patients have diabetes, but only **0.3% of diabetics have NLD**
- F > M
- Rx: low-dose ASA, nicotinamide, topical or IL steroids, fibrinolytics, pentoxifylline, and surgical treatments

Multiple endocrine neoplasia (MEN)

Cutaneous findings and associations

- Type I (Wermer syndrome): **pituitary** gland adenomas, **parathyroid** tumors, and **pancreatic** tumors; tuberous sclerosis-like skin changes (collagenomas, facial angiofibromas, leukodermic macules, gingival papules, CALMs, lipomas)
- Type IIa (Sipple syndrome): **parathyroid** adenomas, **medullary thyroid** carcinoma, **pheochromocytoma,** notalgia paresthetica, and macular/lichen amyloidosis
- Type IIb/III (multiple mucosal neuroma syndrome): **mucosal neuromas, medullary thyroid** carcinoma, **pheochromocytoma**, GI ganglioneuromatosis, marfanoid habitus, nodular/thickened lips
- Most important mucocutaneous changes (Boards Fodder!):
  - MEN 1 = **TS-like** changes
  - MEN 2a = **amyloid**
  - MEN 2b = mucosal **neuromas, marfanoid** features

Genetics

- AD
- Type I: **MEN1** (encodes menin, a tumor suppressor)
- Types IIa and IIb/III: **RET** protooncogene (encodes a tyrosine receptor kinase)

Infections more common in diabetes

- Erythrasma
- Furuncles/carbuncles
- Candidiasis: angular cheilitis, median rhomboid glossitis, chronic paronychia, erosio interdigitalis blastomycetica, genital infections, and intertrigo
- Other bacterial and fungal infections: group B strep, mucormycosis, pseudomonas causing malignant external otitis media

THYROID DISEASE

Graves' disease

Cutaneous findings

- Velvety, smooth, or moist skin; palmar erythema; facial flushing
- Localized or generalized hyperpigmentation
- Fine hair; mild but diffuse alopecia
- Koilonychia, onycholysis, and clubbing from **thyroid acropachy**
- Vitiligo (7%)
- Pretibial myxedema: **indurated** red-brown **pretibial** plaques (> posterior external forearms > other sites) (Fig. 10.5)
  - Affects 3%–5% of patients with Graves' disease
  - Often occurs after surgical treatment of Graves' disease
  - A/w exophthalmos, thyroid acropachy, clubbing, and trachyonychia
- Thyroid dermopathy: symmetric, nonpitting, yellow to red-brown, waxy papules, nodules, and plaques on upper/lower extremities
  - Rx: topical and IL steroids
  - A/w hyperthyroidism

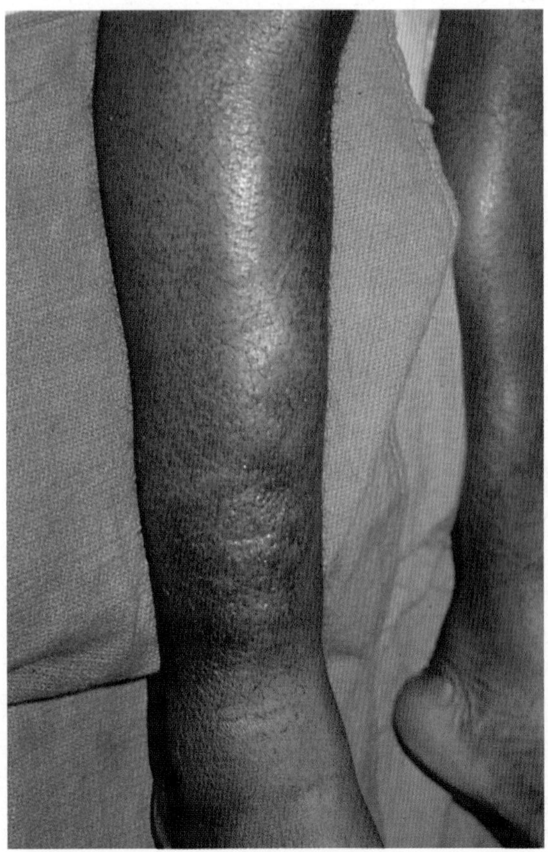

Fig. 10.5 Pretibial myxedema on the lower extremities. (From Brinster NK, Liu V, Diwan AH, McKee PH. *Dermatopathology: A Volume in the High Yield Pathology Series*. Philadelphia: Elsevier, 2011.)

Hypothyroidism

Cutaneous findings

- Coarse, dry, scaly, cold, boggy, and edematous skin
- **Generalized** myxedema
- Dull, **brittle**, and **coarse hair**; diffuse alopecia
- **Madarosis** (loss of eyebrows/eyelashes), hypohidrosis, onycholysis, and striated/brittle/slow-growing nails
- Cutaneous pallor or **yellowing of skin** secondary to carotenemia
- Thickened skin with enlargement of the lips and tongue, cutis verticis gyrata, onycholysis
- Periorbital infiltration 2° to deposits of mucopolysaccharides

Thyroid cancer

Cutaneous findings

- **Papillary** thyroid carcinoma is most common type to present as a skin metastasis

Associations/comments

- Thyroid cancer is a/w multiple syndromes:
  - Medullary thyroid carcinoma: MEN IIA, MEN IIB, and Birt-Hogg-Dubé
  - Follicular thyroid carcinoma: Cowden syndrome

OTHER DISEASES

Addison disease

- **Diffuse hyperpigmentation** (accentuated in sun-exposed areas, trauma/pressure sites, and scars) secondary to adrenocorticotropic hormone (ACTH) secretion; fibrosis and calcification of cartilage; ↓ ambisexual hair in postpubertal women; palmar crease darkening; eruptive onset of multiple nevi
- Due to adrenal insufficiency; can be part of polyglandular autoimmune syndrome I and II

Cushing syndrome

- Thin atrophic skin, easy bruising and poor wound healing, violaceous **striae**, **buffalo hump, moon facies**, steroid-induced acne, hypertrichosis, thinning of scalp hair

10.3 GASTROENTEROLOGY

Bannayan-Riley-Ruvalcaba syndrome

Cutaneous findings

- Macrocephaly, **lipomas**, **penile lentigines,** and **vascular malformations**

Genetics

- AD, mutation in **PTEN gene** (encodes protein phosphatase); affects mTOR pathway

Associations/comments

- Mild phenotypic variant of Cowden syndrome (much lower risk of visceral malignancy)
- A/w intestinal hamartomatous polyposis

Blue rubber bleb nevus syndrome

Cutaneous findings

- Multiple soft blue-purple subcutaneous "blebs" (**venous malformations**) mainly on trunk and arms; may be a/w nocturnal pain

Genetics

- Sporadic (>AD); most patients have mutations in *TEK* gene (encodes TIE2, an endothelial cell tyrosine kinase receptor)

Associations/comments

- Most important and common internal manifestation = GI venous malformations (blue blebs) → **GI hemorrhage (potentially fatal);** vascular malformations can also occur in CNS, lungs
- **Skin lesions precede GI** involvement (birth vs. early adulthood, respectively) → early recognition of skin changes is important!

Bowel-associated dermatosis-arthritis syndrome (BADAS, bowel bypass syndrome)

Cutaneous findings

- Erythematous macules and patches with overlying **papulovesicles and pustules on proximal extremities and trunk**; nodular panniculitis

Associations/comments

- p/w fevers, chills, malaise, polyarthritis, tenosynovitis, and skin findings
- Due to **bowel bacterial overgrowth** → complement activation → deposition of antibody complexes in skin/synovium
- 20% are a/w jejunoileal **bypass surgery** for obesity
- May be a/w inflammatory bowel disease (**IBD**)
- Rx: **antibiotics** (tetracyclines, quinolones, metronidazole, and macrolides) and topical steroids; consider surgical revision of bowel bypass if severe

Cirrhosis

- Spider angiomas, **palmar erythema**, gynecomastia, Terry nails (liver failure), Muehrcke's nails (hypoalbuminemia), pruritus, and **jaundice**

Cowden syndrome (PTEN hamartoma syndrome [PTHS])

Cutaneous findings

- Facial **trichilemmomas**, **oral papillomas (tongue, gingivae** most commonly), palmoplantar keratoses, multiple lipomas, **sclerotic fibromas** (pathognomonic), and **penile lentigines**

Genetics

- AD, mutation in **PTEN** (encodes protein phosphatase); affects mTOR pathway

Associations/comments

- A/w **hamartomatous GI polyps and fibrocystic breast disease**
- Lifetime risk of cancer: **B**reast (85%; often bilateral) > **T**hyroid (35%; follicular most common) **> E**ndometrial
- Mnemonic: "**BET** on cancer with Cowden syndrome"
- **Dysplastic gangliocytoma** of cerebellum (**Lhermitte-Duclos** disease)—neurologic part of Cowden syndrome; is a hamartoma that leads to cerebellar ataxia, macrocephaly, and ↑ intracranial pressure
- **PTEN hamartoma syndrome (PTHS)**: umbrella term encompassing Cowden syndrome, Bannayan-Riley-Ruvalcaba syndrome, PTEN-related Proteus syndrome, and Proteus-like syndrome; all diseases have overlapping features

Cronkhite-Canada syndrome

Cutaneous findings

- Lentiginous **hypermelanosis, alopecia, and nail thinning**

Associations/comments

- A/w **nonhereditary adenomatous polyposis**, **diarrhea**/malabsorption (leading to weight loss), edema, and abdominal pain
- No ↑ risk of cancer

Degos disease (malignant atrophic papulosis)

Cutaneous findings

- Eruption of multiple papules with **porcelain-white** center and **erythematous rim** (early lesions) → **atrophic ivory scars (late lesions)**; most commonly upper extremities, trunk

Associations/comments

- **Is an occlusive vasculopathy** of small arteries w/ **poor prognosis** (exception: skin-limited form has good prognosis)
- A/w **GI perforation** (most common and most severe complication; occurs in 50% of cases; high mortality) > CNS disease; rarely pleuritis or pericarditis
- May be related to lupus erythematosus or antiphospholipid antibody syndrome

Dermatitis herpetiformis (Duhring disease)

Cutaneous findings

- Symmetric **itchy papulovesicles** w/ overlying erosions on **extensor extremities**, scalp, nuchal area, and **buttocks**

Genetics

- A/w **HLA-DQw2** > **HLA-DQ8** > other cited haplotypes (HLA-A1, HLA-B8, HLA-DR3)

Associations/comments

- Very strong association with **gluten-sensitive enteropathy/celiac disease**
- Poor adherence to gluten-free diet → ↑ risk **GI lymphoma**
- Laryngeal involvement can → hoarseness
- A/w thyroid disease

Gardner syndrome (phenotypic variant of familial adenomatous polyposis syndrome)

Cutaneous findings

- **Multiple epidermoid cysts** (often hybrid cysts w/ focal pilomatrical differentiation), **multiple pilomatricomas**, **multiple lipomas**, desmoid tumors (15%), fibromas, **jaw osteomas**, and **odontogenic cysts**

Genetics

- AD mutation in **APC gene** (normally functions to downregulate **β-catenin**)

Associations/comments

- A/w many neoplasms: **colorectal** (~100%) carcinoma
- A/w congenital hypertrophy of retinal pigment epithelium)
- **Syndromes a/w multiple pilomatricomas**: Gardner, Rubenstein-Taybi, myotonic dystrophy
- **Syndromes a/w multiple lipomas**: Gardner, Bannayan-Riley-Ruvalcaba, and MEN-I

Hemochromatosis

Cutaneous findings

- Generalized **bronze** hyperpigmentation increased in sun-exposed areas, koilonychia, icthyosis, mucous membrane pigmentation (20%), alopecia, pruritus, leg ulceration in those with CVD

Genetics

- **Four genes cause AR form**
  - **HFE gene** (**C282Y** most common), hemojuvelin and hepcidin (juvenile-onset), transferrin 2 receptor (adult-onset)
- One gene, ferroportin, causes AD form

Associations/comments

- A/w **CHF**, excess iron stores, cardiac dysfunction, supraventricular arrhythmias, diabetes mellitus, arthropathy, **cirrhosis**, and hepatocellular carcinoma
- Rx: **phlebotomy** (first line) and chelation (second line)

Hepatitis B and C

Cutaneous findings

- <u>Most important hepatitis B-associated diseases</u>:
  - Gianotti-Crosti (**B** > C)
  - Classic PAN (**B** > C)
  - erythema nodosum (**B** > C)
- <u>Most important hepatitis C-associated diseases</u>:
  - Necrolytic acral erythema (**C**)
  - Erosive oral lichen planus (**C**)
  - Cryoglobulinemia types 2 and 3 (**C** > B)
  - Porphyria cutanea tarda (**C** >B)
  - Cutaneous PAN (**C** > B)
  - Sarcoidosis a/w IFN or ribavirin (**C** > B)
  - Cutaneous B-cell lymphoma, xerostomia (C > B)
  - Autoimmune thyroid disease (C > B)

Associations/comments

- **Other associated diseases (Hep B = C)**: erythema multiforme, pruritus, urticarial vasculitis, urticaria

Inflammatory bowel disease

Cutaneous findings and associations

- A/w erythema nodosum, urticarial vasculitis, hidradenitis suppurativa (HS), small vessel vasculitis, PAN, BADAS, **PG**, neutrophilic dermatosis, pyostomatitis vegetans, aphthous ulcers, granulomatous infiltrates, fissures, fistulas (perianal in Crohn disease), **metastatic Crohn disease** (granulomatous involvement of skin noncontiguous from GI tract), and **epidermolysis bullosa acquisita**

Primary biliary cirrhosis

Cutaneous findings

- **Pruritus**, jaundice, diffuse hyperpigmentation, xanthomas, LP and lichenoid eruptions

Associations/comments

- Autoimmune disease strongly a/w **antimitochondrial antibodies** (>90%)
- F > M (9:1)
- Osteoporosis is common complication
- Rx: **ursodiol**, colchicine, methotrexate, and transplant

Peutz-Jeghers syndrome

Cutaneous findings

- Mucosal (> cutaneous) melanotic macules

Genetics

- AD, mutation of serine/threonine protein kinase (**STK11**/ LKB1) tumor suppressor gene

Associations/comments

- Benign hamartomatous polyps of the digestive tract (minimal malignant potential); a/w ↑ risk of intussusception and hemorrhage
- Most important associated malignancies: **GI** (small intestine, colon, stomach) > **breast** > **pancreatic** > **ovary** > **lung**

Pseudoxanthoma elasticum (PXE)

Cutaneous findings

- Yellow papules/plaques in **intertriginous** areas, along with redundant, lax skin (Fig. 10.6) (**"plucked chicken skin"**)

Genetics

- AR; mutation in **ABCC6** gene (ABC transporter/ATPase involved in multidrug resistance)

Associations/comments

- A/w **GI hemorrhage**, **angioid streaks** (small breaks in **Bruch membrane**), HTN, **premature atherosclerosis**, **MI**, uterine hemorrhage, and vascular calcification
  - Angioid streaks a/w: PXE, Paget bone disease, sickle cell anemia, and lead poisoning

Pyoderma gangrenosum

Cutaneous findings

- Violaceous nodule or hemorrhagic pustule that progresses to an ulcer with **undermined purpuric borders** (Fig. 10.7); ulcer base may be purulent and hemorrhagic with necrotic eschar; ulcers heal with **cribriform scaring**; most commonly affects **lower extremities**

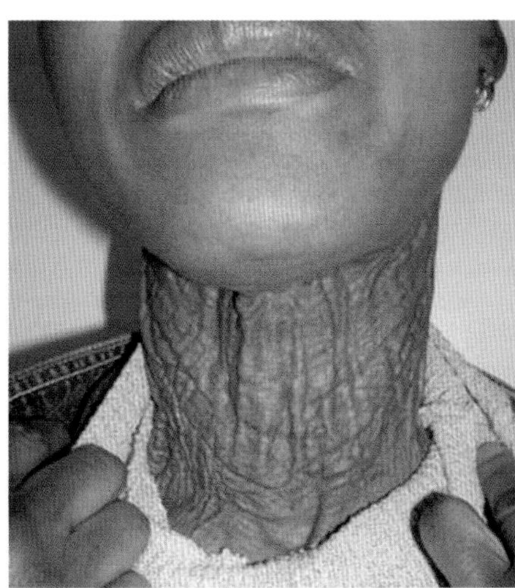

Fig. 10.6 Lax skin and redundant folds on the anterior neck of a patient with pseudoxanthoma elasticum. (From Akram H, Sewell MD, Cheng LHH. Pseudoxanthoma elasticum. *Br J Oral Maxillofac Surg.* 2008;46[3]:237–238.)

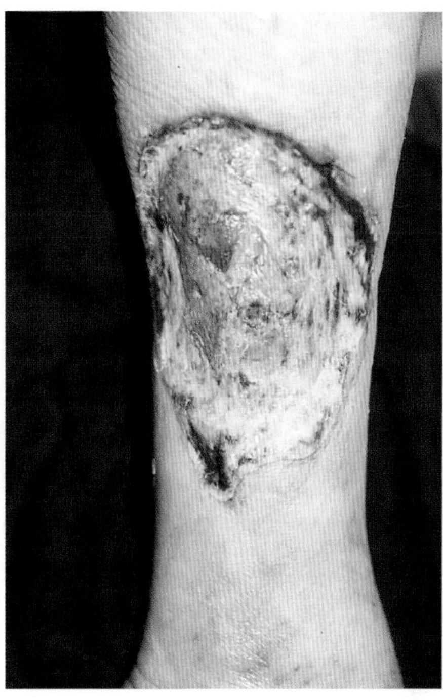

Fig. 10.7 Pyoderma gangrenosum on the lower extremity of a patient with ulcerative colitis. (From Brinster NK, Liu V, Diwan AH, McKee PH. *Dermatopathology: A Volume in the High Yield Pathology Series*. Philadelphia: Elsevier, 2011.)

Associations/comments

- A/w **IBD (ulcerative colitis** > Crohn disease), rheumatoid arthritis, HS, and **myeloid blood dyscrasias**
- Can show **pathergy**

Pyodermatitis/pyostomatitis vegetans

Cutaneous findings

- Pustules and ulcerations on **lips**, **buccal mucosa** (Fig. 10.8), and **skin folds**
- Often a/w pyoderma gangrenosum

Associations/comments

- Almost always a/w **IBD** (**ulcerative colitis** > Crohn disease)
- Rx: treat underlying IBD; may use topical steroids or tacrolimus for local control

Muir-Torre syndrome (phenotypic variant of Lynch syndrome)

Cutaneous findings

- **Multiple sebaceous neoplasms**: sebaceous adenoma, sebaceoma, and sebaceous carcinomas
- Multiple **keratoacanthomas** (often w/ sebaceous differentiation)

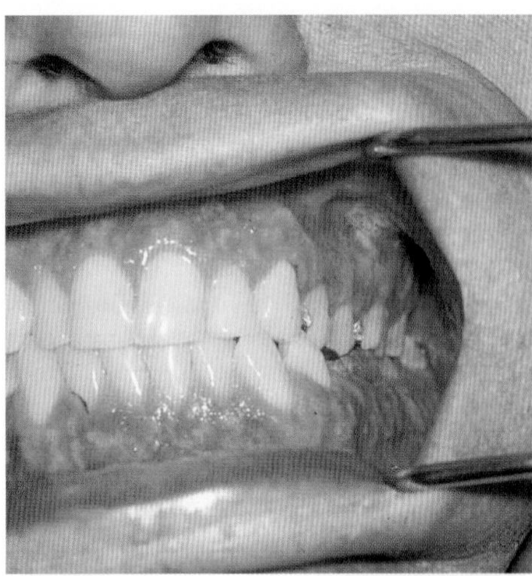

Fig. 10.8 Patient with pyostomatitis vegetans exhibiting erythematous oral mucosa with overlying yellow pustules. (From Islam NM, Bhattacharyya I, Cohen DM. Common oral manifestations of systemic disease. *Otolaryngol Clin North Am.* 2011;44[1]:161–182.)

Genetics

- AD, mutations in **mismatch repair genes** → microsatellite instability; most common mutations: **MSH2 (90%)** > MSH6, MLH1, and PMS-2

Associations/comments

- Cancer associations: **colon (most common, 50%)** > **GU** (second most common) > gastric, ovarian, endometrial cancers, and lymphoma
- **Extrafacial** sebaceous neoplasms are very strongly a/w Muir-Torre (more so than facial lesions)
- **Keratoacanthomas** w/ sebaceous differentiation strongly a/w Muir-Torre

Scleroderma (systemic sclerosis)

Cutaneous findings

- Early **bilateral edema of hands** progressing to **acrosclerosis**, dermal sclerosis (most commonly arms and head/neck); Raynaud phenomenon w/ digital infarction, **ventral pterygium**, facial telangiectasias (esp. CREST variant), and **"salt-and-pepper" dyspigmentation; dermoscopy** of nail folds show **dilated capillary loops w/ surrounding avascular areas**

Associations/comments

- Dermal sclerosis as a result of **TGF-β** (and endothelin-1, PDGF, IL-4, and connective tissue growth factor)
- Most commonly a/w **esophageal dysmotility and pulmonary fibrosis** (up to 60%)
- Anti-topoisomerase I (**Scl-70**): a/w diffuse SSc and **pulmonary fibrosis**
- **Anticentromere** antibodies: a/w CREST syndrome (lcSSc), and ↓ pulmonary, cardiac, and renal involvement
- **Anti-PM/Scl** antibodies: a/w polymyositis-scleroderma overlap syndrome

Scurvy (vitamin C deficiency)

Cutaneous findings

- **Perifollicular petechiae and purpura**, **"corkscrew hairs,"** follicular hyperkeratosis, **gingivitis**, conjunctival hemorrhage, anemia (from GI blood loss), woody edema, and difficulty walking (Fig. 10.9)

Associations/comments

- Four H's: hemorrhagic signs, hyperkeratosis of hair follicles, hypochondriasis, and hematologic abnormalities
- A/w fad diets, malnutrition, and alcoholism
- Vitamin C (ascorbic acid) is **cofactor for lysyl hydroxylase and prolyl hydroxylase** (required for collagen hydroxylation and subsequent cross-linking) → **defective collagen cross-linking** → bone deformities, vascular fragility, poor wound healing, and aforementioned skin findings

Spider angioma

- Red macule or papule with vascular extensions, typically planar
- Occurs secondary to **hyperestrinism**
- Develops in at least 75% of those with **cirrhosis**; also can occur with **pregnancy** and **oral contraceptive** use

Wilson disease (hepatolenticular degeneration)

Cutaneous findings

- **Kayser-Fleischer** rings, **blue lunulae**, **pretibial hyperpigmentation,** and skin changes of cirrhosis

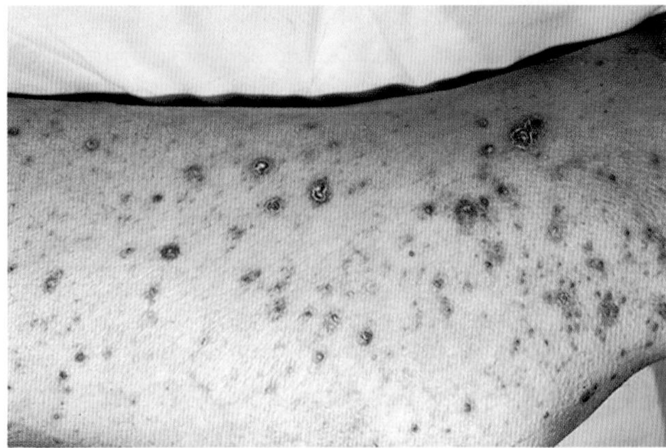

Fig. 10.9 Perifollicular purpura and follicular hyperkeratosis seen in scurvy. (From Demidovich CW. Cutaneous signs of nutritional disturbances. In: Fitzpatrick JE, Morelli JG, eds. *Dermatology Secrets Plus.* 5th ed. Philadelphia: Elsevier; 2016:357–362.)

Genetics

- AR mutation in **ATP7B**

Associations/comments

- Defects in **copper metabolism** → deposition in liver and subsequent **liver failure**
- Neuropsychiatric symptoms common
- **Ceruloplasmin** levels low
- Kayser-Fleischer rings as a result of copper deposition in **Descemet membrane** (cornea)
- Rx: **penicillamine**, trientine, zinc supplementation, or liver transplantation

10.4 NEUROLOGY

- Darier disease has been a/w **mild intellectual disability**, epilepsy, encephalopathy, depression, and **schizophrenia**
- Bullous pemphigoid has been associated with several neurological conditions, most commonly **dementia**, stroke, multiple sclerosis, epilepsy, **Parkinson disease**, Shy-Drager syndrome, and amyotrophic lateral sclerosis
- See Pediatric Dermatology **(Chapter 4)** for review of NF, basal cell nevus syndrome (Gorlin-Goltz syndrome), ataxia-telangiectasia syndrome, xeroderma pigmentosum, Sjögren-Larsson syndrome, Refsum disease, Cockayne syndrome, incontinentia pigmenti, Keratitis Icthyosis Deafness syndrome, Vohwinkel syndrome, Björnstad syndrome, photosensitivity, ichthyosis, brittle hair, intellectual impairment, decreased fertility and short stature, and Menkes disease

10.5 RENAL

Birt-Hogg-Dubé syndrome (see cardiopulmonary section of this chapter)

- **Multiple renal carcinomas (15%**, most commonly chromophobe renal carcinoma and oncocytoma)

Calciphylaxis

Cutaneous findings

- p/w painful **"stellate"** or **retiform** purpuric plaques on **lower legs** → indurated, **necrotic**, **ulcerative** plaques

Associations/comments

- Due to small-to-medium **vessel calcification + thrombosis**
- Most commonly occurs in setting of **end-stage renal disease** (a/w ↑ calcium-phosphate product)
- Other causes: diabetes mellitus and **hyperparathyroidism**
- A/w secondary infections and sepsis; **high mortality**
- Rx: treat underlying renal failure, partial parathyroidectomy, debride necrotic tissue, sodium thiosulfate, hyperbaric oxygen, tissue-plasminogen activator, parathyroidectomy (in refractory cases), and treat underlying infections

End-stage renal disease (ESRD)

Cutaneous findings

- Pale color, **yellowing of skin** secondary to deposition of carotenoids and urochrome, photodistributed hyperpigmentation, ecchymoses, xerosis, and **Lindsay's (half-and-half)** nails

Associations/comments

- **Pruritus**, **calciphylaxis**, metastatic calcification, **nephrogenic fibrosing dermopathy (NFD)/nephrogenic systemic fibrosis (NSF**; a/w gadolinium exposure), perforating diseases, uremic frost, pseudoporphyria, and PCT

Henoch-Schönlein purpura

Cutaneous findings

- Leukocytoclastic vasculitis (legs and buttocks most commonly)

Associations/comments

- May be a/w **IgA glomerulonephritis**
- Most common in prepubescent children; majority of patients have **preceding upper respiratory tract infection (URTI)/pharyngitis; group A** *Streptococcus* is the most common associated infection
- p/w **abdominal pain**, fever, headache, scrotal pain/edema, **arthritis**, and **transient renal insufficiency** (may have chronic renal insufficiency in up to 10%–20%, but only 2% develop ESRD)

Nail-patella syndrome (iliac horn disease and HOOD syndrome = hereditary onycho-osteodysplasia)

Cutaneous findings

- Hypoplasia of nails (**fingernails** > toenails; **thumb** most severely affected), **triangular lunulae,** webbing of the elbows

Genetics

- AD; **LMX1B** gene mutation (regulates collagen synthesis)

Associations/comments

- A/w **focal segmental glomerulosclerosis** (seen in 40%, fatal in 10%; important to treat early to prevent renal failure), **absence/hypoplasia of patella (90%)**, **iliac horns** (**pathognomonic** exostoses of iliac bone of pelvis, seen in 80%; asymptomatic)

- Classic eye finding: **Lester iris** (~50%; hyperpigmentation of pupillary margin of iris)

Nephrogenic Systemic Fibrosis (NSF)

Cutaneous findings

- Woody, indurated plaques most commonly on **legs** (>trunk) with **"peau d'orange"** appearance → cobblestoning, puckering/linear banding over time; **face is spared;** yellow papules on palms

Associations/comments

- Can have systemic fibrosis affecting the heart, lungs, and skeletal muscle
- All patients have history of exposure to **gadolinium-based MRI contrast dye** (highest risk w/ **Omniscan**, Magnevist, and Optimark) in setting of **renal insufficiency** (chronic > acute)
- Important eye finding—**yellow scleral plaques**

Polyarteritis nodosa

Cutaneous findings

- Dermal/**SQ nodules**, necrotizing vasculitis, and **livedo reticularis**

Associations/comments

- Ten diagnostic criteria associated with systemic PAN: livedo racemosa, polymorphonuclear arteritis, leg pain/myopathy, **mono/polyneuropathy**, +HBV serology, weight loss > 4 kg, testicular pain/tenderness, diastolic BP > 90 mm Hg, elevated BUN/creatinine, arteriographic abnormality
- Classic associations: **renal artery aneurysms** and HTN; also a/w hepatitis B > C

Reed syndrome (familial cutaneous leiomyomas)

Cutaneous findings

- Multiple cutaneous painful **pilar leiomyomas**, genital leiomyomas, angioleiomyomas, and uterine leiomyomas

Genetics

- AD; **fumarate hydratase** gene mutation (fumarate hydratase is an enzyme involved in **citric acid/Krebs cycle** of cellular respiration)

Associations/comments

- ↑ Risk of **renal cell carcinoma (RCC)** (15% lifetime risk) and renal cysts

Tuberous sclerosis

Cutaneous findings

- Facial angiofibromas in butterfly distribution (**adenoma sebaceum**), periungual and subungual angiofibromas (**Koenen tumors**), **ash leaf** macules, **shagreen** patch (back/neck most common), CALMs, oral papillomatosis, gingival hyperplasia

Genetics

- AD; caused by mutations in **TSC1** (**hamartin**) and **TSC2** (**tuberin**)

Associations/comments

- A/w **renal angiomyolipomas**, CNS tumors (giant cell astrocytoma, cortical tubers, subependymal nodules), intellectual disability, seizures, **cardiac rhabdomyomas**, and ocular lesions (**coloboma** and phakoma)

10.6 PARANEOPLASTIC SYNDROMES

Acquired angioedema (AAE)

Cutaneous findings

- Painless, nonpitting, edema of the skin; **no associated urticaria**

Associations/comments

- Caused by ↓ **C1-INH** activity (common to **all** forms of hereditary angioedema [HAE] and AAE)
- Both types AAE (AAE1 and AAE2) have ↓ **C1q** (distinguishes from HAE) and ↓ **C2/C4**
  - AAE type 1: a/w **lymphoproliferative disease** (lymphomas and **monoclonal gammopathy of undetermined significance**)
  - AAE type 2: a/w **autoimmune disease**
  - Idiopathic form

Acquired ichthyosis

Cutaneous findings

- Adherent **polygonal** scale/keratosis on **lower extremities** (favors extensors); **spares flexural creases**; may also see fine scaling of trunk and extremities, carotenemia, and diffuse alopecia

Associations/comments

- Most commonly a/w **Hodgkin and non-Hodgkin lymphoma**
- Other associations: sarcoidosis, lupus, hypothyroidism, drugs, lymphoma, breast and lung cancer, mycosis fungoides, multiple myeloma

- Usually diagnosed after malignancy and course follows that of underlying malignancy
- Drug-induced ichthyosis can occur secondary to nicotinic acid, statins, triparanol, butyrophenones

Acrokeratosis paraneoplastica (Bazex syndrome)

Cutaneous findings

- Initially p/w **symmetric** erythematous to **violaceous psoriasiform** plaques on **nasal bridge, helices, distal extremities,** +/– PPK; eruption gradually extends proximally to knees, legs, arms, and scalp (Fig. 10.10)
- Other clinical findings include xanthonychia, subungual hyperkeratosis, onycholysis, and **horizontal and longitudinal nail ridging** (seen in 75%)

Associations/comments

- Most commonly a/w cancer of **upper aerodigestive tract** (oral cavity, pharynx, larynx, esophagus)
- Can clinically resemble psoriasis (involvement of helices and nose is a clue to Bazex)
- M > F; average age = 40
- Skin findings precede the diagnosis by 2 to 6 months

Alopecia neoplastica

- **Localized scarring alopecia** due to dermal infiltration by metastatic carcinoma
- A/w metastatic breast cancer

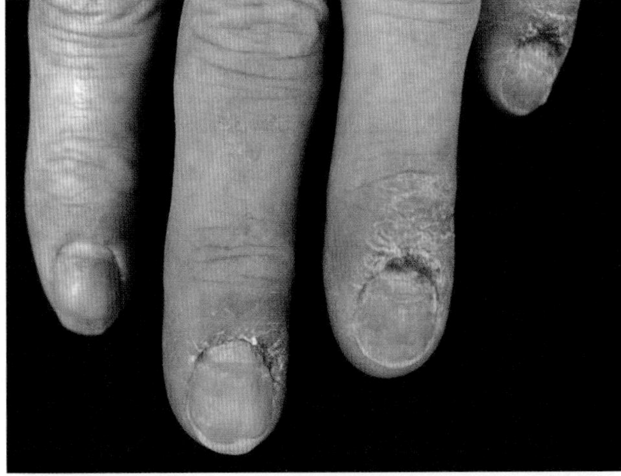

Fig. 10.10 Nail dystrophy and erythematous to violaceous plaques in a patient with Bazex syndrome. (From Antonovich DD, Thiers BH, Callen JP. Dermatologic manifestations of internal malignancy. In: Rigel DS, Robinson JK, Ross M, et al., eds. *Cancer of the Skin*. 2nd ed. Philadelphia: Elsevier; 2011:367–378.)

Anti-epiligrin cicatricial pemphigoid

Cutaneous findings

- Severe, scarring **mucocutaneous** bullous disease affecting mouth, eyes (e.g., conjunctival erosions), genitalia, and skin

Associations/comments

- Antibodies target **laminin 5** (typically α3 subunit)
- A/w variety of **adenocarcinomas (GI and lung >** gynecologic and GU > others)

Carcinoid syndrome

Cutaneous findings

- Head, neck, and upper trunk **flushing** with scarlet color and mottled red patches; **pellagra-like dermatitis**; sclerodermoid changes in advanced disease, +/– cyanosis

Associations/comments

- Systemic symptoms: **diarrhea**, dyspnea, **wheezing**, and bronchospasm
- ↑ **5-HIAA** levels in urine
- **Metastasis to liver** is typically required for **midgut tumors** to produce carcinoid syndrome
- The **appendix** is the most common location for primary carcinoid tumors, which rarely metastasize to the liver (and thus rarely cause carcinoid syndrome)
- **Bronchial and gastric** carcinoid tumors may cause flushing in **absence of liver metastases**
- A/w right-sided cardiac valvular fibrosis (60%)

Carcinoma en cuirasse/carcinoma erysipeloides

Cutaneous findings

- Carcinoma en cuirasse: indurated skin w/ orange peel-like (**peau d'orange**) appearance
- Carcinoma erysipeloides: well-demarcated, raised red plaque
- Both typically present on the chest wall, but can also involve axilla and upper extremities

Associations/comments

- Due to **metastatic breast carcinoma** infiltration into lymphatic vessels → lymphedematous skin changes (erythema, indurtion)

Cryglobulinemia type I

Cutaneous findings

- Retiform purpura and necrosis on **cool acral sites**; acral cyanosis and livedo reticularis

- A/w follicular hyperkeratotic spicules of central face (esp. nose)

Associations/comments

- Due to **monoclonal gammopathy** (typically in the form of a plasma cell dyscrasia such as multiple myeloma, B-cell lymphoma, or Waldenström macroglobulinemia)
- Histology: vessels plugged with pink proteinaceous material (immunoglobulins)

Cutaneous metastases

Cutaneous findings

- Erythematous and violaceous painless papules and nodules

Associations/comments

- A/w poor prognosis
- Cutaneous metastases occur most commonly from **breast cancer** (women) and **lung cancer** (men)
  - Among common malignancies, breast carcinoma is the most likely and prostate carcinoma is the least likely to metastasize to the skin
  - Other cancers with a high cutaneous metastatic potential include colon, melanoma, and larynx/oral cavity/nasal sinus
- Metastases from **renal carcinoma** appear as **highly vascular papules and nodules** on the head/neck

Dermatomyositis

Cutaneous findings

- Classic DM findings (heliotrope sign, Gottron papules, poikiloderma, dilated capillary loops, diffuse/scaly/ erythematous alopecia)

Associations/comments

- Most commonly a/w **ovarian cancer**
- Other associated malignancies: lung, colorectal, pancreatic, and non-Hodgkin lymphoma
- Malignancy is mainly associated with **adult-onset DM** (up to 40% of patients); ANA(−) DM also has strong malignancy association; anti-TIF1 and anti-NXP2 antibodies are associated with significantly increased malignancy risk

Ectopic ACTH syndrome

Cutaneous findings

- Generalized hyperpigmentation

Associations/comments

- Secondary to tumor production of ACTH (often **small cell carcinoma of the lung**)
- May show features of Cushing syndrome

Erythema gyratum repens

Cutaneous findings

- Widespread **serpiginous, polycyclic**, and pruriginous erythema with desquamating edges that produce concentric figures (**"woodgrain"** pattern) (Fig. 10.11)
- Spares hands and feet

Associations/comments

- **Lung cancer** is most commonly associated malignancy (>esophageal and breast)
- Usually **precedes** detection of primary malignancy and resolves w/ treatment of underlying malignancy
- Average age = 60s; M > F (2:1)
- Plaques expand rapidly (~1 cm/day)

Erythroderma

Cutaneous findings

- Widespread erythema of total body w/ overlying scale; usually spares palms and soles

Associations/comments

- May have alopecia, nail dystrophy, and ectropion
- Underlying **leukemias** and **lymphomas** (e.g. Sezary syndrome)

Extramammary paget disease (EMPD)

Cutaneous findings

- Red and white macerated/eroded plaques (**"strawberries and cream"**) located around the anal verge and below dentate line (Fig. 10.12); most common sites are **vulva** (women) and **perianal** regions (men)

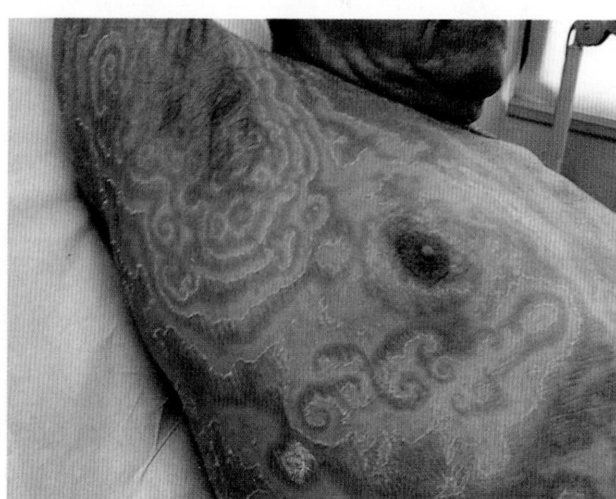

Fig. 10.11 Erythematous, serpiginous, and polycyclic patches with scale and desquamation in a patient with erythema gyratum repens. (From De La Torre-Lugo EM, Sánchez JL. Erythema gyratum repens. *J Am Acad Dermatol.* 2011;64[5]:e89–e90.)

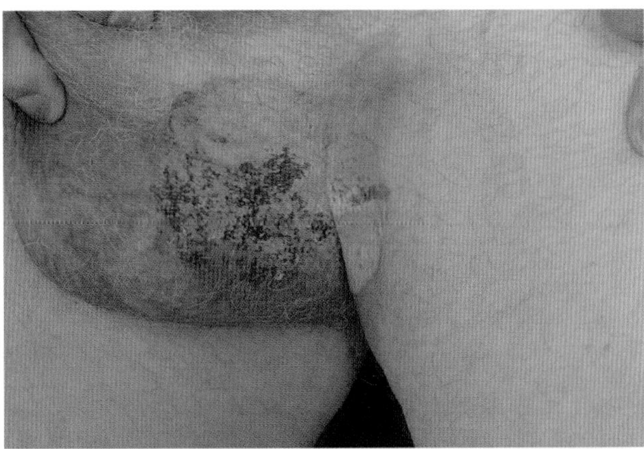

Fig. 10.12 Extramammary Paget disease of the left inguinal crease and scrotum. (From Virich G, Gudi V, Canal A. Extramammary Paget's disease—occupational exposure to used engine oil and a new skin grafting technique. *J Plast Reconstr Aesthet Surg.* 2008;61[12]:1528–1529.)

Associations/comments

- **Primary EMPD (>75%)**: primary cutaneous adenocarcinoma; likely derived from **Toker cells** or cutaneous adnexal glandular epithelium (sweat glands); immunophenotype: **CK7$^+$**, **GCFDP-15$^+$**, and CK20$^-$
- **Secondary EMPD (25%)**: may be as a result of direct extension **or** epidermotropic metastases of underlying **GI/GU** (> prostate, ovarian, and endometrial) adenocarcinoma; immunophenotype: CK7$^{+/-}$, GCFDP-15$^-$, and **CK20$^+$**
- **High rate of recurrence**, even w/ Mohs (because it is difficult to see individual Paget cells on frozen H&E sections); Mohs with CK7 immunostaining has improved cure rates (>95%); may try CO_2 laser ablation, imiquimod, or 5-FU; lymph node dissection + radiation in cases w/ multiple lymph node metases
- 5× ↑ risk of internal malignancy w/ **perianal** EMPD versus vulvar and penoscrotal

Familial atypical mole and multiple melanoma syndrome

Cutaneous findings

- NIH consensus criteria:
  - Numerous (>50) melanocytic nevi, some of which are clinically dysplastic
  - Some nevi are histologically atypical
  - Family history of melanoma in one or more first-degree relatives

Associations/comments

- AD; **CDKN2A** gene mutation (encodes two separate tumor suppressor proteins: **p16 (INK4)** and **p14/ARF**)
- **p16 (INK4) inhibits CDK4** → preventing phosphorylation of RB1 → inhibits release of transcription factors that induce S phase progression (thus, mutations in CDKN2A → inappropriate G1 to S phase progression and cellular proliferation)
- **p14/ARF inhibits** MDM2 (normally degrades p53) → in normal state p14 indirectly increases p53 expression
- ↑ Risk of **pancreatic cancer**

Howel-Evans syndrome (tylosis with esophageal carcinoma [TOC])

Cutaneous findings

- **Diffuse waxy keratoderma** of high pressure areas on plantar surface (i.e., heel, ball of foot), oral leukokeratosis

Associations/comments

- AD, mutation of "**TOC gene**" on chromosome 17q25 (gene renamed RHBDF2)
- A/w **esophageal carcinoma**

Hypertrichosis lanuginosa acquisita ("malignant down")

Cutaneous findings

- Sudden onset of long, thin, soft, **lanugo-like hair** initially on the face and ears, which can spread in craniocaudal manner (Fig. 10.13)

Associations/comments

- A/w **lung**, **colorectal**, and breast cancer; anorexia nervosa
- F > M (3:1); average age 40 to 70 years
- Tumor treatment usually leads to regression of hair growth

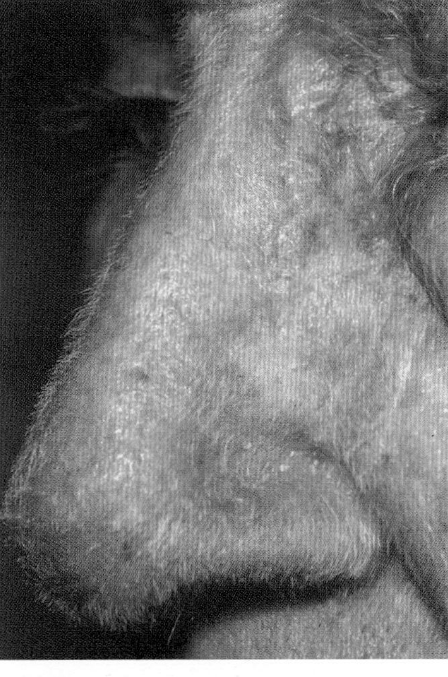

Fig. 10.13 Increased lanugo hair on the nose and face of a man with underlying metastatic prostate cancer. (From Wyatt JP, Anderson HF, Greer KE, Cordoro KM. Acquired hypertrichosis lanuginosa as a presenting sign of metastatic prostate cancer with rapid resolution after treatment. *J Am Acad Dermatol.* 2007;56(2 suppl):S45–S47.)

Juvenile xanthogranuloma + NF-1

Associations/comments

- **Triple association** w/ juvenile xanthogranuloma, NF-1, and **juvenile myelomonocytic leukemia**

Sign of Leser-Trélat

Cutaneous findings

- Sudden increase in the size and number of seborrheic keratoses

Associations/comments

- Most commonly a/w underlying **gastric adenocarcinoma** (>colon, breast, others)
- A/w pruritus and inflammation; may improve with treatment of underlying malignancy
- May be a/w **AN** and **tripe palms**
- Can also occur in erythrodermic patients without malignancy

Malignant acanthosis nigricans

Cutaneous findings

- Sudden onset with extensive and severe lesions; p/w symmetric hyperpigmented velvety plaques typically in intertriginous and flexural areas, glossitis

Associations/comments

- Typically a/w **GI** (esp. stomach) and GU cancers
- Can occur simultaneously, before, or after cancer diagnosis and can have associated weight loss
- Improves with treatment of underlying malignancy
- 25% of patients also have **tripe palms** (tripe palms in absence of AN is more commonly a/w **lung cancer**)

Multicentric reticulohistiocytosis

Cutaneous findings

- Multiple red to red-brown, nontender papules and nodules primarily on **dorsal hands** and **nail folds** with a **"coral-beaded"** appearance; face (esp. ears and perinasal) is second most common site

Associations/comments

- Up to 50% have **arthritis mutilans**
- 25%–33% have **underlying malignancy** (no specific internal malignancy favored); skin eruption usually **precedes** diagnosis of internal malignancy

Necrolytic migratory erythema (NME)

Cutaneous findings

- Arcuate and polycyclic, erosive, erythematous patches +/− vesicles/bullae often on **genital region**, **buttocks/anal region**, lower extremities, and intertriginous areas (Fig. 10.14)

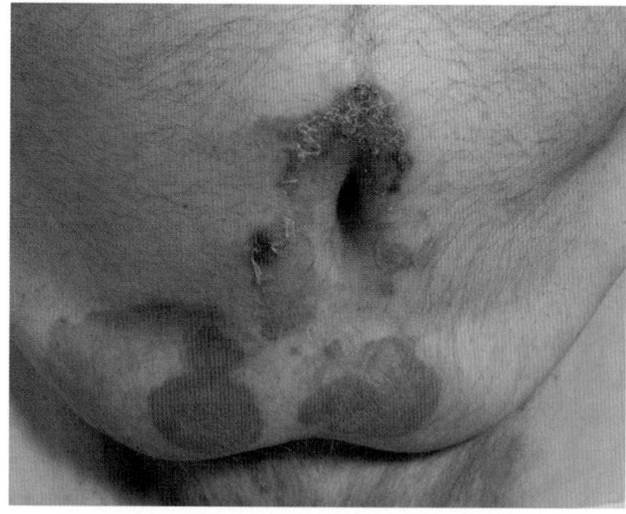

Fig. 10.14 Erythematous, scaly plaques on lower abdomen of patient with necrolytic migratory erythema. (From Michels G, Nierhoff D, Steffen HM. Necrolytic migratory erythema due to glucagonoma. *Clin Gastroenterol Hepatol.* 2010;8[8]:A18.)

Associations/comments

- **Glucagonoma** syndrome consists of NME, glucose intolerance, weight loss, glossitis, and glucagon-secreting carcinoma, angular cheilitis
- A/w **pancreatic islet cell** carcinoma (**α-2 glucagon**)

Necrobiotic xanthogranuloma

Cutaneous findings

- Indurated **yellow plaques** w/ frequent **ulceration** and necrosis (Fig. 10.15); most commonly **periorbital**

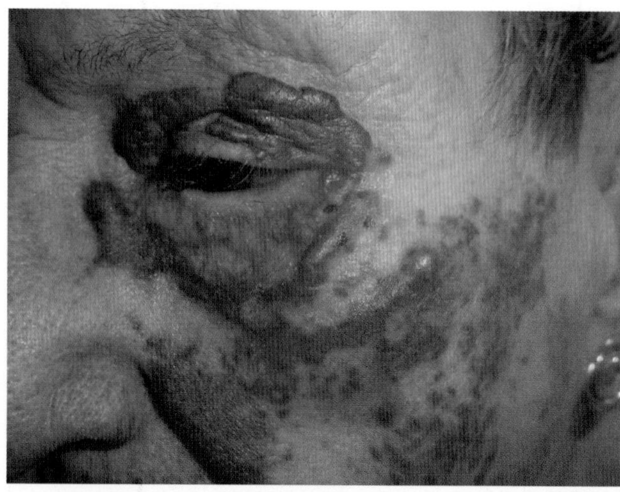

Fig. 10.15 Red-brown papules and plaques on the periorbital skin and cheek in a patient with necrobiotic xanthogranuloma. (From Brinster NK, Liu V, Diwan AH, McKee PH. *Dermatopathology: A Volume in the High Yield Pathology Series.* Philadelphia: Elsevier, 2011.)

Associations/comments

- A/w **paraproteinemia** (most often **IgG-κ**); occasionally a/w multiple myeloma and other lymphoproliferative malignancies

Paget disease of the breast

- Eczematous and psoriasiform plaques of the nipple
- Almost always a/w underlying **ductal breast carcinoma**

Paraneoplastic pemphigus

Cutaneous findings

- **Severe erosive** disease of mucous membranes leading to painful oral stomatitis; **polymorphous bullous skin eruption** (individual lesions may resemble erythema multiforme, lichen planus, pemphigus vulgaris, or bullous pemphigoid) (Fig. 10.16)

Associations/comments

- 90% mortality; most common causes of death: **underlying malignancy**, **bronchiolitis obliterans**, and **sepsis**
- Most commonly a/w **non-Hodgkin lymphoma** or chronic lymphocytic leukemia
- Other associated malignancies: **Castleman** disease (most common association in **children and Asians**), **thymoma**, **sarcoma**
- No sex predominance; usually affects ages 45 to 70 years

Pityriasis rotunda

Cutaneous findings

- Multiple well-defined **circular** hyperpigmented and hypopigmented scaly patches, usually on the **trunk/buttocks**

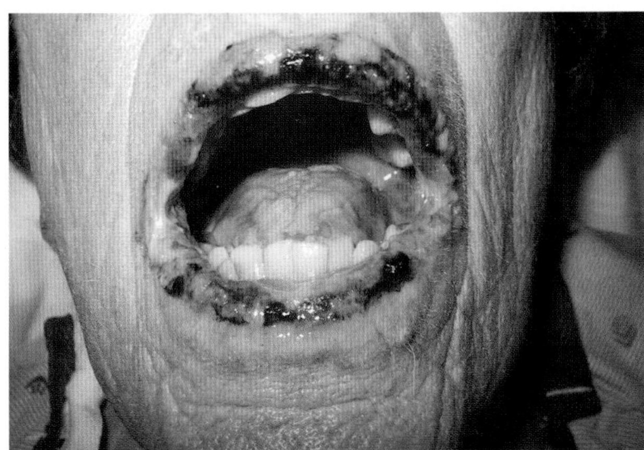

Fig. 10.16 Erosive and pustular hemorrhagic ulcers on the lips, tongue, and oropharynx of a patient with paraneoplastic pemphigus. (Courtesy of M. Avram, MD; Harvard Medical School, Boston, Massachusetts. In: Brinster NK, Liu V, Diwan AH, McKee PH. *Dermatopathology: A Volume in the High Yield Pathology Series*. Philadelphia: Elsevier, 2011.)

Associations/comments

- Two types: type I in Blacks and Asians with less than 30 hyperpigmented patches +/–systemic disease; type II in Caucasians with hypopigmented patches and no internal disease
- Most strongly a/w **hepatocellular carcinoma (type I > type II)**
- Other associated conditions: tuberculosis, leprosy, and liver and lung disease; gastric and esophageal carcinoma, leukemia, and lymphoma

Plane xanthoma

Cutaneous findings

- Yellow patches and thin plaques (Fig. 10.17)
- Tends to affect trunk, periorbital skin, and body folds

Associations/comments

- Often a/w **paraproteinemia**, multiple myeloma, and lymphoproliferative malignancies

POEMS Syndrome (Crow-Fukase syndrome)

Cutaneous findings

- **P**: Polyneuropathy (distal → proximal motor and sensory)
- **O**: Organomegaly
- **E**: Endocrinopathy (hypogonadism #1)
- **M**: *M*-protein (**IgG and IgA** light chains)
- **S**: Skin changes
  - Most common cutaneous findings: **hyperpigmentation** (90%), lower extremity edema > **hypertrichosis** (80%), **sclerodermoid** changes > **glomeruloid hemangiomas**, cherry angiomas, and nail changes (leukonychia, clubbing) > acrocyanosis and Raynaud phenomenon, hyperhidrosis

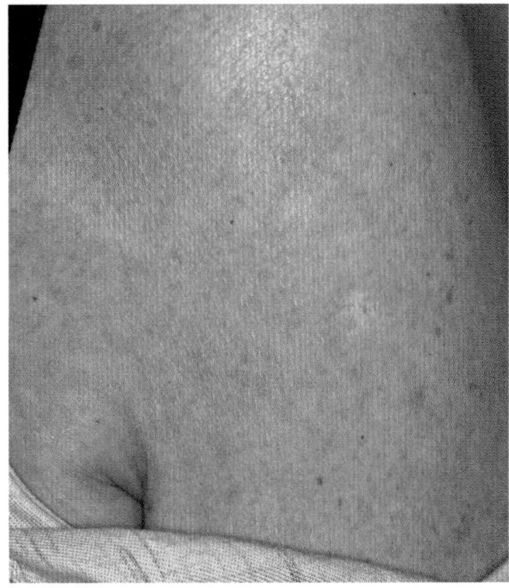

Fig. 10.17 Large, thin, yellow-orange plaque in a patient with monoclonal gammopathy. (Courtesy of Whitney High, MD, JD. In: Bolognia JL, Schaffer JV, Duncan KO, Ko CJ. *Dermatology Essentials*. Philadelphia: Elsevier; 2014.)

Associations/comments

- **Always a/w plasma cell dyscrasia**: Waldenström macroglobulinemia, **osteosclerotic myeloma**, MGUS, and **Castleman** disease
- ↑↑ **VEGF** levels
- Other associated findings include pulmonary effusions, ascites, peripheral edema, polycythemia, and thrombocytosis

Primary systemic amyloidosis (AL amyloidosis)

Cutaneous findings

- Discussed in cardiopulmonary section

Associations/comments

- Monoclonal gammopathy; most commonly due to **plasma cell dyscrasia > multiple myeloma**
- As a result of deposition of light chains (AL) in various tissues

Schnitzler syndrome

- Chronic urticaria in patient with fever, **arthralgias**, hepatosplenomegaly, and **bone pain**
- A/w **IgM-κ paraproteinemia** and lymphoplasmacytic malignancies

Scleromyxedema

- Widespread, firm, **waxy papules** often arranged in **linear** fashion; sclerodermoid skin changes; **leonine facies**
- Invariably a/w paraproteinemia (most commonly **IgGλ light chains**); progresses to multiple myeloma in 10%

Sister Mary Joseph nodule

Cutaneous findings

- Palpable nodule at **umbilicus** secondary to metastatic tumor

Associations/comments

- Typical source is malignancy of pelvis or abdomen including colon, ovarian, pancreatic, uterine, and gastric cancer
- Has also been a/w breast cancer

Sweet syndrome

Cutaneous findings

- **"Juicy" red-violaceous** papules/plaques that can have overlying pustules and pseudovesicles; favors **head/neck**, and **upper extremities**

Associations/comments

- **F** > M (except in cases a/w underlying malignancy, where M = F)
- Malignancy-associated Sweet syndrome: commonly p/w fever, malaise, leukopenia, anemia, thrombocytopenia, absence of arthralgia; histiocytoid or subcutaneous histopathology
- A/w **IBD**, URTI, malignancy (**most common is** acute myeloid leukemia), and polycythemia vera
- Rx: steroids, potassium iodide, clofazimine, and colchicine

Tripe palms

Cutaneous findings

- Yellow, velvety, diffuse palmar hyperkeratosis with accentuated dermatoglyphic patterns (Fig. 10.18)

Associations/comments

- **Tripe palms + Acanthosis nigricans → gastric cancer** (most common)
- **Tripe palms alone → lung cancer** (most common)

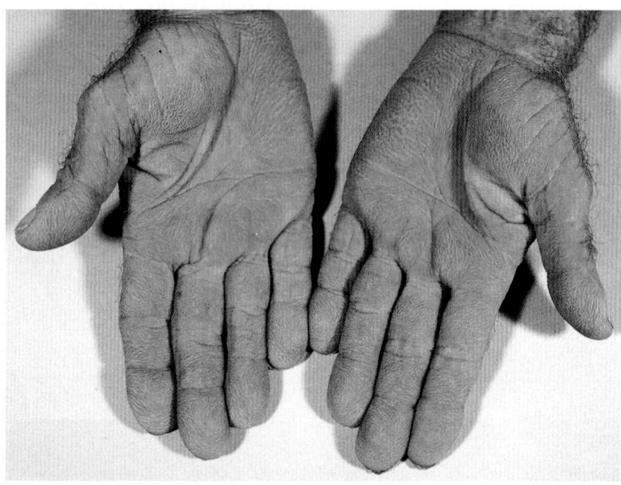

Fig. 10.18 Tripe palms. (Courtesy of Jon Dyer, MD, Columbia, Missouri. In: Callen JP, Jorizzo JL, Zone JJ, Piette WW, Rosenbach MA, Vleugels RA. *Dermatological Signs of Systemic Disease*, 5th Ed. Philadelphia: Elsevier; 2017, p 131–140.)

11 Epidemiology, Statistics, Study Design, Public Health Principles, and Billing

Jonathan I. Silverberg and Alexander Maley

CONTENTS LIST

11.1 EPIDEMIOLOGIC DEFINITIONS
11.2 EPIDEMIOLOGIC PRINCIPLES
11.3 TYPES OF STUDIES AND THEIR LIMITATIONS
11.4 TYPES OF BIAS
11.5 MAINTENANCE OF CERTIFICATION FOR THE AMERICAN BOARD OF DERMATOLOGY
11.6 BILLING

11.1 EPIDEMIOLOGIC DEFINITIONS

- Prevalence—total number of cases/total at-risk population, most often stated as a percentage
- Incidence—number of new cases/total at-risk population, most often stated as a percentage
  - Cumulative incidence is expressed over a given time frame
  - Incidence rate is the cumulative incidence divided by the time frame
- Precision—how consistently repeated are the assays of a test (reliability)
- Validity—how close an assay of a test comes to the truth (accuracy)

11.2 EPIDEMIOLOGIC PRINCIPLES

- Calculations using 2 × 2 tables
- For the word problems you will encounter, a 2 × 2 table can usually be constructed by identifying:
  - **Exposure**—the baseline characteristics of the study population
    - a. An intervention, for example, drug administration, educational session
    - b. Assessment of a risk, for example, smoking
    - c. For studies on diagnostic test accuracy—consider the test results as the exposure
  - **Outcome**—what happens during the study
    - a. A response to the intervention
    - b. Development of disease after exposure
    - c. For studies on diagnostic test accuracy—consider outcome, the true presence or absence of disease (Table 11.1)
- Often one of these variables will not be given in the question stem and must be calculated from the given variables. a + b + c + d will always equal the total number of study subjects.
- For assessing diagnostic test accuracy:
  - Sensitivity—proportion of correctly identified positive results, that is, true-positive rate
    - a/ a + c
    - If a test with high sensitivity is negative, the disease is very likely to be absent because there are very few false negatives
  - Specificity—proportion of correctly identified negative results, that is, true-negative rate
    - d/b + d
    - If a test with high specificity is positive, the disease is very likely to be present because there are very few false positives

Table 11.1 The True Presence or Absence of Disease

Exposure	Present	Absent
Exposed	a	b
Nonexposed	c	d

- Positive predictive value—likelihood that a person with a positive test result actually has the disease
  - a/a + b
  - **More likely to be high for diseases with a high prevalence**
- Negative predictive value—the likelihood that a person with a negative test result does not have the disease
  - d/c + d
  - More likely to be low for diseases with high prevalence
- The null hypothesis is the assumption that there is no difference between two groups being studied. After conducting the correct type of statistical testing, the null hypothesis may be rejected or accepted. A **type I error (false positive)** is the incorrect rejection of a true null hypothesis. The **type I error rate is alpha**, which is the threshold set for statistical significance. An arbitrary threshold of 0.05 (equivalent to a false-positive rate of 5%) is commonly used in studies. If the *P* value calculated from the data set is less than or equal to the alpha level, then the result of the data is considered significant and the null hypothesis is rejected. The probability of making at least one type I error increases with the number of tests performed. For example, pair-wise independent comparisons among three groups with a significance level of 0.05 for each test actually results in a 14.3% chance of making one or more type I errors. A **type II error (false negative)** is the incorrect acceptance of a false null hypothesis. The **type II error rate is beta**, which is related to the power of the test (power = 1-beta). The larger the power of the test, the less likely the test is to produce a false positive. The power of the test is frequently increased by increasing the number of test subjects.

11.3 TYPES OF STUDIES AND THEIR LIMITATIONS (TABLE 11.2 AND FIG. 11.1)

- Descriptive studies
  - Case reports, case series—offer the lowest level of evidence in favor of an intervention, but are very low

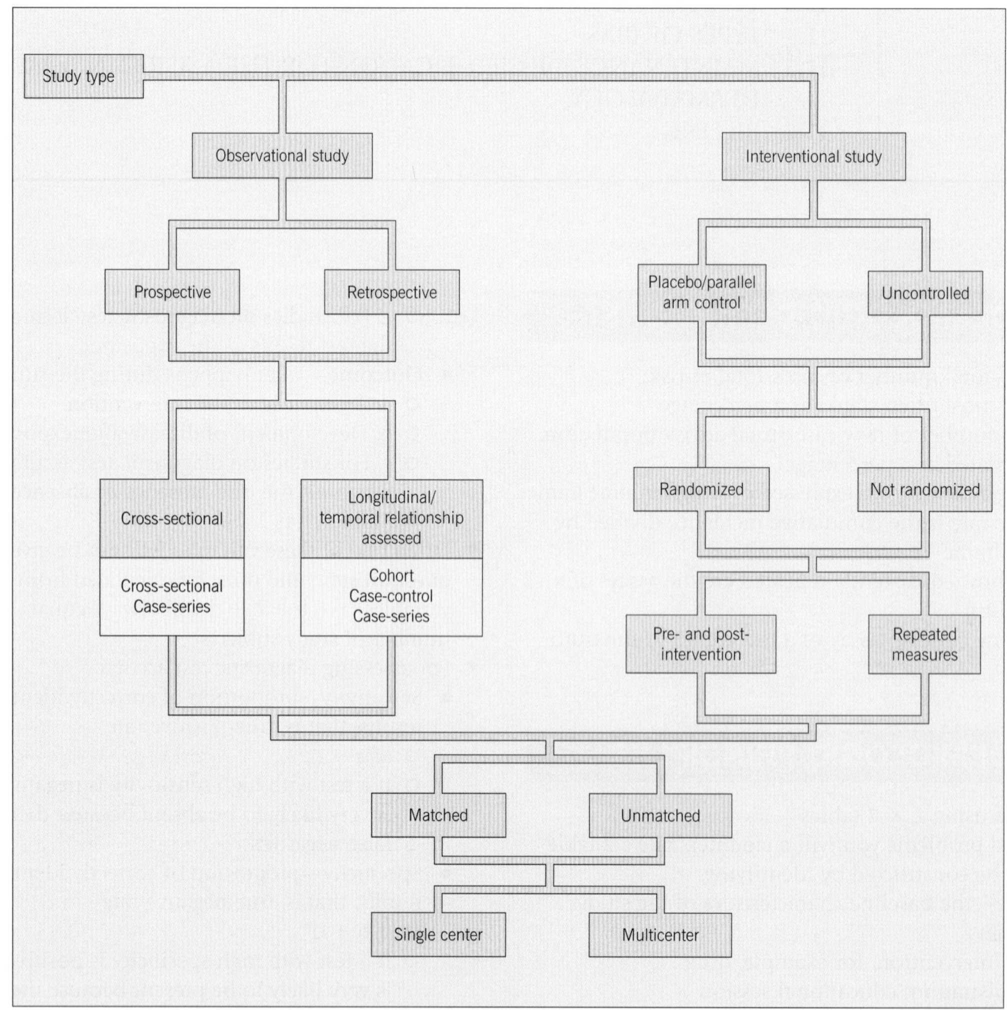

Fig. 11.1 Study designs. (Redrawn from Silverberg JI. Study designs in dermatology: a review for the clinical dermatologist. J Am Acad Dermatol. 2015;73[5]:721–731.)

Table 11.2 Study Designs

Design[a]	Definition	Level of Evidence USPSTF[b]	JAAD	Pros	Cons
Meta-analysis[c]	Statistical analysis of the combined results of multiple randomized, well-controlled trials	I (highest)	IA (highest)	Ability to qualitatively evaluate multiple studies; increases the numbers of subjects and statistical power; results may be generalized to the multiple cohorts represented by each individual study	Only as good as the individual studies included for analysis; questionable validity of estimates of the effect size for an intervention or association because of inherent differences of included studies
Randomized controlled study[d]	Randomized controlled studies compare ≥ 2 treatment groups, whose members are randomly selected, for a subsequent outcome	I (highest)	IB	Better *a priori* planning; better quality data; randomization; blinding of subjects and observers when used	Expensive; more time to complete; difficulty enrolling large numbers of subjects; dropout bias; limited generalizability
Controlled trial/ quasiexperiment	Controlled trials compare ≥ 2 treatment groups, whose members are not randomly selected, for a subsequent outcome	II-1	IIA		
Cohort analysis	Cohort studies compare between exposed and unexposed subjects for a subsequent outcome	II-2	III	Practical if exposure is rare; able to show a temporal relationship; able to determine the true incidence of an outcome	Expensive when prospective; more time to complete when prospective; impractical if outcome is rare; difficulty enrolling large number of subjects; dropout bias
Case-control analysis[e–g]	Case-control studies compare between subjects with and without a particular outcome for a preceding exposure	II-2	III	Inexpensive; less time to complete; practical if outcome is rare	Less rigorous *a priori* planning; poorer data quality; inability to control for confounding factors; observational bias; selection bias; recall bias; impractical if the exposure is rare; unable to show temporal/ causal relationship; unable to determine incidence of an outcome
Case series/single-arm trial	Report of multiple clinical cases or subjects with a finding	II-3	IV (lowest)	Inexpensive	
Case report	Individual report of a clinical case or finding	III (lowest)	IV (lowest)		Anecdotal

JAAD, Journal of the American Academy of Dermatology; USPSTF, *United States Preventive Services Task Force.*
[a]*References for reviews of a particular study design in dermatology are included where available.*
[b]*US Preventive Services Task Force.* Guide to clinical preventive services report of the U.S. Preventive Services Task Force. *Washington, DC: The Task Force; 1989.*
[c]*Rothman KJ, Greenland S, Lash TL.* Modern epidemiology. *Philadelphia: Lippincott Williams & Wilkins; 2008.*
[d]*Hill AB. The environment and disease: association or causation?* Proc Royal Soc Med. *1965;58:295–300.*
[e]*Heacock H, Rivers J. Assessing scientific data: the case-control study as it applies to dermatology part 1; the case control method.* J Cutan Med Surg. *1997;1:151–154.*
[f]*Heacock H, Rivers J. Assessing scientific data: the case-control study as it applies to dermatology part 2; interpreting the results.* J Cutan Med Surg. *1997;2:35–40.*
[g]*Bigby M. Odds ratios and relative risks.* Arch Dermatol. *2000;136:770–771.*
From Silverberg JI. Study designs in dermatology: a review for the clinical dermatologist. J Am Acad Dermatol. *2015;73(5):721–731.*

cost and often provide sentinel observation (e.g., phocomelia in thalidomide use)
- Cross-sectional survey—a type of **observational study** that provides information on a study sample at a single time point. Cross-sectional studies lack temporal information related to exposures and outcomes.

- Analytic studies
  - Case-control study
    - Type of **observational study** where two existing groups differing in already-known outcomes (e.g., disease vs. healthy) are retrospectively compared to see if the two groups have differences with regard to a suspected exposure
    - Example: identify end-stage renal disease (ESRD) patients with nephrogenic systemic fibrosis (NSF; = known outcome) and a group of ESRD patients without NSF and see if there is a difference between the two groups with regard to exposure to a certain type of MRI contrast agent (= suspected exposure)

- Advantages: **cheaper and faster** to conduct than cohort studies or randomized controlled trials (RCTs; since retrospective); especially useful for investigating **rare diseases** (since it takes a long time to accrue enough patients with rare diseases in prospective cohort studies or RCTs)
- An **odds ratio** can be calculated, which identifies the magnitude of the risk or protection afforded by the exposure
  - If the confidence interval is < 1, protective; includes 1 if no discernible effect; if > 1 increased risk

- Cohort—a type of **observational study** where two populations are defined upon the basis of exposure to a variable of interest (exposed and unexposed groups) and then compared to see if there is a difference in terms of risk of developing an outcome of interest (e.g., disease)
  - Prospective—exposure status is identified before outcome
    - Example: identify two groups of people that are matched in every way (income, socioeconomic status, etc.) except that one group frequently uses tanning beds (= **exposure**). Then monitor these groups over time to see if the two groups have different skin cancer rates (= **disease or outcome**)
    - **Relative risk** can be calculated
      - ➔ If the confidence interval is < 1 = protective; if it includes 1 = no discernible effect; if > 1 = increased risk
  - Retrospective—data on exposure is obtained from medical records, and records are followed to see outcomes
    - Example: retrieve all biopsies of nevi with severe cytologic atypia and look for new melanoma incidence documented in 10 years after diagnosis
    - Relative risk can be calculated

- RCT
  - Type of **interventional study** where study participants are randomly assigned to either a treatment group (group that receives the drug or intervention being investigated) or control group (do not receive the intervention being studied). The two groups are compared to see if there is a difference in outcomes (e.g., disease control, mortality rate, etc.)
  - **Gold standard** for clinical trials, because the randomization minimizes selection bias and potentially confounding variables
  - Example: patients with delusions of parasitosis are randomly assigned to receive either a new study drug (intervention group), or a placebo (control group). They are then compared to see if there is a difference in outcomes (e.g., disease control, improved QOL, etc.)
- Meta-analysis
  - Meta-analyses attempt to pool the data from all available studies to reach a conclusion
  - A well-conducted meta-analysis based on multiple high-quality RCTs is the best evidence for or against an intervention (i.e., preferable to a single RCT)

11.4 TYPES OF BIAS (TABLE 11.3)

- Biases that affect one arm of a study and not the other may affect the study results; their effect will either be to make it more likely find an effect that is not true, or to make it less likely to find an effect that is true; bias that affects both arms of a study may affect the study's generalizability
- **Selection bias**—the bias toward enrolling patients that do not represent the entire population of patients or controls; in referral centers, the selection bias may be toward more severe disease, called spectrum bias; in nonrandomized studies, physicians may preferentially enroll sicker patients in treatment arms
- Information bias
  - Misclassification—occurs when the case definition cannot accurately differentiate between affected and unaffected persons
  - **Recall**—affects case-control studies where patients with a disease may be more likely to recall an exposure even though both groups received the exposure equally
  - Lead time—in observational studies, when a patient with a disease found earlier in its natural course appears to have a longer survival (either with or without treatment) due only to the time they are known to have the disease, and not because of a difference in response to treatment or a naturally slower progressing disease
  - Observer bias—unconscious assumptions or preconceptions of researchers that affect study design and results
  - **Loss to follow-up**—affects cohort studies when more patients are lost to follow-up preferentially from one group
- **Confounding**
  - When a third, and untested, variable exists that provides a probable explanation of the perceived association between the tested outcome and the exposure
    - This variable must be associated with the exposure, with a risk factor, and/or be independent of the pathway from the exposure to the disease

11.5 MAINTENANCE OF CERTIFICATION FOR THE AMERICAN BOARD OF DERMATOLOGY

- See Table 11.4.

11.6 BILLING

- Evaluation and management codes (E/M)
  - The 2021 guidelines are focused on **medical decision making**. Time is defined as the total time spent on the day of the encouter (Table 11.5)
- A **global period** is the time after a procedure is performed. The global period begins the day after the procedure day. Managing complications that arise as a result of that procedure (e.g., bleeding, postoperative

Table 11.3 Types of Bias in Research Studies

Bias	Definition	How to Avoid
Ascertainment or sampling bias	Systematic error introduced by the sampling method; study sample is not representative of the target population	Random sampling; population-based sampling to include all sociodemographic levels; random allocation to an intervention
Attrition or transfer bias	Systematic differences between groups in withdrawals from a study; outcome data are not available; may be caused by treatment failure or disease resolution	Minimize loss to follow-up by offering convenient office hours, personalized patient contact via phone/email, and investigator visits to the patient's home
Confounding	Association between an exposure and outcome is caused by a third variable that is correlated to both	Matching cases and controls by the confounding factor; stratified and multivariate regression analyses
Data-snooping bias	Performing a large number of statistical tests increases the type I error rate; so-called "fishing expedition"	Hypothesis-driven testing rather than data-driven testing; correction for multiple comparisons
Detection bias	Systematic differences between groups in how outcomes are determined	Blinding
Exposure misclassification	Measurement error because of poorly defined exposures or if proxies of exposure are used	Use "criterion standard" assessment and objective tests; correct for differential misclassification between groups
Funding bias	Systematic preference toward performing funded studies; tendency of the research to support the study's sponsor	Investigator-initiated and unfunded research studies
Hawthorne effect	Systematic differences in behavior or response in a subject who knows they are being investigated	Placebo group
Information or measurement bias	Systematic error in measurement of an outcome or exposure	Standardized measurements and instruments and use of multiple data points for improved accuracy
Interviewer or observer bias	Systematic difference between how information is solicited, recorded, or interpreted	Blinding
Lead-time bias	Systematic error because of cases being detected at different stages of disease; early detection does not equal improved survival	Correction for lead-time and length bias (often very challenging)
Nonresponse bias	Some subjects may not participate or respond to questionnaires because of various personal factors	Assess for systematic differences between responders and nonresponders; data interpolation techniques for nonresponders
Outcome misclassification	Measurement error related to poorly defined outcomes or if proxies of outcome are used	Use "criterion standard" assessment and objective tests; correct for differential misclassification between groups
Performance bias	Systematic differences between groups in the care that is provided, or in exposure to factors other than the interventions of interest	Blinding; giving equal attention and care to all study groups
Procedural bias	Systematic error introduced by the interview or questionnaire being administered with too much pressure on participants	Not imposing time constraints or incentivizing rushing through the questionnaire
Recall bias	Systematic difference between how events or experiences are remembered; better recall of recent or more serious events than those occurring a long time ago; patients suffering from disease are able to recall events more easily than healthy subjects	Confirmation of self-reported exposures and outcomes using the medical record
Reporting bias	Systematic differences between reported and unreported findings; only significant findings get published	Reporting of negative findings
Selection bias	Systematic differences between baseline characteristics of the groups that are compared	Randomization
Self-improvement effect	Some disorders are self-limiting and may improve independent of an intervention	Placebo group; longitudinal study design that accounts for waxing and waning disease course
Type III error	Solving the wrong problem precisely	Improved communication between investigator and statistician

From Silverberg JI. Study designs in dermatology: a review for the clinical dermatologist. J Am Acad Dermatol. *2015;73(5):721–731.*

Table 11.4 Maintenance of Certification for the American Board of Dermatology

Yearly	3× Per 10 Years	2× Per 10 Years	Every 10 Years
25 AMA level 1 credits	100 self-assessment questions	Practice improvement activities	Maintenance of certification examination (CertLink periodic examinations are an alternative) and patient safety module
License attestation			
Annual fee			

Table 11.5 2021 Coding

Code	Level of MDM (Requires two third elements)	Number and Complexity of Problems Addressed	Amount/Complexity of Data Reviewed	Risk of Complications or Morbidity of Patient Management
99202 (15–29 min)/99212 (10–19 min)	Straightforward	1 limited or minor problem	Minimal or none	Minimal risk of morbidity from additional diagnostic testing or treatment
99203 (30–44 min)/99213 (20–29 min)	Low	2 or more self-limited or minor problems; or 1 stable chronic illness; or 1 acute, uncomplicated illness or injury	Must meet ½ category requirements Category 1: Tests and documents Any combination of two from the following: • Review of prior external note(s) from each unique source; • Review of the result(s) of each unique test; • Ordering of each unique test Category 2: Assessment requiring an independent historian(s)	Low risk of morbidity from additional diagnostic testing or treatment
99204 (45–59 min)/99214 (30–39 min)	Moderate	1 or more chronic illnesses with exacerbation, progression, or side effects of treatment; or 2 or more stable chronic illnesses; or 1 undiagnosed new problem with uncertain prognosis; or 1 acute illness with systemic symptoms; or 1 acute complicated injury	Must meet requirements for 1/3 categories Category 1: Tests, documents, or independent historian(s) • Any combination of 3 from the following: • Review of prior external note(s) from each unique source; • Review of the result(s) of each unique test; • Ordering of each unique test; • Assessment requiring an independent historian(s) Category 2: Independent interpretation of tests • Independent interpretation of a test performed by another physician/other qualified health care professional (not separately reported); Category 3: Discussion of management or test interpretation • Discussion of management or test interpretation with external physician/ other qualified health care professional\appropriate source (not separately reported)	Moderate risk of morbidity from additional diagnostic testing or treatment Examples: • Prescription drug management • Decision regarding minor surgery with identified patient or procedure risk factors • Decision regarding elective major surgery without identified patient or procedure risk factors • Diagnosis or treatment significantly limited by social determinants of health
99205 (60–74 min)/99215 (40–54 min)	High	1 or more chronic illnesses with severe exacerbation, progression, or side effects of treatment; or 1 acute or chronic illness or injury that poses a threat to life or bodily function	Must meet requirements of 2/3 categories Category 1: Tests, documents, or independent historian(s) • Any combination of three from the following: • Review of prior external note(s) from each unique source; • Review of the result(s) of each unique test; • Ordering of each unique test; • Assessment requiring an independent historian(s) Category 2: Independent interpretation of tests • Independent interpretation of a test performed by another physician/other qualified health care professional (not separately reported); Category 3: Discussion of management or test interpretation • Discussion of management or test interpretation with external physician/ other qualified health care professional/appropriate source (not separately reported)	High risk of morbidity from additional diagnostic testing or treatment Examples: • Drug therapy requiring intensive monitoring for toxicity • Decision regarding elective major surgery with identified patient or procedure risk factors • Decision regarding emergency major surgery • Decision regarding hospitalization • Decision not to resuscitate or to deescalate care because of poor prognosis

Modified from American Medical Association. CPT E/M office revisions level of medical decision making (MDM); 2021. https://www.ama-assn.org/system/files/2019-06/cpt-revised-mdm-grid.pdf.

infection) that fall within a global period are not reimbursed
  - **10-Day global period:** all destruction, excision, and linear repair codes
  - **90-Day global period:** all flap (tissue transfer or rearrangement) and graft codes
- Modifiers—coding numbers added to denote additional service provided on day of service
  - 25—significant, separately identifiable **E/M** service by the same provider on the same day of the procedure or other service
    - The history and physical exam is included in every procedure code, if a patient comes in for one problem which requires a procedure, a separate E/M code is not billed
    - If a procedure is performed during an office visit in which a separate problem with its own history and exam is also addressed, then a 25 modifier is placed on the E/M code (e.g., a patient has a new rash in addition to having a skin lesion that requires a biopsy)
      - Example (1) a patient presents with an erythematous pearly papule on the ear, a biopsy is performed. The correct coding would be for the ear biopsy procedure code **without** an E/M code
      - Example (2) a patient presents with an erythematous pearly papule on the ear, a biopsy is performed. The patient also complains of erythematous plaques on the elbows and knees for which a diagnosis of psoriasis is made and a topical steroid is prescribed. The correct coding would be the E/M code + 25 modifier and the ear biopsy procedure code
  - 59—procedure or service was distinct or separate from other services performed on the same day, applied to **procedure codes** not E/M codes
    - Two distinct procedures are performed on the same day: either two different procedures (cryosurgery + biopsy), two different sites or lesions (biopsy of ear, biopsy of chest)
  - 24—unrelated **E/M** service by the same physician **during a postoperative global period.** If a patient returns to the original provider during a global period with a new problem, unrelated to the procedure that was performed, a 24 modifier is used
    - A patient returns 3 days after an excision of a basal cell carcinoma with a new rash that requires an exam and medical management → -24 modifier should be added to the E/M visit code
  - 79—separate and **unrelated** procedure during a global period. Analogous to the 59 modifier but used **during global** periods
    - A patient returns 3 days after an excision of a basal cell carcinoma with a new skin lesion that is then biopsied → -79 modifier should be added to the biopsy code
  - 57—separately identifiable **E/M** service related to the decision to perform a procedure with a 90-day period
    - Example: History is taken, exam is performed on patient with large basal cell of the face and it is decided to proceed with **Mohs surgery with flap or graft repair, performed all on the same day →** should bill E/M code with -57 modifier in addition to the Mohs code and repair code
  - 58—staged or related procedure or service by the same physician during the postoperative (global) period
    - Example: "**slow Mohs**" (staged excisions over many days), **takedown of an interpolation flap** or a re-excision of a malignancy for margins within the previous procedure's global period → -58 modifier should be added to the second procedure's CPT code
  - Other modifiers:
    - 50—bilateral procedure during one encounter (e.g., application of bilateral unna boots, NOT biopsy of left arm and right arm)
    - GC—office visit or procedure was performed by resident under supervision of an attending
    - GT—visit was performed using live telemedicine
    - GQ—visit was performed using store and forward telemedicine
- Special procedural definitions
  - Shave removal: sharp removal transversely through dermis, without extension into fat
  - Excision: requires a full-thickness removal (through the dermis and into the fat)

Index

Page numbers followed by "*f*" indicate figures, "*t*" indicate tables, and "*b*" indicate boxes.

A
A- and U-serrated pattern, 402*f*
AA. *see* Alopecia areata (AA)
AAE. *see* Acquired angioedema (AAE)
Absorption spectra, 484*f*
Acantholytic disorders, 429*t*
Acanthosis nigricans, 402–414*t*
Accessory digit, 402–414*t*
Accessory nipple, 402–414*t*
Accessory tragus, 234*t*, 402–414*t*
ACD. *see* Angiokeratoma corporis diffusum (ACD)
Acitinic keratoses (AKs), 57
Acitretin, 53*t*
for pityriasis rubra pilaris, 84
ACLE. *see* Acute cutaneous lupus (ACLE)
Acne, in setting of endocrinologic abnormality, 178
Acne associated syndromes, 179
Acne conglobata, 177
Acne cosmetica, 178
Acne excoriée (de jeunes filles), 177
Acne fulminans, 177
Acne inversa. *see* Hidradenitis suppurativa (acne inversa)
Acne keloidalis, 182
Acne keloidalis nuchae, 217, 402–414*t*
Acne mechanica, 177
Acne vulgaris, 175*t*, 176–177
Acneiform eruptions, 179
Acquired angioedema (AAE), 520
Acquired cutis laxa, 272
Acquired digital fibrokeratoma, 402–414*t*
Acquired ichthyosis, 520–521
Acquired melanocytic nevus, 348
Acral erythema, 513
Acral fibrokeratoma, 376
Acral nevus, 389*f*
Acral peeling skin syndrome, 282*t*
Acrocephalosyndactyly. *see* Apert syndrome (acrocephalosyndactyly)
Acrodermatitis chronica atrophicans, 317*t*
Acrodermatitis continua of Hallopeau, 81
Acrodermatitis enteropathica, 258–261
Acrokeratosis paraneoplastica, 521
Acrokeratosis verruciformis of Hopf, 338*t*
Acropustulosis of infancy, 290
Actinic keratosis, 339, 398*f*
Actinic prurigo, 186, 281–289
Actinomycosis, 309, 402–414*t*
Acute cutaneous lupus (ACLE), 126
Acute exanthem, of primary HIV infection, 301
Acute febrile mucocutaneous lymph node syndrome. *see* Kawasaki disease
Acute febrile neutrophilic dermatosis. *see* Sweet's syndrome
Acute generalized exanthematous pustulosis (AGEP), 73
Acute graft-*versus*-host disease, 417*f*
Acute hemorrhagic edema of infancy, 198–199
triggers of, 198*t*
Acute meningococcemia, 311, 314*f*
Acute myeloid leukemia, 417*f*
Acyclovir, 62
AD. *see* Atopic dermatitis (AD)
AD cutis laxa, 270
Adalimumab, 52, 53*t*
Adaptive immunity, 18
Addison's disease, 514
Adenoid cystic carcinoma, 356, 359
Adherens junctions, 1, 3*f*
Adipocytic tumors, 436*t*
Adnexal neoplasms, 351
Adult forms, 250
Adult onset Still's disease, 141–142
Adult T-cell leukemia/lymphoma (ATLL), 370–371
AEC. *see* Ankyloblepharon-ectodermal dysplasia-clefting syndrome (AEC)
African trypanosomiasis, 331
AFX. *see* Atypical fibroxanthoma (AFX)
AGA. *see* Androgenetic alopecia (AGA)
AGEP. *see* Acute generalized exanthematous pustulosis (AGEP)
Aggressive digital papillary adenocarcinoma, 355, 358–359
Aggressive epidermotropic cytotoxic ($CD8^+$) T-cell lymphoma, 373
Airborne allergic contact dermatitis, 90
AKs. *see* Acitinic keratoses (AKs)
Alagille syndrome, 263
Alkaptonuria, 263
Allergic contact dermatitis, 90
specific contactants of, 91–92, 93–95*t*
Allergic granulomatous angiitis, 505
Allylamines, 64
Alopecia, 74–78*t*
Alopecia areata (AA), 215, 402–414*t*
Alopecia mucinosa, 370*f*
Alopecia neoplastica, 521
Alopecias, 216
Alpha1-antitrypsin deficiency panniculitis, 211
Alternative pathway, 20
Aluminum chloride, 70
Amalgam tattoo, 402–414*t*
Amblyomma, 334
American Board of Dermatology, maintenance of certification for, 530, 531*t*
American trypanosomiasis, 331, 331*f*
Aminolevulinic acid, 66
Amiodarone, 74–78*t*
Amniotic band syndrome, 234*t*
AMPs. *see* Antimicrobial proteins (AMPs)
Amyloid, 395–396*t*, 402–414*t*
Amyloidoses, 188–189
cutaneous, 183*t*
ANA. *see* Antinuclear antibodies (ANA)
Anagen effluvium, 215
Analytic studies, 529–530
Anaphylaxis, 72
ANCA positive vasculitis, 200–203, 200*t*, 201*t*
Androgen inhibitors, 68–69
Androgenetic alopecia (AGA), 212–215
Angioedema, 72, 166–169
Angiofibroma, 376, 402–414*t*
Angiokeratoma, 379
Angiokeratoma corporis diffusum (ACD), 255
Angioleiomyoma, 368, 368*f*
Angiolipoma, 382, 384*f*, 402–414*t*
Angiolymphoid hyperplasia, 435*t*
with eosinophils, 379, 379*f*
Angioma serpiginosum, 256*t*
Angiosarcoma, 381–382, 381*f*, 402–414*t*, 437*f*
Anhidrosis, 183
Ankyloblepharon-ectodermal dysplasia-clefting syndrome (AEC), 261
Ankylosing spondylitis, psoriasis and, 82
Annular elastolytic giant cell granuloma, 153
Anthralin, for psoriasis, 82
Anthrax, 309–310
Antiandrogens, 68–69
Anti-angiogenesis (VEGEF) inhibitors, 74–78*t*
Antibiotics, for prevention of surgical site infections, 479*t*
Antibody molecule, 21
structure of, 23*f*
Anti-epiligrin cicatricial pemphigoid, 521
Antifungal agents, 63–65
Antihistamines, 39–40
Antimalarial agents, 50–51
Antimalarials, 74–78*t*
Antimicrobial agents, 57–65
Antimicrobial peptides, 18*t*
Antimicrobial proteins (AMPs), 20
Antinuclear antibodies (ANA), 119–120, 120–121*t*
Antiparasitic agents, 65, 65*t*
Antiphospholipid syndrome (APLS), 207
Anti-psychotics and anti-depressants, 74–78*t*
Antiretroviral-associated lipodystrophy, 303–304
Antiseptics, 459*t*
Antiviral agents, 62–63
Antoni A, 392–394*t*
Antoni B, 392–394*t*
Apert syndrome (acrocephalosyndactyly), 179
Aphthous stomatitis, 301–302

Aplasia cutis congenita, 234t
APLS. *see* Antiphospholipid syndrome (APLS)
Apocrine glands, 10
Apocrine miliaria. *see* Fox-Fordyce disease (apocrine miliaria)
Apremilast, 53t
Apremilast (Otezla), 46
Aquagenic pruritus and aquadynia, 190
AR cutis laxa, 263
ARCL type II, 270
Arteriovenous malformations (AVMs), 254–255, 402–414t
Arthritis mutilans, psoriasis and, 82
Artifacts, 398t
Ascertainment or sampling bias, 531t
Ashy dermatosis. *see* Erythema dyschromicum perstans (ashy dermatosis)
Aspergillosis, 328f
Asteatotic dermatitis (eczema craquele), 89
Asteroid bodies, 392–394t
Ataxia telangiectasia, 256t
ATLL. *see* Adult T-cell leukemia/lymphoma (ATLL)
Atopic dermatitis (AD), 86–89
  clinical features of, 86–89
  epidemiology of, 86
  erythroderma and, 85
  histopathology of, 88
  laboratory testing for, 88
  pathogenesis of, 86–87
  prognosis/clinical course of, 87–88
  regional variants of, 88
  treatment of, 88–89
Atopic triad, 86
Atrichia with papules, 259–261t
Atrophie blanche. *see* Livedoid vasculopathy
Attenuated androgens, 69
Attrition or transfer bias, 531t
Atypical fibroxanthoma (AFX), 375–376, 375f
Atypical (dysplastic) melanocytic nevus, 348
Auramine-rhodamine, 395–396t
Auricle, pseudocyst of, 344
Auriculotemporal nerve syndrome (Frey syndrome), 192
Auspitz sign, 82
Autoimmune connective tissue disease (CTD), 96
  erythema multiforme, 96–97, 97f
  fixed drug eruption, 101
  graft-*versus*-host disease, 101–103, 102f
  pityriasis lichenoides, 100, 100f
  SJS/TEN, 98, 99t
Autoimmune diseases, 119–120
Autoimmune subepidermal blistering diseases, 110–116, 110f, 111t
Autoinflammatory disorders, 269–271t, 269–271
  epidemiology of, 269
  histopathology of, 271
  pathogenesis of, 269
  prognosis/clinical course of, 271
  treatment of, 271
Autosensitization (id reaction and disseminated eczema), 95–96
Axillary granular parakeratosis, 85f
Azathioprine, 47–48
Azelaic acid, 58
Azithromycin, 59–60
Azoles, 63–64
AZT (zidovudine), 74–78t

B

B cells, 20–21
B lymphocyte, 397t
Bacillary angiomatosis, 313f
Bacitracin, 57–58
Bacterial folliculitis, 305
Bacterial infections, 304–318
BADAS. *see* Bowel-associated dermatosis-arthritis syndrome (BADAS)
Balloon cell nevus, 346, 402–414t
Balloon cells, 392–394t
Banana bodies, 392–394t
Bannayan-Riley-Ruvalcaba syndrome, 244t, 514–515
Bartonella, 303–304, 312t
Basal cell carcinoma, 339, 342–343, 343b, 343t, 384
Basal cell nevus syndrome, 248
Basement membrane zone (BMZ), 7, 7f, 8t
Basic science, 1–38
BCL2, 21
Bean bag cells, 392–394t
Becker's melanosis, 348
Beckwith-Wiedemann syndrome, 252
Behçet's disease, 171–172, 171f, 505
Benign acanthosis nigricans, 512
Benign cephalic histiocytosis, 163f
Benign vascular lesions, 378–380
Benzoyl peroxide, 58
Benzylamines, 64
Bias, types of, 530
  in research studies, 531t
Bilateral advancement flap, 468f, 469f
Biliary pruritus, 189
Bilobed flap, 467–468t
Bimatoprost, 67
Biopsy, 426t
Biotinidase deficiency and multiple carboxylase deficiency, 261–262
Birbeck granules, 392–394t
Birt-Hogg-Dube syndrome, 248–249, 505–506, 519
  fibrofolliculomas in, 506f
  trichodiscomas, 506f
Bite-induced infections, 316
Bites and stings, 296
Biting and stinging insects, 333–334
Blastomycosis, 325f, 402–414t
Bleomycin, 62–63
Blindness, laser safety and, 484
Blistering diseases, 107–118, 118t
Blistering distal dactylitis, 307
BLK and LP-like keratosis. *see* Lichenoid keratosis
Bloom syndrome, 277
Blue nevus, 345–346, 425f
Blue rubber bleb nevus syndrome, 253, 515
BMZ. *see* Basement membrane zone (BMZ)
Body dysmorphic disorder, 191
Bohn's nodules, 231t
Borderline vascular neoplasms, 380–381
Borrelia, 317t
Borrelial lymphocytoma, 317t
Botryomycosis, 306, 306f
Botulinum toxin, 70, 488, 489f
  different forms of, 489t
  injection dosing of, 491t
Bowel bypass syndrome, 515
Bowel-associated dermatosis-arthritis syndrome (BADAS), 172, 515
Bowenoid papulosis, 294–295
Bowen's disease, 339–340, 387f, 402–414t, 425t
Brachioradial pruritus, 191
BRAF inhibitors, 55
Branchial cleft cyst, 344, 402–414t
Breast adenocarcinoma, metastatic, 402–414t
Brentuximab vedotin, 57
Brimonidine, 67
Broadband UVB, 66
Brodalumab, 53t
Bromhidrosis, 183–184
Bromoderma and Iododerma, 74–78t
Bronchogenic cyst, 344, 402–414t
Brooke-Spiegler syndrome, 249, 353
Brucellosis, 314
Bullous diabeticorum, 512
Bullous impetigo, 304, 402–414t
Bullous pemphigoid, 110–113, 111t, 112b, 112f, 116f, 402–414t
Bullous systemic lupus erythematosus, 114, 129f
Burning mouth syndrome, 191
Burow's advancement flap, 469f
Buschke-Lowenstein tumor, 295
Buschke-Ollendorf syndrome, 267
Butenafine, 64

C

Café-au- lait macule (CALM), 345
Calcinosis cutis, 402–414t
Calciphylaxis, 402–414t, 519
Calcipotriene and calcitriol, 69
Calcium, 395–396t
CALM. *see* Café-au- lait macule (CALM)
Cantharidin, 63
Capillary malformations, 251–252
Caput succedaneum, 230t
Carcinoid syndrome, 521
Carcinoma en cuirasse/carcinoma erysipeloides, 507
Cardio-facio-cutaneous syndrome (CFC), 506
Cardiopulmonary disease, 505–512
Cardiovascular disease, 505–512
Carney complex, 244t, 506
Carotenemia, 512
CARP. *see* Confluent and reticulated papillomatosis (CARP)
Carvajal syndrome, 506
Caterpillar bodies, 392–394t
Cathelicidins, 20
Cavernous hemangioma, 378
CBG. *see* Cortisol-binding globulin (CBG)
CCLE. *see* Chronic cutaneous lupus erythematosus (CCLE)
CD4+ T cell, 21, 22
CD8+ T cell, 22, 28
CDEs. *see* Cutaneous drug eruptions (CDEs)
Cell-rich pemphigoid, differential diagnosis of, 401t
Cells of significance, 20–28
Cellular blue nevus, 402–414t
Cellular engineering and gene therapy, 35
Cellular neurothekeoma, 365, 402–414t
Cellulitis, 308
Central centrifugal cicatricial alopecia, 216
Central hypothyroidism, 42
Centrofacial lentiginosis, 244t
Cephalohematoma, 230t
Cephalosporins, 59
Ceramide, 2
Certolizumab, 53t
Certolizumab pegol, 52
Cervical nerves, sensory innervation of, 445t
Cetirizine, 39
CFC. *see* Cardio-facio-cutaneous syndrome (CFC)
CGH. *see* Comparative genomic hybridization (CGH)
Chalazion clamp, 454
Chanarin-Dorfman syndrome, 282t
Chancroid, 319t
Chédiak-Higashi syndrome (CHS), 241t
Chemical irritant contact dermatitis, 91
Chemical peels, 498
Chemokines, 23–24
Chemotherapy, 74–78t
Chemotherapy recall, 74–78t
Chikungunya virus, 300
CHILD syndrome. *see* Congenital hemidysplasia with ichthyosiform erythroderma and limb defects (CHILD) syndrome
Childhood forms, 250
Chloracne, 178
Chlorambucil, 50
Chlorpheniramine, 39
Cholesterol clefts, 392–394t
Chondrodermatitis nodularis helicis (CNH), 402–414t
Chromhidrosis, 184
Chromoblastomycosis, 402–414t
Chromophore, 482t
  thermal relaxation times of, 482t
Chromosomal abnormalities, cutaneous findings in patients with, 290
Chronic cutaneous lupus erythematosus (CCLE), 122–126, 123f
Chronic meningococcemia, 311
Chronic mucocutaneous candidiasis, 239–240
Chronic plaque psoriasis, 81
Chronic radiation dermatitis, 429f
Chronic recurrent multifocal osteomyelitis. *see* SAPHO (chronic recurrent multifocal osteomyelitis)
CHS. *see* Chédiak-Higashi syndrome (CHS)
Churg-Strauss syndrome, 202–203, 202t, 505
Cicatricial (scarring) alopecia, 213–214t, 216–218
Cicatricial pemphigoid. *see* Mucous membrane pemphigoid (MMP)
Ciclopirox olamine, 64
Cidofovir, 62

CIE. *see* Congenital ichthyosiform erythroderma (CIE)
Cirrhosis, 515
Clarithromycin, 60
Classical pathway, 20
Clear cell acanthoma, 338*t*, 384*f*, 402–414*t*, 415*f*
Clear cell hidradenoma, 402–414*t*
Clindamycin, 61
Clofazimine, 69, 74–78*t*
Clostridium skin infections, 310–311
Clothing dermatitis, 90
Clotrimazole, 64
Clouston syndrome, 258
Clustered regularly interspaced palindromic repeats (CRISPR), 35, 36*f*
CNH. *see* Chondrodermatitis nodularis helicis (CNH)
Cnidarians, 335*f*, 336
Cobb syndrome, 254–255
Coccidioidomycosis, 327*f*, 402–414*t*, 422*f*
Cockayne syndrome, 277
Coining, 191
Colchicine, 69
Cold injuries, 184–185
Collagens, 8, 395–396*t*
Colloid milium, 438*f*
Colloidal iron, 395–396*t*
Colon adenocarcinoma, metastatic, 402–414*t*
Coma blister, 402–414*t*
Comparative genomic hybridization (CGH), 30–31*t*
Complement activation pathways, 21*f*
Complement pathways, 20, 22*t*
Complex cystic proliferations, 424*t*
Complex regional pain syndrome/reflex sympathetic dystrophy, 191
Confluent and reticulated papillomatosis (CARP), 86, 86*f*
Confounding, 531*t*
Confounding bias, 530
Congenital atrichia with papules, 216
Congenital candidiasis, 238*f*
Congenital CMV, 236*t*
Congenital contractual arachnodactyly, 268
Congenital dermal melanocytosis, 345
Congenital erythropoietic porphyria, 187*f*
Congenital hemidysplasia with ichthyosiform erythroderma and limb defects (CHILD) syndrome, 282*t*
Congenital ichthyosiform erythroderma (CIE), 282*t*
Congenital lymphedema, 254
Congenital malalignment of great toenails, 258
Congenital melanocytic nevus, 347–348
Congenital milia, 231*t*
Congenital nevus, 402–414*t*
Congenital rests of the neck, 234*t*
Congenital rubella, 236*t*
Congenital self-healing collodion baby, 282*t*
Congenital smooth muscle hamartoma, 232–233*t*
Congenital syphilis, 236*t*
Congenital toxoplasmosis, 236*t*
Connective tissue, abnormalities of, 149, 151*t*
Connective tissue diseases (CTDs)
  laboratory studies, 119–122
  and sclerosing dermopathies, 119–149
    acute cutaneous lupus, 126
    adult onset Still's disease, 141–142
    chronic cutaneous lupus erythematosus, 122–126, 123*f*
    cutaneous lupus erythematosus, 122–126, 123*t*, 125*f*
    dermatomyositis, 132–135, 133*f*, 134*b*
    eosinophilic fasciitis, 147–148
    lupus-related diseases, 132
    mixed connective tissue disease, 138
    morphea, 142–144, 142*f*, 143*f*, 145*f*
    nephrogenic systemic fibrosis, 148–149, 148*f*
    relapsing polychondritis, 137–138, 137*f*
    rheumatoid arthritis, 138–140, 139*f*, 140*f*
    SCLE-like syndromes, 127–128
    Sjögren syndrome, 135–137
    subacute cutaneous lupus erythematosus, 126, 126*f*
    systemic lupus erythematosus, 129–131
Connective tissue diseases *(Continued)*
    systemic-onset juvenile idiopathic arthritis, 140–141, 141*f*
Connective tissue nevus (CTN), 232–233*t*, 378, 378*f*
Connexin 26 (GJB2), 2*t*
Connexin 30 (GJB6), 2*t*
Connexin 30.3 (GJB 4), 2*t*
Connexin 31 (GJB 3), 2*t*
Conradi-Hünermann-Happle syndrome, 282*t*
Contact dermatitis, 89–92
  clinical features of, 90
  epidemiology of, 89
  histopathology of, 90
  laboratory testing of, 90–91
  pathogenesis of, 89–90
  specific contactants of, 91–92
  treatment of, 91
Contact urticaria (CU), 96
Co-reaction, in contact dermatitis, 90
Cornification, disorders of, 278–281, 282*t*, 287*f*, 289*f*
Cornified cell envelope, 2, 5*f*
Corticosteroids (CS), 42–46, 74–78*t*
  adverse effects, 39
  adverse effects (systemic), 43–44
  clinical use of, 44–45
  contraindications of, 44
  monitoring of, 45–46
  pharmacology key points, 42–43, 43*t*
  pregnancy in, 44
  for psoriasis, 81
Cortisol-binding globulin (CBG), 43
Corynebacterial skin infections, 308
Cosmeceuticals, 497
Cosmeceuticals, nutraceuticals, and supplements, 496*t*
Cosmetic dermal fillers, 74–78*t*
Cosmetic dermatology, 481–504
  botulinum toxin, 488, 489*f*
    different forms of, 489*t*
    injection dosing of, 491*t*
  cosmeceuticals, 497
  dermal fillers, 489*t*, 491
  fat reduction, 491, 494
  hair transplantation, 498
  lasers, 481
    continuous, 481
    depth of optical penetration by, 483*f*
    light sources of, 485–486, 485*t*
    pulsed, 481
    quality switched, 481
    quasicontinuous, 481
    resurfacing, 486, 486*t*
    safety of, 484
    terminology of, 482*t*
  liposuction, 494
  nutraceuticals, 497
  sclerotherapy, 494
Cosmetics dermatitis, 90
Costello syndrome, 507
Coumadin-induced skin necrosis, 74–78*t*
COVID-19, 301
Cowden syndrome, 249, 515
Cowdry A body, 392–394*t*
Cowdry B body, 392–394*t*
Cowpox, 300
Crescent excision, 461
Crisaborole, 46
CRISPR. *see* Clustered regularly interspaced palindromic repeats (CRISPR)
Cronkhite-Canada syndrome, 244*t*, 515
Cross-reaction, in contact dermatitis, 90
Cryoglobulinemia type I, 402–414*t*, 521–522
Cryoglobulinemias, 205–206, 206*t*
Cryolipolysis, 494*t*
Cryopyrin-associated periodic syndromes, 269–271*t*
Cryosurgery, 461
Cryptococcus, 402–414*t*
CS. *see* Corticosteroids (CS)
CTN. *see* Connective tissue nevus (CTN)
CU. *see* Contact urticaria (CU)
Cumulative incidence, 527
Cupping, 191
Cushing's syndrome, 514
Cutaneous amebiasis, 333
Cutaneous B-cell lymphomas, 374*t*
Cutaneous burns, laser safety and, 484
Cutaneous Crohn's disease, 154–156, 156*f*
Cutaneous drug eruptions (CDEs), 71
Cutaneous effects, 44
Cutaneous lupus erythematosus, 123*t*, 125*f*, 126
Cutaneous mastocytosis, 290–291
Cutaneous metastases, 522
Cutaneous neurology, 9–10
Cutaneous polyarteritis nodosa, 437*f*
Cutaneous small vessel vasculitis, 196–200, 197*t*
  treatment approach for, 197*t*
  triggers of, 196*t*
Cutaneous vasculature, 9
Cutaneous warts, 293
Cutis laxa, 507
Cutis laxa/generalized elastolysis, 263–264, 263*f*
Cutis marmorata telangiectatica congenita, 255, 255*f*
Cyclophosphamide, 50
Cyclosporine, 48, 53*t*
Cylindroma, 354, 354*f*, 357, 402–414*t*
CYP isoforms, 71
Cyproheptadine, 39
Cysticercosis, 333
Cysts, 343
Cytochrome P-450 system, drug interactions and, 70–71
Cytokines, 18, 19*t*
Cytomegalovirus, 299
Cytotoxic agents, 49–50
β-Catenin, 2*t*

D
Danazol, 69
Danger triangle, 444
Dapsone, 51
Daptomycin, 62
Darier's disease (keratosis follicularis), 116–117, 402–414*t*, 432*f*
Darier's sign, 250–251
Data-snooping bias, 531*t*
DCMO. *see* Diffuse capillary malformation with overgrowth (DCMO)
DDD. *see* Dowling-Degos disease (DDD)
De Barsy syndrome, 270
Deep penetrating nevus, 347, 347*f*, 402–414*t*
Degos disease, 515
Dendritic cells, 27
Dendritic histiocytes, 6
Deoxyribonucleic acid (DNA), 15
Depositional and calcification disorders, 193*t*
Dermacentor, 334
Dermal dendritic cells, 397*t*
Dermal duct tumor, 356–357
Dermal fibrous and elastic tissue, abnormalities of, 149
Dermal fillers, 488, 489*t*
Dermal melanocytosis, 232–233*t*, 345, 402–414*t*
Dermal melanosis, 233*f*
Dermal papilla, 10
Dermatitis
  lichenoid interface, 421*t*
  vacuolar interface, 419*t*
Dermatitis herpetiformis (Duhring's disease), 114–115, 117*f*, 401*f*, 402–414*t*, 516
Dermatofibroma, 373–374, 386*f*, 387, 402–414*t*
Dermatofibrosarcoma protuberans (DFSP), 374–375, 375*f*, 402–414*t*
Dermatofibrosis lenticularis disseminata, 279
Dermatology, oncologic agents in, 54–57
Dermatomyofibroma, 376
Dermatomyositis (DM), 132–135, 133*f*, 134*b*, 402–414*t*, 415*f*, 507, 522
Dermatopathology, 391–442
  diagnoses at a glance, 415, 402–414*t*
  essential concepts in, 391
  high yield differential diagnoses, 415
  immediate pattern recognition diagnoses, 439*t*
Dermatopharmacology, 39–78
Dermatoses of pregnancy, 212, 213*t*
Dermatosis papulosa nigra, 338*t*

Dermis, 7–13, 416*t*, 437*t*
blue balls in, 425*t*
dermal cells, 7–8
structural components and cell biology of, 8–13
Dermoid cyst, 343
Dermoscopic patterns of melanocytic lesions, 387
Dermoscopy, 384–387, 389*f*
Dermpath bodies, 392–394*t*
Descriptive studies, 528–529
Desloratadine, 39
Desmocollin 1, 2*t*
Desmocollin 2, 2*t*
Desmocollin 3, 2*t*
Desmoglein 1, 2*t*
Desmoglein 3, 2*t*
Desmoglein 4, 2*t*
Desmoplakin, 2*t*
Desmoplastic trichilemmoma, 362
Desmoplastic trichoepithelioma, 361, 361*f*, 423*f*
Desmosomes, 1
Detection bias, 531*t*
DFSP. *see* Dermatofibrosarcoma protuberans (DFSP)
Diabetes, 512
infections common in, 513
Diabetic dermopathy, 513
Diaper dermatitis, 289
DIF. *see* Direct immunofluorescence (DIF)
Diffuse capillary malformation with overgrowth (DCMO), 252–253
Digital mucous cyst, 402–414*t*
DIHS. *see* Drug-induced hypersensitivity syndrome/drug reaction with eosinophilia and systemic symptoms (DIHS/DRESS)
Diltiazem, 74–78*t*
Diphenhydramine, 39
Direct immunofluorescence (DIF), 33
Discoid lupus, 427*f*
Discoid lupus erythematosus (DLE), 123*f*
Dissecting cellulitis of the scalp, 217, 212*f*
Disseminate and recurrent infundibulofolliculitis, 181
Disulfide bonding, 13
DLE. *see* Discoid lupus erythematosus (DLE)
DM. *see* Dermatomyositis (DM)
DNA. *see* Deoxyribonucleic acid (DNA)
DNA sequencing, 31–32
Donor sites, 473*t*
Donovan bodies, 392–394*t*
Dose, 17
Dowling-Degos disease (DDD), 243
Doxepin, 40
DRESS. *see* Drug-induced hypersensitivity syndrome/drug reaction with eosinophilia and systemic symptoms (DIHS/DRESS)
Drug reactions, 71–74, 184
angioedema, 166–169
immunologic, 158–159*t*
urticaria, 166–168
Drug-induced acne, 179
Drug-induced hypersensitivity syndrome/drug reaction with eosinophilia and systemic symptoms (DIHS/DRESS), 72, 73*t*, 304
Drug-induced pigmentary changes, 74
Drug-induced pruritus, 190
Drug-induced Sweet syndrome, 74–78*t*
Duhring's disease, 516. *see also* Dermatitis herpetiformis (Duhring's disease)
Dupilumab, 54
Dutcher body, 392–394*t*
Dyschromatosis symmetrica hereditaria, 243
Dyschromatosis universalis hereditaria, 243
Dyskeratosis congenita, 243
Dysplastic nevus, 402–414*t*
β-Defensins, 20

E
EAC. *see* Erythema annulare centrifugum (EAC)
Ear
nerve innervation of, 445–446*t*
sensory innervation of, 448*t*
EB simplex, 248*f*
E-cadherin, 2*t*
Eccrine glands, 10
Eccrine poroma, 352*f*
Eccrine syringofibroadenoma, 428*f*
Echinocandins, 64–65
Echinoderms, 336
ECM. *see* Extracellular matrix (ECM)
Econazole, 64
Ecthyma, 307
Ecthyma contagiosum, 300
Ecthyma gangrenosum, 311
Ectodermal dysplasias, 257–258
as a result of *p63* mutation, 258
Ectopic ACTH syndrome, 522
Ectrodactyly ectodermal dysplasia-cleft lip/palate syndrome (EEC), 261
Eczema craquele. *see* Asteatotic dermatitis (eczema craquele)
Eczema herpeticum, 295
Eczematous dermatoses, 86–96
asteatotic dermatitis, 89
atopic dermatitis, 88
autosensitization, 95–96
contact dermatitis, 89–92
contact urticaria, 96
nummular dermatitis, 89
progesterone dermatitis, 89
stasis dermatitis, 92–95
EDS. *see* Ehlers-Danlos syndrome (EDS)
EEC. *see* Ectrodactyly ectodermal dysplasia-cleft lip/palate syndrome (EEC)
Efinaconazole, 64
Eflornithine, 67
EGFR inhibitors, 74–78*t*
EGR. *see* Erythema gyratum repens (EGR)
Ehlers-Danlos syndrome (EDS), 265–266, 266*t*
classic form, 507
vascular form, 508
Elastic fibers, 8–9, 395–396*t*
Elastosis perforans serpiginosa (EPS), 402–414*t*
Electrical hemostasis, 460*t*
bipolar circuits, 458–459
biterminal devices, 459–460
methods of, 459–460, 460*t*
monopolar circuits, 458–459
monoterminal devices, 459–460
Electrocautery, 460, 460*t*
Electrocoagulation, 460, 460*t*
Electrodesiccation, 460, 460*t*
Electrofulguration, 460, 460*t*
Electrosection, 460, 460*t*
Elejalde syndrome, 236
ELISA. *see* Enzyme-linked immunosorbent assay (ELISA)
Embolia cutis medicamentosa, 74–78*t*
EN. *see* Erythema nodosum (EN)
Encephalocele, 234*t*
End stage renal disease (ESRD), 519
Endocarditis, 508
Endocrine, 512–513
Endocrine mucin-producing sweat gland carcinoma, 356
Endometriosis
cutaneous, 402–414*t*
of umbilicus, 440*f*
Endothelial cells, 397*t*
Energy, 482*t*
Enzyme-linked immunosorbent assay (ELISA), 30–31*t*, 34–35
Eosinophilic cellulitis. *see* Well's syndrome
Eosinophilic disorders, 172–173
eosinophilic folliculitis, 172
granuloma faciale, 172
hypereosinophilic syndrome, 172–173
papuloerythroderma of Ofuji, 172
Wells' syndrome, 172
Eosinophilic fasciitis (aka Shulman syndrome), 147–148
Eosinophilic folliculitis, 172, 181
Eosinophilic pustulosis/folliculitis, 231*t*, 301
Eosinophils, 27, 27*t*
Ephelides, 344–345
Epidemiology, 527–534
Epidermal cells, 4–6
Epidermal nevus, 338–339
Epidermis, 1–6, 13
cellular biology of, 1–4
layers of, 4*t*
Epidermodysplasia verruciformis, 293, 294*f*, 402–414*t*
Epidermoid cyst, 343, 424*t*
Epidermolysis bullosa, 116, 244–248
Epidermolysis bullosa acquisita, 114, 116*f*
Epidermolytic hyperkeratosis, 402–414*t*
Epidermolytic ichthyosis, 282*t*
Epithelial carcinomas, 400*t*
Epithelial immunostains, 398*t*
Epithelioid cell histiocytoma, 376
Epithelioid hemangioma, 379, 402–414*t*
EPS. *see* Elastosis perforans serpiginosa (EPS)
Epstein pearls, 231*t*
Epstein-Barr virus, 299*t*
Eruptive xanthomas, 402–414*t*
Erysipelas, 307, 307*f*
Erysipeloid, 310
Erythema ab igne, 184
Erythema annulare centrifugum (EAC), 173, 402–414*t*
Erythema dyschromicum perstans (ashy dermatosis), 105
Erythema elevatum diutinum, 199–200, 302
with fibrosis, 436*f*
triggers of, 199*t*
Erythema gyratum repens (EGR), 174, 174*f*, 522
Erythema induratum/nodular vasculitis, 211, 402–414*t*
Erythema infectiosum, 231–235, 238*f*
Erythema marginatum, 173
Erythema migrans, 174
Erythema multiforme, 96–97, 97*f*, 402–414*t*
Erythema nodosum (EN), 210–211, 402–414*t*
Erythema toxicum neonatorum, 231*t*
Erythematotelangiectatic (vascular) rosacea, 149–153
Erythrasma, 308
Erythroderma, 85–86, 508, 522
causes of, 85*b*
Erythrodermic psoriasis, 81
Erythrokeratodermia variabilis, 282*t*
Erythromelalgia, 210
Erythromycin, 59
ESRD. *see* End stage renal disease (ESRD)
Etanercept, 52, 53*t*
Exanthem subitum, 238
Excimer laser, 66
Exogen, 13
Exposure misclassification, 531*t*
Exposure time, 17
Extracellular matrix (ECM), 8–9
Extracorporeal photochemotherapy, 66
Extramammary Paget disease, 522–523, 523*f*
Extranodal NK/T-cell lymphoma, nasal type, 373
Extravasation reactions, 74–78*t*

F
Fabry disease, 259, 508
Face, sensory innervation of, 452*f*
Facial artery, 443
surgical anatomy of, 443–444
Factitial dermatitis/dermatitis artefacta, 190
Famciclovir and penciclovir, 62
Familial adenomatous polyposis syndrome, 516
Familial atypical mole and multiple melanoma syndrome, 523
Familial benign chronic pemphigus. *see* Hailey-Hailey disease (familial benign chronic pemphigus)
Familial cold autoinflammatory syndrome, 269–271*t*
Familial cutaneous leiomyomas, 520
Familial dysautonomia/Riley-Day syndrome, 192
Familial Mediterranean fever, 269–271*t*
Fat reduction, 494, 494*t*
FDE. *see* Fixed drug eruption (FDE)
Fexofenadine, 39
FFPE. *see* Formalin-fixed, paraffin-embedded (FFPE)
Fibroblastic proliferations, 376–378
Fibroblasts, 397*t*
Fibrofolliculoma, 359, 360*f*, 402–414*t*
in Birt-Hogg-Dube syndrome, 506*f*
Fibrohistiocytic neoplasms, 373–374

Fibromatosis, 377, 436*t*
Fibrous hamartoma of infancy, 377–378
Figurate erythemas, 173–174
  erythema annulare centrifugum, 173
  erythema gyratum repens, 174, 174*f*
  erythema marginatum, 173
  erythema migrans, 174
  flushing, 174, 175*b*
Filamentous bacteria, 309
Finasteride and dutasteride, 68
Fingers, nerve innervation of, 445–446*t*
Fire hazard, laser safety and, 484
FISH. *see* Fluorescence in situ hybridization (FISH)
Fixed drug eruption (FDE), 101
Flagellate eruptions, 74–78*t*
Flaps, 463–467
  anatomy of, 464*f*
  category of, 466*t*
Flegel disease, 339
Floret cells, 392–394*t*
Fluconazole, 63
Fluence, 481, 482*t*
Fluorescence in situ hybridization (FISH), 30–31*t*, 32–33
Fluoroquinolones, 60
Flushing, 174, 175*b*
Focal dermal hypoplasia, 268, 268*f*
Follicular and eccrine/apocrine disorders, 176–184
  acne associated syndromes, 179
  acne conglobata, 177
  acne cosmetica, 178
  acne excoriée, 177
  acne fulminans, 177
  acne in setting of endocrinologic abnormality, 178
  acne mechanica, 177
  acne vulgaris, 176, 175*t*
  acneiform eruptions, 179
  anhidrosis, 183
  Apert syndrome, 179
  bromhidrosis, 183–184
  chloracne, 178
  chromhidrosis, 184
  drug-induced acne, 179
  follicular occlusion tetrad, 182
  folliculitis, 181–182
  Fox-Fordyce disease, 184
  granulomatous rosacea, 180
  HAIR-AN (hyper androgenism, insulin resistance, acanthosis nigricans), 179
  hyperhidrosis, 183
  hypohidrosis, 183
  infantile acne, 177–178
  lupus miliaris disseminatus faciei, 180
  miliaria, 176*t*, 183
  neonatal acne, 177
  PAPA (pyogenic arthritis, pyoderma gangrenosum, acne conglobata), 179
  perioral/periorificial dermatitis, 180–181
  pomade acne, 178
  pyoderma faciale, 180
  radiation acne, 178
  rosacea, 179–180
  SAPHO (chronic recurrent multifocal osteomyelitis), 179
  solid facial edema in acne, 177
  solid facial edema in rosacea, 180
  transverse nasal crease, 178
Follicular hyperkeratosis, in scurvy, 518*f*
Follicular infundibulum, tumor of, 362–363
Follicular microanatomy, 11*f*
Follicular mucinosis, 402–414*t*
Follicular occlusion tetrad, 182
Folliculitis, 181–182
  acne keloidalis, 217
  disseminate and recurrent infundibulofolliculitis, 181
  eosinophilic folliculitis, 181
  Gram-negative folliculitis, 181
  hot tub folliculitis, 181
  pseudofolliculitis barbae, 181
  superficial folliculitis, 181
Folliculitis decalvans, 217, 402–414*t*
Folliculo-sebaceous-apocrine hamartomas, 359–360
Fong disease, 290
Fontana-Masson (silver stain), 395–396*t*
Foot
  nerve innervation of, 445–446*t*
  sensory innervation of, 447*f*
Forceps, 454
Foreign body reactions, 157, 159*t*
Formalin-fixed, paraffin-embedded (FFPE), 34
Foscarnet, 62
Fox-Fordyce disease (apocrine miliaria), 184
Free-living amoeba, 333
Frey syndrome. *see* Auriculotemporal nerve syndrome (Frey syndrome)
Fucosidosis, 255
Funding bias, 531*t*
Fungal diseases, 322–323

G
Gap junctions, 1
Gardner syndrome, 249–250, 516
Gardner-Diamond syndrome, 190
Gastroenterology, 514–519
Gastrointestinal effects, 44
Gene silencing, 16–17
General dermatology, 79–228
General laser boards fodder, 484–485
Generalized essential telangiectasia, 256*t*
Generalized pustular psoriasis, 81
Genital herpes, 295
Genital leiomyoma, 368
Genital warts, 294
Gentamicin, 58
German measles, 230–231
Gianotti Crosti syndrome, 239, 239*f*
Giant cell arteritis. *see* Temporal arteritis (giant cell arteritis)
Giant cell tumor of tendon sheath, 378, 402–414*t*, 440*f*
Gingival hypertrophy, 74–78*t*
Glanders, 314
Glatiramer acetate, 74–78*t*
Glomeruloid hemangioma, 380
Glomus bodies, 392–394*t*
Glomus cells, 7
Glomus tumor/glomangioma, 380, 380*f*, 402–414*t*
Glucocorticoid effects, 44
Glycopyrrolate, 70
GM1 gangliosidosis, 259
Gnathosomiasis, 333
Golimumab, 52
Goltz syndrome, 268, 268*f*
Gonorrhea, 299*t*
Gorham-Stout disease, 254
Gout, 402–414*t*, 430*t*
Gradle scissors, 454
Graft-*versus*-host disease (GVHD), 101–103, 102*f*
Grafts, 472–473
  in soft tissue reconstruction, 472*t*
Gram-negative skin infections, 310–311
Gram-positive skin infections, 304–310
Granular cell tumor, 365–366, 366*f*, 402–414*t*
Granuloma annulare, 149–153, 152*f*, 402–414*t*, 416*f*, 512
Granuloma faciale, 172, 200, 402–414*t*, 436*f*
Granuloma inguinale, 299*t*
Granulomatosis with polyangiitis, 511
Granulomatous dermatitides, histologic features of, 433*t*
Granulomatous disorders, 430*t*
Granulomatous rosacea, 180
Granulomatous/histocytic disorders, 149–161, 158–159*t*
  histiocytosis, 161, 162*t*
  non-infectious granulomas, 149–157, 158*f*
    annular elastolytic giant cell granuloma, 153
    cutaneous Crohn's disease, 154–156, 156*f*
    foreign body reactions, 157, 159*t*
    granuloma annulare, 149–153, 152*f*
    interstitial granulomatous dermatitis and arthritis, 153, 153*t*
    interstitial granulomatous drug eruption, 153
    necrobiosis lipoidica, 153–154, 154*f*, 155*f*
Granulomatous/histocytic disorders *(Continued)*
    necrobiotic xanthogranuloma, 154, 155*f*
    palisaded neutrophilic granulomatous dermatitis, 153, 153*t*
  sarcoidosis, 156–157, 156*f*, 157*f*, 157*t*
Graves' disease, 514
Green nail syndrome, 310
Griscelli syndrome (GS), 241*t*
Griseofulvin, 64
GS. *see* Griscelli syndrome (GS)
Guarnieri body, 392–394*t*
Guselkumab, 53*t*
Guttate psoriasis, 81, 402–414*t*, 431*f*
GVHD. *see* Graft-*versus*-host disease (GVHD)

H
H. influenzae cellulitis, 315
H syndrome, 290
Hailey-Hailey disease (familial benign chronic pemphigus), 118, 118*f*, 402–414*t*, 432*f*
Hair, 10–13, 11*t*
  nail, and mucosal disorders, 212–220
  and nails, disorders of, 255–258
Hair collar sign, 234*t*
Hair cycle, 11*t*, 13
Hair follicle neoplasms, 359–360
Hair follicle stem cells, 13
Hair reduction lasers, 485–486, 485*t*
Hair shaft abnormalities, 217*t*, 218
Hair transplantation, 498
HAIR-AN (hyper androgenism, insulin resistance, acanthosis nigricans), 179
Halo nevus, 346, 402–414*t*
Halo scalp ring, 230*t*
Hamartomas, 351, 359–360
Hand
  nerve innervation of, 445–446*t*
  sensory innervation of, 447*f*
Hand-foot skin reaction (HFSR), 74–78*t*
Hand-foot-and mouth disease, 238–239
Hansen's disease, 322*t*
Harlequin ichthyosis, 282*t*
Hartnup disease, 262
Hawthorne effect, 531*t*
Head and neck
  motor innervation of, 445*t*
  sensory innervation of, 445*t*
  surgical anatomy of, 443–444
Heavy metals, 74–78*t*
Hematolymphoid neoplasms, 368–370
Hemochromatosis, 516
Hemorrhage, 387
Henderson-Paterson bodies, 392–394*t*
Henoch-Schönlein purpura (HSP), 519
Heparin-induced skin necrosis (heparin-induced thrombocytopenia with thrombosis syndrome), 74–78*t*
Heparin/LMWH, 74–78*t*
Hepatitis B, 516
Hepatitis C, 516
Herald patch, 84
Hereditary benign telangiectasia, 256*t*
Hereditary dyschromatoses, 243
Hereditary hemorrhagic telangiectasia, 256*t*, 508–509
  patient with, 508*f*
Hereditary onycho osteo dysplasia, 519–520
Hermansky-Pudlak syndrome, 241–242
Herpes gestationis, 402–414*t*
Herpes zoster, 302–303
  treatment of, 298
HES. *see* Hypereosinophilic syndrome (HES)
HFSR. *see* Hand-foot skin reaction (HFSR)
Hibernoma, 382, 402–414*t*
Hidradenitis suppurativa (acne inversa), 182
Hidradenoma, 351–352, 352*f*, 356, 402–414*t*
Hidradenoma papilliferum (HPAP), 354, 354*f*, 358
Hidroacanthoma simplex, 356, 402–414*t*, 425*t*
Hidrocystoma, 344, 402–414*t*
Hidrotic ectodermal dysplasia, 257–258
Hirsutism, 217*f*, 218–220
Histiocytes, 397*t*, 399*f*
Histiocytosis, 161, 162*t*

Histoplasmosis, 325*f*, 402–414*t*
HIV and cutaneous malignancies, 303
HIV photodermatitis, 302
HIV/AIDS dermatology, 301–304
HIV-associated dermatoses, 301–302, 303–304*t*, 304*t*
Hobnail hemangioma, 379–380, 380*f*
Homocystinuria, 262, 509
Hori's nevus, 345
Hot tub folliculitis, 181
Howel-Evans syndrome, 523
HPA axis suppression, 43, 43*b*
HPAP. *see* Hidradenoma papilliferum (HPAP)
HPV. *see* Human papillomavirus (HPV)
HSP. *see* Henoch-Schönlein purpura (HSP)
Human herpesviruses, 295–299
Human papillomavirus (HPV), 293–295
Hunter syndrome, 263
Hutchinson-Gilford progeria, 275–276
Hyalohyphomycosis, 402–414*t*
Hyaluronic acid fillers, 491
Hydroa vacciniforme, 281
Hydroquinone, 67, 74–78*t*
Hydroxyurea, 50
Hydroxyzine, 39
Hypereosinophilic syndrome (HES), 172–173
Hyperhidrosis, 183
Hyperlipoproteinemias, 165*t*, 509
Hypermobile EDS, 275
Hyperpigmentation, 242–243
  disorders of, 227–228
Hypertrichosis, 218–220
Hypertrichosis lanuginosa acquisita, 523
Hypo-/depigmentation, 240–242
Hypohidrosis, 183
Hypohidrotic ectodermal dysplasia, 257–258, 257*f*
Hypopigmentation and depigmentation, disorders of, 220–227
Hypothyroidism, 514

I
IBD. *see* Inflammatory bowel disease (IBD)
Ibrutinib, 57
Ichthyosis en confetti, 282*t*
Ichthyosis follicularis-atrichia-photophobia (IFAP) syndrome, 282*t*
Ichthyosis hystrix Curth-Macklin, 282*t*
Ichthyosis vulgaris, 282*t*, 402–414*t*
Idiopathic erythroderma, 86
IF. *see* Immunofluorescence (IF)
IGDA. *see* Interstitial granulomatous dermatitis and arthritis (IGDA)
IHC. *see* Immunohistochemistry (IHC)
II F. *see* Indirect immunofluorescence (II F)
IL-1 inhibitors, 54
IL-2 reactions, 74–78*t*
IL-17 inhibitors, 53–54
IL-23 inhibitors, 53
Iliac horn disease, 519–520
Imatinib, 74–78*t*
Imatinib mesylate, 56–57
Immune reconstitution inflammatory syndrome (IRIS), 303, 304*t*
Immunofluorescence (IF), 33–34
Immunofluorescence staining (direct), 30–31*t*
Immunofluorescence staining (indirect), 30–31*t*
Immunohistochemistry (IHC), 30–31*t*, 34, 35*f*
Immunologic mediators, 18–20
Immunology, 18–28
Immunomodulators, 74–78*t*
Immunomodulatory agents, 46–54
Immunostains, by cell type, 397*t*
Impetigo, 304–305
Impetigo herpetiformis, 82
Implantable electronic devices, 461
Incidence, 527
  rate, 527
Inclusion body fibromatosis, 376–377, 377*f*
Incontinentia pigmenti (IP), 274–275, 274*f*, 274*t*, 275*t*, 402–414*t*
Indirect immunofluorescence (II F), 33–34
Infantile acne, 177–178
Infantile digital fibromatosis, 402–414*t*
Infantile hemangioma, 379
Infantile systemic hyalinosis (ISH), and juvenile hyaline fibromatosis (JHF), 267
Infections, common in diabetes, 513
Infectious dermatoses, 302–303
Infectious disease, 293–336
Inflammation of AKs, 74–78*t*
Inflammation of DSAP, 74–78*t*
Inflammation of SKs, 74–78*t*
Inflammatory bowel disease (IBD), 516
Inflammatory dermatoses, 301–302
Inflammatory phase, 13–14
Infliximab, 52, 53*t*
Information bias, 530
Information or measurement bias, 531*t*
Inhalation of biohazardous plume, laser safety and, 484
Inherited blistering diseases, 116–118
  Darier's disease (keratosis follicularis), 116–117
  epidermolysis bullosa, 116
  Hailey-Hailey disease (familial benign chronic pemphigus), 118*f*
Inherited connective tissue disorders, 263–269
Inherited metabolic and nutritional disorders, 258–263
Inherited pigmentary disorders, 240–243
Injection-site reactions, 304
Ink spot lentigo, 387
Innate immunity, 18
Innate lymphoid cells, 24
Innate *vs.* adaptive immunity, 18
Integrins, 23
Intercellular junction proteins, 2*t*
Interface dermatitis, 96–107
Interferon reactions, 74–78*t*
Internal disease, cutaneous manifestations of, 505–526
Interpolation flaps, 467–468*t*
Interstitial granulomatous dermatitis and arthritis (IGDA), 153, 153*t*
Interstitial granulomatous drug eruption, 153
Intertriginous/axillary granular parakeratosis, 85
Interviewer or observer bias, 531*t*
Intralesional CS, 45
Intramuscular CS, 44
Intravascular papillary endothelial hyperplasia, 378–379, 402–414*t*
Invasive cutaneous squamous cell carcinoma, 340–341
Inverted follicular keratosis, 338*t*, 402–414*t*
Iodoquinol, 58
Ipilimumab, 56
IRIS. *see* Immune reconstitution inflammatory syndrome (IRIS)
Iris scissors, 454
Irradiance, 482*t*
Irradiance/power (watts), 17
Irritant contact dermatitis, 90
  specific contactants of, 91
Isotretinoin, for pityriasis rubra pilaris, 84
Itraconazole, 63
IVIG, 70
Ixekizumab, 53*t*

J
Jackson-Lawler, 260
Jadassohn-Lewandowski, 260
Janus kinase inhibitors, 46–47
Jessner's lymphocytic infiltrate of skin, 132, 132*f*
Juvenile plantar dermatosis, 289–290
Juvenile spring eruption, 289
Juvenile xanthogranuloma, 163*f*, 402–414*t*
JXG + NF1, 524

K
Kamino bodies, 392–394*t*
Kaposi sarcoma, 380–381, 381*f*, 402–414*t*, 426*f*
Kaposiform hemangioendothelioma, 380
Kasabach-Merritt phenomenon, 250–251
Kawasaki disease, 203*f*, 204–205, 509
Keloid, 402–414*t*
Kenogen, 13
Keratin granuloma, 402–414*t*
Keratinocytes, 4, 397*t*
Keratinocytic neoplasms, 337–338
Keratins, 4, 8*t*
Keratitis ichthyosis-deafness (KID) syndrome, 282*t*
Keratoacanthoma, 341–342, 386*f*
  subungual, 341
Keratosis follicularis. *see* Darier's disease (keratosis follicularis)
Keratosis lichenoides chronica (KLC), 105
Ketoconazole, 63
KIT and BCR-ABL inhibitors, 74–78*t*
Kitamura, reticulate acropigmentation of, 243
KLC. *see* Keratosis lichenoides chronica (KLC)
Klippel-Trenaunay syndrome, 252
Koilocytes, 392–394*t*
Koplik spot, 230
Krause end bulbs, 9

L
LABD/CBDC. *see* Linear IgA bullous dermatosis/chronic bullous disease of childhood (LABD/CBDC)
Labial/angular artery, cutaneous danger zones of, 450*t*
Lamellar ichthyosis, 282*t*
Lamina densa, 7
Lamina lucida, 7
Langerhans cell histiocytosis, 161, 161*f*, 402–414*t*
Langerhans cell sarcoma, 161
Langerhans cells, 6, 27, 397*t*
Langer's lines, 443
Langhans giant cells, 392–394*t*
Large cell acanthoma, 338*t*
Large vessel vasculitis, 205
Lasers, 481
  continuous, 481
  depth of optical penetration by, 483*f*
  light sources of, 485–486, 485*t*
  pulsed, 481
  quality switched, 481
  quasicontinuous, 481
  resurfacing, 486, 486*t*
  terminology of, 482*t*
Laugier-Hunziker syndrome, 244*t*
LBT. *see* Lupus band test (LBT)
Lead-time bias, 531*t*
Lebrikizumab, 54
Lectin pathway, 20
Leder (chloracetate esterase), 395–396*t*
Legius syndrome, 275*t*
Leiomyoma, 367*f*, 402–414*t*
Leiomyosarcoma (LMS), 368, 368*b*
Leishmaniasis, 330*f*, 402–414*t*
Lentigines, atrial (and cutaneous) myxomas, blue nevi (LAMB) syndrome, 506
Lentiginoses syndromes, 243, 244*f*, 244*t*
Lentigo simplex, 345
LEOPARD syndrome, 244*t*, 509
Lepidopterism, 333–334
Leprosy, 321*t*, 402–414*t*
Lesch-Nyhan syndrome, 262
Leser-Trelat, sign of, 524
Leukemia cutis, 373, 402–414*t*
Leukopenia, 42
Levocetirizine, 39
Lichen myxedematosus, 431*f*
Lichen nitidus, 105, 402–414*t*
Lichen planopilaris, 216–217, 402–414*t*
Lichen planus, 103–105, 104*t*, 402–414*t*
Lichen planus pigmentosus, of face, 222*f*, 227
Lichen sclerosis, 106
Lichen sclerosus, 402–414*t*
Lichen simplex chronicus, 402–414*t*
Lichen striatus, 106, 402–414*t*
Lichenoid drug eruptions, 104
Lichenoid interface dermatitis, 103–107
  erythema dyschromicum perstans, 105
  keratosis lichenoides chronica, 105
  lichen nitidus, 105
  lichen planus, 103–105, 104*t*
  lichen sclerosis, 106
  lichen striatus, 106
  lichenoid keratosis, 105

Lichenoid keratosis, 105, 338t
Linear IgA bullous dermatosis/chronic bullous disease of childhood (LABD/CBDC), 113–114, 114f, 117f
Lines of Blaschko, pigmented macules along, 227f
Linezolid, 61
Lip pits, 234t
Lip wedge excision, 462
Lipid effects, 44
Lipids, 395–396t
Lipodermatosclerosis, 212, 402–414t
Lipodystrophies, 210–212
Lipoid proteinosis, 267, 440f
Lipoma, 382
Liposuction, 494
Listeria, 310
Livedo reticularis (LR), 210
Livedoid vasculopathy, 207f, 208, 402–414t
LMS. *see* Leiomyosarcoma (LMS)
Lobomycosis, 402–414t
Lobular capillary hemangioma, 379, 402–414t
Local anesthetics, 451t
  differential diagnosis of, 456t
  in surgery, 450–454
Localized scleroderma. *see* Morphea
Louis-Bar syndrome, 256t
Louse-borne relapsing fever, 317t
LR. *see* Livedo reticularis (LR)
Luliconazole, 64
Lupus, 402–414t
Lupus band test (LBT), 120–122
Lupus erythematosus, 427f
Lupus erythematosus panniculitis/profundus, 124f
Lupus miliaris disseminatus faciei, 180
Lupus profundus/panniculitis, 402–414t
Lupus-related diseases, 132
Lyell's syndrome. *see* SJS/TEN (Lyell's syndrome)
Lyme disease, 316, 317t
Lymphangioma, 402–414t
Lymphatic malformations, 253–254
Lymphatic system, surgical anatomy of, 444
Lymphatics, 397t
Lymphocyte subsets, 24t
Lymphocytes, 21–24, 24t
Lymphogranuloma venereum, 299t
Lymphomatoid granulomatosis, 509–510
Lymphomatoid papulosis (LyP), 371–372, 371f, 402–414t
Lynch syndrome, 517–518
LyP. *see* Lymphomatoid papulosis (LyP)

M
MAC. *see* Microcystic adnexal carcinoma (MAC)
Macrocystic lymphatic malformations, 253–254
Macrolides, 59–60
Macrophages, 397t
Maffucci syndrome, 253
Major histocompatibility complex, 28
  -associated diseases, 28
  class I molecules present antigens, 28
  class II molecules present antigens, 28
MAL. *see* Methyl aminolevulinate (MAL)
Malakoplakia, 314–315
Malignant acanthosis nigricans, 524
Malignant atrophic papulosis, 515
Malignant histiocytic disorders, 161
Malignant otitis externa, 310
Malignant peripheral nerve sheath tumor, 366
Mandibular nerve, sensory innervation of, 445t
Marfan syndrome (MFS), 266–267, 510
Marginal mandibular nerve, cutaneous danger zones of, 450t
MAS. *see* McCune Albright syndrome (MAS)
Mass spectrometry, 30–31t
Masson trichrome, 395–396t
Masson's tumor, 378–379
Mast cell stains, 395–396t
Mast cells, 27, 27t, 397t
Mastocytoma, 402–414t
Maxillary artery, 443
Maxillary nerve, sensory innervation of, 445t
Mayo scissors, 454
McCune Albright syndrome (MAS), 242–243, 242f
Mechanical injuries, 187–188
Mechanical irritant contact dermatitis, 91
Mechlorethamine hydrochloride, 57
MED. *see* Minimal erythema dose (MED)
Median raphe cyst, 344
Medium vessel vasculitis, 203–205
Medlar bodies, 392–394t
Meissner's corpuscle, 9
MEK inhibitors, 55, 74–78t
Melanin, 4, 395–396t
Melanocytes, 4, 397t
Melanocytic lesions
  examples of, 387
  global patterns of, 387–388t
Melanocytic neoplasms, 344–345
Melanoma, 349–351, 389f, 402–414t
  classification of, 350t
  epidemiology of, 349
  histologic features of, 349
  pathogenesis of, 349
  prognosis of, 349
  risk factors of, 349
  site specific criteria of, 388t
  stage groupings for, 350t
  subtypes of, 349
  treatment of, 349–351
Melanonychia, 74–78t
Melioidosis, 314
Membranous aplasia cutis, 235f
MEN. *see* Multiple endocrine neoplasia (MEN)
Meningocele, 234t
Meralgia paresthetica, 191
Merkel cell carcinoma, 366–367, 402–414t
Merkel cells, 6, 397t
Merkel nerve ending, 9
Mesotherapy, 494t
Messenger RNA (mRNA), 15
Meta-analysis, 530
Metastases, 505–526
Methotrexate, 48–49, 53t
Methyl aminolevulinate (MAL), 66
Methyl green pyronin, 395–396t
Metronidazole, 58
Metzenbaum scissors, 454
Mevalonate kinase deficiency/hyper-IgD syndrome, 269–271t
MFS. *see* Marfan syndrome (MFS)
Michaelis- Gutmann body, 392–394t
Miconazole, 64
Microbial stains, 395–396t
Microcystic adnexal carcinoma (MAC), 355, 358, 402–414t, 419f
Microcystic lymphatic malformations, 253, 254f
Microscopic polyangiitis (MPA), 202, 202t
MIDAS syndrome, 290
Midline cervical cleft, 234t
Miescher's radial granuloma, 392–394t
Mikulicz cells, 392–394t
Miliaria, 176t, 183
Miliaria crystallina, 231t
Miliaria rubra, 231t
Mineralocorticoid effects, 44
Minimal erythema dose (MED), 17
Minocycline, 74–78t
Miscellaneous agents, 67–70
Miscellaneous pediatric dermatologic disorders, 281–291
Mites, 334–335
Mixed connective tissue disease, 138
Mixed cryoglobulinemia, 200
Mixed tumor (chondroid syringoma), 353, 353f, 402–414t
MMP. *see* Mucous membrane pemphigoid (MMP)
MMS. *see* Mohs micrographic surgery (MMS)
Mogamulizumab, 57
Mohs appropriate use criteria, 463b
Mohs micrographic surgery (MMS), 463
Mohs surgery, 463
Molluscum contagiosum, 300, 303
Monilethrix, 259–261t
Monoclonal gammopathies, 525f
  of dermatologic interest, 161–164, 164t
Monogenic periodic fever syndromes, 269–271t
Mononuclear phagocytes, 25
Morbilliform, 72
Morphea, 142–144, 142f, 143f, 145f, 430f
Motor innervation, surgical anatomy of, 444
Motor nerve injury, cutaneous danger zones of, 450t
Movat's pentachrome, 395–396t
MPA. *see* Microscopic polyangiitis (MPA)
M-plasty, 461, 462f
mRNA. *see* Messenger RNA (mRNA)
mTOR inhibitors, 74–78t
Mucicarmine, 395–396t
Mucinous carcinoma, 402–414t
  primary cutaneous, 356f, 359
Muckle-Wells syndrome, 269–271t
Mucocele, 402–414t
Mucocutaneous, 42
Mucosal disorders, 212–220, 223–224t
Mucosal melanotic macule, 345
Mucositis, 74–78t
Mucous membrane pemphigoid (MMP), 113, 113f
Muir-Torre syndrome, 517–518
Mulberry cells, 392–394t
Multicentric reticulohistiocytosis, 163f, 524
Multinucleate cell angiohistiocytoma, 376
Multiple endocrine neoplasia (MEN), 249, 513
Multiple hamartoma syndrome, 516
Mupirocin, 58
Muscular effects, 44
Musculoskeletal/vascular effects, 44
Mycetoma, 324f
Mycobacterial infections, 318–320
Mycophenolate mofetil, 49
Mycosis fungoides, 368–370, 369f, 370f, 402–414t
  clinical features of, 368
  clinical variants of, 380–381
  epidemiology of, 368
  histology of, 368
  staging of, 372
Myofibroblasts, 397t
Myofibroma, 378, 402–414t, 440f
Myopericytoma, 402–414t
Myrmecia, 424f
Myxoid liposarcoma, 402–414t
Myxoid/round cell liposarcoma, 382

N
Naegeli-Franchescetti-Jadassohn syndrome (NFJS)/ dermatopathia pigmentosa reticularis (DPR), 243
Naftifine, 64
Nail, 13, 13t
  surgery of, 477–479
Nail disorders, 218–219t, 220, 222f
Nail dystrophy, 521f
Nail hyperpigmentation (melanonychia), 74–78t
Nail-patella syndrome, 290, 519–520
Narrowband UVB, 66
Nasal glioma, 234t
Nasolabial/melolabial transposition flap, 471f
Natural killer cells, 397t
Naxos syndrome, 510
NCCN treatment guidelines, 349–351
Necrobiosis lipoidica, 153–154, 154f, 155f
Necrobiosis lipoidica diabeticorum (NLD), 153–154, 402–414t, 513, 513f
Necrobiotic xanthogranuloma (NXG), 154, 155f, 434f, 524–525
Necrolytic migratory erythema (NME), 524, 524f
Necrotizing fasciitis, 308
Needle drivers, 454
Neisseria meningitidis, 311–314
Nemolizumab, 54
Neomycin, 58
Neonatal acne, 177
Neonatal dermatology, 229, 230f, 230t, 231t, 232f, 234t, 236t, 245–247t
Neonatal herpes simplex virus, 238f
Neonatal lupus erythematosus (NLE), 510
Neonatal pustular melanosis, 231t
Neonatal-onset multisystem inflammatory disease (NOMID/chronic infantile neurological cutaneous articular (CINCA) syndrome, 269–271t

Neoplasms
of adipocytic lineage, 382
with follicular germinative differentiation, 360–361
with follicular matrix differentiation, 361–362
with follicular sheath (trichilemmal) differentiation, 362
with Pagetoid Scatter, 400*t*
with superficial follicular (isthmus and infundibular) differentiation, 362–363
Neoplastic dermatology, 337–390
premalignant/malignant, 339–343
Nephrogenic fibrosing dermopathy, 519. *see also* Nephrogenic systemic fibrosis (NSF)
Nephrogenic systemic fibrosis (NSF), 148–149, 148*f*, 149*t*, 402–414*t*, 520
Nerve sheath myxoma, 365, 402–414*t*
Nerves, 397*t*
Netherton syndrome, 282*t*
Neural crest-derived melanin-producing dendritic cells, 4
Neural neoplasms, 364
Neural tumors, 435*t*
Neuroblastoma, 367
Neurocutaneous syndromes, 271–275
Neurodermatology, 189–192
Neurofibroma, 365, 402–414*t*, 420*f*
Neurofibromatosis (NF), 271–273, 271*b*, 275*t*
Neurofibromatosis type 1, 275*t*
Neurofibromatosis type 2, 275*t*
Neurologic changes, 44
Neurology, 519
Neuropathic ulcers, 512
Neurothekeoma, 365, 365*f*
Neurotic excoriations, 190
Neutral lipid storage disease with ichthyosis, 282*t*
Neutrophilic dermatoses, 169–172
Behcet's disease, 171–172, 171*f*
bowel-associated dermatosis arthritis syndrome, 172
of dorsal hands, 170
pyoderma gangrenosum, 170–171
Sweet's syndrome, 169–170, 169*f*
Neutrophilic eccrine hidradenitis of childhood, 291
Neutrophils, 27–28, 397*t*
Nevi, atrial (and cutaneous) myxomas, ephelides (NAME) syndrome, 506
Nevus araneus, 256*t*
Nevus comedonicus, 339
Nevus of Ito, 345
Nevus of Ota, 345
Nevus sebaceus, 360, 402–414*t*
Nevus simplex, 232–233*t*
Nevus spilus/speckled lentiginous nevus, 348
Next-generation DNA sequencing, 30–31*t*
Next-generation sequencing methodology, 31, 34*f*
NF. *see* Neurofibromatosis (NF)
NF1, 510
Nicotinamide, 69
NK cells, 24–25
NLD. *see* Necrobiosis lipoidica diabeticorum (NLD)
NLE. *see* Neonatal lupus erythematosus (NLE)
NLRP12-associated periodic syndrome (NAPS12), 269–271*t*
NME. *see* Necrolytic migratory erythema (NME)
Nocardiosis, 309, 309*b*, 309*t*
Nodular amyloid, 402–414*t*, 438*f*
Nodular fasciitis, 377, 377*f*, 402–414*t*
Nonbullous impetigo, 304
Non-immunologic contact urticaria, 91
Non-infectious granulomas, 149–157, 158*f*, 435*f*
Non-langerhans cell histiocytoses, 161
Nonmelanocytic lesions, dermoscopic features of, 384–387
Nonresponse bias, 531*t*
Non-scarring alopecia, 212–216
Nonvenereal spirochete infections, 316
Nonvenereal treponematoses, 316–318, 317*t*
Notalgia paresthetica, 191
NSF. *see* Nephrogenic systemic fibrosis (NSF)
Nummular dermatitis, 89
Nutraceuticals, 497
Nutritional deficiency, 402–414*t*, 420*f*
Nutritional disorders, in dermatology, 192–193
NXG. *see* Necrobiotic xanthogranuloma (NXG)
Nystatin, 64

O
Occipital horn syndrome, 270, 507
Occlusive vascular disorders, 433*t*
Occlusive/moisture-retentive wound dressings, 479*t*
Occupational allergic contact dermatitis, 90
Ochronosis, 402–414*t*
OCPs, 74–78*t*
Ocular effects, 44
Ocular rosacea, 180
Oculocutaneous albinism, 230*t*, 240, 240*t*
Odland bodies, 2
Oligoarthritis, psoriasis and, 82
Omalizumab, 54
Omphalomesenteric duct cyst, 344
Oncologic agents, in dermatology, 54–57
Onychomycosis, 322
Onychoosteodysplasia, 290
Ophthalmic artery, 443–444
Ophthalmic nerve, sensory innervation of, 445*t*
Opportunistic infections, 44
Opportunistic systemic mycoses, 326
Oral erythromycin, for pityriasis rosea, 85
Oral hairy leukoplakia, 298
Oral stomatitis, 90
Oral warts, 295
Osler-Weber-Rendu syndrome, 256*t*
Osteogenesis imperfect, 264–265
Osteoma cutis, 402–414*t*
Osteopoikilosis, 279
Otitis externa, 310
Outcome misclassification, 531*t*
Oxybutynin, 70
Oxymetazoline, 67

P
Pachyonychia congenita, 257*f*, 289*f*
Pacinian corpuscle, 9
Paget disease of the breast, 525
Pagetoid, 425*t*
Paget's disease, 402–414*t*
Paisley Tie, 423*f*
Palisaded encapsulated neuroma, 364, 402–414*t*
Palisaded neutrophilic granulomatous dermatitis (PNGD), 153, 153*t*
Palmoplantar keratodermas (PPKS), 192
Palmoplantar pustulosis, 81
PAN. *see* Polyarteritis nodosa (PAN)
Pancreatic fat necrosis, 402–414*t*
Pancreatic panniculitis, 211–212, 437*f*
Panniculitides, 210–212, 434*t*
Panniculitis, secondary to external factors, 212
PAPA (pyogenic arthritis, pyoderma gangrenosum, acne conglobata), 179
Papillary eccrine adenoma (PEA), 354, 355*f*
Papillary endothelial hyperplasia, 417*f*
Papillary mesenchymal bodies, 392–394*t*
Papuloerythroderma of Ofuji, 172
Papulopustular (inflammatory) rosacea, 180
Papulosquamous dermatoses, 79–86
confluent and reticulated papillomatosis, 86, 86*f*
erythroderma, 86
intertriginous/axillary granular parakeratosis, 85
pityriasis rosea, 84–85
pityriasis rubra pilaris, 82–84
psoriasis, 79–82
seborrheic dermatitis, 84
Paracoccidioidomycosis, 326, 327*f*, 402–414*t*
Paraneoplastic pemphigus, 109–110, 116*f*, 525
Paraneoplastic syndromes, 520–526
Parasites and other creatures, 329
Parasitic infections, 329
Parkes-Weber syndrome, 254
Paronychia and periungual pyogenic granulomas, 74–78*t*
Parotid duct, cutaneous danger zones of, 450*t*
PAS. *see* Periodic acid Schiff (PAS)
Pattern recognition receptors, 18–19
PCMC. *see* Primary cutaneous mucinous carcinoma (PCMC)
PCR. *see* Polymerase chain reaction (PCR)
PD-1 inhibitors, 56
PDT. *see* Photodynamic therapy (PDT)
PEA. *see* Papillary eccrine adenoma (PEA)
Pediatric dermatology, 229–292, 275*t*
Pediatric effects, 44
Pelvis/sacral syndrome, 250, 250*f*
Pemphigoid group, 110–113, 117*f*
bullous pemphigoid, 110–113, 111*t*, 112*b*, 112*f*
bullous systemic lupus erythematosus, 114
dermatitis herpetiformis, 114–115
epidermolysis bullosa acquisita, 114, 116*f*
linear IgA bullous dermatosis/chronic bullous disease of childhood, 113–114, 114*f*
mucous membrane pemphigoid, 113, 113*f*
Pemphigus, 107, 107*b*
Pemphigus erythematosus, 402–414*t*
Pemphigus foliaceus, 108–109, 108*f*, 109*f*, 109*t*, 402–414*t*
Pemphigus vegetans, 402–414*t*
Pemphigus vulgaris, 107–108, 108*b*, 108*f*, 402–414*t*
Penicillins, 58–59
Penis, nerve innervation of, 445–446*t*
Pentoxifylline, 69
Perforating diseases, 149, 151*t*
Performance bias, 531*t*
Perianal streptococcal skin infection, 307
Perifollicular purpura, in scurvy, 518*f*
Perifolliculitis capitis abscedens et suffodiens, 217
Periodic acid Schiff (PAS), 395–396*t*
Perioral/periorificial dermatitis, 180–181
Periungual fibrous nodules, 274*f*
Pernio, 402–414*t*
Peroneal nerve blocks, 453*f*
Peutz-Jeghers syndrome, 244*t*, 516–517
PG. *see* Pyoderma gangrenosum (PG)
PHACE syndrome, 250
PHACES syndrome, 510
Phakomatosis pigmentokeratotica, 251–252
Phakomatosis pigmentovascularis, 251
Phenylketonuria, 262
Phosphotungstic acid hematoxylin (PTAH), 395–396*t*
Photoaging, 185
Photodermatoses, 184–188
and other physical dermatoses, 184–188
cold injuries, 184–185
erythema ab igne, 184
mechanical injuries, 187–188
photoaging, 185
sunburns and pigment darkening, 185
thermal burns, 184
Photodynamic therapy (PDT), 66–67
Photosensitive drug reactions, 73
Photosensitivity, 74–78*t*
Phototherapy, 65–67
Phymatous rosacea, 180
Phytophotodermatitis, 92, 92*f*
Piebaldism, 242
Pigmentary alteration, 304
Pigmentary disorders, 220–228
Pigmented purpuric dermatosis, 402–414*t*
Pigmented spindle cell nevus of Reed, 347, 402–414*t*
Pilar leiomyoma, 367–368, 367*f*
Pili torti, 259–261*t*
Pilomatricoma, 361–362, 361*f*, 402–414*t*
Pilonidal cyst, 182
Pimecrolimus and tacrolimus, 70
Pitted keratolysis, 308
Pityriasis lichenoides, 100, 100*f*, 421*f*
Pityriasis rosea, 84–85, 402–414*t*, 432*f*
Pityriasis rotunda, 525
Pityriasis rubra pilaris (PRP), 82–84, 402–414*t*, 420*f*
additional boards factoids in, 82
clinical features of, 83–84, 83*f*, 84*f*
histopathology of, 82
pathogenesis/epidemiology of, 82
prognosis/clinical course of, 84
treatment of, 82
Plague, 315
Plakophilin, 2*t*

Plane xanthoma, 525
Plasma cells, 397*t*
Plasmacytoid dendritic cells, 397*t*
Pleomorphic fibroma, 376
Pleomorphic lipoma, 402–414*t*
PNGD. *see* Palisaded neutrophilic granulomatous dermatitis (PNGD)
Podophyllin and podofilox, 63
POEMS syndrome, 525–526
Polar and borderline leprosy, 299*t*
Polarity, summary of, 465*t*
Polyarteritis nodosa (PAN), 202*f*, 203–204, 203*t*, 402–414*t*, 520
Polycythemia vera, 189
Polymerase chain reaction (PCR), 29, 30–31*t*
Polymicrobial Gram-positive skin infections, 308
Polymyxin B, 58
Pomade acne, 178
Porokeratosis, 338, 339*f*, 402–414*t*
Porokeratotic eccrine ostial and dermal duct nevus, 338
Poroma (classic juxtaepidermal type), 356, 402–414*t*
Porphyria cutanea tarda, 117*f*
Posaconazole, 64
Posterior tibial, 453*f*
Potassium iodide, 69
Potassium permanganate ($KMnO_4$), 395–396*t*
Power, 482*t*
Poxviruses, 299–300
PPKS. *see* Palmoplantar keratodermas (PPKS)
Precision, 527
Precooling, 482
Pretibial myxedema, 402–414*t*, 514*f*
Prevalence, 527
Primary biliary cirrhosis, 516
Primary cicatricial alopecia, 216
Primary cutaneous ALCL (anaplastic large cell lymphoma), 372
Primary cutaneous B-cell neoplasms, 373
Primary cutaneous CD4-positive small/medium pleomorphic T-cell lymphoma, 373
Primary cutaneous mucinous carcinoma (PCMC), 359
Primary cutaneous γ/δ T-cell lymphoma, 373
Primary immunodeficiency disorders (PIDS) with cutaneous manifestations, 278, 278*t*
Primary systemic amyloidosis (AL amyloidosis), 510–511, 526
Procedural bias, 531*t*
Profilaggrin, 2
Progeria (Hutchinson-Gilford progeria), 511
Progesterone dermatitis, 89
Progressive symmetric erythrokeratoderma, 282*t*
Prolidase deficiency, 263
Proliferating pilar (trichilemmal) tumor, 363, 402–414*t*
Proliferative phase, 14
Promethazine, 39
Prostaglandin analogs, 74–78*t*
Prostate cancer, 523*f*
Proteus syndrome, 252
Protothecosis, 402–414*t*
Protozoa and worms, 329–331
PRP. *see* Pityriasis rubra pilaris (PRP)
Prurigo nodularis, 190
Pruritic papular eruption, 302
Pruritus, mediators of, 189
Pruritus ani, 189
Pruritus scroti/vulvae, 189
Psammoma body, 392–394*t*
Pseudoangiosarcoma, 378–379
Pseudoatrophoderma colli, 86
Pseudofolliculitis barbae, 181
Pseudolymphoma, 74–78*t*
Pseudomonal folliculitis, 305, 310
Pseudomonal pyoderma, 310
Pseudomonas hot-foot syndrome, 310
Pseudoxanthoma elasticum (PXE), 264, 264*f*, 402–414*t*, 517, 517*f*
Psoralen plus UVA (PUVA), 66
Psoralens, 74–78*t*
Psoriasiform mycosis fungoides, 420*f*
Psoriasis, 79–82, 402–414*t*, 427–428*t*, 511
  additional boards factoids in, 82
  clinical features of, 81–82
  epidemiology of, 79
  erythroderma and, 85–86
  histopathology of, 82
  pathogenesis of, 79–81, 80*f*
  prognosis/clinical course of, 82
  treatment of, 82
Psychiatric agents, 67–68
Psychiatric changes, 44
Psychodermatology, 189–192
PTAH. *see* Phosphotungstic acid hematoxylin (PTAH)
Public health
  billing, 530–533
  definitions of, 527
  epidemiologic principles, 527–528
  epidemiology, statistics, study design and principles of, 527–534
  presence or absence of disease in, 528*t*
  types of studies and limitations in, 528–530
Pulse IV CS, 44–45
Pulse width, 482*t*
Pustular psoriasis, 402–414*t*
Pustulo-ovoid bodies of Milian, 392–394*t*
PUVA. *see* Psoralen plus UVA (PUVA)
PXE. *see* Pseudoxanthoma elasticum (PXE)
Pyoderma faciale (rosacea fulminans), 180
Pyoderma gangrenosum (PG), 170–171, 517
Pyodermatitis, 517
Pyogenic granuloma, 386*f*
Pyomyositis, 306
Pyostomatitis vegetans, 517, 518*f*

Q
Quantitative reverse transcriptase PCR (qRT-PCR), 29, 30–31*t*
Quinupristin and dalfopristin, 62

R
Radiation acne, 178
Radiation dermatitis, 402–414*t*
Radiation enhancement and recall, 74–78*t*
Radiation-induced EM, 74–78*t*
Radiofrequency devices, 494*t*
RAF inhibitors, 74–78*t*
Rat-bite fever, 315
Reactive perforating collagenosis (RPC), 402–414*t*
Recall bias, 531*t*
Recessive dystrophic epidermolysis bullosa, 248*f*
Recurrent melanocytic nevus, 346
Recurrent nevus, 402–414*t*
Red man syndrome, 74–78*t*
Reed's syndrome, 520
Reed-Sternberg cells, 392–394*t*
Refsum disease, 282*t*
Relapsing polychondritis, 137–138, 137*f*, 511
Relaxed skin tension lines, 443
Remodeling phase, 14–15
Renal (clear) cell carcinoma, 402–414*t*
Renal cell carcinoma, metastatic, 402–414*t*, 419*f*
Renal diseases, 519
Reporting bias, 531*t*
Restrictive dermopathy, 268–269
Resurfacing lasers, 486, 486*t*
Retapamulin, 58
Reticular erythematous mucinosis, 132
Reticulate acropigmentation of Kitamura, 243
Reticulohistiocytoma, 402–414*t*
Retinoid-like effect, 304
Retinoids, 40–42
  contraindications of, 42
  interactions of, 42
  mechanism of, 40–42, 40*t*, 41*t*
  SEs of systemic, 42
  side effects of, 42
Reverse transcription PCR (RT-PCR), 30–31*t*
Rheumatic fever, 511
Rheumatoid arthritis, 138–140, 139*f*, 140*f*
  psoriasis and, 82
Rheumatoid nodules, 402–414*t*, 435*f*
Rhinoscleroma, 315, 402–414*t*
Rhinosporidiosis, 402–414*t*, 422*f*
Rhombic flap, 467–468*t*
Ribonucleic acid (RNA), 14
Ribosomal RNA (rRNA), 15, 29–31, 30–31*t*
Rickettsia, 311, 313–314*t*
Rifampin, 61
Risankizumab, 53*t*
Rituximab, 54
RNA. *see* Ribonucleic acid (RNA)
RNA interference (RNAi), 16–17
RNA microarray, 30–31*t*
RNA sequencing, 30–31*t*, 32
RNAi. *see* RNA interference (RNAi)
Rocha-Lima bodies, 392–394*t*
Romidepsin, 57
Rosacea, 179–180
  subtypes of, 180
  variants, 180
Rosacea fulminans. *see* Pyoderma faciale (rosacea fulminans)
Rotation flaps, 466–467*t*
Rothmund-Thomson syndrome, 277
Rowell's syndrome, 129
RPC. *see* Reactive perforating collagenosis (RPC)
rRNA. *see* Ribosomal RNA (rRNA)
RT-PCR. *see* Reverse transcription PCR (RT-PCR)
Rubella, 230–231
Rubeola, 229–230
Rubinstein-Taybi syndrome, 258, 259–261*t*, 261*f*
Ruffini corpuscle, 9
Russell bodies, 392–394*t*
Ruxolitinib (Jakafi/Jakavi), 46

S
Salmonellosis, 315
Salt-split skin, immunofluorescence microscopy of, 402*f*
Sanger DNA sequencing, 30–31*t*, 31, 33*f*
SAPHO (chronic recurrent multifocal osteomyelitis), 179
Sarcoidosis, 156–157, 156*f*, 157*f*, 157*t*, 402–414*t*, 435*f*, 511
Scabies, 402–414*t*
Scalp, dissecting cellulitis of, and acne conglobata, 182
Scalp dysesthesia/burning scalp syndrome, 191
Scalp pruritus, 189
Scalpel handles, 454
Scar, 402–414*t*
  prevention, 476–477
    nonsurgical modalities, 476–477
    overview of, 476
    surgical modalities, 477
Scarlet fever, 307
Schaumann bodies, 392–394*t*
Schnitzler syndrome, 526
Schöpf-Schulz-Passarge, 258
Schwannoma, 364, 365*f*, 402–414*t*
Scissors, 454
SCLE. *see* Subacute cutaneous lupus erythematosus (SCLE)
SCLE-like syndromes, 127–128
Scleredema, 402–414*t*, 429*f*
Scleredema diabeticorum, 512–513
Sclerema neonatorum, 230*t*
Scleroderma, 144–147, 518
Scleromyxedema, 402–414*t*, 431*f*, 526
Sclerosing lipogranuloma/paraffinoma, 402–414*t*
Sclerosing panniculitis, 211*f*
Sclerosing solutions, characteristics of, 494*t*
Sclerosing sweat duct carcinoma, 355
Sclerosing/fibrosing skin disorders, 150*t*
Sclerotherapy, 494
Sclerotic fibroma, 376
Scorpions, 334–335
Scurvy, 518, 518*f*
Seabather's eruption, 332, 332*f*
Sebaceoma, 363
Sebaceous adenoma, 363, 363*f*, 402–414*t*
Sebaceous carcinoma, 363, 364*f*, 402–414*t*
Sebaceous glands, 10, 397*t*
Sebaceous hyperplasia, 363
Sebaceous proliferations, 363

Seborrheic dermatitis, 84, 402–414*t*
Seborrheic keratosis, 337–338, 338*t*, 384
Secondary cicatricial alopecia, 216
Secukinumab, 53*t*
Sedative antihistamines, for atopic dermatitis, 89
Selectins, 22–23
Selection bias, 530, 531*t*
Selective photothermolysis, 481
Selenium sulfide, 64
Self-improvement effect, 531*t*
Sensory nerves, surgical anatomy of, 444
Serum sickness eruption, 74–78*t*
Serum sickness-like eruption, 74–78*t*
Sexually transmitted bacterial infections, 318
Sezary cells, 392–394*t*
Sezary syndrome, 370
Shoe dermatitis, 90
Short interfering RNA (siRNA), 15
Shoulder parakeratosis, 84
Shulman syndrome. *see* Eosinophilic fasciitis (aka Shulman syndrome)
Signet ring cells, 392–394*t*
Silver nitrate, 395–396*t*
Silver sulfadiazine, 58
Silvery hair syndromes, 240–241, 281*f*
Sinecatechins, 63
siRNA. *see* Short interfering RNA (siRNA)
Sister Mary Joseph nodule, 526
Sjögren syndrome (SjS), 135–137
Sjögren-Larsson syndrome, 282*t*
SjS. *see* Sjögren syndrome (SjS)
SJS/TEN (Lyell's syndrome), 98, 99*t*
Skin
  embryology of, 13, 14*t*
  genetics, 15–17, 16*t*
    genome, basic cell biology of, 15–16
    inheritance patterns, 16–17
  normal, 415*t*
    features of, 391*t*
  stem cell biology, 13
  structure and function of, 1–13
  surgical anatomy of, 443–444
  ultraviolet light in, 17
  wound healing, 13–15
Skin tumors, 385*t*
SLE. *see* Systemic lupus erythematosus (SLE)
Small to medium vessel vasculitis, 200–203
Smallpox, 299
Smooth muscle, 397*t*, 436*t*
  neoplasms, 367–368
Sodium sulfacetamide, 58
Soft tissue reconstruction, 472*t*
Solar lentigo, 345
Solid facial edema
  in acne, 177
  in rosacea, 180
Sonidegib, 54–55
SPAP. *see* Syringocystadenoma papilliferum (SPAP)
Spider angioma, 256*t*, 518
Spiders, 334–335, 335*f*
Spinal accessory nerve, cutaneous danger zones of, 450*t*
Spindle cell neoplasms, 400*t*
Spindle cell/pleomorphic lipoma, 382, 384*f*
Spiradenoma, 353–354, 353*f*, 357, 402–414*t*
Spironolactone, 68
Spitz nevus, 346–347, 402–414*t*
S-plasty, 461
Spongiotic disorders, 427–428*t*
Sporotrichosis, 402–414*t*
Spot size, 482*t*
SPTCL. *see* Subcutaneous panniculitis-like T-cell lymphoma (SPTCL)
Squamous cell carcinoma, 384
Squamous cell carcinoma in situ, 384
SSSS. *see* Staphylococcal scalded skin syndrome (SSSS)
Staphylococcal scalded skin syndrome (SSSS), 305, 305*f*
Staphylococcal skin infections, 304–306
Staphylococcal toxic shock syndrome (S-TSS), 306
Stasis dermatitis, 92–95, 402–414*t*
Steatocystoma, 344, 402–414*t*
Steiner (silver stain), 395–396*t*
Stem cells, 1–2
Steroid sulfatase deficiency, 282*t*
Stiff skin syndrome, 269
Still's disease. *see* Systemic-onset juvenile idiopathic arthritis (Still's disease)
Stratum basale, 1–2
Stratum corneum, 2–4
Stratum granulosum, 2
Stratum spinosum, 2
Streptococcal skin infections, 307
S-TSS. *see* Staphylococcal toxic shock syndrome (S-TSS)
Stucco keratosis, 338*t*
Sturge-Weber syndrome, 251, 251*f*
Subacute cutaneous lupus erythematosus (SCLE), 126, 126*f*, 427*f*
Subcutaneous fat necrosis, 230*t*
  of newborn, 402–414*t*
Subcutaneous mycoses, 323
Subcutaneous panniculitis-like T-cell lymphoma (SPTCL), 372–373, 402–414*t*
Subgaleal hematoma, 230*t*
Sublamina densa, 7
Sunburn cells, 392–394*t*
Sunburns and pigment darkening, 185
Sun's nevus, 345
Sunscreens, 67
Supercut scissors, 454
Superficial epidermolytic ichthyosis, 282*t*
Superficial folliculitis, 181
Superficial musculoaponeurotic system (SMAS), surgical anatomy of, 444
Superficial mycoses, 322–323
Superficial temporal artery, 443
Supernumerary digit, 402–414*t*
Supernumerary nipple, 402–414*t*
Supratrochlear artery, cutaneous danger zones of, 450*t*
Sural nerve blocks, 453*f*
Surgery
  anatomy, 443–444
  antisepsis, 458, 459*t*
  complications, 460, 473–476
  dermatologic, 443–480
  excisions, 461–462
  fire hazards, 460–461
  instruments and needles, 454–455
    scalpel, 454
    scissors, 454
  local anesthetics, 450–454, 451*t*
  of nail, 477–479
  perioperative pain control, 450–454
  prophylaxis algorithm for, 475*f*
  suture techniques, 455
    cuticular suturing, 455
    knots, 455
    subcuticular suturing, 455
  wound closure materials, 455–458
Suture, 398*t*
  granuloma, 402–414*t*
  specific properties of, 472*t*
  techniques, 455
    cuticular suturing, 455
    knots, 455
    subcuticular suturing, 455
  types of, 456*t*
    absorbable, 456*t*, 457*t*, 472*t*
    monofilament, 456*t*
    multifilament, 456*t*
    natural, 456*t*
    nonabsorbable, 456*t*
    synthetic, 456*t*
Sweat gland neoplasms, high-yield dermatopathologic features of, 356–359
Sweat glands, 397*t*
Sweet's syndrome, 169–170, 169*f*, 402–414*t*, 526
Swimmer's itch, 332
Symmetrical drug-related intertriginous and flexural exanthem, 74–78*t*
Syphilis, 299*t*, 318*f*, 402–414*t*
Syringocystadenoma papilliferum (SPAP), 354, 355*f*, 402–414*t*
Syringofibroadenoma, 355, 358
Syringoma, 352–353, 357, 402–414*t*, 422*f*
Systemic allergic contact dermatitis, 90
Systemic antibacterial agents, 58–62
Systemic lupus erythematosus (SLE), 129–131, 511
Systemic mycoses, 326, 327*f*
Systemic sclerosis. *see* Scleroderma
Systemic-onset juvenile idiopathic arthritis (Still's disease), 140–141, 141*f*

T
T cells, 21–24
TAA. *see* Tubular apocrine adenoma (TAA)
Takayasu's arteritis, 205, 206*t*
TALENs. *see* Transcription activator-like effector nucleases (TALENs)
Talimogene, 57
Talon noir, 402–414*t*
Targetoid hemosiderotic hemangioma, 379–380
Tattoo (lead), 402–414*t*
Tattoo removal lasers, 486–488, 488*t*
Tavaborole, 65
T-cell receptor (TCR) gene rearrangement, 30–31*t*
TCIs. *see* Topical calcineurin inhibitors (TCIs)
TCR gene rearrangement. *see* T-cell receptor (TCR) gene rearrangement
TE. *see* Telogen effluvium (TE)
TEC. *see* Toxic erythema of chemotherapy (TEC)
Telangiectasia, 208–210
Telangiectasia macularis eruptiva perstans, 425*f*
Telogen effluvium (TE), 215, 215*b*
Temporal arteritis (giant cell arteritis), 205
Temporal nerve, cutaneous danger zones of, 450*t*
Temporal triangular alopecia, 216, 259–261*t*
Tendon, giant cell tumor of, 378
Teratogenicity, 42
Terbinafine, 64
Terminality, summary of, 465*t*
Tetracyclines, 60–61
Th2 cells, 22
Th17 cells, 22
Thalidomide, 70
T-helper 1 (Th1) cells, 21
Thermal burns, 184
Thermal relaxation time, 481, 482*t*
Thioflavin T, 395–396*t*
Thrombosis, 206–208
Thrombotic syndromes, 206–208
Thyroglossal duct cyst, 344
Thyroid cancer, 514
Thyroid disease, 514
Tick-borne relapsing fever, 317*t*
Ticks, 334–335, 334*f*
Tight junctions, 1
Tildrakizumab, 53*t*
Tinea capitis, 322
Tinea corporis, 402–414*t*
Tinea versicolor, 402–414*t*
Tissue acquisition and processing, 28
T-lymphocytes, 397*t*
TNF-α inhibitors, 52
Toes, nerve innervation of, 445–446*t*
Tofacitinib (Xeljanz), 46
Toll-like receptors, 18, 20*t*
Toluidine blue, 395–396*t*
Tongue, nerve innervation of, 445–446*t*
Topical anesthetics, 453
Topical antibacterial agents, 57–63
Topical azoles, for seborrheic dermatitis, 84
Topical calcineurin inhibitors (TCIs), 70
Topical cosmetic agents, 67
Topical CS, 45
Touraine's syndrome, 244*t*
Touton giant cells, 392–394*t*
Toxic epidermal necrolysis-like lupus erythematosus, 129
Toxic epidermal necrosis, 99*f*
Toxic erythema of chemotherapy (TEC), 74–78*t*
Traction alopecia, 218
Tralokinumab, 54
Transcription activator-like effector nucleases (TALENs), 35

Transfer RNA (tRNA), 15
Transient amplifying cells, 1–2
Transposition flaps, 467–468*t*
Transverse nasal crease, 178
TRAPS. *see* Tumor necrosis factor receptor-associated periodic syndrome/familial Hibernian fever (TRAPS)
Traumatic neuroma, 364
Traumatic/amputation neuroma, 402–414*t*
Treatment-associated dermatoses, 303–304
Trichilemmal (pilar) cyst, 343
Trichilemmoma, 362, 362*f*, 402–414*t*
Trichoadenoma (of Nikolowski), 363
Trichoblastoma, 361*f*
Trichodiscomas, in Birt-Hogg-Dube syndrome, 506*f*
Trichoepithelioma, 360–361, 402–414*t*, 423*f*
Trichofolliculoma, 359, 359*f*, 402–414*t*
Trichorhinophalangeal syndrome, 290
Trichorrhexis nodosa, 259–261*t*, 261*f*
Trichothiodystrophy, 277–278
Trichotillomania, 215, 402–414*t*
Trigeminal nerve, sensory innervation of, 445*t*
Trigeminal trophic syndrome, 191
Trimethoprim-sulfamethoxazole, 61
Tripe palms, 526, 526*f*
tRNA. *see* Transfer RNA (tRNA)
Tryptase, 395–396*t*
TSC. *see* Tuberous sclerosis complex (TSC)
TSGs. *see* Tumor suppressor genes (TSGs)
Tuberous sclerosis, 275*t*, 520
Tuberous sclerosis complex (TSC), 273, 273*t*, 274*f*, 274*t*
Tubular apocrine adenoma (TAA), 358
Tufted angioma, 380
Tularemia, 315, 315*b*
Tumescent liposuction, 494*t*
Tumor necrosis factor receptor-associated periodic syndrome/familial Hibernian fever (TRAPS), 269–271*t*
Tumor suppressor genes (TSGs), 16–17
Tumor syndromes, 248–250
Tungiasis, 329*f*
Tylosis with esophageal carcinoma, 523
Type III error, 531*t*
Tyrosine kinase inhibitors, 56, 74–78*t*

U
Ulcers, 194, 194*t*
Ulnar nerve, cutaneous danger zones of, 450*t*
Ulnar nerve blocks, 453*f*
Ultraviolet light, 17, 17*f*
Umbilical granuloma, 234*t*
Umbilicus, developmental anomalies of, 234*t*
Uncombable hair (pili trianguli et canaliculi), 259–261*t*
Unilateral laterothoracic exanthem, 239
Unilateral nevoid telangiectasia, 256*t*
Urticaria, 72, 166–168
Urticarial vasculitis, 199
  causes of, 199*t*
  systemic involvement in, 199*t*
  treatment approach for, 199*t*
Ustekinumab, 52–53, 53*t*
UVA-1, 66
UVA modalities, 66
UVB modalities, 66

V
V advancement flap, 470*f*
Vaccines containing aluminum, 74–78*t*
Vacuolar interface dermatitis, 96–103
Valacyclovir, 62
Validity, 527
Vancomycin, 59
Vascular disorders, 194–210, 206*t*
  characterized by telangiectasias, 256*t*
Vascular EDS, 275
Vascular lasers, 485
Vascular lesions, 387
Vascular malformations, 251–255, 382
Vascular neoplasms, 381–382, 381*f*
Vascular proliferations, 378–380
Vascular tumors, 435*t*
Vasculitides, 194–210, 195–196*t*
Vasculopathies, 194–210
  and other vasculitides, 208
Vellus hair cyst, 344, 402–414*t*
Venous lake, 208
Venous malformations, 253
Venous system, surgical anatomy of, 444
Verhoeff-van Gieson (VVG), 395–396*t*
Verocay bodies, 392–394*t*
Verruca plana, 402–414*t*, 424*f*
Verruciform xanthoma, 402–414*t*, 441*f*
Verrucous carcinoma, 341, 342*f*, 402–414*t*, 424*f*
Vibrio vulnificus, 315–316
Viral diseases, 293–301
Viral exanthems, 229–240
Viral hepatitis infection, dermatologic manifestations of, 301, 301*t*
Viral-associated trichodysplasia of immunosuppression, 301
Virchow cells, 392–394*t*
Vismodegib, 54–55
Vitamin D_3 analogs, 69
Vitamin B12, 74–78*t*
Vitamin deficiencies and excesses, 188*t*
Vitamin K, 74–78*t*
Von Hansemann cells, 392–394*t*
Von Kossa, 395–396*t*
von Recklinghausen's neurofibromatosis, 272*f*
Voriconazole, 63–64
Vorinostat, 57
VVG. *see* Verhoeff van Gieson (VVG)

W
Waardenburg syndrome, 242, 242*t*
Warthin-Starry (silver stain), 395–396*t*
Warty dyskeratoma, 339, 339*f*, 402–414*t*
Waveforms, 460
Wavelength, 481, 482*t*
Wegener's granulomatosis, 200*f*, 511
Weibel-Palade bodies, 392–394*t*
Weird endophytic neoplasms, 421*t*
Well-differentiated liposarcoma, 382
Well's syndrome, 129, 392–394*t*, 402–414*t*
Werner syndrome, 276
Westcott scissors, 454
Western blot, 30–31*t*
Wilson disease, 518–519
Wooly hair, 259–261*t*
Woronoff ring, 82
Wound, classification of, 474*t*
Wound dressings, 479*t*
Wound healing, 13–15
  phases of, 13–15

X
Xanthelasma, 402–414*t*
Xanthoma disseminatum, 164*f*
Xanthomas, 164–166, 164*f*
Xeroderma pigmentosum, 276, 277*f*
XLR mutations in ectodysplasin (ED1), 260

Y
Y advancement flap, 470*f*
Yellow nail syndrome, 512

Z
ZFNs. *see* Zinc-finger nucleases (ZFNs)
Zinc deficiency, 262*f*
Zinc-finger nucleases (ZFNs), 35
Zinsser-Engman-Cole syndrome, 243
Zoon's balanitis, 402–414*t*
Zygomatic nerve, cutaneous danger zones of, 450*t*
Zygomycosis, 328*f*, 402–414*t*